Nonprescription Product Therapeutics

the pharmacist as triage expert   forces that shape

the nonprescription product market   plaque-induced

diseases: caries and gingivitis   oral problems   g

digress   motion sickness   intestinal gas discomfo

bloating and flatulence   lactose intolerance

colic   constipation   diarrhea   pinworm   hemorrhoid

allergic rhinitis   the common cold   and rela

conditions   humidity deficit   asthma   headache an

other minor pains   menstrual discomfort   injuri

muscles, ligaments   and tendons   low back pai

obesity   fatigue and drowsiness   sleep disturb

Nonprescription Product Therapeutics

W. STEVEN PRAY, B.S., M.P.H., Ph.D.

Registered Pharmacist (1973–present)

Professor, Nonprescription Products and Devices (1976–present)

Southwestern Oklahoma State University

Weatherford, Oklahoma

Contributing Editor, U.S. Pharmacist (1988–present)

Member, NAPLEX Review Committee (1987–present)

LIPPINCOTT WILLIAMS & WILKINS

A **Wolters Kluwer** Company

Philadelphia • Baltimore • New York • London
Buenos Aires • Hong Kong • Sydney • Tokyo

Editor: Donna Balado
Managing Editor. Jennifer Schmidt
Marketing Manager: Tara Williams
Development Editor: Daniel V. Edson
Project Editor: Paula C. Williams
Design Coordinator: Mario Fernandez

351 West Camden Street
Baltimore, Maryland 21201-2436 USA

530 Walnut Street
Philadelphia, Pennsylvania 19106-3621 USA

Printed in the United States of America

First Edition

Library of Congress Cataloging-in-Publication Data

Pray, W. Steven.
     Nonprescription product therapeutics / W. Steven Pray. — 1st ed.
          p.   cm.
     Includes bibliographical references and index.
     ISBN 0-683-30126-8 (alk. paper)
     1. Drugs, Nonprescription. I. Title.
     [DNLM: 1. Drugs, Non-Prescription—therapeutic use. QV 772 P921n 1999]
     RM671.A1P69   1999
     615′ .1—dc21
     DNLM/DLC
for Library of Congress   98-22505
                                                                                      CIP

To purchase additional copies of this book, call our customer service department at **(800) 638-3030** or fax orders to **(301) 824-7390.** For other book services, including chapter reprints and large quantity sales, ask for the Special Sales Department. International customers should call **(301) 714-2324.**

Visit Lippincott Williams & Wilkins on the Internet: http://www.lww.com. Lippincott Williams & Wilkins customer service representatives are available from 8:30 AM to 6:00 PM, EST.

                                                                          00 01 02
                                                                       2 3 4 5 6 7 8 9 10

This book is dedicated to my wife, Carole L. Pray; my children, Joshua Jameson and Gabriel Elijah Pray; and our families, Walter L. and Flossie W. Pray, Odis and Leona Grayson, and Waymon, Sheila, and Shelly Peterson.

Preface

Nonprescription Product Therapeutics, a textbook for pharmacy students and practitioners, presents a clear discussion of self-treatable medical conditions. It has been written with four goals in mind:

- To serve the needs of students and professors by drawing on the skills gained from more than two decades of teaching students and recommending nonprescription products and devices to patients.
- To serve the needs of future and practicing retail pharmacists by reflecting the knowledge and skills gained from more than two decades of work in retail pharmacy. I know from thousands of patient-counseling sessions exactly what the concerns of the patients are and how the pharmacist can best address them in the relatively public area of the retail pharmacy.
- To uphold the highest precepts of science by continually stressing the validity of the FDA's Over-the-Counter (OTC) review process, which has brought us a body of safe and effective nonprescription products and has clarified fully which medical conditions are self-treatable.
- To educate future professionals for the expanding role of the pharmacist. The concept of pharmaceutical care mandates that the pharmacist expand the professional responsibility beyond products, structures, and pharmacology to encompass patients and their medical conditions. As a result, the concept of the "OTC course" has grown to cover a much wider range of the self-treatable conditions and the therapeutic decisions made in the entire process of patient triage (described in Chapter 1), many of which involve nonprescription products.

ORGANIZATIONAL PHILOSOPHY

The study of nonprescription products is an eclectic discipline. The conditions that can be safely self-treated are a diverse group, and they can be categorized in numerous ways. Conditions that can be self-treated might be classified according to their etiology such as infectious conditions (e.g., athlete's foot and warts), genetic conditions (e.g., psoriasis, hair loss, and Type 1 diabetes), accidents (e.g., burns, minor cuts, and sprains), conditions caused by unhealthy lifestyle choices (e.g., sunburn and smoking), and conditions of neglect (e.g., gingivitis). However, this approach would leave many conditions uncategorized. For instance, where would one place obesity, dry eye, and gastroesophageal reflux, which are combinations of genetic and environmental problems?

I chose the *systems* approach to categorize conditions that can be self-treated. While not perfect, this categorization does have certain advantages. For instance, it allows the instructor and student to cover the conditions in a coherent method (e.g., gastrointestinal, respiratory, dermatologic, etc.). Also, when the patient presents with a certain condition (e.g., dermatologic), the pharmacist may more easily draw together the possible recognition factors because they are studied in logical groupings. The major sections of the book are as follows:

- The Pharmacist and Nonprescription Drug Products
- Oral and Gastrointestinal Conditions
- Respiratory Conditions

- Pain Conditions
- Miscellaneous Internal Conditions
- Ophthalmic/Otic Conditions
- Dermatologic Conditions
- Miscellaneous Medical Conditions and Situations
- Topics Related to Self-Care Therapeutics

CHAPTER STRUCTURE

The organization of the chapters provides pharmacy students and pharmacists with a logical method of recommending nonprescription products and devices. Because patients often ask for help with a medical problem such as motion sickness, chapter titles have been chosen to indicate the conditions described within them. Some chapters incorporate what is known as a "regional diagnosis" (e.g., foot problems). Other chapters reflect an etiologic agent (e.g., fungal skin infections).

All chapters that address medical conditions use standard headings (when relevant) presented in the following order:

- **Prevalence** allows pharmacists to gauge the probability of patients approaching to ask about the condition.
- **Epidemiology** helps pharmacists assess patients for variables that might help confirm the presence of the condition. The traditional scope of practice of the hospital-based clinical pharmacist includes such activities as amassing lab data and monitoring the patient accordingly. In retail practice, however, pharmacists are usually presented with patients for whom no such data can be obtained. Further, community pharmacists cannot order laboratory tests. Therefore, pharmacists must rely on less obvious information to recognize minor conditions. Knowledge of the epidemiology of minor medical conditions facilitates their recognition. For instance, the pharmacist's index of suspicion for tinea pedis (athlete's foot) should be high in a postpubertal male but low in a prepubertal female.
- **Etiology** allows the pharmacist to understand the cause of the conditions, whether infectious, genetic, or traumatic. Since the patient often wishes to know how the condition occurred, this section allows the pharmacist to describe these various etiologic processes with the patient.
- **Transmission** is included for many infectious conditions and infestations so the pharmacist can understand the possible routes by which the patient contracted the condition (e.g., pinworm, warts).
- **Manifestations** describes the various signs and symptoms that are expected with the typical presentation of each condition.
- **Specific Considerations** includes discussion on topics specific to that medical condition.
- **Prognosis** is included in some cases to allow the pharmacist to describe to the patient the consequences of failure to treat the condition appropriately.
- **Complications** are included in some cases to describe complications that may occur with the condition so their presence may be ascertained at the time of presentation.
- **Treatment** begins with general treatment guidelines. The concept of nonprescription products and devices follows, along with the various FDA-mandated labeling information to help ensure safe and effective usage of the ingredient(s). When appropriate, nonpharmacologic therapies and other professional treatments are discussed.
- **Prevention** is discussed, if appropriate, so that the pharmacist may provide helpful information on preventing future occurrences.

PEDAGOGIC FEATURES

Most chapters include numerous special pedagogic features that enhance the book's mission as the primary reference and teaching resource on nonprescription products and devices:

- **Case Studies** 👤 Two or more per chapter, titled "At the Counter." The cases focus on real-life scenarios, providing a structured method to carry out patient triage. The case studies illustrate pharmacists making the various triage decisions (e.g., recommend a product; recommend referral to a medical professional).

- **Patient Assessment Algorithms,** one or more for most chapters, provide a logical, reasoned approach to the triage decision. The algorithms allow the pharmacist to clearly identify which patients require referral to another medical professional, as well as to recommend ingredients and formulations when appropriate.

- **Counseling Tips** 🖐 highlight information that the patient should be given during a counseling session (shown by icon plus italicized text).

- **Warnings** ⚠ provide information on dangerous or life-threatening ingredients, actions, situations, etc. (shown by icon plus boldfaced italicized text).

- **Key Terms** (boldface text) are defined directly following each term.

- **"Focus On" sidebars** present information that is important to the topic but that requires encapsulation in a separate area to enhance delivery and readability of the primary narrative.

- **"A Pharmacist's Journal"** describes true pharmacy experiences (an unusual feature in a pharmacy text), reflecting the cornucopia of retail pharmacy practice situations—humorous, tragic, horrifying, ironic. As I relate these incidents in my class, my students often tell me that these instances reveal the pitfalls of practice and bring home the value of having a professor who is also an actively practicing retail pharmacist. Occasionally, relevant patient encounters from published literature are included in this feature.

ART AND TABLES

To illustrate the textbook, **figures** have been chosen that will enhance the reader's understanding of the medical condition and its treatment. This textbook is not a primer in physiology and assumes that pharmacy students have a grasp of both anatomy and physiology, acquired during prerequisites to a nonprescription products course. Readers who discover that certain aspects of anatomy or physiology are unclear should consult a basic text.

To provide examples of nonprescription products, **product tables** are included throughout the textbook. The intent, however, is not to present seemingly endless tables of nonprescription products' trade names. Thousands of products could have been listed, but such a list would forever be incomplete because of the dynamic nature of industry. Furthermore, any such list is outdated as soon as it is published since manufacturers frequently change concentrations, strengths, and trade names. I contend that students should not be unduly focused on products, ingredients, and concentrations at the expense of the patient and the conditions about which he or she is concerned. In general, the product tables in this textbook are composed of well-established products and products needed to support the narrative (such as products with which pharmacists should be familiar).

SPECIAL INCLUSIONS/EXCLUSIONS

Special concern about ensuring that readers of this text have access to the best information on the safety and effectiveness of nonprescription products has motivated the inclusion of five appendices.

- Appendix 1: FDA-Labeled Lower Age Limits for Use of Nonprescription Products
- Appendix 2: FDA-Labeled Time Limits for Use of Nonprescription Products
- Appendix 3: FDA-Labeled Contraindications for Use of Nonprescription Products
- Appendix 4: FDA-Labeled Drug Interactions and Concurrent Use Precautions with Nonprescription Products
- Appendix 5: Miscellaneous FDA-Labeled Precautions with Use of Nonprescription Products

Information on ostomy care and contact lenses is not included. In my experience, ostomy care is a subject best left to the enterostomal therapist except when pharmacists are able to attend workshops that detail the various appliances and their accessories. (The scope and breadth of this information is beyond the scope of an introductory textbook.) Contact lens products present an uncomfortable situation for pharmacists. The patient's questions are often very specific (such as, "Can I use this rewetting solution with my gas-permeable lens?"), but manufacturers seldom supply this information to pharmacies. Further, contact lens products change frequently as new technology becomes available. In the face of incomplete information, pharmacists risk making incorrect recommendations that might damage some contact lenses. The most prudent approach is referral to the patient's ophthalmic care provider.

CLASS TESTED

My required course in nonprescription products and devices is taught three times a year as a full-semester, 4-hour course. Because we teach to smaller classes three times yearly, I have shared information with pharmacy students over 45 cycles. During this large number of teaching cycles, I have amassed a sizable amount of course material. This material, popularly known as "Dr. Pray's Notebook," is purchased at the bookstore at the beginning of the semester. Many students have told me that they take their notebooks to work, shelving them permanently with references required by the state Board of Pharmacy. Some former students contact our university bookstore to obtain updated notebooks through the mail. This course material forms the basis for *Nonprescription Product Therapeutics*.

SUMMARY

In summary, this textbook provides a comprehensive overview of the conditions treatable with nonprescription products without becoming mired in minutia about the products themselves. In a single volume, *Nonprescription Product Therapeutics* presents the sum total of the knowledge I have gleaned from two decades of recommending nonprescription products and two decades of clarifying them for pharmacy students and pharmacists, as well as the result of numerous literature reviews undertaken for the professional presentations I have given (more than 70 live presentations, radio broadcasts, and nationally televised satellite broadcasts to pharmacists, pharmaceutical industry personnel, dental hygienists, and lay audiences), as well as the articles I have written (more than 170 published articles related to medical conditions, pharmacy practice, and dental hygiene).

W. Steven Pray, B.S., M.P.H., Ph.D.
Registered Pharmacist
Professor, Nonprescription Products and Devices
School of Pharmacy
Southwestern Oklahoma State University
Weatherford, Oklahoma

Acknowledgments

A textbook such as *Nonprescription Product Therapeutics* cannot be developed without the cooperation and contributions of a host of individuals and groups. I am indebted to them all and am pleased to be given the opportunity to provide some recognition to them, however inadequate. It is vital to note that every effort has been made to ensure that all information in *Nonprescription Product Therapeutics* is correct. The responsibility for any errors that remain is borne solely by the author, who would welcome a chance to correct them in the second edition, if the reader would be so kind as to notify him or the publishers.

My colleagues have been most patient with me during my educational journey and the rigors of writing *Nonprescription Product Therapeutics.* I appreciate their comradeship, including David Coates, R.Ph., Ph.D.; Tom W. Davis, R.Ph., M.D.; Michael Deimling, R.Ph., Ph.D.; Ed Fisher, R.Ph., Ph.D.; Norman Foster, R.Ph.; Benny French, R.Ph., Ph.D.; ElGenia French, R.Ph, Pharm.D.; Barry Gales, R.Ph., Pharm.D.; Mark Gales, R.Ph., Pharm.D.; Patti Harper, M.B.A.; Pete Huerta, R.Ph., Ph.D.; Jaques Landry, R.Ph., Pharm.D.; Scott Long, R.Ph., Ph.D.; Sara Marquis, R.Ph., Pharm.D.; Nina Morris, R.Ph., Pharm.D.; Charles Nithman, R.Ph., Pharm.D.; Gus Ortega, R.Ph., Ph.D.; Richard Philips, R.Ph., M.S.; Shelly Prince, R.Ph., Ph.D.; Les Ramos, R.Ph., Ph.D.; Peter Ratto, R.Ph., Ph.D.; Keith Reichmann, R.Ph., Ph.D.; Dana R. Pierce, R.Ph., Pharm.D.; Jim Scruggs, R.Ph., Ph.D.; Penny Skaehill, R.Ph., Pharm.D.; Lynne Studier, R.N., B.S.; Susan Thiessen, M.A.; Dennis Thompson, R.Ph., Pharm.D.; Floyd Ulrich, R.Ph., Ph.D.; Virgil Van Dusen, R.Ph., J.D.; Edward Wanek, R.Ph., Ph.D.; Neal Weber, Ph.D.; and Ben Welch, R.Ph., Pharm.D. I have learned much from them and salute them for their contributions to the pharmacy program of which I am a part. I appreciate having an excellent working relationship with these fine professionals.

Various colleagues across the country have served as national "sounding boards" during discussions of nonprescription products. Their input has helped me refine my thought processes and serves as an invaluable touchstone. They include Dennis Worthen, Ph.D.; Nicholas Popovich, R.Ph., Ph.D.; Gail Newton, R.Ph., Ph.D.; Henry Palmer, R.Ph., Ph.D.; Doug Pisano, M.S.; Janet Engle, Pharm.D.; Timothy Covington, Pharm.D.; J. David Harvill; and Marty Cohen.

My colleagues and friends from the National Association of Boards of Pharmacy and the NAPLEX Review Committee have helped keep my knowledge and skills sharp as we have constructed the NAPLEX for the last decade. Similarly, the staff of *U.S. Pharmacist* have been most helpful in the past decade as I have written my monthly column, "Consult Your Pharmacist."

The various members of administration at Southwestern Oklahoma State University have allowed me unparalleled latitude to develop this specialty and to carry out the necessary literature reviews that underlie *Nonprescription Product Therapeutics.* I appreciate the leadership of present and former deans Walter L. Dickison, R.Ph., Ph.D.; Bernard G. Keller, R.Ph., Ph.D.; H.F. Timmons, Ph.D.; David Bergman, R.Ph., Ph.D., as well as Former Associate Dean Edward C. Christensen, R.Ph., M.S.; Assistant Dean David Ralph, R.Ph., Ph.D.; former Department Chair (Pharmaceutics) William G. Waggoner, R.Ph., Ph.D.; and former Department Chair (Pharmaceutical Sciences) and presently Dean, School of Arts & Sciences Vilas Prabhu, Ph.D. The book could not have been developed without the cooperation of former University President Leonard Campbell, Ed.D.;

present President Joe Anna Hibler, Ed.D.; former Vice President for Academic Affairs Bob Brown, Ed.D.; present Vice President for Academic Affairs William Kermis; and present Executive Vice President for Administration John Hays.

My students are a constant reminder of the inexhaustible curiosity that youth possess. Their insights are refreshing; their questions serve to keep me ever sharp. Encouragement to write *Nonprescription Product Therapeutics* from many students helped me in the difficult decision to begin the process.

The patients whom I am able to treat as I work part-time are silent partners in the creation of *Nonprescription Product Therapeutics*. They are the source from which spring the real-life stories related in this text. Without them, this textbook would be irrelevant. I hope that their needs are better served when students study the text and apply its principles in their own careers.

Every part of *Nonprescription Product Therapeutics* underwent a review with the kind cooperation of a bevy of faculty, a pharmacist, and student reviewers. As of this writing, their names are unknown to me for purposes of maintaining the blinded nature of the review. Nevertheless, I would like to express my profound appreciation for the many hours of work that this project entailed. The text was improved by their suggestions.

The personnel at Lippincott Williams & Wilkins have been a source of encouragement and assistance. They include Donna Balado (my Acquisitions Editor), Jennifer Schmidt (Associate Managing Editor), Nancy Evans (Editorial Director), Paula Williams (Project Editor), Susan Kimner (Managing Editor), Christine Kushner (Senior Marketing Manager), Danielle Jablonski (Editorial Assistant), Tara Williams (Associate Marketing Manager), and Victoria Vaughn (Senior Managing Editor).

The secretarial staff for the School of Pharmacy and School of Health Sciences have been of invaluable assistance in helping me with the various chores associated with production of this text, including Ms. Margie Vincent, Ms. Lyanna Schultz, and Ms. Janice Hix.

Three individuals provided assistance in production of *Nonprescription Product Therapeutics*. They are Dan Edson, my Development Editor, who spent many hundreds of hours making sure that the text was in a proper format. Through the exhaustive processes of his edits, he provided the guidance that allowed me to organize each chapter consistently.

Christina Logan served as my right hand in retyping each chapter during the final phase of the developmental edit. She instituted the majority of Dan's excellent suggestions for improvement.

Matthew Chansky of Chansky, Inc., was the illustrator chosen for the project. His ability to translate my rough drawings into finely honed illustrations allows the reader to more easily grasp the fine points covered in the text.

Contents

The Pharmacist and Nonprescription Drug Products

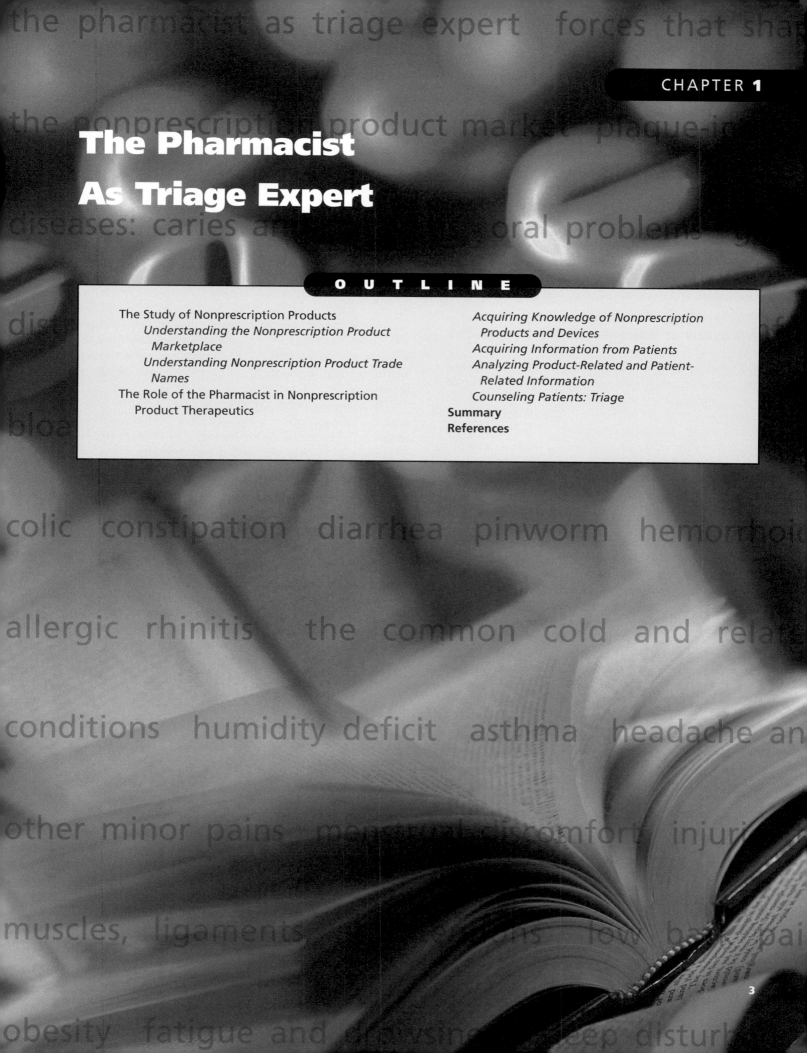

The Pharmacist As Triage Expert

O U T L I N E

Since 1977 the Gallup Polling organization has asked the public to rank the honesty and ethical standards of twenty-six professions. Pharmacists have topped the list (which includes physicians, clergy, dentists, and engineers) for 9 of the 20 years, and in 1997 scored higher than any other profession ever has, with 69% of Americans ranking the pharmacist as "high" or "very high."[1] One of the key ingredients in this high opinion undoubtedly is the pharmacist's broad knowledge of medications and willingness to share this knowledge through effective counseling with patients. Patients see the pharmacist as the expert in prescription medications, but also seek out pharmacist advice about nonprescription medications (also known as over-the-counter, or "OTC" medications).

THE STUDY OF NONPRESCRIPTION PRODUCTS

The study of nonprescription products and the conditions they treat is challenging and extremely rewarding. The challenge springs from the vast knowledge required to effectively recommend products for patients. The reward arises from the knowledge that pharmacists can use their knowledge of nonprescription medications to render vitally important advice to patients regarding health-care problems.

The study of nonprescription products is not yet a **pure science** or basic science (a focus area with its own specialized body of information), but rather an **applied study** (a focus area with a knowledge base drawn from many disparate areas). At the present time the status of the study of nonprescription products is similar to the status of pharmacology and pharmacy administration several decades ago. Both of these disciplines were originally considered to be applied sciences; eventually, however, each discipline amassed a body of knowledge sufficient for it to emerge as a basic science.

Because the study of nonprescription products incorporates information from multiple pharmacy disciplines, this text incorporates information from multiple knowledge bases:

- Pharmacology—The mechanisms of action of nonprescription products
- Medicinal chemistry—Patient risk of certain medication groups (e.g., potential allergies to "caine" anesthetics)
- Pharmaceutics—The relative advantages of nonprescription dosage forms (e.g., vaginal creams, foams, suppositories, and films)
- Toxicology—The short- and long-term impact of ingredients (e.g., short-term toxicity of nasal decongestants and long-term toxicity arising from abuse of stimulant laxatives)
- Pharmacy administration—Product marketing (e.g., certain products that are heavily advertised but lack proof of safety and/or efficacy)
- Ethics—The decision to recommend ingredients that lack proof of safety and/or efficacy
- Pharmaceutical jurisprudence—The legality of pediatric dosing charts, sales of Schedule V OTCs, and the FDA review of OTC products

Discussions of the various disease conditions that are considered self-treatable by the Food and Drug Administration (FDA) incorporates such general medical knowledge areas as anatomy, physiology, epidemiology, pathogenesis, and differential diagnosis (recognition). A complete curriculum on nonprescription products must also encompass such medical/scientific specialty disciplines as bacteriology, botany, dentistry, dermatology, dietetics, emergency medicine, endocrinology, endodontics, entomology, environmental health, family planning, gastroenterology, geriatrics, gynecology, internal medicine, microbiology, mycology, ophthalmology, otorhinolaryngology, parasitology, pediatrics, periodontics, podiatry, proctology, public health, pulmonary medicine, rheumatology, sports medicine, and virology. While the pharmacist cannot become intimately familiar with this dazzling array of sciences, he or she must be cognizant of the minor disease conditions that fall within the purview of each discipline (e.g., hemorrhoids as a self-treatable aspect of proctology).

The nonprescription curriculum is not static, but mutable, and must change as new nonprescription products become available. When minoxidil was limited to prescription use, for example, pharmacists only needed the knowledge to counsel patients on physician-supervised use. The availability of nonprescription minoxidil, however, required pharmacists to further expand their knowledge base. Pharmacists were required to become aware of other causes of hair loss to refer patients for care if the suspected cause was not treatable by the product. Thus, differential recognition (known as differential diagnosis to the physician) of baldness was added to the responsibilities of the pharmacist. *Patient counseling must also include the consequences of product use beyond restrictions that appear on the OTC label.*

Despite the inherent difficulties in learning the intricacies of the nonprescription product market, the knowledge of nonprescription products will yield great benefit. Patients who are able to fully utilize self-care interventions not only can benefit from reduced pain and suffering and/or improved health, they also can avoid costly and unnecessary physician visits. Research shows that nonprescription products save patients an estimated $20 billion yearly.[2]

Understanding the Nonprescription Product Marketplace

The nonprescription product marketplace is difficult to understand because of several factors:

- The massive number of products marketed as nonprescription items
- The difficulty in understanding nonprescription product trade names

NUMBERS OF PRODUCTS

An estimated 300,000 nonprescription products are currently marketed in the United States.[3] The market for nonprescription medications and health-and-beauty aids is $41.9

billion.[3] Understanding the sheer number of nonprescription products and the many conditions they treat can be overwhelming for consumers.

NUMBER OF RETAIL OUTLETS

With few exceptions nonprescription drug products and related devices can be purchased at any retail outlet willing to stock them. Thus patients may find OTC drugs for sale in pharmacies, nonpharmacy food and department stores, convenience stores, gasoline and service stations, health-food stores, dress shops, variety centers, hotel lobbies, airport shops, train stations, and in vending machines located at strategic points throughout the country.[4] Therefore, the patient may purchase nonprescription products in locations that have no medical professional to help with purchases.

A number of pharmacists and other health-care professionals have at one time opposed nonpharmacy sales, suggesting instead that the sale of nonprescription products be limited to pharmacies, but no action along these lines has been taken by any legal body.[5,6] No clear mechanism exists at the state level for such restrictions. The FDA conceivably could enact such legislation, but political pressures undoubtedly would prevent the FDA from enacting any regulation limiting venues for sales of nonprescription products, so the situation will probably not change.

Understanding Nonprescription Product Trade Names

To gain market share, manufacturers of nonprescription products and devices attempt to portray their products as superior to the competition. Before 1972 manufacturers could claim superiority based on unique ingredients or purported therapeutic benefit. The FDA OTC-product review (initiated in 1972) drastically reduced the freedom of manufacturers to make claims for products by requiring manufacturers to prove safety and efficacy for ingredients and by ensuring that labeling claims were valid. (See Chapter 2, Forces That Shape the Nonprescription Product Market.) As a result, nonprescription products that survived the FDA review began to be more and more similar, and product manufacturers found it increasingly more difficult to gain a competitive edge over other manufacturers.

One marketing strategy employed by pharmaceutical product manufacturers to increase (or hold) market share has been to build consumer brand loyalty. Pharmaceutical manufacturers spend many millions of advertising dollars each year on specific brand names. As a consequence, many brand names have become very familiar to the average consumer. A popular marketing tactic has been to use these established brand names to carry other products, a practice known as "creating line extensions."[7,8] Manufacturers wager that consumer loyalty to a familiar brand such as Bayer, Robitussin, or Tylenol will carry over into purchase of entirely new—and different—products that carry these names such as a Bayer Select line of products, Maalox Anti-Gas, or Mylanta Natural Fiber Supplement (some of these examples

have been discontinued). Manufacturers sometimes even use the familiar trade name as an adjective such as a store coupon that boasted, "Finally, Robitussin Relief For Your *Cold*!" (Because a wide variety of products carry the Robitussin trade name, this sales tactic can be confusing to patients, who may not know which Robitussin product actually gives the promised relief.)[9]

Brand loyalty is so important that manufacturers often retain a familiar trade name in spite of formula changes—as in the case of Donnagel, Kaopectate, or Caladryl. This can be problematic, because the older trade name may convey misleading connotations regarding older ingredients that are no longer present.[10] Table 1.1 presents several examples of brand name confusion that may require judicious counseling by the pharmacist to clarify patients' misconceptions.

THE ROLE OF THE PHARMACIST IN NONPRESCRIPTION PRODUCT THERAPEUTICS

Most nonprescription products and devices are advertised directly to potential patients, bypassing pharmacists.[11,12] While there is a popular move on the part of pharmacy organizations and professional journals to add the pharmacist to the label of these products (e.g., "Ask your doctor or pharmacist if . . . "), it is opposed by industry and physicians.[13] The American Medical Association commented that placing pharmacists on the label would "inappropriately place the pharmacist in a position for which he or she is not qualified, is likely to be confusing to patients, and may adversely impact the health of some patients."[14] The Nonprescription Drug Manufacturers Association registered its opposition to a specific reference to pharmacists by stating that "A broader reference to any 'health professional' would be more appropriate and more practical than the listing of many different health professionals."[15] Thus it is incumbent on pharmacists to create entry points for patient counseling in the sale of nonprescription products. Pharmacists can increase the opportunities for patient counseling by taking the following steps:

1. Pharmacists must first acquire a full working knowledge of nonprescription products.
2. Pharmacists must attempt to gather information from patients (or caregivers) through an interview process, which may include several types of assessment.
3. Pharmacists must analyze the information by considering all product-related and patient-related factors that are appropriate.
4. Pharmacists must counsel patients about the problem(s) presented.

This approach is utilized in the case studies included in this textbook (Fig. 1.1).

Counseling patients should include a recommendation from the pharmacist on the optimal action to take. This recommendation—which could be not to treat, to refer, or to self-treat—is known as patient **triage** (a French term meaning "to

Table 1.1. Examples of Confusing Nonprescription Drug Product Brand Names

PRODUCT	REASON FOR CONFUSION
Americaine	Available as a spray for surface anesthesia in minor cuts and burns or an aerosol spray for hemorrhoids
Bayer	May indicate a product for sinus pain, nighttime pain, a head cold, or menstrual problems
Boil-Ease	Trade name implies that it will cure boils
Borofax	No longer contains boric acid
Caladryl	Diphenhydramine removed, but trade name not changed
Creomulsion	Product once contained ipecac; ipecac removed, but trade name not changed
Donnagel	Belladonna alkaloids not present as implied in the name
Duofilm	Changed from Rx to an OTC, formula changed; trade name not changed
Dramamine II	Contains meclizine, rather than dimenhydrinate, as in Dramamine
Fungi-Nail	Trade name implies that it will cure fungal nail conditions
Hypo Tears	One product is a solution, another is an ophthalmic ointment
Kaopectate	No longer contains kaolin or pectin, as implied in the name
Legatrin PM	Original Legatrin contained quinine; formula changed, trade name retained with minor change. Patient may still purchase it for nocturnal leg cramps
Maalox	May refer to an antacid or antiflatulent
Mile's Nervine	The original product contained toxic bromides; bromides were removed. Product now contains diphenhydramine; trade name unchanged
Modane	Danthron removed, trade name not changed
Mycitracin Plus Pain Reliever	"Plus" denotes the addition of a local anesthetic to the original Mycitracin, but package is similar to Mycitracin
Mylanta	May refer to an antacid, antiflatulent, or H2 blocker
Neosporin Plus Cream	Does not contain bacitracin, while Neosporin Plus Ointment does
Outgro	Trade name implies it will cure ingrown toenails
Phazyme	No longer contains enzymes
pHisoDerm	Trade name similar to pHisoHex, a product which is prescription only
Progaine	Trade name very similar to Rogaine
Red Cross Toothache Medicine	Trade name implies it will cure toothache, and that it carries American Red Cross endorsement
Robitussin	May refer to a product containing guaifenesin, dextromethorphan, or a combination of these plus other ingredients
Sinulin	Belladonna alkaloids removed for safety; trade name unchanged
Stye	Trade name implies that it will cure sties
Swim-Ear	Trade name implies it will cure swimmer's ear
Tavist Sinus	"Tavist" traditionally referred to the presence of clemastine fumarate, but this product does not contain clemastine
Thum	Trade name implies it will cure thumb sucking
Trichotine	Trade name implies activity against *Trichomonas*
Tums	Available as an antacid and a calcium supplement, which contains 2.5 times more elemental calcium than the antacid
Tylenol	Trade name may refer to an analgesic, cold medication, influenza medication, or a sinus product
Unisom	Some Unisom products contain doxylamine, but some contain diphenhydramine

From Pray WS. Confusion in the OTC marketplace. US Pharm 20(1) 16, 1995.

sort.") Used in medicine decades ago to describe the care of battlefield casualties and casualties of mass disasters, the term is now being applied to the process by which pharmacists make a decision regarding patient care with nonprescription products.[16-18]

This step-by-step approach leading to a triage decision allows pharmacists to utilize a structured method for creating valid and useful entry points in nonprescription product counseling. Importantly, the actual patient counseling should not take an undue amount of time. Patients initially may seem to resist nonprescription counseling sessions that are more than several minutes long, but once pharmacists demonstrate concern for their problems, most patients will devote more time to the purchase. Nevertheless, *pharmacists still must strive to collect information rapidly, analyze incisively, and counsel succinctly.*

Acquiring Knowledge of Nonprescription Products and Devices

Knowledge about nonprescription products can be gained using several sources:

- Formal coursework
- Attending continuing-education lectures
- Reading periodicals such as the *Federal Register*
- Analyzing nonprescription product labels

FORMAL COURSEWORK
Knowledge of nonprescription products and devices is growing in importance to pharmacists. For this reason pharmacy students should strive to complete a university course dedicated to nonprescription products and devices.

Unfortunately, courses with nonprescription products and devices as the main emphasis are not offered by some pharmacy schools.[19] Approximately two-thirds of the pharmacy schools that do offer a course on nonprescription products only give it elective status. Some schools fragment information on nonprescription products by including it in other courses, which deemphasizes the importance of this discipline.

CONTINUING EDUCATION
Even pharmacists with a strong background in nonprescription products may discover that information that was once timely has become outdated. Written or live continuing-education courses that cover nonprescription products and devices can be one of the best options for maintaining a current storehouse of knowledge, although they are a piecemeal method of learning.

THE *FEDERAL REGISTER*
Published each working day of the year, the *Federal Register* reports the work of many governmental agencies. Reading the *Federal Register* can help pharmacists keep current with federal deliberations concerning nonprescription products

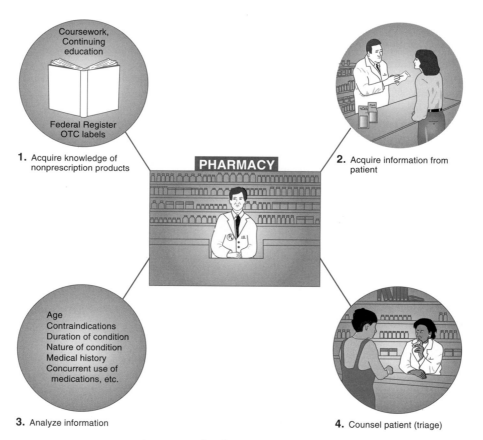

Figure 1.1. The pharmacist as triage expert.

and devices.[20] Print copies of the *Federal Register* may be perused at repository libraries, and it can be accessed for a fee through several Internet sites (e.g., http://cos.gdb.org/repos/fr/fr-intro.html).

NONPRESCRIPTION PRODUCT LABELS

Product labels on nonprescription products provide considerable information. At least 40% of Americans who take both prescription and nonprescription medications do not read the labels each time the medications are taken.[21] Further, the labels are not easily read by those with visual problems. Also, United States citizens who do not speak English cannot read the labels.

The FDA has proposed a reworking of the nonprescription products label. The agency gathered comments from many interested parties such as the Nonprescription Drug Manufacturers Association. The new label would provide information to the consumer in a more standard format than previously available.[22] The consumer should be more readily able to access the label information. As of this writing, the agency is in the midst of preparing the final rule on nonprescription product labeling.[23]

The redesigned labels would use the bold headings shown in the subsections below.

Ingredients

The FDA proposal requires the heading, **Active Ingredient [in each dosage unit]** or **Active Ingredients [in each dosage unit]**, followed by **Purpose.** The active ingredient(s) would consist of the established name of each ingredient, listed in alphabetical order. The dosage unit would be tablet, capsule, suppository, or concentration per 5 mL (for standardization purposes). If the product should be a topical product marketed without a discrete dosage unit, the dosage unit would not be required.

The "purpose" section of the label would be an accurate statement of the general pharmacologic category(ies) or principal intended action(s) of each ingredient, as contained in applicable OTC drug monographs (Table 1.2). The proposal mandates inclusion of sodium, magnesium, calcium, and potassium content if a single recommended dose of the product contains 5 mg or more of sodium, 8 mg or more of magnesium, 20 mg or more of calcium, or 5 mg or more of potassium.[24]

Inactive Ingredients

Pharmacists should also be knowledgeable about inactive ingredients in nonprescription products, some of which can produce seizures, headaches, bronchospasm, and diarrhea (in pediatric patients).[25] Nonprescription drug products are not required to list inactive ingredients at this time (although many manufacturers voluntarily do so) and will not be required to provide this information on the new labels.[22] Should manufacturers choose to include information on inactive ingredients, it would be placed just after the list of active ingredients.

Uses

The uses of the nonprescription product will be on the label, as shown in Table 1.2, following the heading, **Uses.**

Warnings

Any specific warning or warnings associated with the ingredient(s) will also be on the label under the current proposal, headed **Warning** or **Warnings.** When applicable, the label will also contain specific subheadings for the warning such as **Allergy Warning** or **Alcohol Warning.** Table 1.2 illustrates the placement of this aspect of the label.

Absolute Contraindications

The proposed format requires contraindications to follow the heading, **Do Not Use.** The agency stressed that contraindications listed are absolute, intended for any situation where patients should avoid use unless a physician has made a prior diagnosis or for situations in which patients are not to use the product under any circumstances, regardless of whether a health professional has been consulted. Contraindication examples include the requirement for a diagnosis of asthma prior to use of nonprescription bronchodilators, interactions involving monoamine oxidase inhibitors, allergies to active or inactive ingredients, and the precaution to obtain immediate medical treatment for all open wounds in or near the eyes prior to use of eyewashes.

Consult a Physician Prior to Use

The labels of *some* nonprescription products contain specific warnings against self-treatment without first consulting a physician. These warnings will be preceded by **"Ask a Doctor Before Use"** followed by a phrase such as **"If You Have," "If You Are,"** or **"If You."** These introductory phrases are used when grammatically appropriate to convey warnings against use with preexisting conditions, for specific symptoms, and for dangerous drug/food interactions. Examples of these warnings are shown in Table 1.2.

Adverse Reactions/Situations To Avoid

In the proposed labeling format, each nonprescription product label may include side effects the patient might expect and substances or activities the patient should avoid while using the product (e.g., drinking alcohol, operating machinery, or driving a car). This information will be preceded by **"When Using This Product:"** as illustrated in Table 1.2.

Discontinuation Alerts

A section of the proposed label would include signs of toxicity and other serious reactions that necessitate immediate discontinuation of the product. These would be preceded by **"Stop Using This Product If:"** followed by the warning. The last line below the warning(s) would contain two sentences, also boldface and indented under the major heading, **(Ask a doctor. These [This] may be signs [a sign] of a serious condition),** as illustrated in Table 1.2. Some required warnings may not fit under any other categories and would appear without a separate heading under this subheading. Examples include the precaution against use if pregnant or breast-feeding and the warning to keep the product out of the reach of children. Sample placement is illustrated in Table 1.2.

Table 1.2. Sample Label for a Fictional Nonprescription Product as Proposed by the FDA[a,b]

ACTIVE INGREDIENTS (IN EACH TABLET):	PURPOSE:
Chlorpheniramine Maleate 2 mg	Antihistamine
Dextromethorphan 15 mg	Cough suppressant
Pseudoephedrine HCl 30 mg	Nasal decongestant

Uses: For the temporary relief of these cold symptoms
*Sneezing   *Nasal congestion, stuffiness
*Runny nose   *Cough

Warning: Children and teenagers should not use this medicine for chicken pox or flu symptoms before a doctor is consulted about Reye syndrome, a rare but serious illness reported to be associated with aspirin.

Do Not Use: this product unless a diagnosis of asthma has been made by a doctor.

Ask a Doctor Before Use:
  If You Have:
  *Heart disease
  *High blood pressure
  *Thyroid disease
  *Diabetes
  *Difficulty in urination due to enlargement of the prostate gland
Ask a Doctor Before Use:
  If You Are:
  *Taking sedatives or tranquilizers
  *On a sodium restricted diet
Ask a Doctor Before Use:
  If You:
  *Have kidney disease
  *Are taking other drugs

When Using This Product:
  *Use caution when driving a motor vehicle or operating machinery.

Stop Using This Product If:
  *Nervousness, dizziness, or sleeplessness occurs.
  Ask a doctor. These may be signs of a serious condition.
If pregnant or breast-feeding, ask a health professional before use. **Keep out of reach of children.** For external use only. If more than used for _____ is accidentally swallowed, get medical help right away.

Directions:
  *Adults and children over 12 years: Take one tablet every 4 to 6 hours as needed. Do not take more than 6 tablets in 24 hours.

Other Information:
  *The combined daily use of a fluoride preventative treatment rinse and a fluoride toothpaste can help reduce the incidence of dental caries.

[a]This sample label includes combinations of information that would not be found together on an actual label, since an attempt has been made to include samples of all types of label requirements. For example, the Reye syndrome warning is not required for any of the ingredients listed in this example. The asterisks above appear as they did in the original *Federal Register* monograph.

[b]The FDA has proposed that each major heading be separated by a horizontal line.

Directions

Directions for use are included under the heading, **Directions,** as illustrated in Table 1.2. The directions must conform to the approved application or to an OTC monograph. (See "The Nonprescription Product Review" in Chapter 2 for information on the FDA monographs and other FDA drug review documents.)

Other Information

Occasionally, an ingredient may require information that does not fit any other heading but is mandatory through an approved marketing application or is optional under an OTC monograph. This information would be included under the heading, **Other Information.** An example is shown in Table 1.2.

Miscellaneous Labeling Issues

The FDA is seeking input on the proper placement of an expiration date.[22] The agency has also determined that headings should not be exclusively in upper case since they are harder to read; accordingly, the proposal specifies a mix of lower case and upper case. The proposed type size will be no smaller than 6 point type to ensure readability.

The FDA recognizes that some packages are marketed with a small inner container and a larger outer package. The agency intended for the newer format to appear only on the outer package, so manufacturers would not be forced to enlarge the inner container. However, since many consumers discard the outer package, the inner container must still include all information in a type size no smaller than 6 point, perhaps in a more compact arrangement.

Acquiring Information from Patients

Patients obtain information about nonprescription products from several sources[26]:

- First—Friends, members of the family, and coworkers
- Second—Advertisements and store coupons
- Third—Physicians
- Fourth—Pharmacists

To help remedy this situation, pharmacists must leave the prescription-filling area and enter the nonprescription product aisles to appear available for patient questions (see "Universal Precautions When Counseling Patients").[27] In the words of one chain-store executive, the line between the "pharmacy and the front of the store should be transparent to the consumer."[28] By talking with patients, pharmacists can attempt to discover why specific products are requested and can collect the information needed for appropriate triage. The types of information elicited during the patient interview should include the reason the patient is requesting a specific product, the age of the patient for whom the product request is made, the duration of the condition, current medical conditions or other patient situations that would contraindicate a certain product, medications currently being taken, history of alcohol use, various demographic variables, past medication use, exact nature of the condition, and a medical history (see "Suspected Child Abuse"). The information may be entered on a form so a record can be kept of the counseling session (see "Patient Information Form").

REASONS FOR REQUESTING A SPECIFIC PRODUCT
Many patients enter pharmacies with a specific product purchase in mind. In many cases they choose their product, purchase it, and leave before a pharmacist has an opportunity to provide counseling. These lost opportunities may result in patients using an inappropriate product.

Pharmacists often are only alerted to situations of *inappropriate* use when receiving a seemingly simple query such as "Where's the Neosporin." While it is tempting to respond, "It's over there by the alcohol," pharmacists should pursue the counseling opportunity. To initiate a counseling session, a pharmacist should leave the area behind the counter and approach the patient to allow a private conversation. Then the pharmacist should attempt to "get behind the question," to discover the presumptions on which the patient has decided that this particular product is appropriate for his or her problem.

The following questions help pharmacists explore the issues involved in preselected purchases:

- Why do you want to buy this product?
- Was this purchase recommended by a friend or relative?
- Did you see an advertisement for this product?
- Have you used this product before for the same problem?
- Did a physician recommend this product? [At least 40% of physicians recommend nonprescription products.[29,30]]
- Does your physician know that you are taking this product [if the product is purchased because the previous supply has been depleted]? Only one-half of physicians ask about use of nonprescription products.[31]
- Do you know the active ingredients in this product?

While interviewing patients, pharmacists sometimes determine that a patient's preselected product is inappropriate.[32] The patient may be misinformed about the situations in which the product may be used safely and effectively; for instance, *if a pharmacist becomes convinced that a purchase poses possible danger to the patient's health, the pharmacist has a professional responsibility to recommend that the product not be purchased.* A negative recommendation, accompanied by a logical, reasoned argument couched in language that the patient can understand, may convince the patient that the pharmacist's advice should be followed.

EXACT NATURE OF THE CONDITION
Patients often voice self-diagnoses before pharmacists can conduct even the most cursory assessments. Patients may have had a prior physician diagnosis or may be guessing. Pharmacists should attempt to confirm patients' diagnoses when possible. When patients have no idea what their problem is, pharmacists should help them discover the cause of their problems.

The pharmacist's ability to recognize conditions is more limited than that of other health professionals for several reasons:

- Many pharmacists have never received formal training in physical assessment, and the methods and techniques are thus somewhat foreign.[33]
- Pharmacists also do not routinely possess the most basic equipment needed for physical assessment (e.g., otoscopes, ophthalmoscopes).
- Pharmacists are required to render judgments without a full spectrum of information. For instance, few retail pharmacists can independently order lab tests and conduct similar investigations. Thus, although trained pharmacists can usually recognize poison ivy dermatitis, for example, differentiating streptococcal pharyngitis from viral causes of a sore throat is difficult without throat assessment equipment and without a throat culture.
- The typical pharmacy does not have a private space where patients can disrobe for assessment. Pharmacist-initiated inspections for pubic lice or hemorrhoids may also open the door to malpractice lawsuits, since the legal grounds for such private examinations are shaky.

Thus, unless disorders can be visually assessed (e.g., warts), pharmacists may be wholly dependent on patients' descriptions.

Pharmacists must understand that the exact natures of patients' problems are often elusive. Thus the major goal of pharmacist-conducted assessment in retail pharmacy is not to pin down sophisticated diagnoses, but to allow pharmacists to gather the information needed to evaluate the patients and to suggest a specific triage option.[34–36] In this regard

(tip) *pharmacists should concentrate on recognizing minor, self-treatable conditions, while referring all other conditions for further diagnosis and testing.* (See "Universal Precautions When Counseling Patients.")

MEDICAL HISTORY

Certain medical conditions can only be self-treated if the patient's medical history is explored. For instance, should a patient present with ophthalmic redness and tearing, the pharmacist should inquire about the medical history. Patients with a history of allergic rhinitis would be expected to experience ophthalmic symptoms such as this and may be directed to self-treat with ophthalmic, antihistamine-decongestant combinations. However, patients who do not have a history of allergy might have viral conjunctivitis.

(tip) *Several categories of nonprescription products require a prior physician/dentist diagnosis before patients can safely use them,* including toothpastes for hypersensitive teeth, vaginal antifungals, and hypertonic sodium chloride solutions. Pharmacists can inquire into patients' medical histories to ensure that they have been diagnosed with dentinal hypersensitivity by a dentist, vaginal fungal infection by a physician or gynecologist, or ocular hypertonicity unrelated to any pathologic condition by an ophthalmologist.

FOCUS ON...

PATIENT INFORMATION FORM

Some pharmacists use patient information forms to elicit information in an orderly manner and to allow it to be recorded for later reference. These have various advantages and disadvantages. While they are useful in reminding the pharmacist of the types of information that should be asked, the patient may be reluctant to provide a name or any other identifying information because of sensitivity about the nature of the condition. However, if the pharmacist explains that the form is to allow better care to be given, the patient may be persuaded to provide the requisite information. One such form is reproduced below:

PATIENT NONPRESCRIPTION TRIAGE RECORD

1. Date_____   Time_____

2. Patient Name_____   Phone_____(Home)_____(Business)

3. Patient Age_____(If more than one patient, use separate form for each patient)

4. Medical History; Current Medical Conditions (Other Than the Reason for Visit)_____
   _____

5. Other Medications Currently Taken (Prescription and Nonprescription)_____
   _____
   _____

6. Patient Gender_____   7. Pregnant   Breast-feeding   (circle if one or both apply)

8. Specific Product Requested?_____(If none, go to #10)

9. Reason for Requesting a Specific Product?_____

10. Description of Condition (as Specific as Possible)_____
    _____

11. Duration of the Condition_____

12. Does Anything Trigger or Worsen the Condition?_____

13. Other medications used for this problem_____

PHARMACIST RECOMMENDATION

A. No product needed (explain why)_____

B. Refer to Another Health Professional (explain)_____

C. Purchase one or more Nonprescription Products or Devices (explain and list

   product(s)/device(s) recommended, if any)_____

PATIENT AGE

The FDA and its advisory panels have established dosing guidelines for most nonprescription products based on patient age. The guidelines specify age cutoffs—that is, the ages below which products should not be used or administered. In some cases age guidelines are simply the result of lack of information regarding product safety; in other cases products pose known hazards below the age cutoff. For instance, children younger than 6 who ingest antihistamines face the risk of paradoxical excitation; similarly, children younger than 3 who ingest antidiarrheals can face life-threatening electrolyte abnormalities.

In general, nonprescription products are not recommended for children younger than 2. Exceptions include ingredients proven safe at these ages such as intraoral local anesthetics for teething and skin protectants for diaper rash.

(tip) *Appendix 1 provides the FDA-recommended age cutoff for most categories of nonprescription medications.*

When counseling the parents or caregivers of a child, the pharmacist should be alert for signs of child abuse or neglect. (See "Suspected Child Abuse.")

Some manufacturers of nonprescription products have chosen to supply dosing charts for certain products—including such potent ingredients as ibuprofen, acetaminophen, pseudoephedrine, antihistamines, and loperamide—that conflict with the FDA-approved age limits. Some manufacturers even suggest that some products can be used to treat newborns. **In the absence of a physician-patient relationship, a pharmacist may incur significant liability should a patient younger than the FDA cutoff suffer an adverse reaction because of using a product the pharmacist recommended.**

DURATION OF THE CONDITION

Some conditions for which self-treatment is allowed are minor and self-limiting conditions that resolve naturally, regardless of whether they are treated. In some cases, however, a condition may reflect underlying pathology that is potentially lethal such as diarrhea and certain types of headache. Thus the FDA often specifies a maximum period for the presence of symptoms that suggest the possibility of a more serious pathology before the patient should see a general practitioner or specialist (e.g., dentist, optometrist, or podiatrist).

(tip) *The maximal periods of self-treatment for various nonprescription products appear in Appendix 2.* These time limitations fall into two categories and must be interpreted cautiously:

- Time limits that signal a maximal safe duration *of the medical condition* before a physician or other practitioner should be consulted
- Time limits for safe use *of a product* before a physician or other practitioner should be seen

The first type of time cutoff can be confusing for patients and professionals. The FDA has not provided sufficient guidance for interpreting the time cutoffs to allow patients to make a logical choice in many cases. The time cutoffs that signal a maximal safe duration for various conditions do not seem to consider the time that has elapsed between the onset of symptoms and when patients enter a pharmacy. For example, patients may be experiencing dehydration and/or electrolyte abnormalities from severe diarrhea of 2 weeks' duration when they enter the pharmacy. The label of the antidiarrheal products cautions, "Do not use for more than 2 days unless directed by a physician" (or similar wording). Patients may believe that self-treatment for another 2 days is recommended by the label, a misconception that—in this example—might be rectified by judicious intervention by a (tip) pharmacist. *It is better to err on the side of patient safety.* For instance, recommend immediate physician consultation for diarrhea that began more than 48 hours before and recommend only 24 hours of self-treatment if the first loose stool was 24 hours prior to the patient's visit to the pharmacy.

The second type of time cutoff is more straightforward. The intent is simply to specify periods beyond which products are not likely to be useful. For example, topical hypopigmenting agents have been given a 3-month time limit because the products probably will have produced a maximal skin lightening effect in that period. Further use would produce little additional benefit, but would not be harmful in most instances. Another example is the 12-week maximal time of self-treatment for wart products during which a wart should have disappeared completely. In these cases the pharmacist can ask the patient if he or she is presently using the product and the duration of use. This helps prevent patients from needlessly applying or ingesting products for extended periods. If the products have not worked as expected in the recommended periods, patients may need to see a physician or other practitioner to ensure that the condition has been diagnosed correctly.

CONTRAINDICATIONS/PRECAUTIONS

(tip) *Many nonprescription products and devices are unsafe when used by certain individuals, as described in Appendix 3.* Contraindications can be based on a number of scenarios:

- A more serious underlying condition may exist—such as a teething baby with fever or nasal congestion, either of which could indicate an infection that should be seen by a physician, not treated with nonprescription products.
- The products could produce adverse reactions in patients such as the ingestion of aspirin by children or teenagers who have or who are recovering from chicken pox, flu symptoms, or flu. (This is an attempt to prevent Reye syndrome.)
- Patients who have a more severe form of the condition should be seen by a physician—such as the warning against use of antiasthmatics for patients who have been hospitalized for asthma.

Because patients can overlook contraindication warnings, pharmacists should discuss them with patients prior to sale.

Despite the vital nature of contraindication information, research indicates that pharmacist counseling in this area needs improvement. For example, in one study researchers asked working pharmacists about storage of insulin and if Contac capsules (which are clearly contraindicated in diabetes) would be good for a summer cold and sniffles.[37] Over 30% of pharmacists queried failed to warn the "patient" about the contraindication.

CONCURRENT USE OF MEDICATIONS AND/OR ALCOHOL

Certain nonprescription products should not be used if the patient is already taking other prescription and/or nonprescription medications. Other nonprescription products caution against concurrent use with alcohol. For example, dextromethorphan, pseudoephedrine, ephedrine, and epinephrine should not be used by patients taking monoamine oxidase inhibitors (MAOIs) or by patients who have stopped taking an MAOI less than 2 weeks previously. In another example labels of antihistamines warn that alcohol can cause drowsiness when consumed concurrently.

DEMOGRAPHIC VARIABLES

Occasionally, demographic variables make certain products inadvisable. For instance, nonprescription diuretics are only approved as safe and effective for menstrually related symptoms. Thus gender disqualifies all males from safely using these products. Male patients who wish to purchase diuretics should be questioned closely regarding their intended use.

In another example, American blacks are rarely infested with head lice (see Chapter 30, Arthropod Stings and Bites, Pediculosis, and Scabies). If black patients request lice products, pharmacists should consider other dermatoses that mimic lice.

Also, some black patients have inappropriately used hypopigmenting agents containing hydroquinone to lighten overall skin color. This unapproved use is unsafe and can lead to a paradoxical darkening of the skin known as exogenous ochronosis (see Chapter 39, Skin Hyperpigmentation). Black patients who wish to purchase skin lightening products should be counseled to ensure that they understand the hazards.

PAST MEDICATION USE

Pharmacists should ask patients what product(s) they have used previously. Answers to this question should yield information on the duration of conditions and could expose the use of undesirable home remedies and unapproved medical products.

Analyzing Product-Related and Patient-Related Information

Once a pharmacist has gathered the necessary information from a patient, the pharmacist must integrate it with knowledge of the capabilities and limitations of the nonprescription products and devices to choose an appropriate triage op-

tion. Considering the following will help work through this analysis:

- In all probability does the patient have the condition he or she thinks he or she has?
- Is the patient's condition self-treatable?
- Do any of the patient-related factors (e.g., age, duration of the condition, etc.) contraindicate self-therapy?
- Is a nonprescription product or device likely to provide benefit for this patient?

Counseling Patients: Triage

The final goal of pharmacist-conducted nonprescription product and device counseling is to ensure that patients are counseled appropriately and triaged correctly. During the analysis phase of the pharmacist's decision-making process, three triage conclusions are possible:

- The patient may not require any product or device at all; the condition will resolve without intervention and is better treated using nonpharmacologic measures (e.g., advising an overweight patient to explore the uses of exercise, portion control, and weight-loss support groups).
- The patient may require an appointment with a physician, dentist, podiatrist, or optometrist.
- The patient may be able to use a safe and effective nonprescription drug product or device.

When pharmacists counsel patients about specific triage decisions, many patients accept the advice without question. Others, however, resist questioning, argue with the pharmacist, and/or ignore the advice. Pharmacists should stress the wisdom of following professional advice, but must recognize that patients are free to act as they wish. After many hours of counseling, most pharmacists will begin to recognize when to discontinue the triage discussion with resistant patients. The following closing comments can help pharmacists disengage gracefully:

- You can take the product if you want, but I'd still see a doctor first.
- If it were my child, I'd take him/her to a doctor.
- If you are going to use the product anyway, please be sure to watch the patient for the reactions I discussed (e.g., for signs of dehydration with diarrhea).
- I don't believe the product will help the problem, but if you're going to use it anyway, be careful to . . . (e.g., watch the severe burn for signs of infection).
- Do you mind if I call you a little later to see if the problem is getting better or worse?
- If you are going to use the product anyway, why don't you call your physician first to see if it sounds appropriate.

The great concern of nontriaged patients is that they will suffer from a serious medical condition, although they still will use a nonprescription product or device rather than make a physician appointment.[38] A study carried out by a chain pharmacy demonstrated that a pharmacist located outside of the dispensing area increased the likelihood of patients selecting proper products and prevented inappropriate treatment when self-therapy was contraindicated and when a visit to a physician was recommended instead.[39]

SUMMARY

The presence of a highly trained professional who can provide counseling on self-care issues—the pharmacist—differentiates the pharmacy from all nonpharmacy retail outlets. Pharmacists who are willing to undertake nonprescription product and device counseling can apply their training to help patients improve the safety, medical effectiveness, and cost effectiveness of self-care therapeutics.

Patients who enter pharmacies often have numerous questions about nonprescription products. It is incumbent on pharmacists to create an atmosphere in which patients feel comfortable asking

(tip) questions. *If patient-pharmacist consultation is not encouraged, then pharmacies lose their primary benefit to consumers over other retail outlets in the sale of nonprescription products.*

To effectively counsel patients on self-care issues, pharmacists should endeavor to carry out several activities:

- Acquire knowledge about nonprescription products and devices themselves. The ingredients in OTC products are often unsafe below certain ages, should not be recommended if a condition has persisted for too long a period, and should not be used in the presence of certain contraindications or if contraindicated when the patient is taking other medications.
- Interview and assess patients to acquire information.

FOCUS ON...

SUSPECTED CHILD ABUSE

According to the National Clearinghouse on Child Abuse and Neglect Information, over 1 million children experience child abuse and/or neglect yearly.[40] This breaks down to 52% who suffer neglect, 25% who experience physical abuse, 13% who undergo sexual abuse, 5% with emotional maltreatment, 3% medical neglect, and 14% miscellaneous forms of maltreatment. (Some children experience multiple types of maltreatment.)

In 1996, Public Law 104–235 (The Child Abuse Prevention and Treatment Act, or CAPTA) defined child abuse as acts resulting in imminent risk of serious harm, death, serious physical or emotional harm, sexual abuse, or exploitation of a child (under the age of 18, unless the state's child protection law carries a different age) by a parent or caretaker (including residential facility employees or staff persons providing out-of-home care) who is responsible for the child's welfare. Withholding medical treatment that would ameliorate or correct life-threatening conditions is defined as failure to respond to the infant's life-threatening conditions by denial of treatment.

Pharmacists may be exposed to child abuse in several ways:

- An abused child may not be taken to a hospital or physician out of fear that X-rays will expose current and past abuse or that a physical exam will expose sexual abuse. Since the pharmacist does not carry out these procedures, the perceived risk of detection of abuse is lower.
- The nonabusing parent/caregiver may express dismay over a child's history of vague aches and pains.
- The child may be seen to have visible bruises, with the abuser requesting external analgesics or heating pads.
- The parent/caregiver may request various bandages and wraps for sprains, muscle tears, or tendon damage incurred during harsh discipline.
- The pharmacist may be asked about products to prevent infection when harsh discipline has broken the skin of the child.
- The pharmacist may be asked to help with burns from such objects as irons or cigarettes.
- The parent/caregiver may request vaginal care products (e.g., douches or vaginal antimonilials) for a child who has contracted an STD, in the mistaken belief that they can prevent a physician visit.
- The parent/caregiver may ask for products to deal with pubic lice in the hair, eyelashes, or eyebrows of young children who have been sexually abused.
- The pharmacist may be asked to help with fecal incontinence in a young child who has undergone anal sexual abuse, leading to lax sphincter.
- The parent/caregiver may ask the pharmacist to supply repeated doses of laxative agents, which may be given to the child to gain medical attention (known as Munchausen by Proxy).
- The pharmacist may receive a request to supply syrup of ipecac or activated charcoal when a parent/caregiver has intentionally fed the child a toxic chemical or medication.
- The parent/caregiver may refuse to treat a child for whom a nonprescription product is clearly indicated (e.g., head lice). While the condition may not be life-threatening in itself, this attitude exposes the possibility of a general neglect.
- The parent/caregiver's description may disclose an emergency situation that mandates referral of the child, but the parent/caregiver does not wish to obtain medical care (e.g., a baby with continual diarrhea that has lasted more than several days).

The typical abuser is a young adult parent in the mid 20s who has not finished high school, is living near or below the poverty level, is depressed and unable to cope with stress, and who has been a victim of violence at one time.

Continued

- Analyze the situation.
- Triage patients: Recommend no action, refer, or recommend a nonprescription product.

More than 50% of child abuse reports emanate from professionals such as educators, law enforcement and justice officials, medical and mental health professionals, social service professionals, and child-care providers. Only 19% originate from the child or relatives of the child.

Should the pharmacist suspect child abuse, it is vital to immediately contact the local child protective services agency or call a state or national hotline number. The National Clearinghouse on Child Abuse and Neglect Information can provide these contacts and can be reached at (800) FYI-3366, or (703) 385-7565 (fax to 703-385-3206) (e-mail to nccanch@calib.com).

FOCUS ON...

UNIVERSAL PRECAUTIONS WHEN COUNSELING PATIENTS

At one time pharmacists and other health-care workers experienced little worry when assessing and working with patients.[41] That attitude changed radically in 1985 with recognition that HIV could be transmitted through needlesticks and contamination with the blood and other body fluids of infected patients.

Hospital personnel and other health-care workers (including students) whose activities involve contact with patients or with their blood and other bodily fluids were required to learn a more strict set of recommendations for preventing transmission of HIV and other bloodborne diseases.[42] These are known as "Universal Blood and Body Fluid Precautions", or "Universal Precautions" for prevention of transmission of HIV, hepatitis B virus, and other bloodborne pathogens. Universal precautions prevent health-care workers from accidental parenteral, mucous membrane, or nonintact skin exposures.

The precautions, which are extensive, are available through Internet access. A few that may apply to the pharmacist who performs triage with nonprescription products are worth special attention, however[41]:

- Barriers should be used to prevent exposure of the pharmacist's skin or mucous membranes when contact with the patient's blood, nonintact skin, or bodily fluids is expected. For instance, if the pharmacist participates in mass screenings involving removing a sample of blood or piercing the skin (e.g., immunizations), gloves must be worn. Should the pharmacist wish to assess dermatologic conditions with broken skin (e.g., dermatitis or athlete's foot), gloves should also be worn. Should the pharmacist assess a wound, gloves must be worn.
- A new pair of gloves is to be used with each patient, and the hands are washed immediately after each pair of gloves is removed.
- Needles should not be recapped, purposely bent or broken, removed from disposable syringes, or manipulated by hand. They should be placed in puncture-resistant containers. These precautions also apply to lancets or other devices used to pierce the skin.
- Should the pharmacist have exudative lesions or weeping dermatitis, all direct patient care should be suspended until the condition resolves.

References

1. Schwartz RM. Pharmacists again top Gallup poll. Am Drugg 215(2):15, 1998.
2. Anon. OTC drugs saved consumers $20 billion in 1996. NDMA Exec Newsletter 10–97: 1, 1997.
3. Snyder K. The state of the OTC marketplace. Drug Topics 141(11):82, 1997.
4. Smith MC. Pharmacists and nonprescription medication: paradox and prospect. Drug Topics 140(2):78, 1996.
5. Weston DR. Canadian pharmacies oppose nonpharmacy OTC sales. Drug Topics 132 (13):13, 1988.
6. Ricker RH. Need to remove nonprescription medications from nonpharmacies (Letter). Am J Hosp Pharm 34:923, 1977.
7. Gannon K. Are all-in-the-family OTC brands misleading? Drug Topics 136(18):50, 1992.
8. Rupp MT, Parker JM. Drug names: when marketing and safety collide. Am Pharm NS33 (5):39, 1993.
9. Pray WS. Confusion in the OTC marketplace. US Pharm 20(1):16, 1995.
10. Conlan MF. Same name, different game. Drug Topics 139 (16):58, 1995.
11. Lauring R. Opportunities in OTC prescribing (Letter)? Am Drugg 213(12):9, 1996.
12. Reynolds WJ. Hey, look me over (Editorial). Drug Topics 135(3):8, 1991.
13. Rubin I. Urgent: write FDA about new OTC labeling. Pharm Times 63(4):19, 1997.
14. Anon. Pharmacists on the OTC label comment deadline nears. The New Independent Fall:4, 1997.
15. Anon. Keep R.Ph.s off OTC labels, NDMA tells FDA. Drug Topics 141(20);28, 1997.
16. Pray WS. When should you recommend an Rx or OTC med to your patrons? US Pharm 14(9):19, 1989.
17. Gasbarro R. The art of triage. Am Drugg 213(2):28, 1996.
18. Snyder K. New role for R.Ph.s: Triage. Drug Topics 140(9): 104, 1996.
19. Palmer H. 1996 OTC teaching survey results. Unpublished research, 1996.
20. Kessler D. FDA chief answers 10 questions on RPhs' expanding health role. Wellcome Trends Pharm 14(3):3, 1992.
21. Anon. 40% of patients on multiple medications don't always read labels. Pharm Times 60(9):1994, 1.
22. Fed Reg 62:9024, 1997.
23. Anon. OTC label study. Weekly Pharm Reports 47(8):1, 1998.

24. Fed Reg 61:17798, 1996.

25. Anon. Reveal inactive ingredients, say pediatricians. Drug Topics 141(4):8, 1997.

26. Gannon K. Where your patients get their information on OTCs. Drug Topics 134(4):32, 1990.

27. Epstein D. How are you doing? Drug Topics 141(12):45, 1997.

28. Gebhart F. Trump card. Drug Topics 139(14):56, 1995.

29. Anon. Docs make more OTC suggestions. Drug Topics 140(18):7, 1996.

30. Snyder K. Study sheds light on doctor recommendations of OTCs. Drug Topics 139(7):37, 1995.

31. Holden MD. Over-the-counter medications. Postgrad Med 91:191, 1992.

32. Pray WS. The pharmacist as self-care advisor. J Am Pharm Assoc NS36:329, 1996.

33. Lober CW. The pharmacist physician (Editorial). J Am Acad Dermatol 13(5Pt1):817, 1985.

34. Hopefl AW. Ethics of diagnosis by pharmacists (Letter). Am J Hosp Pharm 47:2659, 1990.

35. Uretsky SD. (Untitled letter). Am J Hosp Pharm 47:2659, 1990.

36. Simonsmeier LM. Pharmacist prohibited from engaging in the practice of medicine. Pharm Times 57(3):90, 1991.

37. Sierralta OE, Scott DM. Pharmacists as nonprescription drug advisors. Am Pharm NS35(5):36, 1995.

38. Cantrill JA, et al. A study to explore the feasibility of using a health diary to monitor therapeutic outcomes from over-the-counter medicines. J Soc Admin Pharm 12(4):190, 1995.

39. Garnett WR. The final frontier: clinical pharmacy practice in community pharmacy settings. Am J Pharm Educ 53:313, 1989.

40. Anon. What is child maltreatment? National Clearinghouse on Child Abuse and Neglect Information. 1998 (February 27) www.calib.com/nccanch/pubs/index.html.

41. Anon. Universal precautions for prevention of transmission of HIV and other bloodborne infections. National Center for Infectious Diseases. 1998 (February 27) www.cdc.gov/ncidod/diseases/hip/universa.htm (Source: MMWR 36(Su02): 001, 1987).

42. Anon. Recommendations for prevention of HIV transmission in health-care settings. 1998 (February 27) aepo-xdv-www.epo.cdc.gov/wonder/prevguid/p0000318/p0000318.him.

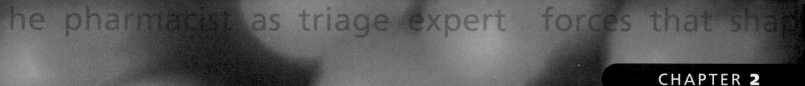

CHAPTER 2

Forces That Shape the Nonprescription Product Market

The nonprescription product market is dynamic and ever-changing, with many older nonprescription drugs discontinued and many new OTC products introduced each year. Some of the new nonprescription products hold special challenges for pharmacists, because they were formerly limited to prescription status. To better understand the forces that shape this volatile market, this chapter examines the regulation of nonprescription drugs, the FDA's OTC review, the Rx-to-OTC switch phenomenon, and the national call for a third class of drugs.

REGULATION OF NONPRESCRIPTION DRUGS AND DEVICES

The Rx Legend

Prior to passage of the 1938 Federal Food, Drug, and Cosmetic Act (FD&C Act) in 1938, the line between prescription and nonprescription products was nonexistent (although the Harrison Narcotic Act of 1914 had made narcotics prescription-only).[1] This legislation required that manufacturers submit a new drug application providing proof of safety prior to marketing medications.[2,3] It also required that adequate directions and warnings be provided on all drug labels, unless the label specifically carried a new prescription legend, "CAUTION: Federal Law Prohibits Dispensing Without Prescription."

There was no actual requirement that any medication carry the legend. As a result manufacturers opted to attempt to provide directions and warnings to allow self-use and were slow to adopt the legend. Thus many dangerous medications were labeled as though safe for self-use, and the distinctions between prescription and nonprescription products remained unclear during the ensuing 2 decades.

The Durham-Humphrey Amendment of 1951

In 1951 the Durham-Humphrey Amendment to the FD&C Act of 1938 attempted to further define nonprescription and prescription medications and to clarify the requirement for the Rx legend.[1,3] Products without the prescription-drug legend became known as "nonlegend" or nonprescription medications, a new class of medications now popularly known as "over-the-counter drugs" or OTCs.

The Kefauver-Harris Amendments of 1962

In 1962 the Kefauver-Harris Amendments to the FD&C Act mandated proof of effectiveness for prescription medications marketed after 1938.[2] (Medications marketed prior to 1938 are known as "grandfathered" drugs because, at that time, they were assigned GRASE [generally recognized as safe and effective] status.)

Medical Device Regulation

In 1976 the Medical Device Amendments to the FD&C Act clarified the marketing requirements of medical devices. According to this amendment manufacturers must notify the FDA at least 90 days before marketing a medical device for the first time.[2] If the application is simple, it is usually approved within the 90 days, although more complicated applications may require more time, causing the manufacturer to wait a longer period before marketing the device.[4]

THE NONPRESCRIPTION PRODUCT REVIEW

The Kefauver-Harris Amendments gave the FDA authority to review nonprescription drugs marketed after 1938 for proof of safety and efficacy. The FDA carefully considered the most appropriate method to use in this review. In 1972 the Food and Drug Administration began the review.[5,6] Because there were an estimated 300,000 nonprescription products to review, the agency quickly realized that the product-by-product method used for prescription products would not be feasible with OTCs. The FDA decided to facilitate the review by placing OTCs into therapeutic classes (e.g., antidiarrheals, antacids, otic products).[7] The subsequent OTC drug review, certainly one of the most comprehensive programs undertaken by FDA, proceeded in three phases[8]:

- Phase 1—Review panels evaluate products. "Advance Notice of Proposed Rulemaking" published for each therapeutic class.
- Phase 2—Deliberations for Category II and III ingredients. "Proposed Rule" or "Tentative Final Monograph" published for each therapeutic class.
- Phase 3—Deliberations continue for Category II and III ingredients. "Final Rule" or "Final Monograph" published for each therapeutic class.

Phases of the Review

PHASE 1
In Phase 1 of the review the FDA appointed an advisory review panel for each therapeutic class.[9,10] The advisory review panels were asked to amass data regarding the safety and efficacy of the ingredients included in products sold for that condition. Panels were made up of representatives from medical and scientific fields as voting members such as physicians, pharmacologists, toxicologists, and pharmacists and other professionals appropriate for that group of products (e.g., dentists or podiatrists).[11] Consumer and industry representatives could be included on panels but only as nonvoting members.[3] FDA employees too could be included on the panels but also not as voting members.

The review panels asked manufacturers to submit products for which review was desired. The advisory panel listed the various ingredients in products sold for that condition and then exhaustively searched for evidence of safety and efficacy. During the reviews the advisory panels examined 20,000 volumes of data concerning 1454 uses of 722 individual ingredients and held 508 meetings.[7,11]

The reviews concluded with the publication of a report, a

proposed rule or proposed monograph known as the "Advance Notice of Proposed Rulemaking," in the *Federal Register*. These evaluations took more than a decade for some product categories, and the last report was not issued until 1983.[12,13] Each advisory panel placed the nonprescription ingredients evaluated into one of three categories[1]:

- Category I: Sufficient evidence of safety and effectiveness
- Category II: Sufficient evidence that the ingredient is unsafe and/or ineffective
- Category III: Insufficient evidence to prove safety and/or effectiveness

The panel also considered such issues as proper labeling claims and the validity of combination products for that therapeutic class.

PHASE 2

Phase 2 for each therapeutic class began with the publication of the "Advance Notice of Proposed Rulemaking." Nonprescription manufacturers were most profoundly affected by the Advance Notice. If the ingredients in a given OTC product were all Category I, they could continue to market it without further work, assuming that their labeling was truthful and correct and conformed to suggested advisory-panel guidelines. However, if a product contained Category II or Category III ingredients, manufacturers had to address potential problems with the product. If a product contained Category II ingredients, but not Category III ingredients, manufacturers were put on notice that there was evidence of ineffectiveness and/or danger to patients. The manufacturers were forced to decide whether to continue to market these ingredients pending further FDA publications or to reformulate.

If a product contained Category III ingredients, manufacturers were allowed to continue to market the product in most instances while considering several options[6]:

- To continue marketing the product pending further review but not to conduct research themselves
- To reformulate to include Category I ingredients
- To undertake research to prove safety and efficacy on their own

If the products were produced in large quantities (e.g, Robitussin), companies often chose the third option. Research had to conform to the highest standards of scientific methodology, including double-blinding, placebo controls, crossovers when appropriate, washout periods, and proper application of the correct statistical test to prove significance in results. The expense of this approach precluded many companies from choosing this option for products that did not justify such a commitment of time and resources.

Any interested party could appear before the FDA during Phase 2 deliberations, including patients or physicians whose favorite products were in jeopardy. Without legitimate research, however, such testimonials received a polite hearing at best, but could not be allowed to alter the outcomes of scientific scrutiny.

Phase 2, which took nearly 15 years for some therapeutic classes, ended for a particular class when the FDA made a decision to terminate information gathering for that therapeutic class. All research submitted during Phase 2 was carefully assessed to decide the safety and efficacy of ingredients. Finally, the agency published in the *Federal Register* a Phase 2 document, known as a "Proposed Rule" or "Tentative Final Monograph." (This document may be referred to using either term; however, there are many other types of rules proposed by the FDA. The tentative final monograph is simply one type of rule proposed by the agency on a wide variety of topics.) The document detailed all comments about the Phase 1 document and presented the new data submitted.

In the Phase 2 documents, the FDA again assigned ingredients to Category I, II, or III. In most cases the FDA agreed with the report of its appointed advisory review panel, but ingredients were reassigned as appropriate.[11] Some ingredients moved from Category III to Category I because manufacturer-sponsored research proved safety and efficacy; other Category III ingredients remained unchanged because no new evidence was submitted or because the research that was done was flawed. (Flawed research such as bias in patient recruitment, insufficient blinding, or use of parametric statistics on nonparametric data was not considered acceptable.[14]) Ingredients also moved from Category I to Category II or Category III because of new information regarding safety. Ingredients originally placed in Category II had already accumulated sufficient evidence of lack of safety and/or efficacy. Thus most manufacturers considered it a waste of time to devote further resources to them, and they seldom, if ever, were reassigned to another category.

Also, the agency addressed the comments that were collected during the Phase 2 period in regard to labeling and combination products and issued preliminary conclusions on these issues.

Publication of the "Tentative Final Monograph" in the *Federal Register* ended Phase 2.

PHASE 3

Phase 3 gave the manufacturers of products containing Category III ingredients further time to either reformulate or design and carry out studies to prove safety and/or efficacy. During this phase the public and health professionals had one last chance to appear before the FDA.

Phase 3 lasted nearly 15 years also. As in Phase 2 the FDA eventually decided that information gathering must conclude for a therapeutic class, subsequently publishing a "Final Rule" that appears in the *Federal Register* in the form of a "Final Monograph."[11] On publication of the "Final Rule" or "Final Monograph" Categories I, II, and III were obsolete, and ingredients were placed in one of only two groups:

- Meets monograph conditions (safe and effective, the former Category I)
- Does not meet monograph conditions (former Categories II and III combined)

The manufacturers were given a period (usually 6 months from publication of the "Final Rule") during which products containing ingredients that did not meet monograph conditions had to be reformulated to contain only fully approved monograph ingredients. Products not reformulated by the end of the allotted time could be seized for adulteration and misbranding. Further, labeling had to conform in regard to indications, claims, hazards, directions for use, dosages, drug interactions, etc. Of course, only the approved combination products could be marketed.

Manufacturers may choose to petition the FDA to amend the final monograph. Such a petition may request that additional ingredients be included or that labeling be modified. Until the amendment is accepted, however, the ingredients cannot be marketed and the labeling cannot be modified.[2]

Criticism of the Review

The FDA OTC review, the first attempt to bring the power of scientific protocol to a poorly regulated group of products, was criticized on several grounds. First was the great amount of time it took. In most cases manufacturers were allowed to continue marketing ingredients in Category II or III pending publication of the Phase 3 document, even though the review process took more than 2 decades to complete. Consequently, consumers were exposed to ingredients that were already proven to be unsafe and/or ineffective or that were of unknown safety and/or efficacy.

To prevent this situation, the FDA could have chosen to force all products known to be lacking safety or efficacy or not yet proven to be safe and efficacious from the market after the publication of the Phase 1 document, and then to permit them to be remarketed only when their ingredients were proven both safe and effective (or they had been reformulated). Erring on the side of the pharmaceutical industry—another criticism—was seen as a compromise of the FDA's function. Specifically, the Congressional General Accounting Office charged that the FDA assigned such a low priority to OTCs that it did not carry out its mandate to protect the public.

One might argue that pharmacists were the last line of defense during the lengthy evaluation and deliberation period, prior to the issuance of the Phase 3 document. This argument assumes, however, that pharmacists were properly informed about category assignments of the various nonprescription ingredients. The *Federal Register* is not on the reading list of most pharmacists, and in practice most pharmacists were poorly informed about the FDA deliberations.[15] Failure to adequately publicize unapproved ingredients led to several decades during which the pharmacy profession was unable to act properly as patient advocates.

In 1995 *U.S. News & World Report* highlighted patient dangers from "FDA-banned pills and potions"—further exposing weaknesses in the drug-review process.[16] Specifically, the publication examined the FDA policy of placing ingredients in nonmonograph status, yet failing to recall them. "Once a ban takes effect, manufacturers are barred from shipping new supplies, but stores legally can sell banned drugs until their own and their wholesalers' inventories run out. It's consumers who remove banned items from drugstore shelves—by buying them." The publication highlighted cases in which consumers had been injured by banned products (e.g., quinine-induced renal failure). *Informed pharmacists should take the initiative to remove unsafe and ineffective products from the shelves*, returning them to the wholesaler for credit if permitted or discarding them if they cannot be returned.

Products Not Reviewed

Nonprescription ingredients marketed prior to 1938 (e.g., phenazopyridine) are sometimes spoken of as being protected from FDA scrutiny because they are "grandfathered."[9] However, personnel within the FDA stress that eventually these grandfathered ingredients will also be examined for safety and efficacy. Further, regardless of whether they were reviewed, the labeling claims of these products must be truthful.

Benefits of the Review

Eventually, when the FDA OTC review is finished (e.g., all amendments settled), pharmacists—and patients—will have assurance that nonprescription products (and combination products) that underwent the review contain ingredients that are both safe and effective for their labeled indications and thus can be recommended with confidence.[17] Further, labels will inform patients about the conditions for safe use, doses, contraindications, warnings, and ingredients. At this point OTC products sold at nonpharmacy outlets can be chosen with confidence also, assuming patients are correct in their self-diagnosis and that they read and understand all label information. FDA rulings should help eliminate deceptive advertising as well.[3] Of course, deceptive advertising and misleading products will always be offered to an unwary public (See Chapter 49, Precautions in Self-Care.)

After the review is complete, prospective manufacturers of nonprescription products may simply examine the pertinent copies of the *Federal Register* to see which ingredients can be included in their products and what information to place on the label. If a manufacturer wishes to market new ingredients, they must be submitted through the New Drug Application process if FDA approval is sought.

CURRENT FDA NONPRESCRIPTION PRODUCT OVERVIEW

The Nonprescription Drug Advisory Committee (NDAC)

The FDA created an Office of Over-the-Counter Drug Evaluation in 1991, to place renewed emphasis on the review of nonprescription drug products.[18] Shortly thereafter, the agency also formed a Nonprescription Drugs Advisory Committee (NDAC) to examine safety and effectiveness issues regarding OTCs. Serving as a replacement for the advisory panels utilized during Phase 1 of the FDA OTC review, which were disbanded as their work was completed, the experts appointed to the NDAC consider issues of importance as they arise.

The FDA OTC Review Process

The FDA OTC review process is ongoing. Final monographs are lacking for some therapeutic classes as of this writing. With the assistance of the NDAC to provide advice on various issues, the FDA is optimistic that the review will proceed in a timely fashion.

THE PRESCRIPTION-TO-NONPRESCRIPTION (RX-TO-OTC) SWITCH

The nonprescription marketplace has been kept in a state of flux for several reasons such as new product introductions and reformulations of established brands. The most exciting impetus to the market, however, has been a phenomenon popularly referred to as the "Rx-to-OTC switch." The Rx-to-OTC switch occurs when an ingredient or product formerly available only by prescription becomes available for nonprescription use.

Methods by Which Prescription Medications Gain OTC Status

Prescription medications may gain nonprescription status by a variety of methods. The discussions below describe the three primary Rx-to-OTC avenues:

* The FDA OTC review
* The "switch regulation"
* Processes related to the New Drug Application (NDA)

THE FDA OTC REVIEW
The FDA OTC review process has allowed some medications to attain nonprescription status, although it has not been utilized in recent years.[1,19] This may have occurred when the advisory panel or the FDA itself decided a prescription medication possessed sufficient safety to allow self-use. Examples of medications that joined the ranks of nonprescription agents through this route include hydrocortisone, diphenhydramine, oxymetazoline, and fluoride dental rinses. Proceedings are not confidential, which compromises manufacturer trade secrets.[20] Lack of confidentiality is one reason manufacturers prefer not to use this method.

THE "SWITCH REGULATION"
The switch regulation, which dates from the 1950s, allows any interested party to petition the FDA to switch any medication to OTC status.[1] Historically, manufacturers have usually been the sponsors. While one manufacturer might petition for a switch, another might not, resulting in Rx and OTC marketing of the same ingredient, a confusing situation. Lack

of confidentiality of the proceedings is a major drawback, so that most manufacturers do not prefer this route to OTC status. The switch regulation was used for dextromethorphan and tolnaftate, but has not been used since 1971.[21]

PROCESSES RELATED TO THE NEW DRUG APPLICATION (NDA)
Processes related to the NDA are the most common paths from Rx to OTC. When a medication is originally approved as a prescription product, a full NDA must be submitted, which can take years and millions of pages of documentation. Following approval of the original NDA, if the manufacturer wishes to change a dosage or formulation, a full NDA may also be required. However, if a minor change is anticipated, the FDA may only request a supplemental NDA that addresses certain issues. If another manufacturer wishes to also market the same product (or one closely related), an abbreviated NDA may be all that is necessary, which is a shorter version of the original NDA submitted by the parent company. Manufacturers may proceed through Rx-to-OTC switching by three methods related to NDAs:

* Submit a full NDA for a medication currently available by prescription, but for a new dosage or formulation such as a lower strength than the Rx version
* Submit a supplemental NDA for a product for which the manufacturer already holds an approved NDA or holds an abbreviated NDA for a closely related product
* Submit an abbreviated NDA for products that are identical to an existing prescription product

If the company is not required to carry out clinical trials, an abbreviated NDA is approvable immediately. If the FDA requires a manufacturer to carry out new and possibly novel research by way of clinical trials (e.g., intravenous animal injections to prove safety for nonprescription status), the company is granted 3 years of marketing exclusivity against competing abbreviated NDAs.[6,22] (This provision of the Drug Price Competition and Patent Term Restoration Act of 1984 helps compensate the sponsor for the costs of the research.[2,21]) Thus other companies cannot market the same ingredient without also carrying out original research until 3 years have elapsed, at which time the ingredient will be eligible for an abbreviated NDA.[23,24]

Marketing exclusivity is a major draw for companies, who have used this method in ever-increasing numbers in the 1990s. Products switched under NDA-related processes include ibuprofen, loperamide, permethrin, vaginal antifungals, Actifed, Rogaine, Nicorette, NicoDerm CQ, Nicotrol, Tagamet HB, Pepcid AC, Zantac 75, Axid AR, and Nasalcrom.

All proceedings related to the NDA are confidential, which the pharmaceutical industry prefers.[20]

Types of Rx-to-OTC Switches

There are two types of Rx to OTC switches, as measured by the ingredient's status after the switch[25]:

* The complete switch
* The partial switch

THE COMPLETE SWITCH

In the complete switch the product becomes nonprescription—all dosage strengths if there were more than one—and no prescription version remains. Examples include Rogaine, vaginal antifungals, pyrantel pamoate for pinworm, Nix for head lice, and both strengths of Nicorette gum for smoking cessation (Fig. 2.1).

THE PARTIAL SWITCH

In the partial switch one or more doses that were formerly prescription become OTC, or lower strengths that were never available on an Rx basis become OTC, but higher doses remain only available through prescription order. Examples include clemastine (Tavist-1 [OTC] contains 1.34 mg of clemastine fumarate per tablet; Tavist Tablets [Rx] contain 2.68 mg each) and naproxen sodium (Aleve [OTC] contains 220 mg naproxen sodium per tablet; Anaprox [Rx] contains 275 mg each). Other examples include ketoprofen, all of the H2-blockers, and ibuprofen. Occasionally, the same strength is simultaneously available in both prescription and nonprescription versions (e.g., Imodium 2 mg capsules and Imodium A-D caplets, Tagamet 200 mg tablets and Tagamet HB 200 caplets) (Fig. 2.2).

Factors Considered in Rx-to-OTC Switch Decisions

The Durham-Humphrey Amendment of 1951 clearly delineated the differences between Rx and OTC medications.

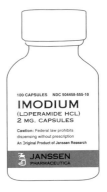
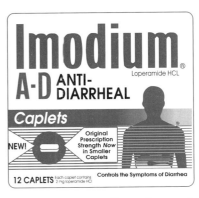

Figure 2.2. Artistic representation of a product marketed simultaneously in prescription (*top*) and nonprescription (*bottom*) versions.

Factors that mandate prescription status include the potential for harm such as unreasonable toxicity, the ability of the patient to understand the method of use or collateral measures necessary for use, and the possibility of patient misuse.[26] The FDA occasionally applies other factors as well. In 1985 the Director of the Office of Drug Standards listed four broad categories of considerations[27]:

- Safety
- Effectiveness
- Labeling
- Other issues

SAFETY

Safety, the first of the four factors, is a relative term, since no medication can be absolutely harmless in all potential patients at all times. Thus a decision of safety for potential nonprescription products focuses on several questions.

Toxicity or Other Potential for Harmful Effect

Overall Safety. The FDA examines the traditional measures of safety and toxicity such as the LD50, pharmacokinetic parameters, potential for drug interactions, carcinogenicity, possible adverse reactions, and safety in subpopulations (e.g., geriatric, pediatric, and pregnant patients).[27,28] Thus medications with high potential for toxicity that must be dosed under medical supervision (e.g., digitalis, phenytoin) are not suitable OTC candidates. The question of overall safety halted the po-

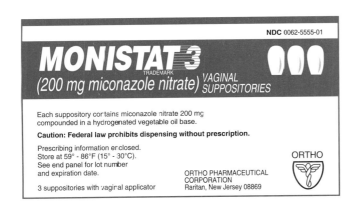

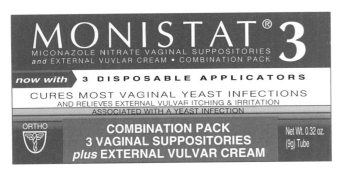

Figure 2.1. Artistic representation of the labels of a product once marketed as a prescription product (*top*), but switched to nonprescription status (*bottom*).

tential switch of terfenadine, for example, which may cause abnormal heart rhythms in patients taking other medications (e.g., ketoconazole, itraconazole, clarithromycin, erythromycin, and troleandomycin). Eventually, the product was withdrawn from the United States market completely.

Two additional illustrations of potential drug interactions help clarify this issue. If an interaction is common or of such serious potential that adequate labeling cannot be developed to allow safe use, the product will retain prescription status. Cholestyramine has been considered for a switch, but an FDA committee member raised the concern about serious interactions with medications such as anticoagulants, digitalis, thyroid supplements, and folic acid.[29] The agency member felt the company had downplayed the potential for such interactions, and the committee denied OTC status.

Cimetidine is another example. Although cimetidine can cause serious drug interactions with theophylline, phenytoin, and anticoagulants, the manufacturer was able to develop labeling that explained the problem clearly enough for the average patient, and the product was approved for OTC status.

Benefit:Risk Ratio. A medication proposed for OTC use should produce a low incidence of adverse reactions when used as directed and when patients are adequately warned against unsafe use.[30] This qualification may also apply in a larger sense to the larger group of potential patients.[28] For instance, topical erythromycin was under consideration for acne at one time. However, there was concern within the FDA that widespread, unsupervised use might cause resistance to develop in the population.[31] The same concern was partly responsible for lack of approval for nonprescription acyclovir for genital herpes.[32]

There also must be little risk that a medication would mask a serious underlying medical disorder. If the medication alleviated the symptoms of this disorder, it might progress without the patient receiving proper treatment. As an example, vomiting is a symptom of many serious problems that require physician screening. Thus nonprescription medication cannot be labeled for relief of vomiting, unless it is related to the minor etiology of motion sickness.

Potential for Abuse/Misuse. If the medication can cause addiction, it has high potential for abuse and is not allowed to be sold OTC. Potential misuse could include sales to those for whom the product is not intended. For instance, OTC nicotine products for smoking cessation were only approved with the understanding that measures to prevent abuse would be instituted. The products cannot be sold to individuals younger than 18, nor can they be placed in a vending machine or in any other retail sales situation where proof of age cannot be verified.

Need for Routine Medical Examinations or Lab Work. If a medication used in a certain condition requires periodic medical examinations to ensure that the medication is helping the condition or lab work to ensure that it is not causing toxicity, it must be disqualified from nonprescription sales

for that condition, or its indications must be limited to other minor conditions that are less serious.[30] For instance, H2-blockers cannot be labeled for treatment of an ulcer, which requires periodic laboratory testing and physician evaluation.

This criterion disqualified metaproterenol from nonprescription status in 1982.[1] At that time the FDA indicated that the ingredient could be marketed OTC, and several manufacturers did so. However, health professionals quickly pointed out that patients with asthma might obtain short-term relief from metaproterenol, delaying physician visits for proper monitoring. After due consideration, the FDA reversed its opinion, forcing manufacturers to withdraw the product from OTC sales and returning it to Rx status.

Method of Use and Collateral Measures Necessary for Use
This criterion encompasses several important questions regarding the condition to be treated:

- Ability of patients to self-diagnose conditions
- Ability of patients to recognize symptoms
- Potential of the condition to be self-treated

Ability of Patients to Self-Diagnose Conditions. Nonprescription products are usually only appropriate for conditions that patients can self-diagnose.[27] This objective has caused manufacturers to go to great lengths to teach patients to self-diagnose certain conditions. For instance, when the FDA contemplated an Rx-to-OTC switch for Rogaine (topical minoxidil for hair loss), one vital point was the ability of the patient to differentiate self-treatable androgenetic baldness from other causes of hair loss. Extensive patient education material in the package insert was deemed sufficient to accomplish this, and the ingredient was approved for nonprescription sales. Conversely, the FDA does not feel that patients can self-diagnose genital herpes, which has caused difficulties in a proposed Rx-to-OTC switch of acyclovir.[32] This switch has not occurred at this time because of these issues.

Ability of Patients to Recognize Symptoms. The underlying cause of some symptoms might not be diagnosable by the patient. For instance, patients may not know the exact cause of headache, muscle ache, or upset stomach. However, as these symptoms do not usually reflect serious underlying pathology, they are considered to be self-treatable when patients can recognize them. For example, internal analgesic products treat headache effectively, even though patients might not be able to identify the specific type of headache.

Potential of the Condition to be Self-Treated. For a condition to be judged as self-treatable, the FDA considers three questions:

- What are the risks to the patient who uses the medication but does not have the condition for which the medication was intended?
- What are the risks to the patient who has the condition and does not seek medical attention but chooses to use the nonprescription medication instead?

- What is the potential length of time the patient might use the nonprescription product before seeking medical attention?

These criteria help ensure that nonprescription products are used primarily for minor conditions that would resolve even if they are not treated (e.g., motion sickness, the common cold). The criteria also help the FDA decide on time limits for self-use prior to seeking medical care. For instance, the male may treat androgenetic alopecia with Rogaine for 12 months before deciding that it does not work. On the other hand, one may only self-treat diarrhea for 2 days prior to seeking medical care. Obviously, the risks of uncontrolled diarrhea are far more serious (even deadly) than the risks of poorly treated androgenetic alopecia.

One notable exception to these criteria should be pointed out.[28] Insulin, a nonprescription product in the U-100 strength, is only available from pharmacies and retail outlets with a pharmacy. This restriction has been the case since insulin was first marketed in the 1920s. Few would argue that Type 1 and Type 2 diabetes mellitus are either self-diagnosable or self-treatable without physician monitoring. Nevertheless, Type 1 diabetics who cannot obtain insulin can become hyperglycemic, which can cause death. Nonprescription insulin sales evidently are allowed to make it easier for diabetics to obtain this crucial drug. Thus insulin is perhaps the most dangerous nonprescription product available, since only moderate overdoses can induce irreversible CNS damage and can cause death from hypoglycemia.

EFFECTIVENESS

Effectiveness is the second of the four factors in Rx-to-OTC switch decisions. For a given product a significant proportion of patients should experience the beneficial effect described on the product's label. (The proposed nonprescription use should be similar or identical to that of the approved prescription version of the product.[27]) If the proposed nonprescription dosage is lower than the Rx version, new studies may be required to prove that this lower dose is still effective.

LABELING

The product must be labeled with adequate directions for proper use.[28] Labeling must be stated clearly, so that "ordinary" patients can understand terminology, including patients with low reading comprehension. Adequate warnings must be developed also, warning patients against:

- Use in dangerous conditions
- Use by patients who are too young to use the product safely
- Unsafe dosages
- Unsafe durations of use
- Use longer than recommended prior to seeking medical attention
- Use in pregnancy and nursing, unless the medication is exempt (such as protectant ingredients applied topically for hemorrhoids)

OTHER ISSUES

The FDA occasionally considers other criteria in approving an Rx-to-OTC switch, even though they may not be part of formal policy. In 1993, for example, an FDA panel attempted to hold a meeting to discuss the possibility of switching oral contraceptives to OTC status.[33] There was an immediate outcry by public groups against any move in this direction. The agency canceled the meeting, citing concerns that they had consulted with too few interest groups such as family planning advocates. Apparently, the deciding factor in canceling the meeting was the social impact of allowing unrestricted sales of a potent and highly effective birth control product. This proposal has never been reopened.

Benefits to the Rx-to-OTC Switch Movement

BENEFITS TO INDUSTRY

Manufacturers can benefit in several ways by switching medications from Rx to OTC status. For example, OTC sales expand the potential market for products that are threatened by patent expiration.[34,35] To illustrate, all four H2-blockers (Axid, Pepcid, Tagamet, and Zantac) had either undergone patent expiration or were nearing those dates. As a result their market share was threatened by the potential introduction of less expensive generic competitors. By converting to OTC sales, the brand names gained new life through new OTC advertising campaigns and the 3-year extended-patent exclusivity for the nonprescription version of the product.[28,36,37] (See: Processes Related to the New Drug Application [NDA]") The sales of products switched from Rx to OTC often double or triple.[38]

Switching to OTC status also allows manufacturers to move into different competitive arenas. As an example, when Merck & Co. introduced Prilosec, a proton-pump inhibitor, it created competition for Pepcid, its H2-blocker. By switching Pepcid to OTC status (while retaining an Rx version) and retaining Rx status for Prilosec, Pepcid AC was allowed to enter the lucrative market for antacid products for gastroesophageal reflux.

BENEFITS TO PATIENTS

Rx-to-OTC switches provide several benefits to patients. Rx-to-OTC switches allow patients to self-treat conditions for which medical advice was once required—such as smoking cessation, androgenetic alopecia, vaginal candidal infections, and ophthalmic complications of allergic rhinitis—and thus gain more control over their health care.[39] Patients also save on the costs of physician visits (even with insurance deductibles which usually range from $10 to $15), reduce time taken from work (possibly with docked pay), and eliminate the need to purchase a prescription product. As a case in point, patients have saved an estimated $150 million yearly since hydrocortisone 1% switched to OTC status.[18]

BENEFITS TO PHARMACY AND PHARMACISTS

As more medications attain OTC status, the role of the pharmacist as a self-care advisor becomes more critical. Labeling for products switched from Rx to OTC is often more complex than with older OTC products because the conditions require more sophisticated skills for recognition. Booklets enclosed with some newly switched products may have many pages, all of which should be read by patients before using the products.

To properly counsel the patients who request recently switched OTC products, pharmacists should ask patients the following questions to ensure that the medications are appropriate[40]:

1. Did a physician recommend that you purchase this medication?
2. How did you hear about this product?
3. Have you ever taken the prescription form of this product?
4. Have you ever had a reaction to this product in its prescription forms?
5. Do you currently have a prescription for this medication that you can get refilled?
6. Do you currently have a prescription for this medication for which refills have been denied by a physician? If so, why?
7. What condition do you intend to treat with this medication?
8. Has this condition ever been medically diagnosed?
9. Do you intend to take this along with any prescription product? (If so, the pharmacist should attempt to ascertain if the Rx product contains the same ingredient(s) as the OTC such as a Motrin prescription plus Nuprin.)
10. What prescription and OTC medications are you currently taking on a daily basis?

Pharmacists should anticipate questions such as the following from patients regarding switched OTC products[40]:

1. Is this safer than it was when it was prescription?
2. Why don't I need a prescription for this now?
3. Can I take/give it in the same amount as my doctor recommended when it was an Rx product (e.g., Children's Motrin)?
4. What is the difference between this product and that product since one tablet is fewer milligrams than the other (e.g., ketoprofen versus ibuprofen versus naproxen)?
5. Why can't I just take four of these tablets to get the same dose as I did when it was a prescription product?
6. Will this cost the same or more?
7. Does this mean that I never have to see my doctor again for this problem (e.g., vaginal fungal infections)?
8. My friend said she has the same problem as I do, but she didn't want to go to the doctor. Can I suggest the use of this product for her because you can get it without a prescription now?
9. I was taking this for [condition], but that's not printed on the label. I know how to use it for that condition, so can't I just treat myself since I can get it without a prescription?
10. Can you keep a record of this on your computer for me?

Problems with the Rx-to-OTC Switch Movement

REIMBURSEMENT PROBLEMS

Patients whose insurance plans provided full coverage for a prescription product usually discover that when the product changes to OTC status, it is no longer covered.[41,42] This is usually also true for patients who rely on Medicaid coverage, which often does not provide coverage for nonprescription products. With a product such as Rogaine, for example, no Rx version remains as an alternate for physicians to prescribe.

PATIENT CONFUSION

The Rx-to-OTC switch can result in confusion for patients because of the following:

- Dual Rx and OTC marketing
- Misperceptions regarding safety
- Misleading advertising
- Lost pharmacist counseling

Dual Rx and OTC Marketing

When simultaneous marketing of Rx and OTC versions of an ingredient is allowed, the OTC version is usually a lower strength. The FDA has considered allowing dual marketing of the same strengths, but the prescription and nonprescription packages would have to differ in size, shape, color, and name labeling and would have to be promoted differently.[43,44]

There are exceptions, however. For example, a certain strength of an ingredient may be suitable for self-treatment for one condition but not for another. Thus ingredients are sold at the same strength in both Rx and OTC forms.[24] For example, meclizine 25 mg is available as an OTC for motion sickness, but only as an Rx product for vertigo. Pharmacists must explain that motion sickness can be safely self-treated, but that vertigo may be caused by any of several serious medical problems that require sophisticated medical testing.

Simultaneous marketing of the same ingredient as an Rx and an OTC can lead to patient confusion, however, regardless of whether the strengths are identical. Patients are understandably confused when they discover that ibuprofen is in Advil and also in Motrin 800 mg, for example. They may feel that the product in nonprescription form allows them to simply take four tablets to duplicate the Rx doses.[45] (In this case, the pharmacist must explain that the only safe dosage is that listed on the label. Taking more than recommended could increase the risk of adverse reactions.)

Misperceptions Regarding Safety

Patients often see nonprescription products as safe in any dose and able to treat virtually any condition. OTC products are usually quite safe when used as directed for their labeled indications, although there is a risk of adverse reactions at even normal doses. Problems such as adverse reactions multiply when patients stray from the intended doses. For example, a patient may decide to use ibuprofen for rheumatoid arthritis, taking incorrect doses far in excess of the maximum duration recommended on the label, possibly resulting in gastric ulceration.

Misleading Advertising

Most consumers have limited medical knowledge, which hampers their ability to evaluate the veracity of advertising campaigns.[46] When products switch to OTC status, sponsors often resort to aggressive marketing, especially when there is strong competition (as with the H2-blockers). The result may be misleading advertising. In 1995 a New York federal court examined advertising for Pepcid AC and Tagamet HB.[47–49] The court ruled that both companies had misled consumers regarding such issues as effectiveness and onset of action. The companies agreed to withdraw or modify the offending ads, but, of course, the ads had been seen by an unknown number of impressionable consumers by that time.

Lost Pharmacist Counseling

FDA-mandated OTC labeling does not specifically recommend that the patient speak with a pharmacist prior to purchase. In fact, the FDA assumes that switched OTC products will be used without any pharmacist involvement.[50] Although pharmacist counseling was considered to be mandatory when these ingredients were prescription items, apparently the FDA feels it has no place in nonprescription sales of the same ingredient. Unfortunately, this deprives patients of the rich storehouse of knowledge pharmacists have amassed when counseling patients on the ingredient as a prescription item.

PHYSICIAN RESISTANCE

Some physicians view the Rx-to-OTC switch as "putting a scalpel in the hands of a child."[51] Often when a nonprescription product switches to OTC status, the specialty journals for physicians in that field predict adverse consequences.[52] For example, when hydrocortisone was proposed for an OTC switch, dermatology literature carried cautions about a patient who misdiagnosed herpes simplex as poison oak dermatitis and applied hydrocortisone. Another patient treated a bacterial infection of the face with hydrocortisone, thinking it was contact dermatitis.[53] In both cases, the infection worsened.

INSUFFICIENT PHARMACIST PREPARATION

Because of the proprietary nature of NDA-related Rx-to-OTC switches, manufacturers are not forced to disclose before product introduction what the approved labeling of a newly switched product will contain. Consequently, the product hits the shelves with the advertising campaign in full swing. Patients might ask questions about warnings, contraindications, drug interactions, durations of use, etc., while pharmacists struggle to become informed about the product. Of course, much of the usage information on new OTC products is in booklets sealed in the package, preventing the pharmacists from reviewing it. The solution is to sacrifice a package, which can be opened, studied, and used in patient counseling.

The problem is worsened for pharmacists when manufacturers cannot ship sufficient product, hampering pharmacists' attempts to obtain labeling. Some companies have tried to inform pharmacists by sending "launch kits" to pharmacies. Timed to coincide with the arrival of the OTC versions of the product, these kits might contain booklets, videotapes, etc.

A THIRD CLASS OF DRUGS

What are the implications when medications switch from Rx-to-OTC status? By abruptly moving a product from Rx to OTC status, the FDA communicates the following message to consumers and the profession: Today this medication is so dangerous that it must be prescribed by a physician; tomorrow you may purchase it from a vending machine in a hotel lobby or gas station whenever you desire.[54] There is no middle ground.

Many health-care professionals and consumers believe it would be more logical to place newly switched products into a different class of medications—essentially a "third class of drugs"—so that newly switched drugs can be monitored more carefully for a few years. Debate continues over this hotly contested proposal, although the FDA has not been supportive. Interestingly, the United States and South Africa are the only countries without such a class of drugs. A third class would only be available in the 65,000 pharmacies nationwide, rather than the 750,000 retail outlets that now sell nonprescription products.[55] (Under the current rules, the OTCs can be bought in one million retail outlets.)

The Pharmacist's Responsibilities with a Third Class of Drugs

Although there has been no clear consensus, the pharmacist's responsibilities with a third class of drugs might include the following:

- Stocking the third-class items behind the counter, with signage announcing their availability, and referring the patient to the pharmacist
- Training supportive personnel not to sell these items without the pharmacist's knowledge and approval
- Conducting counseling appropriate to ensure that the product is indicated
- Demonstrating use of the product to the patient

The Various Proposals for a Third Class of Drugs

Proponents of a third class of drugs have offered two methods by which it might be accomplished.

- A fixed class: A class for permanent placement of switched OTCs, medications that would never be placed into another class.
- A transition class: A "way-station" class where Rx-to-OTC drugs would remain for 2 to 5 years.[56] During this period the FDA should be notified of any adverse reactions. At the end of the transition period the agency would consider any adverse reactions reported and decide whether to move to full OTC sale status. Proponents of this approach argue that it could actually increase the number of OTC products available to patients. Further, they assert that it would reduce drug misuse since patients would receive

pharmacist counseling (since counseling would be mandatory prior to sale to determine whether the product is indicated). Also, proponents point out that a transition class could lower health-care costs by freeing physicians to spend more time with seriously ill patients because more minor ailments could be treated by pharmacists.

Supporters of a Third Class of Drugs

THE NATIONAL ASSOCIATION OF BOARDS OF PHARMACY (NABP)
The NABP passed a resolution in 1995 calling for legislation to create the third class.[57] This was a unanimous vote despite a recommendation from the executive committee against the measure, citing concerns that it would restrain consumer choice.

THE PHARMACISTS PLANNING SERVICE, INC. (PPSI)
The PPSI, a pharmacy advocacy group, petitioned the FDA to place ipecac, promethazine, hydrocortisone 1%, metaproterenol, phenylpropanolamine, and naproxen into a third class in 1991.[55] In 1995 the group presented a series of citizens' petitions in support of a third class of drugs to the FDA.[58,59]

The PPSI has charged that opponents of a third class of drugs are ignoring health problems associated with OTC-Rx interactions, as well as OTC products such as phenylpropanolamine, ephedrine, and ibuprofen. The PPSI has pointed out that OTC packaging is ineffective in conveying warnings.[58] The PPSI initially asked for a pharmacist-only class, but it now is seeking approval for a transitional class.

CONSUMER GROUPS
The National Consumers League (NCL), an organization that backed the establishment of the FDA in the early 1900s, strongly supports the third class.[58,60] The NCL is joined by the Consumer Federation of America, the Consumers Union, the National Insurance Consumer Federation, and the Public Health Citizen's Health Research Group.[61]

PHARMACISTS
Pharmacists as a whole back the concept of a third class. Understandably, pharmacy is seen by opponents as a special interest desirous of a monopoly to boost their profits at the expense of other retailers, who now enjoy a significant portion of the OTC market.[28,61–63]

THE NATIONAL COMMUNITY PHARMACISTS ASSOCIATION (NCPA)
The NCPA (formerly the National Association of Retail Druggists or NARD) passed a resolution calling for an interim drug category in 1982 (to be known as a "pharmacist legend" class) and has supported the concept since that time.[54,65] A NARD spokesperson suggested that a transition class would create a "buffer" period during which pharmacists can learn about newly switched medications before they are sold in locations with no health professional.

OTHER PROFESSIONAL ASSOCIATIONS
The American Pharmaceutical Association (APhA) and the American College of Apothecaries support a concept of the third class of drugs.[66,67]

Opponents of a Third Class of Drugs

THE FDA
The FDA, which has opposed a third class for many years, denied petitions from consumers and the NCPA (then known as NARD) for a third class in 1984.[55] The FDA contends that proponents have yet to show justification for a third class of drugs.[68] The FDA maintains that all OTC drugs are supposed to be properly labeled for safe and effective use and stresses that the agency acts appropriately when products do not provide proper information for safe and effective use.[68]

The FDA insists it lacks the authority to establish the third class, but given the power of the FDA, that position is debatable.[58]

THE CONSUMER HEALTHCARE PRODUCTS ASSOCIATION
This manufacturers organization (formerly known as the Proprietary Association and the Nonprescription Drug Manufacturers Association or NDMA) is understandably against anything that might restrain consumers in buying their products.[55,69] In a 1990 position paper the NDMA stated their objections as follows[70]:

- Druggists (the term used by this organization) would have a monopoly, denying consumers the right to buy safe products at convenient locations of their own choice and at competitive prices and also denying general merchants (grocery stores, discount stores, department stores, and convenience stores, etc.) the right to sell these safe products.
- The restrictions imposed on a third class would result in increased costs and inconvenience to consumers by removing these products from grocery, discount, and convenience stores and other general retail outlets without any public health benefits.
- The concept had been rejected by the FDA.
- The concept had been rejected by the American Medical Association (AMA). (See "The American Medical Association [AMA]".)

An NDMA spokesman stated in 1992 that drugs are either safe for self-treatment or not, adding that the current two-tiered system is suitable.[58]

A former FDA commissioner has charged that drug manufacturers are concerned that the third class would cut into profits. The NDMA rebutted this charge, stating that the issue is consumer access.[55] The NDMA also cited the 1995 finding by the General Accounting Office (GAO) that a third class of drugs is not needed.[65] (See "The General Accounting Office [GAO]".)

THE GENERAL ACCOUNTING OFFICE (GAO)
The GAO, the chief investigating arm of the U.S. Congress, looked at the third class issue in 10 countries and decided that the success of the third class is tied to the role of pharmacists in the drug distribution system.[71] The GAO also determined, however, that, in countries with a third class of drugs, pharmacists often gather incomplete information on patient symptoms and histories and that pharmacist counseling was infrequent and incomplete.[72] Further, safeguards to

prevent drug misuse were circumvented. The GAO also stated that a third class of drugs would saddle pharmacists with time-consuming, costly tasks such as recording patient symptoms and medical conditions, names of practitioners who recommended products, amount of product purchased, patients' experiences with given products (including efficacy, side effects, and interactions with foods and drugs), and medical conditions.[65]

As a result of its investigation, the GAO concluded in 1995 that the need for a third class was not demonstrated.[55,73] The agency did note that the then-emerging concept of pharmaceutical care might change these views, but that it had not yet been implemented sufficiently to know its impact on OTCs.

THE AMERICAN MEDICAL ASSOCIATION (AMA)

The AMA passed a resolution against the third class in 1984. The organization has maintained that position ever since. The view of physicians is typified by a dermatologist who pointed out the lack of clinical diagnostic skills in pharmacists, the inability of the pharmacist to physically examine patients, and the difficulty the pharmacist would have in keeping complete medical records.[74]

OTHER OPPONENTS

The third class is opposed by companies and associations in the retail food, retail merchants, and direct selling industries, chambers of commerce, senior citizens' organizations, labor unions, farm organizations, the U.S. Department of Justice (on antitrust grounds), Congress, state legislatures, federal and state courts, and the Association of State Attorneys General.[67] Advertising agencies and television networks, which subsist on convincing consumers to buy OTC products through direct-to-consumer OTC ads, understandably are also opposed to the revenue loss that would result from the third class.

THE FUTURE OF A THIRD CLASS OF DRUGS

The outlook is not bright for a third class of drugs. Ironically, however, some pharmacists are voluntarily creating a third class by placing certain medications behind the counter such as asthma medications and laxatives abused by anorexics. Unfortunately, this gesture is meaningless when patients can simply go next door to buy the products in question. The action may even be counterproductive if it results in patients shopping at nonpharmacist outlets where counseling is not an option.

An alternative is for concerned pharmacists to place newly switched products under a sign that states: "This product has recently been released for use without a prescription. Your pharmacist would like to discuss the safe and effective use of the product if you have not yet used it without a prescription."[75]

SUMMARY

The FDA began an exhaustive process of review for most nonprescription product ingredients in 1972. During this three-phase process, which has taken close to three decades, drug manufacturers submitted evidence of ingredient safety and effectiveness. After data on drug ingredients were reviewed by expert advisory panels and FDA staff, the FDA specified the drug ingredients that pharmacists can recommend with confidence. The FDA also specified labeling requirements for nonprescription products. The FDA OTC review is ongoing, with new information emerging each year.

A large number of ingredients have become available to the consumer for self-care through a process known as the Rx-to-OTC switch. In some cases entirely new categories of nonprescription products have been created (e.g., vaginal antifungals, smoking cessation products, and androgenetic alopecia treatment). For these conditions patients often require more sophisticated counseling than was the case with older products.

Because of the dangers inherent in switching medications directly from tight prescription control to unrestricted sales, many groups have called for a third class of drugs, medicine that might be restricted to sales by a pharmacist. The concept is strongly supported by pharmacists and various pharmacy groups, but is vigorously opposed by physicians, the FDA, and those who manufacture nonprescription drug products.

References

1. Sherman M, Strauss S. How drugs are moved from Rx to OTC status. US Pharm 13(6):69, 1988.
2. Anon. An Introduction to FDA Drug Regulation: 1993, National Association of Boards of Pharmacy, Park Ridge, IL.
3. Hodes B. Nonprescription drugs: An overview. Int J Health Serv 4:125, 1974.
4. Nordenberg T. FDA and medical devices. FDA Consumer 30(10):6, 1996.
5. Anon. Safety and effectiveness of over-the-counter drugs: The FDA's OTC drug review. Pediatrics 59:309, 1977.
6. Fredd SB. The OTC drug approval process. Am J Gastroenterol 85:12, 1990.
7. Feldmann EG. New era for nonprescription drugs. J Pharm Sci 72:1373, 1983.
8. Fisher GM. The need for regulatory uniformity for over-the-counter products. Food Drug Cosm Law J 38:383, 1983.
9. Farley D. Benefit vs. risk: How FDA approved new drugs. FDA Consumer Special Report 2:23, 1995.
10. Gilbertson WE. The OTC drug review—Switch without regulation of application. Drug Infor J 19:101, 1985.
11. Baumgartner KC. A historical examination of the FDA's review of the safety and effectiveness of over-the-counter drugs. Food Drug Cosm Law J 43:463, 1988.
12. Hayes AHH Jr. Accomplishments at FDA and a look toward the future. Food Drug Cosm Law J 38:64, 1983.
13. Becker RH. Is the over-the-counter drug review program still viable? Food Drug Cosm Law J 38:349, 1983.
14. Pray WS. The pharmacist as self-care advisor. J Am Pharm Assoc NS36:329, 1996.
15. Anon. How many pharmacists see the Federal Register? Wellcome Trends in Pharm 14(2):13, 1992.
16. Podolsky D, et al. Questionable medicine. U.S. News and World Report 118(19):101, 1995.

17. Scarlett T. The legal and administrative effects of final over-the-counter monographs. Food Drug Cosm Law J 39:152, 1984.

18. Bachrach EE. The FDA's new over-the-counter drug office and advisory committee: An industry perspective. Food Drug Law J 48:563, 1993.

19. Hecht A. Drugs that are Rx no more. FDA Consumer 17(6): 23, 1983.

20. Mahinka SP, Bierman ME. Direct-to-OTC marketing of drugs. Possible approaches. Food Drug Law J 50:49, 1993.

21. Rice TF. Physicians' Desk Reference for Nonprescription Drugs, 17th Ed.: 1996, Medical Economics Co, Montvale, NJ.

22. Waldholz M. Nonprescription drug industry urges more prescription-to-nonprescription switches. Am J Hosp Pharm 46:1512, 1989.

23. Bewley PD. Switching—The triple threat from Tylenol to ibuprofen. Drug Infor J 19:95, 1985.

24. DeSimone EM II. Rx to OTC—Special counseling concerns. US Pharm 20(1):37, 1995.

25. Latz LM. Prescription to over-the-counter drug switches. Food Drug Law J 48:567, 1993.

26. Segal M. Rx to OTC—The switch is on. FDA Consumer 25(2):9, 1991.

27. Rheinstein PH. Criteria used by the FDA to determine what classes of drugs are appropriate switch candidates. Drug Infor J 19:139, 1985.

28. Hutt PB. A legal framework for future decisions on transferring drugs from prescription to nonprescription status. Food Drug Cosm Law J 37:427, 1982.

29. Barnett AA. OTC status denied to cholestyramine. Pharm Today 1(16):14, 1995.

30. Rachanow GM. The switch of drugs from prescription to over-the-counter status. Food Drug Cosm Law J 39:201, 1984.

31. Anon. Topical erythromycin OTC switch rejected. Weekly Pharm Reports 43(48):3, 1994.

32. Anon. No OTC switch for acyclovir. Drug Topics 139(2):7, 1995.

33. Anon. FDA cancels meeting on making the pill an OTC. Drug Topics 137(3):5, 1993.

34. Gannon K. Why Rx manufacturers would want to make the switch to OTC. Drug Topics 134(12):36, 1990.

35. Helwick C. Are Rx-to-OTC switches fending off generic attacks? Drug Topics Supplement 140(March):30s, 1996.

36. Haverkost LF. How industry assesses and picks suitable candidates for switch. Drug Infor J 19:133, 1985.

37. Hutt PB. Drugs for self-medication in the future: Their source and the social, political, and regulatory climate. Drug Infor J 19:195, 1985.

38. Whitney DW. Product liability issues for the expanding OTC drug category. Food Drug Law J 48:321, 1993.

39. Anon. Rx-to-OTC switch driven by many factors. NDMA Exec Newsletter 24–96:3, 1996.

40. Newton G, Popovich NG, Pray WS. Rx-to-OTC switches: From prescription to self-care. J Am Pharm Assoc NS36:489, 1996.

41. Snyder K. A better deal? Drug Topics 140(6):41, 1996.

42. Gannon K. Rx-to-OTC switches could be a mixed blessing for R.Ph.s. Drug Topics 134(30):31, 1990.

43. Anon. Double trouble? Drug Topics 133(24):5, 1989.

44. Conlan MF. FDA may move to allow sale of drugs as both Rx and OTC. Drug Topics 133(51):51, 1989.

45. Rheingold PD. The expanding liability of the drug manufacturer to the consumer. Food Drug Cosm Law J 40:135, 1985.

46. Guerard C. The impact of advertising and its regulation—A Federal Trade Commission perspective. Drug Infor J 19:163, 1985.

47. Anon. Antacid war goes to court. Drug Topics 139(18):7, 1995.

48. Anon. Heartburn judgment. Drug Topics 139(21):30, 1995.

49. Anon. Tagamet, Pepcid seek ad injunctions. Am Drugg 212(6):1, 1995.

50. Gebhart F. Off the hook. Drug Topics 140(14):42, 1996.

51. Vickery DM. A medical perspective. Drug Infor J 19:155, 1985.

52. Ciccone PE. Introduction and commentary. Drug Infor J 19:85, 1985.

53. Zoeller J. In a class of their own? Am Drugg 204(4):39, 1991.

54. Lessing M. The OTC drug phenomenon: Double-edged clinical implications. Milit Med 152:557, 1987.

55. Blank C. Is this the right time for a third class of drugs? Drug Topics 141(11):106, 1997.

56. Penna RP. A transitional category: How APhA's policy would work. Am Pharm NS25:46, 1985.

57. Ukens C. Class act—NABP backs third class of drugs. Drug Topics 139(10):13, 1995.

58. Gebhart F. FDA nixes third class of drugs once again. Drug Topics 136(16):69, 1992.

59. Anon. PPSI petitions FDA for third class of drugs. Pharm Times 58(8):125, 1992.

60. Anon. Consumers join APhA in seeking third class of medications. Am Pharm NS31:474, 1991.

61. Ukens C. New hope for third class, but the going is still slow. Drug Topics 135(21):12, 1991.

62. Bectel MQ. The Rx-to-OTC switch: Good for pharmacy. Am Pharm NS24:184, 1984.

63. Denysyk OS. How do pharmacists approach the OTC area? Drug Topics 130(20):64, 1986.

64. Gannon K. Rx-to-OTC switches raise new call for third class. Drug Topics 133(48):48, 1989.

65. Schwartz RM. GAO frowns on third drug class. Am Drugg 212(6):18, 1995.

66. Marshall RP. A transition category of drugs: win-win-win-win? Am Pharm NS32:828, 1992.

67. Fisher GM. Third class of drugs-A current view. Food Drug Cosm Law J 46:583, 1991.

68. Anon. Nix to third class. Drug Topics 136(2):5, 1992.

69. Anon. An interview with Charles A. Pergola. Am Pharm NS24:86, 1984.

70. Anon. Position paper—Third class of drugs. Nonprescription Drug Manufacturers Assoc, 1990.

71. Anon. Third class of drugs' success is tied to role of pharmacists. Weekly Pharm Reports 44(36):4, 1995.

72. Anon. Pharmacist-controlled class. Weekly Pharm Reports 44(35):1, 1995.

73. Anon. GAO rejects third class of drugs. NDMA Exec Newsletter #19–95:2, 1995.

74. Lober CW. The pharmacist physician. J Am Acad Dermatol 13:5 Pt 1:817,1985.

75. White JP. Third class of drugs opens up first-class feud. Drug Topics 128(18):38, 1984.

Oral and Gastrointestinal Conditions

Plaque-Induced Diseases:
Caries and Gingivitis

AT THE COUNTER

A patient, appearing to be in his mid 40s, tells the pharmacist that his gums bleed when he brushes his teeth and asks if any nonprescription medications will stop the bleeding.

Interview/Patient Assessment

The patient states that his toothbrush is bloody after brushing. He is taking no medications and has no chronic diseases. He specifically asks if brushing more often will help.

Pharmacist's Analysis

1. What problems could lead to bleeding gums?
2. If gingivitis is the cause of gingival bleeding, what should the pharmacist do?
3. What nonprescription products/devices would be appropriate for self-care?

Among other things (e.g., blood dyscrasias and anticoagulant therapy), bleeding gums can indicate gingivitis caused by inadequate oral hygiene.

Patient Counseling

The pharmacist should refer the patient to a dentist or periodontist for evaluation, since he may also have periodontitis or gingival recession, which will require professional care. The pharmacist should explain that these professionals will likely point out the importance of routine care—brushing, flossing, periodontal cleansing, etc.—and may suggest the use of specific products, nonprescription medications, and/or prescription medications. Finally, the pharmacist should offer to assist the patient further after he has seen a dentist or periodontist.

The last 2 decades have been an innovative period for oral-care products. New toothbrushes and toothpaste formulations and a wide array of cleansing devices have been marketed. Oral hygiene is vital to prevent two medical conditions, **caries** (erosion of the teeth, usually caused by exposure to bacteria and their acids, also known as cavities) and **gingivitis** (inflammation of the gingiva or gums).

Regular cleansing of the teeth is vitally important to remove **plaque** (a gelatinous matrix that is responsible for caries and gingivitis) and to prevent the formation of **calculus or tartar** (a calcified material that adheres tightly to teeth). Both caries and gingivitis are preventable with proper oral hygiene and the use of fluoride. (See Figure 3.1 to review tooth and gum anatomy.)

Pharmacies sell a multitude of nonprescription items related to oral hygiene and cavity prevention. These products range from toothbrushes and picks that mechanically remove plaque to medicated mouthwashes and toothpastes that help treat gingivitis. Ideally, patients will purchase these items as a part of a total oral-hygiene program recommended by dentists, dental hygienists, or periodontists. In these cases pharmacists may help patients locate the proper products when the pharmacy stocks them or may order them when it does not.

Occasionally, patients will request ancillary devices (such as periodontal aids and disclosing solutions or tablets), which are marketed mainly to the dental community and are provided to the patient by the dental office just after the patient is trained in their use. Pharmacists may need to contact patients' oral-care practitioners to locate sources for these items. (After repeated requests, a pharmacy may choose to add some of these items to its permanent stock.)

Patients who do not visit the dentist regularly suffer from piecemeal dental care (see "A Pharmacist's Journal: What's Wrong with My Gums?"). Although these patients may brush

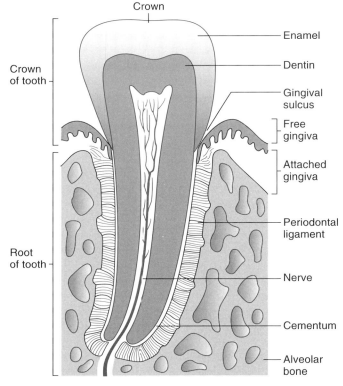

Figure 3.1. The anatomy of the oral area includes the tooth, its crown and root, the gingival structures, and the associated elements of the periodontium.

more or less regularly, they also may be quite susceptible to the latest, highly advertised device such as a special new toothbrush. Unless they understand the need for regular flossing and outlining of the gums using a **periodontal** (related to the tissues of the periodontium) aid, they may be receiving a false sense of security from purchase and use of the new device. Patients could have advanced periodontal disease and not be aware of the virtues of a total oral-care program supervised by a dental professional. *It is incumbent on the pharmacist to recommend that the patient consult an oral-care practitioner to see whether his total care is appropriate and whether any new device would be helpful for his unique situation.*

This chapter is concerned with the value of regular cleansing of the teeth to prevent the two most common plaque-induced diseases, caries and gingivitis. In Chapter 4 gingival diseases other than gingivitis (such as canker sores and gingival injury) are covered. Chapter 4 does not describe prevention of caries, but discusses caries as a possible cause of dental pain.

CARIES AND GINGIVITIS

PREVALENCE OF CARIES AND GINGIVITIS

The number of individuals with the two most common plaque-induced diseases, caries and gingivitis, is extremely high, even in developed countries.[2] In one United States study, for example, all subjects had visible plaque.[3] In fact, because of the high rate of plaque-induced disease, tooth decay is exceeded only by the common cold as the most common health problem in this country.[4] Interestingly, the incidence of caries in the United States has declined steadily over the past 2 decades, although the decline is attributed to the increased use of fluoride dentifrices and the widespread fluoridation of water, rather than improved oral hygiene.[5–8]

Gingivitis, the other common plaque-induced disease, is so common that the term "normal gingiva" has lost its meaning.[6] The normal state of the gingiva is one of neglect, so that "normal" gingiva are diseased, inflamed, and bleeding (Fig. 3.2). As many as 85% of all individuals over the age of 40 experience gingival disease, ranging from mild gingival inflammation to severe periodontal disease (Fig. 3.3).[9] Periodontal disease affects 50% of white adults and 75% of nonwhite adults.[10] At least 90% of geriatric patients suffer from periodontitis.[10]

EPIDEMIOLOGY OF CARIES AND GINGIVITIS

Since plaque-induced diseases mainly result from oral cleansing deficiencies, a discussion of the epidemiology of plaque-induced diseases focuses on the individuals whose oral-care habits are neglectful. While figures vary widely, as many as 30 to 40% of Americans may not receive regular dental care.[6] As might be expected, individuals with higher incomes and educational levels are more likely to visit their dental professional on a regular basis.[11] Of course, there are many reasons that patients do not visit the dentist.

Inadequate finances have a significant impact on dental care. Studies confirm that as many as 40% of Americans lack dental insurance.[6,12,13] Even with insurance coverage, the patient may be unable to afford the copayment required by the plan. Many individuals whose resources are strained only seek medical care when they can no longer overlook or cope with an acute problem.

Other patients may possess the resources, but lack the motivation to seek regular professional dental care. Some fail to understand the concept of prevention as it applies to dental care, seeking care only when pain is overwhelming. Motivation to visit the dentist may also be dampened by dental anxiety or phobia, a major problem for as many as 35 million Americans.[14,15] These patients may be committed to the idea of prevention in general, but remain unable to seek dental care because of crippling fear. Anxious and phobic people typically experience nausea and general discomfort prior to an appointment.[14,16] Other symptoms are those of the "fight or flight" response, including tachycardia, tachypnea, hypersalivation, and perspiration.

A final group of patients lack access to dental care for one of several reasons. Some are unable to keep an appointment

A Pharmacist's Journal

"What's Wrong with My Gums?"

A 34-year-old male patient complained of marked gingival recession, inflammation of the gums, and ulceration of the buccal attached gingiva and adjacent alveolar mucosa in the maxillary right quadrant.[93] He also exhibited some loss of interproximal hard and soft tissue. Plaque control was quite good, and the patient stated that he used the softest toothbrush available. However, on closer questioning, he mentioned that he had been given a bottle of Xylocaine Viscous. He used this to anesthetize the area before "brushing away the infected tissue." He then revealed that he started using a stiffer toothbrush that was "as hard as steel wool." The final diagnosis was factitious gingival injury. On cessation of Xylocaine Viscous and all mechanical oral-hygiene measures, the site was well healed, but he was informed that gingival grafting might be required.

because of physical limitations or lack of transportation. Others do not have the capability to make an appointment because of cognitive deficits such as depression or dementia.

Aside from the factors that prevent regular dental checkups, gingival disease reflects certain other epidemiologic trends:

- The oral cleansing habits of males, for instance, are generally inferior to females, so the incidence of severe gingivitis is higher in men.[17,18]
- Patients with diabetes mellitus have impaired gingival blood flow that worsens gingival disease.[9,19]
- Older patients develop gingivitis more rapidly than younger patients.[20]
- Tobacco use worsens deposition of plaque and mitigates against efforts at plaque removal.[21,22]
- Gingival recession is more common in people who use smokeless tobacco, with the lesions being located at the exact spot where the patient places the tobacco in the mouth (such as between the lower lip and the gum tissue).[23]

ETIOLOGY OF CARIES AND GINGIVITIS

Within a matter of a few minutes after thorough cleansing, the teeth are covered with a coating known as the pellicle.[1] This does not contain organisms, but is composed of the by-products of saliva and gingival fluid (such as glycoproteins, polypeptides, and lipids).

As time passes during the day, bacteria normally found in the mouth adhere to the pellicle. Just as growth occurs in a Petri dish, the warmth and moisture of the mouth allow organisms adhering to the pellicle to grow and reproduce, forming a series of microcolonies that eventually cover all tooth surfaces. This is the gel-like matrix known as plaque.[2] Unless it is removed, plaque may contain as many as 10^8 organisms per milligram. Diseased gingiva may contain as much as 200 mg of plaque.

Normally, the patient removes plaque as the teeth are

FOCUS ON...

ORAL ANATOMY

To understand the importance of hygiene and the development of caries and gingivitis, a brief review of anatomy may be necessary.

ANATOMY OF THE TOOTH

The tooth is divided into two general sections:

- The visible part of the tooth that extends above the gingival line is the crown.[1] The crown is covered by enamel, the hardest part of the human body, composed of hydroxyapatite crystals. Beneath the crown is a softer material known as dentin, which contains collagen in addition to hydroxyapatite.
- The portion of the tooth that is embedded in the bony socket of the maxilla or mandible is known as the root. The root is covered by cementum, a substance that is softer than either enamel or dentin.

ANATOMY OF THE GINGIVA

The gingiva (gums) is a membrane that is normally tightly attached to the underlying alveolar bone and is therefore known as attached gingiva.[1] Normal gingiva appear pink in all areas because of the underlying circulation of oxygenated hemoglobin. Healthy gingiva also have margins with a "knife-edge" appearance, denoting healthy noninflamed tissues. The depth of the sulcus should not exceed 2 to 3 mm. Healthy gingiva do not bleed and are not painful.

THE ANATOMY OF THE PERIODONTIUM

The teeth are supported in their bony sockets by the periodontium, a multipart anatomic entity that allows teeth to absorb the shock of chewing and that is composed of six elements:

- Alveolar bone is the bone that lines the socket into which the tooth is fitted.
- Cementum, the material that covers the root, is arranged around the root in layers.
- Periodontal ligament is a set of many connective tissue fibers that extend from the cementum to the alveolar bone, providing a tight attachment of the tooth to bone. They suspend the tooth in the alveolar socket and allow it to resist the forces that occur during chewing.
- The dentogingival junction is composed of the tooth surface and the inner cellular layers of the gingiva. In the healthy patient it forms a tight seal that protects the periodontal ligament, cementum, and alveolar bone from the foods and other substances found in the mouth.
- The free margin of the gingiva is an outward growth from the attached gingiva. This free gingival margin encircles all teeth.
- The gingival sulcus (or gingival crevice) is a slitlike space between the tooth and the free margin of the gingiva.

---

cleaned, but if plaque is allowed to remain, the organisms in **supragingival plaque** (plaque above the gingival line) undergo a predictable succession:

- Initially, plaque organisms are Gram-positive cocci, primarily streptococci. Plaque is able to adhere to tooth surfaces as a result of the glutinous polysaccharides that streptococci produce from dietary sucrose.
- By the third or fourth day, filamentous organisms replace the cocci.[24,25] These organisms are able to undergo inter-

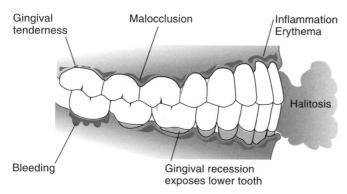

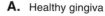

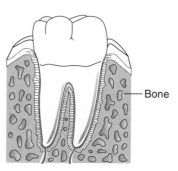

Figure 3.2. Gingivitis and periodontal disease result in numerous oral problems.

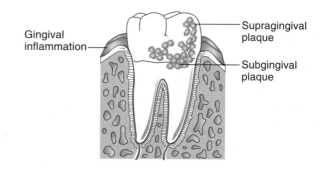

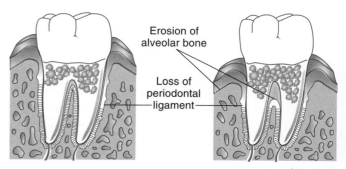

Figure 3.3. Periodontal disease is characterized by gingival inflammation and recession and loss of periodontal ligament, causing tooth mobility and tooth loss.

nal calcification, producing calcium phosphate that is the substance known as calculus. Calculus acts as a retention matrix for bacteria and their toxins, helping prevent cleansing of these organisms.

- On days 6 to 10, Gram-negative organisms and anaerobic organisms colonize the area.

The amount of plaque in the mouth varies according to location. Supragingival plaque accumulation is more common in neglected areas such as the gingival margins, in the subgingival crevices around the teeth, in **interproximal** (between the teeth) spaces, in deep pits and fissures, and on teeth with orthodontic appliances. Should plaque not be removed thoroughly from these areas, growth can extend to the subgingival (below the gumline) areas.

Once plaque has hardened to form calculus, the patient's ability to cleanse is further compromised. Plaque is relatively soft and nonmineralized and may be removed through proper use of appliances. However, calculus is a mineral deposit on teeth that is only removable through a dental visit. The patient must strive to disrupt the plaque colonies prior to their mineralization as calculus.

Plaque and Caries

Caries result when a triad of factors is present:

- The bacteria found in dental plaque
- Dietary carbohydrate (especially sucrose) to serve as a bacterial substrate
- A susceptible host tooth

The specific plaque organism that induces caries is currently thought to be *Streptococcus mutans,* an efficient producer of the acids that dissolve tooth enamel and cause the typical caries lesion.[2,4,26] When plaque is exposed to sugars and starches—even briefly—its pH decreases rapidly, remaining at that low level for many hours.[26] Plaque microorganisms such as *S. mutans* accomplish this pH drop through fermentation of sugars, producing acidic by-products.[27] (Sucrose seems to be the most destructive

sugar, partially because it is frequently ingested, but also because it is able to specifically act as a substrate for glycan synthesis by the mutans streptococci.[26,28–30]) Also carbohydrate ingestion induces the shift of plaque organisms to more dangerous acidogenic species.

Although the calcium hydroxyapatite of which enamel is composed is quite durable, a sufficiently low pH can erode it. As acidogenic organisms are allowed to proliferate in calculus, the pH falls to 5.5 and below. This pH favors dissolution of calcium hydroxyapatite, which forms carious lesions.

Plaque and Gingivitis

Gingivitis is inflammation of the marginal gingiva or **papillary** (the projections of gingiva between the teeth) gingiva in response to the action of plaque bacteria on the gums.[31]

Researchers believe that plaque bacteria release numerous toxins and enzymes that directly irritate gingival tissue, producing the characteristic symptoms of gingivitis that include the following[5]:

- A magenta or bluish color, denoting impaired circulation
- Tender, sensitive gingiva
- Inflammation
- Bleeding in response to eating, brushing, or flossing; spontaneous bleeding from the gums
- A sulcular depth exceeding 4 mm when measured by a periodontal probe

All of these symptoms indicate that the patient's oral-care regimen is inadequate. Gingivitis is reversible in many cases.[5] When gingival damage is not halted or reversed, the result is **periodontitis** (inflammation of the periodontium; destruction of the collagen fibers in the periodontal ligament), a severe condition that is not reversible.[5,31] With periodontitis, also known as periodontal disease, inflammation and infection have extended downward from the dentogingival junction to involve the periodontal ligament, cementum, and perhaps alveolar bone. As much as 60 to 70% of the collagen can be destroyed. This pernicious process reduces the normally firm attachment of the tooth in alveolar bone. A space known as the periodontal pocket forms around the tooth.[24,32] This is the intermediate stage in a vicious cycle:

- The patient fails to remove supragingival plaque.
- Calculus forms, which contributes to the further growth of plaque.[33]
- Plaque extends to subgingival areas, where cleansing cannot be effectively accomplished.[34]
- The patient develops a set of organisms known as unattached plaque, a group of motile, Gram-negative bacteria which extend deeply into the gingival crevice.
- The patient develops subgingival calculus.
- Calculus irritates the free gingival margin due to its rough, mineralized nature.
- Irritation of tissues from calculus causes gingival recession, with widening of the gingival crevice.
- As the gingival crevice widens, calculus extends further downward, causing further destruction of the periodontium.
- The tooth becomes loosened in alveolar bone as the firm attachment is eroded.
- As the tooth becomes mobile, plaque and calculus extend further downward, until the alveolar bone is destroyed.

FOCUS ON...

PLAQUE AND HALITOSIS

Halitosis (bad breath) may have several causes, but 90% of cases originate in the oral cavity (e.g., periodontal disease, poor oral hygiene, food residues, faulty dental restorations).[35–37] The balance of cases are caused by systemic disease such as carcinoma, diabetes, hepatic failure, or renal failure.[38]

Halitosis is common, especially on awakening.[39] Unlike caries and gingivitis, it is usually only an embarrassment. Many people perceive the problem as much worse than it actually is.[40] Its cause is the action of oral bacteria with the production of volatile sulfur compounds.[36] While bacteria of plaque are one source, bacteria on the surface of the tongue are also responsible for the problem. In these cases the patient might ask a dentist for a tongue-cleaning device.[41]

- Eventually, the pressures of chewing and further alveolar destruction result in loss of the affected teeth.

With the fluoride-driven reduction in the incidence of caries, periodontal disease is the leading cause of tooth loss in adults.

Plaque and periodontal disease may also be responsible for halitosis. (See "Plaque and Halitosis.")

TREATMENT OF CARIES AND GINGIVITIS

See "Treatment of Caries" and "Treatment and Prevention of Gingivitis."

PREVENTION OF CARIES AND GINGIVITIS

See "Prevention of Caries" and "Treatment and Prevention of Gingivitis."

CARIES

See preceding text for prevalence, epidemiology, and etiology of caries and gingivitis.

TREATMENT OF CARIES

Treatment of caries is the professional responsibility of a dentist. Pharmacists who suspect that a patient has active caries must stress the need for immediate care to prevent caries from progressing more deeply into the tooth. Lack of care can damage a tooth irreparably, possibly necessitating tooth extraction or a root canal.

PREVENTION OF CARIES

The Role of Fluoride in Prevention of Caries

Because of its role in reducing the incidence of caries, fluoride stands as one of the four great public health advances of the twentieth century (along with pasteurization of milk, chlorination of water, and immunizations). When a patient is given fluoride, the chemical is thought to decrease the risk of caries by three methods:

- Reducing the solubility of dental enamel through conversion of hydroxyapatite to fluoroapatite, which makes it more acid-resistant
- Enhancing remineralization of dental enamel
- Interfering in the growth and function of dental plaque bacteria

The Role of Plaque Control in Prevention of Caries

The patient is able to control plaque through two methods: prompt removal or prevention of plaque buildup. Overwhelming evidence exists that plaque removal reduces caries.[4,5]

PLAQUE REMOVAL
Patient devices for home care such as new toothpaste formulations, a wide variety of manual and electric toothbrush designs, and specialty dental flosses have proliferated rapidly in the preceding decade. With this bewildering array of products, one would think that the battle against caries and gingivitis would be short-lived. Unfortunately, it is not sufficient to simply brush, floss, and use an interdental device.[42] These self-care practices must be carried out skillfully.[43–45]

It is important to note, further, that using fluoride in home care (e.g., toothpaste with fluoride) and drinking fluoridated water does not compensate for poor oral hygiene. The preventive effect of fluoride will be less pronounced unless the patient follows other dietary advice—the most critical being the frequency and nature of carbohydrate ingestion. After a meal, food residue remains on the dorsum of the tongue and in other sites within the oral cavity. From these locations the residue slowly solubilizes, releasing a continual nutrient bath that allows plaque bacteria to proliferate.[11,30] Thus prompt cleansing after ingestion of carbohydrates is essential.

As discussed above, because of finances, fears, or availability, professional dental care is not an option for everyone. For people who do not obtain professional dental care, the only recourse for plaque control is self-care. Even conscientious individuals who do obtain regular professional care must undertake a rigorous regimen of self-care, including tooth brushing with fluoridated toothpastes and flossing to prevent problems between appointments.[16,46]

Another important component of home care is the use of periodontal cleaning aids, also known as interdental cleaning devices. These auxiliary devices are often recommended by dentists and periodontists to clean the gingival sulcus more thoroughly than either toothbrushing or flossing can do.[47]

Despite understanding the importance of daily home care

Patient Assessment Algorithm 3.1. Plaque

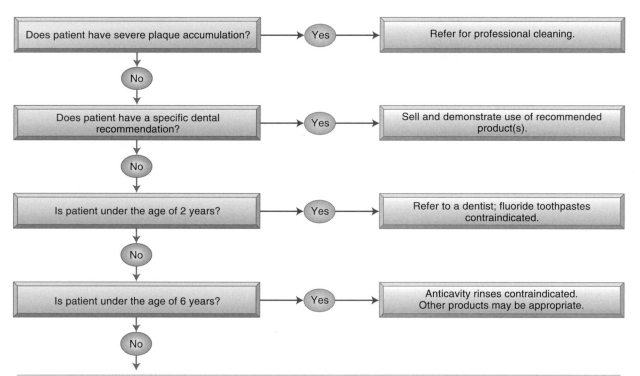

Does patient have severe plaque accumulation? → Yes → Refer for professional cleaning.

No ↓

Does patient have a specific dental recommendation? → Yes → Sell and demonstrate use of recommended product(s).

No ↓

Is patient under the age of 2 years? → Yes → Refer to a dentist; fluoride toothpastes contraindicated.

No ↓

Is patient under the age of 6 years? → Yes → Anticavity rinses contraindicated. Other products may be appropriate.

No ↓

Recommend the patient brush after meals and at bedtime with a brush with soft, rounded bristles, using a fluoride-containing, low-abrasive toothpaste; daily use of floss and a periodontal cleaning device should also be recommended. Consider also anticavity rinses, plaque-disclosing devices for training, tartar-control toothpastes or gingivitis-preventives, and such mechanical devices as oral irrigators or sonic toothbrushes. Also consider chemical plaque preventives (e.g., cetylpyridinium chloride mouthwash or triclosan toothpaste).

in plaque control, many people do not comply.[12] Although surveys reveal that most people brush regularly, less than one-third use interdental cleaning devices, and as few as 3 to 18% floss.[47] The individuals most likely to carry out basic self-care include the more highly educated, and those of higher income.[12,47] Those with higher incomes are also less likely to have caries because of advanced dental techniques such as the professional application of sealing materials that fill the pits and fissures of the teeth, preventing food and plaque from colonizing those hard-to-clean surfaces. (See Patient Assessment Algorithm 3.1.)

Toothbrushes and Nonmedicated Toothpastes

Toothbrushing is a useful method of mechanically cleaning plaque from the teeth. Toothbrushing has two major functions:

- Removing food debris from recent meals and snacks
- Disrupting the bacterial colonies that grow as plaque on tooth surfaces

Pharmacists are generally not trained to provide toothbrushing instructions, and time is usually too limited to allow anything more than a superficial discussion of oral hygiene in any case. Patients must be given proper instruction on intraoral cleansing by the dental care practitioner, a process that often includes the use of audiovisual aids, dental mirrors, and the services of a dental hygienist. In particular, patients must be aware that trauma to the gingiva caused by excessive brushing can result in severe problems such as dental hypersensitivity. (See "Correct Brushing Technique" and "Dangers of Wet Toothbrushes.")

A patient's dentist or hygienist should advise them about the type of bristle to be used. However, there are several pieces of general advice:

CORRECT BRUSHING TECHNIQUE

The toothbrush is held in the hand and placed at a 45° angle against the gingiva as shown in the figure.[48,49] The brush is moved gently back and forth in several strokes that cover one-half of the tooth at a time. The patient should feel the bristles moving along and slightly below the gingival line. This method should be used to clean the outside and upper chewing surfaces of the teeth. The end of the toothbrush can be angled to use a gentle up-and-down stroke to clean the inner surfaces of the teeth. Individuals who have never been given instructions for appropriate brushing may neglect the areas just below the gumline, the lingual (inner) surfaces, and the back molars. Nevertheless, although a properly wielded toothbrush in the hands of a trained patient does a fairly good job of cleaning buccal (outer) and lingual tooth surfaces, it is inefficient for **proximal** (next to each other) tooth surfaces, which underscores the need for the various ancillary devices such as floss. As a final step in brushing, the patient might brush the tongue, which may help prevent halitosis. The patient should brush after meals and at bedtime, unless the dental care practitioner has recommended a different regimen. The toothbrush should be changed every 3 to 4 months at the outside, although changing it every few weeks may help reduce the incidence of infections.

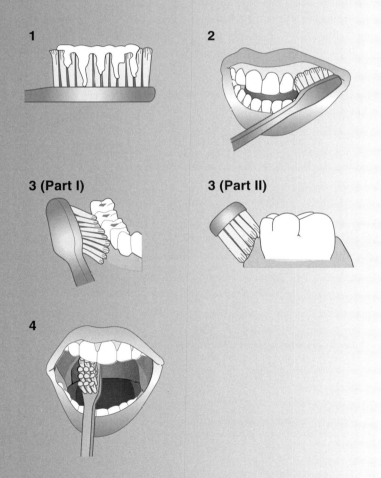

Proper brushing: (1) Place toothpaste on the brush so it moves downward into the bristles. (2) Place the brush in the mouth at a 45° angle. (3) Brush gently in an up-and-down motion, making sure the brush moves downward into the sulcus. (4) Use the toe of the brush to clean the inner surfaces.

- Choose the commonly available toothbrushes that have synthetic bristles, rather than natural bristles.
- Avoid hard bristles. They may damage the gingiva, causing them to recede below the normal gumline. The hard bristles then can abrade the softer cementum of the root, perhaps producing damage to the nerve (see "A Pharmacist's Journal: What's Wrong With My Gums?").
- Medium bristle brushes should only be chosen under the advice of a dentist.
- Unless otherwise advised, choose a toothbrush that has the softest bristle available.
- Bristles come in several types such as rounded or polished. The dentist may have a specific recommendation. The American Dental Association recommends round-ended bristles, however.[50]
- Toothbrush handles and heads are available in several configurations. The patient should try several and choose one that allows him or her to reach the tooth surfaces most easily. The size of the brush itself should allow comfortable brushing.
- Toothbrush heads are also available in a wide variety of sizes. There may be more rows of bristles in a certain brush, or the head may be made of plastic with a configuration that encircles the tooth. The patient's dentist may have a specific recommendation.

Various studies have assessed the efficacy of ultrasonic and powered brushes.[51,52] Generally, they might be used for patients who brush too vigorously, causing gingival or enamel damage. Their attributes are quite variable, so that the patient should be advised to check with the dental practitioner prior to choosing a specific product. The ADA has given its Seal of Acceptance (see "The American Dental Association [ADA] Seal of Acceptance") to the following powered toothbrushes[53]:

- Emjoi Action Toothbrush
- Conair Interplak Power Toothbrushes (seven models)
- Braun Oral-B Plaque Removers
- Butler G•U•M Plaque Remover
- Johnson & Johnson Hapica Powered Brush
- Teledyne Plaque Control 3000
- Teledyne SenSonic Plaque Removal Instruments (four models)

- Windmere Plak Trac

Patients may choose from a wide variety of toothpastes.

tip When the patient chooses toothpastes that are not fluoridated or otherwise medicated, the pastes add little to the mechanical effect of toothbrushing other than freshening the inside of the mouth. (See "A Pharmacist's Journal: I Need a White Toothpaste.")

Fluoridated Products

Fluoridation of water has been hailed as one of the four great mass preventive public-health measures (along with pasteurization of milk, chlorination of water, and immunization against disease).[54,55] Fluoride exerts beneficial effects by converting hydroxyapatite in dental enamel to fluoroapatite, which reduces its solubility and makes it more resistant to acid etching. It also interferes with the functions of dental plaque bacteria (e.g., *Streptococcus mutans,* lactobacilli) and helps remineralization of early carious lesions. By halting and reversing carious lesions, fluoride is beneficial for adults as well as children, and the overwhelming evidence is in favor of fluoridation as the primary method of caries prevention.[54,56,57]

The most cost-effective and efficient method of enhancing dental health is the addition of fluoride to water.[57] When added to community water in a concentration of 0.7 to 1.2 parts per million, fluoride can reduce caries by 50% or more. Numerous studies show an indirect relationship of fluoride in community water to the number of decayed, missing, and filled teeth (DMFT)—that is, communities with less fluoride in water have greater numbers of DMFT.[58,59] Epidemiologists also point to the results of migrant studies. People who move from fluoridated water communities to those with nonfluoridated water suffer more cavities after the move, but their DMFT scores remain lower than those who lived in the nonfluoridated water communities all of their lives.[60,61]

Communities that cease fluoridation of water also experience increases in caries. The Scottish city of Stranaer experienced a 21% increase in the costs of dental treatment after stopping fluoride. The cost of tooth restoration caused by cavities rose by 115%.[62]

In 1980 the Public Health Service listed 12 dental-health

A Pharmacist's Journal

"I Need a White Toothpaste."

A young man approached me in a retail pharmacy and asked for a white toothpaste. I asked whether he wanted fluoridated or nonfluoridated. He said, "I don't care, I just want it to be white." He also didn't care whether it provided whitening or antisensitivity actions. I asked why it was so important that it be white. He said he was moving out of his apartment and had heard that white toothpaste will cover all of the nail holes in his walls so his landlord would return his full security deposit.

objectives that the nation should meet by 1990.[63] One of these was that 95% of the United States population that drinks community water should have optimal fluoride levels added. At present, however, less than 70% of the population benefits from fluoridated water.[64] The federal government cannot legislate fluoridation, so that the decision to fluoridate water rests with individual cities through community referendums. Unfortunately, opponents of fluoridation incorrectly assert that it is ineffective and that it causes medical conditions.[54] When a city vote is imminent, pharmacies can serve as a health resource center during the campaign to help counter the opponents of water fluoridation. The pharmacist should also remember that some families choose not to use community water, opting to ingest nonfluoridated, bottled water instead. For these families, the issue of supplemental fluoride becomes more important.

Toothpastes that are nonfluoridated do little for caries prevention, as discussed above. Fluoridated toothpastes, although not as effective as fluoridated water, are an excellent method of applying fluoride to the teeth. Everyone can benefit from fluoridated toothpaste, but it is especially important for those living in communities with nonfluoridated water or those drinking water from wells or other sources.[65] These medicated dentifrices can reduce the incidence of caries by 25 to 40% compared with nonfluoridated toothpaste.[66] *Children must be monitored carefully when*

Table 3.1. Representative Anticavity Rinses	
PRODUCT	SELECTED INGREDIENTS/COMMENTS
Reach ACT Rinse	Sodium fluoride 0.05%; cetylpyridinium chloride; a special measuring device at the top of the bottle facilitates dose measurement
Reach ACT Rinse for Kids	Sodium fluoride 0.05%; cetylpyridinium chloride; a special measuring device at the top of the bottle facilitates dose measurement
Phos-Flur Anti-Cavity Fluoride Rinse	Sodium fluoride 0.044%

Table 3.2. Representative Dental Flosses	
PRODUCT	SELECTED INGREDIENTS/COMMENTS
Colgate Total Floss	Mint waxed, no-shred floss
Dr. Du-More's Flosser	A toothpick-like holder with approx. 0.75 inch of floss suspended between two arms at one end
Glide Floss	Nonshred floss; mint or regular
Glide Tape	Nonshred tape for a large cleaning surface
Oral-B Flosses	Available as waxed, mint waxed, waxed with fluoride
Oral-B Mint Tape	Waxed with fluoride
Oral-B SuperFloss	Three-section floss; stiffened end to thread under appliances, regular floss, and a spongy floss to clean around appliances and in wide spaces
Oral-B Ultra Floss	Floss is composed of a network of spongy fibers rather than straight nylon strands; it stretches to fit into tight spaces
Reach Dentotape	Large cleaning surface, unflavored or mint
Reach Floss	Available as waxed, unwaxed, cinnamon waxed, mint waxed, mint unwaxed
Reach Floss Easy Slide	Shred-proof floss
Reach Floss for Kids	Grape-flavored woven floss
Reach Gentle Gum Care Baking Soda Floss	Woven floss; gentle to gums
Reach Gentle Gum Care Fluoride Floss	Woven floss; gentle to gums
Reach Gentle Gum Care Fresh Mint	Woven floss; gentle to gums

using fluoride toothpaste to ensure that they do not swallow it and ingest fluoride above the levels required for proper supplementation.[67–69] *Fluoride is toxic in excessive doses.* For this reason the FDA requires a warning label to parents to monitor use of fluoridated toothpastes in children under the age of 6 and does not allow use for those under the age of 2 at all.[70,71]

Anticavity Rinses

Nonprescription fluoride rinses synergize the effects of fluoride toothpastes when both are used (Table 3.1 for representative fluoride anticavity rinses). The FDA allows manufacturers to include a label that states, "The combined daily use of a fluoride rinse and a fluoride toothpaste can aid in reducing the incidence of dental caries."[72] The FDA also requires the label to caution users about the increased risk of swallowing mouthrinses compared with toothpastes. Other labeling information includes the following[70,71]:

- Mouthrinses are not to be used by patients younger than 6 without a specific dentist or physician recommendation.
- Mouthrinses should not be used by patients younger than 12 without adult supervision.
- Patients should use the mouthrinses once daily, after brushing with toothpaste.
- Patients should vigorously swish approximately 10 mL of mouthrinse around and between the teeth for 1 minute and then expectorate.
- Patients must not swallow mouthrinse.
- Patients should not eat or drink for 30 minutes after using mouthrinse.

Dental Flosses

Daily flossing is another cornerstone in proper oral hygiene (Table 3.2). Regular and correct flossing can reduce the percentage of plaque on teeth and the incidence of gingival bleeding (Fig. 3.4).

Dental floss reaches the **interproximal** (between the adjoining tooth surfaces) surfaces that are inaccessible to toothbrush bristles. (See "Correct Flossing Technique.") Gentle flossing also helps reach back molars and slightly below the gumline of the areas between the teeth.

Some people become discouraged when they first begin flossing because the floss seems to constantly break or shred. This can occur when teeth are extremely tightly spaced. Fortunately, special flosses and flossing aids are available that help patients floss despite having "tight contacts." Flosses are available in package sizes from 50 to 200 yards. Floss varieties include the following:

- Plain, unwaxed floss—suitable for patients with no special problem
- Waxed floss—passes more easily between tight teeth without shredding or breaking
- Extrafine floss—helps with tight contacts
- Mint-flavored or cinnamon-flavored flosses—leave a pleasant intraoral aftertaste (may be available as waxed and/or extrafine)

- Flosses for children—have a flavor such as bubble gum
- Dental tape—suitable for broad surface cleansing

Patients who are asked to begin a flossing regimen often offer several reasons why they cannot comply. One is the inability to master the rather intricate manipulation of floss required to work it between each set of teeth. As with tooth brushing, patients are best trained by a dentist or hygienist, who should ensure that they understand the pressures required to force the floss between their teeth and also that they can tell the difference between the pressure needed to clean the gums and the dangerous pressures that actually cut the gums. Several picture-aided articles can be found in pharmacy periodicals or public libraries.[73–75] The patient should not floss with too great a force since gums and teeth can be traumatized.

Patients also complain that their mouth is too small to permit entry by the fingers. Devices are available that facilitate flossing. For example, with the Butler G•U•M Flossmate, which is a Y-shaped forklike tool, the patient threads floss over each leg of the "Y" then uses the tool to work floss between the teeth. This device also is useful for patients who only have the use of one hand or arm and for caregivers who have to floss the teeth of another, such as an elderly parent

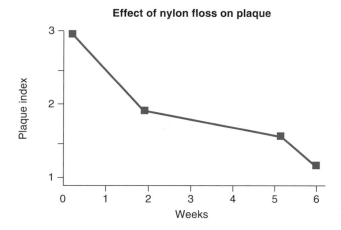

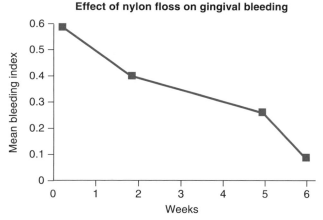

Figure 3.4. Use of dental floss reduces the percentage of plaque on teeth and the incidence of gingival bleeding.

or small child. The Glide Floss Holder is a similar device.

Several companies also market small plastic handles with a short length of floss prethreaded between two protrusions. Patients with normal and widely spaced teeth may be able to use these, but they are impractical for patients with tight contacts, who customarily shred and break floss.

Floss aids are marketed that help patients whose contacts are so tight that they absolutely prohibit the patient from moving the floss down between the teeth without floss breakage. Two of these products—Eze-Thru Floss Threaders and BridgeAid—are soft, flexible plastic loops with a short arm. Patients "thread" the floss through a loop and then pull the arm through the teeth at the gumline and use the arm to pull the loops and floss through. Once the floss has been threaded between the teeth, the patient then removes the loop and moves the floss up and down in the characteristic cleaning motion. The floss is then simply pulled out of the interdental space and the loop is used to thread the next interdental area, repeating the process at any place in the mouth where it is necessary. (If only one or two spots in the mouth cannot be flossed, calculus or a filling may be protruding into the interdental space. A dentist may be able to remedy these problems.)

Patients with caps, bridges, or orthodontic appliances may be unable to use floss. Orthodontists can suggest a mix of other techniques to permit plaque removal.

Periodontal Aids

While toothbrushing cleans broad, nonproximal tooth surfaces fairly well, and flossing can clean proximal tooth surfaces, **sulcular** areas (between the gum and the tooth) may not be adequately cleaned with brushing and flossing. As a result, food particles may remain in the oral cavity, which promotes bacterial growth and lytic ferment, slowly eroding the periodontium that holds teeth in place. To ensure that the sulcular area is properly cleaned, some periodontists consider the use of a periodontal aid as fundamental to gingival health (Table 3.3). Generally, patients are directed to use the periodontal aid

FOCUS ON . . .

CORRECT FLOSSING TECHNIQUE

The patient should pull out and break off approximately 18 inches of floss.[48] As shown in the figure, just enough floss is wound around the middle fingers of one hand to anchor it. Enough of the long section of floss is wound around the other middle finger to anchor it. The hand holding the shorter section will take up the floss as it is used. The floss is pinched between the thumb and first finger. There should be at least 1 to 2 inches of floss between the fingers. Holding the floss tightly between the thumbs and fingers, the patient should attempt to gently move the floss between the first interdental space to be cleaned. A back-and-forth motion is used for tight contacts. However, the floss should not be allowed to snap between the teeth because gingival damage can occur. With the floss between the teeth, the patient curves it into a "C" shape around the first tooth. A sliding motion allows the floss to be gently moved up and down that interdental space and moved below the gumline of the first tooth. Then the gumline of the adjacent tooth is cleaned. This method is repeated on all teeth, including the back side of the last molars. As the floss becomes dirty or shreds, the patient takes up the older section, releasing floss from the longer section, maintaining the 1- to 2-inch distance between the fingers.

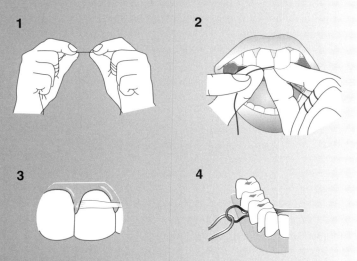

Proper flossing: (1) A short piece of floss is placed between the thumb and first finger. (2) The floss is gently passed between all tooth spaces. (3) Scrape the floss gently up and down along the tooth and below the gumline of each tooth. (4) Use a floss threader for extremely tight contacts.

once daily to cleanse sulcular areas and prevent gingival recession and tooth loss.

The typical periodontal aid is a handle that allows the patient to insert the end of a toothpick or a brush. Following tightening of the toothpick, the patient uses the end of the toothpick to outline all gums (both lingual and buccal surfaces), moving up and down all interdental tooth surfaces and cleaning behind the back molars. A simple toothpick could serve as a periodontal aid, but most people using it do so in an improper manner. This also applies to certain plastic or wooden devices (e.g., Stim-U-Dent) that claim to remove plaque. It is too difficult to move these devices to the areas requiring cleansing. The periodontal aid takes care of this problem.

Table 3.3. Representative Periodontal Aids

PRODUCT	COMMENTS
Brushpicks	Long toothpick-shaped polypropylene plastic pick with a triangular end and cleaning bristles at the other end
Dental Pik Tartar Remover	Handle with a curved plastic tip
Dr. Du-More's Plaq-U-Pick	Plastic pick with a tapered end
Oral-B Interdental Kit	A handle that accepts small tapered or conical brushes
OraPik	Handle with a curved metal hook at one end
OraPik Traveler	Smaller version of the OraPik
Perio-aid	Plastic handle with an end that threads down on a short length of a toothpick
ProPicks	Plastic pick with a 45° angle at one end
Proxabrush	A handle that accepts small tapered or conical brushes
Proxabrush Trav-Ler	A handle with a small prefitted brush protruding from one end
Proxabrush Gum Stimulator	Metal handle with the end fitted to accept rubber tips
Stim-U-Dent Plaque Removers Mint Flavor	Wooden pick with one tapered end

Table 3.4. Representative Plaque-Disclosing Agents and Aids

PRODUCT	SELECTED INGREDIENTS/COMMENTS
Butler G•U•M Mouth Mirror	A handle with a small, round mirror on one end to allow the patient to visualize plaque
Red-Cote tablets	Chewable tablet containing red dye
Red-Cote Dental Disclosing Solution	Solution containing D&C red #28, 1.5%

Table 3.5. Representative Tartar-Control Dentifrices

PRODUCT	SELECTED INGREDIENTS
Aim Tartar Control Toothpaste	Sodium monofluorophosphate 0.14%, zinc citrate trihydrate
Aquafresh Tartar Control Toothpaste	0.13% fluoride from sodium fluoride, tetrapotassium pyrophosphate, tetrasodium pyrophosphate
Close-Up Tartar Control Mint Gel	Sodium monofluorophosphate 0.14%, zinc citrate trihydrate
Colgate Tartar Control Fluoride Toothpaste	Sodium fluoride 0.15%, tetrasodium pyrophosphate
Crest Tartar Protection Toothpaste	Sodium fluoride 0.15%, tetrapotassium pyrophosphate, disodium pyrophosphate, tetrasodium pyrophosphate
Pepsodent Tartar Control	Sodium fluoride 0.14%, zinc citrate trihydrate

Table 3.6. Representative Products Promoted for Whitening the Teeth

PRODUCT	SELECTED INGREDIENTS/COMMENTS
Aquafresh Whitening Toothpaste	0.15% fluoride from sodium fluoride, hydrated silica
Colgate Platinum Toothpaste	Sodium monofluorophosphate 0.76%, hydrated silica
Pearl Drops Tooth Polish	Sodium monofluorophosphate (unlabeled concentration), calcium pyrophosphate, hydrated silica
Pearl Drops Whitening Toothpaste with Baking Soda	Sodium fluoride (unlabeled concentration), sodium bicarbonate, hydrated silica, tetrasodium pyrophosphate, tetrapotassium pyrophosphate
Plus+ White Toothpaste	Sodium monofluorophosphate (unlabeled concentration), hydrated silica
Rembrandt Toothpaste	0.15% fluoride from sodium monofluorophosphate, papain, citric acid, dicalcium phosphate dihydrate
Ultra Brite	Sodium monofluorophosphate (unlabeled concentration), hydrated silica, alumina

Another periodontal aid is the Butler Gum Stimulator, which is a metal handle with a pointed rubber tip that fits over the end to allow periodontal stimulation and cleansing. Replacement tips are available.

Other periodontal aids are metal or nylon handles into which the patient inserts a small cylindrical or conical brush. Patients use them to brush in otherwise hard-to-reach areas. Pharmacies can order replacement handles and brushes separately.

Some dentists discourage the use of periodontal aids, relying instead on other products (e.g., oral irrigators) to cleanse sulcular areas. The pharmacist should urge the patient to follow the advice of his practitioner. Aggressive cleaning with periodontal aids could damage the gingiva.

Plaque-Disclosing Agents

Dentist and hygienists sometimes use plaque-disclosing agents to show patients areas of the mouth that they have neglected with their routine intraoral care. The purple or red solution, which is swished in the mouth and then expectorated, selectively stains plaque and calculus. With the aid of a dental mirror, the dentist or hygienist can demonstrate to patients the hand movements needed to clean those areas. Table 3.4 lists several plaque-disclosing agents that are available for home use.

Tartar-Control Dentifrices

The manufacturers of various toothpastes and rinses claim their products prevent plaque and gum disease. The FDA re-

FOCUS ON...

DANGERS OF WET TOOTHBRUSHES

A study of the toothbrushes of healthy individuals and patients with mouth and throat infections by an oral pathologist revealed pathologic bacteria on the toothbrushes of patients with infections.[79] After the infected group started using new toothbrushes every few weeks, their infections quickly cleared up.

The researcher determined that a new toothbrush is infected heavily within 17 to 35 days. This rapid contamination rate is caused by a number of factors:

- Toothbrushes are kept in warm bathrooms.
- Toothbrushes can be wetted several times daily, providing a moist environment conducive to the growth of organisms.
- Toothbrushes are continually enriched with food particles from the mouth.

The researcher suggested that mouth infections would be easier to overcome if toothbrushes were changed every few weeks, and if individuals alternate between two brushes, so the brushes have a better chance of drying between uses.

quires data to back up these claims since, by claiming to treat or prevent disease and affect structure or function of the body, they are therefore classified as drugs.[76]

Tartar-control toothpastes similarly claim to be able to chemically dissolve tartar as the patient brushes through the use of various chemicals (Table 3.5). The FDA has not yet ruled on the efficacy of these claims. Until that time pharmacists should advise patients that these products will not substitute for a total program of oral care. Further, the consumer who wishes to use a fluoridated product should examine these products carefully to ensure that they do contain fluoride.

Abrasive Dentifrices

Toothpastes employ an abrasive to mechanically remove dental plaque, stain, and debris from tooth surfaces. The ef-

Table 3.7. Representative Products for Plaque/Gingivitis

PRODUCT	SELECTED INGREDIENTS/COMMENTS
Cepacol Mouthwash/Gargle	Cetylpyridinium chloride 0.05%, alcohol 14%
Colgate Total Toothpaste	Sodium fluoride 0.24%, triclosan 0.3%, hydrated silica; FDA-approved for preventing plaque, caries, and gingivitis
Crest Gum Care Toothpaste	Stannous fluoride (0.15% fluoride ion), hydrated silica, sodium gluconate, stannous chloride
Mentadent Gum Care	Zinc citrate trihydrate 0.2%, sodium fluoride (0.15% fluoride ion) (efficacy unknown)
Plax Original Flavor Rinse	Sorbitol, 8.7% alcohol, tetrasodium pyrophosphate (efficacy unknown)

A Pharmacist's Journal

"Help My Loose Teeth."

While working in a retail pharmacy, I was approached by a young man who asked if the pharmacy carried anything for "loose teeth." When I asked him to elaborate further, the young man volunteered to demonstrate his problem. He grasped one incisor between a forefinger and thumb and wiggled it back and forth. He further stated that all of his teeth were that loose. He also stated that because he worked two jobs, he simply did not have time to brush his teeth at all. I explained that there are no nonprescription products for loose teeth and that he was in imminent danger of losing all of his teeth, and I encouraged him to seek advanced periodontal care immediately.

fectiveness of toothpaste depends partially on the difference in hardness between surface debris and the tooth. Debris should be removed before tooth damage occurs. Most toothpastes have a moderate level of abrasives such as dicalcium phosphate, silica, calcium carbonate, calcium pyrophosphate, or alumina.[71] Sample products containing silica ingredients or other formulae, specifically focusing on dental staining, are listed in Table 3.6.

Abrasives should only be applied to the tooth crown, which is protected somewhat by enamel. Enamel is 10 to 20 times as hard as the root portion of the tooth, for instance, which is composed of a thin layer of cementum over dentin. If the root portion of the tooth has become exposed because of gingival recession, the use of high-abrasive toothpaste can actually remove tooth substance. Thus older patients with receding gums are at higher risk of dental damage from high-abrasive toothpastes.[77]

Miscellaneous Oral Cleansing Devices

A number of other devices are useful for oral cleaning. Manufacturers of oral irrigators claim that their products, which direct a spray of water into the mouth, help patients clean their teeth. (The intensity of the spray can be adjusted.) The patient's dentist can recommend an optimal product and can give the precautions that would apply to the patient's particular situation. For instance, use of the device can cause transient bacteremia, which could be dangerous in patients with rheumatic heart disease or those with prosthetic heart valves.[78]

Patients may also purchase handles with stainless-steel tips to allow home removal of tartar (calculus) such as the Dental Pik. Patients can cause permanent damage to the enamel of the tooth through unsupervised use of metallic instruments on the teeth.

Manufacturers of home tooth cleaners (e.g., The Doctor's Tooth Polisher) claim that patients can use rotary polishers and tooth polish to clean their teeth at home. Pharmacists should advise patients to seek professional dental help for cleaning the teeth of calculus rather than assuming that they can achieve decent results at home. (See "Dangers of Tooth-Bleaching Products.")

PLAQUE PREVENTIVES

Recently, a Plaque Subcommittee of the FDA has been active in examining the role of oral products in plaque prevention. Two ingredients have been found safe and effective in preventing plaque. One, cetylpyridinium chloride, is found in Cepacol Antiseptic Mouthwash.[80] Another, triclosan, is found in a toothpaste, Colgate Total, which also contains fluoride (Table 3.7).[81,82] Experimental evidence indicates that stabilized stannous fluoride toothpastes such as Crest Gum Care also provide anticaries action and inhibition of gingivitis.[83–85] The hypothesized mechanism against gingivitis is a direct reduction of the virulence of plaque organisms by lowering the metabolism of the organisms, which slows the development of the gingivitis-producing metabolic by-products.

GINGIVITIS

See the preceding text for prevalence, epidemiology, and etiology of caries and gingivitis.

PREVENTION AND TREATMENT OF GINGIVITIS

Professional plaque removal can reverse the gingivitis that is present at the time of a dental visit.[4,5] Gingivitis that is ignored can proceed to irreversible periodontitis, which can result in significant tooth mobility and possible loss of teeth.[5] Unfortunately, while topical and systemic fluorides can compensate for poor oral hygiene, there is no corresponding barrier to the development of gingivitis. As a result, as many as 50% of adults suffer from gingivitis—and many people with gingivitis are both unaware of its presence and its long-term significance. (See "A Pharmacist's Journal: Help My Loose Teeth.")

While treatment of caries consists of well-known dental interventions and topical or oral fluorides, therapy of existing gingivitis/periodontitis is not as well delineated. A dental visit and professional cleaning can reverse the problem, however.[5] The patient should also maintain excellent oral hygiene, which provides better periodontal health.[32] Plaque preventives may have a role in the prevention of gingivitis. See "Plaque Preventives." (See Patient Assessment Algorithm 3.2.)

FOCUS ON...

DANGERS OF TOOTH-BLEACHING PRODUCTS

Listen to advertising and you might conclude that tooth whiteness is the major index of popularity among peers. (Some individuals have even used white paint in attempts to become socially acceptable.) Teeth-whitening products include high-abrasive toothpastes and bleaches. The high-abrasive toothpastes, which promise to remove stains from teeth, can damage tooth enamel. Pharmacists should advise patients to use caution with high-abrasive toothpastes. (See "Abrasive Dentifrices.") (See "A Pharmacist's Journal: I Like Comet.")

Bleaching products can be highly dangerous. (Bleaches are considered to be drugs by the FDA since they act by altering tooth structure.)[86] In 1991 Dr. Chakwan Siew, head of the American Dental Association Research Institute's Department of Toxicology at the time, stressed that the hydrogen peroxide these products contain had not been proven safe for this use.[87] Hydrogen peroxide has documented mutagenic potential when used in other situations, it boosts the effects of known carcinogens, it may harm periodontal tissues with prolonged use, and it can delay wound healing.

Some tooth-whitening products used a three-step system, with an acidic rinse included as one of the steps. The acids "microetch" or scratch the teeth, creating pores that are then filled in with a "polishing paste" containing white pigment. The white pigment is often titanium dioxide, the ingredient in white typewriter-correction fluids and white paint. The paint does not provide a long-lasting effect, however, yet the enamel has undergone permanent damage. As an example, a young patient who purchased a three-step whitening system in a food store suffered severe loss of tooth enamel when using it.[88]

The FDA has stated that hydrogen peroxide bleaches and three-step whiteners cannot be marketed legally without approval. Also, they must go through the NDA process to prove safety and efficacy.[89,90] No NDA had been submitted as of early 1992, when sales were mushrooming. Until the FDA takes strong action, some companies continue marketing these products, as seen in the table.

Representative Tooth Bleaching Products

PRODUCT	SELECTED INGREDIENTS/COMMENTS
Natural White Original Tooth Whitening System	A 3-part system; a conditioning prerinse with vinegar; an oxygenation bleaching gel with hydrogen peroxide; a pigmentation polishing cream with hydrated silica, titanium dioxide
Natural White Rapid Tooth Enamel Whitening System	A 3-part system; a prewhitening toothpaste with hydrated silica, titanium dioxide; a whitening gel with hydrogen peroxide, ammonium hydroxide; an oral rinse neutralizer with sodium bicarbonate, sodium hydroxide
Perfect Smile Tooth Whitening System	A 3-part system; ingredients are not labeled on the package, but are concealed on tubes inside the tamper-proof container

A Pharmacist's Journal

"I Like Comet."

After my lecture on the dangers of tooth-whitening products, a student told me that he uses Comet to attain white teeth. I asked "Doesn't the use of Comet cause you any concern?"—intending him to address the issue of using this harsh toilet bowl and sink cleanser on relatively soft dental enamel. He misunderstood my question as concern regarding systemic toxicity and answered, "No, I spit it out into the sink as I brush so I won't swallow any." The question of toxicity is secondary; even if he is able to expectorate all of the product, each use still results in irreversible damage to dental enamel.

FOCUS ON...

THE AMERICAN DENTAL ASSOCIATION (ADA) SEAL OF ACCEPTANCE

The Seal of Acceptance is awarded by the ADA to certain products that meet its requirements.[91,92] Approximately 350 companies voluntarily participate in the program by submitting the following information on their products:

- Objective data from clinical and/or laboratory studies that support safety, effectiveness, and promotional claims
- Clinical trials that have been conducted in accordance with ADA guidelines and procedures
- Evidence that manufacturing and laboratory facilities have proper supervision and can produce products that are pure and uniform, in compliance with Good Manufacturing Processes
- All advertising, promotional claims, and patient education materials, for assessing their truthfulness
- Ingredient lists and other pertinent information

At least 1300 products carry the ADA seal, about 30% of which are sold directly to patients. The remainder are used or prescribed by dentists. Patients and pharmacists have an added degree of assurance that these products are actually safe and effective for their labeled indication(s).

Patient Assessment Algorithm 3.2. Gingivitis

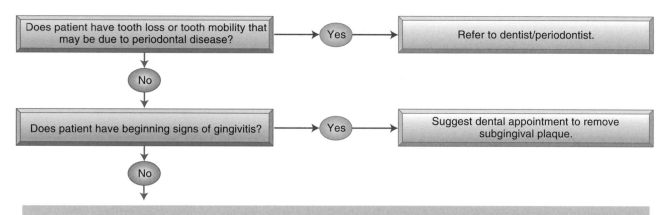

AT THE COUNTER

A mother with a 3-year-old girl says that she wants to start flossing the child's teeth, but doesn't know how to do it.

Interview/Patient Assessment

She has flossed her own teeth daily for about 10 years. The child's teeth appear to be tightly spaced in both the lower and upper jaws. Several teeth have not yet erupted.

Pharmacist's Analysis

1. Is flossing safe for a child of this age?
2. How often should the child's teeth be flossed?
3. What types of floss would facilitate the child's care?

4. What other devices would help the mother care for her child's teeth?

There are no general or specific contraindications for flossing.

Patient Counseling

The mother should be encouraged to floss her child's teeth once daily. She could be shown a waxed floss for initial use, to prevent shredding and tearing of the floss. She might also be shown one of the floss extenders (e.g., Floss Tip). Since the mother has a history of successful self-flossing, she does not need to be shown the method of flossing.

SUMMARY

Proper oral care is one of the most important routine health precautions patients can take to enhance the quality of life in later years. A properly motivated and trained patient can keep his teeth free of cavities and properly and firmly fixed in the bony sockets for a lifetime. Neglect leads to decayed and filled teeth that are lost from the gums, compromising mastication and nutritional status.

Steps in plaque removal include brushing with fluoridated toothpastes, using anticavity rinses, flossing, using periodontal aids, and checking teeth with plaque-disclosing agents. Gingivitis can be prevented through the use of such products as stabilized stannous fluoride toothpastes. Self-care devices must be used correctly, however, or teeth and /or gums can be damaged. Potentially dangerous products such as metallic, home-use, tartar-removal aids and tooth whiteners containing high abrasive levels or dangerous concentrations of hydrogen peroxide must be avoided.

References

1. Pray WS. The Pharmacist's Role in Oral Health Care, 1996, University of Kentucky College of Pharmacy, Lexington, KY.
2. Larmas M. Plaque-mediated disease. Ann NY Acad Sci 694:252, 1993.
3. Van Dyke TE. New agents in the chemical control of plaque and gingivitis—Reaction paper. J Dent Res 71:1457, 1992.
4. Duckworth RM. The science behind caries prevention. Int Dent J 43(6 Suppl 1):529, 1993.
5. Johnson NW. Hygiene and health: The value of antiplaque agents in promoting oral health. Int Dent J 43(4 Suppl 1):375, 1993.
6. White BA. An overview of oral health care status, resources, and care delivery. J Dent Educ 58:285, 1994.
7. Nourjah P, Horowitz AM, Wagener DK. Factors associated with the use of fluoride supplements and fluoride dentifrice by infants and toddlers. J Public Health Dent 54:47, 1994.
8. Stamm JW. The value of dentifrices and mouthrinses in caries prevention. Int Dent J 43(6 Suppl 1):517, 1993.
9. Delawter DE. Oral hygiene and diabetes. Md Med J 39:487, 1990.
10. Hubbard TM. Periodontal disease and the family physician. Am Fam Physician 44:487, 1991.
11. Blinkhorn AS. Factors affecting the compliance of patients with preventive dental regimens. Int Dent J 43(3 Suppl 1):294, 1993.
12. Lang WP, Farghaly MM, Ronis DL. The relation of preventive dental behaviors to periodontal health status. J Clin Periodontol 21:194, 1994.
13. Dental health of school children—Oregon, 1991–1992. MMWR 42:887, 1993.
14. Smyth JS. Some problems of dental treatment. Part 1. Patient anxiety: Some correlates and sex differences. Aust Dent J 38:354, 1993.
15. Milgrom P, Weinstein P. Dental fears in general practice: New guidelines for assessment and treatment. Int Dent J 43(3 Suppl 1):288, 1993.
16. De Jongh A, et al. Cognitive correlates of dental anxiety. J Dent Res 73:561, 1994.
17. Omar SM, Pitts NB. Oral hygiene, gingivitis and periodontal status of Libyan school children. Community Dent Health 8:329, 1991.
18. Addy M, et al. The effect of toothbrushing frequency, toothbrushing hand, sex and social class on the incidence of plaque, gingivitis and pocketing in adolescents: a longitudinal cohort study. Community Dent Health 7:237, 1990.
19. Safkan-Seppalla B, Ainamo J. Periodontal conditions in insulin-dependent diabetes mellitus. J Clin Periodontol 19:24, 1992.
20. Fransson C, Berglundh T, Lindhe J. The effect of age on the development of gingivitis. Clinical, microbiological and histological findings. J Clin Periodontol 23:379, 1996.
21. Ismail AI, Lewis DW. Periodic health examination, 1993 up-

date: 3. Periodontal disease: classification, diagnosis, risk factors and prevention. Can Med Assoc J 149:1409, 1993.

22. Bergstrom J. Oral hygiene compliance and gingivitis expression in cigarette smokers. Scand J Dent Res 98:497, 1990.

23. Cummings KM, et al. Use of smokeless tobacco in a group of professional baseball players. J Behav Med 12:559, 1989.

24. Robinson PJ. Gingivitis: A prelude to periodontitis? J Clin Dent 6 Spec No:41, 1995.

25. Riviere GR, et al. Periodontal status and detection frequency of bacteria at sites of periodontal health and gingivitis. J Periodontol 67:109, 1996.

26. Navia JM. Carbohydrates and dental health. Am J Clin Nutr 59(3 Suppl):719S, 1994.

27. McMahon J, Parnell WR, Spears GFS. Diet and dental caries in preschool children. Eur J Clin Nutr 47:297, 1993.

28. van Houte J. Role of micro-organisms in caries etiology. J Dent Res 73:672, 1994.

29. Woodward M, Walker ARP. Sugar consumption and dental caries: Evidence from 90 countries. Br Dent J 176:297, 1994.

30. Lingström P, et al. Effect of frequent consumption of starchy food items on enamel and dentin demineralization and on plaque pH *in situ*. J Dent Res 73:652, 1994.

31. Praytino SW, Addy M, Wade WG. Does gingivitis lead to periodontitis in young adults? Lancet 342:471, 1993.

32. Lang WP, Ronis DL, Farghaly MM. Preventive behaviors as correlates of periodontal health status. J Public Health Dent 55:10, 1995.

33. Ramberg P, Axelsson P, Lindhe J. Plaque formation at healthy and inflamed gingival sites in young individuals. J Clin Periodontol 22:85, 1995.

34. Daly CG, Highfield JE. Effect of localized experimental gingivitis on early supragingival plaque accumulation. J Clin Periodontol 23:160, 1996.

35. Scully C, Porter S, Greenman J. What to do about halitosis. BMJ 308:217, 1994.

36. Spielman AI, Bivona P, Rifkin BR. Halitosis. A common oral problem. NY State Dent J 62:36, 1996.

37. Iwakura M, et al. Clinical characteristics of halitosis: Difference in two patient groups with primary and secondary complaints of halitosis. J Dent Res 73:1568, 1994.

38. Replogle WH, Beebe DK. Halitosis. Am Fam Physician 53:1215, 1996.

39. Eli I, et al. The complaint of oral malodor: Possible psychopathological aspects. Psychosom Med 58:156, 1996.

40. Richter JL. Diagnosis and treatment of halitosis. Compend Contin Educ Dent 17:370, 1996.

41. Bosy A, et al. Relationship of oral malodor to periodontitis: Evidence of independence in discrete subpopulations. J Periodontol 65:37, 1994.

42. Stolze K, Bay L. Comparison of a manual and a new electric toothbrush for controlling plaque and gingivitis. J Clin Periodontol 21:86, 1994.

43. Kleisner J, Imfeld T. Evaluation of the efficacy of interdental cleaning devices. J Clin Periodontol 20:707, 1993.

44. Berry JH. Home care, health care. J Am Dent Assoc 125:146, 1994.

45. Etty EJ, et al. Influence of oral hygiene on early enamel caries. Caries Res 28:132, 1994.

46. Anon. Success is in the flossing, not the type of dental floss (Editorial). NY State Dent J 60:49, 1994.

47. Payne BJ, Locker D. Preventive oral health behaviors in a multi-cultural population: The North York oral health promotion survey. J Can Dent Assoc 60:129, 1994.

48. Anon. Cleaning your teeth and gums. http://www.ada.org/consumer/clean.html. 1997.

49. Anon. How to brush your teeth. http://www.ada.org/consumer/radio/970721.html. 1997.

50. Anon. When to change your toothbrush. http://www.ada.org/consumer/radio/970623.html. 1997.

51. Terezhalmy GT, et al. Clinical evaluation of the effect of an ultrasonic toothbrush on plaque, gingivitis, and gingival bleeding: A six-month study. J Prosthet Dent 73:97, 1995.

52. Bader H, Williams R. Clinical and laboratory evaluation of powered electric toothbrushes: Comparative efficacy of two powered brushing instruments in furcations and interproximal areas. J Clin Dent 8:91, 1997.

53. Anon. ADA seal of acceptance: Toothbrushes, powered. http://www.ada.org/p&s/seal/cons/ccat-013.html. 1998.

54. Editorial. Fluoridation then and now. Am J Public Health 79:561, 1989.

55. Musto RJ. Fluoridation: Why is it not more widely adopted? Can Med Assoc J 137:705, 1987.

56. Editorial. Fluoride and oral health: A story of achievements and challenges. J Am Dent Assoc 118:529, 1989.

57. Levy SM, et al. American Association of Public Health Dentistry: Recommendations for teaching about the prescription of dietary fluoride supplement. J Public Health Dent 49:237, 1989.

58. Anon. Dental caries and dental fluorosis. Nutr Rev 46:317, 1988.

59. Szpunar SM, Burt BA. Dental caries, fluorosis, and fluoride exposure in Michigan schoolchildren. J Dent Res 67:802, 1988.

60. dos Santos MN, Cury JA. Dental plaque fluoride is lower after discontinuation of water fluoridation. Caries Res 22:316, 1988.

61. Burt BA, et al. Dental benefits of limited exposure to fluoridated water in childhood. J Dent Res 61:1322, 1986.

62. Attwood D, Blinkhorn AS. Trends in dental health of ten-year-old schoolchildren in South-West Scotland after cessation of water fluoridation. Lancet 2(8605):266, 1988.

63. Anon. Progress toward achieving the national 1990 objectives for fluoridation and dental health. MMWR 37:578, 1988.

64. Schultz D. Fluoride. FDA Consumer 26:34, 1992.

65. Hattab FN. The state of fluorides in toothpastes. J Dent 17:47, 1989.

66. Beiswanger BB, et al. A clinical evaluation of the relative cariostatic effect of dentifrices containing sodium fluoride or sodium monofluorophosphate. ASDC J Dent Child 56:270, 1989.

67. Evans DJ. Fluoride supplements (Letter). Br Dent J 167:225, 1989.

68. Brown RH. Fluorides and the prevention of dental caries. Part II: The case for water fluoridation. N Z Dent J 85:8, 1989.

69. Simard PL, et al. The ingestion of fluoride dentifrice by young children. ASDC J Dent Child 88:177, 1989.

70. Anticaries drug products for over-the-counter human use: Tentative final monograph. Fed Reg 50:39854, 1985.

71. Fed Reg 60:52474, 1995.

72. Anon. FDA Consumer 19:2, 1985/1986.

73. Anon. The best ways to put your money where your mouth is. Consumer Reports 49:129, 1984.

74. Borger JA. How to floss properly in order to preserve that healthy smile. Pharmacy Times 49:42, 1983.

75. McGregor TD, Nelson LA. Oral health care. II. Patient education. Am Pharm 27:57, 1987.

76. Anon. Drug clams on toothpaste, mouthwash. FDA Consumer 24:5, 1990.

77. Fed Reg 45:20676. 1980.

78. Nelson LA, et al. Oral health care products. Am Drugg 195:103, 1986.

79. Anon. Med World News 27:68, 1986.

80. Anon. Cetylpyridinium chloride gets category I status. NDMA Exec Newsletter 10–97:5, 1997.

81. Anon. FDA approves triclosan to prevent gingivitis, plaque and cavities. NDMA Exec Newsletter 16–97:2, 1997.

82. Anon. First toothpaste approved for reducing gum disease. FDA Consumer 31(7):4, 1997.

83. Axelsson P. Current role of pharmaceuticals in prevention of caries and periodontal disease. Int Dent J 43:473, 1993.

84. Stephen KW. Dentifrices: Recent clinical findings and implications for use. Int Dent J 43(6 Suppl 1):549, 1993.

85. Wei SHY, Yiu CKY. Mouthrinses: Recent clinical findings and implications for use. Int Dent J 43(6 Suppl 1):541, 1993.

86. Anon. Pharm Times 58:51, 1992.

87. Berry JH. What about whiteners? Pharm Times 57:33, 1991.

88. Anon. Exercise extreme caution in purchasing tooth whitening products. Drug Store News 13:69, 1991.

89. Anon. The Green Sheet 40:1, 1991.

90. Anon. Some teeth whiteners are drugs. FDA Consumer 26:2, 1992.

91. Anon. Products with the ADA seal of acceptance. http://www.ada.org/p&s/seal/tc-seal.html. 1997.

92. Anon. The American Dental Association seal of acceptance. http://www.ada.org/consumer/adaseal.html. 1997.

93. Raab FJ, Young LL. Episodic factitious gingival injury secondary to topical anesthesia: A case report. J Periodontol 62:402, 1991.

Oral Problems

Almost everyone suffers from oral discomfort during their lifetime. Complaints range from easily treatable conditions such as dry mouth and teething pain to more troublesome complaints such as toothache. The typical pharmacy has a large oral-products section with items that can provide relief for many of these problems.

Chapter 3 covered plaque and its role in the development of caries and gingivitis. It describes the prevention of caries. This chapter also discusses caries, but focuses on the condition as a possible cause of toothache.

PART 1: XEROSTOMIA

Xerostomia, a condition in which the mouth is excessively dry, has a number of causes (see "Etiology of Xerostomia"). While it may be only a minor annoyance for most patients, in its most extreme form it may cause decayed teeth, difficulty in speaking, and hamper eating and swallowing. (To taste substances in the oral cavity, they must be soluble in water.[1] Saliva allows taste to occur.)

Saliva also lubricates the oral cavity, facilitating mastication, swallowing, and speaking. **Hyposalivation** (low levels of saliva) can compromise these functions, producing **dysphagia** (difficulty in eating) and **dysphonia** (difficulty in speaking).

Saliva protects tooth surfaces from oral acids and alkalies through the buffering effects of its bicarbonate, phosphate, and protein components.[2] In addition, the teeth and oral mucosa are cleansed of organisms and food debris through the mechanical cleansing of salivary flow. Saliva also remineralizes teeth to limit the extension of caries.[3] A reduction of

saliva can result in rampant caries and secondary periodontal infection.

Saliva helps maintain proper hydration by preventing dryness of the oral mucosa.[4] As dehydration occurs, reduced salivary flow signals dehydration, triggering the thirst reflex. The glycoproteins and mucoids in saliva form a protective coating over the oral mucosa, similar to that protecting the gastric mucosa from acid.[5] The buffering components of saliva protect the esophagus from acid-induced injury during bouts of acid reflux.

Sialometry (salivary flow measurement) can indicate salivary gland hypofunction.[6] However, criteria for assessment of salivary gland function vary. The circadian cycle regulates salivary flow, so that a series of salivary flow examinations should be conducted at identical times on successive days, ideally in early mornings.[7] Patients should fast overnight and brush the teeth only with water the morning of the examination. Saliva is collected using the resting or stimulated techniques.[8,9]

PREVALENCE OF XEROSTOMIA

While xerostomia is often referred to as a common condition, and elderly patients are the focus of most studies, its true prevalence is unknown. In one study, at least 16% of 70-year-old men and 25% of women the same age had symptoms related to dry mouth.[10] In hospitalized patients, 27% of males and 52% of females had xerostomia.[10] Twenty-nine percent of adults attending a family health center volunteered that they suffered from xerostomia and related symptoms when specifically questioned.[11]

EPIDEMIOLOGY OF XEROSTOMIA

The axiom that salivary production decreases with age has several possible causes.[7–9] The well-known increase of medications with aging is probably the reason that so many studies demonstrate an age-related decrease.[7,12,13] The increased risk of **Sjögren's syndrome** (a medical condition causing dry mouth, dry eyes, and a connective tissue disorder, usually rheumatoid arthritis), hypertension, and Type II diabetes mellitus with age contributes to the relationship between age and xerostomia.[14,15]

ETIOLOGY OF XEROSTOMIA

Rather than being a discrete illness, xerostomia is a manifestation of disordered salivary production or transportation. The term "primary xerostomia" refers to the condition when it is induced by a pathologic lesion in the salivary glands (Fig. 4.1).[14,16] Within this framework, "secondary xerostomia"—which can indicate many underlying disorders—is the diagnosis when no salivary lesion can be demonstrated.

Duct Obstruction

In rare instances, a **sialolith** (a small obstruction of the salivary ducts) reduces or blocks salivary flow (Fig. 4.1). Inflam-

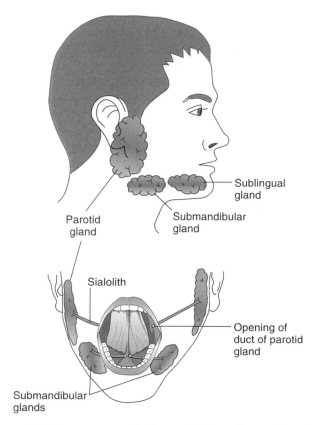

Figure 4.1. There are several salivary glands, as illustrated in this drawing. A sialolith has been shown in one location.

mation of the ducts caused by viral infections also can obstruct the ducts, but immunization against mumps has made this uncommon. Bacterial infections producing duct obstruction are seen in sialolithiasis.[15]

Irradiation

Approximately 30,000 to 50,000 patients yearly suffer radiation injury to the salivary glands.[8] (It is often impossible to radiate primary tumor sites [e.g., the head and neck] with curative dosages while sparing the salivary glands.) When malignancies involve the upper aerodigestive tract, major and minor salivary glands are commonly included in the radiation ports. Following their exposure to radiation, dissection of the glands reveals necrosis and fibrosis. Radiation-induced xerostomia is usually permanent, although in some cases if limited function returns, it is never at the preradiation levels.[12,17] The times to necrosis and recovery vary, depending on the radiation dose received.

Other Medical Conditions

Quite often, xerostomia is secondary to another medical condition. For example, dry mouth is one of the triad of characteristic symptoms of Sjögren's syndrome.[7,18] The single most common disease affecting the salivary glands, Sjögren's syndrome causes progressive and irreversible xerostomia.[8,12] This chronic inflammatory disease of the exocrine glands is caused by the presence of antibodies directed against the parenchymal cells of the glands.[7,8] The condition—which has a 9:1 female:male ratio—primarily affects postmenopausal females.[2,8] The prevalence in the United States is 2 million patients overall.

Xerostomia may also result from the HIV complex, hypertension, cystic fibrosis, systemic lupus erythematosus, Crohn's disease, primary biliary cirrhosis, graft versus host disease, and dehydration secondary to reduced water intake or increased output, as in diarrhea.[7,8,16,19] Since xerostomia can be produced by dehydration secondary to polyuria, it may be the presenting feature of diabetes mellitus.[8,13,14,20]

Medication-Induced Xerostomia

Dry mouth is one of the most common adverse reactions of medications.[21–23] In fact, the reason that xerostomia is so common in hypertension and depression may be the **xerogenic** (causing xerostomia) medications taken for those conditions.[7]

Medications can induce xerostomia through inhibition of parasympathetic impulses or autonomic ganglia, or via stimulation of the sympathetic nervous system.[20,24] At least 400 medications produce xerostomia; therefore, a careful review of medications is an integral part of the differential diagnostic process.[7,16] Xerogenic medications include antihypertensives, anorectics, anticholinergics, antihistamines, anticonvulsants, antiparkinson agents, bronchodilators, antipsychotics, antidepressants, and tranquilizers.[7,8,24] Signs and symptoms of xerostomia have been reported both during monotherapy and combination therapy when patients are receiving diuretics. A review of medications must include nonprescription products such as antihistamines, which may also be causal.[12]

Medication-induced xerostomia is often reversible, since medications usually do not cause permanent salivary gland damage.[7] Pharmacists must be aware that dry mouth prompts some patients to reduce dosages or discontinue their medications altogether, which could be detrimental. Patients should be advised to consult a physician, who may need to empirically substitute other medications in an attempt to optimize therapy and minimize this adverse reaction.[8]

Miscellaneous Causes

Emotions such as fear, excitement, and anxiety, as well as psychologic problems (e.g., neuroses, organic brain disorders, depression), can incite xerostomia.[9,15] **Orthognathic surgery** (wiring the jaws together) also can result in dry mouth.[7,9] High-protein diets, anemias, vitamin A, and ascorbate deficiency have all been identified as possible etiologies, as has prolonged mouth breathing, especially in children.[21]

COMPLICATIONS OF XEROSTOMIA

Hyposalivation compromises mastication because it makes it difficult to form a bolus of food between the tongue and palate. Patients especially notice this when eating and swallowing dry foods such as crackers or biscuits.[11] Hyposalivation often causes **hypogeusia** (lowered taste sensation) or **ageusia** (inability to taste substances), which affects appetite and nutrition.[14,25] Also, speech can be affected so severely by xerostomia that it is difficult or impossible to speak for any length of time.[8] Xerostomia may be more troublesome at night, to the point of affecting sleep.[17]

Oral epithelium (the tissue inside the mouth) can atrophy with continual xerostomia, possibly resulting in mucositis, inflammation, fissuring, cracks at the corners of the mouth, ulceration, and intraoral discomfort.[5,6,17] With xerostomia, intraoral and tongue surfaces can burn and tingle, or feel pasty or sticky.[11] Patients who are **edentulous** (lacking teeth) cannot retain their dentures with dry mouth and undergo increased denture trauma, resulting in soreness and ulcers.[4,22] Xerostomic patients wearing intraoral prosthetic devices exhibit similar problems.[16,17] Xerostomia causes changes in oral microflora that predispose patients to oral candidiasis, and infection of the pharynx and salivary glands.[8,14,24]

Without the buffering and cleansing actions of saliva, tooth surfaces can erode from decalcification and decay, which can result in rampant caries on the entire cervical area of the teeth and increased attrition and periodontal disease.[8,24] Part of the increase in caries is caused by overgrowth of pathogenic bacteria such as *Lactobacillus* and *Streptococcus mutans*.[14,16]

Chronic marginal gingivitis, gingival recession, and periodontitis are also caused by xerstomia.[16] Xerostomia patients should practice meticulous oral hygiene and should visit a dentist frequently.[14]

TREATMENT OF XEROSTOMIA

Treatment Guidelines

Patients should first eliminate factors that cause dry mouth. For example:

- Tobacco worsens xerostomia and should be avoided.[14,26]
- Drugs of abuse (e.g., marijuana, cocaine, alcohol, caffeine in the form of carbonated beverages, coffee, and tea) also must be eliminated.[14]
- Nonprescription products containing CNS stimulants (e.g., pseudoephedrine and phenylpropanolamine) or antihistamines may cause dry mouth.
- Mouthwashes containing alcohol dry the mouth.
- Although some people use mouth swabs containing lemon extract to moisten the mouth, the acid in these products contributes to tooth decay. They should be avoided.

Increasing the amount of fluid consumed with each meal also helps cope with dry mouth. *Patients should sip water after every bite of solid food.* Taking excess water along when eating out facilitates this, since one does not have to repeatedly signal restaurant personnel.[27,28] As an alternative, the patient may request a pitcher of water upon being seated. Patients may experience relief from yogurt, ice cubes in gauze inside the cheek, or butter, margarine, or vegetable oil placed inside the mouth.

Mastication itself stimulates salivary flow. Thus pharmacists should advise patients to eat foods that require chewing such as carrots and celery rather than soft-texture food, and to eat moist food, rather than dry, bulky food. Spicy or acidic foods should be avoided since they may burn the tissues or damage the teeth more severely in the presence of xerostomia.

The treatment regimen for xerostomia depends on patient's ability to produce saliva. If salivary function is eradicated completely, stimulants are not efficacious, and the patients should use saliva substitutes instead. If some salivary function remains, both salivary stimulants and saliva substitutes are potentially helpful.[14]

Chewing gum or paraffin wax provides gustatory and/or masticatory stimulation of salivary flow.[29] Pharmacists should recommend chewing gum with low amounts of fermentable sugars or nonfermentable sweeteners (e.g., xylitol as in the product XyliFresh gum) to help prevent caries. Sucking on oral lozenges or hard candy can also be helpful, but pressure and osmolarity from the chronic use of lozenges or candy can result in oral mucosal damage.[30] Patients must choose sugarless candies so tooth structures are not further compromised.[14]

While citric acid 2% serves as a salivary stimulant, long-term and repeated contact with the teeth causes demineralization, resulting in dental erosion.[31] Actual **sialagogues** (salivary stimulants) such as oral pilocarpine are prescription products.[32]

Nonprescription Medications

Available without a prescription, saliva substitutes are more effective than plain water. Some products attempt to mimic saliva content by including glycoproteins in gel formulations. They usually also contain carboxymethylcellulose and/or mucins for lubrication and viscosity, electrolytes for buffering and remineralization (e.g., calcium, phosphate), a sugar (e.g., xylitol or sorbitol) to sweeten, flavoring agents, and preservatives. Saliva substitutes last about 30 minutes when they are used prior to meals.

Mucin-based saliva substitutes seem to have a longer duration of action and are less irritating to mucosa than glycoprotein-based formulas.[32] Their taste is superior to carboxymethylcellulose products and their rheologic properties more closely mimic natural saliva. Commercially available saliva substitutes are listed in Table 4.1. The FDA asked the manufacturers of these products to submit safety/efficacy data in 1991.[33] As of this writing, the evaluations have not yet appeared.

Because dry mouth may be part of a larger problem of inadequate moisture, patients might also experience dry eyes, dry skin, and dryness in the nostrils, notably in the cold, dry winter months.[14] *Pharmacists should advise patients noticing widespread dryness related to the seasons that a steam vaporizer or cool-mist humidifier in the house and workplace should help relieve the overall problem of bodily dryness, including dry mouth.*[3,12,33] (See Chapter 16, Humidity Deficit.)

PART 2: PROBLEMS AFFECTING THE GINGIVA AND INTRAORAL SOFT TISSUES

MINOR GINGIVAL AND INTRAORAL INJURY

Gums and intraoral tissues are exposed to many potentially harmful environmental insults such as very hot and very cold food and drink and hard and/or sharp substances that are eaten or placed in the mouth (e.g., toothpicks), any of which can result in burns and cuts. Gums and intraoral tissues also suffer from bacterial infections from decaying food, teething, braces, and denture abrasions. Unless they are promptly dealt with, the teeth may be affected, or an abscess may develop.

See "Treatment of Gingival and Intraoral Tissue Discomfort."

Table 4.1. Representative Saliva Substitutes[a]

Mouth Kote

Optimoist Oral Moisturizer

Oral Balance

Roxane Saliva Substitute

Salivart

[a]These products are a mixture of many ingredients, which may include sorbitol, sodium carboxymethylcellulose, electrolytes, and preservatives.

RECURRENT APHTHOUS STOMATITIS (RAU)

Recurrent aphthous ulcerations (RAUs)—also known as aphthous ulcers, aphthous stomatitis, and, to the lay public, canker sores—are defined as deep craters that extend through the entire thickness of the oral surface epithelium and involve underlying connective tissue (Fig. 4.2).[34] RAUs appear on intraoral surfaces that are not attached to bone, such as the inside linings of the cheek, lips, and tongue.[35,36] They are not usually found on the gums or top of the mouth.[37,38] Although the term "aphthous" actually denotes any ulceration, it refers exclusively to ulcerations of the oral cavity when used medically.[34]

RAUs comprise over 80% of recurrent oral ulcers. However, there are two additional types of recurrent oral ulcers that the pharmacist should refer to the physician[39]:

- Major recurrent aphthae. A painful, 1- to 3-cm lesion, major recurrent aphthae persists for 6 weeks to 20 or more years. It usually scars, unlike the minor canker sore.[40–42]
- Herpetiform ulcers. Although they resemble herpes, herpetiform ulcers are not caused by an infectious agent.[43,44] As many as 100 ulcers, each measuring 1 to 3 mm in diameter, appear throughout the oral cavity in crops.[42] Lesions also coalesce to form large, irregularly shaped ulcers. The lesions, which occur more often in females, last for 7 to 10 days.

Since major recurrent aphthae and herpetiform ulcers are relatively uncommon—and not treatable with nonprescription products in any case—the balance of this discussion will focus on the pharmacist-recognizable canker sore.

A set of four appearance-related factors confirm the recognition of a canker sore[43]:

- Roundish
- Shallow-cratered
- Regular border surrounded by a red halo
- Interior white-yellow pseudomembranous covering

There is currently no better diagnostic method of recognizing canker sore than use of these criteria.

Although the size is variable, RAUs typically are 5 to 10 millimeters (about 1/2 inch) in diameter with a raised, erythematous, distinct border. Canker sores are found on any intraoral surface other than the hard palate and the tissue over the alveolar bone. They do not form blisters and, if patients have several, they do not coalesce. Canker sores generally last for 7 to 14 days and heal without scarring.[42,43]

PREVALENCE OF RECURRENT APHTHOUS STOMATITIS (RAU)

In one large-scale survey, more than 10% of United States adults reported at least one oral lesion. Inflammatory ulcers, the category that includes RAU, was the seventh most common type of lesion in that survey. RAU affects 20 to 55% of all Americans at one time or another.[34,45]

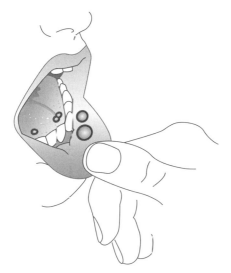

Figure 4.2. The canker sore is a roundish, shallow crater with a regular border surrounded by a red halo and with an interior, white-yellow, pseudomembranous covering. These are typical locations.

EPIDEMIOLOGY OF RECURRENT APHTHOUS STOMATITIS (RAU)

RAU affects both genders and all ages. In one survey, 50% of females and 40% of males experienced two or more episodes of RAU during their lifetime. Twenty-five percent of each sex had suffered an occurrence during the previous year. RAUs, which can develop at any age, have a strong genetic link.[35,39] Children with both parents affected have a 90% chance of also experiencing RAU; if no parent suffers from them, there is only a 10% chance that the children will.[43]

ETIOLOGY OF RECURRENT APHTHOUS STOMATITIS (RAU)

RAU is of unknown etiology, although a great deal of research has focused on its cause.[34] Since the etiology is unknown, research into the most effective treatments for RAU has been hampered. Despite the lack of knowledge concerning causation, however, investigators have revealed provocative information on RAU. For instance, the etiology of RAU may be multifactorial since the localized death of surface tissue with RAU could result from several of the conditions discussed below, all of which injure oral mucosa. It does seem certain that RAUs are not contagious.

Oral Trauma

Some patients notice that RAUs develop on high-trauma sites such as the side of the tongue or the inside lower lip.[45] Patients may relate a recent history of accidental self-inflicted bites of the lip or cheeks, dental or oral surgery, dental impressions, dental injections, or toothbrush injury.[34,35]

Infective Agents

Some researchers hypothesize that bacteria (e.g., streptococci) colonize an initial oral lesion to produce RAUs; the ulceration may occur because the organisms are pathogenic or because the host is allergic to them.[43] On the other hand, such factors as the recurrent nature of the lesions and their similarity to herpes labialis suggest a viral pathology; however, the location, course of the disease, and recurrence patterns are wholly different.[45,46]

At this time, infectious causes of canker sores are not thought to be primarily causal in and of themselves.

Nutritional Factors

Limited or single-case studies have led investigators to explore deficiencies of iron, vitamin B12, folic acid, and zinc in the etiology of RAU.[35,47–49] Supplementation of the suspected nutrient generally does not support these theories, however.[34] In fact, deficiencies in RAU patients may be secondary to the ulceration.

RAU also may be the result of food allergies.[39,50] Eliminating the foods patients are allergic to, however, although effective for the occasional patient, is not recommended for most patients.

Systemic Disease

Chronic mucosal ulcerations are associated with the acute leukemias and other blood dyscrasias.[43] Researchers have attempted to prove that RAU is a symptom of other systemic diseases such as Crohn's disease, Behçet's disease, Sweet's syndrome, cyclic neutropenia, immunodeficiencies (including AIDS), and *Giardia lamblia* infection, but evidence is contradictory at best.[39,51–53]

Other Factors

Anecdotal evidence suggests that periods of stress correlate with appearance and severity of canker sore lesions.[34,45,54] Stress is indeed a well-known factor in gastric stress ulcer, so the concept of stress influencing mucosal ulceration is in place. However, controlled studies using stress measurements do not support an association between stress and RAU.[35,54] Also, merely *having* canker sores produces stress.

Studies of female patients reveal an increase in number and severity of RAU during the premenstrual phase of the menstrual cycle and total clearing of the lesions during pregnancy.[35,45]

PROGNOSIS OF RECURRENT APHTHOUS STOMATITIS (RAU)

Pharmacists should advise patients that no therapy can guarantee a lifelong cure of minor RAU. The canker sore is normally an innocent lesion, but it can be sufficiently painful to make it difficult to eat, drink, and/or talk, particularly for patients with more than three or four canker sores in the mouth at one time. The following guidelines can help minimize the impact of RAUs[45]:

- Avoid potato chips, crackers, and other foods with sharp edges, which can cause more pain for the canker sore.
- Avoid spicy foods, pineapple, citrus fruits, and chocolate.
- Sip acidic juices and soft drinks though a straw to lessen contact with the canker sore and avoid the resultant pain.

TREATMENT OF RECURRENT APHTHOUS STOMATITIS (RAU)

See "Treatment of Gingival and Intraoral Tissue Discomfort."

See above for background on minor gingival and intraoral injury and for prevalence, epidemiology, etiology, and prognosis of recurrent aphthous stomatitis (RAU).

(Patient Assessment Algorithm 4.1 illustrates the steps used in treating the patient with an oral lesion such as RAU.)

TREATMENT OF GINGIVAL AND INTRAORAL TISSUE DISCOMFORT

Treatment Guidelines

If pharmacists feel certain that patients do not have serious conditions such as oral cancer, they may recommend any

Patient Assessment Algorithm 4.1. Oral Lesions

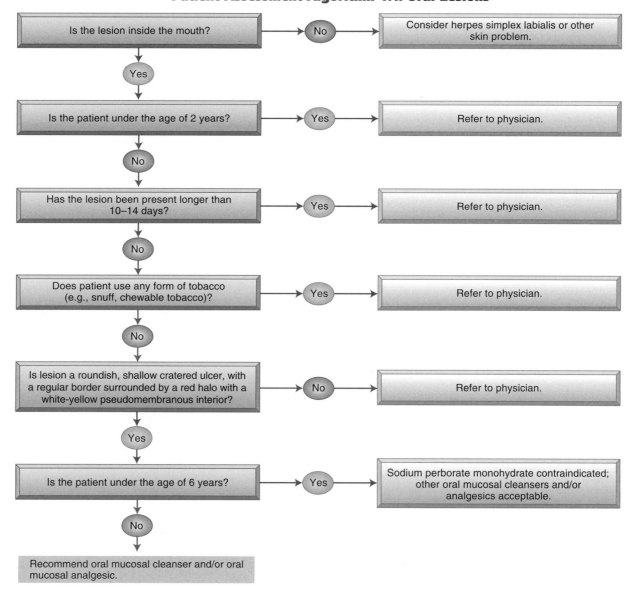

combination of gingival protectants, oral mucosal cleansing products, and oral mucosal analgesics (see "A Pharmacist's Journal: The Stuck Upper Plate").

Nonprescription Medications

GINGIVAL PROTECTANTS

These pharmacologically inert products adhere to gums to provide a protective coating, insulating the injury or RAU against further irritation. Benzoin compound and benzoin tincture are the only approved ingredients.[55] However, a product known as Orabase Plain is alleged to protect mucosa, although the ingredients were not reviewed by the FDA and the status of the product is questionable.

Orthodontists have long provided their patients with strips of wax to serve as gingival protectants. A patient with newly installed braces simply works the wax into the appliances so that sharp edges or wires do not abrade the oral mucosa. Wax can be ordered by pharmacies as Butler Orthodontic Wax.

ORAL MUCOSAL CLEANSING PRODUCTS

While seriously and persistently painful gums should prompt a dentist consultation, minor wounds and RAU can be cleansed with a number of products (Table 4.2). These medications, which are swished and spit out, should not be used longer than 1 week.[33] The four approved ingredients are:

- Sodium perborate monohydrate
- Carbamide peroxide
- Hydrogen peroxide
- Sodium bicarbonate

Sodium Perborate Monohydrate

In solution, sodium perborate monohydrate forms hydrogen peroxide and sodium perborate.[33,56,57] Boron comprises 10.8% of the molecule known as sodium perborate monohydrate. A leading toxicology text states that the toxicologic aspects of the sodium perborates cannot be distinguished from those of sodium borate and boric acid.[56] One unit-of-use package of buffered sodium perborate monohydrate oral rinse contains approximately 0.13 g of boron. If used QID as directed, and inadvertently swallowed, the patient would consume 0.52 g of boron, six times the amount safe for daily ingestion. Boric acid absorption is rapid from the mucous membranes of the mouth, throat, and GI tract. Symptoms of poisoning from boron derivatives include nausea/vomiting, diarrhea, and epigastric pain. Vomiting is often persistent, and vomitus and feces may contain blood. Both vomitus and stools may have a blue-green color. Weakness, lethargy, headache, restlessness, irritability, tremors, and intermittent convulsions with subsequent depression of the CNS occur. Skin eruptions and kidney and liver damage have also been reported. Because of this, the FDA review panel recommended Category II status for these oral products in 1979.[57] In 1982 another panel recommended that all OTC products containing boric acid for topical use on the mucous membranes of the mouth and throat be condemned.[56] However, in 1983 the FDA reclassified the ingredient as Category I for use as an oral wound cleanser, citing the company's assertions that:

- Many of the references on boron toxicity are related to the use of boric acid misused as antiseptics.
- Reports discussing irritating effects of the molecule actually referred to sodium perborate; properly used sodium perborate monohydrate does not cause these problems.
- A considerable difference of opinion exists regarding the toxicity of boron in humans.
- The FDA admitted that some reports suggest that boron is more toxic in children than adults and that children are more likely to swallow a mouthrinse, the basis for the warnings on the packages.[58]

In allowing boron-containing products to remain on the market, the FDA assumed correct patient use. Approval is based

---

A Pharmacist's Journal

The Stuck Upper Plate

While studying intraoral problems, a student mentioned that he was once a dental corpsman in the armed services. The dentist asked him to help remove a serviceman's upper plate, which was stuck on the patient's palate. With both of them working, they finally managed to loosen and remove the upper plate. As the dentist looked into the patient's mouth, he noticed blisters covering the roof of his mouth. He asked the patient how long he had the blisters. The patient said about 2 weeks, adding that they were painful. The dentist asked what he thought they were, and the patient responded: "I think I know what they are. You see, I don't have time to eat lunch, so before I leave the house in the morning, I take out my upper plate, stick a piece of bologna on top of it, put it in my mouth, and suck on the bologna all day!"

Table 4.2. Representative Oral Mucosal Cleansers

PRODUCT	SELECTED INGREDIENTS/COMMENTS
Amosan Oral Wound Cleanser	Sodium perborate monohydrate (amount unlabeled)
Cank-Aid	Carbamide peroxide 10%, glycerol
Gly-Oxide	Carbamide peroxide 10%, glycerin
Orajel Perioseptic Spot Treatment Oral Cleanser	Carbamide peroxide 15%, anhydrous glycerin
Peroxyl Antiseptic Dental Rinse	Hydrogen peroxide 1.5%
Proxigel	Carbamide peroxide 10%, glycerin

on labeling that states, "Do not swallow; spit out. Do not use under 6 years old; use under 12 only with supervision." Pharmacists must reinforce the usage directions when selling boron-containing products.

Carbamide Peroxide

Carbamide peroxide in anhydrous glycerin breaks down in the mouth to H_2O_2, which separates into water and oxygen. The effervescence of the oxygen cleanses.

The patient places several drops directly on the affected area, allows them to remain in place for 1 minute, then expectorates. The products can be used up to four times daily, after meals and at bedtime. Children under 12 should be supervised; children younger than 2 should not use them.

Hydrogen Peroxide

The cleansing agent of hydrogen peroxide is free oxygen. The approved concentration is 3%, because higher amounts could damage mucosa and cause black, hairy tongue.[33]

Hydrogen peroxide solutions may be formulated as drops or mouthrinse. In either case, the product is applied to the affected area, held for 1 minute, then expectorated. Age restrictions are the same as for carbamide peroxide.

Sodium Bicarbonate

Sodium bicarbonate (baking soda) was also given Category I status by the FDA for use as a gingival wound cleanser.[33] For patients older than 2 years, 1/2 to 1 teaspoonful in 1/2 glass of water can be swished around the mouth for at least 1 minute and then expectorated, up to four times daily. Children under 12 should be supervised.

ORAL MUCOSAL ANALGESICS

Oral mucosal analgesics can provide temporary relief of pain caused by minor irritation or injury of the mouth and gums; sore mouth, sore throat, minor pain; canker sores; minor dental procedures; and minor irritation caused by dentures or orthodontic appliances (Table 4.3).[55] They have a use limit of 1 week, to be communicated by this warning: "If sore mouth symptoms do not improve in 7 days, or if irritation, pain or redness persist or worsen or if swelling, rash or fever develop, see a dentist or doctor."[33] The age cutoff is 2 years. Category I ingredients include benzocaine, phenol, benzyl alcohol, dyclonine, hexylresorcinol, and menthol.[33] Most of the products currently targeted for these problems contain benzocaine. (Oral mucosal analgesics specifically marketed for relief of sore throat are discussed in Chapter 15, The Common Cold.)

Benzocaine in a 5 to 20% concentration applied up to four times daily provides a relief onset within seconds that may last for 5 to 10 minutes. However, it acts on surface cells only, so that deep-seated pain is not relieved. It may be used for patients as young as 4 months.[33]

PART 3: TEETHING PAIN

Teething pain is caused by the pressure of the teeth erupting through the gum surface. Incidentally, the discomfort is not confined to infants and young children; adults also experience teething pain when their third molars ("wisdom teeth") begin their upward migration. Figure 4.3 indicates the ages at which teeth typically come in.

Benzocaine 5 to 20% and phenol are approved by the FDA for infants and children 4 months of age and older.[33,55] The medication should not be applied more than four times daily (or as directed by a dentist or physician).

Table 4.4 lists representative products targeted for teething, although any product with an effective amount of benzocaine would also be helpful in relieving teething pain. Alcohol produces an unpleasant oral sensation, so that products containing it should be avoided. Figure 4.3 presents the ages at which teeth typically come in.

When recommending products such as those listed in Table 4.4, the pharmacist should ascertain whether the child also has fever or nasal congestion. These are not symptoms of teething and may indicate the presence of infection. If fever or nasal congestion are present, the caregiver should contact a physician for proper care. No product should be used for children younger than 4 months[33] (see "Home Remedies for Teething Pain").

Table 4.3. Representative Oral Mucosal Analgesics

PRODUCT	SELECTED INGREDIENTS/COMMENTS
Anbesol Regular Strength Liquid or Gel	Benzocaine 6.4%, phenol 0.5%
Anbesol Maximum Strength Liquid	Benzocaine 20%, alcohol 60%
Benzodent Cream	Benzocaine 20%, eugenol
Orajel Denture	Benzocaine 10%, menthol, methyl salicylate
Orabase-B	Benzocaine 20%; plasticized hydrocarbon gel vehicle adheres to oral mucosa
Orajel Mouth-Aid	Benzocaine 20%, benzalkonium chloride 0.02%, zinc chloride 0.1%, allantoin

PART 4: PROBLEMS AFFECTING THE TEETH

TOOTHACHE

Toothache is a common cause of severe pain.[59] Some patients with toothache visit an emergency room, although many patients first attempt to purchase a nonprescription product.[60] Quite often, patients avoid visiting a dentist until the last minute because of dental phobia and hope that the pharmacist can provide a product that will allow them to further avoid the dentist.

PREVALENCE OF TOOTHACHE

Information on the prevalence of toothache is sparse, although a study of older Floridians revealed that 29% had experienced one or more dental problems.[61] In one study of individuals chosen randomly, 20 to 30% of respondents revealed that they had experienced pain or distress from dental-related pain in the previous 3 months, of which a good proportion could be toothache.[62] Said to be one of the most common causes of severe pain, toothache causes 1 million lost nights of sleep yearly in the United Kingdom.[59]

EPIDEMIOLOGY OF TOOTHACHE

A study of dental patients with pain showed that the average age for dental pain was 54 years.[59] Women in the study visited the clinic at a rate three times that of men.

Toothache is in many cases the result of neglect, and dental phobia (see Chapter 3) is the cause of much dental neglect.[61,62] For instance, 86% of those with toothache would not seek treatment.[63]

ETIOLOGY OF TOOTHACHE

Toothache is a symptom rather than a disease in itself. As such, it can be produced by a wide variety of underlying disorders.

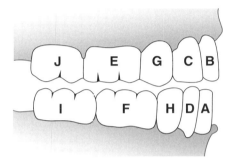

A:	Central incisors (bottom)	6–10 months
B:	Central incisors (top)	8–12 months
C:	Lateral incisors (top)	9–13 months
D:	Lateral incisors (bottom)	10–16 months
E:	First molar (top)	13–19 months
F:	First molar (bottom)	14–18 months
G:	Cuspid (upper)	16–22 months
H:	Cuspid (lower)	17–23 months
I:	Second molar (lower)	23–31 months
J:	Second molar (upper)	25–33 months

Figure 4.3. Teething pain may occur at different locations, depending on which teeth are erupting. This chart illustrates the times of eruptions of the primary ("baby") teeth.

Dental Neglect

Toothache often results from dental neglect, usually the failure to cleanse the teeth properly coupled with improper fluoride supplementation. Because of dental neglect, enamel begins to erode, producing pain when the eroded cavity reaches the dentin. Early complaints include intermittent pain and cold sensitivity. The degree of pain, which varies with the degree of caries progression, is caused by penetration through enamel into the dental pulp.[60] Eventually, it becomes constant and severe.

If pulpitis is caught at the reversible stage, a dentist can restore a damaged tooth.[64] However, if the damage proceeds to irreversible pulpitis, a pulpectomy (root canal) is mandatory. Patients who refuse to undergo the procedure can suffer in-

Table 4.4. Representative Products for Teething Pain

PRODUCT	SELECTED INGREDIENTS
Baby Anbesol	Benzocaine 7.5%, alcohol free
Baby Orajel	Benzocaine 7.5%, alcohol free
Baby Orajel Nighttime Formula	Benzocaine 10%, alcohol free
Orabase Baby	Benzocaine 7.5%, alcohol free

fection and necrosis of the pulp. The resulting abscess causes pain, fever, malaise, and leukocytosis.

A dentist visit is also mandatory for the following conditions[60,65]:

- An abscess
- Caries
- A cracked tooth[65]

All of these cases must be seen immediately by the dentist.

Atypical Odontalgia

Atypical odontalgia (AO), most common in females aged 40 to 60, is characterized as severe, throbbing pain in teeth that are radiologically and clinically normal.[66] While the pain is often present in several oral areas simultaneously, it may be located in only a single maxillary molar or premolar. Referral to a dentist is mandatory.

AO is often associated with emotional problems, hypotensive therapy, and excessive oral hygiene. The pharmacist might suspect AO in female patients with pain described above who also have a history of multiple dental procedures to relieve the pain.

Other Conditions

The necessity for differential diagnosis to rule out conditions that shall not be self treated presents a compelling reason for pharmacists to refer patients with tooth pain. Other conditions that may be responsible for tooth pain include:

- Sinus infection or inflammation may cause continuous dull toothache, with a perception that the tooth feels pushed out. This most often occurs with a maxillary sinus infection, causing pain in the maxillary teeth on the affected side. An x-ray that reveals inflammation of the sinus confirms the diagnosis. The pain worsens with seasonal changes, allergies, or barometric pressure changes—all of which indicate a sinus condition. (In two cases, tooth pain was the sole discomfort or presenting symptom of this condition.[67,68])
- Lymphoma
- Sickle cell disease[69]
- Headache. Migraine causes tooth pain described as dull and throbbing, occurring once or more weekly.[70] Cluster

headache causes toothache in 53% of patients. One important characteristic often seen with cluster headache is a peak frequency of attacks between 4:00 AM and 10:00 AM. Cluster headache pain is one of the few pain syndromes that wakes a person from sleep.

- Temporomandibular joint (TMJ) disorder pain may be indistinguishable from toothache. With TMJ, the pain is referred from trigger points such as certain portions of the masseter muscles.
- Bruxism, also a known cause of pain in the teeth, has been pointed to as a possible explanation of the phenomenon of tooth pain occurring during bereavement.
- Sand trapped between the teeth from eating poorly washed clams or other seafood can cause toothache.[71]
- A galvanic reaction occurring when two different metallic restoration materials such as a silver-chromium nonprecious crown and a silver-mercury amalgam.[60] If they are in adjacent teeth, the pain can be persistent or sharp. If they are in opposition, and only contact each other with speech or eating, the patient will complain of sharp pain.

In one survey, 21% of patients experienced dental pain of unknown origin.[62]

TREATMENT OF TOOTHACHE

Treatment Guidelines

Toothache is a symptom that inevitably requires dentist intervention. Nonprescription products applied topically to the tooth are either of unknown effectiveness or can cause further damage to the root. Internal products may provide

Patient Assessment Algorithm 4.2. Toothache

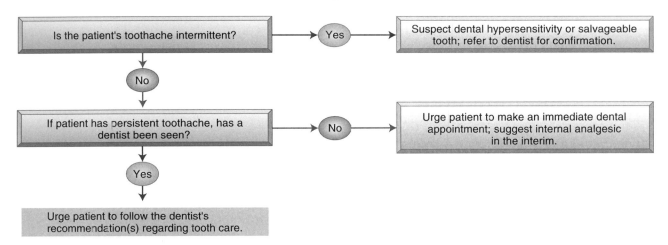

relief while the patient is awaiting the appointment, but will not allow a patient to neglect appropriate dental care. (Patient Assessment Algorithm 4.2 illustrates the steps used in treating the patient with toothache.)

Nonprescription Medications

Currently marketed nonprescription products are labeled for application directly into an open tooth cavity (Table 4.5). These products have two drawbacks, however:

- They contain irritating chemicals such as eugenol or clove oil. They can further irritate nerves that have become exposed through neglect. Exposed dental pulp is very susceptible to irritation caused by placing these chemicals directly into the cavity.
- The chemicals dehydrate dentin. Dehydration is damaging because it increases the permeability of the dentinal tubular contents. Opening dentinal tubules may worsen nerve damage.[55]

Inflammation of the pulp caused by an improperly maintained tooth or a cavity can be divided into two stages, reversible and irreversible. When the nerve damage is still reversible, proper dental care can save the tooth. However, additive irritation or dentinal dehydration caused by eugenol or clove oil can accelerate the process of nerve damage, con-

verting reversible damage to irreversible damage. The tooth has then been rendered nonviable through application of the toothache remedy and must be extracted or subjected to a root canal. Consequently, any agent that irritates or dehydrates dentin is considered unsafe if applied during the reversible stage of pulp disease. (Toothache remedies contain caustic preparations that will burn the oral mucosa, but oral mucosal burns heal rapidly, so the consequences of the burns are usually minimal. The real danger is that of nerve damage to teeth.)

Further, it is irrational to place any substance in a tooth cavity that may occlude the opening through which an abscess may drain allowing fluid and gas to escape.[33] Cotton balls soaked with medication—as supplied in one toothache remedy—are occlusive agents. Occlusion of the cavity in this manner may intensify pain and promote the spread of infection to deeper tissues.

An FDA advisory panel assigned oral pain products was fully aware of the above information, but classified toothache remedies containing eugenol as Category I in the first phase of the OTC product review.[57] In its Phase 2 document, however, the FDA responded to comments about eugenol.[33] The comments reiterated that eugenol damages viable tooth pulp and that consumers might actually place it on teeth with viable pulp or even on open cavities from which fillings have

Table 4.5. Representative Topical Toothache Products	
PRODUCT	SELECTED INGREDIENTS/COMMENTS
Maximum Strength Orajel Liquid	Benzocaine 20%, not proven effective for toothache
Orajel P.M.	Benzocaine 20%, menthol, methyl salicylate, not proven effective for toothache
Orajel Regular Strength	Benzocaine 10%, not proven effective for toothache
Red Cross Toothache Medication	85% eugenol, tweezers, cotton pellets; can be damaging to dental nerves

been lost. In either case, the known irritant activity of eugenol could compromise pulp vitality. In response, the FDA proposed Category III status for eugenol 85 to 87% toothache drops.

If eugenol eventually gains Category I status, it would be labeled with a time cutoff for home use of 7 days and warnings that patients younger than 12 must be supervised and that it must not be used for patients younger than 2. The following procedure should be followed to use products containing eugenol:

1. Rinse the tooth with water to flush out debris.
2. Moisten a cotton ball from the kit with 1 to 2 drops of the product.
3. Using the tweezers in the kit, place the eugenol-soaked cotton pellet into the cavity for 1 minute, then remove. Do not allow the product to contact gums.

Further, if eugenol is finally approved, the FDA will restrict use to teeth with persistent, throbbing pain (indicating irreversible damage of tooth pulp). Labeling should warn against use in teeth with occasional, intermittent pain, since this indicates reversible damage. Thus, if eugenol is ever approved, the only tooth that the pharmacist should permit the patient to self-treat is one damaged so badly that it will have to be extracted or subjected to root canal.

Other toothache remedies contain benzocaine, which is presently Category III for toothache.[33] While it does not irritate or dehydrate teeth like eugenol, there is insufficient data to show any effect when benzocaine is applied directly to dental nerve tissue in the cavity of a tooth. Thus patients using products containing benzocaine are further procrastinating, avoiding the dental care necessary to prevent tooth loss.

The pharmacist has a difficult task when patients with toothache ask for help. S/he must dissuade the patient from use of any topical product for toothache. This includes the use of home remedies such as clove oil, which contains eugenol. Another dangerous home remedy is an aspirin tablet placed next to a painful tooth, which burns the mucosa as it dissolves.[36] (The burn appears as a diffuse white patch of coagulated tissue. Healing usually proceeds quickly after the topical aspirin therapy is discontinued.)

Patients may gain temporary relief from naproxen, ibuprofen, or other nonprescription internal analgesics, but pharmacists must inform patients that an immediate dental appointment is necessary if they have any desire to preserve the viability of the tooth. Should the tooth be beyond repair, an extraction or root canal can be scheduled to ease the pain much more effectively than with the use of topical eugenol or benzocaine.

LOST FILLINGS, LOOSE CROWNS

Pharmacists should refer patients with these problems to the dentist for an emergency appointment. Most dentists are able to work in previous patients when emergency work such

as this is needed. A major review of common dental emergencies does not mention any role for such home dental kits.[60]

Dentemp, a nonprescription product advertised in pharmacy journals, is promoted to provide fast, temporary relief of pain and discomfort, replace lost fillings, and temporarily cement loose caps and crowns. Patients are instructed to mix a packet of zinc oxide powder (2 g) with the contents of a tube of eugenol (1 mL) to make a ball of wetted powder that is placed into the cavity (in the case of a lost filling), or used to cement a loose crown or inlay. While the status of a filling or crown cement was not explored by any FDA panel, the eugenol present in the product could irreversibly damage pulp, converting a salvageable tooth to one requiring extraction. Thus, although the company cautions the patient to see a dentist for permanent work to be performed, it may be too late to save the tooth.

DENTAL HYPERSENSITIVITY

Dental (or dentinal) **hypersensitivity** (a condition in which one or more teeth are exquisitely sensitive to certain triggers such as cold) is a common cause of pain associated with the teeth.[72] A dentist must diagnose hypersensitive teeth to rule out more serious conditions that might require dental work.[55] If nonprescription products are used without dentist diagnosis of dental hypersensitivity, patients may not receive proper restorative care for injured teeth.

PREVALENCE OF DENTAL HYPERSENSITIVITY

Although reliable epidemiologic data are lacking, it appears possible that from 8 to 30% of adults with teeth may experience the condition.[72–74] (The wide variation from 8 to 30% may be the result of the different methods used to diagnose dental hypersensitivity.) Market survey data suggest that 40 million adults are affected, with 10 million chronic sufferers.[75,76]

EPIDEMIOLOGY OF DENTAL HYPERSENSITIVITY

Researchers hypothesize that the incidence of dental hypersensitivity is rising because of the increase in the life span and the rising average age of the United States population.[77] Further, the widely successful push for fluoridation of community water supplies is also a contributory factor. Fluoride has allowed an ever-growing percentage of the population to keep their natural teeth until death. Thus teeth in the United States are asked to perform their various duties and undergo regular cleansing regimens for more years than perhaps at any time in the past.

Age-stratified studies support these explanations for dental hypersensitivity. The age range for dental hypersensitivity is generally 15 to 69, but the most common ages are from 20 to 40, peaking at the end of the third decade.[72,78]

As many as 23.4% of chemical plant workers exposed to acidic or other enamel-etching vapors suffer dental hypersensitivity as an occupational hazard.[72,77]

Dental hypersensitivity affects females to a slightly higher degree than males.[72] The author of one study demonstrating this gender preference related it to the documented more intensive grooming habits of females.[76]

ETIOLOGY OF DENTAL HYPERSENSITIVITY

The etiology of dental hypersensitivity involves the physiology behind the condition, its triggers, and underlying pathology.

The Hydrodynamic Theory

The hydrodynamic theory of dental hypersensitivity has gained widespread acceptance as the primary etiologic mechanism for the disorder.[73,79] This theory flows from several underlying assumptions:

- Each tooth contains dentinal tubules that connect the dentin-enamel junction to the dental pulp (Fig. 4.4).[72] Dentinal tubules are microscopic, each containing a protoplasmic fluid, which can be forced by certain stimuli or triggers to recede from the pulp or move nearer to it.[80–82]
- The tubules are normally occluded on the dental surface, protecting the dental pulp. Pain of dental hypersensitivity begins when the tubules are exposed by erosion (e.g., caused by ingestion of acidic foods or drinks), periodontal therapy, abrasion, or gingival recession (e.g., caused by vigorous brushing and cleansing of the teeth), because **dentin** (a softer layer of tooth substance below dental enamel) has patency directly to the pulp through the dental tubules.
- Various stimuli such as cold, heat, pressure, and hyperosmotic solutions can cause movement of fluid in the tubules. Movement of fluid within the dentinal tubules stimulates mechanoreceptors in the pulpal-dentinal area, perhaps through deformation of odontoblasts that line the periphery of the pulp.[83] Because the pulpal nerve fibers are interwoven with the odontoblasts, the fluid-induced disturbance of the odontoblasts stretches or compresses nerve fibers, causing pain.

The hydrodynamic theory explains how various pain triggers induce dental hypersensitivity.[84–87] Thermal stimuli trigger pain through expansion (e.g., after drinking hot substances) or contraction of the intratubular fluid. Contraction causes greater sensitivity than heat. (Ingestion of cold foods and beverages is the single most common trigger of dental hypersensitivity.[78,85]) An air blast directly on the tooth causes a thermal stimulus, since the air blast from a dental instrument is generally set at 65 to 70°F.[85] The air blast also results in a fluid movement into the space vacated by the evaporated fluid, which is interpreted as pain.[88]

During routine cleaning regimens, the patient touches, scratches, and applies pressure to teeth with brushes, floss, and periodontal aids. Touch, scratch, and pressure induce pain by physically displacing the fluid. Osmotic pressure such as from a strong sugar solution placed in the oral cavity causes a net fluid shift from the tubules into the oral cavity.

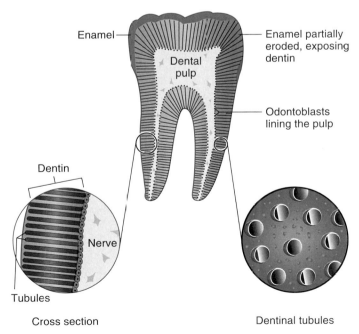

Figure 4.4. The hydrodynamic theory of dentinal hypersensitivity hypothesizes that fluid inside small dentinal tubules moves against odontoblasts lining the dental pulp, causing pain.

Oral Hygiene

Reduced oral hygiene does not appear to contribute to dental hypersensitivity. In fact, the opposite appears true.[85] Teeth with the lowest plaque exhibit the highest sensitivity.[72] Accordingly, canines and premolars, the most thoroughly cleaned teeth, are most often hypersensitive. Likewise, buccal gingiva are most likely to recede as a result of overenthusiastic brushing, and the buccal tooth surfaces are most often hypersensitive.[72,76] Conversely, lingual surfaces are most neglected and the least likely surfaces to exhibit hypersensitivity.

The relationship between vigorous cleaning and hypersensitivity may be caused by the smear layer, a 0.5-micrometer organic film of microcrystalline debris that normally covers dental tubules.[85] The smear layer can be removed by overly aggressive brushing and by ingesting acidic foods and beverages.[72] Removing this film opens the dentinal tubules, causing dental hypersensitivity (as in the hydrodynamic theory).

Dental Procedures

Various dental procedures can cause dental hypersensitivity, perhaps also by disrupting the smear layer. For example, periodontal procedures that expose dentin to the oral environment (e.g., root planing and removal of cementum, plaque, and calculus) can produce an iatrogenic root sensitivity.[79] Postrestoration pain is also a common, but short-term source of discomfort.[85,89]

Miscellaneous Causes

Other causes of dental hypersensitivity include gastroesophageal reflux disease (which increases oral acidity), bruxism, occlusal trauma due to biting, and various kinds of tooth damage such as incomplete fracture and chipped enamel.[72,83] *OTC products are not indicated for dental hypersensitivity caused by actual tooth injury.*

PROGNOSIS OF DENTAL HYPERSENSITIVITY

Usually, pain resulting from dental hypersensitivity only occurs when affected teeth contact pain triggers.[72] This makes it different from persistent toothache, but on the other hand makes it similar to intermittent toothache, which is often continually painful until the tooth is repaired or removed. When it is not caused by actual tooth damage (e.g., chipped enamel), hypersensitivity undergoes spontaneous remission in 20 to 45% of patients in 4 to 8 weeks.[83] Dental hypersensitivity following root planing usually becomes less noticeable within 2 to 3 weeks.

TREATMENT OF DENTAL HYPERSENSITIVITY

Treatment Guidelines

According to the hydrodynamic theory, occlusion of exposed dentinal tubules would help alleviate the condition.[90,91]

Brushing with any toothpaste causes deposition of toothpaste ingredients (e.g., abrasive silica particles) in the tubules.[72,75] This approach has great potential. Poiseuille's law states that if the particles can reduce the radius of a dentinal tubule by 50%, it will reduce fluid flow through that tubule to one-sixteenth of the original value.[85,92,93] (Patient Assessment Algorithm 4.3 illustrates the steps used in treating the patient with dental hypersensitivity.)

Nonprescription Medications

Toothpastes intended for dental hypersensitivity are FDA-regulated nonprescription products and must meet the same standards for safety and efficacy as all nonprescription products (Table 4.6).[75] Thus these products must desensitize teeth to a significantly greater extent than the same toothpaste without the active desensitizing ingredient. Two mechanisms of desensitizing teeth are denaturation of the superficial ends of nerve endings in dentin, or stimulation of dentin formation. Other mechanisms are the crystallization of the inside of the tubules and the formation of a precipitate at the entrance of the tubules.[87]

To use these products properly, patients should brush with a soft-bristle toothbrush, for at least 1 minute twice daily (morning and evening), using about an inch of toothpaste. Patients should contact all areas where teeth are sensitive. Four weeks is the maximum time the patient may use these products without a professional examination. The FDA-labeled age cutoff is 12.[33]

The FDA requires this warning on packages of toothpastes intended for dental hypersensitivity: "Sensitive teeth may indicate a serious problem that may need prompt care by a dentist. See a dentist if the problem persists or worsens." Therefore, if the problem persists for more than 4 weeks or worsens, an appointment with a dental professional is indicated. *Toothpastes for hypersensitive teeth might not contain fluoride; thus, the patient may need to use fluoridated toothpastes at the same time as these are used.*

POTASSIUM NITRATE

Potassium nitrate, hypothesized to act directly on sensory pulpal nerves, is the only approved ingredient for reduction of dental hypersensitivity.[33,75] Once sensory nerve fiber membranes have been depolarized, excess potassium from the toothpaste will prevent repolarization, decreasing pain.[87]

The FDA proposed in 1992 that potassium nitrate can be combined with any safe and effective fluoride in toothpastes formulated for dental hypersensitivity.[94] The fluoride is solely for caries prevention, not for reducing dental hypersensitivity (see "Fluorides").

STRONTIUM CHLORIDE

The only other ingredient once marketed in the United States is strontium chloride. Researchers hypothesize that it undergoes dental calcium-strontium exchange, which forms a crystallized strontium-apatite complex.[75,83] The FDA placed strontium chloride in Category III, although products containing it may still be marketed.

Patient Assessment Algorithm 4.3. Dental Hypersensitivity

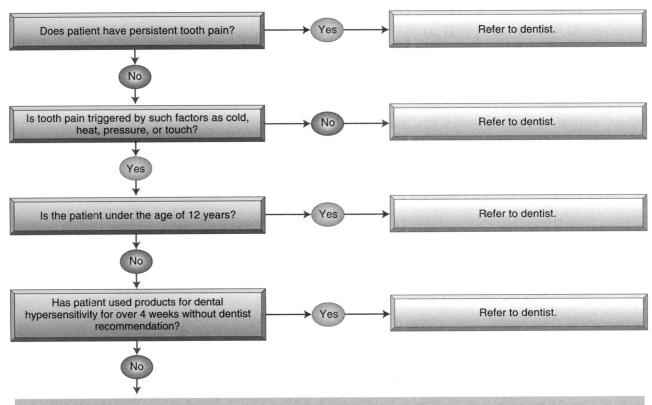

Table 4.6. Representative Toothpastes for Dental Hypersensitivity

PRODUCT	SELECTED INGREDIENTS
Aquafresh Sensitive	Potassium nitrate 5%, 0.15% fluoride from sodium fluoride, hydrated silica
Crest Sensitivity Protection	Potassium nitrate 5%, sodium fluoride 0.15%, hydrated silica
Dental Care Sensitive Formula	Potassium nitrate 5%, sodium fluoride 0.243%, baking soda
Sensodyne Extra Whitening	Potassium nitrate, sodium monofluorophosphate (unlabeled concentrations), hydrated silica
Sensodyne Fresh Mint	Potassium nitrate, sodium monofluorophosphate (unlabeled concentrations), silica
Sensodyne Tartar Control	Potassium nitrate, sodium monofluorophosphate (unlabeled concentrations), silica, tetrapotassium pyrophosphate

FLUORIDES

Desensitization has been attempted unsuccessfully with various fluorides.[83,95] For example, sodium fluoride has excellent dental affinity and may form a tubule-occluding precipitate of insoluble calcium fluoride, but many patients still experience dental hypersensitivity despite widespread use of fluoride-containing dentifrice that permits them to obtain optimal oral concentrations of fluoride.[75] Calcium fluoride may form a crystal, but it is too small to effectively occlude the tubules.

PREVENTION OF DENTAL HYPERSENSITIVITY

The diet may contribute to dental hypersensitivity. Acidic foods and drinks erode dental enamel and open the smear layer.[83,91] *Pharmacists should advise all patients to avoid acidic foods and beverages* such as (from most acidic to least acidic), ginger ale, limes, or lemons and their juices, wine, cranberry sauce, coffee, vinegar, pickles, Coca-Cola, Pepsi-Cola, oranges/juice, plums, cider, grapefruit juice, apples, rhubarb, raspberries, root beer, relish, grapefruit, strawberries, fruit jams/jellies, Orange Crush, peaches, sauerkraut, blueberries, pineapples/juice, cherries, and grapes.[96]

Because oral hygiene also affects dental hypersensitivity, pharmacists should counsel patients about the hazards of overzealous brushing. *Patients prone to dental hypersensitivity should use the softest bristle brush available* to help prevent recession and hypersensitivity and brush no more than twice daily. When brushing, patients should avoid excessive force and never use toothpastes with a high abrasive nature (even though they may promise more whitening power).[72] (Note that individuals usually brush harder on the side opposite the hand holding the brush: right-handers brush the left side more aggressively, left handers brush the right side more aggressively.[72,76]) The patient should also avoid brushing teeth immediately after eating the acidic foods identified above, since dental tubules are more likely to be open at those times. A wait of an hour or so should be sufficient to allow the smear layer to reestablish itself.

PART 5: PROBLEMS AFFECTING THE LIPS

HERPES SIMPLEX LABIALIS

An infectious disease, herpes simplex labialis is characterized by fever blisters on the lips, and occasionally inside the mouth (Fig. 4.5).

Herpes simplex labialis, also called "cold sore" and "fever blister," usually occurs on the outer surface of the lips along the area known as the vermilion border or around or inside of the nostrils.[97] When they occur inside the mouth, they affect nonmovable parts of the mouth such as the gums and roof of the mouth. Patients often experience a prodrome, which consists of various paresthesias such as tightness, soreness, burning, or swelling, before the first blisters form.[98] When the blisters rupture, they often grow together to form a large exudative lesion. Also, the skin can crack and separate and become painful during eating, drinking, or talking. Eventually scabs form, and complete healing occurs in 10 to 14 days without scarring.[98]

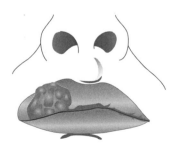

Figure 4.5. The cold sore (herpes simplex labialis) is a viral lesion that often occurs along the outer surface of the lips, or around or inside the nostrils.

PREVALENCE OF HERPES SIMPLEX LABIALIS

At least 70% of children show evidence of past herpes simplex virus (HSV) type 1 infection, by age 14.[99] In a study of fourth-year college students, 46% had a history of HSV-1.[100] HSV type 2, commonly associated with genital herpes, may also be responsible for oral lesions, just as HSV type 1 may be responsible for genital lesions, both caused by oral-genital sexual practices.[97,101]

EPIDEMIOLOGY OF HERPES SIMPLEX LABIALIS

Differences in infectivity in subsections of the population reflect different behaviors and circumstances (e.g., having children in day care as opposed to being childless, sharing a musical instrument in the band room, dating many people) rather than any inherent immunity to the virus. In one examination of children in day care, twice as many males as females were infected.[101] The percentage of the population infected increased with age, as expected, since it is an infectious disease from which one cannot be cured. The number of blacks and whites affected is approximately equal.[101]

ETIOLOGY OF HERPES SIMPLEX LABIALIS

Herpes simplex labialis is usually caused by HSV type 1, which has no other host but man.[98]

An intact oral epithelium is the best defense against HSV infection.[97] When the virus contacts injured epithelium, it invades nerves innervating the area and migrates to sensory ganglia (e.g., trigeminal nerve ganglia), where it establishes latency for the life of the individual.[98] Affected individuals can transfer the virus to **fomites** (inanimate objects that can carry an infectious agent to other people when they handle or touch it) or directly to others, both when symptomatic and asymptomatic. (Fomites include anything that contacts lesions or carries saliva such as glasses or drinking straws.[98]) Direct transfer includes mouth-to-mouth contact, in the transfer of HSV type 1, or oral-genital sex, in the case of HSV type 2. As many as 10% of adults shed HSV type 1 in saliva periodically.[97] *Infected individuals must never kiss others while lesions are present.* Infected children must be taught never to share drinking glasses or straws. (Fomite transfer is probably the cause of the high transmission rates—as high as 84%—observed in day care.[99,102] *Affected individuals also must avoid touching the lesions, as they may inadvertently transfer the virus to other people, or to objects that others might touch.* Further, HSV is able to survive for several hours on surfaces.

The incubation period of HSV type 1 following inoculation averages 7 days.[97] Once an individual is infected, attacks can potentially continue throughout life, although the incidence drops after the age of 35. Recurrence rates range from 16 to 45%.[97] While some individuals never have another recurrence, 6% suffer another attack within 1 week, and 13% within 2 weeks. HSV type 1 cannot be eliminated, since it remains dormant between attacks, usually in the trigeminal nerve ganglia. *To prevent the virus from activating, patients should avoid certain stimuli, including sunlight, tanning booths, emotional stress or excitement, fatigue, chilling, and windburn.*[97,103] Since an increase in body temperature is an important cause, the patient should wear sunscreens and large hats to reduce exposure to sunlight. Other possible triggers include fever, illness, injury, the menstrual cycle, and dental work.[98] When lesions appear in the absence of a specific trigger, some researchers propose that the patient suffered transient immunodepression.[97,104]

TREATMENT OF HERPES SIMPLEX LABIALIS

Treatment Guidelines

The prescription ingredient acyclovir, which is quite effective in treating HSV, was once considered for nonprescription sale. Concerns about the development of viral resistance have so far caused its rejection by the FDA.

Ingredients such as ether and salicylic acid, used in some products sold for treating herpes simplex labialis, have not yet been proven safe and effective for use in fever blisters.

Tannic acid, also found in some products promoted for fever blisters, has received a great deal of FDA attention. In 1978, the FDA review panel for OTC skin protectants ex-

amined its use in sprays, jellies, and solutions applied to severe burns.[105] Its use has occasionally resulted in toxic hepatitis within 36 hours and death from central liver necrosis from 80 to 130 hours later. The 1978 report also mentioned that it is used in burns because of its astringent effect. It precipitates protein, having little action on intact skin. But when applied to abraded skin, it precipitates a protein-tannate film that serves as a mechanical cover. This report placed it in Category II because of documented hepatotoxicity and obsolete indications in burn therapy.

Subsequently, a 1982 report from the FDA panel on external analgesics described the use of tannic acid for treating fever blisters.[103] The report stressed that the protein-tannate film it produces may encourage bacterial growth beneath the protein-tannate crust. The FDA tentatively decided that application to a small area would be safe, but that efficacy data was lacking, resulting in a Category III assignment. In 1983, the FDA followed up the 1978 report by affirming the Category II status for burns; the FDA also stated that the film or crust formed over abraded tissue does provide a suitable medium under which bacterial growth may flourish.[106]

In 1990, the FDA revisited the use of tannic acid as an astringent in fever blister products.[107,108] In particular, the FDA noted that the usual site of fever blisters is at the junction of the mucous membrane, and the primary herpetic infection in nonimmune persons manifests itself by vesicles on the mucous membranes of the mouth. The FDA expressed concern about absorption through the mucous membranes, as well as oral in-

Table 4.7. Representative Products for Herpes Simplex Labialis

PRODUCT	SELECTED INGREDIENTS/COMMENTS
Blistex	Phenol 0.5%, camphor 0.5%, allantoin 1%, menthol 0.6%
Campho-Phenique Cold Sore Gel	Phenol 4.7%, camphor 10.8%
Camphor Spirit	Camphor (concentration unlabeled, but excessive; extremely hazardous if ingested); also contains 84% alcohol
Carmex	Menthol, camphor, alum, salicylic acid (unlabeled concentrations), phenol; salicylic acid may produce damage to lips; alum not proven safe or effective for this use
ChapStick Medicated	Petrolatum 41%, camphor 0.6%, menthol 0.5%, phenol (concentration unlabeled)
Herpecin-L	Padimate-O, allantoin; efficacy of a sunscreen in fever blister protection unproven (concentrations unlabeled)
Lactinex Tablets or Granules	*Lactobacillus acidophilus* and *Lactobacillus bulgaricus*; unproven efficacy for herpes simplex
Lysine Oral Tablets	Unproven efficacy for herpes simplex
Orajel CoverMed	Dyclonine HCl 1%, allantoin 0.5%
SensoGARD Gel	Benzocaine 20%
Tanac No Sting Liquid	Benzocaine 10%
Viractin Cream	Tetracaine 2%
Zilactin	Benzyl alcohol 10%

Table 4.8. Representative Products for Chapped Lips

PRODUCT	SELECTED INGREDIENTS/COMMENTS
Blistex Regular Lip Balm	Padimate O 6.6%, oxybenzone 2.5%, dimethicone 2%
ChapStick Lip Balm	Petrolatum 44%, padimate O 0.1%, lanolin
Vaseline Lip Therapy	White petrolatum

gestion that may occur when the product is applied in proximity to the mouth. The FDA noted that because of the necessity for frequent applications of medication, oral ingestion could result in toxic levels of intake.

Further, the FDA in 1990 questioned the use of astringents in fever blisters—in particular whether lesions should be dried out or kept moist. When astringents dry the area, fissuring can result, which renders the cracked lesion more susceptible to secondary bacterial infection, can delay healing, and usually increases discomfort. In fact, astringents may fractionate the herpes simplex virus, causing the emergence of resistant strains. Accordingly, the FDA assigned tannic acid a Category III rating for safety in fever blister products. Most major brands have been reformulated to remove tannic acid, but older boxes and some generic products may still contain it—these products should not be sold.

Health-food stores and magazines tout the effectiveness of internally ingested lysine for fever blisters. Similarly, people have used systemic antidiarrheals containing lactobacillus in an attempt to help deal with fever blisters. The FDA has reviewed data on lysine and lactobacillus and concluded that there is no evidence to establish their efficacy in the treatment of fever blisters.[109–111] Patients should be advised that no internal product is effective for fever blisters.

Nonprescription Medications

Safe and effective nonprescription interventions currently available include products containing external analgesics-anesthetics (e.g., benzocaine, benzyl alcohol, camphor, dibucaine, diphenhydramine, dyclonine, juniper tar, lidocaine, menthol, phenol, pramoxine, resorcinol, tetracaine) and pro-

FOCUS ON...

WARNING: SALICYLIC ACID POTENTIALLY HARMFUL

Carmex, which contains salicylic acid (the amount unspecified on the label) is labeled as being helpful for cold sores, fever blisters, and chapped lips. Because of the salicylic acid, however, Carmex could initiate a harmful chain of events.

Salicylic acid commonly is used to eat away corns, calluses, and warts. Salicylic acid eats away the outermost layer of the skin, the stratum corneum, a protective layer of dead skin cells. While this process may be safe on external skin, it can be dangerous on the lips, because the stratum corneum of the lips is thin (even absent in some individuals). The lips do not react as external skin and are much more prone to suffer keratolytic damage. Anecdotal accounts describe lip peeling following use of Carmex. In 1.8 to 3% concentrations, salicylic acid can cause keratolysis in 7 to 10 days; in higher concentrations it can cause keratolysis in 2 to 3 days.[112]

The scenario for lip damage should be obvious: If Carmex applied for a minor case of chapped lips causes peeling, the patient might unknowingly use more product. Since Carmex also contains menthol, phenol, and camphor, it could anesthetize the discomfort caused as the acid eats the outer skin surfaces away. Clearly, removing the outer layer of the skin when treating a cold sore or fever blister would not be beneficial.

The manufacturer claims that the salicylic acid concentration is "way below 1%," but cannot be revealed since it is a trade secret.[113] The manufacturer also claims that the FDA does not require concentrations to be on the label "in this country." (The FDA has stated that all ingredients listed as active ingredients on the label must have the concentration listed clearly on the label.[114]) Until the product formulation is changed to include only ingredients that are proven safe and efficacious, prudent pharmacists would be well-advised not to sell this product.

tectants such as allantoin, calamine, petrolatum, zinc oxide, and cocoa butter (Table 4.7). Protectants help soften the skin to prevent cracking and relieve dryness. Note that Carmex, which contains salicylic acid, could be harmful (see "Warning: Salicylic Acid Potentially Harmful").

PREVENTION OF HERPES SIMPLEX LABIALIS

For prevention of attacks of herpes simplex labialis through avoidance of triggering factors, see Etiology of Herpes Simplex Labialis. Some products contain sunscreens to be applied to the lips in fever blister prevention. However, there is no evidence to demonstrate that topically applied sunscreens prevent the occurrence of ultraviolet light-induced herpes labialis.[32,107]

CHAPPED LIPS

Several lip balms are available to soothe chapped, dry, and cracking lips, essentially a skin protectant action. Skin protectants such as petrolatum (e.g., Vaseline Lip Therapy) or allantoin, found in several lip products as listed in Table 4.8, are safe and effective.[106] Lip products containing sunscreens to prevent sun-induced lip damage are discussed in Chapter 33, Sun-Induced Skin Damage.

See "Warning: Salicylic Acid Potentially Harmful."

SUMMARY

Oral problems cause significant discomfort for patients. Xerostomia (dry mouth), which produces significant difficulty with mastication and can lead to caries and intraoral tissue degeneration, may be helped with use of saliva substitutes.

RAUs (canker sores), a condition of uncertain etiology, result in significant pain for as long as 2 weeks but resolve without scarring. While RAUs are present, pharmacists may recommend such helpful products as oral mucosal cleansing agents and oral mucosal analgesics.

Teething is extremely uncomfortable for a baby and often results in sleepless nights. The pain caused by erupting teeth can be alleviated by topical anesthetic agents.

Toothache is a problem often seen by the pharmacist. Too often, the patient goal is immediate relief, without seeing a dentist. While the pharmacist may recommend systemic analgesic agents, no topical product is safe. Patients with toothache must be urged to obtain an immediate appointment with a dentist to discover the reason for the pain.

Dental hypersensitivity may have serious or benign causes. Serious causes must be ruled out by a dentist before the patient can freely use nonprescription medications such as potassium nitrate–containing toothpastes.

Herpes simplex labialis is a viral condition that results from an initial penetration of tissue by the virus. As it cannot be cured, pharmacist advice must include avoidance of triggers that allow the virus to lose dormancy such as exposure to the sun or tanning booths (UV light). Once the virus has manifested, treatment includes external analgesics-anesthetics and protectants.

AT THE COUNTER

 A middle-aged female patient asks for a product for dental pain.

Interview/Patient Assessment

When the pharmacist questions her about the duration of pain, she says that she has had sensitivity to cold in several teeth for 3 or 4 years. Her dentist says she has sensitive teeth and she should ask for a product to help it.

Pharmacist's Analysis

1. Do this patient's gender and age provide any clue to the cause of her dental discomfort?
2. What would the pharmacist's action be if she had not seen a dentist?
3. What should the pharmacist recommend for her dental pain?

The patient's age and gender signal dental hypersensitivity. If she had not previously seen a dentist, she would need to be referred for evaluation. However, she has previously been screened by a dental professional and given a diagnosis of dental hypersensitivity.

Patient Counseling

The pharmacist is free to recommend any of several products containing potassium nitrate, which is safe and effective for this usage. The pharmacist should cover all of the usage guidelines prior to sale to ensure that they are clearly understood.

 A patient in his early 20s asks the pharmacist for something for a canker sore.

Interview/Patient Assessment

The pharmacist asks how long it has been present, and the patient states that he began to notice it about 1 month ago. The patient denies use of any medications, but admits to usage of smokeless tobacco. The patient pulls out the lower lip to show the lesion inside the lip to the pharmacist. It has notched margins and appears to penetrate the tissue deeply, with a necrotic center.

Pharmacist's Analysis

1. Why should the pharmacist suspect that the lesion is not a canker sore?
2. What is the significance of the patient's history of smokeless tobacco use?
3. Should the pharmacist recommend a nonprescription product?

The patient cannot treat an intraoral lesion that exceeds 1 week in duration. This duration of this patient's lesion, coupled with the history of smokeless tobacco, indicates the possibility of oral carcinoma. Further, the lesion does not resemble a canker sore in appearance.

Patient Counseling

The patient must be referred to a physician for full evaluation.

References

1. Anon. Dry mouth and functions of saliva. Practitioner 234: 605, 1990.
2. Herrera JL. Saliva: Its role in health and disease. J Clin Gastroenterol 10:569, 1988.
3. Glass BJ. Drug-induced xerostomia as a cause of glossodynia. Ear Nose Throat J 68:776, 1989.
4. Aagaard A, et al. Comparison between new saliva stimulants in patients with dry mouth: A placebo-controlled double-blind crossover study. J Oral Pathol Med 21:376, 1992.
5. Korsten MA, et al. Chronic xerostomia increases esophageal acid exposure and is associated with esophageal injury. Am J Med 90:701, 1991.
6. Navazesh M, et al. Clinical criteria for the diagnosis of salivary gland hypofunction. J Dent Res 71:1363, 1992.
7. Sreebny LM. Recognition and treatment of salivary induced conditions. Int Dent J 39:197, 1989.
8. Crockett DN. Xerostomia: The missing diagnosis? Aust Dent J 38:114, 1993.
9. Butt GM. Drug-induced xerostomia. J Can Dent Assoc 57:391, 1991.
10. Björnström M, et al. Comparison between saliva stimulants and saliva substitutes in patients with symptoms related to dry mouth. Swed Dent J 14:153, 1990.
11. Sreebny LM, Valdini A. Xerostomia. Part I: Relationship to other oral symptoms and salivary gland hypofunction. Oral Surg Oral Med Oral Pathol 66:451, 1988.
12. McDonald E, Marino C. Dry mouth: Diagnosing and treating its multiple causes. Geriatrics 46:61, 1991.
13. Sreebny LM, et al. Xerostomia. Part II: Relationship to nonoral symptoms, drugs and diseases. Oral Surg Oral Med Oral Pathol 68:419, 1989.
14. Navazesh M. Xerostomia in the aged. Dent Clin North Am 33:75, 1989.
15. Papas AS. Caries prevalence in xerostomic individuals. J Can Dent Assoc 59:171, 1993.
16. Sciubba JJ, Mandel ID. Sjogren's syndrome. NY State Dent J 58:39, 1992.
17. Kusler Dl, Rambur BA. Treatment for radiation-induced xerostomia. Cancer Nurs 15:191, 1992.
18. Vissink A, et al. The causes and consequences of hyposalivation. Ear Nose Throat J 67:166, 1988.
19. Risheim H, Arbeberg P. Salivary stimulation by chewing gum and lozenges in rheumatic patients with xerostomia. Scand J Dent Res 101:40, 1993.
20. Anon. Causes of dry mouth. Practitioner 234:610, 1990.
21. Enwonwu CO. Ascorbate status and xerostomia. Med Hypotheses 39:53, 1991.
22. Olsson H, Axéll T. Objective and subjective efficacy of saliva substitutes containing mucin and carboxymethylcellulose. Scand J Dent Res 99:316, 1991.
23. Nederfors T, et al. Oral mucosal friction and subjective perception of dry mouth in relation to salivary secretion. Scand J Dent Res 101:44, 1993.
24. Persson RE, et al. Differences in salivary flow rates in elderly subjects using xerostomic medications. Oral Surg Oral Med Oral Pathol 72:42, 1991.
25. Rhodus NL. The association of xerostomia and inadequate intake in older adults. J Am Diet Assoc 90:1688, 1990.
26. Van Dis ML. What to do about dry mouth. J Am Dent Assoc 122:100, 1991.
27. Joensuu H, et al. Pilocarpine and carbacholine in treatment of radiation-induced xerostomia. Radiother Oncol 26:33, 1993.
28. Anon. Management of dry mouth and halitosis. Practitioner 234:618, 1990.
29. Odusola F. Chewing gum as aid in treatment of hyposalivation. NY State Dent J 57:28, 1991.
30. Brundage S. Use of lozenges may cause dry mouth. Postgrad Med 85:35, 1989.
31. Anon. (Editorial). Xerostomia. Lancet 1:884, 1989.
32. Jacob RFK. Management of xerostomia in the irradiated patient. Clin Plast Surg 20:507, 1993.
33. Fed Reg 56:48301, 1991.
34. Drinnan AJ, Fischman SL. Controversies in oral medicine. Dent Clin North Am 34:159, 1990.
35. Conklin RJ, Blasberg B. Common inflammatory diseases of the mouth. Int J Dermatol 30:323, 1991.
36. Levin Sl, Johns ME. Lesions of the oral mucous membranes. Otolaryngol Clin North Am 19:87, 1986.
37. Colvard M, Kuo P. Managing aphthous ulcers: Laser treatment applied. J Am Dent Assoc 122:51, 1991.
38. Rosenstein DI, et al. Treating recurrent aphthous ulcers in patients with AIDS. J Am Dent Assoc 122:65, 1991.
39. Porter SR, Scully C. Aphthous stomatitis—an overview of aetiopathogenesis and management. Clin Exp Dermatol 16:235, 1991.
40. Brown RS, et al. Combination immunosuppressant and topical steroid therapy for treatment of recurrent major aphthae. Oral Surg Oral Med Oral Pathol 69:42, 1990.
41. Phelan JA, et al. Major-aphthous-like ulcers in patients with AIDS. Oral Surg Oral Med Oral Pathol 71:68, 1991.
42. Scully C, Porter SR. Recurrent aphthous stomatitis: Current concepts of etiology, pathogenesis and management. J Oral Pathol Med 18:21, 1989.
43. Meiller TF, et al. Effect of an antimicrobial mouthrinse on recurrent aphthous ulcerations. Oral Surg Oral Med Oral Pathol 72:425, 1991.
44. Grinspan D, et al. Treatment of aphthae with thalidomide. J Am Acad Dermatol 20:1060, 1989.
45. Anon. Treating canker sores. ASDC J Dent Child 58:90, 1991.
46. Pedersen A. Are recurrent oral aphthous ulcers of viral etiology? Med Hypotheses 36:206, 1991.
47. Nolan A, et al. Recurrent aphthous ulceration: Vitamin B1, B2, and B6 status and response to replacement therapy. J Oral Pathol Med 20:389, 1991.
48. Rogers III RS, Hutton KP. Screening for haematinic deficiencies in patients with recurrent aphthous stomatitis. Australas J Dermatol 27:98, 1986.
49. Palopoli J, Waxman J. Recurrent aphthous stomatitis and vitamin B12 deficiency. South Med J 83:475, 1990.
50. Nolan A, et al. Recurrent aphthous ulceration and food sensitivity. J Oral Pathol Med 20:473, 1991.
51. Endre L. Recurrent aphthous ulceration with zinc deficiency and cellular immune deficiency. Oral Surg Oral Med Oral Pathol 72:559, 1991.
52. Grant SCD, et al. Aphthous ulceration as a presentation of *Giardia lamblia* infection. Br Dent J 166:457, 1989.
53. Dundar S. Recurrent aphthous stomatitis (Letter). Australas J Dermatol 28:143, 1987.
54. Pedersen A. Psychologic stress and recurrent aphthous ulceration. J Oral Pathol Med 18:119, 1989.
55. Fed Reg 47:22711, 1982.
56. Fed Reg 47:22760, 1982.

57. Fed Reg 44:63269, 1979.

58. Fed Reg 48:33983, 1983.

59. Goss AN. Dental patients in a general pain clinic. Oral Surg Oral Med Oral Pathol 65:663, 1988.

60. Klokkevold P. Common dental emergencies. Emerg Med Clin North Am 7:29, 1989.

61. Gilbert GH, Heft MW, Duncan RP. Oral signs, symptoms, and behaviors in older Floridians. J Public Health Dent 53:151, 1993.

62. Bailit HL. The prevalence of dental pain and anxiety. NY State Dent J 53:27, 1987.

63. Reisine ST. The effects of pain and oral health on the quality of life. Commun Dent Health 5:63, 1988.

64. Comer RW, et al. Dental emergencies. Postgrad Med 85:63, 1989.

65. Reeh ES, El Deeb ME. Referred pain of muscular origin resembling endodontic involvement. Oral Surg Oral Med Oral Pathol 71:223, 1991.

66. Reik L. Atypical odontalgia: A localized form of atypical face pain. Headache 24:222, 1984.

67. Kant KS. Pain referred to teeth as the sole discomfort in undiagnosed mediastinal lymphoma: Report of case. J Am Dent Assoc 118:587, 1989.

68. Bavitz JB, Patterson DW, Sorensen S. Non-Hodgkin's lymphoma disguised as odontogenic pain. J Am Dent Assoc 123:99, 1992.

69. O'Rourke C, Mitropoulos C. Orofacial pain in patients with sickle cell disease. Br Dent J 169:130, 1990.

70. Graff-Radford S. Headache problems that can present as toothache. Dent Clin North Am 35:155, 1991.

71. Gallin DM. "The clam syndrome," dental pain of unusual etiology. NY State Dent J 57:41, 1991.

72. Addy M. Etiology and clinical implications of dentine hypersensitivity. Dent Clin North Am 34:503, 1990.

73. Rosenthal MW. Historic review of the management of tooth hypersensitivity. Dent Clin North Am 34:403, 1990.

74. Muzzin KB, Johnson R. Effects of potassium oxalate on dentin hypersensitivity in vivo. J Periodontol 60:151, 1989.

75. Kanapka JA. Over-the-counter dentifrices in the treatment of tooth hypersensitivity. Dent Clin North Am 34:545, 1990.

76. Addy M, et al. Dentine hypersensitivity: The distribution of recession, sensitivity and plaque. J Dent 15:242, 1987.

77. Guo-hua L, Morimoto M. Magnesium sulphate as a new desensitizing agent. J Oral Rehab 18:363, 1991.

78. Clark GE, Troulos ES. Designing hypersensitivity clinical studies. Dent Clin North Am 34:531, 1990.

79. Markowitz K, Kim S. Hypersensitive teeth. Dent Clin North Am 34:491, 1990.

80. Sena FJ. Dentinal permeability in assessing therapeutic agents. Dent Clin North Am 34:475, 1990.

81. Yoshiyama M. Transmission electron microscopic characterization of hypersensitive human radicular dentin. J Dent Res 69:1293, 1990.

82. Absi EG, et al. Dentine hypersensitivity. J Clin Periodontol 16:190, 1989.

83. Trowbridge HO, Silver DR. A review of current approaches to in-office management of tooth hypersensitivity. Dent Clin North Am 34:561, 1990.

84. Curro FA. Tooth hypersensitivity in the spectrum of pain. Dent Clin North Am 34:429, 1990.

85. Pashley DH. Mechanisms of dentin sensitivity. Dent Clin North Am 34:449, 1990.

86. Kleinberg I, et al. Methods of measuring tooth hypersensitivity. Dent Clin North Am 34:515, 1990.

87. Reinhart TC, et al. The effectiveness of a patient-applied tooth desensitizing gel. J Clin Periodontol 17:123, 1990.

88. Närhi M. The neurophysiology of the teeth. Dent Clin North Am 34:439, 1990.

89. Borgmeijer PJ, et al. The prevalence of postoperative sensitivity in teeth restored with Class II composite resin potentials. ASDC J Dent Child 58:378, 1991.

90. Addy M, Mostafa P. Dentine hypersensitivity. II. Effects produced by the uptake in vitro of toothpastes onto dentine. J Oral Rehab 16:35, 1989.

91. Cuenin MF, et al. An in vivo study of dentin sensitivity: The relation of dentin sensitivity and the patency of dentin tubules. J Periodontol 62:668, 1991.

92. Addy A, Mostafa P. Dentine hypersensitivity. I. Effects produced by the uptake in vitro of metal ions, fluoride and formaldehyde onto dentine. J Oral Rehab 15:575, 1988.

93. Kerns DG, et al. Dentinal tubule occlusion and root hypersensitivity. J Periodontol 62:421, 1991.

94. Fed Reg 57:20114, 1992.

95. McFall WT Jr., Hamrick SW. Clinical effectiveness of a dentifrice containing fluoride and a citrate buffer system for treatment of dentinal sensitivity. J Periodontol 58:701, 1987.

96. Clark DC, et al. The influence of frequent ingestion of acids in the diet on treatment for dentin sensitivity. J Can Dent Assoc 56:1101, 1990.

97. Scully C. Orofacial herpes simplex infections: Current concepts in the epidemiology, pathogenesis, and treatment, and disorders in which the virus may be implicated. Oral Surg Oral Med Oral Path 68:701, 1989.

98. Blondeau JM. Herpes simplex virus infection: What to look for. What to do! J Can Dent Assoc 56:785, 1990.

99. Schmitt DL. Herpes simplex type 1 infections in group day care. Pediatr Infect Dis J 10:729, 1991.

100. Gibson JJ, et al. A cross-sectional study of herpes simplex virus types 1 and 2 in college students: occurrence and determinants of infection. J Infect Dis 162:306, 1990.

101. McKenna JG, et al. Cold sores and safer sex (Letter). Lancet 338:632, 1991.

102. Kuzushima K, et al. Clinical manifestations of primary herpes simplex virus type 1 infection in a closed community. Pediatrics 87:152, 1991.

103. Fed Reg 47:39417, 1982.

104. Rosenstein DI, Chiodo GT. Recurrent herpes simplex virus and the acceleration of the wasting syndrome: Report of a case. J Am Dent Assoc 43(Suppl):43S, 1989.

105. Fed Reg 43:34627, 1978.

106. Fed Reg 48:6819, 1983.

107. Fed Reg 55:3361, 1990.

108. Fed Reg 55:3370, 1990.

109. Fed Reg 47:501, 1982.

110. Fed Reg 50:25155, 1985.

111. Fed Reg 57:29165, 1992.

112. Fed Reg 45:65609, 1980.

113. Telephone call, Carma Laboratories (unnamed company personnel): 11/15/93.

114. Telephone call, Food and Drug Administration (Michael Benson): 11/15/93.

Gastric Distress

Patients with gastric distress present with symptoms of conditions ranging from gastroesophageal reflux disease (GERD) to peptic ulcer. Nonprescription products are not indicated for treatment of peptic ulcer, but the pharmacist can recommend nonprescription products to treat minor gastric distress symptoms such as **heartburn** (a burning feeling that the patient feels in the area of the heart, usually caused by gastroesophageal reflux), sour stomach, acid indigestion, and upset stomach.[1] Quite often, these are symptoms of gastroesophageal reflux disease, but they may also reflect nonreflux gastric distress such as **gastritis** (inflammation of the lining of the stomach).

Patients also experience stomach distress when they have eaten too much food in combination with alcohol. Hangover also causes unpleasant gastric effects.

To review the anatomy of the gastrointestinal tract, see Figure 5.1.

PART 1: GASTROESOPHAGEAL REFLUX DISEASE (GERD) AND NONREFLUX GASTRIC DISTRESS

GASTROESOPHAGEAL REFLUX DISEASE (GERD)

GERD, popularly referred to as heartburn, is a **retrograde** (backward, against normal flow) movement of stomach contents into the esophagus.[2,3] This abnormal **orad** (toward the oral cavity) movement of contents would be vomiting if the stomach contents exited the mouth, but in GERD they do not. The underlying cause is usually a problem with the integrity of the lower esophageal sphincter (LES), which normally acts to keep stomach contents in the stomach[4] (Fig. 5.2).

PREVALENCE OF GERD

Most authors assert that GERD is common, but few quote hard data, partly because of difficulty in defining the disease.[5] As many as 7% of people experience daily episodes of reflux.[6,7] An estimated 10 to 20% of the population of the United States experiences GERD that is serious enough to require regular ingestion of medications.[8,9] Perhaps as many as 50% of the population experiences scattered episodes.[9] Because of either the pressure of the gravid uterus or hormonal causes, as many as 50% of pregnant females suffer from GERD.[10]

EPIDEMIOLOGY OF GERD

When a pharmacist suspects that a patient's symptoms are the result of esophageal reflux, the pharmacist should assess the patient for predisposing factors (such as those discussed below) and urge him or her to modify these factors when possible.

Obesity

Obesity is perhaps the only predisposing factor for GERD that can be voluntarily modified to reduce risk, although objective supporting data are scanty at best.[11,12] Theoretically, obesity increases intraabdominal pressure, which may overwhelm the tonicity of the LES, allowing reflux.[13] Other theories advanced to explain the correlation of weight with reflux are that obese persons have increased esophageal transit and subnormal LES pressures.[14] (Of course, clothing that fits tightly around the waist should be avoided in patients of all weight categories, since it could produce reflux in patients through the same mechanism.)

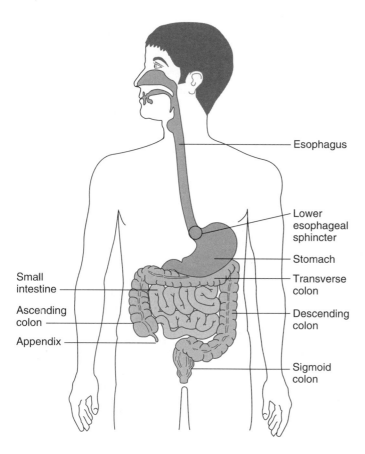

Figure 5.1. The anatomy of the gastrointestinal tract.

Pregnancy

Pregnancy is a significant risk factor for GERD. As many as 50 to 80% of females have complained of GERD-type symptoms during the later stages of pregnancy, especially after the fourth month.[10,15–17] GERD during pregnancy frequently has been attributed to pressure of the gravid uterus on the stomach; however, this supposition was disproven in a novel study in which **tense ascites** (ascites in which the abdomen is highly distended) was used as a model of pseudopregnancy.[18] The adult men in the study did not suffer a higher incidence of reflux, despite high intraabdominal pressures caused by the ascites. Some research suggests that hormonal changes may also directly lower the pressure of the LES.[19]

Hiatal Hernia

Physiologically and clinically, hiatal hernia is a more severe condition than GERD. In this condition the upper portion of the stomach (including the LES) herniates or slides upward through the diaphragm into the thoracic cavity.[20,21] Not all patients with hiatal hernia exhibit GERD, and most patients with GERD do not have hiatal hernia, but it is nonetheless clear that the two can be related.[22] In some patients the hiatal hernia may inhibit closure of the LES or act as a trap for gastric fluids, allowing gastric fluids to bathe esophageal mucosa when the patient is supine.[8] Surgical repair of the hiatal hernia may be necessary in those patients to eradicate GERD.

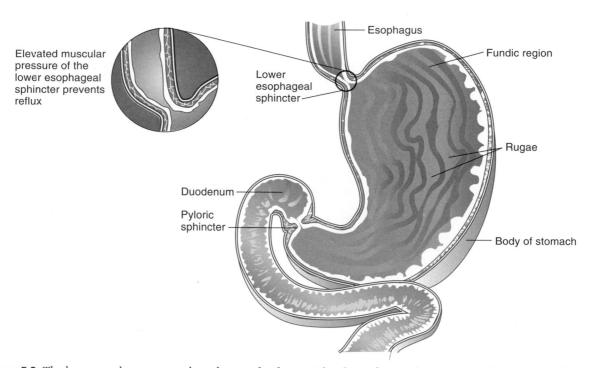

Figure 5.2. The lower esophagus, stomach, and upper duodenum. The elevated muscular pressure of the lower esophageal sphincter prevents reflux.

ETIOLOGY OF GERD

The etiology of GERD can be studied from two aspects:

- Aggressive factors, which promote the development of GERD
- Defensive factors, which help prevent GERD

See Figure 5.3 for a summary of these factors.

Aggressive Factors (Promote GERD)

Physiologists and others who study the pathogenesis of GERD find it helpful to explore the factors that increase the likelihood of tissue damage when the condition occurs—the aggressive factors. The aggressive factors (and defensive factors—see below) are similar to those for peptic ulcer. However, since damage occurs primarily in the esophagus, the balancing of aggressive and defensive factors is not identical to that occurring in peptic ulcer.

Acid, a primary aggressive factor, injures esophageal tissues through denaturation of protein.[10] However, **pepsin** (the major digestive enzyme for protein found in the gastric fluids) produces **reflux esophagitis** (inflammation of the esophagus) through digestion of mucosal protein and undoubtedly contributes to the symptoms of GERD.[23] Bile acids and pancreatic enzymes worsen the damage by causing proteolysis when they are present in the **refluxate** (refluxed material).[10,23,24] Bile acids and pancreatic enzymes can enter the stomach if patients suffer from **duodenogastric reflux** (backward movement of materials from the duodenum to the stomach), and if patients have undergone gastric surgery.[8,25] The role of bile acids and pancreatic enzymes in GERD is underscored by the fact that some patients experience esophagitis despite achlorhydria (e.g., following total gastrectomy).[6]

Defensive Factors (Prevent GERD)

Fortunately, many people never experience reflux because the factors that prevent its occurrence (known as defensive factors) are dynamic and highly active.

LOWER ESOPHAGEAL SPHINCTER

While the pathogenesis of GERD is thought to be multifactorial, the anatomic area primarily important in prevention of the condition is the sphincter that separates the stomach from the esophagus.[8] This band of circular smooth muscle, known as the lower esophageal sphincter (LES), under normal conditions acts as a barrier to keep gastric contents in the stomach.[26] Basal LES pressure varies between individuals, as well as in the same individual during a typical day, but for healthy patients its tone is sufficient to prevent reflux.[13] The act of swallowing triggers waves of esophageal peristalsis, which appropriately relaxes LES tone so the bolus of food may be admitted to the stomach.[3,7,20] The LES then returns to a resting tone that should be sufficient to prevent reflux under most conditions.[26]

ESOPHAGEAL CLEARING

Reflux of gastric contents may not cause injury to esophageal epithelium if refluxate is promptly returned to the stomach.[27] The duration of exposure is determined by the process known as esophageal clearance.[23] (Fig. 5.4 illustrates normal esophageal acid clearance.) Clearance to the stomach is aided by gravity and may take several minutes as esophageal peristalsis occurs.[8,23] Research has demonstrated that as many as 40 to 50% of GERD patients suffer from lower esophageal dysmotility.[6,26]

SALIVA

While esophageal clearing acts to clear the esophagus of injurious chemicals, bicarbonate in saliva acts as a natural antacid to return esophageal pH to normal.[24,28] Without saliva the residual acid that remains following peristalsis could still cause damage and discomfort. Thus esophageal peristalsis and adequate saliva work together as defensive factors against tissue damage.[8,26] Understandably, patients with xerostomia experience heightened tissue damage caused by reflux.[7,23] (See Chapter 4, Oral Problems.)

TISSUE RESISTANCE

Inherent resistance of esophageal tissues to injury by acid is an additional line of defense against reflux-induced injury.[13]

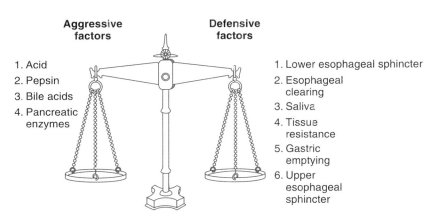

Aggressive factors

1. Acid
2. Pepsin
3. Bile acids
4. Pancreatic enzymes

Defensive factors

1. Lower esophageal sphincter
2. Esophageal clearing
3. Saliva
4. Tissue resistance
5. Gastric emptying
6. Upper esophageal sphincter

Figure 5.3. Gastroesophageal reflux is worsened by the aggressive factors, while the patient's defensive factors work to protect against gastroesophageal reflux disease (GERD).

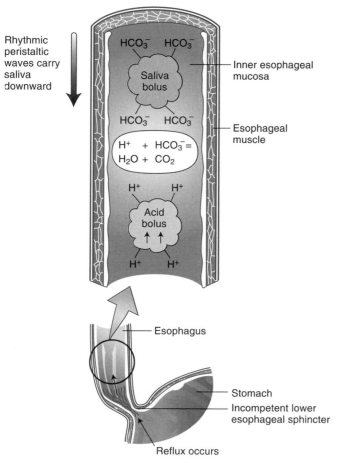

Rhythmic peristaltic waves carry saliva downward

HCO_3^- HCO_3^-

Saliva bolus

Inner esophageal mucosa

HCO_3^- HCO_3^-

Esophageal muscle

$H^+ + HCO_3^- = H_2O + CO_2$

H^+ H^+

Acid bolus

H^+ H^+

Esophagus

Stomach

Incompetent lower esophageal sphincter

Reflux occurs

Figure 5.4. When reflux occurs, the bicarbonate in saliva acts to neutralize refluxed acids.

Esophageal epithelium consists of stratified squamous epithelium with a surface coating of mucus, which helps prevent chemical or mechanical injury.[8,26] Esophageal epithelium also regenerates rapidly to repair injury when it does occur.[26] However, these protective mechanisms may be weakened by age, nutrition, or other factors.[8]

GASTRIC EMPTYING

Injurious refluxate is composed of gastric contents; thus the more rapidly gastric contents move from the stomach to the intestinal tract, the less likely they are to reflux.[29] In fact, delayed gastric emptying of solid meals has been shown to contribute to higher rates of esophagitis.[30] Gastric emptying is delayed through ingestion of meals that are high in fats, or when patients are in a supine position.[26] Research also suggests that the high incidence of GERD in pregnancy is the result of hampered motility caused by increased levels of circulating female sex hormones.[15,16,19]

UPPER ESOPHAGEAL SPHINCTER

The upper esophageal sphincter (UES), an area of elevated muscle tone near the top of the esophagus, may or may not prevent reflux.[25] The UES does prevent esophagopharyngeal reflux and subsequent aspiration, however.[31] Research found a decreased UES pressure in reflux patients.[25]

MANIFESTATIONS OF GERD

General Considerations

Patients suffering from GERD typically can recite numerous complaints that the condition causes. Should a pharmacist be unsure from the symptoms that a specific patient has reflux, physician referral for confirmation is advisable. While the physician can choose several tests to confirm GERD, they generally are time-consuming, invasive, painful and/or expensive. Tests for GERD include endoscopy, barium swallow, and the Bernstein test. In the latter, 0.1N hydrochloric acid and normal saline are dripped alternately into the esophageal area; GERD is confirmed if symptoms begin when the acid is passed through the nasogastric tube and then remit when normal saline is infused.

Rather than using tests, physicians often suggest that a "careful history is the most useful diagnostic tool . . ."[23] Likewise, full knowledge of symptomatology can guide the pharmacist in tentative recognition of GERD to allow initial therapy with a nonprescription product, with physician referral if symptoms persist.[28]

Regurgitation is **pathognomonic** (leading to a sure diagnosis) for GERD and points the way to recognition of the condition. Patients may be asked if they experience **waterbrash phenomenon** (fluids rushing into the mouth), a reflex hypersalivation induced by acid reflux into the esophagus.[6,7,26,28] Many of the signs and symptoms of the condition do not result until the refluxate produces damage.[28]

Some individuals do not perceive actual regurgitation. For them, the initial symptom is often chest pain induced by esophageal injury, which may or may not be recognized as heartburn. (Heartburn is said to be the classic and most common symptom of GERD.[9,32])

The individual with chest pain is understandably concerned about the presence of coronary artery disease.[1] In fact, impulses in afferent sensory nerves from the heart and from the esophagus travel via the same nerve roots. Patients describe GERD pain as tight, gripping, or viselike and often state that it radiates to the left arm, shoulder, or neck. It may have occurred in relation to exercise and may be relieved by nitroglycerin.

Since the quality, location, radiation, and character of the pain cannot serve as criteria for differentiating GERD from myocardial infarction (MI), pharmacists must consider that individuals who suspect they have indigestion may be suffering an MI.[3] This confusion also highlights the importance of recognizing risk factors for both conditions in the individual being counseled. If an MI is suspected, hospital procedures can confirm either diagnosis.[13] Of course, both disorders may coexist, further complicating the clinical picture.[32] In fact, GERD can precipitate anginal pain.[6]

Patients may also describe swallowing problems such as **dysphagia** (difficulty in swallowing) or **odynophagia** (pain when swallowing) as symptoms of GERD.[32] These can be caused by damage to the esophageal muscle resulting from acute inflammation. Continued exposure to refluxate also may cause bleeding resulting from esophageal ulceration, scarring, and stricture.[17,32] It is axiomatic that any patient presenting to the pharmacist with a history of bleeding from the esophagus, stomach, lungs, or any other source must be referred immediately to rule out such potentially devastating problems as esophageal cancer.

Other regional problems are common. For instance, the throat feels tight and may be chronically sore.[28,32,33] In addition, nonspecific chronic pharyngitis may be accompanied by chronic laryngitis, which the patient describes as hoarseness.[9,34] These problems may be so severe that the patient experiences choking spells.[35]

Esophageal damage may also result in "globus hystericus."[36] In this condition patients interpret damaged esophageal tissue as an object in the throat and may resort to frequent dry swallowing or throat clearing to move the nonexistent obstruction from the esophagus to the stomach.[35] Because of its etiology, this maneuver will be unsuccessful. Patients also may relate a history of environmental stress and varying degrees of anxiety. Antacid regimens resolve the problem for many patients.[9,32,35]

Swallowing ceases during sleep. For this reason refluxate does not remain in the esophagus, but is often aspirated from the pharyngeal areas into the airways. Even small amounts of gastric acid aspirated into the tracheobronchial tree can cause pulmonary complications. Cough is the most minor of these (resulting from the chemical tracheobronchitis), but aspirated refluxate can also produce aspiration pneumonia, **bronchiectasis** (chronic dilation of bronchi), abscess, wheezing, laryngospasm, **hemoptysis** (spitting up of blood from the lungs), **atelectasis** (pulmonary collapse), globus hystericus, and asthmatic symptoms.[37–39] If the refluxate also contains vegetable particles from a nighttime snack, granulomatous interstitial pulmonary fibrosis may also occur.[3]

Determinants of Severity of GERD

Most patients with GERD suffer mild symptoms at sporadic intervals.[40] They usually do not need medical assistance. A smaller group of patients seek help for minor symptoms, but do not suffer complications. The most severely affected group is a small one that may require medical treatment for such complications as stricture or bleeding.

The volume of refluxate and its contents are primary determinants of the severity of the condition and of a particular episode. More damaging episodes occur when the refluxate contains bile acids and pancreatic enzymes.[8,23]

The length of time that the refluxate is in contact with esophageal tissue is also important. Most patients reflexively swallow when reflux occurs. The rapid removal of the refluxate coupled with the buffering capacity of saliva act to prevent tissue damage. Patients who experience reflux when asleep often awaken briefly to swallow. However, should patients not be awakened by the episodes, the swallowing reflex will not occur. Thus refluxate is allowed a prolonged time in which to damage esophageal mucosa.[26] For this reason

prescription and nonprescription sleeping aids are counterproductive for patients with GERD.

COMPLICATIONS OF GERD

If GERD is not appropriately addressed, serious problems can result. Death is uncommon, but has occurred with acid aspiration resulting from pulmonary injury.[37] Further, GERD may be a causal or contributory factor in sudden infant death syndrome.[23,41]

Esophageal scarring can lead to stricture and mild problems such as dysphagia, as previously described.[7] The development of Barrett's esophagus, however, is a more severe esophageal complication.[42] In this condition the normal squamous mucosa of the esophagus is replaced by **columnar epithelium** (tall cells with an arrangement resembling numerous aligned columns), perhaps induced by long-term reflux. While its exact etiology is controversial, Barrett's esophagus is found in 12% of reflux patients and at least 33% of those with esophagitis.[7,28] Patients with Barrett's esophagus suffer more severe disease and experience a higher incidence of esophageal stricture than patients without this condition.[24] Also, the abnormal tissue apparently has a greater propensity to develop into adenocarcinoma, and at the time of diagnosis of Barrett's esophagus at least 10% of patients already have adenocarcinoma.[24,28,43] One-third of all esophageal cancers arise from Barrett's esophagus.

The potential sequelae arising from stricture and from the development of Barrett's esophagus constitute extremely potent arguments for preventing and treating GERD.

TREATMENT OF GERD

Treatment of GERD is divided into three levels[29]:

1. The vast majority of patients are helped by conservative, first-level therapy, involving lifestyle modifications and the use of nonprescription medications.
2. Patients for whom these measures fail to provide relief proceed to second-level therapy, involving prescription medications (e.g., omeprazole or cisapride).
3. Patients not helped by prescription interventions may undergo surgery.

As pharmacists are usually involved at only the first level of therapy for reflux, the other two will not be discussed. However, patients should be referred for more advanced treatment if conservative therapy does not produce remission of symptoms fairly rapidly.

See "Treatment of Gastroesophageal Reflux and Nonreflux Gastric Distress."

PREVENTION OF GERD

For many patients, GERD can be prevented by dietary and lifestyle modifications. Pharmacists should discuss these preventive measures with GERD patients.

81

Dietary Modification

Dietary modification consists of modifying the timing and volume of meals and avoiding certain foods and drinks.

Gastric distension worsens reflux, since the pressure caused by a distended stomach may overcome the LES tone by serving as a potent stimulus for LES relaxation.[2,43] Thus GERD sufferers are advised to eat a greater number of smaller meals rather than the typical three large meals.[43] Further, the last meal should be light and fully completed at least 3 to 5 hours prior to bedtime.[23,28] GERD patients also may find it helpful to eat more slowly to minimize the output of gastric acids.[44]

High-fat foods impair lower esophageal sphincter function and should be avoided in favor of more protein-rich foods.[26] *Foods that irritate the esophagus, perhaps because of inherent acidity and/or hyperosmolarity, include citrus juices (e.g., orange, grapefruit), soft drinks (with or without caffeine), beer, liquor, milk, and tomato products or foods using spicy tomato bases (e.g., pizza).*[23,26,43] Pepper also is a direct irritant.[26] Even hot liquids have been implicated in the problem, but this may be because liquids in general reflux more readily than solid foods.[32,35]

Although carminatives (e.g., peppermint, spearmint) are thought to soothe the stomach after a meal, they induce reflux by impairing sphincter function and should be avoided.[6,26] Other nonfood candies such as chewing gum, hard candy, breath fresheners, lozenges, and cough drops should be avoided in reflux patients since they tend to increase stomach acids, but do not buffer the acid as actual food does.[35]

Chocolate, which is high in fats and contains methylxanthines, also impairs sphincter function.[3,26,35] (Methylxanthines relax smooth muscle.[43]) Xanthines are also found in tea, coffee, and caffeinated soft drinks. Since caffeine itself is a xanthine, the GERD sufferer would be well advised to avoid all foods, drinks, medications, and other products that contain it. Caffeine also stimulates the stomach to increase acid output.[44]

Carbonated beverages in general are unwise for the GERD patient. Following ingestion of 10 to 12 ounces of a typical carbonated drink, normal bodily movement can produce gas from residual carbonation. If sufficient gas is produced, it can be ejected through the LES, carrying damaging refluxate with it. Burping to relieve the pressure buildup can also induce GERD. Carbonated beverages containing caffeine act through numerous mechanisms to produce GERD.

Tobacco

Nicotine, which directly lowers LES pressure, promotes duodenogastric reflux, increases the frequency of GERD episodes, impairs esophageal clearance, and increases bile acids in gastric contents, should be avoided completely.[26,43] This prohibition includes smokeless tobacco and passive smoke exposure.[11] In one study 92% of GERD patients were found to be smokers.[35]

Alcohol

Alcohol increases secretion of stomach acids, lowers LES pressure, and may have a direct irritant effect.[24,28] It also inhibits awakening during the night through its sedative effect, which may worsen damage caused by nocturnal reflux.

Postural Interventions

Preventing nocturnal reflux can require major postural intervention. When patients are recumbent, gravity no longer facilitates gastric retention.[45] Therefore, *GERD patients have long been advised to raise the head of the bed with wooden or concrete blocks or bricks approximately 6 to 10 inches high.*[3,11] An angle of 30° must be attained for effectiveness.[23] Should this be impractical or unacceptable to the patient or spouse/partner, the patient might gain relief by elevating the head and upper body with two or more pillows, although this is less effective than elevation of the whole bed.[28,29] An alternative is sleeping on a foam wedge, which has been found to be equivalent to bed elevation.[46]

Patients should also avoid slumping, bending at the waist, kneeling, and wearing constricting garments.[10,26,27] All of these actions place excessive pressure on gastric contents and promote reflux.[35]

NONREFLUX GASTRIC DISTRESS

While many episodes of gastric distress are related to GERD, not all are. Some gastric distress is simply caused by eating foods that do not agree with the individual or overeating. In these cases the problem may be gastric irritation or gastric hyperacidity, causing simple gastritis (Fig. 5.5). Identification of reflux is relatively simple because of the partial reflux of gastric contents. Conversely, proper recognition of

---

FOCUS ON...

MEDICATIONS AND REFLUX

Medications that cause xerostomia act to worsen episodes of reflux by preventing salivary buffering of refluxate. For a discussion of these medications, see Chapter 4.

Medications that directly decrease LES tone include theophylline, caffeine, calcium channel blockers, β-adrenergic antagonists, progesterone derivatives, α-adrenergic antagonists, dopamine, diazepam, morphine, and anticholinergics.[26,35,43] Also, because of their acidity, vitamin C and aspirin also should be avoided.[35]

Patients who are taking a reflux-inducing medication should be referred to a physician for a benefit-to-risk analysis to determine whether to reduce the dose of the offending medication, discontinue the medication, or simply accept the inevitability of reflux.

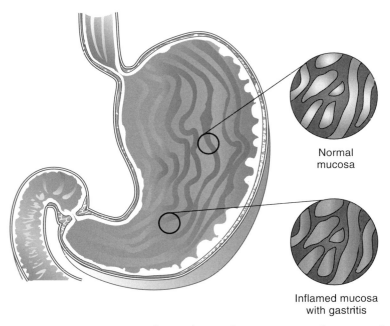

Normal
mucosa

Inflamed mucosa
with gastritis

Figure 5.5. Gastritis is a condition wherein the gastric mucosa becomes inflamed.

more vague complaints is based only on the patients' verbal descriptions of their problems. In any case, as long as the pharmacist is satisfied that a given patient's complaint is a minor one, nonprescription products may also be recommended for them.

See "Treatment of Gastroesophageal Reflux and Nonreflux Gastric Distress."

GASTROESOPHAGEAL REFLUX DISEASE (GERD) AND NONREFLUX GASTRIC DISTRESS

See above for prevalence, epidemiology, manifestations, complications, and prevention of GERD and for background on nonreflux gastric distress.

TREATMENT OF GASTROESOPHAGEAL REFLUX AND NONREFLUX GASTRIC DISTRESS

Treatment Guidelines

Pharmacists can recommend either antacids or histamine-2 blocking agents or antagonists (H2-blockers) for minor conditions of gastric distress (see Patient Assessment Algorithms 5.1 and 5.2). FDA-approved symptoms include "heartburn, sour stomach, acid indigestion, and upset stomach associated with these symptoms."[47,48]

To ensure that patients do not use nonprescription antacids and H2-blockers to treat a chronic condition requiring physician evaluation, the label on these nonprescrip-

tion products should advise that they cannot be used longer than a 2-week period without physician approval. *The 2-week time limit begins with the onset of the gastric distress, not when a patient approaches a pharmacist for a recommendation.* Thus pharmacists must ask patients how long they have experienced discomfort. Patients who have suffered for more than 14 days must be referred since the nonprescription product is contraindicated.

Nonprescription antacids and H2-blockers should also be reserved for minor problems such as heartburn, sour stomach, acid indigestion, and upset stomach. If patients experience any serious symptoms in addition to gastric distress—such as continuous vomiting, diarrhea, extreme discomfort or gastrointestinal pain, vomiting of blood (perhaps resembling coffee grounds in the vomitus), fever, or passage of blood in the stool—which can indicate an active ulcer, a physician must be consulted.[48] Extreme symptoms such as severe or persistent pain, vomiting, anorexia, weight loss, or dysphagia require urgent diagnosis to rule out cancer.[49]

Nonprescription Medications

NONPRESCRIPTION ANTACIDS

Virtually all physicians who discuss GERD therapy stress the usefulness of antacids, although some advise limiting their use to mild to moderate cases.[3,6,7,10,23,24,35,40,43] Antacids decrease acidic damage from reflux, reduce the number of reflux episodes and quantity of refluxate, and may increase LES tone.[23] The FDA does not allow the wording "gastroesophageal reflux disease" on nonprescription antacid labels, but heartburn, the commonly accepted synonym for reflux,

Patient Assessment Algorithm 5.1. Gastric Distress

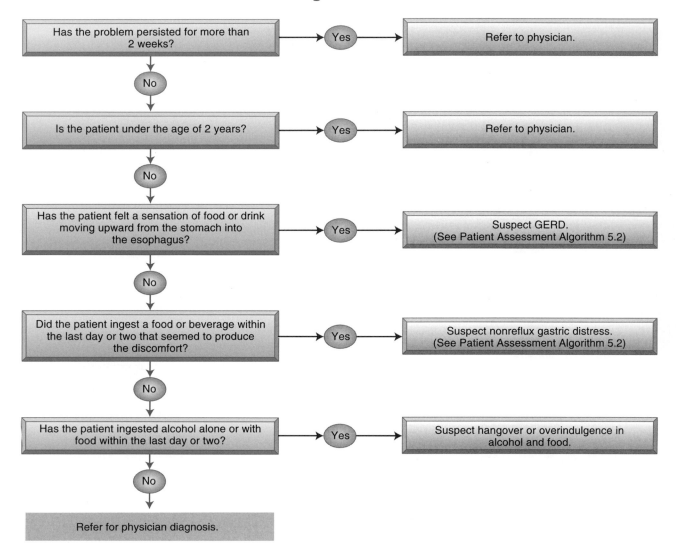

is permitted.[50] The major FDA lay publication also describes GERD fully and recommends antacids for the problem.[44]

Several antacid ingredients are safe and effective for self-use, including certain salts of magnesium, aluminum, and calcium.[47] The adverse effects of some ingredients are more troubling than others, but in any case therapy is empirical. If a patient tries one product but dislikes the flavor or experiences adverse reactions, he may try another nonprescription antacid, as long as the 2-week time limit on self-treatment has not yet been exceeded.

Other ingredients may be added to antacids. For instance, simethicone is sometimes included as an antiflatulent. (See Chapter 7, Intestinal Gas Discomfort: Bloating and Flatulence.) Also, alginates are sometimes included to help alleviate gastroesophageal reflux.

Antacid products must not be given to patients younger than 2. (In one case a hospitalized 17-day-old infant given Gaviscon suffered aluminum toxicity, possibly because citric acid in the formula enhanced aluminum absorption.[51])

Antacid products must be labeled with a drug interaction precaution, but it is a vague statement about "any prescription drugs"[52] (see "Drug Interactions").

Ingredients in Nonprescription Antacids

Sodium Bicarbonate. The approved dose of sodium bicarbonate (commonly called baking soda) as an antacid is 200 mEq (under the age of 60) or 100 mEq (60 or older). While it is potent and rapid acting, its effect abates quickly, making it unsuitable for long-term relief.[48] Sodium bicarbonate can raise the pH of the gastric contents so much that the body reacts by producing more acid, a phenomenon known as acid rebound.[53] Sodium bicarbonate is soluble in body fluids, and its ready absorption can increase the patient's sodium load.

🔵 For this reason *sodium bicarbonate is not to be recommended for patients on sodium-restricted diets.* Packages for products containing more than 5 mEq of sodium per maximum recommended daily dose must carry this warning:

Patient Assessment Algorithm 5.2. Gastroesophageal Reflux Disease and Nonreflux Gastric Distress

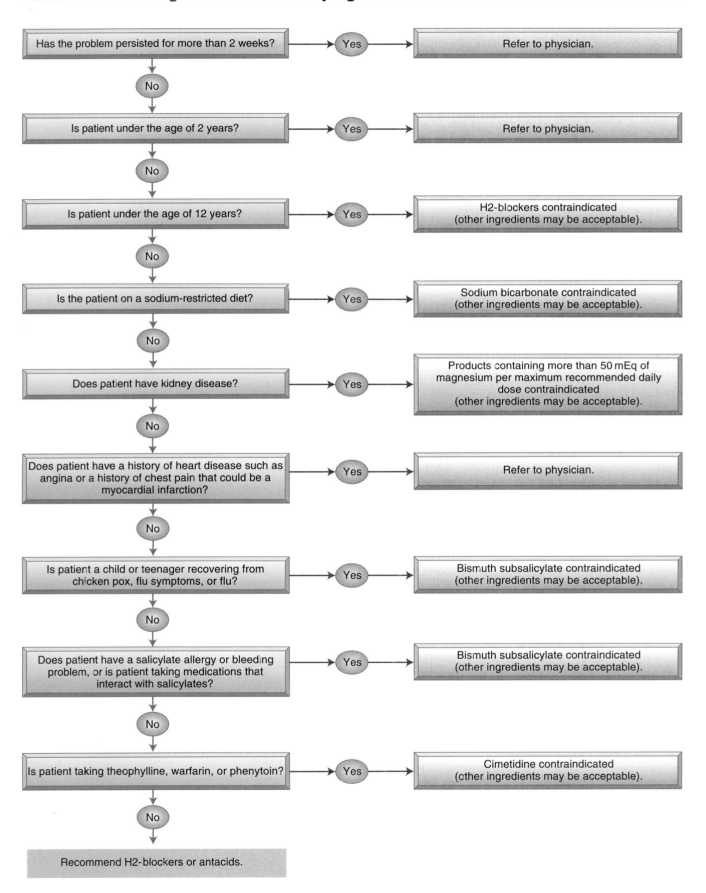

"Do not use this product except under the advice and supervision of a physician if you are on a sodium-restricted diet."[54] For patients taking diuretics, pregnant patients, and patients with a tendency to fluid overload, sodium bicarbonate should be recommended cautiously.

Sodium bicarbonate can cause **systemic alkalosis** (an alkaline shift of the body's normal pH balance).[53] It is also a known contributor to milk-alkali syndrome, in which the patient suffers simultaneously from systemic alkalosis, hypercalcemia, and renal failure. The syndrome has been associated with ingestion of sodium bicarbonate and milk.[53]

Ingesting sodium bicarbonate after a large meal can cause excess carbon dioxide, resulting in gastric distension and even stomach-wall perforation.[55] The risk of perforation is enhanced if the product is effervescent. (Residual food remaining after repair of a perforation can result in abscesses several years later.[56]) In an incident on national news, a man ingested a bowl of homemade chili, two martinis, and a glass of wine.[57] When he awoke with indigestion, he placed a spoonful of baking soda in a glass of water and drank it. The patient, who claimed that the baking soda caused a nearly fatal gastric explosion, required six surgeries to recover from the incident. The manufacturer of the baking soda denied responsibility. The patient's attempts to force the product from the market failed. In light of its drawbacks, the use of sodium bicarbonate as an antacid is considered obsolete by many clinicians.

Sodium bicarbonate is a primary component of two products labeled for acid indigestion with headache (Table 5.1).

Bromo-Seltzer, which combines sodium bicarbonate and citric acid (both of which combine to form sodium citrate in solution) with acetaminophen, and Alka-Seltzer, which combines sodium bicarbonate and citric acid with aspirin. In solution these become sodium citrate and sodium acetylsalicylate. Aspirin has well-known adverse effects on the gastric mucosa, so its use in a product labeled for gastritis is puzzling (see "Combination Products").

Calcium Carbonate. The most potent antacid ingredient, calcium carbonate, is also rapid acting, but with a more prolonged action than sodium bicarbonate (Table 5.2).[53] Unfortunately, because of its relatively high potency, calcium carbonate may also cause rebound and milk-alkali syndrome.[58,59] The latter is of importance because calcium carbonate supplies calcium and produces alkalosis. Since the use of calcium carbonate is far more common than sodium bicarbonate, *pharmacists must be aware that calcium carbonate can cause rebound and milk-alkali syndrome when recommending calcium carbonate products.* Symptoms of the milk-alkali syndrome include hypercalcemia, alkalosis, irritability, headache, vertigo, nausea, vomiting, weakness, and myalgia. Neurologic changes and renal dysfunction may also occur. In one case report four patients with mild, asymptomatic renal failure ingested nonprescription antacids containing calcium in 4- to 8-g doses.[60] All four became severely hypercalcemic, but did recover with hospitalization and proper treatment. Overuse in patients with normal renal function can also result

Table 5.1. Representative Antacids Containing Sodium Bicarbonate

PRODUCT	SELECTED INGREDIENTS/COMMENTS
Original Alka-Seltzer	Sodium bicarbonate 1916 mg, citric acid 1000 mg, aspirin 325 mg (an effervescent tablet that forms sodium citrate in water)
Bromo-Seltzer	Per ¾ capful: sodium bicarbonate 2781 mg, citric acid 2224 mg, acetaminophen 325 mg (a powder that forms sodium citrate when dissolved)

Table 5.2. Representative Calcium Carbonate Single-Entity Antacids

PRODUCT	SELECTED INGREDIENTS
Alka-Mints Tablets	Calcium carbonate 850 mg
Childrens' Mylanta Suspension	Per 5 mL: calcium carbonate 400 mg
Chooz Gum	Calcium carbonate 500 mg
Titralac Tablets	Calcium carbonate 420 mg
Tums Tablets	Calcium carbonate 500 mg
Tums E-X Tablets Extra Strength	Calcium carbonate 750 mg
Tums Ultra Tablets	Calcium carbonate 1000 mg

in carbonate kidney stones or hypercalcemia, with symptoms such as nausea and vomiting, polyuria, and epigastric pain.[61,62] Constipation may occur with normal doses.

Magnesium Salts. Magnesium-containing antacids are less potent than sodium bicarbonate or calcium carbonate. Within the group itself, the hydroxide salt has the highest potency.

The magnesium salts cause osmotic diarrhea in as many as 4 to 76% of patients.[63] (This characteristic of magnesium is used to advantage in certain laxatives.) Patients who overuse these products could suffer electrolyte imbalance.

Magnesium antacid ingredients generally are not absorbed; any small amounts absorbed are cleared rapidly renally. However, *in renal failure patients, hypermagnesemia can occur rapidly.* (Symptoms of hypermagnesemia include hypotension, nausea, vomiting, muscle paralysis, respiratory depression, depressed reflexes, and coma.) As an example, a 62-year-old man admitted to the hospital for resection of a squamous cell carcinoma of the tongue was prescribed 30 mL of Maalox alternating with 30 mL of Mylanta every 2 hours.[64] Over the next several days, he developed diarrhea, dehydration, hypotension with a blood pressure of 86/50 mm Hg, oliguria, mental confusion, combativeness, and a marked decrease in deep tendon reflexes. On discontinuation of antacids and fluid supplementation, his serum magnesium returned from a high of 5.5 mg% to a normal value of 2.1 mg%. This high dose prescribed by a physician highlights the importance of pharmacists showing patients the maximum doses listed on the bottles.

Kidney stones may also result from the use of magnesium salts. Products containing more than 50 mEq of Mg per maximum recommended daily dose must have this warning: "Do not use this product except under the advice and supervision of a physician if you have kidney disease."

Magnesium-containing antacids given to a low-birth-weight infant resulted in intestinal perforation, underlining the prohibition against antacid use under the age of 2. The infant suffered hypermagnesemia, hypocalcemia, and fecaliths in the peritoneal cavity (which were presumed to be magnesium bezoars).[65]

Magnesium hydroxide is the single, active ingredient in the products listed in Table 5.3.

Aluminum Salts. Aluminum salts have the lowest neutralizing capacity of all of the antacids. In addition, they have a number of significant disadvantages. *Aluminum salts are constipating, and repeated doses may cause intestinal obstruction in elderly patients.*[66]

Aluminum salts (other than aluminum phosphate) bind with dietary phosphate, which can be used to advantage in a patient with hyperphosphatemia secondary to renal failure. In these patients aluminum phosphate can be fecally excreted.[67] In a normal patient, however, this effect could lead to hypophosphatemia with symptoms of anorexia, weakness, and malaise, culminating in death.[68] The loss of phosphate, coupled with aluminum-induced loss of calcium and fluoride, can weaken bone and lead to osteomalacia or osteoporosis, perhaps causing fracture of bones.[69] (Symptoms of osteomalacia include bone pain, malaise, and muscular weakness.[70]) The problem is also seen with magnesium-aluminum combinations.[70,71] Chronic use may lead to accumulation of aluminum, especially in patients with chronic renal failure.[72,73] Aluminum has been linked to Alzheimer's senile dementia; although the FDA ruled in 1984 that the data supporting this association were weak, nonprescription sales of aluminum-containing antacids are still permitted.[62,67]

Representative products containing aluminum as a single-entity antacid ingredient are listed in Table 5.4.

Magaldrate. Magaldrate, the active ingredient in Riopan, is a chemical combination of aluminum and magnesium hydroxides and sulfates, with both the advantages and disadvantages of each. The regular-strength suspension con-

Table 5.3. Representative Single-Entity Products Containing Magnesium	
PRODUCT	SELECTED INGREDIENTS
Phillips MOM Tablets	Magnesium hydroxide 311 mg
Phillips MOM Suspension	Per 5 mL: magnesium hydroxide 400 mg

Table 5.4. Representative Single-Entity Products Containing Aluminum	
PRODUCT	SELECTED INGREDIENTS/COMMENTS
Amphojel Tablets	Aluminum hydroxide as dried gel 600 mg
ALternaGEL Suspension	Per 5 mL: aluminum hydroxide dried gel 600 mg
Basaljel Suspension	Per 5 mL: aluminum carbonate equivalent to 400 mg of aluminum hydroxide

tains 130 mg of magnesium/5 mL and 63 mg of aluminum/ 5 mL. These amounts are doubled in the extra-strength suspension.

Bismuth Subsalicylate. Bismuth subsalicylate is labeled for heartburn and indigestion. Procter & Gamble, the major marketer, stresses that it works by coating the mucosa; however, the FDA does not consider it to be an antacid. In addition, bismuth subsalicylate has several important precautions in its use (see "Treatment of Upset Stomach Caused by Overindulgence in Food and Alcohol").

Combination Products. Many manufacturers combine antacids to produce better effects than single-entity products (Table 5.5). The FDA also allows antacids to be combined with aspirin or acetaminophen. These combinations will be labeled for the temporary relief of occasional minor aches and pains, etc., coupled with acid indigestion, although there is a risk to recommending aspirin in stomach problems, as previously mentioned.[74]

Points to Consider When Choosing an Antacid

Dosage Form. Antacids in tablet form are more convenient to use when away from home.[63] *Tablets must be chewed thoroughly to obtain an optimal effect.* If they are not completely chewed, bowel obstruction could result since they are not absorbed to any extent.

Suspensions are more efficacious because they cover a greater surface area.

The objectionable taste of antacid liquids may be helped by refrigeration, although they must not be frozen.

Optimal Dosing Regimen. Antacids will neutralize stomach acids for up to 3 hours if taken 1 hour after meals.[75] If taken without food, antacids neutralize for only 20 to 40 minutes.

Drug Interactions. Antacids may cause drug interactions through several mechanisms. The increase in stomach pH enhances absorption of salicylates, indomethacin, naproxen, pseudoephedrine, and levodopa.[76] However, the effectiveness of tetracycline, digoxin, phenytoin, chlorpromazine, and isoniazid is impaired.

Aluminum hydroxide delays gastric emptying, slowing absorption of indomethacin, isoniazid, barbiturates, and some benzodiazepines. Patients should space tetracycline doses 1 to 2 hours apart from antacids (other than sodium bicarbonate).[53,62] If taken with enteric-coated medications, antacids may cause gastric release. This could cause premature dissolution of Dulcolax tablets, with gastric spasms.

The aforementioned drug interaction warning label that must appear on antacids provides little information: "Drug Interaction Precaution: Antacids may interact with certain

Table 5.5. Representative Antacid Combinations

PRODUCT	SELECTED INGREDIENTS/COMMENTS
Advanced Formula Di-Gel Tablets	Calcium carbonate 280 mg, magnesium hydroxide 128 mg, simethicone 20 mg
Aludrox Suspension	Per 5 mL: aluminum hydroxide gel 307 mg, magnesium hydroxide 103 mg
Maalox Extra Strength Antacid/ Anti-Gas Suspension	Per 5 mL: magnesium hydroxide 450 mg, aluminum hydroxide (as dried gel) 500 mg, simethicone 40 mg
Maalox Suspension	Per 5 mL: magnesium hydroxide 200 mg, aluminum hydroxide (as dried gel) 225 mg
Mylanta Double Strength Tablets	Calcium carbonate 700 mg, magnesium hydroxide 300 mg
Mylanta Gelcaps	Calcium carbonate 550 mg, magnesium hydroxide 125 mg; contains two of the most potent antacids; calcium constipation balances magnesium laxation
Mylanta Suspension	Per 5 mL: aluminum hydroxide (as dried gel) 200 mg, magnesium hydroxide 200 mg, simethicone 20 mg
Riopan Plus Double Strength Suspension	Per 5 mL: magaldrate 1080 mg, simethicone 40 mg
Rolaids Tablets	Calcium carbonate 550 mg, magnesium hydroxide 110 mg
Tempo Tablets	Calcium carbonate 414 mg, aluminum hydroxide 133 mg, magnesium hydroxide 81 mg, simethicone 20 mg
Titralac Plus Tablets	Calcium carbonate 420 mg, simethicone 21 mg
Tylenol Headache Plus Caplets	Calcium carbonate 250 mg, acetaminophen 500 mg; FDA-approved for the dual problems of upset stomach and pain

prescription drugs. If you are presently taking a prescription drug, do not take this product without checking with your physician or other health professional."[51,76,78]

ALGINATES

Some products sold for stomach problems also contain alginates in addition to antacids (Table 5.6).[10,28] Alginic acid is said to react with saliva to form a viscous raft of nonirritating material that floats atop stomach contents.[2,13,26,35] When reflux occurs, refluxate consists of the nonirritant material, rather than acids and enzymes.[16,23,29] The material also may present an actual barrier to reflux.[7] *This mechanism of alginates likely is only helpful if a patient is upright.*[6] The tablets must be chewed prior to swallowing to allow the foam to form fully.[10] Alginate-containing products should not be used with other antacids that contain simethicone in the formulation as the simethicone will cause the bubbles of the foam to coalesce, directly inhibiting its purported action.[10] Although results are encouraging in some studies, to date they are insufficient for the FDA to approve the novel mechanism.[78]

Speaking specifically to the alginate combination Gaviscon, the FDA denied the manufacturer's petition to include alginic acid as an approved nonprescription antacid and to allow the labeling claim of "floating."[79] The product is currently being sold under a New Drug Application (NDA), which recognizes it as an antacid for the relief of heartburn. Alginates are considered inactive ingredients under this ruling; the claim of floating was found to lack evidence of effectiveness. The company also is not permitted to suggest on the label that the floating property contributes uniquely to the product's effectiveness. In their lay publication (*FDA Consumer*) describing therapy of reflux with nonprescription products, the FDA significantly omitted any mention of alginates.[44]

HISTAMINE-2 BLOCKING AGENTS (H2-BLOCKERS)

The introduction of the powerful H2-blockers as nonprescription products in the mid 1990s revolutionized nonprescription therapy of both gastroesophageal reflux disease and nonreflux gastric distress (Table 5.7). Where antacids only neutralize acid that has already been produced (and may be causing symptoms), the H2-blockers actually prevent acid production.

Product similarities include the following:

- Available in a dose that is one-half of the lowest available prescription dosage unit (with the exception of Tagamet HB 200 in which a 200 mg prescription strength of Tagamet remains available)
- Contraindicated for children under the age of 12[80–83]
- Dosed up to twice daily
- Limited to use for 2 weeks after onset of symptoms

Product differences include the following:

- Varying product effectiveness
- The time of onset varies in preventing the problem:
  -Pepcid AC is taken 60 minutes before the meal.
  -Axid AR is taken right before eating or up to 60 minutes before eating.
  -Tagamet HB taken right before eating or up to 30 minutes before eating.
- All four products can treat active symptoms. However, Zantac 75 is the only one of the four that cannot be labeled for prevention prior to eating a problem-causing meal.
- Varying duration (Table 5.7)

The manufacturers of Tagamet HB were required by the FDA to warn patients taking theophylline, warfarin, and phenytoin not to use the product. The remaining three products do not carry these warnings.

PART 2: UPSET STOMACH CAUSED BY OVERINDULGENCE IN FOOD AND ALCOHOL

PREVALENCE OF UPSET STOMACH CAUSED BY OVERINDULGENCE IN FOOD AND ALCOHOL

The prevalence of this condition is unknown, although the number of consultations in a typical pharmacy suggest it is common.

Table 5.6. Representative Alginate/Antacid Combinations

PRODUCT	SELECTED INGREDIENTS
Gaviscon Regular Strength Suspension	Per 15 mL: aluminum hydroxide 95 mg, magnesium carbonate 358 mg, sodium alginate
Gaviscon Extra Strength Suspension	Per 10 mL: aluminum hydroxide 508 mg, magnesium carbonate 475 mg, sodium alginate
Gaviscon Regular Strength Tablets	Aluminum hydroxide 80 mg, magnesium trisilicate 20 mg, alginic acid, sodium bicarbonate
Gaviscon Extra Strength Tablets	Aluminum hydroxide 160 mg, magnesium carbonate 105 mg, alginic acid, sodium bicarbonate

Table 5.7. Comparison of Nonprescription H2-blockers

ATTRIBUTE	PEPCID AC MYLANTA•AR	TAGAMET HB 200[a]	ZANTAC 75	AXID AR
OTC date	June 1995	August 1995	April 1996	June 1996
Contents	10 mg Famotidine	200 mg Cimetidine	75 mg Ranitidine	75 mg Nizatidine
Lower age cutoff	12	12	12	12
Dosage	1 tablet up to BID	1 tablet up to BID	1 tablet up to BID	1 tablet up to BID
For prevention?	1 tab 60 minutes before problem-causing meal	1 tab 0–30 minutes ac[b]	Not labeled at present[b]	1 tab 0–60 minutes ac before problem-causing meal
Treats active symptoms?	Yes	Yes	Yes	Yes
Max. time for self-use	2 weeks	2 weeks	2 weeks	2 weeks
Duration of effect	Up to 9 hours[b]	6–6.5 hours[b]	8–12 hours[b]	Variable, no definite figure given by product specialist[b]
Drug interaction warnings?	No	Theophylline (Theo-Dur, Theo-24, Uniphyl), warfarin (Coumadin), Phenytoin (Dilantin)	No	No

[a]Originally a 100-mg tablet. Increased to 200 mg in November 1996.

[b]Information gained from company's toll-free lines: Pepcid AC (800-755-4008), Tagamet HB (800-482-4394), Zantac 75 (800-223-0182), Axid AR(800-555-AXID), Mylanta A•R (800-469-5268).

MANIFESTATIONS OF UPSET STOMACH CAUSED BY OVERINDULGENCE IN FOOD AND ALCOHOL

The FDA describes this syndrome, which is different from a simple hangover, as nausea, heartburn, and fullness (gas), possibly in combination with other symptoms. The symptoms begin within about 1 hour of the overindulgence and can persist for as long as 24 hours.[84]

TREATMENT OF UPSET STOMACH CAUSED BY OVERINDULGENCE IN FOOD AND ALCOHOL

Treatment Guidelines

Usually, this is a minor condition that will resolve as soon as the effects of the alcohol abate and/or the food is processed. However, should the patient wish relief, several nonprescription medications may be helpful.

Nonprescription Medications

Representative products containing ingredients approved for treatment of upset stomach caused by overindulgence in food and alcohol are listed in Table 5.8. Bismuth subsalicylate was given Category I status in treatment of this syndrome, as were sodium citrate in solution and antacids in combination with internal analgesics.

 Sodium bicarbonate should be avoided for treatment of overindulgence because of its propensity to cause gastric rupture, especially when the organ is already distended.[55] In 1994 the FDA disallowed any labeling referring to overindulgence in food and drink for sodium bicarbonate products that are dissolved in liquid before ingestion. The agency specifically cited gastric dilatation and rupture, as well as its propensity to cause systemic metabolic alkalosis, milk-alkali syndrome, and increased sodium load.[85]

One disadvantage in recommending bismuth subsalicylate is the salicylate content. The recommended adult dose results in administration of 258 mg of salicylate.[86] If the patient takes the product every 30 minutes up to 8 doses daily as directed, the salicylate received is 2064 mg.[87] As much as 97% of this salicylate is absorbed. Thus a Reye's syndrome warning is appropriate, as is a caution to watch patients who have ingested the product for salicylate toxicity. Further, it should be given carefully to young children, to individuals with salicylate sensitivity or bleeding disorders (e.g., hemophilia), and to patients taking medications that interact with salicylates (e.g., anticoagulants, antidiabetics, or products for gout or arthritis).

The Reye's syndrome warning has taken several forms over the years. In 1993 the FDA proposed this revised warning for oral and rectal aspirin products: "Children and teenagers who have or are recovering from chicken pox, flu symptoms, or flu should NOT use this product. If nausea, vomiting, or fever occur, consult a doctor because these symptoms could be an early sign of Reye's syndrome, a rare but serious illness."[88]

Following the death of a 6-year-old child in 1989, the FDA proposed also requiring a warning on all bismuth

Table 5.8. Representative Products for Upset Stomach Due to Overindulgence in Food and Alcohol

PRODUCT	SELECTED INGREDIENTS/COMMENTS
Original Alka-Seltzer	Sodium bicarconate 1916 mg, citric acid 1000 mg, aspirin 325 mg (an effervescent tablet that forms sodium citrate in water)
Bromo-Seltzer	Per ¾ capful; sodium bicarbonate 2781 mg, citric acid 2224 mg, acetaminophen 325 mg (a powder that, when dissolved, forms sodium citrate)
Pepto-Bismol Caplets	Bismuth subsalicylate 262 mg
Pepto-Bismol Chewable Tablets	Bismuth subsalicylate 262 mg
Pepto-Bismol Suspension	Per 15 mL: bismuth subsalicylate 262 mg
Pepto-Bismol Maximum Strength Suspension	Per 15 mL: bismuth subsalicylate 525 mg

subsalicylate products (including the generics). The FDA stated that the product had been given to the child for flu-like symptoms, diarrhea, and nausea.[88]

Another problem with recommending bismuth subsalicylate products is bismuth toxicity. An adult taking the daily recommended dose of this product receives 2424 mg of bismuth daily.[87] Even though bismuth is poorly absorbed, unlike salicylate, toxicity can occur. Symptoms of excessive bismuth ingestion include apathy, mild ataxia, and headaches in the early phases, progressing to myoclonic jerks, dysarthria, severe confusion, hallucinations, epileptic seizures, and even death. Fortunately, there are few cases of encephalopathy related to therapeutic uses of currently available nonprescription bismuth preparations.

Bismuth salts react with hydrogen sulfide produced by anaerobic bacteria in the colon to produce bismuth sulfide, which is highly insoluble.[86] Since it is a black salt, it discolors the stools. The tongue may also become discolored as a result of a reaction with sulfides produced by oral bacteria. Patients can become alarmed, but the darkening is harmless.

PART 3: HANGOVER

Hangover is a syndrome that occurs after ingestion of large amounts of alcohol.

MANIFESTATIONS OF HANGOVER

Hangover includes gastrointestinal, neurologic, and metabolic symptoms such as nausea, heartburn, thirst, tremor, disturbances of equilibrium, fatigue, generalized aches and pains, headache, dullness, depression, and irritability.[84]

TREATMENT OF HANGOVER

Treatment Guidelines

Hangover is generally an acute, self-limiting condition. However, a person may experience symptoms for several days, either as a result of excessive and physically harmful consump-

tion of alcohol or as a result of the alcohol aggravating some other disease or condition. For this reason nonprescription products for treating hangover have a 2-day cutoff.[89] If symptoms persist longer than this period, the individual should cease reliance on these products and seek medical guidance.

Nonprescription Medications

Combination products are preferable for symptoms. For instance, internal analgesics alleviate headache and minor aches and pains, antacids relieve gastric distress, and caffeine helps fatigue and drowsiness associated with the hangover. Products containing activated charcoal are not effective for this indication.[90] *Sodium bicarbonate in a dosage form meant to be dissolved in a liquid cannot be labeled with this indication because of the possibility of gastric rupture.*[85]

Internal analgesics, antacids, and caffeine may be combined for hangover, with one exception. Since caffeine is a proven stimulator of gastric acid secretion, it is irrational to combine caffeine with an antacid.[89] Products intended to relieve hangover symptoms are listed in Table 5.9.

No nonprescription product can be marketed with the claim of minimizing or preventing hangover. Such products would be ineffective and might encourage someone to drive under the influence.[91]

PART 4: PEPTIC ULCER

Pharmacists should be familiar with peptic ulcer since many patients will attempt to purchase nonprescription products to treat a previously diagnosed or suspected ulcer. In those cases pharmacists should refer patients for proper care if symptoms of peptic ulcer are apparent. For that reason this section will focus more on the role of medications and the symptoms of the condition rather than on etiology and non-medication-related epidemiologic factors.

PREVALENCE OF PEPTIC ULCER

Approximately 10 to 15% of males and 4 to 15% of females will develop peptic ulcer disease (PUD) at least once during their

Table 5.9. Representative Products for Relief of Hangover Symptoms	
PRODUCT	SELECTED INGREDIENTS
Dr. Seltzer's Hangover Helper Caplets	Calcium carbonate 500 mg, aspirin 450 mg, acetaminophen 288 mg, thiamin 250 mg, caffeine 64 mg
XS Hangover Relief	Per 15 mL: calcium citrate 1250 mg, acetaminophen 1000 mg, magnesium trisilicate 750 mg, calcium carbonate 350 mg, caffeine 200 mg

life.[92] It is estimated that PUD affects more than 4 million patients yearly; perhaps 100,000 patients have bleeding PUD each year.[93]

EPIDEMIOLOGY OF PEPTIC ULCER: THE ROLE OF MEDICATIONS

Despite their benefits in arthritis, the use of nonsteroidal, antiinflammatory (NSAIDs) medications is associated with significant morbidity and mortality as a result of peptic ulceration.[94] A great deal of research links long-term NSAID use to peptic ulcer disease and its complications.[75] Indeed, the prevalence of peptic ulceration in patients receiving NSAIDs lies between 17 and 31%. Gastric erosions were observed endoscopically in another 50% of subjects taking aspirin or other NSAIDs for 1 month.[75] NSAIDS reduce mucosal prostaglandin levels, particularly in the stomach, an impairment of gastric cytoprotective factors that produces a spectrum of injury ranging from hemorrhages and petechiae to erosions and ulcers.[75,95] It has been suggested that elderly patients who smoke are most likely to suffer from this problem, perhaps because of the additive effect of cigarettes.

Corticosteroids, too, have been implicated in the development, reactivation, perforation, hemorrhage, and delayed healing of peptic ulcers. Corticosteroid-induced ulcer occurs in less than 2% of patients, leading most practitioners not to recommend routine concomitant administration of antacids with corticosteroids.

MANIFESTATIONS OF PEPTIC ULCER

Figure 5.6 indicates common sites of peptic ulcers. Also see "A Pharmacist's Journal: Convulsive Ulcer?"

Dyspepsia

The patient with peptic ulcer often complains of nausea and vomiting.[96] Symptoms may be severe enough to lead to anorexia. (A malignancy may be suspected in elderly patients unless this cause of anorexia is discovered.[97])

FOCUS ON...

HANGOVER PREVENTION AND TREATMENT HOME REMEDIES

Alcohol exacts a terrible economic and physical toll on people when used excessively. Alcohol abusers often attempt to prevent and/or treat hangovers. For instance, conventional wisdom holds that hangovers can be minimized if one does not mix drinks or if one eats a lot (supposedly to absorb the alcohol) or drinks milk. None of these are true. Strangely enough, some individuals who awaken with a hangover treat it with another alcoholic drink (the hair of the dog)! None of this substitutes for either total abstinence or good sense and moderation when drinking. Further, these remedies can be dangerous: The individual who attempts to drive drunk in the mistaken belief that food has absorbed the alcohol could cause injury or death.

Fullness and bloating may also be a component of the condition.[96]

Epigastric Pain

Patients present with recurrent, epigastric, postprandial pain and heartburn.[28] Both symptoms often exhibit a periodic pattern roughly corresponding to the clinical evolution of the disease, which is marked by repeated exacerbations and remissions.[96]

Pain associated with duodenal ulcer is usually localized at a specific point in the central or upper right quadrant of the epigastrum.[98] It manifests more frequently when the patient is fasting. Thus sleeping patients often awaken 2 to 4 hours after the last food ingestion. A light snack at this time may stop the discomfort.

PROGNOSIS OF PEPTIC ULCER DISEASE

Peptic ulcer disease is chronic and recurring. Historically, 2% of patients will die from complications of peptic ulcer disease.[42] At least 15 to 20% of patients will bleed. Fully 6% of ulcers will perforate—the second most common complication of PUD in the elderly.[97,99]

TREATMENT OF PEPTIC ULCER

Treatment Guidelines

There are four therapeutic goals in the treatment of peptic ulcer:
1. Control of symptoms
2. Promotion of ulcer healing

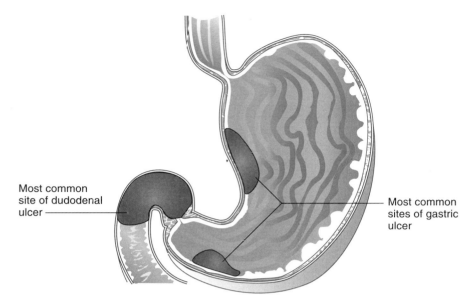

Figure 5.6. Common sites of peptic ulcer.

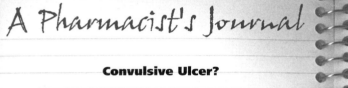

Convulsive Ulcer?

As I approached a woman appearing to be in her mid 50s at the antacid section, she turned and asked me if an antacid product was good for an ulcer. I explained that the products were only for upset stomach and reflux and not for an ulcer. She said, "It's all right for me to use an antacid, though, because I just have a convulsive ulcer." I asked her if that was a previously diagnosed con-dition, and she said yes, it had been diagnosed several years before, but was cured and now it had come back. I asked whether it was actually called by another name such as duodenal, gastric, or peptic ulcer. She said, "No I just had a convulsive or compulsive ulcer, I can't remember which one." I mentioned that in any case no nonprescription product would be allowed for treatment of an ulcer and asked that she visit her physician.

3. Preventing recurrence
4. Preventing complications

Lifestyle modifications such as diet control, cessation of smoking and alcohol ingestion, and avoidance of irritants also should be encouraged by the physician.[96] The choice of therapy is determined by efficacy, adverse reactions, cost, and convenience.

Nonprescription Medications

Antacids have had a long-standing role in the management of dyspepsia and peptic ulceration.[63,100] (See "Nonprescription Antacids" and Table 5.1.) Generally, antacids are prescribed for the relief of symptoms, although not all controlled studies show that they are better than placebo. Moreover, the adverse effects of antacids limit their usefulness in this regard.[101,102]

Additionally, the dosages of antacids required are so high (far in excess of the safe doses for self-treatment) that the pharmacist should not recommend antacids for ulcer therapy.

The role of H2-blockers in treating peptic ulcer is critically important when they are used as prescription medications. However, *H2-blockers are not indicated for peptic ulcer therapy when labeled as nonprescription products.* Pharmacists would be remiss in recommending their use in a patient with peptic ulcer since such a patient would not be properly supervised nor would the progress of the ulcer be monitored.

AT THE COUNTER

 A young man of about 19 examining products in the gastric section asks the pharmacist for assistance.

Interview/Patient Assessment

The patient has had stomach upset for about 1 week. He denies use of any medications and does not have any health conditions. He confirms that occasionally he feels an unpleasant material coming back up out of his stomach and afterward it burns for several hours. When the pharmacist asks him about recent lifestyle changes, he mentions that he just began a part-time job to ease his school finances. He works the midnight shift at a local convenience store. To keep himself awake, he drinks 10 to 12 caffeinated carbonated beverages each night. Previously, he had only ingested one or two daily.

Pharmacist's Analysis

1. What is this young man's problem?
2. What is the significance of his recent lifestyle change?

3. How does his intake of caffeinated carbonated beverages affect his condition?
4. Would a nonprescription product be appropriate?

This patient apparently suffers from gastroesophageal reflux disease. The condition is probably a result of his new job because his sleep patterns and eating patterns have been altered. The major contributing factor is most likely his heavy caffeine and carbonation intake: the caffeine worsens GERD, and the carbonation produces gas in the stomach.

Patient Counseling

The pharmacist has several treatment options. Since he is over the age of 12, an H2-blocker would be appropriate therapy. As an alternative, antacids or alginates also would be appropriate, but these products only combat acid that is already present, while the H2-blockers reduce acid production. With either option he may only self-treat the problem for one additional week. Should it persist beyond that time, a physician visit is necessary. In any case he should be advised to reduce his caffeine intake.

SUMMARY

The pharmacist plays an important role in assisting patients in the recognition of gastroesophageal reflux disease and several other minor gastric conditions (e.g., hangover, nonreflux gastric distress).

Gastroesophageal reflux is a common condition in which gastric contents reflux through the lower esophageal sphincter, causing discomfort and possibly damaging the esophagus. Antacids, H2-blockers, and alginates are effective in varying degrees at preventing esophageal damage. There are also several nonpharmacologic interventions that pharmacists can suggest to prevent GERD.

A recent switch of H2-blockers from prescription to nonprescription status has left many consumers confused about their indications. Although their nonprescription indications do not include self-treatment of ulcer, patients have attempted to do this. Therefore, the pharmacist must ensure that patients with peptic ulcer do not attempt self-treatment with nonprescription products.

A major challenge in treatment of gastric distress is taking the time to differentiate self-treatable conditions from more serious conditions such as peptic ulcer. Further, if a myocardial infarction is suspected to be GERD, and a patient is sent home with nothing more than a bottle of antacid tablets, serious harm could result. For this reason pharmacists must be especially careful to refer patients whose symptoms are not clearly minor and self-treatable.

References

1. Tew S, et al. The illness behavior of patients with gastroesophageal reflux disease with and without endoscopic esophagitis. Dis Esophagus 10:9, 1997.
2. Cochran EB, et al. Gastroesophageal reflux in the pediatric population. Hosp Pharm 22:1053, 1987.
3. Waterfall WE, et al. Gastroesophageal reflux: Clinical presentations, diagnosis and management. Can Med Assoc J 135: 1101, 1986.
4. Xie P, et al. Frequency of esophageal reflux events induced by pharyngeal water stimulation in young and elderly subjects. Am J Physiol 272 (2 Pt 1):G233, 1997.
5. Fuchs KH, et al. Specificity and sensitivity of objective diagnosis of gastroesophageal reflux disease. Surgery 102:575, 1987.
6. Rex DK. Gastroesophageal reflux disease in adults: Pathophysiology, diagnosis and management. J Fam Pract 35:673, 1992.
7. Morton LS, Fromkes JJ. Gastroesophageal reflux disease: Diagnosis and medical therapy. Geriatrics 48:60, 1993.
8. Dodds WJ. The pathogenesis of gastroesophageal reflux disease. Am J Roentgenol 151:49, 1988.
9. Castell DO. Gastroesophageal reflux—the great imitator (Editorial). West J Med 149:81, 1988.
10. Navab F, Texter EC Jr. Gastroesophageal reflux. Arch Intern Med 145:329, 1985.
11. Dent J. Long-term aims of treatment of reflux disease, and the role of non-drug measures. Digestion 51(Suppl 1):30, 1992.
12. Kjellin A, et al. Gastroesophageal reflux in obese patients is not reduced by weight reduction. Scand J Gastroenterol 31: 1047, 1996.
13. Murphy DW, Castell DO. Pathogenesis and treatment of gastroesophageal reflux disease. Med Times 115:27, 1987.

14. Hagen J, et al. Gastroesophageal reflux in the massively obese. Int Surg 72:1, 1987.
15. Baron TH, et al. Gastrointestinal motility disorders during pregnancy. Ann Intern Med 118:366, 1993.
16. Baron TH, Richter JE. Gastroesophageal reflux disease in pregnancy. Gastroenterol Clin North Am 21:777, 1992.
17. Calhoun BC. Gastrointestinal disorders in pregnancy. Obstet Gynecol Clin North Am 19:733, 1992.
18. Van Thiel DH, Wald A. Evidence refuting a role for increasing abdominal pressure in the pathogenesis of heartburn associated with pregnancy. Am J Obstet Gynecol 140:420, 1981.
19. Marrero JM, et al. Determinants of pregnancy heartburn. Br J Obstet Gynaecol 99:731, 1992.
20. Guggenbichler JP, Menardi G. Conservative treatment of gastroesophageal reflux and hiatus hernia. Prog Pediatr Surg 18:78, 1985.
21. Skinner DB. Pathophysiology of gastroesophageal reflux. Ann Surg 202:546, 1985.
22. Isolauri J, et al. Natural course of gastroesophageal reflux disease: 17–22 year follow-up of 60 patients. Am J Gastroenterol 92:37, 1997.
23. Blount BW. Gastroesophageal reflux in children. Am Fam Physician 37:201, 1988.
24. Kleinman MS. Gastroesophageal reflux disease. Hosp Pract 20:40I, 1985.
25. Weirauch TR. Gastro-oesophageal reflux—pathogenesis and clinical implications. Eur J Pediatr 144:215, 1985.
26. Mold JW, Rankin RA. Symptomatic gastroesophageal reflux in the elderly. J Am Geriatr Soc 35:649, 1987.
27. Maddern GJ, Jamieson GG. Oesophageal emptying in patients with gastro-oesophageal reflux. Br J Surg 73:615, 1986.
28. Ward PH, et al. Complications of gastroesophageal reflux. West J Med 149:58, 1988.
29. O'Connor KW. Gastroesophageal reflux: An update. Indiana Med 78:188, 1985.
30. Benini L, et al. Gastric emptying and dyspeptic symptoms in patients with gastroesophageal reflux. Am J Gastroenterol 91:1351, 1996.
31. Stacher G. Oesophageal motility, oesophageal transit and gastro-oesophageal reflux—a methodological review. Hepatogastroenterology 32:299, 1985.
32. Rogers AI. Diagnosis of reflux esophagitis. Pract Gastroenterol 10:1, 1986.
33. Anon. Nonspecific pharyngitis and laryngitis (Editorial). Lancet 1:512, 1983.
34. Brzana RJ, Koch KL. Gastroesophageal reflux disease presenting with intractable nausea. Ann Intern Med 126:704, 1997.
35. Olson NR. The problem of gastroesophageal reflux. Otolaryngol Clin North Am 19:119, 1986.
36. Locke GR III, et al. Prevalence and clinical spectrum of gastroesophageal reflux: A population-based study in Olmsted County, Minnesota. Gastroenterology 112:1448, 1997.
37. Gonzalez ER, Castell DO. Respiratory complications of gastroesophageal reflux. Am Fam Physician 37:169, 1988.
38. Campo S, et al. Esophageal dysmotility and gastroesophageal reflux in intrinsic asthma. Dig Dis Sci 42:1184, 1997.
39. Fonkalsrud EW, Ament ME. Gastroesophageal reflux in childhood. Curr Probl Surg 33:1, 1996.
40. Sontag SJ. The medical management of reflux esophagitis. Gastroenterol Clin North Am 19:683, 1990.
41. Tirosh E, Jaffe M. Apnea of infancy, seizures, and gastroesophageal reflux: An important bur infrequent association. J Child Neurol 11:98, 1996.
42. Csendes A, et al. Prevalence of *Helicobacter pylori* infection in 190 control subjects and in 236 patients with gastroesophageal reflux, erosive esophagitis or Barrett's esophagus. Dis Esophagus 10:38, 1997.
43. Richter JE. A critical review of current medical therapy for gastroesophageal reflux disease. J Clin Gastroenterol 8(Suppl 1):72, 1986.
44. Cramer T. When do you need an antacid. FDA Consumer 26:19, 1992.
45. Dhiman RK, et al. Inclusion of supine period in short-duration pH monitoring is essential in diagnosis of gastroesophageal reflux disease. Dig Dis Sci 41:764, 1996.
46. Hamilton JW, et al. Sleeping on a wedge diminishes expo-sure of the esophagus to refluxed acid. Dig Dis Sci 33:518, 1988.
47. Fed Reg 47:38481, 1982.
48. Cramer T. When do you need an antacid? FDA Consumer 26:19, 1992.
49. Brown C, Rees WDW. Dyspepsia in general practice. BMJ 300:829, 1990.
50. Antacid Drug Products for Over-the-Counter Human Use; Amendment to Antacid Final Monograph; Proposed Rule. Fed Reg 59:5059, 1994.
51. Puntis JWL, et al. Raised plasma aluminum in an infant on antacid (Letter). Lancet 2:923, 1989.
52. Fed Reg 58:45203, 1993.
53. Texter EC. A critical look at the clinical use of antacids in acid-peptic disease and gastric acid rebound. Am J Gastroenterol 84:97, 1989.
54. Fed Reg 39:19861, 1974.
55. Fordtran JS, et al. Gas production after reaction of sodium bicarbonate and hydrochloric acid. Gastroenterology 87:1014, 1984.
56. Brismar B, et al. Stomach rupture following ingestion of sodium bicarbonate. Acta Chir Scand Suppl 530:97, 1986.
57. Anon. Baking soda blamed. The Daily Oklahoman: 6 (9/26/91).
58. Newmark K, Nugent P. Milk-alkali syndrome. Postgrad Med 93:149, 1993.
59. Hade JE, Spiro HM. Calcium and acid rebound: A reappraisal. J Clin Gastroenterol 15:37, 1992.
60. French JK, et al. NZ Med J 99:322, 1986.
61. Fed Reg 38:8713, 1973.
62. Todd B. Antacid alert. Geriatr Nurs 10:278, 1989.
63. Porro GB, Parente F. Antacids for duodenal ulcer: current role. Scand J Gastroenterol Suppl 174:48, 1990.
64. Agarwal BN, Robertson FM. Metabolic alkalosis and hypermagnesemia following "non-absorbable" antacid therapy. Del Med J 58:531, 1986.
65. Brand JM, Greer FR. Hypermagnesemia and intestinal perforation following antacid administration in a premature infant. Pediatrics 85:121, 1990.
66. Fenner L. When digestive juices corrode, you've got an ulcer. FDA Consumer 18:22, 1984.
67. Spencer H, Kramer L. Antacid-induced calcium loss (Editorial). Arch Intern Med 143:657, 1983.
68. Saadeh G, et al. Antacid-induced osteomalacia. Cleve Clin J Med 54:214, 1987.
69. Neumann L, Jensen BG. Osteomalacia from Al and Mg antacids. Acta Orthop Scand 60:361, 1989.

70. Carmichael KA, et al. Osteomalacia and osteitis fibrosa in a man ingesting aluminum hydroxide antacid. Am J Med 76: 1137, 1984.

71. Harmelin Dl, et al. Antacid-induced phosphate depletion syndrome presenting as nephrolithiasis. Aust NZ J Med 20:803, 1990.

72. Ittel TH, et al. Hyperaluminaemia in critically ill patients: Role of antacid therapy and impaired renal function. Eur J Clin Invest 21:96, 1991.

73. Florent C, et al. Morphologic and ultrastructural effects of Maalox TC on human gastric and duodenal mucosa. J Clin Gastroenterol 13(Suppl 1):S139, 1991.

74. Fed Reg 53:46189, 1988.

75. Wilson DE. Gastroduodenal ulcers: Causes, diagnosis, prevention, and treatment. Compr Ther 16:43, 1990.

76. Hecht A. Mixing antacids and Rx drugs can spell t-r-o-u-b-l-e. FDA Consumer 20:9, 1986.

77. Fed Reg 51:27341, 1986.

78. Buts JP, et al. Double-blind controlled study on the efficacy of sodium alginate (Gaviscon) in reducing gastroesophageal reflux assessed by 24h continuous pH monitoring in infants and children. Eur J Pediatr 146:156, 1987.

79. Antacid drug products for over-the-counter human use: Final classification of category III antacid ingredients and labeling claims. Federal Register 52:33576, 1987.

80. Trade Package, Pepcid AC (undated).

81. Trade Package, Tagamet HB: 1995.

82. Trade Package, Zantac 75: 1995.

83. Trade Package, Axid AR (undated).

84. Fed Reg 47:43539, 1982.

85. Fed Reg 59:5067, 1994.

86. Gorbach SL. Bismuth therapy in gastrointestinal diseases. Gastroenterology 99:863, 1990.

87. DuPont HL. Bismuth subsalicylate in the treatment and prevention of diarrhea disease. Drug Intell Clin Pharm 21:687, 1987.

88. Fed Reg 58:26885, 1993.

89. Fed Reg 56:66761, 1991.

90. Fed Reg 56:66741, 1991.

91. Fed Reg 48:32872, 1983.

92. Dukes G. The importance of maintenance therapy in the management of duodenal ulcer disease. Glaxo Inc., Research Triangle Park, 1991.

93. National Institutes of Health. Therapeutic endoscopy and bleeding ulcers. Conn Med 54:22, 1990.

94. Smedley FH. Non-steroidal anti-inflammatory drug ingestion: retrospective study of 272 bleeding or perforated peptic ulcers. Postgrad Med J 65:892, 1989.

95. Sciessel R, et al. Mechanisms of stress ulceration and implications for treatment. Gastroenterol Clin North Am 19:101, 1990.

96. Dukes G. The importance of nocturnal gastric acid secretion in peptic ulcer disease. Glaxo Inc., Research Triangle Park, 1990.

97. Gilinsky NH. Peptic ulcer disease in the elderly. Gastroenterol Clin North Am 19:255, 199.0

98. Magni G, et al. Pain and personality in duodenal ulcer: A preliminary report. Psychol Rep 66:763, 1990.

99. Englund R, Fisher R. Survival following perforation of peptic ulcer. Aust NZ J Surg 60:795, 1990.

100. Weberg R, et al. Comparisons of low-dose antacids, cimetidine, and placebo on 24-hour intragastric acidity in healthy volunteers. Dig Dis Sci 37:1810, 1992.

101. Freston JW. Overview of medical therapy of peptic ulcer disease. Gastroenterol Clin North Am 19:121, 1990.

102. Walt RP, Langman MJS. Antacids and ulcer healing. Drugs 42:205, 1991.

Motion Sickness

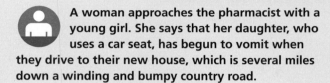

AT THE COUNTER

A woman approaches the pharmacist with a young girl. She says that her daughter, who uses a car seat, has begun to vomit when they drive to their new house, which is several miles down a winding and bumpy country road.

Interview/Patient Assessment

The mother states that this has happened several times in the past week. She would like a product for motion sickness. The daughter is 18 months old and has been taking Bactrim for an ear infection for the past several months. The mother would like to know if the Marezine she saw advertised would be effective.

Pharmacist's Analysis

1. Is motion sickness the most likely cause of vomiting?
2. What is the significance of the new home?
3. What contribution does the Bactrim play, if any?
4. Is Marezine indicated for the child?

Motion sickness is a distinct possibility as a cause of this child's vomiting. Because she is buckled into a car seat, it is difficult for her to see out, a situation that causes neural mismatch for many children. Bactrim (co-trimoxazole) can cause nausea and vomiting, but the fact that she is vomiting only when she travels argues against Bactrim as a cause. No motion sickness product is safe for self-treatment for children under the age of 2, however. Marezine cannot be recommended under the age of 6.

Patient Counseling

The prudent pharmacist will refer the child to her pediatrician for evaluation. Additionally, the pharmacist may offer tips to prevent motion sickness such as the purchase of a car seat that is high enough to allow the child to see out of the window of the moving car.

Motion sickness, a self-limiting condition, is a minor annoyance for many and is debilitating for others. (In addition, it can be a major nuisance such as when one has invested a large sum of money in a cruise and experiences disabling symptoms.) The range of nonprescription products available for treating and preventing this troubling condition is limited, but they are effective if used correctly. (See "Nausea.")

PREVALENCE OF MOTION SICKNESS

The condition popularly known as motion sickness (also sea sickness, space sickness, *mal de mer* [sickness of the sea]) can affect any individual in any type of moving vehicle—land conveyance, watercraft, aircraft, or spacecraft.[1,2] No one with a normal sense of balance is immune.[3] Tests show that individuals who have never suffered from motion sickness invariably begin to experience the symptoms when they are exposed to certain types of motion for a sufficient period.[2,4]

Motion sickness is not peculiar to man. Researchers have routinely induced motion sickness symptoms in several animals (e.g., dogs and squirrel monkeys).[1,5] Even codfish transported in water over rough conditions can be made to vomit from the motion.[6] Humans present a wide range of susceptibility, however, so that some individuals never experience motion sickness.[7] The fact that some people have never had motion sickness leads to the widespread misconception that the condition is all in the sufferer's mind.

One survey revealed that 90% of the population has suffered from motion sickness at one time. Special subgroups of the population report incidences as follows:[4,8–11]

- Naval crew in normal seas (10 to 30%)
- Experienced naval crew members (15 to 60%)
- Patients at a geriatric day hospital (19%)
- Passengers on ferries (29%)
- Military student pilots (38%)
- Astronauts and cosmonauts (50 to 60%)
- Naval crew during the worst seas (50 to 90%)
- Inexperienced sailors (60 to 90%)

EPIDEMIOLOGY OF MOTION SICKNESS

Infants rarely suffer symptoms of motion sickness; the greatest incidence occurs from ages 2 to 12.[6] After age 12 the incidence of motion sickness gradually declines; above age 50 it is considered rare because of the phenomenon of adaptation discussed below.[12]

Motion sickness exhibits a gender preference, with three females affected for every two males.[13,14] The reason is unknown.

Obviously, motion sickness has a sharp occupational correlation, with individuals exposed to provocative motion (such as one whose job requires being a passenger in rough seas) more likely to experience discomfort than those whose jobs are sedentary (such as one who works in an office).

For some reason individuals who are more physically fit seem to be more susceptible to motion sickness than those who are out of shape.[15]

ETIOLOGY OF MOTION SICKNESS

Research to clarify the etiology of motion sickness has revealed that patients whose inner ear is non-functional do not experience motion sickness, while patients with a normal inner ear do. The role of the inner ear in the genesis of motion sickness has been incorporated by researchers into a larger hypothesis known as the neural-mismatch or sensory-conflict theory.[1,16,17]

According to the neural-mismatch theory, sensory cues regarding movement are provided by input from three body systems:

- The visual system in which the eyes tell the body whether movement is occurring
- The **proprioceptive systems** (sensory nerve terminals that give information concerning movement and position of the body, based on input from the muscles, tendons, and other internal tissues), which are extremely important in an individual's ability to sense motion[2,10,18]
- The **vestibular system** (the semicircular canals and the **otolith apparatus** [small calcium-like stones in the inner ear that help sense motion])

Generally, when an individual is subjected to motion, the visual system registers motion, matching the input from the proprioceptive and vestibular systems, and motion sickness does not occur. (See Fig. 6.1 for a description of the three types of input and how they relate to the neural mismatch theory.) However, certain types of motion generate discordant information from receptors in the three systems, information at odds with past experience. Thus the neural mismatch or sensory conflict theory suggests that individuals experience a critical mismatch or conflict when visual and/or proprioceptive input does not match input from the inner ear that gauges actual movement. Researchers believe that a sequence of responses culminating in motion sickness occurs as a result of this sensory mismatch, as illustrated in Figure 6.2.[9]

When investigators compare the relative importance of vestibular versus visual cues, vestibular cues are given equal importance in the genesis of motion sickness. Thus motion sickness usually occurs when the body is moved, but the visual field remains still.[1,4] For example, when riding in a car, the eyes indicate that a person is stationary, but the proprioceptive and vestibular systems register the movement of the vehicle (Fig. 6.2). This insistence that the body is in motion despite the evidence of the eyes is the classical sensory conflict.

FOCUS ON...

NAUSEA

Nausea is the unpleasant sensation that one is about to vomit. It usually does precede vomiting, but may not. Nausea is a component of motion sickness and may be prevented or treated with the FDA-approved motion sickness medications, as may the other symptoms that accompany motion sickness.

 Importantly, *there is no safe and effective nonprescription ingredient for nausea resulting from causes other than motion sickness,* including the following:

- The administration of nauseogenic medications (e.g., digitalis, theophylline, metronidazole, nicotine gum, naproxen)
- Infection with a rotavirus or other agent causing gastroenteritis
- Food poisoning
- Undergoing an intensely revolting experience (e.g., witnessing an automobile accident, seeing a dead animal, or witnessing another person regurgitate)

Active research is proceeding on Emetrol, a product that has been advertised for nausea for many years, although it has not yet been proven safe and effective for nausea. The ingredients—dextrose 1.87 g, fructose 1.87 g, and phosphoric acid 21.5 mg in each 5 mL—are safe for nondiabetic patients, so patients can be assured of a relative lack of toxicity. However, pharmacists who recommend the product to patients whose nausea is clearly not related to motion sickness should explain the potential morbidity associated with the nauseogenic conditions and the possible need to visit a physician for appropriate care (e.g., antibiotic therapy for gastroenteritis).

The theory further explains why voluntary movements (e.g., running, jumping, or dancing) do not produce motion sickness.[1] In these cases the visual, vestibular, and proprioceptive systems are all in agreement. In other words, the motion is appropriate and in harmony with the feelings delivered to the vestibular system. One exception, however, is skiing, which may produce motion sickness in susceptible individuals.[19]

The neural-mismatch theory also explains a reversed type of sensory conflict seen when the body is still but the visual field shows significant movement. An example is watching a movie with an automobile chase scene filmed by an in-car camera in a theater with wide screens (Fig. 6.2).[17] Patrons watching these scenes may feel uncomfortable and may unconsciously lean into the turns. The latter response is an attempt to match the proprioceptive system to the visual input. The maneuver may help prevent motion sickness, because sustained viewing of scenes such as these can produce all of the symptoms of classical motion sickness. Immersion in virtual reality equipment also causes this type of motion sickness since the individual wears goggles that totally obscure vision and show repeated movements that the body is not in fact experiencing.[20]

This "reverse" motion sickness was also implicated in one report of gastroenterology fellows who were required to view slides that were moved rapidly through a teaching microscope with a large viewing screen.[21] Many of the fellows suffered symptoms identical to motion sickness as they attempted to see the details of the slides. Once the genesis of

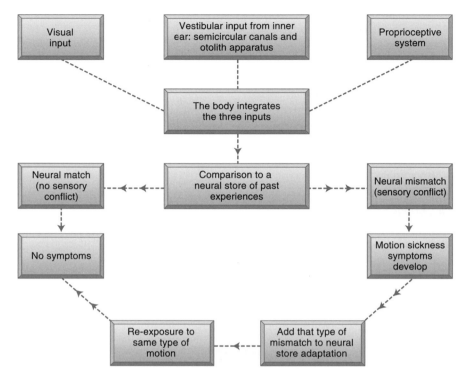

Figure 6.1. The "neural-mismatch" or "sensory-conflict" theory of motion sickness hypothesizes that input from the visual, vestibular, and proprioceptive systems does not match, leading to symptoms. With repeated mismatches of a certain type, however, an individual may adapt so that symptoms do not occur.

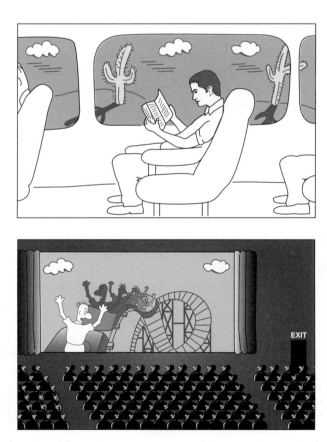

Figure 6.2. The two typical types of motion sickness. In one a person reads in a moving car. In the second a theater audience watches a chase scene with many up-and-down sequences filmed with an in-car camera.

the symptoms was discovered, the professor moved the slides more slowly. All symptoms resolved in the students. A similar situation was reported in a word-processor user who experienced nausea when letters scrolled across the screen.[22]

Experienced military pilots training in flight simulators equipped with wide-field-of-view, computer-generated displays outside the windows complain of motion sickness, even though there is no motion to stimulate the vestibular organs.[1] New glasses that cause significant visual distortion when compared to the previous lenses can also produce motion-sickness symptoms during the initial days of wear.[1]

MANIFESTATIONS OF MOTION SICKNESS

The classical symptom of motion sickness is vomiting. However, other symptoms such as the following develop first[2,14,16,23,24]:

- A feeling of malaise or apathy
- Pallor
- Yawning
- Feeling restless
- Feeling warm
- Drowsiness
- Belching
- Excessive salivation
- Flatulence
- Breaking into a cold sweat
- Headaches

Generally, patients become aware of their stomach and its contents, lose their appetite, and develop nausea.[23] (See "Nausea" above.) The nausea usually progresses gradually to retching and vomiting, the final stage of motion sickness for most sufferers. Vomiting may bring full relief; however, the patient may vomit repeatedly with repeated stimulus. In cases of continued vomiting, motion sickness may result in prostration, severe headache, dehydration, and electrolyte imbalance.[25]

SPECIFIC CONSIDERATIONS OF MOTION SICKNESS

As shown in Figure 6.3, there are three types of linear motion (forward and back, up and down, and side-to-side) and three types of rotational motion about the axes (roll, pitch, and yaw). Investigators have explored the quality of the particular motion as a possible variable, delineating the effects of the six possible types of movement.[26] The type of motion most likely to produce symptoms of motion sickness is up-and-down motion coupled with pitch (the bow of the ship dipping and rising). In other words, the head is undergoing rotation about one axis (pitch) and is simultaneously rotated about another axis (e.g., moving up and down).[14,27]

However, motion alone cannot explain why some individuals suffer motion sickness and others escape unscathed.[12]

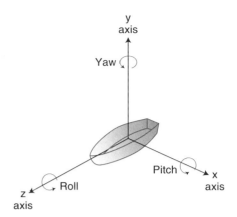

Figure 6.3. A seacraft experiences rotational motion around three axes, known as roll, pitch, and yaw.

As discussed below, various factors impact the effect of motion, as does an individual's adaptation to motion.

Factors Contributing to Motion Sickness

A person in control of a vehicle apparently has some degree of immunity to motion sickness.[28] The driver of an automobile and pilot of an aircraft, for example, are less likely to suffer than passengers.[29]

The duration of motion is also important. The longer the motion is sustained, the more likely the symptoms.

Food and drink also contribute to the incidence of motion sickness. In one study individuals who consumed more than two alcoholic drinks suffered less. On the other hand, patients suffering from motion sickness often complain about odors and seek cool, fresh air. Spicy foods and their associated aromas may worsen the situation.[6,12]

Fear and anxiety, too, increase the incidence of motion sickness.[30,31] Patients with a history of the condition may even become ill when contemplating an upcoming trip or when viewing the plane or ship.[6]

Adaptation to Motion

Several observations support the theory that individuals can develop tolerance to motion. For instance, previous experience in a particular motion environment usually confers a degree of immunity to motion sickness for that motion.[28] People who frequently travel on ships, for example, suffer from motion sickness less than those who rarely do so.[29] In addition, individuals exposed to constant nauseogenic motion find that symptoms often disappear after 2 or 3 days.[32]

Experts theorize that these repeated patterns of sensory mismatch are eventually added to a neural store of motion patterns.[9,10] Thus individuals update previously stored motion-association cues while learning that the body may indeed move in that pattern even though the visual field shows no movement. This adaptation may explain the decreasing incidence of motion sickness with age: as people expand their modes of travel, they are able to accommodate more types of sensory mismatch.

Adaptation to motion, while desirable to a traveler, is unfortunately the cause of a related problem, mal de debarque-ment syndrome.[2] In this case individuals may experience persistent feelings of motion for as long as several days after a sea voyage—even a voyage as short as 3 hours. This phenomenon has also been seen after train travel and space flight.

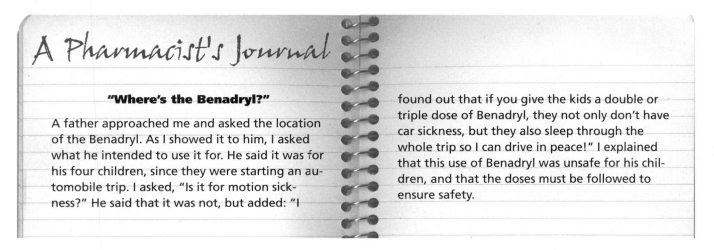

A Pharmacist's Journal

"Where's the Benadryl?"

A father approached me and asked the location of the Benadryl. As I showed it to him, I asked what he intended to use it for. He said it was for his four children, since they were starting an automobile trip. I asked, "Is it for motion sickness?" He said that it was not, but added: "I found out that if you give the kids a double or triple dose of Benadryl, they not only don't have car sickness, but they also sleep through the whole trip so I can drive in peace!" I explained that this use of Benadryl was unsafe for his children, and that the doses must be followed to ensure safety.

Patient Assessment Algorithm 6.1. Motion Sickness

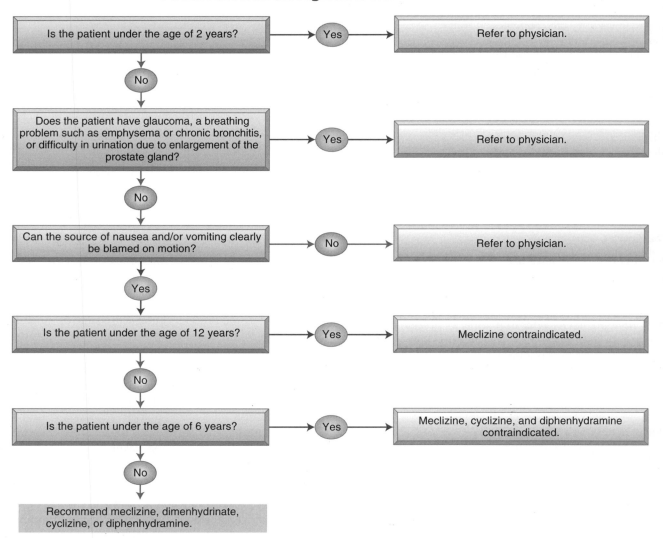

Table 6.1. Representative Motion Sickness Products

PRODUCT	SELECTED INGREDIENTS
Bonine Tablets	Meclizine 25 mg[a]
Diphenhydramine Tablets and Liquid	No product presently labeled for motion sickness[b]
Dramamine Less Drowsy Formula Tablets	Meclizine 25 mg[a]
Dramamine Liquid[b]	Per 5mL: Dimenhydrinate 12.5 mg, alcohol 5%
Dramamine Original Formula Tablets	Dimenhydrinate 50 mg[c]
Marezine Tablets	Cyclizine 50 mg[d]

[a]The dosage for meclizine is 25–50 mg once daily (12 and over, with a daily maximum of 150 mg); there is no dose under 12.

[b]The dosages for diphenhydramine are 25–50 mg q4–6h (12 and over, with a daily maximum of 300 mg); 12.5–25 mg q4–6h (6 through 11, with a daily maximum of 150 mg); there is no dose under 6.

[c]The dosages for dimenhydrinate are 50–100 mg q4–6h (12 and over, with a daily maximum of 400 mg); 25–50 mg q6–8h (6 through 11, with a daily maximum of 150 mg); 12.5–25 mg q6–8h (2 through 5, with a daily maximum of 75 mg).

[d]The dosages for cyclizine are 50 mg q4–6h (12 and over, with a daily maximum of 200 mg); 25 mg q6–8h (6 through 11, with a daily maximum of 75 mg); there is no dose under 6.

Impact of Motion Sickness

While motion sickness rarely causes severe health complications, the discomfort it produces can interfere with the sophisticated skills required of certain employees.[33–35] Further, anti–motion-sickness medications can reduce vigilance and alertness, which could lead to accidents. Ideal therapy would eliminate the annoying symptoms without producing adverse effects.

FOCUS ON...

GINGER AND MOTION SICKNESS

Although ginger has been used as a folk remedy against seasickness and is occasionally included in nonprescription drug products, it does not lessen the incidence of nausea or vertigo associated with motion sickness.[39,40] Ginger is a potent thromboxane synthetase inhibitor and could affect testosterone binding in the fetus if used by a pregnant woman.[41] This could lead to an adverse effect on sex steroid differentiation of the fetal brain.

TREATMENT OF MOTION SICKNESS

Treatment Guidelines

Patients often complain of nausea and vomiting. Pharmacists must discover whether patients have undergone recent motion. If there is no history of any provoking motion, nonprescription products are contraindicated. *These medications are not effective in treating or preventing nausea or vomiting resulting from other causes.*[27] (See "A Pharmacist's Journal: Where's the Benadryl?") Patients taking medications known to induce nausea, for example, should be referred to a physician to balance the risk versus benefit. (Patient Assessment Algorithm 6.1.)

Nonprescription Medications

Several antihistamines (e.g., cyclizine, dimenhydrinate, diphenhydramine, and meclizine) have been judged safe and effective by the FDA in motion sickness (Table 6.1). These nonprescription products can prevent motion sickness (see "Prevention of Motion Sickness") and reduce the severity of nausea, vomiting, and dizziness associated with motion sickness.[36]

In 1993 the FDA slightly changed the contraindications for nonprescription motion sickness products. The label warning now must read, *"Do not take this product, unless directed by a doctor, if you have a breathing problem such as emphysema or chronic bronchitis, or if you have glaucoma or difficulty in urination due to enlargement of the prostate gland."*[37]

Additional precautions include the following: "Use caution when driving a motor vehicle or operating heavy machinery."[36] If the product contains cyclizine or meclizine, it must state: "May cause drowsiness; alcohol, sedatives, and tranquilizers may increase the drowsiness effect. Do not take this product if you are taking sedatives or tranquilizers without first consulting your doctor." If the product contains dimenhydrinate or diphenhydramine, the warning above is the same, except it must state "marked" drowsiness in the first sentence. At this time, no manufacturer of diphenhydramine labels their product for motion sickness.

Nonpharmacologic Therapies

Alternative therapies such as acupressure bands have been proven ineffective for treating or preventing motion sickness[38] (see "Ginger and Motion Sickness").

AT THE COUNTER

A female patient about 20 asks what product she can take for an upcoming airplane trip that her college marching band is taking.

Interview/Patient Assessment

She suffered from periodic bouts of carsickness until she reached the age of 10 or 11 and thinks she may not need any product at all, but is anxious not to experience the problem in front of her friends. The only medication she is taking is triphasic birth-control tablets.

Pharmacist's Analysis

1. Do plane flights provoke motion sickness?
2. Since she no longer becomes carsick, is she likely to experience motion sickness of a plane flight?
3. Do her birth-control tablets present any problem with her therapy?
4. Which product, if any, should be recommended?

Plane flight presents unique motions to the body that are different from car travel. Thus, even though she has accommodated to travel via automobile, the plane may induce airsickness.

Patient Counseling

The medications pharmacists can recommend should be used cautiously with other central-nervous-system depressants, but are not contraindicated with birth-control tablets. At her age any product would be appropriate, although the 24-hour duration of meclizine makes it more convenient to take. Since dimenhydrinate and diphenhydramine cause marked drowsiness, they perhaps should be avoided. Whichever product she chooses, she may take it 30 minutes prior to departure if she wishes to prevent the problem. If she wishes to wait until symptoms occur, she may take the product as soon as she feels ill, although this is not as effective as prevention.

PREVENTION OF MOTION SICKNESS

Prevention of motion sickness is the preferred method of dealing with the condition. Nonprescription products are also helpful in prevention of the condition, but they must be taken at least 30 minutes prior to departure. Other interventions such as acupressure bands and devices have not been proven effective for prevention of motion sickness.

The neural mismatch theory is the basis for many preventive tips for motion sickness. These tips, which help travelers reconcile visual input with vestibular input to overcome the neural mismatch, include the following[6,16]:

- Immobilize the head or body, or shift the field of vision to include objects outside the vehicle.
- Sit where there is minimal motion such as over the wings of a plane, in the front seat of a car, and amidship or on the deck (rather than below deck) of a boat.
- Brace the head against the headrest to prevent head motion.
- Lie on the back, in a semirecumbent position, keeping the head as still as possible.
- Raise children in the car seat so that they can see out of the windows.
- Look outside the windows of a car. Looking only at the inside of the car worsens motion sickness.
- On a sea voyage choose a cabin with a porthole to gain an outside view.
- Avoid reading in a car.

SUMMARY

Motion sickness is thought to be caused by an imbalance between the visual organs and input from the proprioceptive system and/or vestibular apparatus. In some cases the body is moving, but the eyes do not perceive motion; in other cases the eyes see motion, but the proprioceptive system and vestibular apparatus cannot register any corresponding movement. These are known as neural-mismatch or sensory-conflict situations. While common, they need not present continuing problems for children or adults. The patient can be taught some commonsense steps to lessen the incidence of motion sickness and can take products to prevent symptoms from occurring. The same products are also effective when the symptoms have already begun. The only ingredients that are proven safe and effective for prevention and treatment of motion sickness are antihistamines.

References

1. Oman CM. Motion sickness: A synthesis and evaluation of the sensory conflict theory. Can J Physiol Pharmacol 68:294, 1990.
2. Noel P, Norris C. Motion sickness. J La State Med Soc 148:7, 1996.
3. Eden D, Zuk Y. Seasickness as a self-fulfilling prophecy: Raising self-efficacy to boost performance at sea. J Appl Psychol 80:628, 1995.
4. Stokoe D, Zuccollo G. Travel sickness in patients attending a geriatric day hospital. Age Aging 14:308, 1985.

5. Takahashi M, Ogata M, Miura M. Teleology of motion sickness. Acta Otolaryngol 115:130, 1995.
6. Rados B. When motion sickness goes along with the ride. FDA Consumer 19:6, 1985.
7. Scherer H, et al. On the origin of interindividual susceptibility to motion sickness. Acta Otolaryngol 117:149, 1997.
8. Parrott AC. Transdermal scopolamine: A review of its effects upon motion sickness, psychological performance, and physiological functioning. Aviat Space Environ Med 60:1, 1989.
9. Shupak A, et al. Vestibulo-ocular reflex as a parameter of seasickness susceptibility. Ann Otol Rhinol Laryngol 99(2 Pt 1):131, 1990.
10. Bagshaw M, Stott JRR. The desensitization of chronically motion sick aircrew in the Royal Air Force. Aviat Space Environ Med 56:1144, 1985.
11. Wood CD, et al. Evaluation of anti–motion sickness drug side effects on performance. Aviat Space Environ Med 56: 310, 1985.
12. Lawther A, Griffin MJ. A survey of the occurrence of motion sickness amongst passengers at sea. Aviat Space Environ Med 59:399, 1988.
13. Turner M, Griffin MJ. Motion sickness incidence during a round-the-world yacht race. Aviat Space Environ Med 66: 849, 1995.
14. Woodman PD, Griffin MJ. Effect of direction of head movement on motion sickness caused by Coriolis stimulation. Aviat Space Environ Med 68:93, 1997.
15. Cheung BSK, et al. Motion sickness susceptibility and aerobic fitness: A longitudinal study. Aviat Space Environ Med 61:201, 1990.
16. Dobie TG, May JG. The effectiveness of a motion sickness counselling programme. Br J Clin Psychol 34(Pt 2):301, 1995.
17. Eyeson-Annan M, et al. Visual and vestibular components of motion sickness. Aviat Space Environ Med 67:955, 1996.
18. Takahashi M, Ogata M, Miura M. The significance of motion sickness in the vestibular system. J Vestib Res 7:179, 1997.
19. Hausler R. Ski sickness. Acta Otolaryngol 115:1, 1995.
20. Regan EC, Ramsey AD. The efficacy of hyoscine hydrobromide in reducing side-effects induced during immersion in virtual reality. Aviat Space Environ Med 67:222, 1996.
21. Patel AS, et al. Microscopy motion sickness (Letter). N Engl J Med 318:1762, 1988.
22. Gillilan RW, Todd D. Vision therapy as a treatment for motion sickness. J Am Optom Assoc 57:456, 1986.
23. Jozsvai EE, Pigeau RA. The effect of autogenic training and biofeedback on motion sickness tolerance. Aviat Space Environ Med 67:963, 1996.
24. Hu S, et al. Motion sickness susceptibility to optokinetic rotation correlates to past history of motion sickness. Aviat Space Environ Med 67:320, 1996.
25. Thornton WE, et al. Gastrointestinal motility in space motion sickness. Aviat Space Environ Med 58(9 Pt 2):A16, 1987.
26. Lawther A, Griffin MJ. The motion of a ship at sea and the consequent motion sickness amongst passengers. Ergonomics 29:535, 1986.
27. Fed Reg 40:12933, 1975.
28. Wood CD, et al. Habituation and motion sickness. J Clin Pharmacol 34:628, 1994.
29. Fontenot C. Advice for the '90s traveler. J La State Med Soc 147:503, 1995.
30. Fox S, Arnon I. Motion sickness and anxiety. Aviat Space Environ Med 59:728, 1988.
31. Dobie TG, et al. An evaluation of cognitive-behavioral therapy for training resistance to visually-induced motion sickness. Aviat Space Environ Med 60:307, 1989.
32. Bouyer LJ, Watt DG. "Torso rotation" experiments. I. Adaptation to motion sickness does not correlate with changes in VOR gain. J Vestib Res 6:367, 1996.
33. Wright MS, Bose CL, Stiles AD. The incidence and effects of motion sickness among medical attendants during transport. J Emerg Med 13:15, 1995.
34. Golding JF, Markey HM. Effect of frequency of horizontal linear oscillation on motion sickness and somatogravic illusion. Aviat Space Environ Med 67:121, 1996.
35. Lindseth G, Lindseth PD. The relationship of diet to airsickness. Aviat Space Environ Med 66:537, 1995.
36. Fed Reg 52:15885, 1987.
37. Fed Reg 58:45215, 1993.
38. Bruce DG, et al. Acupressure and motion sickness. Aviat Space Environ Med 61:361, 1990.
39. Grøntved A, et al. Ginger root against seasickness. Acta Otolaryngol 105:45, 1988.
40. Holtmann S, et al. The anti–motion sickness mechanism of ginger. Acta Otolaryngol 108:168, 1989.
41. Backon J. Ginger in preventing nausea and vomiting of pregnancy: A caveat due to its thromboxane synthetase activity and effect on testosterone binding (Letter). Eur J Obstet Gynecol Reprod Biol 42:163, 1991.

CHAPTER 7

Intestinal Gas Discomfort: Bloating and Flatulence

A young man who appears to be in his late 20s approaches the pharmacist with a bottle of simethicone tablets. He asks whether the product is for gas.

Interview/Patient Assessment

The pharmacist answers affirmatively, then questions the patient further. The young man says that for the past few months he has had bouts of constipation, during which his gas seems to worsen, alternating with episodes of diarrhea that last for several days. The gas is also fairly painful during the diarrheal episodes. His abdomen is often distended, with frequent rumbling caused by the entrapped gas. He is taking no medications on a regular basis and has no diagnosed health problems.

Pharmacist's Analysis

1. Are the patient's symptoms consistent with a minor, self-treatable complaint?

2. What are the possible causes of this patient's complaint?
3. What should the pharmacist recommend for this patient?

This patient presents with troubling symptoms, of which gas is only one aspect. The reason for constipation alternating with diarrhea could be the result of underlying problems such as irritable bowel syndrome, food allergies, lactose intolerance, or fecal impaction. Some of these are self-treatable, but others are not.

Patient Counseling

The patient should be questioned about such symptoms as blood in the stools, passing mucus, and involuntary staining. Unless further questioning can help the pharmacist rule out more serious conditions, he should be referred for a medical evaluation.

When patients complain of bloating, they could be referring to excess intestinal gas, but they also may be experiencing abdominal swelling from other causes. (Actual abdominal pain may indicate serious diseases such as colon cancer, so these symptoms should be screened by a physician.[1–3]) Discomfort from bloating and intestinal gas can be so acute the patients experience an increase in girth and cannot fasten clothing about the waist.[4]

PREVALENCE OF BLOATING AND INTESTINAL GAS

Although not well documented, bloating and **flatulence** (excessive air or other gas in the stomach and/or intestines) are two of the most common complaints encountered by medical personnel.[5]

A study of triathletes showed that 48% complained of flatulence.[6] A full 74.4% of bulimic patients and 90% of anorectics complained of bloating and flatulence.[7,8] Eighty-three percent of lactose-intolerant children experienced bloating and 44% experienced flatulence.[9] The relative paucity of prevalence data for the general population undoubtedly reflects the fact that discussions about bloating and flatulence are not considered to be "polite."

EPIDEMIOLOGY OF BLOATING AND INTESTINAL GAS

Data on the epidemiology of bloating is scarce. However, it is well known that women complain of abdominal disten-

tion caused by intestinal gas prior to menses and at menopause.[10]

Air Swallowing

Bloating also may refer to **eructation** (belching of air). It is normal to expel a small amount of air orally following a meal.[11] Some individuals, however, complain of excessive burping and feel that it is related to a total picture of gaseousness. Actually, in most cases air that is burped has been swallowed. Some patients with stomach problems or intestinal gas react by sucking in air and producing a noisy burp. They may even be unaware that they are causing their own belching by swallowing air. These patients may compound their problems because some of the swallowed air is retained in the body, leading to further discomfort and further belching.[12] Patients caught in this cycle are often those with nervous, tense, and anxious personality types.

Excessive belching occasionally results from other causes such as excessive talking, gum chewing, or ill-fitting dentures.[11] It may also be caused by an underlying disease. For this reason a physician should be consulted for any excessive belching.

Medical Conditions

Lactose intolerance (See Chapter 9) and other food allergies/intolerances can cause bloating and flatulence, usually coupled with diarrhea and related gastrointestinal (GI) complaints.[13–16] Several other medical conditions also cause excess flatus:

- Patients with irritable bowel syndrome often have abdominal distention and excess flatus as their major complaints.[2]

- Subacute intestinal obstruction—a medical emergency—must also be considered in patients with excess flatus.
- Giardiasis, peptic ulcer disease, and **cholelithiasis** (concretions in the gallbladder or bile ducts) are possible.[17,18]

Malabsorption syndromes—such as celiac disease (sprue) or pancreatic insufficiency—allow unabsorbed nutrients to pass through the intestines, possibly resulting in bacterial fermentation and excess gas.[19] Both the mechanisms and symptoms are similar to lactose intolerance.

Some patients with cancer undergo laryngeal removal, which inhibits normal speech. With one technique used to produce speech, the patients are taught to speak by taking air into the esophagus and stomach, then expelling it while they form words with the mouth and tongue. Unfortunately, patients are usually unable to eliminate all of the air vocally, resulting in flatulence.

ETIOLOGY OF BLOATING AND INTESTINAL GAS

Several kinds of problems can cause bloating and excessive intestinal gas, including ingestion of legumes and other flatulogenic foods and the use of certain sweeteners. In addition, some medications have been implicated in producing excessive gas (see "Medications and Flatulence").

Normal Parameters for Intestinal Gas

The average individual normally has 150 to 200 mL of gas or less in the stomach and colon at any one time.[22,23] An average fasting gas volume is 100 mL (range = 30 to 200 mL) with a maximum of about 50 mL in the stomach. The amount expelled in average individuals is 476 to 1491 mL daily.[24,25] People experience 10 to 18 gas elimination episodes daily.[11,20,26] Gas in excess of these normal values may be construed by the sufferer to be excessive flatulence.

Sensitivity to Gas Movement

Not all complaints of bloating can be ascribed to amounts of gas that exceed these averages noted above.[27] Other factors must be taken into consideration. For example, in some patients the rectum is abnormally sensitive to normal amounts of liquid or gas.[28] With these patients problems stem from an increased consciousness of intestinal contraction and an exquisite sensitivity to overall gas movement.[27] These patients also may suffer from retrograde movement of intestinal gas.[29]

A study compared 12 patients with chronic complaints of gas to a control group of patients without these problems. Gastrointestinal gas volumes in both groups were equal. However, when gas was infused into the intestines of both

FOCUS ON...

MEDICATIONS AND FLATULENCE

Bulk laxative products containing fermentable carbohydrate (e.g., psyllium) can cause flatulence as an adverse reaction.[20,21] (The nonfermentable bulk laxative methylcellulose does not.) The dietary supplement Lactinex, which is not approved for any use, also causes flatulence. Prescription medications that may cause flatulence include certain antibiotics (e.g., oral carbenicillin or cephalexin and parenteral piperacillin or ticarcillin), NSAIDs (e.g., ibuprofen, ketoprofen, naproxen, piroxicam), quinolones (e.g., ciprofloxacin, norfloxacin), nicotine gum, lactulose, and cholestyramine.[21]

groups, the group bothered by gas was found to suffer from abnormal motility resulting in disordered passage of gas through the bowel, with a more painful response to overall gas volume.[29]

Sources and Composition of Gas

Clues to the causes of excess flatulence can come from analysis of the gases. Gas originates from swallowed atmospheric air, bicarbonate neutralization of stomach acids, diffusion of gases into the intestine from blood, and bacterial fermentation (Fig. 7.1).[30]

In regard to swallowed atmospheric air, a small amount of gas accompanies each mouthful of food, but passes from the stomach to the colon within 20 minutes.[27] The composition of expelled gas reflects the composition of ambient air in the patient who habitually swallows air. Ambient air contains approximately 78% nitrogen, while expelled air may contain 17 to 80% nitrogen.[22,23] While nitrogen is the major bowel gas for virtually all individuals, another source is diffusion from the blood into the bowel lumen. Thus using nitrogen as an indicator of the amount of swallowed air is difficult. Also, although ambient air contains about 21% oxygen, flatus typically contains less than 10%, presumably because of rapid utilization by bacteria.[30]

Intraluminal gas production results from bacterial fermentation/metabolism producing the three remaining major bowel gases: hydrogen, carbon dioxide, and methane (Fig. 7.2).[10] Although human newborns (and lab animals grown in sterile environments) do not produce methane or hydrogen, within hours of birth (or introduction of the lab animal to ambient air) both gases are detected in animal experiments.[19] Evidently, bacteria are the sole sources of these gases.[31]

Carbon dioxide is produced as a by-product of bicarbonate acidification of intestinal secretions.[22,23] Acid utilized in this reaction may come from the gastric mucosa or from fat digestion resulting in release of fatty acids. Several liters of carbon dioxide may be formed in the duodenum after a meal, although its rapid absorption by the body prevents painful distention.

Methane is produced by about one-third of the population of the United States.[10] It is seldom a component of gas in humans before age 2. Subsequently, however, about 30% of North American and European individuals harbor

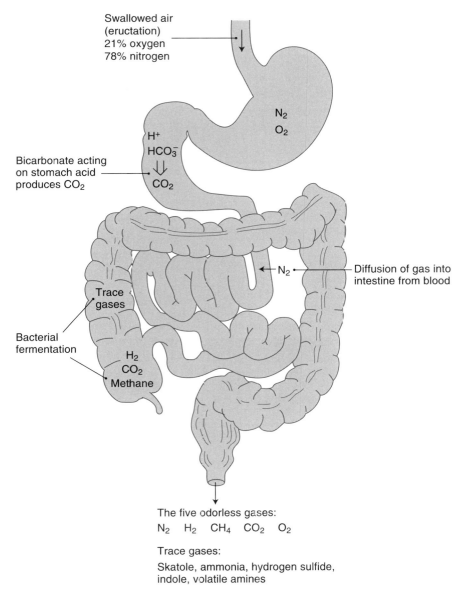

Swallowed air
(eructation)
21% oxygen
78% nitrogen

N_2
O_2

H^+
HCO_3^-

Bicarbonate acting
on stomach acid
produces CO_2

CO_2

N_2 — Diffusion of gas into
intestine from blood

Trace
gases

Bacterial
fermentation

H_2
CO_2
Methane

The five odorless gases:
N_2 H_2 CH_4 CO_2 O_2

Trace gases:
Skatole, ammonia, hydrogen sulfide,
indole, volatile amines

Figure 7.1. The sources and composition of intestinal gas.

methane-producing anaerobes such as *Methobacterium rumenatium* and *Methanobrevibacter smithii.*[29] The tendency to harbor these organisms is familial[10]: when both parents produce methane, 92% of children do also. Fully 84% of individuals with siblings who produce methane also do so, whereas only 18% of individuals without methane-producing siblings do so.

Methane is of clinical importance because methane-laden stools are more likely to float than stools containing other gases.[29] Although floating stools are a time-honored sign of **steatorrhea** (passage of large amounts of fats in the feces), one investigation found that fat content had no role in determining whether stools from healthy subjects float. The tendency to float was instead dependent on methane content.[32]

Methane is also a possible marker for colorectal cancer. Ninety-one percent of patients with colon cancer produce methane, while only 30% of control patients do so.[33] While the exact significance of this finding is unknown, methane may indicate a colonic environment that is conducive to carcinoma.

The five odorless gases already mentioned comprise over 99% of intestinal gas.[23] The well-known odor of flatus is due to trace gases (e.g., skatole, ammonia, hydrogen sulfide, indole, and volatile amines), as well as short-chain fatty acids, which can be detected by humans in amounts as low as one part per 100 million.[10,22,29] Their source is generally either colonic anaerobic bacteria or the diet.[30,34]

Legumes As Sources of Gas

The foods most blamed for gaseous episodes are the legumes. Beans contain the indigestible oligosaccharides raffinose, stachyose, and verbascose (Fig. 7.3).[33] Raffinose and stachyose are also found in the cellulose outer coatings of the seeds of legumes such as chickpeas, lentils, navy beans, string beans, and soy beans.[33] These oligosaccharides pass through

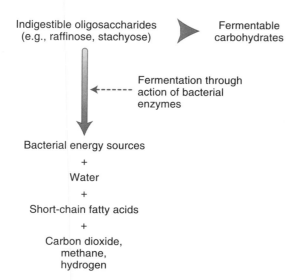

Figure 7.2. The process by which bacteria utilize indigestible oligosaccharides as a nutrient source, producing metabolic by-products, including gases.

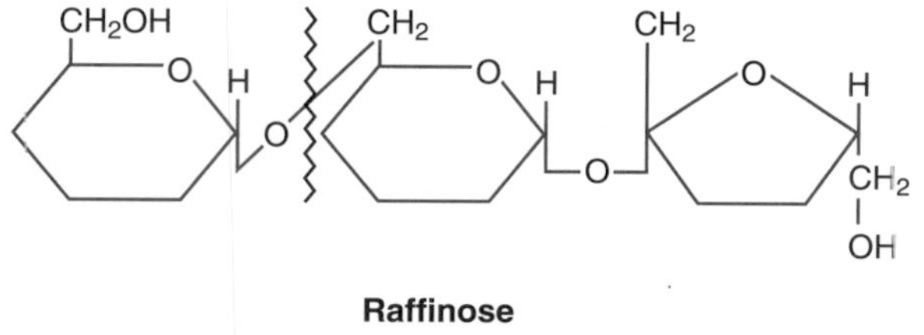

Raffinose

Figure 7.3. The site of action of the enzyme alpha-galactosidase (Beano) on raffinose, an oligosaccharide found in beans and other foods.

the body, reaching the colon in a form utilizable by colonic bacteria. As the bacteria feed on them, they produce gas as a by-product. Researchers are attempting to produce a variety of bean that does not contain these oligosaccharides. This research, using the California small white bean, has not yet been successful.

Other Foods As Sources of Gas

A large group of diverse foods have also been charged with causing intestinal gas because of the indigestible carbohydrates (e.g., fructo-oligosaccharides) they contain; this group includes artichokes, asparagus, broccoli, Brussels sprouts, cabbage, carrots, cauliflower, celery, corn, cucumber, eggplant, lettuce, onions, peas, potatoes, and squash.[10,11,29] Cereals and grain products such as bran, barley, wheat flour, rye, rice, and oats may add to the problem. Some authors add chili (perhaps because of its spices and beans), nuts, and seeds to the list.

Foods that contain air may not be appreciated as sources of intestinal gas. For instance, much of an apple is air.[10] Foods that have air whipped into them (e.g., milkshakes and whipped cream) would be obvious targets for elimination

from the diet. Carbonated beverages such as soft drinks and beer also contain a good deal of air that may contribute to gaseousness. Finally, fatty foods may slow the movement of gas through the person by slowing intestinal transit time, increasing the bloated feeling.

Sweeteners

Several sweeteners can cause gas because of their poor absorption. Fructose has been used as the preferred sweetener by the two largest soda manufacturers in a number of their drinks.[11] However, some patients cannot absorb it well, resulting in complaints of cramping, diarrhea, and flatulence. Sorbitol and mannitol serve as sweeteners in some sugar-free products.[22] They also produce diarrhea, gas, and bloating in some people.[35–37] Individuals afflicted with intestinal gas would be well advised to search product labels for sweetener sources of flatulence.

COMPLICATIONS OF BLOATING AND INTESTINAL GAS

For most patients bloating presents only minor discomfort, and flatulence is socially embarrassing, but nothing more. For others the psychologic effects of bloating or excess gas are devastating, and they may suffer intense social embarrassment.[38] Patients may suffer such a severe fear of passing gas that they voluntarily withdraw from social contacts and give up lucrative careers.[39,40]

Occasionally, patients may even fear that flatulence indicates a dread disease such as cancer.[11] Fortunately, excess gas seldom is caused by a serious organic disease.

Excessive intestinal gas can cause clinical problems. A gas-distended bowel increases the risk of gut necrosis or perforation following a mechanical bowel obstruction. Also, explosions during **electrocautery** (directing a high-frequency electrical current through tissue) have been traced to ignition of the methane and hydrogen gases of flatus during polypectomy when an electric current is passed through the polyp.[11]

Individuals with intraabdominal gas may notice an increasing sensation of discomfort when flying in a pressurized airplane. Large shifts in the pressure of ambient air can cause trapped gas to expand, a phenomenon known as "trapped gas dysbarism."[41]

TREATMENT OF BLOATING AND INTESTINAL GAS

Treatment Guidelines

Patients complaining about bloating or gas are usually most concerned about excess flatus, a socially embarrassing topic for which there is a paucity of information available to the patient. Patients may request information about gaseousness, its various causes, and possible interventions. (See Patient Assessment Algorithm 7.1.)

Patient Assessment Algorithm 7.1. Bloating and Flatulence

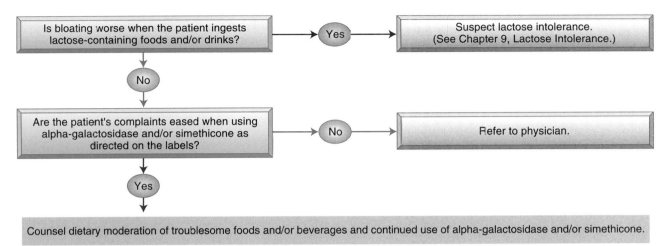

Nonprescription Medications

ALPHA-GALACTOSIDASE

A product known as Beano tablets or liquid may be helpful in the prevention of gas (Table 7.1).[11] Beano contains alpha-galactosidase, which degrades the oligosaccharides that cause gaseousness into easily digestible sugars such as sucrose and glucose. The patient swallows or chews two to three tablets with the first bite of food or adds three to eight drops to the first spoonful. This quantity usually takes care of an entire serving. Because heat will inactivate Beano (hot food should cool to less than 130°F before adding it), Beano cannot be added to food while it is cooking. (See "A Pharmacist's Journal: 'I Can Eat Chili!'")

A preliminary FDA opinion held that the product would not have to go through the FDA nonprescription review process as it is a natural enzyme acting on foods. However, the FDA may still require the product to prove efficacy. In one such study patients were fed two meals of meatless chili at two different times, once with Beano and once without Beano. When the meal was ingested with Beano, the number of flatus events was significantly less.[42]

Since it is produced from the mold *Aspergillus niger*, perhaps one individual in 1000 may experience an allergic reaction to Beano such as stomach upset or skin rash. *Penicillin-sensitive individuals are at higher risk for allergy.*[43]

SIMETHICONE

Simethicone is a defoaming agent that was used in endoscopic procedures to clear small bubbles that obscured the visual field when bile mixed with infused air.[11] That use led to the theory that it might also alter the elasticity of interfaces of mucus-embedded bubbles in the GI tract, thus allowing the gas bubbles to coalesce. In this form gas is more easily eliminated as belching or flatus.

Simethicone does not produce any systemic adverse reactions since it is not absorbed at all from the GI tract.[29] Simethicone is currently the only OTC antiflatulent recognized by

the FDA as safe and effective (Table 7.1).[44] It relieves symptoms of bloating, pressure, fullness, or stuffed feeling caused by gas. There is no specific lower age limit for its safe use. While it is referred to as an antiflatulent, this is not exactly a correct term. The person must still eliminate the excess gas. The product facilitates passage of gas through the GI tract, allowing the patient to more effectively eliminate large pockets at one time.

ACTIVATED CHARCOAL

Activated charcoal has received some support in the literature for reducing the number of flatus events and improving symptoms of gaseousness.[23,29] However, the weight of evidence is far from overwhelming.[11,28] Additionally, activated charcoal has not been approved for symptoms of gas by the FDA nonprescription review process.[45] Therefore, manufacturers of combination products containing simethicone and charcoal cannot claim that the products provide any benefit other than that solely resulting from the simethicone. These combinations are not FDA-approved.

Nonpharmacologic Therapies

LIFESTYLE MODIFICATIONS

Individuals who chew gum or tobacco usually swallow small amounts of air. Likewise, smokers usually swallow air whether they inhale or not.[11] Controlling these habits may be helpful in preventing gas.

Posture may also have an impact on bloating and flatulence. Drinking or eating while lying down prevents gas in the stomach from escaping through the esophagus for elimination through burping.[10,22] Trapped air must then pass through the intestines. Thus *individuals should remain upright for several hours after each meal.*

DIETARY INTERVENTIONS

Individuals bothered by gas might find relief simply by avoiding troublesome foods. Since lactose intolerance causes flat-

Table 7.1. Representative Products for Intestinal Gas Discomfort: Bloating and Flatulence	
PRODUCT	SELECTED INGREDIENTS/COMMENTS
Beano Solution	Per 5 drops: alpha-galactosidase 150 units
Beano Tablets	Alpha-galactosidase 150 units
Gas-X Tablets	Simethicone 80 mg
Gas-X Extra Strength Tablets	Simethicone 125 mg
Infant's Mylicon Drops	Per 0.3 mL, simethicone 20 mg
Infant's Mylicon Drops Non-Staining	Per 0.3 mL, simethicone 20 mg
Maalox Anti-Gas Extra Strength Tablets	Simethicone 150 mg
Mylanta Gas Tablets	Simethicone 62.5 mg
Mylanta Gas Maximum Strength Tablets	Simethicone 125 mg
Phazyme Drops for Infants	Per 0.6 mL, simethicone 40 mg
Phazyme Softgels Extra Strength	Simethicone 125 mg
Phazyme Softgels Maximum Strength	Simethicone 166 mg

A Pharmacist's Journal

"I Can Eat Chili!"

An older woman was hovering in the vicinity of the gastrointestinal products, so I approached her and asked if I could help her. She picked up a bottle of Beano liquid and said, "I hope you never run out of this stuff. I have been able to eat chili again for the first time in 20 years." She actually began to cry as she continued, "You can't imagine what it's like to have such stomach problems that you have to deny yourself one of your favorite foods. And then, to be able to eat it again after all this time . . . ." I assured her that we would always try to keep the product in stock.

ulence (See Chapter 9, Lactose Intolerance), the individual with this problem should either reduce the amount of lactose ingested or use products containing a lactase enzyme to aid indigestion of the lactose.[11] Carbonated beverages (soft drinks and beer) can cause excess gas to be swallowed, as can chewing gum and sucking on hard candies.[11] All should be avoided. Rapid eating can cause more air to be swallowed; patients should take care to eat slowly and masticate the food thoroughly.

CARMINATIVES

Carminatives (medications such as peppermint, which reduce the pressure of the lower esophageal sphincter, allowing the person to belch) have been recommended for many years to help alleviate gaseousness and bloating after a meal.[11] However, they worsen the problem of gastroesophageal reflux. Additionally, they have never been found effective in preventing excessive gas or easing its passage through the GI tract.[28]

SUMMARY

Bloating can result in flatulence that, for most people, can be a minor annoyance. However, because of dietary or medical problems, some individuals experience real discomfort from these conditions and acute embarrassment when flatulence occurs at socially inappropriate times. For these patients pharmacists can give excellent advice regarding dietary and

AT THE COUNTER

 A male in his mid 30s asks the pharmacist to help him with his gas problem.

Interview/Patient Assessment

He is especially bothered when he eats "Mexican food" because it causes embarrassing flatulence for the next day or two. He denies use of medications and says he has no other health problems. He is not bothered appreciably by gas at any other times.

Pharmacist's Analysis

1. What is the probable cause of this man's gas?
2. What intervention(s) can the pharmacist recommend?
3. How should the patient use products available to deal with the gas?

The fact that he only has problems in conjunction with a certain type of food implicates that food. Typical "Mexican food" may include possibly flatulogenic foods such as peppers, onions, refried beans, and lettuce.

Patient Counseling

The pharmacist should suggest moderation of these foods, coupled with judicious use of Beano and simethicone products. Use of Beano at the time of ingestion can help prevent gas production, and use of simethicone after ingestion can ease passage of gas through the bowel. Should these fail to ease the symptoms, the patient may need to completely eliminate the suspected foods from his diet.

---

lifestyle modifications to reduce bloating and flatulence. Bloating may be caused by air swallowing and medical conditions, as well as numerous components of the diet. The diet may be modified to eliminate or reduce the flatulogenic foods and beverages. Should this be ineffective, patients may choose to ingest a product containing alpha-galactosidase when foods containing oligosaccharides (e.g., legumes) are eaten. (This enzyme breaks down the complex starches, allowing them to be digested.) Simethicone is also effective for relieving bloating by easing the passage and excretion of flatus.

References

1. Curless R, et al. Comparison of gastrointestinal symptoms in colorectal carcinoma patients and community controls with respect to gas. Gut 35:1267, 1994.
2. Heitkemper MM, et al. Daily gastrointestinal symptoms in women with and without a diagnosis of IBS. Dig Dis Sci 40:1511, 199.5
3. Hyams JS. Intestinal gas in childhood (Editorial). Curr Opin Pediatr 8:467, 1996.
4. Sullivan SN. A prospective study of unexplained visible abdominal bloating. NZ Med J 107:428, 1994.
5. Tawfik C, et al. A simple radiological method to estimate the quantity of bowel gas. Am J Gastroenterol 86:599, 1991.
6. Rehrer NJ, et al. Gastrointestinal complaints in relation to dietary intake in triathletes. Int J Sport Nutr 2:48, 1992.
7. Chami TN, et al. Gastrointestinal symptoms in bulimia nervosa: Effects of treatment. Am J Gastroenterol 90:88, 1995.
8. Kamal N, et al. Delayed gastrointestinal transit times in anorexia nervosa and bulimia nervosa. Gastroenterology 101:1320, 1991.
9. Medow MS, et al. Beta-galactosidase tablets in the treatment of lactose intolerance in pediatrics. Am J Dis Child 144:1261, 1990.
10. Bouchier IAD. Flatulence. Practitioner 224:373, 1980.
11. Clearfield HR. Clinical intestinal gas syndromes. Prim Care 23:621, 1996.
12. Lundell LR, Myers JC, Jamieson GG. Delayed gastric emptying and its relationship to symptoms of "gas float" after antireflux surgery. Eur J Surg 160:161, 1994.
13. Hermans MMH, et al. The relationship between lactose intolerance test results and symptoms of lactose intolerance. Am J Gastroenterol 92:981, 1997.
14. Hammer HF, et al. Evaluation of the pathogenesis of flatulence and abdominal cramps in patients with lactose malabsorption. Wein Klin Wochenschr 108:175, 1996.
15. Webster RB, DiPalma JA, Gremse DA. Lactose maldigestion and recurrent abdominal pain in children. Dig Dis Sci 40:1506, 1995.
16. Gudmand-Hyer E. The clinical significance of disaccharide maldigestion. Am J Clin Nutr 59(Suppl 3):735S, 1994.
17. Bartes T, et al. Influence of cholecystectomy on symptoms. Br J Surg 78:964, 1991.
18. Egbert AM. Gallstone symptoms. Postgrad Med 90:119, 1991.
19. Levine AS. The relationship of diet to intestinal gas. J Med Soc NJ 76:921, 1979.
20. Levitt MD, Furne J, Olsson S. The relation of passage of gas and abdominal bloating to colonic gas production. Ann Intern Med 124:422, 1996.
21. McEvoy GK, ed. AHFS 97 Drug Information: Bethesda, MD: American Society of Health-System Pharmacists, 1997.
22. Altman DF. Downwind update—A discourse on matters gaseous. West J Med 145:502, 1986.
23. Hall RG Jr, et al. Effects of orally administered activated charcoal on intestinal gas. Am J Gastroenterol 75:192, 1981.
24. Tomlin J, Lowis C, Read NW. Investigation of normal flatus production in healthy volunteers. Gut 32:665, 1991.
25. Furne JK, Levitt MD. Factors influencing frequency of flatus emission by healthy subjects. Dig Dis Sci 41:1631, 1996.
26. Bassotti G, et al. Flatus-related colorectal and anal motor events. Dig Dis Sci 41:335, 1996.

27. Sferra TJ, Heitlinger LA. Gastrointestinal gas formation and infantile colic. Pediatr Clin North Am 43:489, 1996.

28. Fardy J, Sullivan S. Gastrointestinal gas. Can Med Assoc J 139: 1137, 1988.

29. Van Ness MM, Cattau EL. Flatulence: Pathophysiology and treatment. Am Fam Physician 31:198, 1985.

30. Suarez F, et al. Insights into human colonic physiology obtained from the study of flatus composition. Am J Physiol 272 (5 Pt 1):G1028, 1997.

31. Cummings JH. Fermentation in the human large intestine: Evidence and implications for health. Lancet 1:1206, 1983.

32. Levitt MD, Duane WC. Floating stools—Flatus versus fat. N Engl J Med 286:973, 1972.

33. Danzl DF. Flatology. J Emerg Med 10:79, 1992.

34. Hammer HF. Colonic hydrogen absorption: Quantification of its effect on hydrogen accumulation caused by bacterial fermentation of carbohydrates. Gut 34:818, 1993.

35. Kajs TM, et al. Influence of a methanogenic flora on the breath H2 and symptom response to ingestion of sorbitol or oat fiber. Am J Gastroenterol 92:89, 1997.

36. Breitenbach RA. "Halloween diarrhea." Postgrad Med 92: 63, 1992.

37. Oberrieder HK, Fryer EB. College students' knowledge and consumption of sorbitol. J Am Diet Assoc 91:715, 1991.

38. Song JY, et al. Anxiety and depression in patients with abdominal bloating. Can J Psychiatry 38:475, 1993.

39. Lyketsos CG. Successful treatment of bowel obsessions with nortriptyline (Letter). Am J Psychiatry 149:573, 1992.

40. Fishbain DA, Goldberg M. Fluoxetine for obsessive fear of loss of control of malodorous flatulence. Psychosomatics 32:105, 1991.

41. Leonard F. You're the flight surgeon. Aviat Space Environ Med 64:668, 1993.

42. Ganiats TG, et al. Does Beano prevent gas? A double-blind crossover study of oral alpha-galactosidase to treat dietary oligosaccharide intolerance. J Fam Pract 39:441, 1994.

43. Anon (leaflet). Recommend Beano. AK Pharma Inc., undated

44. Fed Reg 53:2715, 1988.

45. Fed Reg 44:8836, 1996.

Infant Colic

AT THE COUNTER

An elderly woman wheels a cart into the pharmacy with a young baby inside. She wants to know about colic.

Interview/Patient Assessment

She cares for the child during the day while her daughter, a single mother, is at work. The child cannot be left at home since the daughter's boyfriend is unreliable because of his drinking and possible drug use. The grandmother is concerned because the 8-month-old child cries for the first few hours after she is dropped off at 7:40 AM. However, she doesn't cry when the grandmother is feeding her during the day. She also asks the pharmacist's advice about several dark marks appearing to be bruises on the child's trunk.

Pharmacist's Analysis

1. Do the child's symptoms appear to be colic?
2. What might be the significance of the crying and marks on the trunk?

3. What is the legal responsibility of the pharmacist in this situation?

Colic usually manifests in the late evening rather than the morning. The child's unstable home life, coupled with possible evidence of abuse (e.g., crying and bruises), should raise the possibility of abuse in the pharmacist's mind, either by the mother or her live-in boyfriend. Any individual who suspects child abuse should report that abuse; in some states failure to report suspected abuse is a prosecutable offense.

Patient Counseling

While it certainly may be unwarranted, the pharmacist must warn the grandmother that the child's situation should be brought to the attention of the authorities because of the child's bruises. Also, the pharmacist should tell her that the baby's symptoms are not indicative of colic.

The word "colic" is derived from the Greek root for "colon," reflecting the early belief that the problem involved the large intestine in some way.[1,2] Colic is usually a minor self-limiting problem of infancy, but nonetheless it can place major stress on the normal parent-child relationship. Fortunately, a number of interventions seem to provide benefit in some cases, including a nonprescription ingredient.

PREVALENCE OF COLIC

Infant colic occurs in 10 to 35% of infants.[1,3-9] Its occurrence in a given infant may be caused by multifactorial etiologies, consisting of a combination of psychologic or functional disorders overlaid with such inciting factors as diet and posture.[10]

EPIDEMIOLOGY OF COLIC

Certain epidemiologic variables can assist in identifying infants that are suffering from colic, including the age of onset. Colic may occur as early as the third day of life, but more often it manifests between the second or third week.[1,6,11] It is most severe at 4 to 6 weeks.[3] Colic occurs more frequently with older mothers and mothers of above-average intelligence and education, although it does not appear to be affected by the mother's employment status.[3,12] Fathers of colicky infants are also more educated than those of noncolicky infants.[13] Birth order may play some role, as colic tends to be more common in firstborn children.[3,12] Babies whose siblings were colicky are also more likely to experience colic. There is no gender difference with colic.[7,13] Also, the incidence of colic is not influenced by a parental history of colic or allergy.[3,13]

ETIOLOGY OF COLIC

Experts have proposed many etiologies for colic, which can be usefully categorized as arising from either gastrointestinal or behavioral-interactional causes.[14]

Intestinal Gas

The observation that infants sometimes experience flatulence during colic episodes has led to the conclusion that the gas is the causative agent.[15,16] Investigators hypothesize that trapped gas in the bowel results in painful intestinal contractions.[17] Gas is normally taken in by the infant as an unavoidable consequence of coordinating suckling with breathing.[11] Should the gas accumulate in the large bowel, as in a constipated infant, a colic episode could be induced as a result.

Gas may also be produced as a result of malabsorption disorders such as lactose intolerance or incomplete digestion of carbohydrate.[14] Undigested lactose and carbohydrates act as substrates for bacterial fermentation.[18] (See "Sources and Composition of Gas" in Chapter 7 for a more complete discussion of intraluminal gas production.) The assumption that gas is a primary causative agent in colic has led to the widespread nonprescription use of the defrothicant simethicone.

Lactose Intolerance

Various investigators have explored the hypothesis that lactose intolerance may be a primary factor in producing gas that triggers colic pain. Some research seems to verify the role of lactose.[19] However, other authors disagree, leading to the viewpoint that the child should not be placed on a lactose-free formula.[15,20,21]

Cow's Milk Allergy

The results of studies that have attempted to pin colic to a true allergy to the proteins or other components of cow's milk are contradictory.[3,6,8,14,11,22] Research that seems to implicate cow's milk is undermined by the fact that babies who are fed breast milk also develop colic, as well as by studies that simply do not show such an association.[4,23,24]

Maternal Diet

Should a mother drink cow's milk, investigators have demonstrated that the whey protein known as beta-lactoglobulin and bovine IgG can be transmitted to the child through the mother's breast milk, causing allergic symptoms that result in colic.[4,5,25] Thus even a child not given cow's milk may eventually develop an allergy to cow's milk proteins found in the mother's breast milk.

Additional research implicates maternal ingestion of cruciferous vegetables (e.g., cabbage, cauliflower, broccoli), onion, and chocolate in causing colic in their breast-fed infants.[26]

Functional Gastrointestinal Disorders

Colic may also be caused by a functional gastrointestinal (GI) problem such as intestinal hypermotility, spasm, and/or spasticity.[5,15,27,28] The immature GI tract may also be inefficient at allowing effective expulsion of gas, a theory that has led to prescribing antispasmodics for the problem, in spite of the fact that evidence to support their efficacy is weak.[6,18] Children with colic have a hypercontractility of the gallbladder not seen in normal controls.[29] Colicky babies of 3 months more often have intestinal colonization with *Clostridium difficile,* although colic itself may predispose to this colonization.[30]

Parental-Child-Environmental Interactions

Some authors suggest that colic is not a true medical condition, but is rather a response of the child to parental behaviors or to the environment.[14,31–33] For instance, a specific infant may have an inherent predisposition to cry more readily, combined with a low sensory threshold.[11,18] When combined with heightened parental tension, anger, impaired coping skills, and lack of training, colic may be the unfortunate result.[11]

Further, simply having a new baby in the house alters the interactions of the other family members; if the new baby has colic, stress levels rise.[3,5,34] Of course, colic increases stress levels even further, creating a vicious cycle of stress leading to colic that increases the stress and thereby further increases the occurrence of colic. Certain parental factors also seem to contribute to the problem. For instance, cigarette smoking increases the incidence of infant colic in breast-fed babies.[35] For the most part, however, attributes of the parent have not been shown to be causal factors in the genesis of colic.[18]

Serious Conditions Misinterpreted As Colic

Clinicians point out the fallacy of ascribing all infant crying to the grab-bag of colic. Specifically, abdominal pain resulting in crying may be caused by other conditions such as pinworm infestation or lead toxicity.[36,37] Additionally, excessive crying may be a marker for child abuse. In one case an infant diagnosed in an emergency department with continual crying was misdiagnosed with colic and discharged.[38] When rushed back to the same hospital 9 hours later, she had expired as a result of shaken-baby syndrome.

MANIFESTATIONS OF COLIC

Some experts question whether colic is a distinct clinical syndrome, or whether infants who suffer from it are perceived to cry excessively when compared with other infants.[18,39–41] In an attempt to sidestep the issue, various definitions have been offered for colic, mostly through quantifying the number and duration of episodes.

A useful definition of colic uses the "rule of 3 times 4."[42] Using this definition, colic has the following characteristics:

1. Usually occurs within the first 3 months of life with an otherwise healthy and well-fed infant, who has violent paroxysms of irritability, unexplained fussing, or full-force crying (which may develop into agonizing screaming)
2. Lasts more than 3 hours a day
3. Occurs on more than 3 days in any one week
4. Continues for at least 3 weeks

A "cry diary" can be a helpful diagnostic tool (Fig 8.1).[31] A parent or caregiver may record episodes of crying, fussiness, and relaxation.[43]

The crying that occurs with colic has become an integral part of the widely accepted definition. However, the colicky infant also exhibits other problems, including pain, as noted by the facial expression, lack of responsiveness to soothing intervention or feeding, and the presence of gastrointestinal symptoms such as gas, abdominal distention and tenseness, **borborygmus** (rumbling intestinal noises produced by the presence of gas), frequent stools (which may be explosive, greenish, or mucoid), vomiting, or regurgitation.[16,27,39,44]

A colicky child may exhibit bizarre changes in body posture; in particular, he may seem to show generalized hypertonicity of the musculature, signified by rolling up into a tight ball with the thighs flexed against the abdomen and the arms drawn tightly inward.[5,7,8,13,14] Then the child may stretch out and stiffen in a spastic manner. During the episode the face may become beet red.

Colic episodes are more likely to occur in the late evening.[5,45] In 80% of infants colic begins between 5:00 and 8:00 PM and terminates by midnight; the remaining 20% of

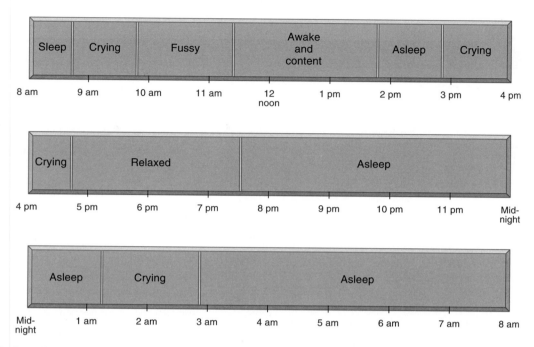

| Sleep | Crying | Fussy | Awake and content | Asleep | Crying |

8 am · 9 am · 10 am · 11 am · 12 noon · 1 pm · 2 pm · 3 pm · 4 pm

| Crying | Relaxed | Asleep |

4 pm · 5 pm · 6 pm · 7 pm · 8 pm · 9 pm · 10 pm · 11 pm · Mid-night

| Asleep | Crying | Asleep |

Mid-night · 1 am · 2 am · 3 am · 4 am · 5 am · 6 am · 7 am · 8 am

Figure 8.1. A daily diary that a parent and/or caregiver may use to chart a baby's activities for a 24-hour period. Excessive crying can help determine if colic is present.

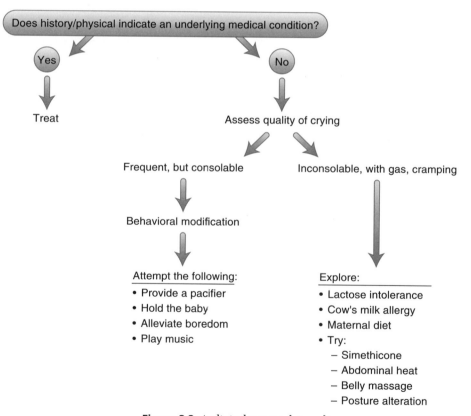

Does history/physical indicate an underlying medical condition?

Yes → Treat

No → Assess quality of crying

Frequent, but consolable → Behavioral modification → Attempt the following:
- Provide a pacifier
- Hold the baby
- Alleviate boredom
- Play music

Inconsolable, with gas, cramping → Explore:
- Lactose intolerance
- Cow's milk allergy
- Maternal diet
- Try:
  - Simethicone
  - Abdominal heat
  - Belly massage
  - Posture alteration

Figure 8.2. A clinical approach to colic.

infants usually begin to show symptoms at 7:00 to 10:00 PM and end at 2:00 AM. A small minority of patients' symptoms may continue for 12 to 15 hours.[5] In about 90% of incidents colic begins when the child is awake.[9] Approximately 90% of the episodes end when the child finally falls asleep.

Should the pharmacist be unsure whether an infant has colic, a referral for a more thorough evaluation is warranted. The physician will first take a careful history and perform a physical examination to rule out organic disorders (Fig. 8.2).[3,11] Beyond this, colic is a diagnosis of exclusion.[7] Colic

Patient Assessment Algorithm 8.1. Colic

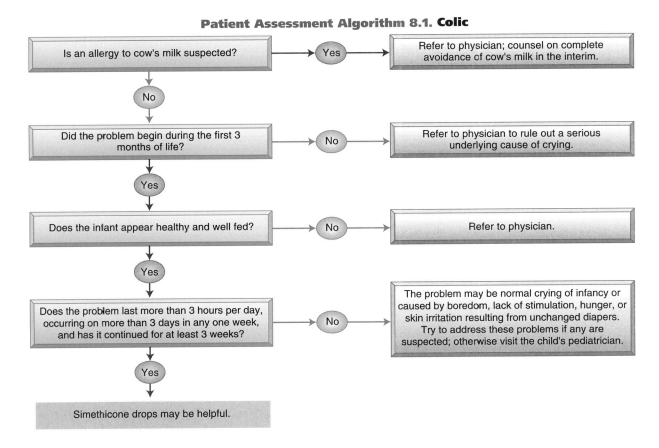

| Is an allergy to cow's milk suspected? | → Yes → | Refer to physician; counsel on complete avoidance of cow's milk in the interim. |

No ↓

| Did the problem begin during the first 3 months of life? | → No → | Refer to physician to rule out a serious underlying cause of crying. |

Yes ↓

| Does the infant appear healthy and well fed? | → No → | Refer to physician. |

Yes ↓

| Does the problem last more than 3 hours per day, occurring on more than 3 days in any one week, and has it continued for at least 3 weeks? | → No → | The problem may be normal crying of infancy or caused by boredom, lack of stimulation, hunger, or skin irritation resulting from unchanged diapers. Try to address these problems if any are suspected; otherwise visit the child's pediatrician. |

Yes ↓

Simethicone drops may be helpful.

Table 8.1. Representative Pediatric Products for Flatulence That May Be Helpful in Infant Colic

PRODUCT	SELECTED INGREDIENTS/COMMENTS
Infant's Mylicon Drops	Per 0.3 mL, simethicone 20 mg
Infant's Mylicon Drops Non-Staining	Per 0.3 mL, simethicone 20 mg
Phazyme Drops for Infants	Per 0.6 mL, simethicone 40 mg

has never been shown to result from organic disease, although some serious medical conditions may mimic colic such as central-nervous-system, cardiovascular, and gastrointestinal disorders.[6,11,18]

TREATMENT OF COLIC

Treatment Guidelines

Colic has no specific cure.[46] Treatments for colic vary according to the underlying etiology being addressed. Advocates of the parent-child-environment interaction model *tip* may choose among several possible therapies. *The baby who is simply bored may benefit through music,*

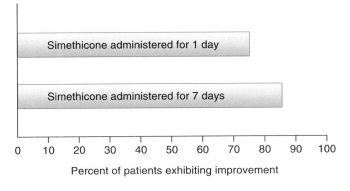

Figure 8.3. The percentage of patients whose infant colic was improved by simethicone drops.

automobile rides, or auditory stimulation.[1,7] The use of a pacifier and holding and walking the infant may also provide relief.[1] (See Patient Assessment Algorithm 8.1.)

Altering the method of breast-feeding may provide benefit. Allowing prolonged feeding at one breast at each feeding produced less colic in infants than allowing the infant to empty both breasts equally at the feeding.[47]

If diet is thought to be the cause, altering the infant's or mother's diet may be effective therapy.[1,27,45,48] Placing mothers of breast-fed infants on low-allergen diets (free of milk, eggs, wheat, nuts, artificial colors, preservatives, and additives) reduced colic appreciably.[49]

If flatulence or abdominal etiologies appear to be causal, a number of actions may relieve colic symptoms:

- Heat applied to the abdomen (e.g., placing the baby in a warm bath for 15 to 20 minutes)
- Belly massage
- Altering the baby's posture during feeding to an upright position to allow gas to be burped more readily[1,2,11,42]
- Administration of 12% sucrose in distilled water[50]

Nonprescription Medications

Medications prescribed to help relieve colic symptoms range from sedatives (e.g., chloral hydrate) to dicyclomine.[5,17,51] However, sedatives do not address the cause of the problem. Also, ***antispasmodics may cause apnea***; thus sedative-antispasmodic combination products are unsafe. (A 1:1 mixture of dimenhydrinate and Donnatal was used for colic in eight infants who as a result suffered cardiorespiratory instability and gastroesophageal reflux.[52]) A few clinicians recommend judicious administration of alcohol to the infant to relieve colonic spasm, but caregivers should be warned not to exceed the amount the physician suggested.[1,11]

Simethicone is frequently given to children with infant colic (Table 8.1). The substance, described as an "inert, nontoxic substance that is virtually nonabsorbed," is safe and effective for treating excess gas in infants and may ease the symptoms of colic in this manner.[3] Although researchers disagree on the effectiveness of simethicone to treat infants, there are no contraindications in its use, and it causes no known adverse reactions.[3]

The various governmental reports that discuss the use of simethicone are silent about its potential nonprescription use in colic.[53–57] However, in one study simethicone reduced colic symptoms in a majority of healthy infants between 2 and 12 weeks of age (Fig 8.3)[3]. This study is counterbalanced by others that show no efficacy.[58]

Should the pharmacist choose to recommend pediatric simethicone drops for infant colic, he or she should keep in mind that the product will not be labeled for colic. When one manufacturer did label a product for colic, it was sent a warning letter from the FDA stating that the FDA was unaware of any substantial scientific evidence that documents the safety and effectiveness of the ingredient for relief of colic symptoms.[59]

SUMMARY

Colic is a self-limited condition that can cause a great deal of discomfort for the child and anxiety for the parents. While several etiologies have been proposed for its occurrence, none has been completely accepted. Suspected causes range from intestinal gas to lactose intolerance, cow's milk allergy, and parental-child interactions. However, the definition of colic is cloudy, hinging on such factors as the duration of crying per episode and the number of episodes. Simethicone

AT THE COUNTER

 A young couple with a 6-week-old child ask about the dose of a pediatric acetaminophen drop for their infant.

Interview/Patient Assessment

The pharmacist discovers that the parents are worried about the infant's crying and associated facial expressions of pain. The crying begins after the child's 6:00 PM feeding, ceasing with the exhausted child finally falling asleep at 11:00 PM or so. The episodes, which occur almost every night, began 1 month before.

Pharmacist's Analysis

1. Do the child's symptoms appear to be colic?

2. Can colic cause pain? Is acetaminophen administration rational?

3. What might the pharmacist recommend?

The child's problem appears to be colic, according to the parameters given in this chapter. Colic can cause pain, but no patient under the age of 2 years should be given acetaminophen unless directed by a physician.

Patient Counseling

The pharmacist should discuss the problem with the child's pediatrician; if colic is suspected, simethicone drops can be recommended, since they have little if any toxicity. Should they fail to relieve the symptoms, however, the parents should be cautioned to make a follow-up appointment with the child's pediatrician.

drops appear to improve the symptoms of colic, even though FDA-approved labeling has not yet been developed.

References

1. Pinyerd BJ. Strategies for consoling the infant with colic: Fact or fiction? J Pediatr Nurs 7:403, 1992.
2. Levine MI. Colic, constipation, and diarrhea—Old symptoms, new approaches. Pediatr Ann 16:765, 1987.
3. Becker N, et al. Mylicon drops in the treatment of infant colic. Clin Ther 10:401, 1988.
4. Clyne PS, Kulczycki A Jr. Human breast milk contains bovine IgG. Relationship to infant colic? Pediatrics 87:439, 1991.
5. Colon AR, Dipalma JS. Colic. Am Fam Physician 40:122, 1989.
6. Keefe MR. Irritable infant syndrome: Theoretical perspectives and practice implications. ANS 10:70, 1988(3).
7. Larson K, Ayllon T. The effects of contingent music and differential reinforcement on infantile colic. Behav Res Ther 28:119, 1990.
8. Forsyth BWC. Colic and the effect of changing formulas: A double-blind, multiple-crossover study. J Pediatr 115:521, 1989.
9. Weissbluth M, Weissbluth L. Colic, sleep inertia, melatonin and circannual rhythms. Med Hypotheses 38:224, 1992.
10. Thomas DB. Of colic and rumbling in the guts. J Paediatr Child Health 31:384, 1995.
11. Adams LM, Davidson M. Present concepts of infant colic. Pediatr Ann 16:817, 1987.
12. Crowcroft NS, Strachan DP. The social origins of infantile colic: Questionnaire study covering 76,747 infants. BMJ 314:1325, 1997.
13. Covington C, et al. Newborn behavioral performance in colic and noncolic infants. Nurs Res 40:292, 1991.
14. Geertsma MA, Hyams JS. Colic—A pain syndrome of infancy? Pediatr Clin North Am 36:905, 1989.
15. Anon. Management of infantile colic. Drug Ther Bull 30:15, 1992.
16. Field PA. A comparison of symptoms used by mothers and nurses to identify an infant with colic. Int J Nurs Stud 31:201, 1994.
17. Sethi KS, Sethi JK. Simethicone in the management of infant colic. Practitioner 232:508, 1988.
18. Miller AR, Barr RG. Infantile colic: Is it a gut issue? Pediatr Clin North Am 38:1407, 1991.
19. Miller JJ, et al. Effect of yeast lactase enzyme on "colic" in infants fed human milk. J Pediatr 117:261, 1990.
20. Laws HF II. Effect of lactase on infantile colic (Letter). J Pediatr 118:993, 1991.
21. Savilahti E, Stahlberg M-R. Lactose tolerance in colicky infants (Letter). J Pediatr 115:333, 1989.
22. Lothe L, Lindberg T. Cow's milk whey protein elicits symptoms of infantile colic in colicky formula-fed infants: A double-blind crossover study. Pediatrics 83:262, 1989.
23. Anon. Is colic in infants associated with diet? Nutr Rev 46:374, 1988.
24. Taubman B. Parental counseling compared with elimination of cow's milk or soy milk protein for the treatment of infant colic syndrome: A randomized trial. Pediatrics 81:756, 1988.
25. Fischer H. Cow milk protein as a cause of infantile colic (Letter). J Pediatr 114:1066, 1989.
26. Lust KD, Brown JE, Thomas W. Maternal intake of cruciferous vegetables and other foods and colic symptoms in exclusively breast-fed infants. J Am Diet Assoc 96:46, 1996.
27. Treem WR, et al. Evaluation of the effect of a fiber-enriched formula on infant colic. J Pediatr 119:695, 1991.
28. Sferra TJ, Heitlinger LA. Gastrointestinal gas formation and infantile colic. Pediatr Clin North Am 43:489, 1996.
29. Lehtonen L, Svedstrom E, Korvenranta H. Gallbladder hypocontractility in infantile colic. Acta Pediatr 83:1174, 1994.
30. Lehtonen L, Korvenranta H, Eerola E. Intestinal microflora in colicky and noncolicky infants: Bacterial cultures and gas-liquid chromatography. J Pediatr Gastroenterol Nutr 19:310, 1994.
31. Treem WR. Infant colic. A pediatric gastroenterologist's perspective. Pediatr Clin North Am 41:1121, 1994.
32. Stein MT. Beyond infant colic. J Dev Behav Pediatr 17:38, 1996.
33. Lehtonen L, Korhonen T, Korvenranta H. Temperament and sleeping patterns in colicky infants during the first year of life. J Dev Behav Pediatr 15:416, 1994.
34. Gurry D. Infantile colic. Aust Fam Physician 23:337, 1994.
35. Matheson I. The effect of smoking on lactation and infantile colic. JAMA 261:42, 1989.
36. Brewster DH. Enterobius vermicularis: A possible cause of intestinal colic? JR Coll Gen Pract 39:387, 1989.
37. Gebeyehu K. (Letter). Pediatr Emerg Care 8:254, 1992.
38. Singer JI, Rosenberg NM. A fatal case of colic. Pediatr Emerg Care 8:171, 1992.
39. Barr RG, et al. The crying of infants with colic: A controlled empirical decision. Pediatrics 90:14, 1992.
40. Barr RG, et al. Carrying as colic "therapy": A randomized controlled trial. Pediatrics 87:623, 1991.
41. Canivet C, et al. Infantile colic—less common than previously estimated? Acta Pediatr 85:454, 1996.
42. Larsen J-H. Infants' colic and belly massage. Practitioner 234:396, 1990.
43. James-Roberts IS, Conroy S, Wilsher K. Bases for maternal perceptions of infant crying and colic behaviour. Arch Dis Child 75:375, 1996.
44. Sampson HA. Infantile colic and food allergy: Fact or fiction? (Editorial). J Pediatr 115:583, 1989.
45. Connor B. Infantile colic. Aust Fam Physician 17:740, 1988.
46. Balon AJ. Management of infantile colic. Am Fam Physician 55:235, 1997.
47. Evans K, Evans R, Simmer K. Effect of the method of breast feeding on breast engorgement, mastitis and infantile colic. Acta Pediatr 84:849, 1995.
48. Holsman P. The role of diet in infant colic. Aust Fam Physician 20:1049, 1991.
49. Hill DJ, et al. A low allergen diet is a significant intervention in infantile colic: Results of a community-based study. J Allergy Clin Immunol 96(6 Pt 1):886, 1995.
50. Markestad T. Use of sucrose as a treatment for infant colic. Arch Dis Child 76:356, 1997.
51. Grunseit F. Evaluation of the efficacy of dicyclomine hydrochloride ('Merbentyl') syrup in the treatment of infant colic. Curr Med Res Opin 5:258, 1977.
52. Hardoin RA, et al. Colic medication and apparent life-threatening events. Clin Pediatr 30:281, 1991.
53. Fed Reg 38:8714, 1973.
54. Fed Reg 38:31260, 1973.

55. Fed Reg 39:19862, 1974.
56. Fed Reg 47:454, 1982.
57. Fed Reg 53:2706, 1988.
58. Metcalf TJ, et al. Simethicone in the treatment of infant colic: A randomized, placebo-controlled, multicenter trial. Pediatrics 94:29, 1994.
59. Anon. Reed & Carnrick's Phazyme Drops. Weekly Pharmacy Reports 40:1, 1991.

Lactose Intolerance

AT THE COUNTER

 A female patient, who appears to be in her late 20s, tells the pharmacist that she is concerned she may have developed lactose intolerance (LI) and asks about tablets that she can take when she drinks milk.

Interview/Patient Assessment

The woman mentions that neither her parents nor her sibling are lactose intolerant. Beginning about 2 months ago, she began noticing gas and abdominal pain several hours after drinking milk with breakfast. Currently, she has several bouts of diarrhea weekly. She also has been nauseated and has vomited several times in the past several weeks. She is certain that she is not pregnant, is taking no medications, and has no diagnosed medical conditions.

Pharmacist's Analysis

1. Do this patient's symptoms suggest LI?
2. Should she be given tablets containing lactase?
3. Should she see a physician?

This patient's problems would indicate LI, except that the vomiting, coupled with the other problems, suggests cow's milk allergy. If this is indeed the case, continuing to ingest milk is extremely dangerous.

Patient Counseling

The patient should be referred to her physician or to an allergist for evaluation. In the meantime she should be advised to abstain from all products containing milk and not attempt to use lactase tablets along with milk.

Lactose intolerance (LI), also known as hypolactasia or lactase deficiency, indicates low lactase activity in the **brush-border** membrane of the small intestine (the outermost layer of the small-intestinal epithelium, composed of many microvilli), specifically in the **microvillous membrane** (membrane of the microvilli, microscopic projections of the cells).[1] Low lactase activity results in the inability to digest lactose, a unique carbohydrate found in the milk of most mammals. (The absorption of lactose is dependent on the enzymatic hydrolysis into two monosaccharides [glucose and galactose].[2] Lactase, a disaccharidase [β-galactosidase] enzyme, performs this breakdown.)[1] LI can cause bloating, gas, diarrhea, and other annoying and possibly uncomfortable symptoms when milk or other dairy products are ingested.

PREVALENCE OF LACTOSE INTOLERANCE (LI)

In general, the prevalence of LI is quite high—perhaps 75% of the world's adult population cannot drink milk or eat lactose-containing foods in amounts over their tolerance without experiencing symptoms.[3,4] The prevalence is higher in some ethnic groups than in others, however (Fig. 9.1). For instance, only about 25% of American adults are severely intolerant.[5] To understand why there is such a remarkable variation in ability to ingest lactose, an understanding of the multiple etiologies of lactose intolerance is necessary.

There are three major types of lactose intolerance:

- Primary LI, a genetically determined reduction in the enzyme needed to digest milk and dairy products after a certain age, is the cause of LI in 70% of the world's population.
- Congenital alactasia, an extremely rare form of lactose intolerance, is present at birth.[1]
- Secondary LI, a common form of LI, occurs secondary to various environmental insults; the remaining 30% of the

world's peoples who can ingest milk and dairy products in adulthood are susceptible to these environmental insults.

EPIDEMIOLOGY OF LACTOSE INTOLERANCE (LI)

Discussion of the epidemiology of LI is confined to the primary and congenital forms of the condition since secondary LI is caused by environmental insults.

Primary Lactose Intolerance (LI)

Primary lactose intolerance (LI), the most common form of LI, is better understood with some knowledge of the development of lactase. Lactase is detectable in the human fetus late in gestation.[1] Levels peak the second or third day after birth and remain high during infancy, when milk is a major component of the diet.[6]

Lactase activity drops off sharply following weaning in all mammals except man.[7] By young adulthood, however, approximately 70% of the world's human population has experienced this lactase dropoff.[7] Thereafter, these individuals suffer from primary LI and cannot ingest lactose-containing foods and drinks over a certain amount without troubling symptoms. The remaining 30% of adult humans are able to digest milk and dairy products as adults, making them the only mammals in whom lactase activity persists into adulthood.[8]

Regarding the reason some humans stand alone among mammals in their ability to digest milk and dairy products as adults, one theory emerges from anthropologic research.[3] According to this theory, early man could not digest lactose as adults. However, about 10,000 years ago, man began to domesticate milk-producing ruminants.[7] Intermittent crop failures caused by drought, disease, or insects and/or the failure of hunter-gatherers resulted in starvation. In desperate efforts to survive, some people fed their families the milk of

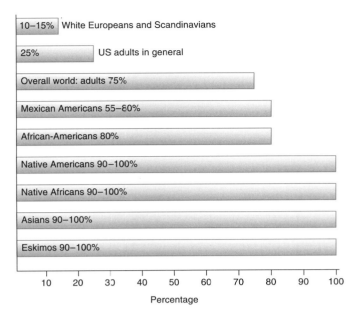

Figure 9.1. The prevalence of lactose intolerance in certain populations.

their domesticated cows. Only those children and adults possessing a genetic mutation allowing them to utilize the milk could survive on that milk. However, over the years—and through periods of famine—their genetic mutation provided a selective advantage that was passed on in the gene pool for an estimated 400 generations.[3]

Only certain races, presumably those descendants of the famine survivors, experience **lactase persistence** (also known as normolactasia, the continuing production of lactase as adults).[1,2] This includes individuals whose ancestors were Northern Europeans, residents of the northwest part of the Indian subcontinent, and those who lived as nomads in the deserts (Bedouins in Jordan and Saudi Arabia).[3] Only 10 to 15% of whites of northwestern European or Scandinavian extraction cannot consume dairy products as adults.[3]

Those whose ancestors did not herd ruminants experience a decline in lactase activity between 2 and 6 years of age in most humans (2 years in residents of Thailand but as high as 10 to 20 years in residents of Finland), until lactase activity is only one-tenth of the pre-dropoff level, so that the amount of lactose they can ingest is quite restricted.[1,7,9] Up to 80% of African-Americans, 55 to 80% of Mexican Americans, and 90 to 100% of Asians, Native Americans, Native Africans, and Eskimos are lactose intolerant.[3,10] None of these subpopulations have a history of ingestion of unfermented milk; ruminants were unavailable to their ancestors. For instance, the pig is the primary domesticated animal in Asia, and it cannot be easily milked by humans.

Congenital Alactasia

A rare form of congenital alactasia also occurs. It has been seen in only in a few dozen patients, the majority in Finland.[3] With this condition infants cannot ingest lactase from birth.[10]

Although the condition was once fatal, soy-based infant formulas can allow infant survival and can also bridge the gap until some infants with congenital alactasia develop sufficient lactase activity to ingest milk.[11]

ETIOLOGY OF SECONDARY LACTOSE INTOLERANCE (LI)

The discussion of etiology of lactose intolerance is confined to secondary lactose intolerance since the primary and congenital forms of the condition are caused by a genetic predisposition.

Secondary LI is the result of nongenetic causes. Conditions that result in extensive mucosal damage can alter the activity of several intestinal disaccharidases, but lactase is the most likely to undergo a decrease in activity. The vulnerability of lactase results from its relatively superficial position among the brush-border enzymes.[12] Its titers of activity are also usually the lowest of these enzymes, making it most vulnerable to secondary depression. The patient with secondary LI may undergo partial or full brush-border regeneration, which eventually allows them to ingest lactose again.[13]

Infections

Secondary LI may follow acute gastroenteritis. Rotavirus infection in infants frequently causes LI, which has fueled speculation that rotavirus has a special affinity for lactase.[10] Invasion of parasites such as hookworm or *Giardia* species may also cause secondary LI by damaging villous architecture. Following acute gastroenteritis, the pharmacist may advise those with LI symptoms of sudden onset to withdraw from dairy products, slowly reintroducing them if they are tolerated.[14]

Other Medical Conditions

Secondary LI may be induced by, and exist concomitantly with, celiac disease (e.g., gluten sensitivity), sprue syndromes, or malnutrition.[1,10]

Surgery

Secondary LI may also result when surgical intervention such as a partial resection of the lactase-rich section of the small intestine causes short bowel syndrome.[10,15] In this case there is insufficient contact between ingested lactose and the remaining brush-border cells.

Gastric reconstructions may produce a dumping syndrome that leads to secondary LI by accelerating the GI transit time. Thus lactase-deficient patients who undergo partial gastrectomy or other gastric or duodenal procedures may find that they now suffer from postsurgical bloating and diarrhea.[16]

Drugs and Alcohol

Antimetabolites, colchicine, tetracyclines, cimetidine, neomycin, kanamycin, and aminosalicylic acid have all caused LI, as has intestinal radiation.[6,13,17] Alcohol ingestion causes gastrointestinal insult, which has produced reversible LI in some heavy drinkers.[18]

MANIFESTATIONS OF LACTOSE INTOLERANCE (LI)

When ingested lactose reaches the small and large intestines, several problems occur. The lactose causes an osmotic pull similar to that caused by the saline laxatives (e.g., magnesium hydroxide). A fluid gradient draws water into the small intestine, resulting in nausea, stomach rumbling (borborygmus), and diarrhea (which may be explosive because of excess gas).[20–22] Bacteria in the bowel ferment the lactose, causing production of excessive hydrogen, organic acids, and carbon dioxide (Fig. 9.2).[2] Thus patients often suffer from dyspepsia, gas, bloating, cramping, and abdominal pain.[1,10,19] Stools may also be watery and frothy and may float because of the high gas content.[23] In the most severe cases the pressure from fluid and gas may defeat normal bowel reflexes and result in involuntary leakage of stool, staining, and incontinence.[6]

SPECIFIC CONSIDERATIONS OF LACTOSE INTOLERANCE (LI)

Differentiating LI from Cow's Milk Allergy

LI is not an allergy to milk, as many patients assume. (True cow's milk allergy is most often caused by the proteins in

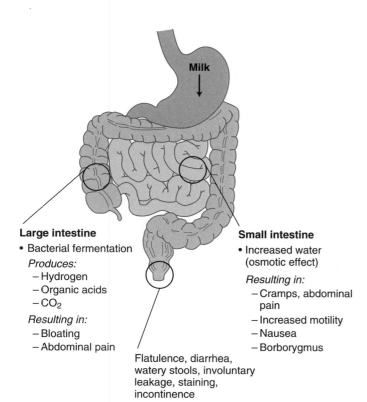

Large intestine
• Bacterial fermentation
Produces:
– Hydrogen
– Organic acids
– CO₂
Resulting in:
– Bloating
– Abdominal pain

Flatulence, diarrhea, watery stools, involuntary leakage, staining, incontinence

Small intestine
• Increased water (osmotic effect)
Resulting in:
– Cramps, abdominal pain
– Increased motility
– Nausea
– Borborygmus

Figure 9.2. The ingestion of lactose produces several bothersome symptoms.

milk.[10]) Confusion exists, however, because some of the symptoms of cow's milk allergy overlap LI symptoms.[10] Most infants with cow's milk allergy experience diarrhea (the most common symptom) and mucus in the stools and may also suffer from colic, abdominal pain, and excessive gas—all symptoms of LI. The second most common symptom of cow's milk allergy is vomiting (especially within 1 hour of eating), and vomiting is not considered to be a common symptom of LI.[24]

Diagnosis of Lactose Intolerance (LI)

Although pharmacists can recognize LI based on the patient's recitation of symptoms produced when milk or dairy foods are ingested, there are several tests physicians can order to confirm the condition[3]:

• Hydrogen breath test. The patient first ingests a measured amount of lactose after an overnight fast.[10] If it reaches the colon unabsorbed, bacterial fermentation generates hydrogen, which in turn is absorbed and exhaled by the lungs.[25] The hydrogen content of the expired air is compared with the amount of lactose ingested. A rise in hydrogen excretion of greater than 20 parts per million is consistent with LI. The hydrogen breath test is more comfortable for the patient (most do not experience diarrhea of abdominal symptoms) and is highly sensitive in the detection of LI, so that it is referred to as the diagnostic test of choice.[10]

• Lactose challenge test. The patient is asked to drink a quart of low-fat or skim milk over a 15-minute period. (Low-fat is used because fat can cause retention of milk in the stomach.) A patient with LI will develop bloating and diarrhea within approximately 4 hours.[26]

• Lactose tolerance test. An initial blood sample is drawn, and then the patient drinks 50 g of lactose. Follow-up blood samples are drawn at 15, 30, 60, 90, and 120 minutes postingestion. LI is probable if the blood glucose does not rise by at least 20 mg% during these tests.[1,27] This test produces an appreciable number of both false-positive and false-negative results.[10]

• Jejunal biopsy. Rarely performed, this invasive test allows direct examination for lactase.[1] Mucosal lactase activity varies from site to site in the same part of the bowel, so that any one test may not be reflective of total bowel lactase activity.[28]

• Stool pH examination. Clinitest, a urine glucose test product, can be used to examine stools for the presence of reducing substances.[20] Large amounts of lactic acid in the stool, creating a pH of less than 5.5, indicate LI.[10]

COMPLICATIONS OF LACTOSE INTOLERANCE (LI)

Nutritional Impact

Lactase persistence into adulthood is advantageous when it does occur. Milk and dairy products contain important nutrients such as phosphorus, magnesium, riboflavin, vitamins A and D, and protein.[7,13] Further, the majority of the dietary calcium of the average United States resident comes from lactose-containing products.[13] Elimination of milk and dairy products may result in poor skeletal growth and osteoporosis.[29,30] Research showed that 76% of women with osteoporosis were lactose intolerant, compared with only 64% of women without osteoporosis who were lactose malabsorbers.[31] Avoidance of milk and dairy products is presumed to have been responsible.

tip *Pharmacists may suggest supplemental calcium for LI patients who must restrict milk and dairy-product intake.* Lactase-deficient patients do not suffer from malabsorption of calcium.[32]

Relationship with Other Medical Conditions

Irritable bowel syndrome and LI have duplicative symptoms. A link between these conditions has been suspected, so that researchers recommend excluding LI before exploring the diagnosis of irritable bowel syndrome.[33] The existence of LI may be linked to either Crohn's disease or recurrent abdominal pain of childhood.[34–37]

TREATMENT OF LACTOSE INTOLERANCE (LI)

Treatment Guidelines

DETERMINATION OF LACTOSE TOLERANCE LEVEL

Patients often recognize that dairy products cause their symptoms and eliminate them from the diet on their own.[5]

Total dairy elimination would be necessary for cow's milk allergy, but is too extreme for many United States citizens with lactose intolerance.[13] Only about 5 to 10% of LI patients in the United States require total lactose restriction.[6] (Patient Assessment Algorithm 9.1.)

Many patients can still ingest some lactose, but do not know when they have exceeded the amount that their remaining lactase activity can metabolize. Once a physician or pharmacist has determined that the patient suffers from LI, the next step is to determine the patient's individual lactose tolerance to increase the patient's comfort level.

To determine the lactose tolerance level, the patient first eliminates all lactose from the diet. The patient must check ingredient labels of all foods searching for such ingredients as milk sugars, casein, caseinate, whey, or nonfat dry-milk solids. These ingredients may be found in milk, cream added to coffee, ice cream, cheese, party dips, bread, butter, baked goods, cereals, salad dressings, candies, baking mixes, sherbets, frozen dairy desserts, puddings, instant potatoes, prepared soups, and some canned and frozen fruits and vegetables.[6,10,23] (A dietitian, if available, might be able to provide a complete list of foods and drinks containing lactose.) (See "Avoidance of Foods and Drinks Containing Lactose.") The patient should also check drug composition with a pharmacist. (See "Avoidance of Medications Containing Lactose.")

After about 3 weeks on the lactose-free diet, the patient should gradually increase lactose-containing foods and

Patient Assessment Algorithm 9.1. Lactose Intolerance

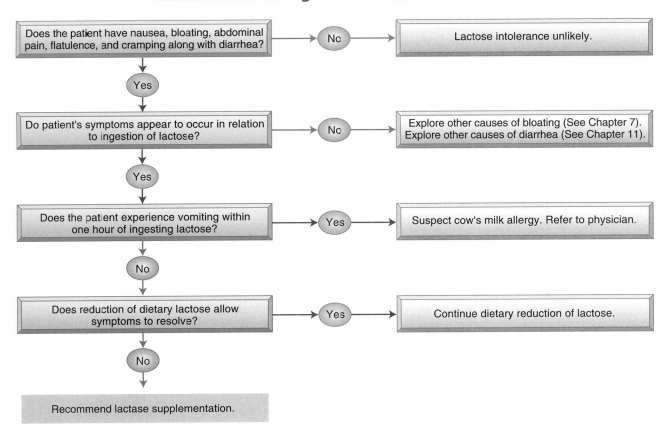

drinks until troubling symptoms begin.[6] For instance, start with 1/4 cup of milk for breakfast. If LI symptoms do not occur, increase the amount to 1/2 cup of milk the following morning. Continue, gradually increasing the amount of milk until symptoms occur. At that point drop back to the previous amount. If a desired breakfast intake is achieved without symptoms, the patient may then set an amount for lunch and supper by repeating the step-up method, while keeping the breakfast amount constant.

Nonprescription Medications

In addition to limiting lactose ingestion, LI patients can also treat LI by supplementing their lactase with lactase-containing medications (Table 9.1). Lactase was not originally required to undergo the FDA OTC review process since the FDA viewed it as a food modifying another food.[40] However, in 1988 the FDA stated that it would examine the efficacy of lactase.[41] The results have not yet been announced.

Lactase derived from the yeast *Kluyveromyces lactis* or *Aspergillis oryzae* may be purchased in several forms—liquid, tablets, and capsules.[3,42] Liquids can be added directly to milk: a ratio of 5 drops per quart produces 70% hydrolysis, 15 drops per quart produces 99% hydrolysis (Fig. 9.3). Alternately, the contents of lactase capsules can be sprinkled into milk (one to two capsules per quart produces appreciable hydrolysis); then the milk is shaken and refrigerated for 24 hours before drinking.[43] In either technique—liquid or capsules—the lactase activity converts the lactose to its component sugars in the carton. Patients have commented that the milk tastes sweeter than normal, although not unpleasantly so.[28]

The drops and the contents of capsules would not work for hard lactose products, of course, such as ice cream or

FOCUS ON...

AVOIDANCE OF FOODS AND DRINKS CONTAINING LACTOSE

When counseling patients, it is helpful to know the estimated content of lactose in various foods. Human milk contains about 7 g of lactose per 100 mL, while cow's milk provides only 4.7 g per 100 mL.[2] The table lists the lactose content of common foods and drinks.[13]

Various Foods and Drinks and Their Approximate Lactose Contents

FOOD OR DRINK	LACTOSE CONTENT (g /100 g)
Low-fat milk	3.8–5.4
Buttermilk	3.8–4.5
Chocolate milk	4.2–5
Acidophilus milk, skim	4.4
Skim milk	5–5.8
Sweetened condensed whole milk	11.4
Dried whole milk	37.5
Yogurt (low-fat)	4.8–5.8
Cheeses	0–5.7
Cottage cheese	2.4–2.9
Cottage cheese, low-fat	3–3.5
Light cream	4
Whipping cream	2.8–3
Butter	1
Orange sherbet	2
Ice cream, French, soft	5.3
Ice cream, regular vanilla	7

FOCUS ON...

AVOIDANCE OF MEDICATIONS CONTAINING LACTOSE

Once the pharmacist becomes aware that a patient suffers from LI, it is prudent to warn the patient about medications containing lactose. Those patients extremely sensitive to lactose may react to the relatively small quantities found as fillers in tablets, capsules, and other dosage forms.[38] Such alternatives as liquids may be preferable.

In one report a patient suffered classic LI symptoms following inhalation of the contents of sodium cromolyn capsules, each of which included only 20 mg of lactose. The authors hypothesized that the symptoms were caused by oral or pharyngeal deposition of the product with subsequent swallowing.[39]

tip *LI patients receiving enteral nutrition, either orally or via nasogastric tube, should also be cautioned about the use of products that contain lactose.*[6] If typical symptoms occur in a patient not previously diagnosed as lactose-intolerant, the pharmacist might alert health-care providers to the possibility of LI. Alternate lactose-free enteral products are available.

cheese.[42] They would also be impractical for meals eaten away from home, as in restaurants.[27,32] In these situations patients may purchase lactase tablets or capsules and ingest them immediately before the dairy product is ingested.[10] The lactase then digests the lactose in the gastrointestinal tract before it can cause symptoms (although the actual location of this digestion is unknown, it is presumed to occur in the stomach and proximal small intestine). Patients must experiment to discover how many tablets or capsules work for a certain amount of lactose-containing food, but generally one to three dosage units are sufficient. (Of course, these products would also work at home for patients who do not wish to pretreat milk in the carton.)

Relatively few studies have compared the efficacy of commercially available formulations. However, one did so by challenging LI patients with 1.5 cups of ice cream.[44] The pa-

Table 9.1. Representative Products for Lactose Intolerance

PRODUCT	SELECTED INGREDIENTS/COMMENTS
Dairy Ease Tablets	Lactase 3000 FCC units
Lactaid Drops	Glycerin water, lactase enzyme (amount specified)
Lactaid Original Caplets	Lactase 3000 FCC units
Lactaid Extra Strength Caplets	Lactase 4500 FCC units
Lactaid Ultra Caplets	Lactase 9000 FCC units

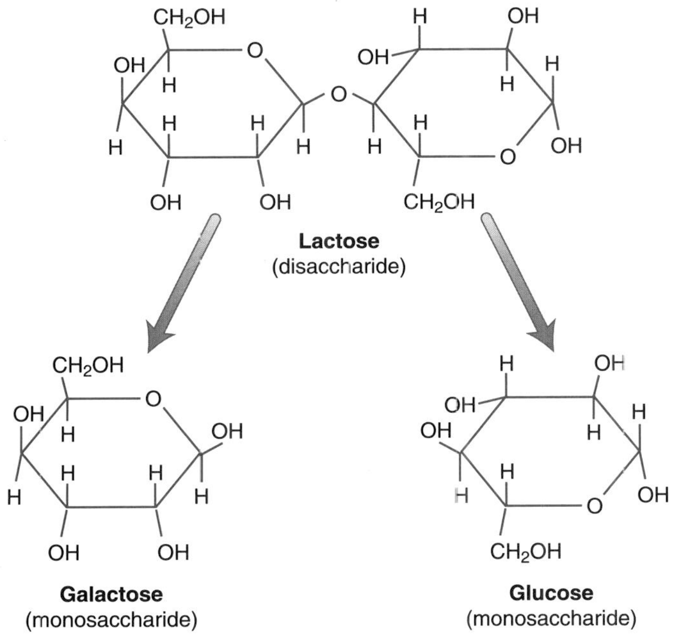

Figure 9.3. Lactase acts on lactose (the disaccharide shown at top) to produce the two monosaccharides galactose and glucose.

Table 9.2. Representative Milk Substitutes for Lactose Intolerance

PRODUCT	COMMENTS
CalciMilk	Lactose-reduced, calcium-fortified milk
Dairy Ease Milk	Lactose-reduced, nonfat milk
Lactaid Lowfat Milk	Lactose-reduced, lowfat milk
Lactaid 100 Nonfat Milk	Lactose-free, nonfat milk
Vitamite	Lactose-free milk substitute

AT THE COUNTER

 A mother asks the pharmacist for help with her 8-year-old son's dietary problem.

Interview/Patient Assessment

He can't seem to drink milk any more without complaining of problems later in school. During the late morning and early afternoon he has bothersome stomach rumbling. His stomach cramping causes him to be excused to go to the bathroom several times each day. If he is too embarrassed to ask, he has staining of his underpants, especially when he also has flatulence. The problem began several months ago. The child and his parents appear to be white. This child is taking no medications and has no diagnosed medical conditions.

Pharmacist's Analysis

1. Is lactose intolerance (LI) a likely cause of this boy's problems?
2. What role does lactose elimination play in his therapy?
3. Is lactase supplementation a possibility for this patient?
4. Should the mother consider supplemental calcium?

These symptoms appear to be caused by LI. The mother might attempt to determine his lactose tolerance level, as outlined in this chapter. However, pending this, he should be placed on a lactose-restricted diet so that his schoolwork does not suffer. Lactase supplementation in the form of tablets could also help.

Patient Counseling

The pharmacist should determine whether the child drinks milk at lunch and should point out that lactase tablets could help prevent problems caused by that ingestion, although he may need to receive lactase tablets from school personnel to satisfy regulations that prohibit self-administration of medications. The pharmacist should also point out the dangers of inadequate calcium intake and should recommend a supplemental calcium product for the child to ensure proper skeletal development. If the problems persist, the patient should see a physician to rule out a more serious disorder.

---

tients received one of three products, in doses and following directions provided by the manufacturers. Lactaid caplets did not reduce any symptom, Dairy Ease chewable tablets reduced pain, and Lactrase capsules reduced both pain and bloating.

As an enzyme, lactase may undergo degradation by stomach acids. However, since lactase-containing products seem to be effective, it may be that the small amounts that survive enzymatic degradation are sufficient for efficacy.

Nonpharmacologic Therapies

Patients may also avoid problems by eating several small meals instead of a few large meals.[6] When a patient wishes to eat a lactose-containing food, eating other food at the same time appears to dilute the lactose and facilitate its enzymatic breakdown.[13,45] Although a dairy product, yogurt (a fermented milk product) may alleviate LI when ingested along with other dairy products.[10,16] Presumably, the cultures used to produce it also produce high quantities of lactase.[13] In preliminary studies yogurt was effective, but some subjects disliked the tartness of unflavored yogurt.[46] Flavored and frozen yogurts were not as effective as plain yogurt, however.

Special lactose-reduced milk products may also allow patients to reach acceptable levels of milk intake without triggering symptoms (Table 9.2).[13] However, cultured milks such as buttermilk are not helpful.[47] Unfermented milk containing *Lactobacillus acidophilus* also does not improve LI.[13]

SUMMARY

LI may be caused by an individual's normal genetic predisposition (primary LI), may be present from birth (congenital alactasia), or may be caused by any one of several environmental insults such as infection, surgery, or ingestion of certain medications (secondary LI). LI symptoms can range from minor to extremely uncomfortable. Pharmacists should counsel patients on such issues as the determination of lactose tolerance level, avoidance of foods and medications containing lactose, and use of lactase supplements. Lactase supplements can be added to milk (for later consumption) or ingested just before eating lactose-containing foods or beverages. Low-lactose or lactose-free milk substitutes also may provide relief for LI patients.

References

1. Sahi T. Hypolactasia and lactase persistence. Scand J Gastroenterol 29(Suppl 202):1, 1994.
2. Arola H, Tamm A. Metabolism of lactose in the human body. Scand J Gastroenterol 29(Suppl 202):21, 1994.
3. Sahi T. Genetics and epidemiology of adult-type hypolactasia. Scand J Gastroenterol 29(Suppl 202):7, 1994.
4. Ferguson A. Mechanisms in adverse reactions to food. The gastrointestinal tract. Allergy 50(20 Suppl):32, 1995.
5. Suarez F, Savaiano DA, Levitt MD. A comparison of symptoms after the consumption of milk or lactose-hydrolyzed milk by people with self-reported severe lactose intolerance. N Engl J Med 333:1, 1995.

6. Englert DM, Guillory JA. For want of lactase. Am J Nurs 86:902, 1986.
7. Anderson B, Vullo C. Did malaria select for primary adult lactase deficiency? Gut 35:1487, 1994.
8. Hertzler SR, Bao-Chau LH, Savaiano DA. How much lactose is low lactose? J Am Diet Assoc 96:243, 1996.
9. Vesa TH, Korpela RA, Sahi T. Tolerance to small amounts of lactose in lactose maldigesters. Am J Clin Nutr 64:197, 1996.
10. Castiglia PT. Lactose intolerance. J Pediatr Health Care 8:36, 1994.
11. Similä S, et al. Use of lactose-hydrolyzed human milk in congenital lactase deficiency. J Pediatr 101:584, 1982.
12. Northrop-Clewes CA, Lunn PG, Downes RM. Lactose maldigestion in breast-feeding Gambian infants. J Pediatr Gastroenterol Nutr 24:257, 1997.
13. Tamm A. Management of lactose intolerance. Scand J Gastroenterol 29(Suppl 202):55, 1994.
14. Szajewska H, et al. Carbohydrate intolerance after acute gastroenteritis—A disappearing problem in Polish children. Acta Paediatr 86:347, 1997.
15. Marteau P, et al. Do patients with short-bowel syndrome need a lactose-free diet? Nutrition 13:13, 1997.
16. Arrigoni E, et al. Tolerance and absorption of lactose from milk and yogurt during short-bowel syndrome in humans. Am J Clin Nutr 60:926, 1994.
17. Fradkin A, et al. Colchicine-induced lactose malabsorption in patients with familial Mediterranean fever. Isr J Med Sci 31:616, 1995.
18. Keshavarzian A, et al. Intestinal-transit and lactose intolerance in chronic alcoholics. Am J Clin Nutr 44:70, 1986.
19. Heikkinen M, et al. Etiology of dyspepsia: Four hundred unselected consecutive patients in general practice. Scand J Gastroenterol 30:519, 1995.
20. Patrick MK. Vomiting and diarrhoea. Aust Fam Physician 23:1913, 1994.
21. Ramkishan D, et al. Prevalence of lactose maldigestion. Dig Dis Sci 39:1519, 1994.
22. Leung AKC, Robson WLM. Evaluating the child with chronic diarrhea. Am Fam Physician 53:635, 1996.
23. Meyers A. Modern management of acute diarrhea and dehydration in children. Am Fam Physician 51:1103, 1995.
24. Walker-Smith JA. Milk intolerance in children. Clin Allergy 16:183, 1986.
25. Hammer HF, et al. Assessment of the influence of hydrogen nonexcretion on the usefulness of the hydrogen breath test and lactose tolerance test. Wien Klin Wochenschr 108:137, 1996.
26. Hermans MM, et al. The relationship between lactose tolerance test results and symptoms of lactose intolerance. Am J Gastroenterol 92:981, 1997.
27. Angelides AG, Davidson M. Lactose intolerance and diarrhea: Are they related? Pediatr Ann 14:62, 1985.
28. Littman A. Lactase deficiency: diagnosis and management. Hosp Pract 22:111, 1987.
29. Suarez FL, Savaiano DA. Lactose digestion and tolerance in adult and elderly Asian-Americans. Am J Clin Nutr 59:1021, 1994.
30. Laroche M, et al. Lactose intolerance and osteoporosis in men. Rev Rheum (Eng Ed) 62:766, 1995.
31. Corazza GR, et al. Lactose intolerance and bone mass in postmenopausal Italian women. Br J Nutr 73:479, 1995.
32. Rosado JL, et al. Enzyme replacement therapy for primary adult lactase deficiency. Gastroenterology 87:1072, 1984.
33. Bohmer CJ, Tuynman HA. The clinical relevance of lactose malabsorption in irritable bowel syndrome. Eur J Gastroenterol Hepatol 8:1013, 1996.
34. Malagelada J-R. Lactose intolerance. N Engl J Med 333:53, 1995.
35. Webster RB, DiPalma JA, Gremse DA. Lactose maldigestion and recurrent abdominal pain in children. Dig Dis Sci 40:1506, 1995.
36. Mishkin B, Yalovsky M, Mishkin S. Increased prevalence of lactose malabsorption in Crohn's disease patients at low risk for lactose malabsorption based on ethnic origin. Am J Gastroenterol 92:1148, 1997.
37. Mishkin S. Dairy sensitivity, lactose malabsorption, and elimination diets in inflammatory bowel disease. Am J Clin Nutr 65:564, 1997.
38. Vaghadia H. Acute abdominal distension in lactase deficiency relieved by metoclopramide. Can Med Assoc J 134:1033, 1986.
39. Brandstetter RD, et al. Lactose intolerance associated with Intal capsules (Letter). N Engl J Med 315:1613, 1986.
40. Fed Reg 49:47384, 1984.
41. Fed Reg 53:2705, 1988.
42. Moskovitz M, et al. Does oral enzyme replacement therapy reverse intestinal lactose malabsorption? Am J Gastroenterol 82:632, 1987.
43. Suarez FL, Savaiano DA, Levitt MD. Review article: The treatment of lactose intolerance. Aliment Pharmacol Ther 9:589, 1995.
44. Ramirez FC, et al. All lactase preparations are not the same: Results of a prospective, randomized, placebo-controlled trial. Am J Gastroenterol 89:566, 1994.
45. Dehkordi N, et al. Lactose malabsorption as influenced by chocolate milk, skim milk, sucrose, whole milk, and lactic cultures. J Am Diet Assoc 95:484, 1995.
46. Onwulata CI, et al. Relative efficiency of yogurt, sweet acidophilus milk, hydrolyzed-lactose milk, and a commercial lactase tablet in alleviating lactose maldigestion. Am J Clin Nutr 49:1233, 1989.
47. Savaiano DA, Kotz C. Recent advances in the management of lactose intolerance. ASDC J Dent Child 56:228, 1989.

Constipation

AT THE COUNTER

A man appearing to be in his mid 20s is looking at different products in the laxative aisle. When the pharmacist approaches, he asks which product is best.

Interview/Patient Assessment

The pharmacist asks exactly what his problem is. He responds, "I'm usually fairly regular, but some days I don't have to go. But I'm not constipated the next day. I just would like to go each morning." In response to further questioning, the patient denies use of any medications and has no chronic health problems. He does not have hemorrhoids or rectal bleeding and does not strain to pass stools. The patient began a second job the month before that requires him to travel during the day. Sometimes he skips lunch, and he also doesn't drink much fluid in a typical day, other than coffee, tea, and caffeinated soft drinks.

Pharmacist's Analysis

1. Do this man's complaints suggest constipation?

2. What is the possible significance of increased travel, skipped meals, and insufficient fluid?
3. Would a nonprescription product be appropriate for this patient?

This patient appears to have simple constipation that may be relieved by lifestyle changes.

Patient Counseling

The patient should first be advised that his stool frequency is in the normal range. Not all patients have bowel movements daily, so that he may be worrying needlessly. Any slight irregularity can probably be easily corrected. The pharmacist should suggest increasing his intake of water or other non-caffeinated beverage, eating bulkier foods, and trying to set aside a few minutes each morning to allow defecation, if needed. There is no clear reason to refer the patient, nor is there a justifiable need for a nonprescription product at this time. A simple bulking agent might also be helpful in increasing stool volume and allowing him to attain some regularity with daily bowel movements if this is his goal.

Constipation is the most common digestion-related complaint in the United States.[1] Patients who say they are constipated may be referring to one or more of the following symptoms that may or may not actually indicate constipation:

- Infrequent stools
- Straining while passing stools
- Stools that are harder or smaller than normal
- Pain when attempting to defecate
- A feeling that the bowel has not been completely emptied after actual or attempted defecation
- A lack of urgency to evacuate[2–5]

Many people have the mistaken idea that one daily bowel movement (BM) is ideal.[6,7] Those few people who are so regulated that they have one bowel movement at the same time each day are actually rare.

Physicians accept a much wider range of BMs as normal. Generally, from as many as three BMs per day to as few as three per week is considered "normal" (Fig. 10.1).[3,8] Three BMs per week is a useful cutoff point for constipation.[9,10] Patients with a frequency below three BMs per week may experience discomfort commonly associated with constipation—lower abdominal discomfort, swelling, low back pain, and bloating—although at least 6% of the general population and 20% of the elderly suffer from painless constipation.[3,9,11]

Most physicians further define constipation as a chronic problem (lasting longer than 6 weeks) with hard stools and/or the inability to pass either hard or soft stools.[2]

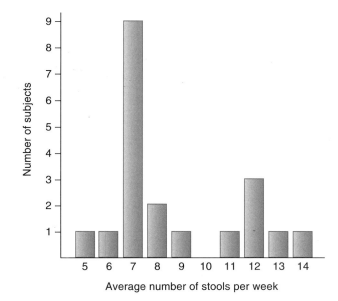

Figure 10.1. Average weekly stool frequencies for 21 healthy subjects.

Some physicians feel that any decrease in the patient's normal stool frequency, even if it is still in the normal range, should be classified as constipation.[12] (See "Dangers of Constipation.")

See Figures 10.2 and 10.3 to review the anatomy of the large intestine and the anorectal region.

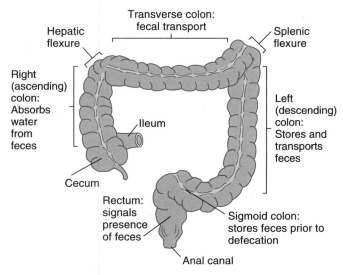

Figure 10.2. The anatomy and functions of the large intestine.

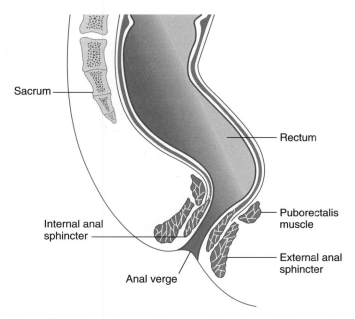

Figure 10.3. The anatomy of the anorectal region and the muscles involved in defecation.

PREVALENCE OF CONSTIPATION

Constipation rarely leads to hospitalization or death, so the prevalence data is not clear.[17,18] Several indicators of its incidence in the United States are available, however:

- Perhaps 2% of people in the United States at any one time consider themselves constipated, a target population of approximately 4.5 million.[2,9,17]
- Physicians average 2.5 million visits for constipation each year.[6]
- Over 3 million prescriptions are written for laxatives each year.
- OTC sales of laxatives were $678 million in 1996.[19]

- At least 40% of patients 65 years of age and above report constipation.[20]
- Constipation is the primary cause of death of more than 20 individuals each year.[9]
- Approximately 900 persons die annually from disorders associated with or related to constipation.[9]
- Constipation was listed as a discharge diagnosis in over 92,000 hospitalizations each year.[10]

EPIDEMIOLOGY OF CONSTIPATION

Knowing the epidemiologic variables related to constipation helps predict the specific patient subgroups most likely to ask a pharmacist for assistance.

Age

Constipation is common in all age groups, although the general public views it as mainly a problem of elderly patients.[21,22] Constipation is often seen as a disorder of elderly patients, partly because elderly patients sometimes complain of constipation when their stools are soft, even though their evacuation frequencies and gut transit times are normal.[23] Infants and children also experience constipation, but there is a marked decrease in the problem after age 10.[17,24]

Although constipation can affect patients of all ages, epidemiologic studies do demonstrate an age-related increase in physician visits. The greatest increase is seen from the 60 to 64 age group to the over-65 age group.[17] The incidence in patients aged 65 to 74 is 4.5%, and it rises to 10.2% in those over 75 (the authors did not provide the incidence for those aged 60 to 64).[1] The strong age relationship has a number of causes including lifelong laxative abuse, immobility, chronic illnesses, medication use, poor nutrition, reduced fluid intake (as opposed to younger patients), and age-related changes in gut motility (decreased colonic contractions).[15,25]

Gender

Constipation shows no gender differences in infants and children. After childhood, females are three times more likely to suffer from constipation than males.[9,17,26] Also, women begin to experience constipation at an earlier age than men and are more likely than men to complain to a physician about the problem.[27]

Race

Complaints of constipation are 1.3 times more prevalent among nonwhites than whites.[10] The condition is especially high in blacks, although no explanation has been offered for this puzzling research finding.

Socioeconomic and Geographic Variables

Constipation is more common in the southern United States, the lowest incidence is seen in the Northeast, and rural patients suffer more than their metropolitan counterparts.[9]

Constipation is also more common in low-income families and those where the family head has a low educational background.[9] The causes of these findings are unknown, although diet may be partially responsible.

Genetic Factors

Epidemiologic variables are often modified by the influence of genetics. Between 38 and 65% of constipated children had an onset before the age of 6 months.[28] Often, constipation is seen in the earliest weeks of life, before epidemiologic variables (e.g., socioeconomic situation) could significantly affect bowel function.

ETIOLOGY OF CONSTIPATION

Lifestyle Causes of Constipation

TRAVEL

Traveling is a particularly common time for constipation to occur.[29] Eating at restaurants usually forces different food choices than when at home. Sitting in a car, plane, or train for hours does not permit exercise. Bathrooms found on the road are sometimes unclean and undesirable. Also, travelers may not want to interrupt their activities to take time for a BM.[11] Obviously, patients must try to observe all normal habits when traveling, but all these factors combine to increase the risk of constipation.

DIET

Inadequate Fluid Intake

Inadequate fluid intake is a major and common cause of constipation. *Unless fluid-restricted (kidney failure, for example), patients should drink at least eight glasses, 8 to 10 ounces each, of noncaffeinated fluids daily (including soup, juices, and/or water).*[2,11] Many older patients do not drink nearly enough fluids because of a decreased thirst response.[3,30]

Inadequate Dietary Fiber

Patients whose diet is low (below 10 to 25 g daily) in dietary fiber may be prone to constipation. Increasing the amount of fiber in the diet is a simple and safe method of avoiding constipation.[2,31] Fiber can shorten the time it takes to pass material through the bowel and can bulk up the stools and make

---

FOCUS ON...

DANGERS OF CONSTIPATION

Most physicians are inadequately trained in the management and evaluation of constipation. Consequently, they often consider constipation a simple complaint that is easy to manage and delegate its treatment to nonphysician members of the health care team.[2,12] However, since constipation can produce direct or indirect morbidity, it should be evaluated carefully.

Elderly patients sometimes believe that constipation will lead to **autointoxication** (a misconception popular in the early 1900's that if feces are left in the bowel more than a short period, toxins will be reabsorbed by the body).[13] Some elderly patients may not eat properly from fear that they will reabsorb toxins from the bowel into the body, contaminating their systems.[2,12]

Straining to pass a stool can decrease coronary, cerebral, and peripheral arterial circulation as a result of changes in intrathoracic pressures, possibly leading to transient ischemic attacks and syncope.[14] Continual straining can also denervate the puborectalis musculature and external anal sphincter, causing further problems (inability to sense the presence of feces; loss of control of the anal sphincter) with passage of stool.

Continued constipation can result in fecal impaction, **megacolon** (dilation of the colon, in this case caused by accumulated feces), or **megarectum** (dilation of the rectum, in this case caused by the accumulation of feces).[12,13] Feces remaining in the distal bowel become progressively dehydrated as a result of colonic absorption of water and salt. Continued peristaltic activity carries further feces to the mass; eventually the material aggregates to form a dehydrated, hardened mass.[15] In some patients, the anal passage often is not capable of relaxing sufficiently to allow this hardened fecal mass to pass. Trapped gas and liquid stool seep around the mass, causing incontinence and paradoxical diarrhea.[3]

If fecal outflow is completely restricted, the lower bowel will stretch to accommodate the continuously accumulating mass. If colonic perforation (toxic megacolon) results, emergency medical treatment will be necessary.

Enemas or suppositories (e.g, hyperosmotic suppositories such as glycerin) are preferred to bulking agents if an impaction is suspected. Surgery must also be considered if these measures are ineffective.[16]

---

them easier to eliminate. Fiber retains water, forming the stool into jellylike masses that ease evacuation (Fig. 10.4).

(tip) *Patients should try to eat at least 10 to 25 g of fiber daily.*
Fibers are found in many foods including grains, beans, oats, and wheat, as well as in certain nonprescription products (e.g., those containing psyllium). (Fiber is not synonymous with roughage.[12] Roughage—as found in most fruits and vegetables—is composed of polysaccharides that do not increase stool bulk through retention of water and are relatively low in fiber.[2] Fiber, on the other hand, is composed of polysaccharides that do increase the bulk of fecal material.) It may take several weeks for a high-fiber diet to achieve full results. Also, patients may notice abdominal discomfort or gas with the first few doses, symptoms that usually stop after a few days.[6,11]

Other Dietary Problems

(tip) *In addition to increasing the amount of dietary fiber, patients should also limit foods that contain little or no fiber (e.g., ice cream, soft drinks, cheese, white bread, and meat) in order to balance the diet with more fiber-rich foods.*

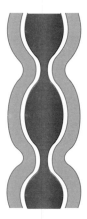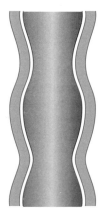

Fecal bolus
resulting from
low-fiber diet:
hard dry stools

Fecal bolus
resulting from
high-fiber diet:
soft bulky stools

Figure 10.4. The benefits of a high-fiber diet: stools are softer and higher in bulk, promoting healthy bowel movements.

Colonic activity is promoted by ingestion of fats, fluids, spices, and both soluble and insoluble fiber.[2]

INADEQUATE EXERCISE

(tip) Aerobic exercises (e.g., walking, jogging, or bicycling) have long been prescribed/recommended to help prevent constipation by promoting bowel motility.[32,33] Compromised mobility that restricts exercise may be another factor promoting constipation in elderly patients.[34] However, the role of exercise has also been debated, with published research indicating that average exercise does not improve gastrointestinal (GI) transit.

PARENT-CHILD INTERACTIONS

The onset of toilet training is traumatic for many children and their caregivers. Children may feel so apprehensive about disappointing their caregivers that they simply refuse to defecate.[15,35] This feeling may be exacerbated when a caregiver cleaning a child while changing diapers expresses disgust and refers to the diaper and child as "dirty."[36] Children with "stool withholding" behavior squeeze the buttocks together tightly, turning red with the effort until the urge to defecate passes. Gentle reassurance may be all that is required.

In older children, constipation may occur with new situations such as a change to a new school with unpleasant bathrooms (e.g., no doors on toilet stalls).[37]

In any of these pediatric cases, prolonged constipation may also lead to **encopresis** (overflow incontinence of stool with staining of underclothing). This paradoxical diarrhea-like condition results when semiliquid stool is forced around the impacted stool in the distal colon.[37] When fecal impaction does occur in a child, the possibility of cystic fibrosis should be explored, since this condition often produces constipation.[15]

LOSS OF THE DEFECATORY REFLEX

When stool passes into the rectum, the body passes a message that the bowels need to be emptied.[2] Some patients suppress this urge to empty the bowels, perhaps because it is not convenient to defecate at that time or place. Eventually (perhaps over several days), the urge disappears altogether.[38,39] Stools become harder and the bowel becomes more full as more and more feces accumulate.[27] Once the problem is taken care of (perhaps with a bulk laxative), the pharmacist may suggest that patients heed the urge to defecate, a process known as bowel retraining.[40,41] (After breakfast [and other meals to a lesser extent], the bowel usually moves more rapidly [this is known as the **gastrocolic reflex**].[37,42] This could be a good time for the patient to set aside a quiet period of several minutes for attempts at defecation.[2,12])

Medical Causes of Constipation

Many medical conditions can cause constipation. For instance, in addition to the conditions discussed below, constipation may be a symptom of hypothyroidism, diverticular disease, depression, anorexia, schizophrenia, or drug abuse (e.g., laxatives, narcotics).[3,43,44]

PREGNANCY

Pregnant women experience a high incidence of constipation for several reasons[43,45]:

- In pregnant women, the uterus pushes against the colon, often pressing the walls together more than normal.
- Pregnant women often do not exercise as much as normal, which may reduce bowel activity.
- Pregnant women usually take vitamins containing iron and calcium, both of which can be constipating.
- Perhaps because of the influence of progesterone, pregnant women suffer from bowel hypomotility.[45]

Pharmacists should exercise caution in recommending laxatives during pregnancy. The patient's obstetrician may prefer a certain product, so that pregnant patients should ask the obstetricians for advice regarding a safe laxative while pregnant (and while breast-feeding). Should the patient's obstetrician have no preference, docusate and bulk-forming agents such as psyllium are usually safe choices. The value of exercise, fluids, and a fiber-rich diet should also be shared with pregnant patients.

NERVE DAMAGE

Females may be constipated because of nerve damage caused by stretch injuries suffered in multiple deliveries.[2,9] Also, large infants delivered vaginally produce the same type of nerve damage, again leading to constipation.

PAIN

Pain during defecation could lead to avoidance and constipation. Painful defecation can be caused by passage of a hard stool, anal fissures, an **anal fistula** (abnormal opening at or near the anus, e.g, opening into the rectum above the internal sphincter), herpes simplex, a perianal abscess, rectal prolapse, pelvic-floor myalgia, or hemorrhoids.[2,11,35] A physician should be consulted if there is any indication that these conditions exist (e.g., presence of involuntary staining, bleeding, protrusion of tissue outside of the anus). Nonprescription hemorrhoidal products are only suitable for the minor pain associated with hemorrhoidal irritation or swelling.

PROLONGED COLON TRANSIT TIME (COLONIC INERTIA)

The average time of passage through the GI tract is 4 days (Fig. 10.5).[2] Colonic dysfunction, which primarily affects female patients, can lead to prolonged colon transit of the fecal bolus, with a subsequent increase in its hardness.[27,46] Conditions slowing transit include reduced activity, dehydration, dementia, Parkinsonism, and stroke.[47] Motility may be stimulated by boosting carbohydrate intake while limiting protein.

MEDICAL CONDITIONS

Many medical conditions can cause constipation. A pharmacist who suspects an association between constipation and a medical condition should refer the patient to a physician for a full evaluation of the underlying disorder.

Carcinoma

Constipation of recent onset associated with discomfort, gaseousness, anorexia, weight loss, malaise, **tenesmus** (painful spasm of the anal sphincter accompanied by involuntary straining to evacuate the bowel, but with passage of little fecal material), and blood in the stool can indicate colorectal carcinoma, especially when the patient is middle-aged or elderly.[3,5] Tumors may produce constipation, either through mechanical obstruction or by metastasizing to the spinal cord.[15] Further, chronic constipation may be a marginal risk factor for colorectal cancer.[8]

Irritable Bowel Syndrome

Irritable bowel syndrome is a common cause of constipation in younger patients.[3,16] Patients experience constipation alternating with diarrhea, cramping abdominal pain, passage of hard or pelletlike stools and mucus, straining to defecate, and a sense of inadequate evacuation.

Diabetes

While a sizable number of diabetics experience intermittent diarrhea, constipation is the most common GI symptom in diabetes, with an incidence of 60%.[11,48] Research indicates that the normal postprandial gastrocolic reflex is diminished or absent in diabetic patients.

Chronic Renal Failure

Fluid volume and electrolyte disturbances secondary to chronic renal failure predispose patients to constipation.

Parkinson's Disease

Patients with Parkinson's suffer from constipation for several reasons, including abnormal gut motility, rigid abdominal muscles, ineffectual diaphragm control, and progressive general immobility.[12] When these are combined with the effect of anticholinergics used in Parkinsonism therapy, the risk of constipation is greatly increased.

MEDICATIONS

When a patient complains of constipation, the pharmacist should ask what medications the patient is taking, since many prescription medications have been implicated. (See "Medications That Can Cause Constipation.") Rather than suggesting use of a nonprescription laxative, the pharmacist should first consider notifying the physician of the problem so the dosage may be adjusted or an alternative therapeutic agent be chosen.[12] If a nonprescription medication is implicated, the pharmacist may choose an alternative ingredient that is less likely to produce constipation.

MANIFESTATIONS OF CONSTIPATION

Early constipation may not produce symptoms, or it may cause lower abdominal cramping, discomfort, or pain resulting from the entrapped gas.[50] The patient may experience a feeling of abdominal swelling caused by the accumulation of

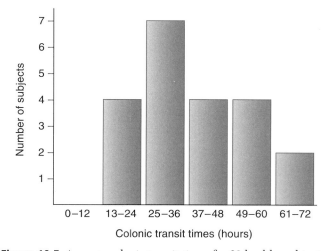

Figure 10.5. Average colonic transit times for 21 healthy subjects.

FOCUS ON . . .

MEDICATIONS THAT CAN CAUSE CONSTIPATION

The list of possible medications that cause constipation is extensive.[49] It includes opiates, anticholinergics, diuretics, NSAIDs, sympathomimetics (e.g., ephedrine, phenylpropanolamine, pseudoephedrine), some antihypertensives, tricyclic antidepressants, MAOIs, anticonvulsants, colestipol, cholestyramine, benzodiazepines, and barbiturates. Nonprescription medications that may be responsible include Schedule V codeine-containing cough syrups, iron supplements and vitamin-mineral combinations containing iron, antihistamines, antacids containing aluminum or calcium, calcium supplements, nonprescription NSAIDs (e.g., ibuprofen, naproxen, ketoprofen), famotidine, nizatidine, and ranitidine.[2,11]

fecal material and gas. Bloating and flatulence may occur as a result of the increased bacterial fermentation.[51] When constipation has resulted in a fecal impaction, the patient may experience paradoxical diarrhea and incontinence as liquid stool seeps around the impaction.

TREATMENT OF CONSTIPATION

Constipation that is not caused by an underlying medical disorder may be treated with various nonprescription medications, as well as with nonpharmacologic therapies, as discussed below. The choice of a particular laxative depends on many variables, including the age, health status, and motivation of the patient. Patient Assessment Algorithm 10.1 illustrates the steps used to determine which agent is optimal to treat constipation.

Treatment Guidelines

GENERAL PRECAUTIONS

Patients under a physician's care for a medical condition such as those listed above (e.g., diabetes, renal failure, thyroid problems), patients taking prescription medications that might cause constipation, and patients who are possible laxative misusers/abusers should be referred to a physician. Pharmacists should also be alert to the following:

- Constipation coupled with abdominal pain, nausea, or vomiting may indicate appendicitis; **using a laxative with appendicitis could cause the appendix to rupture, a medical emergency.** (See "A Pharmacist's Journal: Will These Laxatives Work for My Son?")

- Rectal bleeding or a sudden change in bowel habits that persists for 2 weeks or more may indicate cancer.[2,52]

- **Colostomates** (patients with an artificially created opening on the surface of the skin through which contents of the large intestine empty) or **ileostomates** (patients with an artificially created opening on the surface of the skin through which contents of the small intestine empty) should be referred to the physician.

- Constipation in a patient following recent abdominal surgery may indicate **ileus** (lack of peristalsis).

tip A patient with a physician recommendation for a specific product should use only the product ordered. A harsh stimulant, for example, may be needed to clean a patient's bowel prior to a procedure such as barium enema or proctosigmoidoscopy. Switching them to a bulk could result in a wasted procedure, with added patient costs, time lost from work, etc.

tip Failure to have a bowel movement following lifestyle modifications and the use of a laxative may indicate a serious condition.[12,52] Patients not benefiting from laxatives should discontinue use and see a physician. Patients should never use any laxative for more than 1 week, unless a physician directs them to do so.[52] (The exception is bulk laxatives, which may be used on a long-term basis by the patient to *prevent* constipation; however, these agents should still not be used for longer than 1 week to *treat* constipation). Laxatives are for occasional use only (with the exception of bulk laxatives as preventive therapy).

tip Should pharmacists suspect that a patient suffers from an eating disorder, laxatives should not be sold. How-

A Pharmacist's Journal

"Will These Laxatives Work for My Son?"

A woman in her 30s approached the counter with a box of Ex-Lax and two Fleet enemas and asked me, "Would these be OK for a child?" I asked how old the child was and she said 8. I asked how long the child had been constipated and she said that he did have a bowel movement the day before. I was in the midst of explaining that the daily bowel movement is not as important as parents think, when she interrupted with, "It's not really that he can't go, it's mainly the pain." I immediately halted and asked her to explain what she meant. She continued, "He began to cramp last night. This morning I let him stay home from school while I

went to work. He was hurting so bad when I got home that he could hardly crawl across the floor to unlock the door for me. His shirt was soaked with sweat from the pain." I described the possibility of appendicitis, with the consequences of not having her son checked by a physician immediately (e.g., overwhelming infection and death). I told her if it were one of my sons I would have him in the emergency room immediately. She replied, "I'll probably take him to the doctor, but I just want to buy these in case we need them." I further advised her that she must be cautious with their use since they can rupture an inflamed appendix and again stressed that the child must be seen by a physician. As too often happens, I heard nothing further.

Patient Assessment Algorithm 10.1. Part 1 Constipation

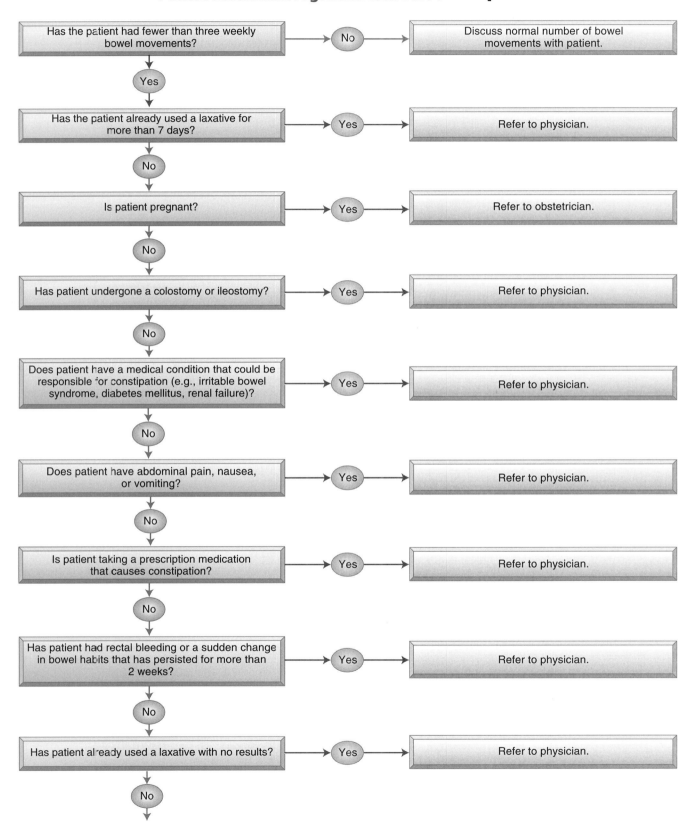

Patient Assessment Algorithm 10.1. Part 2 Constipation

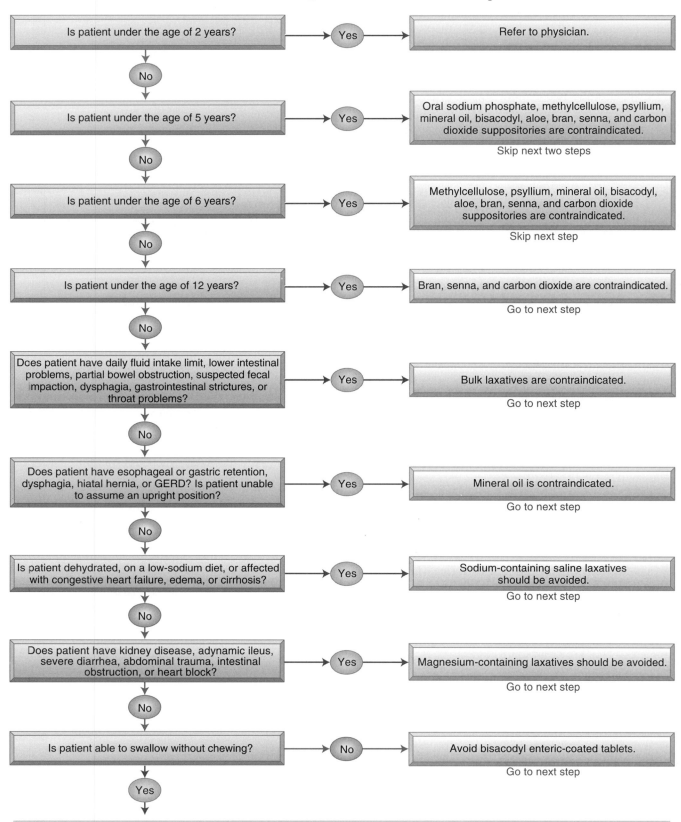

ever, repeat abusers are often as-tute enough to bypass the phar-macist and purchase the products from a cashier. For this reason, the pharmacy may choose to keep the products behind the counter, with a note notifying potential purchasers to ask the pharmacist for help. Laxative abuse is a sig-nificant feature of anorexia-bulimia syndrome.[53,54] (See "Lax-ative Abuse.")

AGE LIMITS FOR LAXATIVE INGREDIENTS

The FDA, which has evaluated the safety of laxatives at different ages, requires the following age-related labeling:

- No laxative can be adminis-tered to a child younger than 2 without a physician's recom-mendation.
- Laxatives safe for children age 2 and older include malt soup extract, polycarbophil, glycerin suppositories, sorbitol, mineral oil enemas, magnesium citrate, magnesium hy-droxide, milk of magnesia, magnesium sulfate, enemas con-taining sodium phosphate, docusate (oral or enema), cas-anthranol, cascara sagrada, castor oil, and phenolphthalein.
- An ingredient safe for children age 5 and older—but not to be recommended for children younger than 5—is oral sodium phosphate.
- Laxatives safe for children age 6 and older—but not to be recommended for children younger than 6—include methylcellulose, psyllium, oral lubricants, bisacodyl (oral and suppositories), and aloe.
- Laxatives safe for patients age 12 and older—but not to be recommended for patients younger than 12—include bran, senna, and carbon-dioxide suppositories.[52]

Nonprescription Medications

BULK LAXATIVES

Bulk laxatives are fiber-replacement products that are taken orally, usually mixed with liquid.

Method of Action of Bulk Laxatives

As mentioned previously, a major cause of constipation in de-veloped countries is a lack of fiber in the diet.[60] Bulk laxatives such as those listed in Table 10.1 replace this missing fiber. (Bulk laxatives are perhaps better termed dietary supple-ments than true laxative drugs.[2,6]) An exception to all other laxatives, bulk laxatives can be used safely for long periods by those who wish to prevent constipation.

When taken orally, bulk laxatives dissolve or swell in the fluids of the digestive tract by attracting water to certain "hydrophilic sites," forming gels that promote healthy

---

FOCUS ON...

LAXATIVE ABUSE

Laxative abuse is a widely recognized problem that may result in constipation or diar-rhea.[55] Abusers usually fall into one of three groups[56]:

- Patients, usually women, with eating disorders who are trying to control their weight
- Young-to-middle-aged persons, usually women, who work in jobs related to medicine
- Children being given laxatives as a form of abuse by their parents (the so-called Polle syndrome).

Abusers often persistently deny laxative use, even when confronted by concrete evidence such as positive urine or stool tests or the discovery of laxatives in their belongings.[57,58]

Although the FDA requires labeling on all laxatives cautioning patients not to use them for longer than 1 week and only to use them occasionally, this warning is often ignored. Overuse can lead to "cathartic colon" and damage to the myenteric ganglion cells. In one series of patients referred for evaluation of diarrhea, 25% were found to be covering up laxative abuse. Authors of another study concluded that at least 15% of patients with di-arrhea of uncertain origin are surreptitious laxative abusers.[59] Laxative abuse also results in constipation because of continued dilation and atony of the colon.[57]

Stimulant laxatives are among the most frequent laxatives abused.[55,57]

BMs.[42,61–63] They increase stool frequency and weight.[64] If the product is meant to be mixed with water, the patient must drink it immediately after adding product to the water. If allowed to stand, the granules will absorb water and swell in the glass, forming a gel.[61] Since most patients would be un-willing to eat this gel with a spoon, the entire dose must be discarded. Patients may take bulk laxatives one to three times daily. (See "Patients Who Should Not Use Bulk Laxatives.")

Patients Who Should Not Use Bulk Laxatives

Bulk laxatives are inappropriate for patients who must limit intake of fluids (e.g., patients with renal disease), patients with lower intestinal problems such as ulcerations or adhe-sions (the bulk may be harder to excrete in these cases), and patients who require prompt or thorough bowel evacuation (e.g., to treat poisonings or in preparation for bowel x-rays, proctoscopy, or bowel surgery). Bulk laxatives also should be avoided in patients with partial bowel obstruction, suspected fecal impaction, dysphagia, gastrointestinal strictures, or throat problems.[22] Finally, bedridden patients usually have colonic distention; bulking agents worsen the distension and may compound the problem.[42]

Time of Action of Bulk Laxatives

More than any other laxatives, bulk laxatives stimulate normal movement of the GI tract. Bulk laxatives do not force an un-natural bowel movement nor increase the number of bowel movements (as do stimulant laxatives).[61] For this reason, the patient should not expect a bowel movement the next morn-ing for a product taken at bedtime. Bulk laxatives take as long as 12 to 72 hours to exert laxation. Pharmacists should tell pa-tients that it may take 3 days of product usage before they are regulated, to prevent patients from becoming disappointed and resorting to use of a less natural laxative.

Table 10.1. Representative Bulk-Forming Laxatives

PRODUCT	SELECTED INGREDIENTS/COMMENTS
Citrucel Orange	Per 19-g heaping tablespoonful dose, 2 g methylcellulose
Citrucel Orange Sugar Free	Per 10.2-g rounded tablespoonful dose, 2 g methylcellulose, aspartame
FiberCon Caplets	Calcium polycarbophil 625 mg equivalent to 500 mg polycarbophil
Konsyl Psyllium Hydrophilic Mucilloid	Per rounded teaspoonful dose, 6 g of psyllium hydrophilic mucilloid
Maltsupex Malt Soup Extract Liquid	Per tablespoonful, the equivalent of 16 g of malt soup extract powder
Metamucil Regular Flavor, Original Texture	Per rounded teaspoonful dose, approx. 3.4 g of 95% pure psyllium husk
Metamucil Orange Flavor, Original Texture	Per rounded tablespoonful dose, approx. 3.4 g of 95% pure psyllium husk
Metamucil Regular Flavor, Smooth Texture, Sugar Free	Per rounded teaspoonful dose, approx. 3.4 g of 95% pure psyllium husk, citric acid, magnesium sulfate
Metamucil Orange Flavor, Smooth Texture, Sugar Free	Per rounded teaspoonful dose, approx. 3.4 g of 95% pure psyllium husk, aspartame, citric acid
Metamucil Orange Flavor, Smooth Texture Packets	Per 12-g packet, 3.4 g pure psyllium husk, citric acid, sodium 3 mg
Metamucil Fiber Wafers, Cinnamon Spice or Apple Crisp	Per 2 wafers, 3.4 g of 95% pure psyllium husk, 6 g of fiber
Perdiem Fiber Therapy	Per 6-g rounded teaspoonful dose, 4.03 g of 100% psyllium
Serutan Granules	Per heaping teaspoonful, 2.5 g psyllium mucilloid

Ingestion of Adequate Water with Bulk Laxatives

The emphatic requirement that the patient consume adequate water along with bulk laxatives is a consequence of their action. They form the gels when they come into contact with water. (Of course, inadequate fluid intake is also a contributing cause of constipation, so the more fluid a patient drinks with the bulk laxative, the more likely he is to have healthy bowel movements in any case.) Products that must be mixed with water should be mixed with 8 to 10 ounces of water, then followed by an additional 8 to 10 ounces of water to ensure optimal activity.

In 1993 the FDA expanded the warning statement and directions comment for polycarbophil, methylcellulose, and psyllium.[65] The revised warning reads: ***"Warnings: Taking this product without adequate fluid may cause it to swell and block your throat or esophagus and may cause choking. Do not take this product if you have difficulty swallowing. If you experience chest pain, vomiting, or difficulty in swallowing or breathing after taking this product, seek immediate medical attention."*** The revised directions read: "Directions: Take this product with at least 8 ounces (a full glass) of water or other fluid. Taking this product without enough liquid may cause choking." This warning was added because of a dangerous diet product that contained guar gum, a bulking agent. Some patients did not consume adequate water with the tablets, causing esophageal obstruction that resulted in hospitalizations and death.

The dangers of esophageal impaction caused by phytobezoars (concretions or masses of fibrous matter such as skin, seeds, and vegetable and fruit residue in the gastrointestinal tract) from bulking agents have been known for decades. For instance, in the early 1950s, two reports appeared that described complete esophageal obstruction when a psyllium product was taken dry, followed by water.[66,67] Later reports also documented that the problem still occurs.[68–70]

A number of reports of intestinal **bezoars** (a concretion found in the GI tract, composed of hair or food materials) caused by bulk laxatives have appeared in the literature, including the following examples:

- A primary colonic bezoar was caused by psyllium, which obstructed the gastric outlet by compression.[71]
- A patient did not have sufficient fruit juice to mix his daily dose of psyllium, so he added a small amount of water and "chewed it down." He suffered gastric outlet and small bowel obstruction caused by the semisolid psyllium.[72]

Drug Interactions of Bulk Laxatives

Patients currently taking such medications as digitalis, warfarin, salicylates, or nitrofurantoin should be cautioned not to take the bulk laxative within 3 hours of the medications because the laxative may reduce effectiveness of the medication.

The manufacturer of Metamucil has voluntarily added the following statement to all of its labels: "Laxatives, including bulk fibers, may affect how well other medicines work. If you are taking a prescription medicine by mouth, take this product at least 2 hours before or 2 hours after the prescribed medicine."[73] This advice could be given by pharmacists to those taking any oral prescription or nonprescription product.

Approved Bulk Laxatives

Products containing a safe and effective bulk laxative will list one of the following in the contents statement: psyllium, bran, calcium polycarbophil, malt soup extract, karaya, or methylcellulose.[52]

Bulk Laxatives and Psyllium Allergies

Psyllium laxatives and psyllium/senna combinations have caused several allergic reactions, including asthmatic attacks, sneezing, watery eyes, skin reactions, wheezing, chest congestion, angioedema, gastrointestinal symptoms, swollen eyelids, red sclera, bronchospasm, and anaphylactic shock.[74] Allergic reactions to psyllium are generally seen in health professionals such as nurses who reconstitute and administer several doses of psyllium laxatives daily. (Therefore, psyllium allergy could be considered an occupational disease.[75]) Patients or caregivers who are highly allergic should avoid mixing these products and should not be in the room when they are mixed, or should wear face masks and use vertical laminar flow biological containment hoods to minimize inhalation.[76]

In a well-documented case, a 45-year-old nurse with a 12-year history of work in a skilled nursing facility visited a physician for allergy consultation after use of Metamucil for constipation.[77] The product caused severe cramping, abdominal pain, and nausea. On questioning, she stated that she suffered from sneezing, runny nose, watery eyes, postnasal drip, headache, fullness and itching in the ears, cough, chest tightness, and wheezing on the days she distributed Metamucil. On her days off and on her days when she did not distribute Metamucil, her symptoms were absent. She coped by using Opticrom, Nasalcrom, and face masks. Her allergists tested her and discovered that nasal resistance increased more than 350% following Metamucil exposure. The authors noted that workers such as this nurse may be regarded as malingerers and added that up to 18% of workers may be allergic to psyllium.

In another case, a nurse who ingested Kellogg's Heartwise cereal suffered an anaphylactic reaction to the psyllium in the product, even though she had not previously ingested psyllium.[78] She had, however, prepared bulk laxatives for patients in a spinal cord unit several years earlier. (Fifteen of 18 allergic reactions to this cereal reported to Kellogg's were in nurses or nursing home employees who dispensed psyllium-containing bulk laxatives.[78])

For patients with suspected heavy occupational psyllium exposure, the pharmacist should recommend an alternate bulking agent.

Utility of Bulk Laxatives

Bulk laxatives are the safest of all of the laxative agents. With the rare exceptions listed above, the health of most patients who complain of constipation would be greatly enhanced if they ingested bulk agents as a routine preventive for constipation. In this regard, the 7-day use limitation on laxatives does not apply, since the agents are being used for preventive purposes, rather than treatment.

Bulk laxatives are also safe and effective for patients who present with actual constipation, if pharmacists are able to convince the patients to consume adequate water and take the products for at least 3 days. However, in this case, the 7-day use limit does apply.

STOOL SOFTENERS (EMOLLIENTS)

Method and Time of Action of Stool Softeners

Stool-softening laxatives employ a surface-active (surfactant) ingredient to help water in the bowel mix with the fecal mass, thereby softening it (Table 10.2).[2,42] The less firm mass is then more easily passed. The only approved stool softener is docusate (formerly known as dioctyl sodium sulfosuccinate), either in the calcium or sodium salt. Pharmacists should advise patients that although docusate may work in as short a period as 12 hours, it could take as long as 72 hours to exert laxation. (See "Enemas" for the use of stool softeners in an enema dosage form.)

When to Recommend Stool Softeners

Stool softeners (i.e., docusate) are useful in patients with hard stools or those who should avoid straining when defecating (e.g., patients with recent rectal surgery or with an abdominal hernia).[2] Some pediatricians consider it the ingredi-

Table 10.2. Representative Stool-Softener (Emollient) Laxatives

PRODUCT	SELECTED INGREDIENTS/COMMENTS
Colace Capsules	Docusate sodium 100 mg
Colace Liquid	Per mL: 10 mg docusate sodium (the company includes a dose for children of 3 to 6 years of age on the package as 2 mL 1–3 times daily)
Dialose Tablets	Docusate sodium 100 mg
Phillips' Liqui-Gels	Docusate sodium 100 mg
Surfak Capsules	Docusate calcium 240 mg

ent of choice in childhood constipation with hard, dry stools although docusate products are not approved for children younger than 2. Docusate is useful for elderly patients because of its low incidence of adverse reactions, although several authors feel that it may not be more effective than a placebo in this subpopulation.[2,21]

Adverse Reactions to Stool Softeners (Docusate)

Adverse effects of docusate use are rare. Occasionally, patients complain of mild, transitory gastrointestinal (GI) cramping pains, a discomfort that may result from the laxation produced by docusate.[71] In addition, some patients experience a generalized dermatologic rash following use of docusate. Also, stool softeners may be hepatotoxic and may enhance absorption of hepatobiliary toxins.[12,42]

Drug Interactions of Stool Softeners (Docusate)

Docusate may increase absorption of medications since it produces a change in the intestinal permeability that lasts a few hours. Pharmacists must be especially wary when patients are taking medications with a narrow therapeutic range, since they may become toxic. ***Never allow concurrent administration with reserpine, digoxin, or warfarin since their therapeutic index is narrow and unanticipated serum increases could be deadly. Also, concurrent administration with mineral oil can result in systemic lipid granulomatosis.***[14] The FDA requires that docusate be labeled with this drug interaction precaution: "Do not take this product if you are presently taking mineral oil, unless directed by a doctor."[79]

Teratogenicity of Stool Softeners (Docusate)

Administration of docusate to pregnant rats resulted in increased fetal resorption and produced significant incidences of fetal malformations, consisting primarily of exencephaly frequently associated with spina bifida and microphthalmia.[79] Skeletal abnormalities included incomplete ossification of cranial bones. However, doses were far in excess of those used in humans. As a result, a scientific review panel cleared docusate in 1993.[79]

MINERAL OIL

Mineral oil is the sole ingredient in the lubricant class of laxatives. The oral form is available as an oil, and an enema form is available (see "Enemas").

Method and Time of Action of Mineral Oil

Mineral oil is the only approved representative of its class, the lubricant laxatives (Table 10.3). Mineral oil works by coating fecal matter with oil, which prevents water from leaving the feces in the large intestine and in turn prevents the fecal mass from forming a semisolid consistency.[2,49] Patients may expect an effect in 6 to 8 hours. Abdominal cramping is not common.[37]

The mineral oil dose for patients 12 and older is 15 to 45 mL and for ages 6 to 12, 5 to 15 mL—either as a single daily dose or in divided doses.[52]

Cautions in the Use of Mineral Oil

While mineral oil may help prevent straining during defecation, its many cautions mitigate against use in almost all cases. During esophageal transit, mineral oil can be aspirated, which can produce acute or chronic lipid pneumonitis, lipoid pneumonia, bibasilar infiltrates, or a localized granuloma resembling a neoplasm.[37,80–84] For this reason, *patients must be upright when taking mineral oil.* Also, patients who are confined to bed or who must remain in a prone, side-lying or supine position must not use it.[83] The patient must be able to raise the top half of the trunk to approximately a 70° angle.

Mineral oil must also be taken 30 to 60 minutes prior to bedtime so that it will not be in the stomach when the patient is lying down, possibly being aspirated. Mineral oil should be avoided in patients with esophageal or gastric retention, dysphagia, hiatal hernia, or GERD, since the risk of aspiration is enhanced in all of these patients. Further, in neurologically or psychologically impaired individuals with swallowing problems, it could be more easily aspirated.[2,12]

Patients using mineral oil may experience rectal itching and leakage of the oil from a competent rectal sphincter. This leakage of oil and feces can be embarrassing, but lowering the dose may help alleviate the problem.[37]

Finally, mineral oil has been found to be carcinogenic in some strains of mice and researchers believe that it could indirectly induce cancer in man through the production of pulmonary fibrosis.[42,85,86]

Drug/Food Interactions of Mineral Oil

The FDA requires the following drug-interaction warning: "Do not take this product if you are currently taking a

Table 10.3. Representative Laxatives Containing Mineral Oil

PRODUCT	SELECTED INGREDIENTS/COMMENTS
Humco Mineral Oil	Heavy mineral oil, USP
Haley's M-O Suspension	Per 5 mL: magnesium hydroxide 301 mg, mineral oil 1.25 mL
Kondremul Plain Emulsion	Mineral oil (amount unlabeled), acacia, benzoic acid, Irish Moss, glycerin
Milkinol Emulsion	Mineral oil (amount unlabeled), emulsifier, BHA
Squibb Mineral Oil	Mineral oil

stool softener laxative."[52] As noted under "Stool Softeners" above, concurrent administration of mineral oil and stool softeners can result in systemic lipid granulomatosis. Although mineral oil may also impair absorption of oral contraceptives and coumarin derivatives, this will not be part of the official labeling.[42]

If mineral oil is taken within 2 hours of a meal, it impairs absorption of fat-soluble vitamins (A,D,E,K).[2] The FDA requires the following warning on all nonprescription containers of mineral oil: "Do not take with meals."[52]

⚠️ The approved FDA label also states that ***mineral oil must not be used by pregnant women. Hemorrhagic disease of the newborn may result from hypovitaminosis K.***

SALINE LAXATIVES
Method and Time of Action of Saline Laxatives
Saline laxatives are sufficiently hyperosmotic/hypertonic in relation to the contents of the GI tract to osmotically draw water into the intestine and keep it there until it reaches the lower bowel and is eliminated, in most cases as a rather watery bowel movement in 6 to 8 hours (Table 10.4).[87] To facilitate this action, patients might be advised to drink a full 8 ounces of water with each dose to prevent dehydration, irritation, and nausea.[42]

Magnesium products may also act through release of cholecystokinin or increase of fecal prostaglandin, although more data is needed to confirm this theory.[42,56] Magnesium does not usually produce abdominal cramping or nocturnal bowel movements, unlike some other laxatives (e.g., stimulants).[87]

Because of the complete catharsis they induce, salines may be used in poisoning cases and are occasionally used in preprocedure, bowel-preparation regimens. This may contribute to a cycle of abuse and habituation.

Cautions in the Use of Saline Laxatives
🛈 Some older patients may be close to dehydration. *By producing watery bowel movements, salines could be dangerous by causing further fluid compromise.*[11]

Sodium-Containing Saline Laxatives
If the product contains more than 5 mEq of sodium in the maximum recommended daily dose, the FDA requires the label to read: "Do not use if on a low-sodium diet unless advised by a physician." *Sodium-containing saline laxatives must be used cautiously, if at all, in patients with* ⚠️ *congestive heart failure, edema, or cirrhosis.* ***Indiscriminate use of sodium-containing saline laxatives has actually caused congestive heart failure.*** If sodium-containing saline laxatives contain phosphates, they must have this label: "Do not use this product if you have kidney disease unless directed by a physician."[52]

Although an oral sodium phosphate product is available, its use is rare compared with the enema form. For this reason, some hazards of sodium phosphate saline laxatives appear under "Enemas."

Magnesium-Containing Saline Laxatives
🛈 *Patients with adynamic ileus, severe diarrhea, abdominal trauma, intestinal obstruction, heart block, and renal failure, and patients needing prolonged catharsis must avoid magnesium-containing saline laxatives.*[88] If the laxative contains more than 50 mEq of magnesium per recommended daily dose, the label must state, "Do not use if you have kidney disease unless advised by a physician." (Excretion of magnesium is retarded in renal failure, causing systemic toxicity.[89])

Safe and effective magnesium-containing laxative compounds include magnesium citrate, magnesium hydroxide, and magnesium sulfate:

- Magnesium citrate (also known as drugstore lemonade) is given in an adult dose of 8 to 10 oz.
- Available in green-colored glass bottles, magnesium citrate should be refrigerated in liquid form to increase palatability and help prevent crystallization. (The label states: "Store at temperatures between 46 and 86°F.")
- Magnesium sulfate (also known as Epsom salts) is approved as a laxative, but pharmacists most often sell it as a soak for sprains and strains to reduce swelling.
- Used as an antacid, magnesium hydroxide in larger doses causes laxation.

A substantial number of instances of hazardous use of magnesium-containing saline laxatives have been documented, including the following examples:

- A man with upper-right-quadrant pain dosed himself with 3 tablespoonfuls of Epsom salts (magnesium sulfate), 1 teaspoonful of Kaopectate, and 15 mg of phenobarbital.[90] He became comatose from magnesium overdose. Hospital

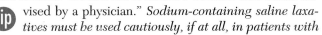

Table 10.4. Representative Saline Laxatives

PRODUCT	SELECTED INGREDIENTS
Citroma	Per fluid ounce: magnesium citrate 1.745 g
Fleet Phospho-Soda Buffered Oral Saline Laxative	Per 5 mL: monophasic sodium phosphate 2.4 g, dibasic sodium phosphate 0.9 g
Humco Epsom Salts	Magnesium sulfate, USP
Phillips' Milk of Magnesia	Per 5 mL: magnesium hydroxide 400 mg

emergency room personnel, unaware that he had taken magnesium, administered oral magnesium citrate solution. He survived without cardiac arrest, despite a serum magnesium of 9.5 mmol/L (normal = 0.7 to 0.95). (Levels exceeding 8 mmol/L generally cause cardiac arrest.)

- A female with normal renal function was given magnesium sulfate in unintentionally high doses (150 mL of a 50% solution every hour for 6 doses) following a suicide attempt.[91] She developed cardiorespiratory arrest as a result of a magnesium level that was 10 times normal. (This incident underlines the fact that magnesium dosing must not exceed the labeled doses. Serum magnesium has also been found to rise after repetitive administration of magnesium citrate in toxic ingestion management situations.[92])

- A 6-week-old infant was given 16 doses (1/3 of a 5 mL teaspoonful) of milk of magnesia in a 48-hour period for constipation.[93] He suffered life-threatening apnea with lethargy, was areflexic, and had a serum magnesium level of 5.85 mmol/L. Within ten hours of admission he was increasingly active, with return of deep tendon reflexes. He recovered and was discharged in 48 hours.

- A 25-day-old baby was given 8 teaspoonfuls a day of milk of magnesia for 1 week.[89] She survived with conservative therapy, which included calcium gluconate and fluids.

Magnesium usage is more likely than bulk and stool softener laxatives to result in diarrhea. Physicians at the Baylor University Department of Internal Medicine, troubled by a group of patients with chronic diarrhea (defined as lasting 1 month or longer), developed a test for diagnosing magnesium-induced diarrhea by examining fecal output of stool magnesium.[94] Twenty-one of 359 patients with chronic diarrhea were found to have an abnormally high fecal concentration of soluble magnesium. Fourteen of the 21 patients admitted to using laxative products containing magnesium; diarrhea ceased for all but one of the 14 patients when magnesium intake was reduced. These 14 patients apparently were simply unaware that magnesium usage was the cause of their problem. (One of the patients in that study was an 8-year-old girl. The girl's mother denied giving the child magnesium hydroxide, but hidden bottles of milk of magnesia were found during a search of the child's hospital room. The child's diarrhea resolved promptly and permanently after a court-ordered separation from the mother. The girl was a victim of abuse known as the Polle syndrome, a type of Munchausen's by proxy.)

STIMULANT LAXATIVES

Stimulant laxatives are taken by the patients in the form of tablets, granules, or liquids. One (bisacodyl) is also available as a suppository and is discussed under "Suppositories."

Method and Time of Action of Stimulant Laxatives

Stimulant laxatives may act through one or more drastic, severe, and nonphysiologic mechanisms (Table 10.5). In general, stimulant laxatives rely on **prodrugs** (nonactive forms of the medication, which require conversion to the active ingredients), which are transformed to an active aglycon and in turn increase colonic motility.[95] Effectively, the bowel is forced to empty its contents.

Recent evidence shows that some stimulant laxatives may also act by forcing the secretion of fluid into the bowel lumen.[45,96] This may include the release of **kinins**, which stimulate chloride secretion in alimentary epithelium.[97]

Whichever action predominates is academic, since they are troublesome laxatives in any case. They do work within 6 to 12 hours, however, when given in oral form. When formulated as suppositories, they have a shorter time of action, as noted under "Suppositories."

Table 10.5. Representative Stimulant Laxatives

PRODUCT	SELECTED INGREDIENTS/COMMENTS
Carter's Laxative Pill	Bisacodyl 5 mg
Dulcolax Tablets	Bisacodyl 5 mg
Correctol Caplets	Bisacodyl 5 mg
ex•lax Pills	Sennosides 25 mg
ex•lax Chocolated Laxative	Sennosides 15 mg
Feen-A-Mint Tablets	Bisacodyl 5 mg
Fleet Laxative Tablets	Bisacodyl 5 mg
Humco Castor Oil	Castor oil, USP
Neoloid Emulsified Castor Oil	Castor oil 36.4% (w/w), preservatives, emulsifying agents, water
Senokot Tablets	Sennosides 8.6 mg
X-Prep Bowel Evacuant Liquid	Per 2.5 ounce bottle, 130 mg sennosides

Cautions in the Use of Stimulant Laxatives
Stimulant Habituation. Used in correct doses for no more than 7 days, stimulant laxatives would not be likely to habituate the patient.[93] However, with misuse, stimulant laxatives cause a vicious cycle of abuse in which a patient becomes dependent on them for the "daily BM." This abuse cycle occurs because stimulant laxatives not only empty the bowel of the contents that were due for excretion on that day, but also usually empty the less distal bowel of contents that would have been emptied with the next BM.[31] Thus, when a patient attempts to defecate the following day, negative results lead him or her to assume that he or she is constipated again. Unless the patient realizes that the stimulant caused the condition, he or she might take another dose of stimulant laxative. The remedy is to stop using the stimulant laxative entirely and allow the bowel to catch up.

Long-term use of stimulant laxatives can lead to damage to bowel tissues. "Cathartic colon," a well-known sequela of long-term use, resembles ulcerative colitis both radiologically and pathologically.[57] With this condition the myenteric plexus suffers structural, permanent damage, with hypertrophy of the muscularis mucosa, smooth muscle atrophy, neural damage, and a dilated featureless appearance on endoscopy.[12,99]

Other Adverse Reactions of Stimulant Laxatives. Other well-known problems related to stimulant laxatives include intestinal griping, abdominal discomfort, cramping, tenesmus, electrolyte abnormalities (e.g., hypokalemia), dehydration, and the production of watery stools.[42,57,58,100] In the most severe reactions caused by short-term use, vomiting, muscle weakness, acidosis, or alkalosis may occur.[55]

Although ammonium urate renal calculi are rare, researchers have documented a series of patients in whom they occurred as the result of abuse of phenolphthalein (an ingredient that has been withdrawn from stimulant laxatives).[101] Apparently, the combination of GI water and electrolyte loss resulted in volume depletion and intracellular acidosis, which stimulated an increase in urinary ammonium. The authors cautioned that other stimulant laxative ingredients could also cause this problem.

Physicians occasionally detect long-term abuse of certain stimulant laxatives (at least 4 months) such as senna, cascara sagrada, and casanthranol during surgery or endoscopy of the colon. Visible light-brown to deep-black pigment on the intestinal wall, (known as pseudomelanosis coli) a well-accepted marker of anthraquinone laxative abuse, is currently not considered pathologically significant and is not a precancerous state.[102] However, it is an alteration of the bowel tissues caused by laxative abuse, usually reversing after 5 to 15 laxative-free months.

In one case of stimulant laxative abuse, a 26-year-old nurse who took 10 times the recommended dose of senna over a sustained period developed hepatitis.[103] The liver function tests improved or deteriorated further as her intake of senna decreased and increased, respectively.

In another case of abuse, a 24-year-old female who weighed nearly 300 pounds took more than 150 tablets of a phenolphthalein laxative each week.[58] Most were ingested on weekends to satisfy her husband, who weighed her every Monday morning. On examination at an emergency department, she was found to be pale with a low hemoglobin and positive stool test for occult blood. On discontinuation of the laxatives, the rectal bleeding ceased.

Medical Use of Stimulant Laxatives
Patients whose physicians have recommended stimulant laxatives to prepare for a medical procedure must follow the physicians' directions exactly. (Generally, however, most other patients could be switched from stimulants to less drastic and safer products.) Stimulant laxatives are probably safe for most patients in the short term; however, FDA approval of stimulants hinged on the often-mistaken supposition that patients would use them for no longer than the labeled cutoff of 1 week. The problem of habituation mentioned above virtually guarantees that many people will use them far longer than 1 week, possibly suffering severe and irreversible damage (e.g., cathartic colon). The prudent pharmacist will avoid recommending stimulant laxatives entirely to prevent this vicious cycle from manifesting.

Problems with Specific Stimulant Laxative Formulations
Anthraquinones. Senna, aloe, cascara sagrada, and its active principle casanthranol fall within this group. All discolor urine pink-to-red or brown-to-black. Anthraquinones also enter the milk of nursing mothers, causing laxation in the infant.[104]

Diphenylmethanes. Bisacodyl and phenolphthalein, which fall within this group, pass in breast milk.[104] Bisacodyl, available as an enteric-coated tablet, carries several FDA-required precautions. For instance, *the following message must appear on all containers of oral bisacodyl: "Do not chew tablets. This product may cause abdominal discomfort, faintness, and cramps. Do not take within 1 hour after taking an antacid or milk. Do not give to people who cannot swallow without chewing."*[52] It should also be avoided in patients taking cimetidine, ranitidine, famotidine, or nizatidine.[42]

Bisacodyl suppositories must be labeled with the following warning: *"This suppository may cause abdominal discomfort, faintness, rectal burning, and mild cramps."* The suppositories work within 15 to 60 minutes.[52] (See "Suppositories.")

Phenolphthalein was removed from laxative products during 1997 and 1998 because of concerns about carcinogenicity. (See "Carcinogenicity of Stimulant Laxatives.")

Castor Oil
This stimulant oil is administered in a dose of 15 mL for constipation and a dose of 15 to 60 mL as a preprocedure, bowel-preparation agent. Castor oil can erode intestinal villi and disorganizes the microvillous surface of the intestinal lumen.[42] Long-term use can lead to nutrient malabsorption.

Note that pregnant women sometimes use castor oil to hasten delivery of an "overdue" baby because of its ability to cause premature uterine contractions.[105] However, **this unapproved use of castor oil is deadly since castor oil can cause amniotic fluid embolism and impaired health of the infant.[106,107]** In at least one case, a physician unwisely advised the expectant mother to use it. *Pharmacists should advise pregnant patients who wish to purchase castor oil that all laxatives (with the possible exception of bulking agents) are unsafe in pregnancy, and castor oil presents unique hazards to her.* (See "A Pharmacist's Journal: Is This the Castor Oil for Airplanes?")

Carcinogenicity of Stimulant Laxatives

Danthron is an anthraquinone laxative that has been removed from the market.[108] Danthron was found to cause intestinal and liver tumors in rodents and was possibly linked to cancer in a human.[109] In 1987 the FDA advised the pharmaceutical industry that it would be unlikely to allow the ingredient to remain on the market with a positive test for carcinogenicity plus two, positive, in vivo studies in rodents that demonstrated carcinogenicity. The companies with products containing danthron issued a swift, voluntary recall. However, other anthraquinone compounds have also been found to exhibit a positive mutagenic effect in some in vitro models. Senna, cascara, and casanthranol could eventually be proven to be carcinogenic.

In mid 1996, the FDA issued a "Talk Paper" relating the findings of a 1995 study that indicated that phenolphthalein can cause tumors in rodents.[110] The FDA also revealed that senna has mutagenic effects. In light of these early warnings, the FDA placed both of those laxatives and three chemically related ingredients (aloe, bisacodyl, and cascara sagrada) into Category III. The FDA allowed the ingredients to remain on the market pending submission of manufacturer-sponsored safety studies, which the agency predicted would be completed in 1998. Subsequently, several manufacturers have switched ingredients to eliminate these suspect chemicals such as phenolphthalein (See "Phenolphthalein" above).

HYPEROSMOTIC LAXATIVES

Hyperosmotic laxatives are a useful group of ingredients that are found in enema form and suppositories (see "Enemas" and "Suppositories") (Table 10.6).

Method and Time of Action of Hyperosmotic Laxatives

Glycerin and sorbitol fall within this group. Given rectally, they exert a hygroscopic and/or local irritant effect, drawing water into the feces and stimulating evacuation.[2,11] Only extremely high oral doses have laxative effects, and the only approved nonprescription use is rectal. For this reason oral glycerin and sorbitol should not be recommended as laxatives. The patient may expect an effect in 15 to 60 minutes. Sorbitol is little used outside of the hospital environment.

Cautions in the Use of Hyperosmotic Laxatives

Adverse effects with rectal use include discomfort, irritation, burning or griping, cramping pain, and tenesmus. An FDA-mandated label on glycerin suppositories warns, "May cause rectal discomfort or a burning sensation."[52]

Glycerin suppositories may be premoistened with water to make insertion more comfortable. They should be inserted high and retained as long as possible. Glycerin suppositories are available in adult shape—the typical suppository shape—or a children's shape—longer and thinner to better match a child's physiology. (As with any nonprescription laxative product, of course, hyperosmotic laxatives are not appropriate for children younger than 2.) For pediatric use, a rectal solution of glycerin is also available, consisting of small individual plastic containers with prelubricated tips, each containing 4 mL of glycerin.

A Pharmacist's Journal

"Is This the Castor Oil for Airplanes?"

A male in his 40s asked me if the bottle of castor oil he was holding was the one that you use for airplanes. I asked, "You mean a laxative to use while you are flying?" He replied, "No, one that I use when I have engine trouble." I attempted to envision what type of aircraft use he proposed (e.g., exhaust problems), when he clarified the issue. He had read in an aircraft magazine that the practice of "dry-torquing" the bolts and screws while reassembling an aircraft engine is dangerous, since tightening the bolts by hand cannot prevent the engine vibrations from eventually loosening the bolts and screws, so that they may fall out in flight. He read that one instead must "wet-torque" the bolts and screws by first soaking them in castor oil, then tightening them while still oily. He advised that the residue remaining locks the bolts and screws in more tightly, so that engine vibration does not loosen them. In any case, he purchased the product, although I have not yet located the article that provides "scientific evidence" of the usefulness of castor oil in securing aircraft bolts.

Table 10.6. Representative Laxatives in Enema or Suppository Form

PRODUCT	SELECTED INGREDIENTS/COMMENTS
Babylax	Per 4 mL applicator: glycerin
Ceo-Two Suppository	Sodium bicarbonate, potassium bitartrate (amounts unlabeled)
Colace Microenema	Per 5 mL applicator: docusate sodium 200 mg
Dulcolax Suppository	Bisacodyl 10 mg
Fleet Bagenema	Kit containing graduated vinyl bag with a 60-inch length of tubing, absorbent pad
Fleet ready-to-use Enema	Per 118 mL delivered dose: monobasic sodium phosphate 19 g, dibasic sodium phosphate 7 g
Fleet ready-to-use Enema for Children	Per 59 mL delivered dose: monobasic sodium phosphate 9.5 g, dibasic sodium phosphate 3.5 g
Fleet ready-to-use Mineral Oil Enema	Per 118 mL delivered dose: mineral oil USP
Fleet Adult Size Glycerin Suppository	Glycerin
Fleet Child Size Glycerin Suppository	Glycerin
Perrigo Adult Size Glycerin Suppository	Glycerin 82.5%

ENEMAS

Enemas are local products that are instilled into the rectum with the use of an enema syringe. Commercially available, preprepared enemas have prelubricated tips and instructional pictures on the box to facilitate use. After the single use, they are disposed of. The patient may also choose an empty bulb with two sizes of nozzles known as an enema syringe. These latter reusable syringes are filled by the patient with a solution that is usually recommended by a physician. (See "A Pharmacist's Journal: What Is a 3-H Enema?")

Method and Time of Action of Enemas

Several of the previously discussed approved laxative ingredients are also active as laxatives when given in enema form (see Table 10.6). The advantages of using enemas to treat constipation is that the medication is directly applied where it is needed, minimizing systemic toxicity and reactions.[111] However, as with other laxatives, enemas are sometimes abused by patients with eating disorders.[3]

The mechanisms of action of enemas generally mirror that of the individual ingredients when administered orally, except that the distension attained when the solution is placed directly into the rectum is another important contributory factor in promoting a bowel movement.[2,6] Importantly, the onset of action is drastically shortened with enemas. For example, mineral oil, saline laxatives, and stool softeners given as enemas act within 2 to 15 minutes. Mineral oil retention enemas have been found to be helpful in disimpaction of hard fecal masses.[2]

Directions for Enema Use

An adult patient should lie on the left side (to facilitate movement into the sigmoid and lower descending colon) with

knees bent or kneel on the bed with head and chest lowered and forward until the left side of the face is resting on the surface of the bed (Fig. 10.6). The patient or person administering the enema should then follow these steps:

1. Insert the lubricated enema nozzle into the rectum with steady pressure, with the nozzle pointed toward navel.
2. Insert the nozzle until it seems that it will go no further.
3. Squeeze the container until the entire dose is expelled.

Patients must resist the natural urge to expel the enema solution at once, which will usually result in failure to evacuate feces. Rather, patients must retain the solution until lower abdominal cramping is definitely felt—perhaps 5 to 7 minutes.

Most pharmacies carry one or more types of enema syringes with their selection of rubber goods. (A child's enema syringe has a 1-ounce bulb, whereas an adult syringe has an 8-ounce bulb.) The tips of these syringes are not lubricated (unlike the syringes in enema kits) and must be lubricated before use. With these syringes, the patient may be directed by a physician to use warm tap water as an enema solution for home use. The water simply distends the rectum to stimulate the defecatory reflex. These syringes are reusable, although they should be thoroughly cleansed and allowed to dry between uses.

Cautions in Enema Use

Chronic enema usage can lead to loss of rectal tone and fecal incontinence.

Patients must be strictly cautioned against the use of soapsuds enemas, sometimes abbreviated on hospital charts as SS enemas.[13,42] Soapsuds enemas were traditional for many years in hospitals and may have provided a laxation because

A Pharmacist's Journal

"What Is a 3-H Enema?"

Working in a hospital on the night shift, I received an order for a "3-H enema" to be given to a female patient the next morning. I could not find the product on our shelves, but suspected the name might be a trade name for another commercially available product. Calls to surrounding hospital and community pharmacies were not helpful, as no other pharmacist was familiar with the product. I could not locate it in any reference or in the wholesaler's list. I finally phoned the physician to discover what the ingredients might be. As I was telling him I had tried to locate the product, he burst into laughter. He finally said, "You mean you've been trying to order a 3-H enema?" I assured him that I had tried diligently to do so. He continued, "I can't believe you've been trying to order that product. Listen,

it's just an abbreviation. I've got this 'old crock' on the third floor. Every day she's been in here she makes me order another enema, and I'm tired of it. I want her to get away from enemas and attempt to defecate on her own. So '3-H enema' is a medical abbreviation for an uncomfortable enema. It means, 'High, Hot, and a Hell-of-a-lot'. In other words, give about 1000 mL of hot tap water. Put the container about 18 inches above the shoulder, and insert the enema tip high into the colon. Maybe next time she'll try to go on her own!" The hazards of introducing excessive fluid with excessive pressure are substantial, and hot water irritates rectal mucosa, perhaps producing bleeding. This old enema method should be discouraged, although the physician in this case was insistent that the nursing personnel administer it as ordered.

---

of an irritant action. However, serious adverse effects have been associated with the fatty acids in the soap, which can be extremely irritating to the delicate rectal mucous membranes.[12] Soap in the rectum and colon can produce inflammation; in more severe cases, **SS enemas have caused ulcerative colitis, fatal gangrene, excessive serosanguinous fluid loss, anaphylaxis, acute hemorrhagic colitis, renal failure, and death.**

Enemas containing magnesium are not commercially available in the Untied States. Their potential toxicity argues against their use in any circumstances. The following cases exemplify adverse affects of magnesium-containing enemas:

- A 25-month-old British child with a long history of constipation was mistakenly given a magnesium sulfate enema containing 32.5 g of magnesium sulfate instead of an SS enema.[112] The child's serum magnesium rose to 7.1 mMol/liter (normal is 0.7 to 0.95 mMol/liter). She became atonic; reflexes ceased. Her pupils became fixed and dilated, and she experienced apnea. Therapy included 20% mannitol and intubation. The child recovered and was discharged after 48 hours.

- A similar situation with a 4-year-old boy resulted in loss of deep tendon reflexes, unconsciousness, and cyanosis.[113] Early administration of 10 mL of 10% calcium gluconate intravenously lowered his serum magnesium from the admission value of 5.87 mMol/liter and normalized his vital signs. He eventually recovered.

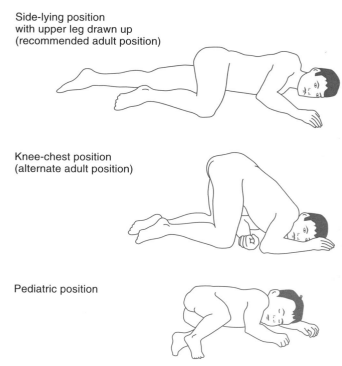

Side-lying position
with upper leg drawn up
(recommended adult position)

Knee-chest position
(alternate adult position)

Pediatric position

Figure 10.6. Positions for administering an enema.

Although the use of commercially available sodium phosphate enemas is said to be "generally standard" in pediatrics, sodium and/or phosphate overload may result from their use.

⚠ *Life-threatening electrolyte abnormalities have occurred in many cases when pediatric patients are given one-half, one, or two pediatric sodium enemas or one or more adult enemas.*[114-120] In many cases, administration of phosphate causes a reciprocal fall in calcium, which results in life-threatening tetany.[121] Therefore the theory that these solutions are not absorbed and are systemically inactive is incorrect. In fact, ions in retained enema solutions are rapidly absorbed and can cause significant, dose-related adverse effects. The following are examples:

- A 4.5-year-old boy with chronic renal failure and other medical problems was given an adult sodium phosphate enema at home. Subsequently, he suffered hypocalcemic tetany, hyperventilation, and tachycardia.[122] He required 3 days in the hospital for his condition to stabilize.
- An 11-month-old infant was given four adult-sized sodium enemas. She suffered a cardiac arrest 2.5 hours later and could not be resuscitated.[123]
- A 5-month-old infant was given one adult Fleet enema because she had not had a bowel movement in 2 days.[124] Within 30 minutes she became lethargic, with increased but shallow respirations. She had no blood pressure, was "glassy-eyed," and suffered constant outpouring of guaiac-positive, gray-colored, liquid stool. She was found to be hyperphosphatemic, hypocalcemic, and acidotic, in addition to suffering from shock. She required aluminum hydroxide gel administration to bind phosphate and IV fluids and a 3-day hospital stay. This case differed from many of the other pediatric cases because she had no previous underlying gastrointestinal or renal disease.

tip *Once again, the lower age limits on nonprescription products such as laxatives are not to be taken lightly.*

tip *Use of hypertonic sodium phosphate enemas in adults is not entirely without risk.* The use of these products is associated with hypocalcemic tetany,[125-127] colonic perforation,[128] and rectal gangrene.[129]

SUPPOSITORIES

Several laxatives are available in suppository form (Table 10.7). One of these formulations—the carbon dioxide suppository—is *only* available as a suppository.

Suppositories are medicated material shaped for easy insertion into an orifice other than the mouth—in this case the anus. Suppositories vary in weight from 2 g for an average adult suppository to about 1 g for a child's dose. The typical adult-shaped dosage form is shaped as a bullet or rocket—a cone with a rounded apex. Investigators have determined that inserting the smaller end first will prevent expulsion and augment effectiveness.[130]

The carbon dioxide suppository, which contains sodium bicarbonate and potassium bitartrate, is premoistened by placing it under tap water for 30 seconds or by soaking it in warm tap water for 10 seconds prior to insertion.[52] After moistening, the carbon dioxide suppository releases 90 to 230 mL of carbon dioxide gas. In the rectum, this gas forces fecal expulsion, generally within 5 to 30 minutes. Patients may complain of rectal discomfort and burning (because of inadequate moistening prior to insertion) and the sudden stretch reflex caused by expanding gas.

The FDA requires the following precaution on the carbon dioxide suppository: "Do not lubricate this laxative with mineral oil or petrolatum prior to rectal insertion."[52] Lubricating a carbon dioxide suppository with these ingredients could retard the product's effectiveness.

LAXATIVE COMBINATIONS

Manufacturers frequently combine laxatives (see Table 10.7). The FDA generally approves of this practice, except in the specific instance cited (e.g., mineral oil and docusate) (See "Mineral Oil" and "Stool Softeners" above). Of course, in combination products (i.e., more than one laxative), patients risk additional adverse reactions.

Nonpharmacologic Therapies

Although scientific data to prove their effectiveness is often sparse, traditional medical wisdom for the treatment of constipation consists of ingesting a high-fiber diet, carrying out

Table 10.7. Representative Combination Laxatives

PRODUCT	SELECTED INGREDIENTS/COMMENTS
Perdiem Overnight Relief	Per 6-g rounded teaspoonful dose, 3.25 g of psyllium, 0.74 g of senna
Senokot S Tablets	Docusate sodium 50 mg, sennosides 8.6 mg
Doxidan Liqui-Gels	Casanthranol 30 mg, docusate sodium 100 mg
Nature's Remedy	Cascara sagrada 150 mg, aloe 100 mg
Peri-Colace Capsules	Casanthranol 30 mg, docusate sodium 100 mg

AT THE COUNTER

 A young mother asks the pharmacist what laxative to use for her child. She is holding a package of Metamucil Fiber Wafers.

Interview/Patient Assessment

The pharmacist determines that her child, who is 4, is not taking any medications and has no diagnosed medical problems. His stools became too hard to pass easily 3 days before.

Pharmacist's Analysis

1. Does the child's problem appear to be constipation?
2. Is the child too young for a laxative?
3. Has the constipation been present too long to allow self-therapy?
4. Which laxatives would be suitable for the child?

The child appears to have simple constipation. He is not too young for self-therapy, and the problem has not persisted too long for self-therapy.

Patient Counseling

Psyllium products are contraindicated under the age of 6, so he should not be given Metamucil. Safe laxatives that could be recommended instead include polycarbophil, glycerin suppositories, and docusate (along with various other less safe alternatives such as some stimulants, salines, and enemas). The pharmacist should advise the woman that should her son fail to defecate after use of one of these products, or should he remain constipated for longer than 1 week from the time the problem began, he should see a physician.

---

mild exercise, and drinking fluids such as juices and water. Patients may be taught manipulative techniques (e.g., insertion of a gloved finger) to facilitate evacuation.[131]

PREVENTION OF CONSTIPATION

Prevention of constipation is optimal.

Many of the prevention steps (in particular, the regular use of bulk laxatives) were fully described above. However, they may be summarized as follows:

- Establish a routine time for defecation (e.g., after breakfast)
- Drink at least eight glasses of noncaffeinated fluids daily
- Increase fiber content of the diet
- Limit intake of foods with little or no fiber
- Limit intake of cheeses and eggs
- Obtain regular aerobic exercise
- Avoid laxatives that cause dependence (e.g., stimulants) and medication-induced constipation

SUMMARY

Constipation is a complex problem. Patients may use the term "constipation" to refer to a number of problems including infrequent stools, straining while passing stools, stools that are harder or smaller than desired, and pain on defecation, but medically constipation generally means fewer than 3 BMs per week. Constipation involves an interplay between lifestyle choices (e.g., exercise, fluid intake, and dietary habits) and other medical or medication-related etiologies (e.g., pregnancy, pain, nerve damage, colonic inertia, carcinoma, irritable bowel syndrome, etc.).

Pharmacists must be alert for patients complaining of constipation who report the following symptoms or situations, and refer these patients to a physician:

- Concomitant abdominal pain, nausea, or vomiting (possible appendicitis)
- Rectal bleeding or a sudden change in bowel habits that persists for 2 weeks or more (possible colorectal carcinoma)
- Colostomate or ileostomate (certain laxatives are contraindicated)
- Recent abdominal surgery (indication of ileus)
- Constipation persisting for more than 1 week
- Eating disorder (laxatives are sometimes used by anorexics/bulimics)

Generally speaking, bulk laxatives are the safest and most physiologically normal products, when ingested with adequate water by nonallergic patients. Stool softeners also have a low incidence of adverse reactions. However, mineral oil can cause several adverse reactions, including aspiration and rectal leakage; saline laxatives can cause dehydration, sodium overload, magnesium overload, and diarrhea; and stimulant laxatives cause habituation, permanent colonic damage, and various other adverse effects. Few patients choose suppositories or enemas. For these reasons, bulk laxatives or stool softeners are the best choices when therapy is required, although increased hydration and increased exercise can effectively eliminate constipation for some patients.

References

1. Sonnenberg A, Koch TR. Epidemiology of constipation in the United States. Dis Colon Rectum 32:1, 1989.
2. Donatelle EP. Constipation: Pathophysiology and treatment. Am Fam Physician 42:1335, 1990.

3. Murray FE, Bliss CM. Geriatric constipation: Brief update on a common problem. Geriatrics 46:64, 1991.

4. Agachan F, et al. A constipation scoring system to simplify evaluation and management of constipated patients. Dis Colon Rectum 39:681, 1996.

5. Ashraf W, et al. An examination of the reliability of reported stool frequency in the diagnosis of idiopathic constipation. Am J Gastroenterol 91:26, 1996.

6. Marshall JB. Chronic constipation in adults. Postgrad Med 88:49, 1990.

7. Lederle FA. Epidemiology of constipation in elderly patients. Drug utilisation and cost-containment strategies. Drug Aging 6:465, 1995.

8. Kune GA, et al. The role of chronic constipation, diarrhea, and laxative use in the etiology of large-bowel cancer. Dis Colon Rectum 31:507, 1988.

9. Johanson JF, et al. Clinical epidemiology of constipation. J Clin Gastroenterol 11:525, 1989.

10. Sandler RS, et al. Demographic and dietary determinants of constipation in the US population. Am J Public Health 80:185, 1990.

11. Tremaine WJ. Chronic constipation: Causes and management. Hosp Pract 25:89, 1990.

12. Castle SC. Constipation: Endemic in the elderly? Med Clin North Am 73:1497, 1989.

13. Alessi CA, Henderson CT. Constipation and fecal impaction in the long-term care patient. Clin Geriatr Med 4:571, 1988.

14. Wald A. Constipation and fecal incontinence in the elderly. Gastroenterol Clin North Am 19:405, 1990.

15. Wrenn K. Fecal impaction. N Engl J Med 321:658, 1989.

16. Kamm MA. Role of surgical treatment in patients with severe constipation. Ann Med 22:435, 1990.

17. Sonnenberg A, Koch TR. Physician visits in the United States for Constipation: 1958 to 1986. Dig Dis Sci 34:606, 1989.

18. Norton C. The causes and nursing management of constipation. Br J Nurs 5:1252, 1996.

19. Snyder K. The state of the OTC marketplace. Drug Topics 141(11): 82, 1997.

20. Talley NJ, et al. Constipation in an elderly community: A study of prevalence and potential risk factors. Am J Gastroenterol 91:19, 1996.

21. Castle SC, et al. Constipation prevention: Empiric use of stool softeners questioned. Geriatrics 46:84, 1991.

22. Kinnunen O, Salokannel J. Comparison of the effects of magnesium hydroxide and a bulk laxative on lipids, carbohydrates, vitamins A and E, and minerals in geriatric hospital patients in the treatment of constipation. J Int Med Res 17:442, 1989.

23. Whitehead WE, et al. Constipation in the elderly living at home. J Am Geriatr Soc 37:423, 1989.

24. Leung AK, Chan PY, Co. HE. Constipation in children. Am Fam Physician 54:611, 1996.

25. Varma JS, et al. Constipation in the elderly. Dis Colon Rectum 31:111, 1988.

26. Herz MJ, et al. Constipation: A different entity for patients and doctors. Fam Pract 13:156, 1996.

27. Snape WJ. The effect of methylcellulose on symptoms of constipation. Clin Ther 11:572, 1989.

28. Pettei MJ. Chronic constipation. Pediatr Ann 16:796, 1987.

29. Murtagh J. Constipation. Aust Fam Physician 19:1693, 1990.

30. Read NW, Celik AF, Katsinelos P. Constipation and incontinence in the elderly. J Clin Gastroenterol 20:61, 1995.

31. Leng-Peschlow E, ed. The rational use of senna. Pharmacology 44(Suppl 1):41, 1992.

32. Camilleri M, et al. Clinical management of intractable constipation. Ann Intern Med 121:520, 1994.

33. Abyad A, Mourad F. Constipation: Common-sense care of the older patient. Geriatrics 51:28, 1996.

34. Romero Y, et al. Constipation and fecal incontinence in the elderly population. Mayo Clin Proc 71:81, 1996.

35. Clayden GS. Constipation in childhood. BMJ 299:1116, 1989.

36. Levine MI. Colic, constipation and diarrhea—Old symptoms, new approaches. Pediatr Ann 16:765, 1987.

37. Gleghorn EE, et al. No-enema therapy for idiopathic constipation and encopresis. Clin Pediatr 30:669, 1991.

38. Klauser AG, et al. Behavioral modification of colonic function. Dig Dis Sci 35:1271, 1990.

39. Wald A. Disorders of defecation and fecal continence. Cleve Clin J Med 56:491, 1989.

40. Spiller R. When fibre fails. BMJ 300:1064, 1990.

41. Loening-Baucke V. Functional constipation. Semin Pediatr Surg 4:26, 1995.

42. Rousseau P. Treatment of constipation in the elderly. Postgrad Med 83:339, 1988.

43. Binder HJ. Use of laxatives in clinical medicine. Pharmacology 36(Suppl 1):226, 1988.

44. Garvey M, et al. Frequency of constipation in major depression. Psychosomatics 31:204, 1990.

45. Godding EW. Laxatives and the special role of senna. Pharmacology 36(Suppl 1):230, 1988.

46. Rantis PC Jr, et al. Chronic constipation—Is the work-up worth the cost? Dis Colon Rectum 40:280, 1997.

47. Devroede G, et al. Idiopathic constipation by colonic dysfunction. Dig Dis Sci 34:1428, 1989.

48. Haines ST. Treating constipation in the patient with diabetes. Diabetes Educ 21:223, 1995.

49. McEvoy GK, ed. AHFS 97 Drug Information: 1997, American Society of Health-System Pharmacists, Bethesda MD.

50. Hall GR, et al. Managing constipation using a research-based protocol. Med Surg Nurs 4:1, 1995.

51. Kock A, et al. Symptoms in chronic constipation. Dis Colon Rectum 40:902, 1997.

52. Fed Reg 50:2123, 1985.

53. Waller DA, et al. Correlates of laxative abuse in bulimia. Hosp Community Psychiatry 41:797, 1990.

54. Gren J, Woolf A. Hypermagnesemia associated with catharsis in a salicylate-intoxicated patient with anorexia nervosa. Ann Emerg Med 18:200, 1989.

55. Mitchell JE, et al. Enema abuse as a clinical feature of bulimia nervosa. Psychosomatics 32:102, 1991.

56. Donowitz M. Magnesium-induced diarrhea and new insights into the pathobiology of diarrhea (Editorial). N Engl J Med 324:1059, 1991.

57. Leng-Peschlow E, ed. Laxative abuse. Pharmacology 44 (Suppl 1):36, 1992.

58. Weiss BD, Wood GA. Laxative abuse causing gastrointestinal bleeding. J Fam Pract 15:177, 1982.

59. Bytzer P, et al. Prevalence of surreptitious laxative abuse in patients with diarrhoea of uncertain origin: A cost benefit analysis of a screening procedure. Gut 30:1379, 1989.

60. McClung HJ, Boyne L, Heitlinger L. Constipation and dietary fiber intake in children. Pediatrics 96(5 Pt 2):999, 1995.

61. Eherer AJ, et al. Effect of psyllium, calcium polycarbophil,

and wheat bran on secretory diarrhea induced by phenolphthalein. Gastroenterol 104:1007, 1993.

62. Tramonte SM, et al. The treatment of chronic constipation in adults. A systematic review. J Gen Intern Med 12:15, 1997.

63. Voderholzer WA, et al. Clinical response to dietary fiber treatment of chronic constipation. Am J Gastroenterol 92:95, 1997.

64. Ashraf W, et al. Effects of psyllium therapy on stool characteristics, colon transit and anorectal function in chronic idiopathic constipation. Aliment Pharmacol Ther 9:639, 1995.

65. Fed Reg 58:45193, 1993.

66. Hinkel CL. Complete obstruction of the esophagus following Serutan® ingestion. JAMA 146:1129, 1951.

67. Melamed A, Marck A. Esophageal obstruction due to Serutan. JAMA 152:318, 1953.

68. Schneider RP. Perdiem causes esophageal impaction and bezoars. South Med J 82:1449, 1989.

69. Lee A, et al. Bulk laxative causing esophageal obstruction. NC Med J 50:489, 1989.

70. Angueira C, Kadakia S. Esophageal and duodenal bezoars from Perdiem (Letter). Gastrointest Endos 39:110, 1993.

71. Agha FP, et al. "Giant colonic bezoar:" A medication bezoar due to psyllium seed husks. Am J Gastroenterol 79:319, 1984.

72. Frohna WJ. Metamucil bezoar: An unusual cause of small bowel obstruction (Letter). Am J Emerg Med 10:393, 1992.

73. Lambert CE. New information about laxative use (Letter). Procter & Gamble, 1996.

74. Marks GB, et al. Asthma and allergy associated with occupational exposure to ispaghula and senna products in a pharmaceutical work force. Am Rev Resp Dis 144:1065, 1991.

75. Arlian LG, et al. Antigenic and allergenic analysis of psyllium seed components. J Allergy Clin Immunol 89:866, 1992.

76. Gillespie BF, Rathbun FJ. Adverse effects of psyllium. Can Med Assoc J 146:16, 1992.

77. Ford MA, et al. Delayed psyllium allergy in three nurses. Hosp Pharm 27:1061, 1992.

78. Lantner RR, et al. Anaphylaxis following ingestion of a psyllium-containing cereal. JAMA 264:2534, 1990.

79. Fed Reg 58:46589, 1993.

80. Paraskevaides EC. Fatal lipid pneumonia and liquid paraffin. Br J Clin Pract 44:509, 1990.

81. Stern EJ. Chronic, progressive bibasilar infiltrates in a woman with constipation. Chest 102:263, 1992.

82. Ferguson GT, Miller YE. Occult mineral oil pneumonitis in anorexia nervosa. West J Med 148:211, 1988.

83. Lauque D, et al. Bronchoalveolar lavage in liquid paraffin pneumonitis. Chest 98:1149, 1990.

84. de Oliveira GA, et al. Radiographic plain film and CT findings in lipoid pneumonia in infants following aspiration of mineral oil used in the treatment of partial small bowel obstruction by Ascaris lumbricoides. Pediatr Radiol 15:157, 1985.

85. Granella M, Clonfero E. The mutagenic activity and polycyclic aromatic hydrocarbon content of mineral oils. Int Arch Occup Environ Health 91:149, 1991.

86. Randell RA. Nasal cancer and mineral oil (Letter). Lancet 335:56, 1990.

87. Donowitz M, Rood RP. Magnesium hydroxide: New insights into the mechanism of its laxative effect and the potential involvement of prostaglandin E2. J Clin Gastroenterol 14:20, 1992.

88. Jones J, et al. Cathartic-induced magnesium toxicity during overdose management. Ann Emerg Med 15:1214, 1986.

89. Mofenson HC, Caraccio TR. Magnesium intoxication in a neonate from oral magnesium hydroxide laxative. J Toxicol Clin Toxicol 29:215, 1991.

90. Gerard SK, et al. Extreme hypermagnesemia caused by an overdose of magnesium-containing cathartics. Ann Emerg Med 17:728, 1988.

91. Smilkstein MJ, et al. Severe hypermagnesemia due to multiple-dose cathartic therapy. West J Med 148:208, 1988.

92. Woodard JA, et al. Serum magnesium concentrations after repetitive magnesium cathartic administration. Am J Emerg Med 8:297, 1990.

93. Alison LH, Bulugahapitiya D. Laxative induced magnesium poisoning in a 6 week old infant. BMJ 300:125, 1990.

94. Fine KD, et al. Diagnosis of magnesium-induced diarrhea. N Engl J Med 324:1012, 1991 .

95. deWitte P, Lemli L. The metabolism of anthranoid laxatives. Hepatogastroenterology 37:601, 1990.

96. Leng-Peschlow E, ed. Modes of action of senna. Pharmacology 44(Suppl 1):16, 1992.

97. Autore G, et al. Kinins and the laxative effect of phenolphthalein. Pharmacol Res 22(Suppl 1):105, 1990.

98. Leng-Peschlow E, ed. Senna and habituation. Pharmacology 44(Suppl 1):30, 1991.

99. Leng-Peschlow E, ed. Senna and damage of the nerve plexus of the intestinal wall. Pharmacology 44(Suppl 1):26, 1992.

100. Sykes NP. A volunteer model for the comparison of laxatives in opioid-related constipation. J Pain Symptom Manage 11:363, 1996.

101. Dick WH. Laxative abuse as a cause for ammonium urate renal stones. J Urol 143:244, 1990.

102. Leng-Peschlow E, ed. Senna and pseudomelanosis coli. Pharmacology 44(Suppl 1):33, 1992.

103. Beuers U, et al. Hepatitis after chronic abuse of senna (Letter). Lancet 337:372, 1991.

104. Nice FJ. Can a breast-feeding mother take medication without harming her infant? MCN 14:27, 1989.

105. Baron TH, et al. Gastrointestinal motility disorders during pregnancy. Ann Intern Med 118:366, 1993.

106. Mitri F, Hofmeyr GJ, van Gelderen CJ. Meconium during labour—Self-medication and other associations. S Afr Med J 71:431, 1987.

107. Steingrub JS, et al. Amniotic fluid embolism associated with castor oil ingestion. Crit Care Med 16:642, 1988.

108. Gilbertson WE, Lessing M. Danthron alarm, FDA response, Crucial OTC drug control. Milit Med 153:487, 1988.

109. Patel PM, et al. Anthraquinone laxatives and human cancer: An association in one case. Postgrad Med J 65:216, 1989.

110. Barnett AA. FDA reclassifies laxative ingredients. Pharm Today 2(6):3, 1996.

111. Campieri M, et al. Role of rectal formulations: Enemas. Scand J Gastroenterol Suppl 172:63, 1990.

112. Ashton MR, et al. Severe magnesium toxicity after magnesium sulphate enema in a chronically constipated child (Letter). BMJ 300:541, 1990.

113. Brown AT, Campbell WAB. Hazards of hypertonic magnesium enema therapy (Letter). Arch Dis Child 53:920, 1978.

114. Honig PJ, Holtzapple PG. Hypocalcemic tetany following hypertonic phosphate enemas. Clin Pediatr 14:678, 1975.

115. Loughnan P, Mullins GC. Brain damage following a hypertonic phosphate enema (Letter). Am J Dis Child 131:1032, 1977.

116. Sotos JF, et al. Hypocalcemic coma following two pediatric phosphate enemas. Pediatrics 60:305, 1977.

117. Davis RF, et al. Hypocalcemia, hyperphosphatemia, and dehydration following a single hypertonic phosphate enema. J Pediatr 90:484, 1977.

118. Forman J, et al. Hypokalemia after hypertonic phosphate enemas. J Pediatr 94:149, 1979.

119. Edmondson S, Almquist TD. Iatrogenic hypocalcemic tetany. Ann Emerg Med 19:938, 1990.

120. McCabe M, et al. Phosphate enemas in childhood: Cause for concern. BMJ 302:1074, 1991.

121. Grosskopf I, et al. Hyperphosphatemia and hypocalcemia induced by hypertonic phosphate enema—An experimental study and review of the literature. Hum Exp Toxicol 10:351, 1991.

122. Oxnard SC, et al. Severe tetany in an azotemic child related to a sodium phosphate enema. Pediatrics 53:105, 1974.

123. Martin RR, et al. Fatal poisoning from sodium phosphate enema. JAMA 257:2190, 1987.

124. Wason S, et al. Severe hyperphosphatemia, hypocalcemia, acidosis, and shock in a 5-month-old child following the administration of an adult Fleet® enema. Ann Emerg Med 68:696, 1989.

125. Korzets A, et al. Life-threatening hyperphosphatemia and hypocalcemic tetany following the use of Fleet enemas. J Am Geriatr Soc 40:620, 1992.

126. Haskell LP. Hypocalcemic tetany induced by hypertonic-phosphate enema (Letter). Lancet 2:1433, 1985.

127. Biberstein M, Parker BA. Enema-induced hyperphosphatemia. Am J Med 79:645, 1985.

128. Bell AM. Colonic perforation with a phosphate enema. JR Soc Med 83:54, 1990.

129. Sweeney JL, et al. Rectal gangrene: A complication of phosphate enema. Med J Aust 144:374, 1986.

130. Abd-El-Maeboud, et al. Rectal suppository: Commonsense and mode of insertion. Lancet 338:798, 1991.

131. Mollen RM, Claassen AT, Kuijpers JH. The evaluation and treatment of functional constipation. Scand J Gastroenterol Suppl 223:8, 1997.

Diarrhea

AT THE COUNTER

 A man with a child in his shopping cart approaches the pharmacist around lunch time and asks for help with diarrhea medications.

Interview/Patient Assessment

The man says that his 4-year-old son has had two loose stools today. His son woke up at 5:00 AM, crying and complaining that his stomach hurt, and had his first loose stool then. He has been cranky and has a fever of 103°. The father wants to know if the attapulgite products are safe for a child of his age. The father says the child has no medical conditions and is taking no medications.

Pharmacist's Analysis

1. Has the diarrhea been present too long to allow self-therapy?

2. Does the child's age preclude self-therapy?
3. Is an attapulgite product suitable for this child?

The child's diarrhea has only been present for 1 day, so could be self-treated. The child is over the age of 3 years, so he could receive an age-appropriate nonprescription product. However, fever is a contraindication for self-therapy of diarrhea.

Patient Counseling

The pharmacist should explain to the father that diarrhea should not be self-treated if the patient has a fever. The child may require antibiotic therapy for a possible infection; therefore, he should be referred to his pediatrician for evaluation.

A disease of worldwide incidence, diarrhea strikes virtually everyone at some point. While it has no universally accepted definition, diarrhea is characterized by increased frequency of defecation, with the stools being loose and watery. Generally, three or more loose stools during a limited period (24 to 48 hours) is perceived to be diarrhea.[1]

Diarrhea is either the leading or second cause of death for all age groups in most developing countries; one study estimates the United States mortality rate at 4.5 million/year.[2,3] American children under 5 experience as many as 325 to 425 diarrhea-related deaths each year.[2] In some years as many as 400 infants have died from diarrhea.[4] Many childhood diarrheal diseases are contracted through day care.[5]

Should diarrhea result in extensive fluid loss, dehydration may result. Since lost fluids contain electrolytes, the patient also may experience hypokalemia, hyponatremia, and other electrolyte imbalances. Dehydration and electrolyte imbalance is potentially deadly if replacement solutions are not given, especially in young and elderly patients.[6]

PREVALENCE OF DIARRHEA

In the United States, children under 5 experience diarrhea an average of two to two and a half times yearly, totaling 2.1 to 3.7 million physician visits and 220,000 hospitalizations, according to one study.[2] Adults in the United States experience a lower rate of diarrhea (1.5 to 1.7 episodes yearly by one study).[7] The higher incidence in children is thought to be related to such fecal-oral activities as crawling at ground level, placing things in the mouth indiscriminately, and wearing diapers.[7]

EPIDEMIOLOGY OF DIARRHEA

Diarrhea is a symptom, not a disease. For that reason the epidemiology of diarrhea mirrors the conditions that cause it. For instance, the epidemiology of diarrhea induced by food intolerance is markedly different from that of diarrhea caused by infectious agents (e.g., traveler's diarrhea, TD). Therefore, epidemiology is an integral part of the discussion of the etiologies of diarrhea below.

ETIOLOGY OF DIARRHEA

Diarrhea is generally classified as either acute or chronic. As discussed below, either acute or chronic diarrhea may be caused by such etiologies as diet, medication, or infections. In addition, however, chronic diarrhea can also result from several serious medical conditions.

Chronic Diarrhea

Diarrhea present for more than 1 month is referred to as chronic.[8] *Since a variety of problems cause chronic diarrhea, patients must always be referred to a physician, unless additional symptoms point to an innocuous etiology such as lactose intolerance.[9]*

Although infectious agents are usually associated with acute diarrhea, they can also cause chronic diarrhea. For instance, viral infections in infants may damage intestinal villi and delay mucosal healing for as long as 2 months, resulting in chronic diarrhea. Bacteria such as *Clostridium difficile* and parasites such as *Giardia lamblia* and *Entamoeba histolytica* can also cause chronic diarrhea.[8,10]

Dietary factors, too, produce chronic diarrhea. Food allergies such as cow's milk allergy can cause diarrhea, along with abdominal pain and vomiting.[11,12] If the allergy is severe, **anaphylaxis** (a severe allergic syndrome resulting in respiratory distress, hypotension and possible death if not immediately treated), skin rash, and bronchospasm may result.[13] Diarrhea is a part of the clinical picture of lactose intolerance, along with gas and abdominal distention.[11,14] If lactose intolerance is suspected, lactase supplementation and/or lactose restriction are the treatments of choice. (See Chapter 9, Lactose Intolerance.)

Cancer of the bowel may signal diarrhea, especially when the episodes of diarrhea alternate with constipation.[14] (Additional symptoms include rectal bleeding, occult blood in the stools, and abdominal pain.[14]) Chronic diarrhea may also be caused by other serious medical conditions such as Crohn's disease, ulcerative colitis, AIDS, diabetes mellitus, endocrine disorders, malabsorption, irritable bowel syndrome, and celiac disease.[14–20]

Various medications can cause diarrhea. However, when diarrhea becomes troublesome, the dosage is usually altered or an alternate agent selected. For this reason they are discussed under "Acute Diarrhea."

Pharmacists should be alert for laxative abuse when counseling patients with chronic (or acute) diarrhea.[14,21] Most patients deny laxative abuse, but it is not uncommon. In one study laxative abuse was identified as the cause of diarrhea in 15% of patients attending a gastroenterology clinic.[22] Laxative abuse should be strongly suspected as a component of the clinical picture in adolescent females who continually experience diarrhea or whose parents seek counseling, for example, after discovering empty laxative packages in the daughter's belongings. (Historically, adolescent girls have a greater tendency toward laxative abuse than other subgroups because of the gender occurrence of anorexia/bulimia.) The diagnosis may require fecal screening. (See Chapter 22, Obesity.) Medical literature contains several cases of parents administering laxatives to their children prior to seeking medical help for the child's diarrhea. In one case the child's diarrhea ceased only after a court-ordered separation from her mother.[23] This mental disorder is termed Polle syndrome (a subcategory of Munchausen by proxy).[24]

Patients complaining of chronic diarrhea must have these various potential diagnoses investigated. Their possibly devastating sequelae generally contraindicate self-therapy with nonprescription products and mandate immediate referral.[25]

Acute Diarrhea

Acute diarrhea has three major causes:

- Infections
- Diet
- Medications[14]

Because pharmacists often must help patients understand the possible causes of acute diarrhea, it is important to fully understand these three major causes.

INFECTIOUS DIARRHEA

The most common cause of diarrhea is an infectious agent.[11] Most deaths and hospitalizations resulting from diarrhea involve an acute infectious diarrhea.

There are several mechanisms by which organisms may produce diarrhea[7,26]:

- Destruction of enteric cells through direct invasion.[27]
- Production of toxins that stimulate fluid and electrolyte secretion, causing watery stools.
- Merging with **enterocytes** (cells of the intestinal tract), injecting cytotoxins into the enterocyte.

The dose of organisms required to overwhelm body defenses varies from 10 to 100 organisms for *Shigella, Giardia lamblia,* and *Entamoeba histolytica* to 10^8 for *Vibrio cholerae* and *Escherichia coli.*[28] However, gastric hypoacidity reduces the numbers needed to produce diarrhea. Thus patients with partial **gastrectomy** (removal of all or part of the stomach) and patients taking antacids or H2-blockers are predisposed to infectious diarrhea.[28] Medications that slow peristalsis (anticholinergics, antihistamines, loperamide, opiates) are generally considered to be counterproductive in infectious diarrhea since they inhibit the elimination of the pathogens, prolonging the symptoms and increasing their severity.[29]

Bacterial Diarrhea

The bacteria causing diarrhea are most often contracted through ingestion of contaminated food or drink, although direct oral-fecal transfer and sexual practices can also be responsible.[28] Thus the pharmacist should ask about ingestion of food at any "risky" event (such as a communal dinner, "pot luck" dinner, or "covered dish" dinner where people untrained in food handling prepare the meal) or recent travel to another country.[11] TD is a subcategory of infectious diarrhea that is solely the result of travel. (See "Traveler's Diarrhea.") Pharmacists often receive questions about the treatment *and* prevention of the condition. Inadequate refrigeration and/or reheating also allows unchecked growth of **diarrheagenic** (capable of causing diarrhea) organisms.

Salmonella organisms may be ingested with infected poultry, eggs, beef, and milk.[27] Salmonellal diarrhea persists for 1 to 4 days, usually accompanied by nausea, vomiting, abdominal pain, fever, and passage of blood and mucus.[14,26] Antimicrobial therapy should be reserved for the elderly, patients with bacteremia, infants, and immunocompromised patients.[27,30,31]

Campylobacter jejuni–induced diarrhea, acquired from undercooked chicken, persists for 1 to 4 days. Fever, crampy abdominal pain, malaise, and profuse watery stools indicate this species.[26,32]

E. coli, the most common cause of traveler's diarrhea, is discussed in "Traveler's Diarrhea." Other bacteria producing diarrhea include *Clostridium, Shigella, Staphylococcus aureus, Vibrio,* and *Yersinia.*[27]

Viral Diarrhea

Viruses account for 70 to 80% of cases of acute gastroenteritis, inducing diarrhea in the majority of cases.[32] Viral diarrhea seldom requires therapy other than electrolyte maintenance and/or replacement when necessary, resolving on its own in most cases.[26]

Rotavirus is the most common viral cause of pediatric gastroenteritis. Rotavirus is contracted through fecal-oral transmission and contaminated water or fomites. Its incidence peaks in the fall in the southwestern United States, moving progressively eastward to reach the Northeast in late winter and spring; the cause of this is unknown.[7] Although it typically affects infants and young children, adults may contract the condition while caring for their affected children.[33] Rotavirus diarrhea is characterized by watery, nonbloody stools accompanied by vomiting and fever, following an incubation period of 24 to 48 hours. It is usually self-limiting, subsiding after 7 to 10 days. However, dehydration may occur.

Norwalk virus, the second most common cause of pediatric gastroenteritis, is also mainly transmitted by the fecal-oral route.[47] Malaise, fever, nausea, vomiting, and abdominal cramps occur along with the diarrhea, which lasts for 24 to 30 hours.[32] Norwalk virus has a different epidemiologic pattern than rotavirus, being more common in late adolescence and adulthood.

Parasite-Induced Diarrhea
Giardia lamblia and *Entamoeba histolytica* are two causes of parasite-induced diarrhea.[48,49] The latter is usually only seen as a cause of traveler's diarrhea, but *Giardia* is contracted through ingestion of water contaminated with animal or human feces containing the cysts.[14,26] Many people are infected with *Giardia* by drinking water from sources with inadequate purification systems, as when drinking from a clear mountain stream while on a hike.[27] Patients who are symptomatic suffer diarrhea, bloating,

FOCUS ON...

TRAVELER'S DIARRHEA

Traveler's diarrhea (TD) is an acute diarrhea caused by bacteria that the patient contacted when traveling, usually to a foreign country.[33] The usual situation is travel from a developed country to a less-developed country. However, it is possible for a patient to contract TD from travel from one location to another in the same country, since the organisms or sanitation in that specific area may be substandard. Approximately 33 to 40% of the 8 million American residents who travel to developing countries will develop TD.[34]

RISK OF DESTINATION

The most important variable for development of TD is the level of risk of the destination. Epidemiologists categorize destinations as follows[35]:

1. High risk—developing countries with tropical and subtropical climates, especially countries with poor sanitary conditions such as some countries in Africa, Asia, Latin America, and the Middle East, as shown on the map

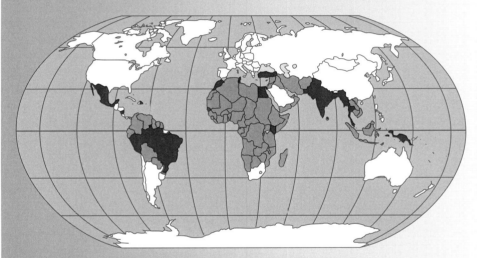

Traveler's diarrhea is proven to be prevalent in certain countries (*blackened*) and thought to be more prevalent in others (*shaded*).

2. Intermediate risk countries—most of southern Europe (e.g., Greece and Spain), the countries of the former Soviet Union, China, and a few Caribbean Islands
3. Low risk—Australia, Canada, northern Europe, Japan, New Zealand, and the United States

The risk of TD is not as simple as the risk level of the destination. The country of origin also influences the risk. Maximal risk occurs when individuals from low-risk areas such as the United States visit high-risk countries such as Mexico.[36] Conversely, travelers from high-risk countries do not suffer TD as frequently when they visit other high-risk countries. For instance, students from Latin America do not suffer TD as often as students from the United States when visiting Mexico.[35] There is little risk of TD when travelers from high-risk areas (e.g., Mexico) visit low-risk areas (e.g., the United States). Evidently, multiple exposures in high-risk countries confer relative immunity. The world map indicates areas of high risk for travelers from low-risk countries.

Continued

abdominal cramps, flatulence, anorexia, and steatorrhea. The prescription product metronidazole is the first line medication.[26]

DIETARY DIARRHEA

Diet can produce diarrhea in many cases. Dietary causes of acute diarrhea include lactose intolerance (See Chapter 9, Lactose Intolerance). Excessive fiber intake may also be responsible, as in a patient ingesting a large amount of sunflower seeds at one time. Drinking large amounts of extremely salty drinks or eating highly salted foods can also cause an osmotic diarrhea. Some enteral diets may cause diarrhea if they are highly osmotic.[50]

MEDICATION-RELATED DIARRHEA

Several groups of medications cause diarrhea, including antibiotics (e.g., ampicillin, cephalosporins, clindamycin, and tetracyclines), antihypertensives, chemotherapeutic agents, colchicine, digitalis, NSAIDs, potassium, propranolol, and quinidine.[14] Diarrhea can be caused by the magnesium in antacids containing magnesium hydroxide or by milk of magnesia, even when they are taken in normal antacid doses.[51,52] A dose reduction may resolve the problem. If it does not, the patient might be urged to consider an antacid containing calcium or an H2-blocker. Laxative abuse can also cause acute diarrhea. (See "Chronic Diarrhea.")

TREATMENT OF DIARRHEA

Treatment Guidelines

Patients often consider diarrhea nothing more than a minor nuisance, but it can be life-threatening. Most deaths resulting from diarrhea in the United States probably could have been prevented if simple guidelines had been followed.[53] Therefore, one of the first tasks of pharmacists is to make patients aware that physician evaluation is needed in

EPIDEMIOLOGY OF TD

Younger adults suffer TD more than older adults. This is explained by a lack of acquired immunity in younger adults and perhaps more daring travel styles and/or eating habits.[36] There is no gender preference for contracting TD.[35]

The risk of TD is also related to the purpose of travel:

- Travelers visiting relatives are at low risk
- Business travelers are at medium risk
- Tourists, students, and convention attendees face the greatest risk

Eating food in private homes rather than restaurants may provide some protection.[35,36] Further, the longer the visit, the greater the risk of developing TD.[35]

ETIOLOGY OF TD

While other organisms may cause TD, as described above, the most common causative agents are the **enterotoxigenic** *E. coli* (organisms that produce toxins that specifically affect intestinal mucosal cells).[36] These organisms are not invasive and do not produce an inflammatory exudate. Enterotoxigenic *E. coli* cause an estimated 40 to 70% of cases of TD, a mild and painless form of the condition. Other *E. coli* (e.g., enteropathogenic, enteroinvasive, and enterohemorrhagic types) cause more severe cases of TD, resulting in pain, fever, and inflammatory exudate.

TRANSMISSION OF TD

TD is not contagious.[35] Sufferers and their secretions present no risk to family and friends. The cause is ingestion of contaminated food or water.[36]

The gastric pH destroys ingested organisms, most within 30 minutes of ingestion. Traveler's diarrhea develops when the traveler ingests a load of organisms that is too large for the defense systems of the body to combat.[36] The risk is directly related to the number of exposures, or dietary mistakes, the traveler makes.[37]

Food may contain organisms that were not destroyed during preparation. Food may also become contaminated by food handlers who have unsatisfactory sanitary habits following bowel movements.[35] For these reasons the traveler should avoid fish, meats, and vegetables that are undercooked, raw, or rare—including salad.[35,38,39] Custards and creamy desserts and pastries, raw eggs, cheese, milk, yogurt, ice cream, and other dairy products are all risky, since they are easily contaminated during preparation and serve as excellent growth media following inoculation.[38] Generally, any dish that is prepared in advance and allowed to stand, such as hot sauces sitting on tables in open containers, also should be avoided.[30] Tap water can be dangerous, even if used to wet a toothbrush.[36] Even ice cubes in drinks are as dangerous as the water and should not be used in drinks.[40] The general rule is: "Boil it, peel it, cook it, or forget it."[41]

Only canned or bottled carbonated beverages, fresh citrus fruits, or drinks made with water that has been boiled should be ingested. Packaged butter and jelly are low risk.[35] Nuts, fruits, and vegetables purchased intact and then shelled or peeled are fairly safe.[35,42] Meat and seafood dishes prepared "well done" and eaten while hot present little danger. Travelers should avoid food from street vendors unless they have seen it boiled for at least five minutes. Some street vendors peel fruit directly in front of customers to ensure that it has not contacted local water, but their hands may be contaminated. Travelers should examine the restrooms in restaurants. If they do not have soap and water, food prepared in that restaurant is suspect.

MANIFESTATIONS OF TD

TD generally begins suddenly, either during the trip or shortly after returning home.[36] Bowel movements may be two or more times the normal daily number.[36] Stools are

Continued

many cases.[54] (See "A Pharmacist's Journal: Diarrhea from New York to Arizona.")

(tip) *Although there are many nonprescription products available for diarrhea, they must not be used if the diarrhea has lasted for more than 2 days.*[25] Although diarrhea that has persisted over 2 days is technically not defined as "chronic," the FDA chose the 2-day cutoff to provide a margin of safety in preventing dehydration. Beyond this time the patient may require laboratory evaluation of fluid and electrolyte status, with possible administration of replacement intravenous fluids.

(tip) Further, *the FDA-labeled age cutoff for diarrhea self-treatment prohibits nonprescription-product recommendations for any patient under age 3.*[25] Patients younger than 3 must see a physician, without exception. Young children are far too susceptible to injury from compromised fluid and electrolyte status to permit self-treatment.

(tip) *Patients with fever must not use antidiarrheals, as this indicates the presence of an infection.*[25] The manufacturers of products containing attapulgite (an adsorbent) have voluntarily added a warning against using those products if there is blood or mucus in the stool.[55] (See "Attapulgite.")

For patients 3 and older who have experienced diarrhea for less than 2 days and do not have contraindications to their use, several nonprescription medications can be used. The nonprescription medications now proven safe and effective for self-treatment of diarrhea are polycarbophil, attapulgite, bismuth subsalicylate, kaolin, and loperamide.[25,56] For an illustration of the steps used in selecting antidiarrheal therapy, see Patient Assessment Algorithm 11.1

Nonprescription Medications

CALCIUM POLYCARBOPHIL
Calcium polycarbophil is a hydrophilic polyacrylic resin that absorbs up to 60 times its weight in water (Table 11.1).[57] The only nonprescription ingredient that is effective for either diarrhea or constipation, calcium polycarbophil can bind water from liquid stools, increasing their consistency.[58] (See "Bulk Laxatives" in Chapter 10, Constipation.) In this regard calcium polycarbophil shares the dangers of bulk laxatives. For

watery and loose and may contain blood. Additional symptoms include abdominal cramps, bloating, nausea, fever, body or joint aches, chills, vomiting, headache, weakness, and anorexia.[36,43]

PROGNOSIS OF TD
The prognosis of TD is excellent, as it is self-limiting in most cases. TD usually improves in 3 to 5 days, even without treatment.[44] Only about 10% of cases last longer than 1 week; only about 5% of the total cases last longer than 1 month.[36,45]

TREATMENT OF TD
Pharmacists may receive questions from returning travelers who have contracted TD. As explained under "treatment guidelines," the FDA recommends a 2-day time limit for self-treatment of diarrhea, a guideline that should be adhered to when treating TD. Patients generally want to stop all bowel movements, but this is counterproductive as TD allows the body to excrete the organisms and their toxins.[29] The physician may treat mild cases with reassurance coupled with mineral and electrolyte replacement, but above all, physicians and pharmacists should avoid medications that decrease motility since they may prolong the illness.

PREVENTION OF TD
Patients at high risk of TD or whose business is critical should be referred to a physician for a prescription for prophylaxis. (See "Prevention of Diarrhea.") These patients include the following:

- Travelers visiting high-risk areas on critical business that could be jeopardized if illness strikes, causing an absence from crucial negotiations
- Travelers with underlying health problems that make them more susceptible to diarrhea (e.g., achlorhydria, dysgammaglobulinemia, and known gastric resection)
- Travelers using H2-blockers or antacids (see "Medication-Related Diarrhea")
- Travelers in whom dehydration could cause medical complications (e.g., those taking diuretics or digitalis)
- Travelers with underlying disease (e.g., diverticulitis).[46]

instance, the warnings and directions to maintain adequate fluid intake to prevent esophageal obstruction must appear on the packages of antidiarrheal products containing calcium polycarbophil. It is only available as tablets that are to be chewed well and not swallowed whole. The adult dose is two chewable 500 mg tablets four times daily (or as needed), but the patient should not exceed eight tablets in any 24-hour period. Children aged 6 to under 12 chew one to two 500 mg tablets three times daily (or as needed), but should not exceed six tablets in 24 hours. Children aged 3 to under 6 years should chew one tablet three times daily (or as needed), but not exceed three tablets in 24 hours.[57]

(tip) *Because of its calcium content, the ingredient should not be taken with prescription antibiotics containing tetracycline.* The few adverse reactions of calcium polycarbophil include occasional epigastric pain and bloating.

ADSORBENTS
Adsorbent agents such as those shown in Table 11.2 alleviate diarrhea by adsorbing toxins, bacteria, and noxious materials (Fig. 11.1). Often patients are directed to take the medica-

A Pharmacist's Journal

Diarrhea from New York to Arizona

A woman appearing to be in her late 60s approached me in the community pharmacy holding a bottle of Imodium A-D. She asked, "Is there anything better than Imodium A-D that I can get without a prescription?" I explained that the product is quite efficacious and often stops diarrhea in one dose. I then asked how many doses she had taken. She replied, "It's not for me. It's for my husband." I asked how many doses he had taken, and she responded, "I've been giving him the Imodium A-D since we left home." I asked how long ago that was. "Well, we left New York driving about three days ago, and we're going to Arizona." I asked how her husband felt. "He's too weak to drive. He hasn't eaten much since we left home." I stressed that her husband must see a physician at once since diarrhea should only be treated for two days, and further, the weakness indicated that he had lost fluids and electrolytes. "He won't go. He's too stubborn and bullheaded." I asked if he could come into the pharmacy so I could persuade him to see a physician in our city's emergency room. "No, he's too weak to walk in. I have him in diapers in the back seat." I then repeated that he was losing fluids and electrolytes with each loose stool. "But I've been giving him ginger ale." I stressed that ginger ale is a poor remedy for diarrhea, and asked about his other health problems. "He's a diabetic and uses insulin and he also has high blood pressure." I described the effects that diabetes and some medications have on normal bowel motility and said that the emergency room physician would probably want to check his medications also.

She appeared defeated, and repeated that her husband "just won't go to the doctor." At that point, I showed her the electrolyte solutions and urged her to try to get him to ingest appreciable amounts. I also mentioned that eventually her husband may have no choice in the matter, since he would become unconscious with inadequate medical attention.

tion after each loose bowel movement, up to a specified daily maximum. Constipation, an adverse reaction, is simply an extension of the pharmacologic effect. *Adsorbents are available as tablets or suspensions. Since adsorbents may also adsorb prescription medications, patients should be advised to stagger doses of medications with the antidiarrheal.* If either the adsorbent or prescription medication is in liquid form, the patient should take the liquid first since it would leave the stomach more rapidly than a solid dosage form.

Attapulgite

OTC manufacturers of attapulgite have voluntarily added these warnings to their products: "Do not take if stools contain blood or mucus. If you are taking a prescription medicine, consult your doctor before taking this product. Drink plenty of clear fluids to help prevent dehydration which may accompany diarrhea."[55] Liquids containing this ingredient must be shaken well before use and should not be refrigerated. Doses vary according to age, with an adult taking two 750-mg caplets after the initial loose stool, and two after each subsequent loose stool, up to a maximum of 12 caplets in 24 hours. Patients aged 6 to 12 should take one caplet initially, and one after each subsequent loose stool, up to a maximum of six caplets in 24 hours. Patients aged 3 to under 6 may use the pediatric suspension, taking 1/2 tablespoonful (300 mg) per dose as directed.

Kaolin-Pectin

Despite having been sold for years for diarrhea, the combination of kaolin and pectin has never been proven effective.[25] Thus, although the trade name may reflect the older kaolin-pectin formulation (e.g., Kaopectate), most nonprescription products were reformulated to contain attapulgite. An FDA advisory committee voted in 1993 that sufficient evidence existed to confirm the effectiveness of kaolin as a single-entity product.[59] A monograph reflecting that vote was expected in the Federal Register in 1994 or 1995, but did not appear.[60] To date no product incorporating it has been marketed.

Bismuth Subsalicylate

An advisory committee to the FDA concluded that bismuth subsalicylate is safe and effective.[61] This decision was based on studies submitted by the company, which verified its efficacy in acute diarrhea, including traveler's diarrhea.[56]

Bismuth subsalicylate is thought to act as an adsorbent and as an astringent, which may decrease secretion of fluid by gastrointestinal (GI) tract walls to make feces more solid. This product was covered thoroughly in the chapter on gastric distress, for which it is also effective. (See Chapter 5, Gastric Distress.) The FDA will require the following label: "This product contains salicylate. Do not take this product with other salicylate-containing products such as aspirin unless

Patient Assessment Algorithm 11.1. **Diarrhea**

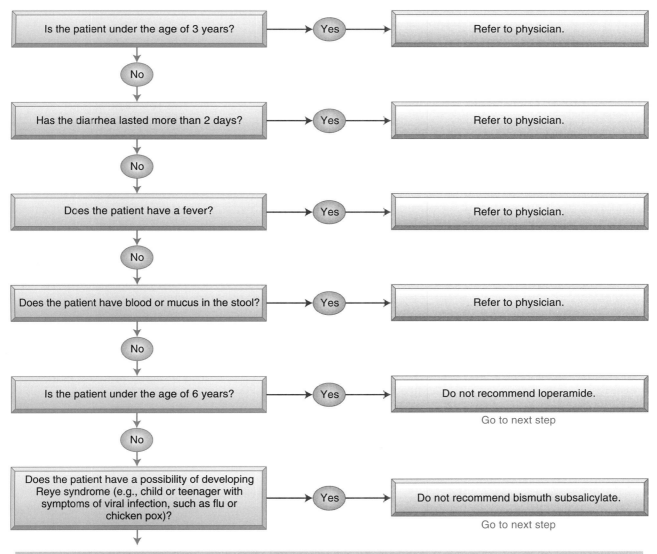

PRODUCT	SELECTED INGREDIENTS
Equalactin Chewable Tablets	Calcium polycarbophil 625 mg (equivalent to 500 mg polycarbophil)
Mitrolan Chewable Tablets	Calcium polycarbophil 625 mg (equivalent to 500 mg polycarbophil)

Table 11.1. Representative Antidiarrheal Products Containing Calcium Polycarbophil

directed by a doctor. If you are taking a drug for anticoagulation (thinning blood), diabetes, gout, or arthritis, do not take this product unless directed by a doctor."[25] The labeling of products containing bismuth subsalicylate will also contain the Reye-syndrome warning described in Chapter 5. The suspension must be shaken well prior to use. If the product contains 262 mg of bismuth subsalicylate per 15 mL, the adult patient should take 30 mL; the child of 9 to 12 should take 15 mL, the patient of 6 to 9 should take 10 mL, and those aged 3 to under 6 should take 5 mL. Doses are repeated every 30 to 60 minutes, to a maximum of 8 doses in any 24-hour period.

LOPERAMIDE

Loperamide is available as liquid or caplets for acute diarrhea, with an initial adult dose of four 5-mL teaspoonfuls

Table 11.2. Representative Adsorbent Antidiarrheal Products

PRODUCT	SELECTED INGREDIENTS
Advanced Formula Kaopectate	Per 15 mL: attapulgite 750 mg
Donnagel Suspension	Per 15 mL: attapulgite, activated 600 mg
Kaopectate Caplets	Attapulgite 750 mg
Kaopectate Children's Liquid	Per 1/2 tablespoonful: attapulgite 300 mg
Pepto-Bismol Caplets	Bismuth subsalicylate 262 mg
Pepto-Bismol Chewable Tablets	Bismuth subsalicylate 262 mg
Pepto-Bismol Suspension	Per 15 mL: bismuth subsalicylate 262 mg
Pepto-Bismol Maximum Strength Suspension	Per 15 mL: bismuth subsalicylate 525 mg
Rheaban Maximum Strength Caplets	Attapulgite, activated 750 mg

after the first loose bowel movement and two teaspoonfuls following each subsequent movement (Table 11.3). The maximum adult amount is 8 teaspoonfuls in any 24-hour period. Liquid dosage forms are clear solutions that do not need to be shaken before use. Caplets are also available.

Patients older than 6 should use the dosage cup packaged with the liquid medication to measure the dose specified. According to FDA guidelines, because of the potential for serious injury and illness, including abdominal distension and ileus, children younger than 6 must not be administered loperamide.[61] In 1993 the Consumer Product Safety Commission required loperamide products to have child-resistant packaging because of the potential serious injury and illness to children younger than 5. Therefore, pharmacists must be especially cautious of the "Professional Dosage Chart" provided by one of the nonprescription manufacturers that specifies dosing down to 2 years of age (24 pounds).

Adverse reactions to loperamide are rare, but can include many gastrointestinal adverse reactions (e.g., nausea, cramps, and dyspepsia), which are possibly related to the medical condition rather than to drug therapy. Loperamide also has reportedly caused drowsiness, dizziness, headache, tinnitus, and dry mouth.

LACTOBACILLUS

Products containing nontoxic strains of *Lactobacillus acidophilus* and *L. bulgaricus* supposedly act by reseeding the bowel, suppressing growth of pathogenic organisms, and helping promote regrowth of normal bowel flora. However, this action has never been proven to benefit diarrhea.[25,35] Because of the increase in bowel organisms, one adverse reaction can be flatulence.

Lactinex, an example of an antidiarrheal product containing lactobacillus, contains living organisms and must be refrigerated (Table 11.4).

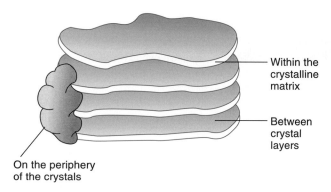

Within the crystalline matrix

Between crystal layers

On the periphery of the crystals

Figure 11.1. Adsorbent antidiarrheals entrap noxious agents in three locations.

ACTIVATED CHARCOAL

Several manufacturers have claimed that activated charcoal has an effect on diarrhea, but this has never been proven (as evidenced by the absence of charcoal from the list of FDA-approved antidiarrheals).[25] Charcocaps, one of the antidiarrheal products containing activated charcoal in a homeopathic formula, lacks proof of efficacy (see Table 11.4). (See Chapter 50, Homeopathy).

REHYDRATION SOLUTIONS

The CDC suggests that many deaths and hospitalizations resulting from rotavirus could be prevented by the early aggressive use of oral rehydration solutions (Table 11.5).[33,62] A diarrhea that originates from the small intestine is watery and high in potassium and bicarbonate; if it originates from the large intestine, it will be pasty or semisolid, with less fluid and electrolytes. A patient who is losing fluid may need fluid and electrolyte replacement, but *many pharmacists feel that a patient who is dehydrated enough to need oral rehydration solutions should use them*

Table 11.3. Representative Antidiarrheal Products Containing Loperamide

PRODUCT	SELECTED INGREDIENTS
Imodium A-D Caplets	Loperamide HCl 2 mg
Imodium A-D Liquid	Per 5 mL: loperamide HCl 1 mg
Imodium Advanced Formula Caplets	Loperamide HCl 2 mg, simethicone 125 mg

Table 11.4. Representative Antidiarrheal Products of Unproven Efficacy

PRODUCT	SELECTED INGREDIENTS/COMMENTS
Charcocaps Homeopathic Formula	Club moss, cinchona bark, sulfur, wood charcoal; ingredients not proven effective
Lactinex Tablets	Whey, lactose, sucrose, evaporated milk, talc, white mineral oil, viable *Lactobacillus acidophilus, Lactobacillus bulgaricus,* beef extract
Lactinex Granules	Whey, evaporated milk, viable *Lactobacillus acidophilus, Lactobacillus bulgaricus,* beef extract

Table 11.5. Representative Products for Rehydration

PRODUCT	SELECTED INGREDIENTS/COMMENTS
Infalyte	Per 1000 mL: sodium 50 mEq, potassium 25 mEq, chloride 45 mEq, citrate 34 mEq, rice syrup solids 30 g, 126 calories; ready-to-use solution
KaoLectrolyte Powder Packets	Per powder packet: sodium 12 mEq, potassium 5 mEq, chloride 10 mEq, citrate 7 mEq, dextrose 5 g, 22 calories; powder packets are to be reconstituted at the time of use
Pedialyte Grape	Per 1000 mL: sodium 45 mEq, potassium 20 mEq, chloride 35 mEq, citrate 30 mEq, dextrose 20 g, fructose 5 g, 100 calories; ready-to-use solution
Pedialyte Unflavored	Per 1000 mL: sodium 45 mEq, potassium 20 mEq, chloride 35 mEq, citrate 30 mEq, dextrose 25 g, 100 calories; ready-to-use solution
Pedialyte Freezer Pops	Per 62.5 mL pop: sodium 2.8 mEq, potassium 1.25 mEq, chloride 2.19 mEq, citrate 1.88 mEq, dextrose 1.56 g, 6.25 calories
Revitalice Freezer Pops	Per 62.5 mL pop: sodium 2.8 mEq, potassium 1.25 mEq, chloride 2.19 mEq, citrate 1.88 mEq, 12 calories

under a physician's supervision only (especially pediatric patients).

Oral rehydration solutions were not subjected to review by the FDA OTC review process. *These products do not reduce the number of stools, nor do they shorten the duration of the condition.*[63] Pharmacists could recommend them as treatment for diarrhea while patients wait to see a physician. The ability of oral rehydration solutions to replace electrolytes along with fluids makes them attractive ancillary items (Fig. 11.2).[4,64,65] One inconvenience is the large size of the bottles:

most are only available in quart sizes; after a bottle is opened, it must be refrigerated to prevent bacterial growth and must be discarded after 48 hours.

Oral rehydration solutions generally contain carbohydrates, sodium, potassium, calcium, magnesium, citrate, chloride, phosphate, sulfate, and bicarbonate.[66] Their caloric content and lack of protein mandates that patients also concurrently receive appropriate nutrition.[67] Some studies conducted to measure the efficacy of glucose against rice-based rehydration solutions have shown rice-based products to be superior.[67–70]

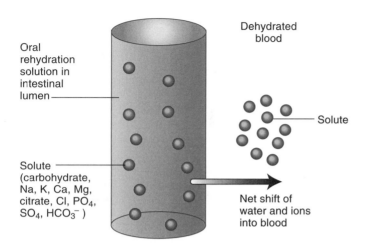

Figure 11.2. Oral rehydration solutions allow a net shift of water and ions from the intestine into the blood to rehydrate the patient.

 Soft drinks should be avoided in diarrhea because of their low electrolyte content and high osmolality, which may worsen diarrhea.[9]

Oral rehydration solutions are contraindicated with the following[17]:

- Signs of shock
- Persistent vomiting (signaling an inability to retain and absorb the solutions)
- Excessive concurrent fluid losses
- An inability to remain hydrated despite use of these fluids
- An inability to drink

- Sodium levels exceeding 160 mmol/L (since the products generally contain high levels of sodium)
- Infants younger than 3 months or weighing less than 4.5 kg

In all of these cases, intravenous rehydration is necessary.

SUMMARY

Diarrhea can be one of the more frightening symptoms the pharmacist is asked to treat. Unfortunately, many patients simply want to stop the bowel movements, disregarding any precautions in use of the nonprescription products. The pharmacist must intervene when appropriate, stressing the potential dangers of fluid and electrolyte depletion and pointing out the precautions associated with the use of nonprescription antidiarrheals. Patients (or caregivers) should never self-treat diarrhea in the following situations:

- Patient age is less than 3 years.
- Duration of diarrhea is more than 2 days.
- The patient also has fever.

Patients may safely self-treat with several nonprescription ingredients, including calcium polycarbophil, attapulgite, kaolin, bismuth subsalicylate, and loperamide. Lactobacillus and activated charcoal have not been proven to be safe and effective for diarrhea.

Rehydration products containing glucose or another carbohydrate in combination with multiple electrolytes may be helpful in preventing dehydration. They may be purchased in the forms of solutions, freezer pops, or powders for reconstitution.

AT THE COUNTER

Two young parents ask about a diarrhea product for their 5-year-old daughter.

Interview/Patient Assessment

The child was given a dose of Imodium A-D when she began having loose stools late the night before. She has no medical conditions and is not taking any medications.

Pharmacist's Analysis

1. Has the child's diarrhea been present too long to allow self-therapy?
2. Is the child too young for self-therapy?
3. Is Imodium A-D a good choice for this child?

The child may be self-treated for 2 days. Thus the pharmacist is still inside the 48-hour time limit and may suggest self-medication.

Patient Counseling

The child is over the age of 3, so she may be self-treated. However, Imodium A-D is not suitable for use under the age of 6. Thus the pharmacist may recommend such ingredients as attapulgite, calcium polycarbophil, kaolin, or bismuth subsalicylate (although the risk of Reye syndrome must be considered if bismuth subsalicylate is recommended). An oral rehydration solution might also be helpful. The parents should be cautioned that the child should see her pediatrician if the diarrhea continues for two nights from the onset of loose stools.

References

1. Baqui AH, et al. Methodological issues in diarrhoeal diseases epidemiology: Definition of diarrhoeal episodes. Int J Epidemiol 20:1057, 1991.
2. Glass RI. Estimates of morbidity and mortality rates for diarrheal diseases in American children. J Pediatr 118:S27, 1991.
3. Plevris JN, Hayes PC. Investigation and management of acute diarrhea. Br J Hosp Med 56:569, 1997.
4. Snyder J. Too many deaths from diarrhea. JAMA 260:3329, 1988.
5. Morrow AL, et al. Risk of enteric infection associated with child day care. Pediatr Ann 20:427, 1991.
6. Sabol VK, Friedenberg FK. Diarrhea. AACN Clin Issues 8:425, 1997.
7. Cohen MB. Etiology and mechanisms of acute infectious diarrhea in infants in the United States. J Pediatr 118:S34, 1991.
8. Baldassano RN, Liacouras CA. Chronic diarrhea. Pediatr Clin North Am 38:667, 1991.
9. Leung AK, Robson WL. Evaluating the child with chronic diarrhea. Am Fam Physician 53:635, 1996.
10. Groschel DH. Clostridium difficile infection. Crit Rev Clin Lab Sci 33:203, 1996.
11. Selby W. Diarrhoea—differential diagnosis. Aust Fam Physician 19:1683, 1990.
12. Tigges BB. Infant formulas: Practical answers for common questions. Nurse Pract 22:70, 1997.
13. James JM, Burks AW. Food-associated gastrointestinal disease. Curr Opin Pediatr 8:471, 1996.
14. Wadle KR. Diarrhea. Nurs Clin North Am 25:901, 1990.
15. Bertomeu A, et al. Chronic diarrhea with normal stool and colonic examinations: Organic or functional? J Clin Gastroenterol 13:531, 1991.
16. Framm SR, Soave R. Agents of diarrhea. Med Clin North Am 81:427, 1997.
17. Camilleri M. Gastrointestinal problems in diabetes. Endocrinol Metab Clin North Am 25:361, 1996.
18. Tanowitz HB, et al. Gastrointestinal manifestations. Med Clin North Am 80:1395, 1996.
19. Verne GN, Cerda JJ. Irritable bowel syndrome. Streamlining the diagnosis. Postgrad Med 102:197, 1997.
20. Reasner CA, Isley WL. Endocrine emergencies. Recognizing clues to classic problems. Postgrad Med 101:231, 1997.
21. Baker EH, Sandle GI. Complications of laxative abuse. Annu Rev Med 47:127, 1996.
22. Bytzer P, et al. Prevalence of surreptitious laxative abuse in patients with diarrhoea of uncertain origin: A cost benefit analysis of a screening procedure. Gut 30:1379, 1989.
23. Fine KD, et al. Diagnosis of magnesium-induced diarrhea. N Engl J Med 324:1012, 1991.
24. Lesaca TG. At mother's mercy: The nightmare of Munchausen syndrome by proxy. W V Med J 91:318, 1995.
25. Fed Reg 51:16137, 1986.
26. Qadri SMH. Infectious diarrhea. Postgrad Med 88:169, 1990.
27. Rubinoff MJ, Field M. Infectious diarrhea. Annu Rev Med 42:403, 1991.
28. Bergquist EJ. The office evaluation of infectious diarrhea. Prim Care 17:853, 1990.
29. Ludan AC. Current management of acute diarrhoeas. Drugs 36:18, 1988.
30. Strum WB. Update on traveler's diarrhea. Postgrad Med 84:163, 1988.
31. Pickering LK. Therapy for acute infectious diarrhea in children. J Pediatr 118:S118, 1991.
32. Grisanti KA, Jaffe DM. Dehydration syndromes. Emerg Clin North Am 9:565, 1991.
33. Anon. MMWR 40:80, 1991.
34. DuPont HL, et al. Prevention of traveler's diarrhea by the tablet formulation of bismuth subsalicylate. JAMA 257:1347, 1987.
35. Feldman M. Southwest internal medicine conference: Traveler's diarrhea. Am J Med Sci 288:136, 1984.
36. Anon. Traveler's diarrhea. NIH Consensus Dev Conf Statement 5:1, 1985.
37. Castelli F, Carosi G. Epidemiology of traveler's diarrhea. Chemotherapy 41(Suppl 1):20, 1995.
38. Lange WR, Kreider S. Traveler's diarrhea. Postgrad Med 77:255, 1985.
39. Lee CC, Lam MS. Foodborne diseases. Singapore Med J 37:197, 1996.
40. Rogers A. Holiday medicine. Pharm J 240:718, 1988.
41. Kozicki M et al. 'Boil it, cook it, peel it or forget it': Does this rule prevent travellers' diarrhoea? Int J Epidemiol 14:169, 1985.
42. Weber SJ, Lefrock JL. Health advice for the international traveler. Am Fam Physician 32:165, 1985.
43. Larson SC. Traveler's diarrhea. Emerg Med Clin North Am 15:179, 1997.
44. Katelaris PH, Farthing MJ. Traveler's diarrhea: Clinical presentation and prognosis. Chemotherapy 41(Suppl 1):40, 1995.
45. DuPont HL, Capsuto EG. Persistent diarrhea in travelers. Clin Infect Dis 22:124, 1996.
46. DuPont HL, et al. Chemotherapy and chemoprophylaxis of traveler's diarrhea. Ann Intern Med 102:260, 1985.
47. Kapikian AZ. Overview of viral gastroenteritis. Arch Virol Suppl 12:7, 1996.
48. Farthing MJ. Giardiasis. Gastroenterol Clin North Am 25:493, 1996.
49. Juckett G. Intestinal protozoa. Am Fam Physician 53:2507, 1996.
50. Mobarhan S, DeMeo M. Diarrhea induced by enteral feeding. Nutr Rev 53:67, 1995.
51. Edes TE, et al. Diarrhea in tube-fed patients: Feeding formula not necessarily the cause. Am J Med 88:91, 1990.
52. Davies NM. Toxicity of nonsteroidal anti-inflammatory drugs in the large intestine. Dis Colon Rectum 38:1311, 1995.
53. Kroser JA, Metz DC. Evaluation of the adult patient with diarrhea. Prim Care 23:629, 1996.
54. Dukes GE. Over-the-counter antidiarrheal medications used for the self-treatment of acute nonspecific diarrhea. Am J Med 88:24S, 1990.
55. Anon. NDMA Defends OTC Antidiarrheals. NDMA Special Report 12–91:1 (4/9/93).
56. Eherer AJ. et al. Effect of psyllium, calcium polycarbophil, and wheat bran on secretory diarrhea induced by phenolphthalein. Gastroenterology 104:1007, 1993.
57. Fed Reg 40:12924, 1975.
58. Anon. OTC antidiarrheals get mixed results. NDMA Executive Newsletter 13–93:2 (4/16/93).
59. Anon. FDA Looks at Labeling. NDMA Executive Newsletter 20–94:2 (6/17/94).

60. Feller MR. Reye warning voluntarily added to Pepto-Bismol labeling (Letter). FDA Consumer 26:7, 1992.

61. Williams DM. Loperamide not for children. Am Pharm 31:614, 1991.

62. Hogan DE. The emergency department approach to diarrhea. Emerg Med Clin North Am 14:673, 1996.

63. Santosham M, et al. Oral rehydration therapy of infantile diarrhea. N Engl J Med 306:1070, 1982.

64. Anon. Cereal-based oral rehydration solutions—Bridging the gap between fluid and food. Lancet 33:219, 1992.

65. Meyers A. Modern management of acute diarrhea and dehydration in children. Am Fam Physician 51:1103, 1995.

66. Mahalanabis D. Current status of oral rehydration as a strategy for the control of diarrhoeal diseases. Indian J Med Res 104:115, 1996.

67. Mohan M, et al. Rice powder oral rehydration solution as an alternative to glucose electrolyte solution. Indian J Med Res 87:234, 1988.

68. Patra FC, et al. Is oral rice electrolyte solution superior to glucose electrolyte solution in infantile diarrhea? Arch Dis Child 57:910, 1982.

69. Molla AM, et al. Rice-based oral rehydration solution decreases the stool volume in acute diarrhoea. Bull World Health Organ 63:751, 1985.

70. Goldberg ED, Saltzman JR. Rice inhibits intestinal secretions. Nutr Rev 54(1 Pt 1):36, 1996.

CHAPTER 12

Pinworm

AT THE COUNTER

 A mother tells the pharmacist that she is concerned that her children might have pinworm infestation.

Interview/Patient Assessment

The pharmacist asks why the mother suspects pinworm infestation. "I notice that my son is always pulling at his pants and scratching the rectal area. He's 3 years old, and I want to give him and his little sister the medicine now. She's 18 months old." The pharmacist asks if the mother has confirmed pinworm infestation in either child. "Yes, because he is always pulling and scratching."

Pharmacist's Analysis

1. Are there other explanations for the child's problems?
2. How might the mother confirm pinworm?
3. Assuming the children have pinworm, is a nonprescription product appropriate?

The child's problems may be symptoms of pinworm. They also may be caused by a nervous habit, an allergy, or lack of cleanliness following bowel movements. Thus the mother's worries may be entirely misplaced.

Patient Counseling

The mother's suspicions should be confirmed by nocturnal examination of the anal area. If the mother is uncomfortable with this method or if it is inconclusive, she may collect a sample of pinworm eggs by touching sticky tape to the anal area. The tape may then be taken to a physician's office for confirmation. Should either method confirm pinworm infestation, the pharmacist may recommend self-treatment with pyrantel pamoate. However, even if pinworm is confirmed in both children, the daughter is too young to allow self-treatment. Thus the younger child requires physician referral.

Man is host to many helminth infestations, ranging in size from microscopic to several feet in length.[1] They include nematodes (*Enterobius, Ascaris, Trichuris, Trichinella, Capillaria*), tapeworms, hookworm, liver fluke, strongyloides, and the worms responsible for filariasis, onchocerciasis (river blindness), schistosomiasis, and dracunculiasis.[2–10] Helminth infestations are rare in developed countries because of sophisticated systems for delivering water and disposing of raw sewage.[11] However, certain patients are at higher risk for these more exotic helminth infestations such as international students and travelers, migrant workers, refugees, homeless persons, and children who have been adopted from a foreign country.[12] Individuals who eat some raw foods such as uncooked pork sausage or other meats or raw fish such as sushi and sashimi also are at higher risk. (Undercooked cod, salmon, or herring can transmit a worm causing a condition known as anisakiasis.[1])

The pinworm is more common than other helminths because it is not spread via waterborne routes. Pinworm (also known as threadworm) infestation—enterobiasis—carries a social stigma and gives many people an uncomfortable feeling because they—or family members—have "worms." However, the condition can be diagnosed by educated caregivers and may be self-treated using nonprescription anthelmintic products.[13]

PREVALENCE OF PINWORM

The pinworm species, *Enterobius vermicularis,* is the most common helminth infestation affecting humans throughout the temperate climates of the world, including the United States and Europe.[14–18] Infestation with this small white nematode is not a reportable disease, so the Centers for Disease Control (CDC) do not compile data on its prevalence.[17] However, experts estimate that as many as 20 to 42 million Americans have pinworms.[19,20] Infestation rates may be as low as 3.4%.[21]

Man is the only host for this species of pinworm, although other species affect other mammals.[14,18,20,22] The pinworm does not mature or germinate in soil at any time in its life cycle.[19]

EPIDEMIOLOGY OF PINWORM INFESTATION

Enterobiasis (infestation with pinworm) exhibits a strong age stratification. Children aged 5 to 14 suffer the highest rates because of the methods by which ova are transmitted.[13,14,19] (See "Transmission of Pinworm.") While infestation rates in adults are approximately 16%, in children they are as high as 50 to 100%.[17,18,23] Group living tends to increase the rate: one study of institutionalized children reported a 66% rate of infection.[24]

Pinworm infestation crosses all socioeconomic lines, but does show a racial division. Whites are at higher risk than blacks and Hispanics.[25] Pinworm occurs in all geographic areas in the United States, both urban and rural. Pinworm infestation appears to be more common in overcrowded conditions and is directly related to bathing and changing underclothing.[19,25–27] Historically, it has been a common parasitic infestation in homosexuals (following amebiasis and giardiasis in frequency).[19,28]

ETIOLOGY OF PINWORM INFESTATION

The human host ingests pinworm eggs through one of the several methods described under "Transmission of Pinworm." After the ova reach the stomach, gastric acids dissolve the outer covering to release minute larvae (140 to 150 micrometers long).[19,22] The larvae hatch in the duodenum, maturing in 15 to 28 days to a length of approximately 5 mm (male) or 13 mm (female) (Fig. 12.1).[19,29] Worms live and mate throughout the length of the bowel, attached to the mucosa of the distal ileum, cecum, proximal ascending colon, or vermiform appendix.[19,30] During the night pregnant females exit the anus to lay eggs, depositing as many as 10,000 ova on the perianal skin.[22,29,31] After laying eggs female pinworms usually die, although they may reenter the individual. The average pinworm life span is 37 to 93 days.[19]

Within 6 hours after being deposited, the ova—or eggs—become infective. They have thick walls that resist desiccation, allowing them to remain infective for up to 20 days.[19,28,32] Their sticky, albuminous outer layer allows the three-sided ova to adhere well to various surfaces.[19] Touching the perianal skin (e.g., by scratching) can loosen the eggs, allowing them to enter the environment.[22,33]

TRANSMISSION OF PINWORM

There are three methods by which individuals contract pinworm (Fig. 12.2):

- Finger-to-mouth
- Inhalation (some of the ova deposit in the oropharynx, from which they are subsequently swallowed)
- Retroinfection[19,26,30,34]

Fingers may become contaminated with pinworms or their eggs in two ways:

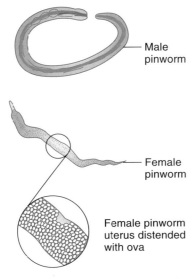

Male pinworm

Female pinworm

Female pinworm uterus distended with ova

Figure 12.1. The male and female pinworm; the female uterus is distended with ova.

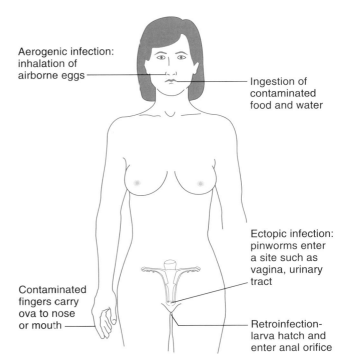

Aerogenic infection: inhalation of airborne eggs

Ingestion of contaminated food and water

Ectopic infection: pinworms enter a site such as vagina, urinary tract

Contaminated fingers carry ova to nose or mouth

Retroinfection-larva hatch and enter anal orifice

Figure 12.2. The methods by which a patient may become infested with pinworm are described in this illustration.

- Host-to-host: infected individuals have large numbers of eggs around the anal area. Scratching the area can contaminate the fingers with eggs. Anus-to-mouth transmission occurs when fingers are placed into the mouth, resulting in reinfection of the same individual.[14,19]
- Host-to-fomite: fingers also may become contaminated through **fomites** (inanimate objects capable of carrying infective agents). Scratching can cause perianal eggs to leave the host's skin and enter the environment.[22,33] Eggs adhere to clothing, bedding, bathroom fixtures, pets, and other objects.[17,19] When objects contaminated with eggs are touched, the eggs stick to fingers and are caught under fingernails. Subsequently, the eggs can contaminate food and infect other individuals.[14]

A person who touches any contaminated object and places the fingers in the mouth transfers the viable eggs to himself. In both of these cases the hand-to-mouth activity of children accounts for their relatively high infestation rates.[17]

The second method of infestation is aerogenic, via inhalation of airborne eggs that fall from bed linen and clothes.[20] As the ova are inhaled, their weight causes them to impact against the mucous membranes of the palate and oropharynx. From there, they are subsequently swallowed.

A final method is retroinfection, which occurs when the pinworm hatches on the **anal verge** (the area where the anal canal joins perianal skin) then reenters that individual's rectum and bowel.[19]

The high transmission rate of pinworm virtually ensures that the first infected patient in the household (the index case) will transmit eggs to each family member in turn, until all are infected.[19,29]

MANIFESTATIONS OF PINWORM INFESTATION

Symptoms of Pinworm Infestation

Pinworms produce symptoms through three mechanisms:

- Mechanical stimulation and irritation
- Allergic reactions
- Rare, accidental movement of the pinworm from its preferred location in the bowel to **ectopic** (found outside of the normal location) sites[19]

Pinworm infestation seldom produces severe problems, and many people are completely asymptomatic.[35,36] The main symptom people expect and recognize is intense perianal itching, which is more common at night when the worm migrates.[17,25] This nocturnal pinworm wandering also causes restless sleep, awakening, nightmares, bedwetting, anorexia, weight loss, irritability, and insomnia.[32,37] Mental development may be affected.[38] Children may complain of nausea or abdominal pain.[19] In rare cases nasal itching may result from the worm migrating to the nares.[37]

Pinworm may cause bowel inflammation such as enterocolitis or ileocolitis, as well as perforation.[39–41] The role of pinworm in causing appendicitis has been debated, with pinworm being found in 2.4% of human appendices.[19,42]

Diagnosis of Pinworm Infestation

Symptoms of pinworm infestation are nonspecific, so patients should not begin therapy until the suspicions of infestation are confirmed.[24] Stool specimen analysis is usually negative since pinworm ova are not released into the fecal stream.[35] A laboratory analysis of fecal material removed during a digital exam and placed onto a slide prepared with normal saline is a more effective method of diagnosis.[19,22]

Some parents or caregivers may wish to make the diagnosis themselves. An hour or so after the child has gone to bed (the females actively lay eggs outside the anus at this time) the parent or caregiver should inspect the child's anal area with a flashlight, looking for actively moving females (approximately 1/4 to 1/2 inch long).[14,17,19] It is difficult for a patient to use this method to self-diagnose because of the awkward nature of self-inspection of the anal opening.

If the parent or caregiver wishes to confirm his or her self-recognition with physician involvement, he or she should follow this procedure:

1. Cover the end of a swab or tongue depressor with double-sided tape or single-sided tape with the sticky side out.[17,19,43] (The tape should be transparent, not frosted.)
2. Touch the tape to several areas surrounding the anal verge in the morning before the child bathes or defecates.[19]
3. Preserve the tape in a glass jar or plastic bag and take it to a physician's office for microscopic evaluation. (Conduct-

ing the test for 3 days increases the chances of a positive diagnosis when the patient actually has pinworm).[44,45]

This method does not allow parent recognition since pinworm eggs are too small to see with the unaided eye. (The double-contoured pinworm egg is asymmetrical, has one flattened side, and averages 55 × 25 micrometers in size.) (Fig. 12.3).[20,46] More than one exam is helpful because a single exam often results in false negatives; five examinations of the same individual detect 99% of infestations.[25]

SPECIFIC CONSIDERATIONS OF PINWORM: ECTOPIC ENTEROBIASIS

Occasionally, pinworms are found in extraintestinal locations, a condition known as ectopic enterobiasis.[16] In some situations the worm may have been able to penetrate the bowel through a defect in the bowel wall. However, the majority of ectopic infections probably have a simpler explanation, since the female pinworm is exclusively responsible for ectopic infections.[37] Researchers theorize that the female pinworm, the only member of the species that migrates, probably mistakes another body orifice for the anus.[25] The human female genital tract is the most common ectopic site, which supports this theory of mistaken retrograde migration.[18,47] Conversely, male humans suffer far fewer ectopic lesions than females, presumably because of lack of a convenient entry site.[48]

Pinworm may ascend the vagina to cause vulvovaginitis.[47,49–51] Pinworm has been found in an inguinal hernia, endometrium, epididymis, myometrium, fallopian tubes, ovaries, and even in the human embryo.[16,18,30,34,52–55] The worm is also able to exit the fallopian tube, entering the peritoneal cavity. The worm may also enter the genitourinary tract, causing burning on micturition and crawling sensations in the urethra.[34] Pinworms have also been found in the conjunctival sac, hernial sac, liver, renal pelvis, prostate, spleen, and the wall of the appendix, although the means by which they gain access to these sites have never been explained.[18,19,48,52,56] Some inhaled ova reach the lungs (rather than being swallowed), where they also produce abscesses.[52]

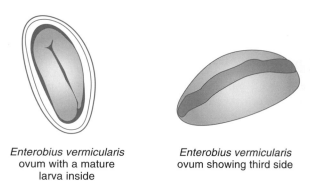

Enterobius vermicularis
ovum with a mature
larva inside

Enterobius vermicularis
ovum showing third side

Figure 12.3. The ova of *Enterobius vermicularis* has a characteristic three-sided appearance.

Pinworm may enter perianal tissues via a crypt to cause cellulitis and unidentified perianal mass.[57]

TREATMENT OF PINWORM

Treatment Guidelines

Once pinworm has occurred in a household, transmission to other members of the household is very likely.[49] Pharmacists should carefully explain the steps that may be taken to help prevent transmission and reinfection:

- Fingernails should be cut short and children should be cautioned against scratching the perianal area since eggs caught under the nails can be transferred to the mouth.[13,17]
- Children must be warned to keep their fingers out of the mouth at all times during treatment, since some physicians think that thumb sucking and fingernail biting may cause reinfection.[19,20]
- During the week following treatment, all family members must wear cotton underpants that are changed twice daily and washed in hot, soapy water.[13,19,20]
- Children's sleeping garments should cover the anus to help prevent scratching this area.[13] Underpants worn underneath the pajamas or closed garments may help prevent anal scratching.[22]
- Daily showers are less likely to promote reinfection than bathtub soaking.[17]
- The toilet seat must be cleaned after each family member uses it.[19,20]
- Furnishings, toys, and similar potential fomites should be disinfected with Lysol.[17]
- The house should also be decontaminated for pinworm eggs by cleaning all bedroom floors with disinfectant soap (e.g., containing triclosan) and water.[17]
- Since the highest concentrations of eggs are likely to be found around the bed itself, this area should be vacuumed thoroughly several times.[19,22] The vacuum filter should retain ova.
- Linens and clothing should be washed using the hottest water available.
- Wash must not be whipped or snapped through the air before washing or after washing (i.e., to remove wrinkles during folding). The pinworm eggs are light and can be blown around the house, where they may land on food or other objects, in drinks, or be inhaled, starting the reinfection process anew.[19,20]

These ancillary steps can help prevent treatment failure. However, pinworm medications only kill adult worms and are ineffective for developing eggs and larvae.[19] Thus any eggs accidentally swallowed at the time the medication is administered or shortly thereafter will mature and cause reinfection within 2 weeks to 2 months.[20] (The duration of the reinfection cycle, from ingestion of eggs to migration of mature, gravid females, is 15 to 43 days.) Ova floating in the atmosphere also contribute to the high failure rate of medications as they can main-

tain viability for up to 20 days.[20] For these reasons some physicians recommend a routine second treatment 2 weeks after the initial treatment.[19,20] Prudent medical practice dictates treatment of all family members.[13] Day-care centers and other sites of group activities should also be notified so that the child's playmates can be assessed.[17,58]

Nonprescription Medication: Pyrantel Pamoate

Regardless of the method by which patients, parents, or caregivers have confirmed pinworm, the treatment is the same— a safe and effective OTC anthelmintic (Table 12.1). Pharmacists must remember that patients infested with pinworm are usually already quite embarrassed and must avoid giving adults or children the feeling that they are unclean or should be ashamed because they have "worms."[19]

Pyrantel pamoate suspension, the only approved nonprescription ingredient, eradicates pinworm through depolarization of muscle, thereby paralyzing the pinworm's contractile hold on the intestinal wall.[14] As the worms fall away, they are carried out of the patient through peristalsis in the feces. *Pyrantel pamoate is suitable for self-treatment unless patients have liver disease, are pregnant, are below the age of 2, or weigh less than 25 pounds.*[59] *(See Patient Assessment Algorithm 12.1 for an illustration of the steps used in counseling the suspected pinworm patient.) The bottles must be agitated thoroughly prior to removal of medication.* At the recommended single OTC dose of 11 mg/kg (up to a maximum of 1 g), adverse effects are rare.[19] Adverse effects, which include gastrointestinal problems such as abdominal cramps, nausea, vomiting, and diarrhea, are probably related to clearing of the worms.[60]

If symptoms of infestation persist, if pinworms are still present after treatment, if any other type of worm is present before or after treatment (e.g., continuing symptoms, presence of visible worms in the stool), if the gastrointestinal reactions persist, or if headache or dizziness occur, patients should consult a physician.[19,59]

PREVENTION OF PINWORM INFESTATION

Prevention of pinworm infestation is difficult, but attention to certain habits can reduce the risk of infection:

- Always clean hands thoroughly after defecation and prior to eating or preparing food.[19] (Pinworm eggs on the hands or under the nails can contaminate food and drink.[14])

Table 12.1 Representative Products for Pinworm Containing Pyrantel Pamoate	
PRODUCT	SELECTED INGREDIENTS
Pin-X Suspension	Per mL: pyrantel pamoate 50 mg
Pin-Rid Suspension	Per mL: pyrantel pamoate 50 mg

Patient Assessment Algorithm 12.1. Pinworm

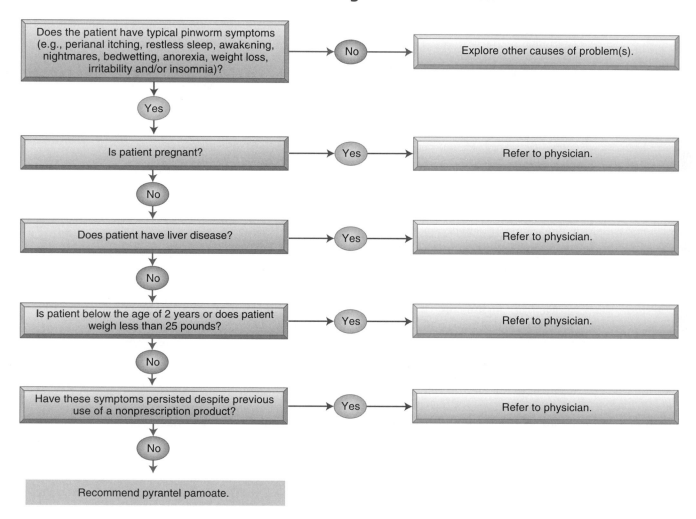

Does the patient have typical pinworm symptoms (e.g., perianal itching, restless sleep, awakening, nightmares, bedwetting, anorexia, weight loss, irritability and/or insomnia)? — No → Explore other causes of problem(s).

Yes ↓

Is patient pregnant? — Yes → Refer to physician.

No ↓

Does patient have liver disease? — Yes → Refer to physician.

No ↓

Is patient below the age of 2 years or does patient weigh less than 25 pounds? — Yes → Refer to physician.

No ↓

Have these symptoms persisted despite previous use of a nonprescription product? — Yes → Refer to physician.

No ↓

Recommend pyrantel pamoate.

AT THE COUNTER

A father asks about dosing a pyrantel pamoate product.

Interview/Patient Assessment

"We've done the night test for pinworm, and our 6-year-old daughter and 9-year-old son both have them. Now my wife and I are starting to imagine that we also have them. How much of this stuff should we use? Should all four of us take the product?

Pharmacist's Analysis

1. Should the parents also be treated?
2. Is pyrantel pamoate suitable for all family members?

3. How do the parents dose the product?

The parents have correctly performed the home diagnostic test for pinworm, confirming the diagnosis in both children.

Patient Counseling

The parents should also be treated because of the nature of transmission. The product is suitable for all family members except patients younger than 2, patients weighing less than 25 pounds, patients who have liver disease, or patients who are pregnant. Dosage is easily calculated by consulting a simple chart on the bottles based on the patient's weight.

- If possible, have children sleep in separate beds to prevent transfer to siblings.
- Use good hygiene practices in bathrooms to prevent the transfer of eggs from cups, toothpaste, doorknobs, and other objects.[14]
- Eggs are not killed by chlorination of water in swimming pools, so never swim with infected siblings or those known to be infected.[19]

SUMMARY

Enterobiasis is caused by a human parasite known as the pinworm. It is the most common helminth infestation in the United States, and it predominantly affects children. Patients contract pinworm through ingestion of eggs, inhalation of eggs, or retroinfection. Although embarrassing, pinworm need not cause undue dismay.

The symptoms of pinworm infestation include rectal itching, restless sleep, awakening, nightmares, bedwetting, anorexia, weight loss, irritability, and insomnia. Pinworm can be diagnosed by the parents or caregivers of a child exhibiting symptoms without the need for physician intervention. Subsequent treatment with pyrantel pamoate can eliminate pinworm. When one resident of a household has pinworm, others are likely to contract it. The spread of pinworm can be prevented by proper attention to basic hygiene such as cleaning the hands thoroughly after bowel movements and before preparing food or drink.

References

1. Segal M. Parasitic invaders and the reluctant human host. FDA Consumer 27(6):7, 1993.
2. Grove DI. Worms in Australia. Med J Aust 159:464, 1993.
3. Reid CJ, Perry FM, Evans N. Dipylidium caninum in an infant. Eur J Pediatr 151:502, 1992.
4. Grencis RK, Cooper ES. Enterobius, trichuris, capillaria, and hookworm including ancylostoma caninum. Gastroenterol Clin North Am 25:579, 1996.
5. Tanowitz HB, Weiss LM, Wittner M. Diagnosis and treatment of common intestinal helminths. II: Common intestinal nematodes. Gastroenterologist 2:39, 1994.
6. Schupf N, et al. Prevalence of intestinal parasite infections among individuals with mental retardation in New York State. Ment Retard 33:84, 1995.
7. Mangali A, et al. Intestinal parasitic infections in Campalagian district, south Sulawesi, Indonesia. Southeast Asian J Trop Med Public Health 24:313, 1993.
8. Hong ST, et al. Immunoblot patterns of clonorchiasis. Korean J Parasitol 35:87, 1997.
9. Brattis N, et al. Differences in cytokine responses to Onchocerca volvulus extract and recombinant Ov33 and OvL3–1 proteins in exposed subjects with various parasitologic and clinical states. J Infect Dis 176:838, 1997.
10. Anon. Trichinosis outbreaks. FDA Consumer 25(4):4, 1991.
11. Bell RG. IgE, allergies and helminth parasites: A new perspective on an old conundrum. Immunol Cell Biol 74:337, 1996.
12. Juckett G. Common intestinal helminths. Am Fam Physician 52:2051, 1995.
13. Harcup J. Tackling threadworms. Prof Care Mother Child 5:15, 1995.
14. Fed Reg 45:59539, 1980.
15. Wagner ED, Eby WC. Pinworm prevalence in California elementary school children, and diagnostic methods. Am J Trop Med Hyg 32:998, 1983.
16. Sun T, et al. Enterobius egg granuloma of the vulva and peritoneum: Review of the literature. Am J Trop Med Hyg 45:249, 1991.
17. Katzman EM. What's the most common helminth infection in the U.S.? MCN 14:193, 1989 .
18. Mondou EN, Gnepp DR. Hepatic granuloma resulting from Enterobius vermicularis. Am J Clin Pathol 91:97, 1989.
19. Russell LJ. The pinworm, Enterobius vermicularis. Prim Care 18:13, 1991.
20. Libbus MK. Enterobiasis. Nurse Pract 8:17, 1983.
21. Dahlstrom JE, Macarthur EB. Enterobius vermicularis: A possible cause of symptoms resembling appendicitis. Aust N Z J Surg 64:692, 1994.
22. Jones JE. Pinworms. Am Fam Physician 38:159, 1988.
23. Hood C. Enterobius vermicularis. Practitioner 233:503, 1989.
24. Novak C, et al. Enterobiasis in the suburbs (Letter). Med J Aust 147:414, 1987.
25. Knuth KR, et al. Pinworm infestation of the genital tract. Am Fam Physician 38:127, 1988.
26. Mahdi NK, Al-Khfaji AA. Prevalence and seasonal variation of enterobiasis in children of Iraq. Southeast Asian J Trop Med Public Health 21:135, 1990.
27. Karrar ZA, Rahim FA. Prevalence and risk factors of parasitic infections among under-five Sudanese children: A community based study. East Afr Med J 72:103, 1995.
28. Fiumara NJ, Tang S. Folliculitis of the buttocks and pinworms. Sex Transm Dis 13:45, 1986.
29. Goldenberg SP, Marignani P. The endoscopic diagnosis of colonic enterobiasis. Gastrointest Endos 36:309, 1990.
30. Wiebe BM. Appendicitis and Enterobius vermicularis. Scand J Gastroenterol 26:336, 1991.
31. Watt P, et al. Enterobiasis in young Australian adults (Letter). Med J Aust 154:496, 1991.
32. Ashford RW, et al. Enterobius vermicularis infection in a children's ward. J Hosp Infect 12:221, 1988.
33. Leach FN. Management of threadworm infection during pregnancy. Arch Dis Child 65:399, 1990.
34. Singh S, Samantaray JC. Topical anthelmintic treatment of recurrent genitourinary enterobiasis (Letter). Genitourin Med 65:284, 1989.
35. Haswell-Elkins MR, et al. The distribution and abundance of Enterobius vermicularis in a South Indian fishing community. Parasitology 95:339, 1987.
36. Kastner T, Selvaggi KA, Cowper R. Pinworm eradication in community residential settings for people with developmental disabilities. Ment Retard 30:237, 1992.
37. Reyes CV, et al. Omental Oxyuriasis: Case Report. Milit Med 149:682, 1984.
38. Bahader SM, et al. Effects of Enterobius vermicularis infection on intelligence quotient (I.Q.) and anthropometric measurements of Egyptian rural children. J Egypt Soc Parasitol 25:183, 1995.

39. Liu LX, et al. Eosinophilic colitis associated with larvae of the pinworm Enterobius vermicularis. Lancet 346:410, 1995.

40. Cacopardo B, et al. Eosinophilic ileocolitis by Enterobius vermicularis: A description of two rare cases. Ital J Gastroenterol Hepatol 29:51, 1997.

41. Patterson LA, et al. Perforation of the ileum secondary to Enterobium vermicularis: Report of a rare case. Mod Pathol 6:781, 1993.

42. Dalimi A, Khoshzaban F. Comparative study of two methods for the diagnosis of Enterobius vermicularis in the appendix. J Helminthol 67:85, 1993.

43. Koltas IS, et al. Serum copper, zinc and magnesium levels in children with enterobiasis. J Trace Elem Med Biol 11:49, 1997.

44. Norhayati M, et al. Enterobius vermicularis infection among children aged 1–8 years in a rural area in Malaysia. Southeast Asian J Trop Med Public Health 25:494, 1994.

45. Kawatu D, Lees RE, Maclachlan RA. Screening for intestinal parasites. Is a single specimen valid? Can Fam Physician 39:1748, 1993.

46. Zaman V. Shape of Enterobius vermicularis ova. Ann Trop Med Parasitol 79:467, 1985.

47. Neri A, et al. Enterobius (Oxyuris) vermicularis of the pelvic peritoneum—A cause of infertility. Eur J Obstet Gynecol Reprod Biol 23:239, 1986.

48. Daly JJ, Baker GF. Pinworm granuloma of the liver. Am J Trop Med Hyg 33:62, 1984.

49. McKay T. Enterobius vermicularis infection causing endometriosis and persistant (sic) vaginal discharge in three siblings (Letter). NZ Med J 102:56, 1989.

50. Chung DI, et al. Live female Enterobius vermicularis in the posterior fornix of the vagina of a Korean woman. Korean J Parasitol 35:67, 1997.

51. O'Brien TJ. Paediatric vulvovaginitis. Australas J Dermatol 36:216, 1995.

52. Mendoza E. et al. Invasion of human embryo by Enterobius vermicularis. Arch Pathol Lab Med 111:761, 1987.

53. McMahon JN, et al. Enterobius granulomas of the uterus, ovary and pelvic peritoneum. Two case reports. Br J Obstet Gynaecol 91:289, 1984.

54. Tornieporth BG, et al. Ectopic enterobiasis: A case report and review. J Infect 24:87, 1992.

55. Kollias G, Kyriakopoulos M, Tiniakos G. Epididymitis from Enterobius vermicularis: Case report. J Urol 147:1114, 1992.

56. Vafai M, Mohit P. Granuloma of the anal canal due to Enterobius vermicularis. Report of a case. Dis Colon Rectum 26:349, 1983.

57. Mattia AR. Perianal mass and recurrent cellulitis due to Enterobius vermicularis. Am J Trop Med Hyg 47:811, 1992.

58. Nunez FA, Hernandez M, Finlay CM. A longitudinal study of Enterobiasis in three day care centers of Havana City. Rev Inst Med Trop Sao Paulo 38:129, 1996.

59. Fed Reg 51:27755, 1986.

60. McEvoy GK, ed. AHFS 97 Drug Information: 1997. Bethesda, MD: American Society of Health-System Pharmacists, 1997.

Hemorrhoids

AT THE COUNTER

 A man in his mid 40s asks the pharmacist for help with nonprescription hemorrhoidal products.

Interview/Patient Assessment

The patient relates a history of rectal burning and discomfort following bowel movements since he was in his late 30s. He denies prolapse, but indicates that he has infrequent bleeding, which lasts for the next several bowel movements only. He relates that the symptoms wax and wane in severity. Symptoms disappear for as long as 2 months, but each time they return, they are worse than before and last for as long as 4 to 5 days before they finally remit. He has used various nonprescription products with varying degrees of success. The symptoms have been present for 2 days this time.

Pharmacist's Analysis

1. Are this patient's symptoms indicative of hemorrhoids?

2. What is the significance of waxing and waning symptoms?
3. What is the significance of bleeding?
4. Should this patient be allowed to self-treat his symptoms?

This patient's symptoms may indicate hemorrhoids. The condition does tend to wax and wane in conjunction with several variables such as diet and straining at the stool. Self-treatment for hemorrhoids, however, is contraindicated when the condition has persisted for longer than 7 days.

Patient Counseling

Even though this episode has only lasted 2 days, the total duration is several years, the criterion that the pharmacist must adhere to. Furthermore, rectal bleeding is an absolute contraindication for use of nonprescription products. The patient must be referred to a proctologist, surgeon, or general practitioner for full evaluation.

Anorectal conditions are common.[1] While there are many such conditions, hemorrhoids are the most common.[2,3] (See "Nonhemorrhoidal Anorectal Conditions.")

Hemorrhoids (known to some laymen as "piles") are a common condition that causes marked disability for a significant number of patients.[5] The definition of hemorrhoids is controversial because of mutually exclusive definitions from different experts. Some experts define hemorrhoids as a normal part of the human anatomy, others as a disease process.[6] The FDA Advisory Panel appointed to study the problem provided this definition: "Hemorrhoids are abnormally large or symptomatic conglomerates of blood vessels, supporting tissues, and overlying mucous membrane or skin of the anorectal area."[7] (Fig. 13.1)

Patient reluctance to discuss anorectal disease is high, partly because of the association with feces.[8] For this reason the pharma-

FOCUS ON...

NONHEMORRHOIDAL ANORECTAL CONDITIONS

Patients may complain of other anorectal conditions that are not hemorrhoidal in nature.

ANAL FISSURE

The anal fissure is a common cause of anorectal pain, being a tear of the skin of the anal canal, usually having occurred during defecation.[2,4] If conservative measures (sitz baths, stool softeners, analgesics) fail to manage anal fissure, surgical correction is the next step.

ANORECTAL/PERIANAL ABSCESS

The anorectal abscess is a painful, inflamed area where organisms have penetrated subcutaneous or submucosal tissues. It is filled with purulent material composed of mixed aerobic-anaerobic organisms requiring surgical incision and drainage. If it is chronic, the patient may develop a **fistula** (an inflamed channel that connects the anorectum to perianal skin; it may discharge feces and pus).[4,7] A physician must be seen for treatment of abscess and/or fistula.

SKIN TAGS

Skin tags are found where hemorrhoidal inflammation has abated somewhat, but the skin has not returned to the preinflammation condition, leaving a small tag. They are usually of no consequence.

RECTAL PROLAPSE

With rectal prolapse, a section of rectal wall moves below the anal canal to protrude from the anus.[5] With complete prolapse, even the anal sphincters protrude. It may occur from excessive straining or exercise.

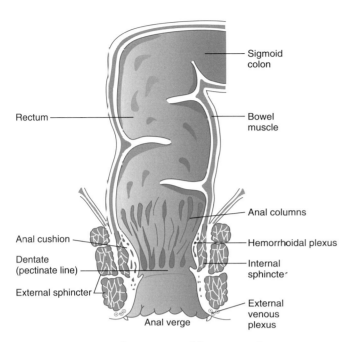

Figure 13.1. The anatomy of the anorectal region.

cist should ensure that other patients cannot overhear the discussion.

PREVALENCE OF HEMORRHOIDS

As many as 20% of the population have symptoms of benign anorectal disease at any one time, and approximately 9% are afflicted with hemorrhoids.[9] As many as one million physician visits occur each year because of hemorrhoids.[10] Up to 80% of both genders will experience symptoms at some time.[5] Age-specific estimates of the incidence of hemorrhoids reveal an increase with age. As many as 50% of individuals older than 50 have hemorrhoids.[5,11–13]

EPIDEMIOLOGY OF HEMORRHOIDS

Age influences the occurrence of hemorrhoids. Although they can occur at any age, they are rare in children and young adults (younger than 20).[13–16] Incidence of hemorrhoids peaks in the 40- to 64-year age group, and they are less common after the age of 65 (when compared with those aged 40 to 64).[17]

Investigators have not found a gender difference in the occurrence of hemorrhoids.[15,18,19] This is puzzling because many women suffer hemorrhoids during pregnancy, and worsening of existing hemorrhoids is common during pregnancy; however, symptoms may disappear entirely after delivery of the infant.[13,15,17,20,21] In males the incidence of hemorrhoids increases with increased socioeconomic level.[18]

Whites are affected with hemorrhoids more than blacks.[18] The problem is more common in rural than urban areas.[13]

Heredity may play a role in predisposing the individual to hemorrhoids.[22] At least 50% of sufferers have a positive fam-

ily history.[15,20] It is not known whether this familial tendency is a result of an inherited anatomic abnormality or to learned habits such as prolonged straining during defecation.[23]

ETIOLOGY OF HEMORRHOIDS

Many factors have been mentioned as contributing to hemorrhoids. For instance, diarrhea may pose considerable risk of developing hemorrhoids.[24,25]

Pathogenesis of Hemorrhoids

Hemorrhoids are thought by many clinicians to be distended veins of the **hemorrhoidal plexus** (the network of interjoining nerves and veins resting on the rectum's posterior and lateral walls).[23,26] (With this theory, the analogy to varicose veins of the legs or esophagus was quite apt.[14])

It is true that hemorrhoids contain dilated veins, but bleeding from hemorrhoids is arterial, as evidenced by its bright red color.[20,22,27,28]

The venous pathology theory has been challenged by detailed anatomic studies that have proved that dilated veins in the hemorrhoidal plexus are normal features of the human anal canal and are found in 80% of neonates, in children, and in every other age group.[14,29,30]

To explain hemorrhoids, studies have focused on anal cushions—submucosal masses containing venous sinusoids (into which arterioles empty) composed of connective tissue and smooth muscle that attaches this mucosa to the muscle wall.[27,31] Anal cushions, which are normal and are found in all patients, seal the anal canal to promote continence.[13,14,32–34] Young patients have well-organized connective-tissue fibers that support the venous sinusoidal vessels. The tissues break down, leading to hemorrhoidal symptoms as people age. Around the age of 30 the cushions and venous sinusoids begin to enlarge, and a section of anal canal tissue slides or descends into the lower anal canal, along with the submucosa, to form prolapsing hemorrhoids (Fig. 13.2).[21,27,29] This has become known as the "sliding mucosal theory."[27,35]

Protrusion of anal cushions with prolapsed internal hemorrhoids

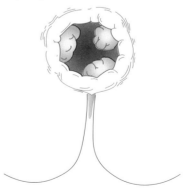

Figure 13.2. When internal hemorrhoids prolapse, the anal cushions are visible.

With this more recent understanding of regional anatomy, the term hemorrhoid can be reserved for an abnormal dilatation of the arteriovenous hemorrhoidal plexus that protrudes into the anal canal lumen.[6,36] (Figure 13.3 indicates common sites of hemorrhoids.)

Hemorrhoid patients may also have an overactive anal sphincter, which contributes to venous congestion by subjecting the cushions to increased shear stress or cellular damage.[13,19] Also, sphincter **hypertonicity** (continual high muscular tone) could be coupled with high resting anal pressures to worsen symptoms.[21,37]

Classification Systems for Hemorrhoids

Hemorrhoids may be classified in several ways, such as prolapsing versus nonprolapsing or external versus internal. In the external versus internal classification the differentiation of external versus internal is based on the location of the dentate (pectinate) line.[38] As shown in Figure 13.1, this landmark is the area where stratified squamous epithelial tissues of the anus become columnar epithelial tissues of the rectal mucosa. Hemorrhoids occurring above the dentate line are internal; those below are external.

Internal hemorrhoids are covered by anal canal mucous membrane. External hemorrhoids are covered by squamous epithelium.[23] Mixed hemorrhoids share features of both types and may occur above and below the dentate line.[13]

Internal hemorrhoids can be further subcategorized by degree of severity:

1. First-degree internal hemorrhoids enlarge but do not prolapse.[15]
2. Second-degree hemorrhoids bleed and prolapse with defecation, but return spontaneously.[40]
3. Third-degree hemorrhoids prolapse with each bowel movement and sometimes with exertion related to work or simply when standing. They can be replaced with manual manipulation.[20]

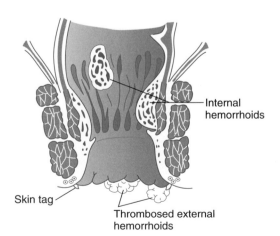

Figure 13.3. The internal hemorrhoid may prolapse below the dentate line; the external hemorrhoid may form a painful thrombosis.

4. Fourth-degree hemorrhoids prolapse irreducibly with thrombosing, profuse bleeding, and great pain.

MANIFESTATIONS OF HEMORRHOIDS

Hemorrhoids are often asymptomatic, which lulls the patient into a false sense of security about the condition.[14,22,26,39] Internal hemorrhoids may be asymptomatic for long periods until prolapse and strangulation occur. Painless bleeding is the most common symptom of internal hemorrhoids.[13,21,22,30,36,40] Eventually, external hemorrhoids may thrombose, which causes pain of sudden onset, perianal irritation, pruritus, and complaints of an uncomfortable rectal mass (an area that is round, purple, tender, and swollen).

Bleeding

Hemorrhoids are named for the Greek words haema (blood) and rhoe (flow).[35] Anal bleeding is the hemorrhoidal symptom that causes the greatest degree of concern for the patient; it is also the symptom that requires the most intense workup to exclude serious underlying pathology (e.g., ulcerative proctitis, Crohn's disease, cavernous hemangioma, colitis, anal fissure, polyps, cancer).[15,20,36,41,42–44] Bleeding is not usually associated with external hemorrhoids.

The nature of the bleeding helps identify the underlying condition. Blood associated with hemorrhoids is bright red and is usually seen on defecation, especially when patients strain to pass constipated stool.[20,30] Rather than being mixed with fecal material, the blood is usually seen on the surface of the toilet water or on the cleansing paper.[21,30] It may also drip slowly from the anus for a short time after defecation.[23,30] In any case, because of the possibility of a more serious condition, anal bleeding is an absolute contraindication for nonprescription products, and patients who report bleeding must be referred to a physician.[45–48]

Hemorrhoidal bleeding caused anemia in at least 0.5 patients per 100,000 seen in a major hospital.[49]

Prolapse

Prolapse is second only to bleeding as a common symptom of internal hemorrhoids, whereas external hemorrhoids are not said to prolapse since they are already located below the dentate line.[32] Prolapse usually precedes bleeding, with the patient neglecting to make a physician appointment until bleeding begins.[32] Prolapse may cause difficulty in cleaning, leading to wetness (from residual feces) or other minor discomforts.[28] For instance, the area may be sore or irritated if prolapse causes passage of mucus.[28] Chronic fecal soiling of perianal skin and fecal soiling of underwear allow prolonged contact of feces (which irritate skin) with sensitive hemorrhoidal skin and can cause excoriation, inflammation, and other discomfort.[20,21]

Prolapsed internal hemorrhoids may return to their normal position.[13] They may also require manual replacement by the patient following each bowel movement. Eventually,

some patients can no longer successfully do this and reluctantly seek care.[50] **_If the irreducible prolapse is not_**
treated, it eventually can become infected and
gangrenous.[36] Nonprescription products cannot provide
relief from prolapse or seepage of feces.[7]

Pain

Pain is not common with hemorrhoids.[13,30] It may be caused
by thrombosis of an external hemorrhoid, as well as with a
prolapsed internal hemorrhoid that has ulcerated or become
gangrenous.[13,21,22,32,51]

Pruritus Ani

Patients may describe pruritus, especially if prolapse with an
internal hemorrhoid or thrombosis with an external hemorrhoid occurs.[15] Anal itch may also be the result of other
causes. (Many patients who have undergone elective hemor-
rhoidectomies find that pruritus persists.[13]) The problem
may regress with education regarding anal hygiene, diet, and
bowel management.[13] For example, patients should wash the
perianal area with mild soap and a soft cloth following bowel
movements.[35] Also, caffeine (e.g., coffee, chocolate, caffeinated beverages), citrus fruits and beverages, carbonated
beverages, cheeses, and spices can all produce rectal burning and itching and should be eliminated from the diet to see
if pruritus ani disappears.[4,35,36]

SPECIFIC CONSIDERATIONS OF
HEMORRHOIDS: CONSTIPATION

Constipation has long been suspected to play a primary
causative role in the development of hemorrhoids. Hemorrhoids are rare in residents of rural Africa (where a high-fiber
diet is common), which has led researchers to the theory that
high crude fiber intake not only promotes normal laxation,
but it also prevents hemorrhoids.[13] Conflicting research,
however, has determined that many patients with symptoms
of hemorrhoids are not constipated, and that many patients
who are constipated do not suffer from hemorrhoids.[19,24]

The causative factor may not be constipation per se but
the act of straining to pass hard stools.[22] Straining increases
the intraabdominal pressure, which may be the underlying
cause of hemorrhoids.[14,17,52] Also, passing hard stool may result in tissue damage.[53] Finally, dried, hard stools engorge
anal blood vessels, resulting in stasis of venous flow and enlargement of the anal cushions.[21,23,35]

Some research indicates that patients with hemorrhoids
spend significantly more time on the toilet during defecation,
are more likely to read during defecation, and are more likely
to strain to pass stool.[54] Thus physicians often stress that constipation—which often results in extended time on the toilet—should be avoided.[53]

The association between constipation and hemorrhoids is
sufficiently compelling that pharmacists should consider the

epidemiologic factors of constipation presented in Chapter
10 when attempting to evaluate patients with symptoms of
hemorrhoids.

TREATMENT OF HEMORRHOIDS

Treatment Guidelines

Treatment of hemorrhoids is divided into several phases:

1. Patients with minor problems should be taught several
   conservative steps that may alleviate hemorrhoidal symptoms (e.g., hygiene and sitz baths).[55] (See "Nonpharmacologic Therapies.")
2. If the simple, nonpharmacologic interventions do not
   help, nonprescription or prescription products may be
   used. (See Patient Assessment Algorithm 13.1.)
3. If a hemorrhoidal problem (e.g., prolapse, bleeding) does
   not resolve, or if it is severe at the time of presentation, a
   physician may choose from among numerous operative
   techniques, including laser or surgical hemorrhoidectomy, sclerotherapy (injection of a medication such as
   phenol into tissues, which produces submucosal scarring
   and atrophy of the hemorrhoid), rubber band ligation
   (bands are placed at the upper end of a hemorrhoid, causing sloughing in 7 to 10 days), cryosurgery (freezing with
   liquid nitrogen), or dilation (digital expansion of the anal
   sphincter).[8,13,56–65]

Nonprescription Medications

Most physicians who discuss treatment of hemorrhoids with
their patients do not include nonprescription products.
Many physicians believe that nonprescription medications
for hemorrhoids are no more than placebos, are unnecessary,
and may be harmful to the anal mucosa.[22,32,35] Some of the
physicians who do recommend nonprescription medications
choose only hydrocortisone products.[23,36]

Despite the practices of physicians, certain nonprescription hemorrhoidal products can relieve specific hemorrhoidal symptoms, and pharmacists are justified in recommending them. See Table 13.1 for specific anorectal
conditions and the ingredients used to relieve them. (See "A
Pharmacist's Journal: Do You Have Rutin?")

The FDA's final monograph for anorectal nonprescription
drug products appeared in 1990.[45] *Because of the lack
of studies involving children and the rarity of hemorrhoids in children, the FDA has determined that hemorrhoidal products may not be recommended for children
younger than 12.*[7] Children with hemorrhoids often have a serious condition such as vena caval or mesenteric obstruction,
cirrhosis, portal hypertension associated with liver disease, or
other causes of venous obstruction, further justification for
the FDA ruling.[7]

*The time limit for self-treatment of anorectal condi-
tions is 7 days.* The FDA OTC Panel that considered
these products determined that cases of hemorrhoids (or

Patient Assessment Algorithm 13.1. Hemorrhoids

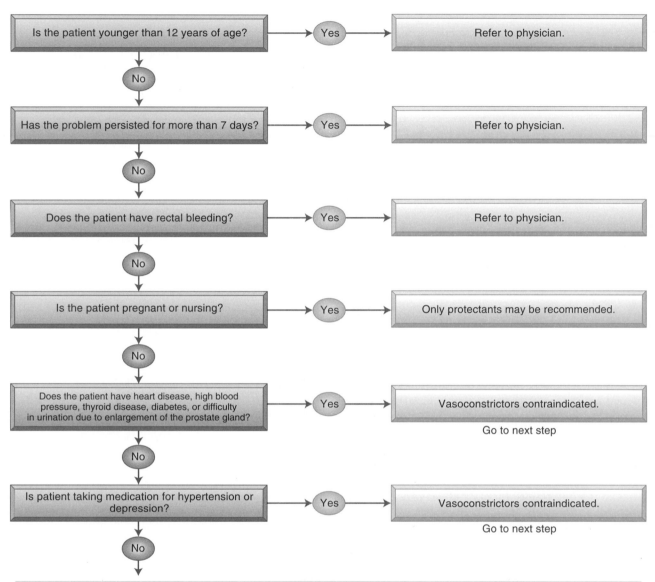

Is the patient younger than 12 years of age? → Yes → Refer to physician.

↓ No

Has the problem persisted for more than 7 days? → Yes → Refer to physician.

↓ No

Does the patient have rectal bleeding? → Yes → Refer to physician.

↓ No

Is the patient pregnant or nursing? → Yes → Only protectants may be recommended.

↓ No

Does the patient have heart disease, high blood pressure, thyroid disease, diabetes, or difficulty in urination due to enlargement of the prostate gland? → Yes → Vasoconstrictors contraindicated.
Go to next step

↓ No

Is patient taking medication for hypertension or depression? → Yes → Vasoconstrictors contraindicated.
Go to next step

↓ No

Recommend products for the specific symptoms that include approved combinations of local anesthetics/analgesics/antipruritics, protectants, astringents, vasoconstrictors, keratolytics, and hydrocortisone, unless contraindicated.

other anorectal conditions) continuing longer than 7 days would require a physician evaluation.[7] In addition, the FDA cautioned that if the condition worsens during the 7-day period, a physician must be consulted.[45]

The labels of hemorrhoidal products caution patients to consult a physician promptly if they experience bleeding. *The labels also advise that products intended only for external use should not be placed into the rectum with the fingers or with any mechanical device or applicator.* (See "A Pharmacist's Journal: How Much Vitamin D Is Too Much?")

Some creams and ointments are packaged with a small tubular tip or dispensing cap (also known as a "pipe") that screws onto the top of the ointment/cream tube. Company labeling may caution the patient that the cap is only to facil-itate application to the lower portion of the anal canal (most companies have shortened the tip to ensure that this is the only area it will reach.) When ingredients are intended for external use only, patients should not use longer applicator tips, which can bypass the lower anal canal and apply the product above the dentate line. With these longer applicators, the holes on the tip and sides of the tube could convert a topical cream or ointment to an internal dosage form, causing potential problems. When used internally, topical creams and ointments share the potential dangers of hemorrhoidal suppositories (which are by design intrarectal products) because they are readily absorbed through the healthy mucous membranes of the rectum. Medications absorbed in this manner might not circulate through the liver for metabolism,

Table 13.1. Anorectal Symptoms and the Ingredients Used to Treat Them

SYMPTOM	INGREDIENTS THAT CAN ALLEVIATE THE SYMPTOM
Pain	Local anesthetics, local analgesics/antipruritics, astringents
Itching	Local anesthetics, vasoconstrictors, local analgesics/antipruritics, keratolytics, hydrocortisone, protectants
Soreness	Local anesthetics
Burning	Local anesthetics, protectants, astringents
Irritation	Local anesthetics, protectants, astringents
Discomfort	Local anesthetics, keratolytics
Dry tissues	Protectants
Itching caused by moist anorectal conditions	Aluminum hydroxide gel, kaolin
Inflammation	Vasoconstrictors

A Pharmacist's Journal

"Do You Have Rutin?"

A woman looking over the hemorrhoidal products asked me, "Do you have rutin?" Rutin is a plant product that was sold for capillary fragility in the 1960s but which has never been proven effective for that condition or for any other symptom or condition. I asked what she wanted rutin for. "It's good for hemorrhoids. My daughter has a bad case of them." I asked where she heard about rutin. "I read that it works." I asked if she had read it in a medical text or article. "No, I read it in one of the newspapers that you pick up at the checkout stand." I explained tactfully that these tabloids were not reliable

sources of medical advice and suggested that her daughter try something besides rutin. "Well, I know what's causing them. She works two jobs and she's on her feet for 16 or more hours every day." I suggested that her daughter call me so I could match a product to her symptoms and describe some other methods of resolving hemorrhoids such as diet and stool habits. However, the daughter never called. It is difficult to convince a patient who is actually present to accept valid medical advice, but it is markedly more difficult when the individual is purchasing a product for someone else.

resulting in potentially dangerous systemic effects.[7] For this reason some hemorrhoidal ingredients are only approved by the FDA for external use—not for intrarectal application. Products with these applicator tips must caution patients to cease use of the tip if insertion causes pain.

Suppositories must carry a warning to remove foil before use. If the product contains ingredients impregnated on a pad, the label should instruct patients to gently apply to the affected area by patting and to then discard the pad.

The FDA maintains that label warnings for pregnant and nursing women are required for nonprescription medications that are intended for systemic absorption or that might be systemically absorbed, rather than those used for a local effect only.[66] By definition, however, since nonprescription

hemorrhoidal products are used only for local effects, they can be used by pregnant or nursing women. Therefore, risk to the fetus or child mandates great precaution for the pregnant or nursing mother.[67]

LOCAL ANESTHETICS

Local anesthetics, which are applied locally as ointments or creams, temporarily relieve pain, itching, soreness, burning, irritation, and/or discomfort (Table 13.2). Products containing benzocaine, benzyl alcohol, dyclonine, lidocaine, and tetracaine may be applied up to six times daily; products containing pramoxine may be applied up to five times daily; and products containing dibucaine may be applied up to three to four times daily. It is irrational to use applicator pipes with

A Pharmacist's Journal

"How Much Vitamin D Is Too Much?"

A woman holding a vitamin product asked, "How much vitamin D is too much?" I showed her that the product in question contained the RDA of vitamin D and stressed that she should not exceed that level. She answered, "I know that, because when I get too much vitamin D, it makes me bleed." I asked her to clarify. "Well, for the past few years, whenever I get too much vitamin D, I bleed out of my hemorrhoids." I asked how long she had experienced rectal bleeding. "Ever since my gall bladder was removed about 5 years ago." I expressed astonish-

ment and asked if she had ever told her physician that she had rectal bleeding. "No, it's only when I get too much vitamin D." I tactfully suggested that vitamin D was probably not responsible, and that her rectal bleeding was an important symptom that needed to be checked immediately. She did not agree and made it fairly clear that I didn't know what I was talking about. At times, in spite of the pharmacist's best effort, patients with dangerous symptoms persist in deluding themselves that there is nothing major that can possibly be wrong with them.

Table 13.2. Representative Products for Anorectal Conditions

PRODUCT	SELECTED INGREDIENTS/COMMENTS
Anusol Ointment	Pramoxine HCl 1%, zinc oxide 12.5%, mineral oil (amount unlabeled)
Anusol Suppositories	Topical starch 51%, benzyl alcohol
Hemorid Creme	Pramoxine HCl 1%, phenylephrine HCl 0.25%, white petrolatum 30%, mineral oil 20%
Hemorid Suppositories	Phenylephrine HCl 0.25%, zinc oxide 11%, hard fat 88.25%
Nupercainal Hemorrhoidal & Anesthetic Ointment	Dibucaine 1%
Preparation H Cream	Phenylephrine HCl 0.25%, shark liver oil 3%, petrolatum 71.9%, mineral oil 14%; box includes an applicator
Preparation H Ointment	Phenylephrine HCl 0.25%, shark liver oil 3%, petrolatum 71.9%, mineral oil 14%; box includes an applicator
Preparation H Suppositories	Shark liver oil 3%, cocoa butter 85.5%
proctoFoam	Pramoxine HCl 1%
Tronolane Cream	Pramoxine HCl 1%
Tucks Clear Gel	Witch hazel 50%, glycerin 10.7%
Tucks Pads	Witch hazel 50%, glycerin, water

any of these ointments or creams (some of these products are packaged with intrarectal pipes) since the mucous membrane lining the rectum does not include sensory nerve fibers. Likewise, intrarectal application of local anesthetics via suppositories is also irrational.[7]

The labels on products containing local anesthetics must carry this warning: "Certain persons can develop allergic reactions to ingredients in this product. If the symptom being treated does not subside or redness, irritation, swelling, pain or other symptoms develop or increase, discontinue use and consult a physician."

ANESTHETICS/ANALGESICS/ANTIPRURITICS

These ingredients, included in products as illustrated in Table 13.2, were actually referred to by the FDA Review Panel as counterirritants, but were later renamed to be analgesic, anesthetic, and antipruritic agents.[7,66] Confusion arises because they are different chemicals from local anesthetics (e.g., benzocaine), although they do produce a degree of anesthesia.

Anesthetics/analgesics/antipruritics relieve pain and itching, and menthol may provide a cooling sensation, all of which can help distract the patient from pain. The ingredients camphor, juniper tar, and menthol should only be applied externally; internal use is irrational since there are no pain fibers in the rectum. They may be applied up to six times daily.

Products containing menthol must carry this warning: "Certain persons can develop allergic reactions to ingredients in this product. If the symptom being treated does not subside or redness, irritation, swelling, pain or other symptoms develop or increase, discontinue use and consult a physician."

PROTECTANTS

Protectants form a protective coating over the skin (see Table 13.2). This protective coating produces the following temporary benefits:

- Prevents drying of tissues
- Protects irritated areas
- Relieves burning
- Relieves skin irritations
- Protects inflamed, irritated anorectal surfaces from abrasion and pain during bowel movements
- Protects inflamed perianal skin

Protectants that may be used internally or externally include cocoa butter, hard fat, lanolin, mineral oil, petrolatum, topical starch, and white petrolatum. Glycerin, another approved protectant, can only be applied externally. Several additional protectant ingredients, including calamine, cod liver oil, shark liver oil, and zinc oxide may be used internally or externally, but must be combined with other protectants as regulated by the FDA.

Aluminum hydroxide gel and kaolin, also approved protectants, relieve itching associated with moist anorectal conditions. Patients using these ingredients should remove any petrolatum or greasy ointment from the itching area prior to application or the ingredients will not adhere.

Protectants may be applied after each bowel movement or as needed, up to six times daily, except petrolatum and white petrolatum, which may be applied liberally to the area as often as necessary.

The FDA allows up to four protectants to be combined in a product, so long as the combined percentage of the protectants is at least 50% of the final product.[66] Further, each protectant must be present in at least 12.5% by weight (however, for shark liver oil and cod liver oil, the 24-hour quantity must provide 10,000 units of vitamin A and 400 units of cholecalciferol).

ASTRINGENTS

Astringents exert a local and limited protein coagulant effect on hemorrhoids. They temporarily protect irritated anorectal areas and temporarily relieve irritation and burning. Astringent ingredients in the final FDA monograph include

calamine and zinc oxide—suitable for internal and external use—and witch hazel (hamamelis water)—suitable for external use only. The astringents may be applied after each bowel movement or as needed up to six times daily. Table 13.2 lists hemorrhoidal products containing protectants.

VASOCONSTRICTORS

Vasoconstrictors temporarily constrict the blood vessels underlying the tissues to which they are applied (see Table 13.2). Thus they temporarily reduce the swelling associated with irritated hemorrhoidal tissues and other anorectal disorders. Approved vasoconstrictors include ephedrine and phenylephrine (both suitable for internal and external use) and epinephrine (only suitable for external use, since it is inactivated by the alkaline secretions of the rectum), all of which may be applied up to four times daily.[7]

tip *Patients must be warned away from vasoconstrictor products if they have heart disease, high blood pressure, thyroid disease (since the effects of hyperthyroidism may be worsened by sympathomimetics), diabetes, or difficulty in urinating as a result of enlargement of the prostate gland, unless directed to use them by a physician.* Patients currently taking prescription medication for high blood pressure and depression also should avoid them. The label of ephedrine-containing hemorrhoidal products will caution that use may cause nervousness, tremor, sleeplessness, nausea, and loss of appetite. If the symptoms persist or worsen when using vasoconstrictors, patients should see a physician.

KERATOLYTICS

Keratolytics (medications that cause desquamation and debridement) would seem to be contraindicated for anorectal nonprescription use since they could potentially erode tissue. However, they are useful in low concentrations to relieve discomfort and itching with hemorrhoids. Approved keratolytics include alcloxa and resorcinol—both suitable for external use only since mucous membranes of the rectum do not contain keratinized outer tissues. Keratolytics may be applied up to six times daily. No leading hemorrhoidal product currently contains keratolytic agents.

Products containing resorcinol must carry this warning: "Certain persons can develop allergic reactions to ingredients in this product. If the symptom being treated does not subside or redness, irritation, swelling, pain, or other symptoms develop or increase, discontinue use and consult a physician." These products must also carry a warning against use on open wounds near the anus. This precaution is meant to prevent absorption of resorcinol, which has caused tinnitus, tachypnea, tachycardia, profuse sweating, methemoglobinemia, circulatory collapse, unconsciousness, and violent convulsions.[7]

HYDROCORTISONE

In 1983 the FDA issued a tentative final monograph that addressed the use of hydrocortisone in anorectal conditions.[68] Proposed labeling included relief of anal itching. In 1988 the FDA required manufacturers to include all of the warnings on hydrocortisone products marketed for anal itch that other anorectal products must carry (e.g., age, contraindications).[69] Hydrocortisone may require as long as 12 hours for onset of relief, but produces a longer-lasting relief than other ingredients. For this reason the pharmacist might recommend an ingredient such as benzocaine for its rapid onset, used concomitantly with hydrocortisone, which provides prolonged duration. Representative products containing hydrocortisone that are specifically targeted for rectal conditions are listed in Table 13.3.

LIVE YEAST-CELL DERIVATIVE

In 1993 the FDA issued a publication addressing the effectiveness of live yeast-cell derivative, an ingredient that some major companies had included in their products for many years.[70] Safety was not an issue, but the studies to date had failed to meet the standards required for full proof of efficacy for its purported actions as a wound-healing agent and its purported ability to relieve pain, swelling, itching, burning, and irritation. In the studies submitted, study personnel rather than subjects appeared to have filled out the forms, a violation of protocol. The FDA ruled that manufacturers must reformulate their products to remove live yeast-cell derivative by September 1994. Also, any claims related to this ingredient would need to be deleted from the packaging.

LAXATIVES

When physicians address the utility of laxatives in hemorrhoids, they most often recommend bulk laxatives or stool softeners (emollients).[28,36] (See Chapter 10, Constipation.) Some physicians, however, feel that regular bowel habits should be achieved through dietary changes and by increasing fluid intake.[35]

Nonpharmacologic Therapies

SITZ BATHS

The sitz bath can relieve minor hemorrhoidal symptoms.[36,53] The sitz bath, which consists of sitting in warm water two to three times daily for 15 to 30 minutes each bath, apparently ameliorates symptoms by decreasing the patient's resting anal pressure.[7,13] (Prolonged bathing should be avoided.[12])

During the sitz bath the patient must not sit on the inflatable rubber rings ("donut cushions"). (See "Donut Cushion.")

ANAL HYGIENE

Simple hygiene measures may alleviate minor symptoms such as washing the anal area with soap and water after each bowel movement.[7,71,72] The soap should be removed to prevent allergic reactions. Also, the area should be blotted dry rather than rubbed to avoid abrading the area further.

DONUT CUSHION

Inflatable and foam "donut cushions" have been sold for many years to provide relief from hemorrhoids. *These devices are generally condemned at all times as they concentrate the pooling of blood in the hemorrhoidal veins.[22]*

PREVENTION OF HEMORRHOIDS

Diet

The possible association of constipation with hemorrhoids has led to recommendations by physicians to increase the amount of fiber in the diet to promote natural laxation.[17,53,71] (Low-residue diets constipate by prolonging transit time.[21]) Such foods as bran, fresh fruits, and vegetables should be increased to soften stools.[14,22,23] By easing passage of stool, high-fiber diets may help decrease symptoms in minor cases of hemorrhoids such as first-degree internal hemorrhoids.[73] Patients should also consume adequate fluids (eight to ten 8-ounce glasses of fluid daily, which may be reduced if such fluid foods as soups are ingested) to help prevent fecal dehydration.[22,30,35] Sedentary lifestyle is also hypothesized to be a causal factor in hemorrhoids, perhaps by inhibiting peristaltic colonic activity.[17]

Reduction of Straining

Physicians stress that patients should not spend too much time attempting to defecate. If defecation has not occurred in perhaps 5 minutes or so, the patient should cease the effort. To this end, physicians suggest removing all reading materials from the bathroom.[13,23,54]

SUMMARY

Hemorrhoids are best defined as abnormal dilations of the arteriovenous hemorrhoidal plexus that protrude into the lumen of the anal canal. Symptoms include bleeding, prolapse, pain, and pruritus ani. Because of the nature of these symptoms, many patients are reluctant to submit to a rectal examination. Thus they tend to self-treat hemorrhoidal conditions that are clearly beyond the scope of nonprescription

Table 13.3. Representative Products for Anorectal Conditions Containing Hydrocortisone

PRODUCT	SELECTED INGREDIENTS
Anusol HC-1	Hydrocortisone acetate equivalent to 1% hydrocortisone
Corticaine Cream	Hydrocortisone 0.5%
Cortizone• 10 External Anal Itch Relief Creme	Hydrocortisone 1%
Preparation H Hydrocortisone 1% Cream	Hydrocortisone 1%

AT THE COUNTER

A patient asks the pharmacist about a hemorrhoid product containing ephedrine.

Interview/Patient Assessment

The patient, a regular customer at the pharmacy, is a female in her early 50s. Her medication profile contains nortriptyline, an oral contraceptive, and Seldane for allergies. Her symptoms have continued for 3 days and consist of burning discomfort after a bowel movement. She has never had the problem before and is unsure if she has hemorrhoids. She denies bleeding and prolapse.

Pharmacist's Analysis

1. Are this patient's symptoms indicative of hemorrhoids?
2. Does her condition require referral to a physician?

3. Is a nonprescription product containing ephedrine suitable for this patient?

This patient's symptoms indicate a minor rectal condition such as early hemorrhoids.

Patient Counseling

Since the problem has only been present for 3 days, she may self-treat for an additional 4 days. Several products may provide relief, but vasoconstrictors should not be recommended for her since she is currently taking a medication for depression, a labeled contraindication to topical vasoconstrictor use. However, products containing hydrocortisone, local anesthetics, protectants, astringents, keratolytics, or antipruritics would all be acceptable for her.

---

therapy. With gentle questioning, the pharmacist can uncover these patients and urge them to make an appointment. Patients should be referred if they are under 12 years of age, if the problem has persisted for longer than 7 days, or if the patient has bleeding. Other patients are in acute discomfort, but can potentially be helped by hemorrhoidal medications. Pharmacists must recognize that many patients are acutely embarrassed at attempts to provide counseling and advice, yet with proper guidance patients can self-treat several of the troubling rectal symptoms caused by hemorrhoids.

Ingredients that provide relief for hemorrhoidal discomfort include the following:

- Local anesthetics—relieve soreness, burning, itching, irritation, pain, and discomfort
- Anesthetics/analgesics/antipruritics—relieve pain and itching
- Protectants—prevent drying of tissues, protect irritated areas, relieve burning and skin irritation, protect tissues from abrasion and pain during bowel movements, and protect inflamed perianal skin
- Astringents—protect irritated anorectal areas and relieve irritation and burning
- Vasoconstrictors—reduce swelling associated with irritated hemorrhoidal tissues and other anorectal disorders
- Keratolytics—relieve discomfort and itching
- Hydrocortisone—relieves anal itching

Table 13.1 provides a cross-reference of symptoms and treatment ingredients.

References

1. Nagle D, Rolandelli RH. Primary care office management of perianal and anal disease. Prim Care 23:609, 1996.
2. Janicke DM, Pundt MR. Anorectal disorders. Emerg Med Clin North Am 14:757, 1996.
3. Mazier WP. Hemorrhoids, fissures, and pruritus ani. Surg Clin North Am 74:1277, 1994.
4. Metcalf A. Anorectal disorders. Five common causes of pain, itching, and bleeding. Postgrad Med 98:81, 1995.
5. Norman DA, et al. Direct current electrotherapy of internal hemorrhoids: An effective, safe and painless outpatient approach. Am J Gastroenterol 84:482, 1989.
6. Haas PA. The prevalence of confusion in the definition of hemorrhoids. Dis Colon Rectum 35:290, 1992.
7. Fed Reg 45:35575, 1980.
8. Pfenninger JL, Surrell J. Nonsurgical treatment options for internal hemorrhoids. Am Fam Physician 52:821, 1995.
9. Nelson RL, et al. Prevalence of benign anorectal disease in a randomly selected population. Dis Colon Rectum 38:341, 1995.
10. Bleday R, et al. Symptomatic hemorrhoids. Current incidence and complications of operative therapy. Dis Colon Rectum 35:477, 1992.
11. Akande B, Esho JO. Relationship between haemorrhoids and prostatism: Results of a prospective study. Eur Urol 16:333, 1989.
12. Ponsky JL, et al. Endoscopic retrograde hemorrhoidal sclerotherapy using 23.4% saline: A preliminary report. Gastrointest Endosc 37:155, 1991.
13. Corman ML. Hemorrhoids. In: Colon and Rectal Surgery. 3rd ed. Philadelphia: JB Lippincott, 1993.
14. Haas PA, et al. The pathogenesis of hemorrhoids. Dis Colon Rectum 27:442, 1984.
15. Dennison AR. Hemorrhoids. Surg Clin North Am 68:1401, 1988.
16. Heaton ND, Howard ER. Symptomatic hemorrhoids and anorectal varices in children with portal hypertension. J Pediatr Surg 27:833, 1992.
17. Johanson JF, Sonnenberg A. Temporal changes in the occur-

rence of hemorrhoids in the United States and England. Dis Colon Rectum 34:585, 1991.

18. Johanson JF, Sonnenberg A. The prevalence of hemorrhoids and chronic constipation. Gastroenterology 98:380, 1990.
19. Gibbons CP, et al. Role of constipation and anal hypertonia in the pathogenesis of haemorrhoids. Br J Surg 75:656, 1988.
20. Dennison AR, et al. The management of hemorrhoids. Am J Gastroenterol 84:475, 1989.
21. Smith LE. Anal hemorrhoids. Neth J Med 37(Suppl 1):S22, 1990.
22. Cocchiara JL. Hemorrhoids. Postgrad Med 89:149, 1991.
23. Schussman LC, Lutz LJ. Outpatient management of hemorrhoids. Prim Care 13:527, 1986.
24. Johanson JF, Sonnenberg A. Constipation is not a risk factor for hemorrhoids: A case-control study of potential etiologic agents. Am J Gastroenterol 89:1981, 1994.
25. Johanson JF. Association of hemorrhoidal disease with diarrheal disorders: Potential pathologic relationship? Dis Colon Rectum 40:215, 1997.
26. Montorsi W. Update on hemorrhoids. Int Surg 74:139, 1989.
27. MacLeod JH. Rational approach to treatment of hemorrhoids based on a theory of etiology. Arch Surg 118:29, 1983.
28. Faulconer HT. Hemorrhoids—Alternative treatments. J Ky Med Assoc 86:617, 1988.
29. Haas PA, Haas GP. The prevalence of hemorrhoids and chronic constipation (Letter). Gastroenterology 99:1856, 1990.
30. Birkett DH. Hemorrhoids—Diagnostic and treatment options. Hosp Pract 23:99,1988.
31. Loder PB, et al. Haemorrhoids: Pathology, pathophysiology and aetiology. Br J Surg 81:946, 1994.
32. Hancock BD. Hemorrhoids. BMJ 304:1042, 1992.
33. Hosking SW, et al. Anorectal varices, haemorrhoids, and portal hypertension. Lancet 1(8634):349, 1989.
34. Denniston GC. Treatment of hemorrhoids (Letter). J Fam Pract 30:360, 1990.
35. Ferguson EF Jr. Alternatives in the treatment of hemorrhoidal disease. South Med J 81:606, 1988.
36. Leff E. Hemorrhoids. Postgrad Med 82:95, 1987.
37. Gorfine SR. Treatment of benign anal disease with topical nitroglycerin. Dis Colon Rectum 38:453, 1995.
38. Zinberg SS, et al. A personal experience in comparing three nonoperative techniques for treating internal hemorrhoids. Am J Gastroenterol 84:488, 1989.
39. Felt-Bersma RJ, et al. Anal sensitivity test: What does it measure and do we need it? Cause or derivative of anorectal complaints. Dis Colon Rectum 40:811, 1997.
40. Standards Task Force, American Society Colon Rectal Surgery. Practice parameters for the treatment of hemorrhoids. Dis Colon Rectum 33:992, 1990.
41. Forde KA. Is there a need to perform full colonoscopy in a middle-age person with episodic bright red blood per rectum and internal hemorrhoids? Am J Gastroenterol 84:1227, 1989.
42. Kishi K, et al. A cavernous hemangioma of the rectum treated as a hemorrhoid for 1 year prior to its diagnosis: Report of a case. Surg Today 24:833, 1994.
43. Machicado GA, Jensen DM. Acute and chronic management of lower gastrointestinal bleeding: Cost-effective approaches. Gastroenterologist 5:189, 1997.
44. Korkis AM, McDougall CJ. Rectal bleeding in some patients less than 50 years of age. Dig Dis Sci 40:1520, 1995.
45. Fed Reg 55:31775, 1990.
46. Nakama H, et al. Immunochemical fecal occult blood test is not suitable for diagnosis of hemorrhoids. Am J Med 102:551, 1997.
47. Nakama H, et al. Clinical diagnostic accuracy of faecal occult blood test for anal diseases. Int J Qual Health Care 9:139, 1997.
48. Graham DJ, Pritchard TJ, Bloom AD. Colonoscopy for intermittent rectal bleeding: Impact on patient management. J Surg Res 54:136, 1993.
49. Kluiber RM, Wolff BG. Evaluation of anemia caused by hemorrhoidal bleeding. Dis Colon Rectum 37:1006, 1994.
50. Iseli A. Office treatment of haemorrhoids and perianal haematoma. Aust Fam Physician 20:284, 1991.
51. Oh C. Acute thrombosed external hemorrhoids. Mt Sinai Med J 56:30, 1989.
52. Read NW, Sun WM. Haemorrhoids, constipation, and hypertensive anal cushions. Lancet 1(8638):610, 1989.
53. Jacob JE. Nonsurgical treatment of hemorrhoids. J SC Med Assoc 83:425, 1987.
54. Dehn TCB, Kettlewell MGW. Haemorrhoids and defaecatory habits. Lancet 1(8628):54, 1989.
55. Nadler LH. Conservative management of hemorrhoids (Letter). Gastrointest Endosc 37:653, 1991.
56. MacRae HM, McLeod RS. Comparison of hemorrhoidal treatment modalities. A meta-analysis. Dis Colon Rectum 38:687, 1995.
57. Polglase AL. Haemorrhoids: A clinical update. Med J Aust 167:85, 1997.
58. Bayer I, Myslovaty B, Picovsky BM. Rubber band ligation of hemorrhoids. Convenient and economic treatment. J Clin Gastroenterol 23:50, 1996.
59. Dennison AR, et al. New thoughts on the aetiology of haemorrhoids and the development of non-operative methods for their management. Minerva Chir 51:209, 1996.
60. Hodgson WJ, Morgan J. Ambulatory hemorrhoidectomy with CO_2 laser. Dis Colon Rectum 38:1265, 1995.
61. Oueidat DM, Jurjus AR. Management of hemorrhoids by rubber band ligation. J Med Liban 42:11, 1994.
62. Wrobleski DE. Rubber band ligation of hemorrhoids. R I Med 78:172, 1995.
63. Ho YH, Seow-Choen F, Goh HS. Haemorrhoidectomy and disordered rectal and anal physiology in patients with prolapsed haemorrhoids. Br J Surg 82:596, 1995.
64. Chia YW, et al. CO2 laser haemorrhoidectomy—Does it alter anorectal function or decrease pain compared to conventional haemorrhoidectomy? Int J Colorectal Dis 10:22, 1995.
65. Arullani A, Cappello G. Diagnosis and current treatment of hemorrhoid disease. Angiology 45(6 Pt 2):560, 1994.
66. Fed Reg 53:30755, 1988.
67. Medich DS, Fazio VW. Hemorrhoids, anal fissure, and carcinoma of the colon, rectum, and anus during pregnancy. Surg Clin North Am 75:77, 1995.
68. Fed Reg 48:5851, 1983.
69. Fed Reg 53:32591, 1988.
70. Fed Reg 58:46745, 1993.
71. Smith RB, Moodie J. Comparative efficacy and tolerability of two ointment and suppository preparations ("Uniroid" and "Proctosedyl") in the treatment of second degree haemorrhoids in general practice. Curr Med Res Opin 11:34, 1988.
72. Sinclair A. Remedies for common family ailments: 9. Haemorrhoids. Prof Care Mother Child 5:161, 1995.
73. Perez-Maranda M, et al. Effect of fiber supplements on internal bleeding hemorrhoids. Hepatogastroenterology 43:1504, 1996.

Respiratory Conditions

Allergic Rhinitis

A mother asks the pharmacist how much of a popular allergy combination product to give her young son.

Interview/Patient Assessment

In response to the pharmacist's questions, the mother gives his age as 8 months. His symptoms include rhinorrhea of several months duration, sneezing, and watery eyes. The pharmacist notes a distinct odor of cigarette smoke on the mother and child. The mother says that the child has not seen a physician for the problem but that another pharmacist told her to use half of the 2-year-old infant's dose on the label for him. Since her son is 1 month older now, she wonders if his dose should increase.

Pharmacist's Analysis

1. Are the child's symptoms consistent with allergic rhinitis?
2. What avoidance and environmental control steps should be advised?

3. What rationale did the other pharmacist use in recommending a nonprescription medication?
4. What should the pharmacist advise for a child of this age?

The child's symptoms are consistent with allergic rhinitis.

Patient Counseling

Prior to recommending medications the pharmacist should attempt to point out the role of allergens in allergic rhinitis, including that of cigarette smoke. Should the parent appear recalcitrant, the pharmacist must also acknowledge that smoking is a difficult habit to break, which may mean that the child will need to use medications. The pharmacist then should explain that no allergy or cold medication is approved as safe for children under the ages of 2–6 if the product contains antihistamines—and explain that the other pharmacist may have used company-provided dosing charts for nonprescription drugs that have a questionable legal status. Because of the child's age, the pharmacist must refer the child to a physician for a dosage determination.

Allergic rhinitis, sometimes referred to as "hay fever," is a common form of allergic airway disease.[1] The morbidity and costs associated with allergic rhinitis are staggering, yet there are safe and effective nonprescription medications that can provide dramatic relief from its symptoms.[2] (See "Differentiation from the Common Cold.")

PREVALENCE OF ALLERGIC RHINITIS

The actual number of allergic rhinitis sufferers is difficult to determine. Not only does severity vary from person to person, but sufferers are motivated to seek help at differing levels of discomfort.[3] The prevalence of allergic rhinitis is perhaps 40% of the American population.[4,5] Allergic rhinitis causes nearly 1 million missed workdays, 1 million missed school days, and over 4 million days of reduced activity.[5] The annual medical cost in the United States is 2 to 4 billion dollars.[6,7]

EPIDEMIOLOGY OF ALLERGIC RHINITIS

Allergic rhinitis is linked to age, which should be expected since the condition is mediated by the immune system and is triggered by repeated exposure.[8] While only about 5 to 9% of children meet full diagnostic criteria for allergic rhinitis, as many as 20 to 30% of adolescents suffer from the condition.[9,10] Incidence peaks in the early teens and then diminishes.[11] About 66% of adult rhinitis patients are younger than 30.[9]

There may also be an inherited tendency to allergic rhinitis.[12] If a child does not have a parent with allergic rhinitis, he or she has only a 10% risk of the condition.[1] However, if one parent has allergic rhinitis, there is a 25% risk, and the risk jumps to 50% if two parents have the condition. Patients who are **atopic** (genetically predisposed to certain conditions with an allergic component such as asthma or dermatitis) tend to experience allergic rhinitis more than those who do not inherit this trait.[1,13,14] There is no gender differentiation in the epidemiology of allergic rhinitis.[11,15]

ETIOLOGY OF ALLERGIC RHINITIS

The pathogenesis of allergic rhinitis involves contact with allergenic substances. As shown in Figure 14.1, when this contact is through inhalation, the nasal mucosal surface is the initial site of attack.[16] Particles such as pollen, animal dander, and molds (all approximately 2 to 60 micrometers in size) are entrapped on the mucous blanket lining the airways, which releases water-soluble proteins that act as allergens.[8,11,17] This results in activation of previously formed IgE antibodies on the surface of **mast cells** (cells that contain histamine and other substances responsible for allergic reactions) in the submucosa and at the epithelial level, producing antigen-antibody cross-linking.[18–20] Linkage of only two cell-bound IgE molecules with allergen is sufficient to trigger a cascade of intracellular enzymatic reactions.[18] The mast cells undergo a process called degranulation, whereby intracellular granules fuse with cell membrane.[10,21] This process releases

A.

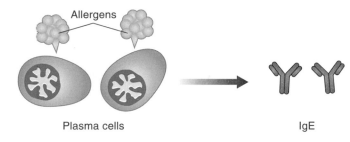

B.

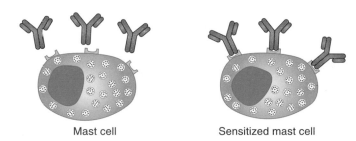

C.

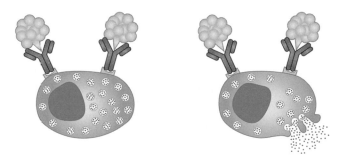

Figure 14.1. The allergen-induced release of histamine that causes allergic rhinitis symptoms. **A.** Allegens (pollen, dust) contact plasma cells, resulting in production of the antibody IgE. **B.** IgE antibodies attach to receptor sites on mast cells. **C.** On subsequent reexposure, allergen links to antibody, causing mast-cell degranulation and histamine release.

potent mediators (e.g., histamine, eosinophil chemotactic factor, neutrophil chemotactic factor, superoxide, kininogenase, and serotonin), which cause vasodilation, mucosal edema, mucus secretion, and stimulation of itch receptors.[16] The mediators also interact with neural elements, mucosal glands, and blood vessels to cause the typical symptoms of allergic rhinitis.

Because of a phenomenon known as nasal priming, decreased amounts of allergen are required to cause symptoms with subsequent exposures.[3] This phenomenon may be the explanation for worsening of symptoms of seasonal rhinitis as a season progresses.

MANIFESTATIONS OF ALLERGIC RHINITIS

Immediate Symptoms

There are four classical symptoms of allergic rhinitis that have a rapid onset following allergen exposure and may be referred to as "immediate symptoms":

- **Rhinorrhea** (nasal discharge)
- Nasal congestion
- Sneezing
- Nasal pruritus[2,10,22]

The symptoms can lead to further problems if allowed to persist. A late-phase reaction that occurs 2 to 11 hours after initial allergen contact in about 50% of patients has also been documented.[8,18] The symptoms duplicate those that the patient originally experienced.

RHINORRHEA
Rhinorrhea usually produces a clear discharge. Frequent blowing and wiping irritate the skin around the nares and may produce skin infections.[23]

NASAL CONGESTION
Congestion that is so severe as to cause total blockage forces the patient to mouth-breathe, which dries the mouth, leads to nasal speech, and produces bad breath.[2,3,24] The congestion may be bilateral or may shift from one nostril to the other every few hours.[8] Dry mouth also lessens the contact time of teeth with saliva, increasing the incidence of cavities.[23] Mouth-breathing throughout much of childhood may abnormally lengthen the midface area since the upper palate matures during this time. This problem is known as "adenoid, atopic, or allergic facies."[25,26] Mouth-breathing can also cause developmental dental problems (e.g., a high, arched palate and marked overbite), leading to difficulty with chewing (malocclusion).[3,23,25] A mouth-breather also must eat with the mouth open, which is uncomfortable and may be the focus of teasing from schoolmates and siblings. Chronic nasal congestion also leads to sinus problems such as sinus ostial occlusion and chronic sinusitis.[11,17] Nasal blockage may result in disrupted sleep, snoring, dry throat, and morning fatigue.[10] **Anosmia** (inability to smell) from congestion interferes with eating habits.[8,10,23]

Eustachian tube obstruction associated with nasal congestion can increase the risk of middle ear disease—for example, serous otitis or chronic ear infections—which may necessitate the placement of tympanostomy tubes.[2,22,23] Patients may complain of tinnitus and popping sounds in the ears.[3,10,17] Hearing difficulties can lead to learning problems.[23]

SNEEZING
Sneezing begins 30 to 60 seconds after inhalation of the allergen.[8] Sneezes occur in paroxysms of as many as 10 to 20 in a row, which can disrupt a child's school day or recreational activities and also makes him the focus of teasing.

NASAL PRURITUS

A continual or intermittent nasal itching, seemingly originating in the posterior nose, can be maddening. To relieve it, the typical sufferer uses the heel of the hand to rub the tip of the nose in an upward direction, a characteristic motion known as the "allergic salute," as illustrated in Figure 14.2.[8,24–26] Repeated often enough, the continual upward pressure can result in a permanent facial deformity (a transverse nasal crease), as illustrated in Figure 14.3.[23–25] The crease is visible as a line appearing about 1/3 of the way up the bridge of the nose, where the cartilage meets nasal bone.[3] Repeated upward rubbing can also stretch tissues upward to produce the "Gothic arch" in which the upper lip and teeth are steadily pushed outward and upward, perhaps resulting in an overbite, also illustrated in Figure 14.2. Children tend to wrinkle the end of the itching nose constantly, which is referred to by allergists as "rabbit nose" or "bunny nose."[24]

Other Manifestations

OPHTHALMIC SYMPTOMS

Various ophthalmic problems are common in allergic rhinitis, but seldom seen in the common cold:

- The allergic shiner, a dark or bluish swelling in the region below the ophthalmic orbit caused by impaired nasal venous outflow, is one example as illustrated in Figure 14.3.[18] Since the congested nasal venous system anastomoses with the infraorbital veins, the allergic shiner reflects stasis in this venous pool.[3]
- Patients also experience a clear watery ophthalmic discharge, **conjunctival injection** (dilation of the conjunctival blood vessels) and photophobia.[8]

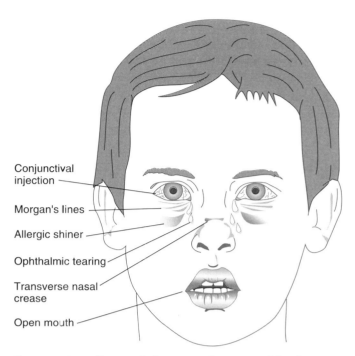

Figure 14.3. As illustrated, this patient has many of the characteristics of a typical allergic-rhinitis sufferer.

- Ophthalmic itching may be so unrelenting that the patient scratches intensely to relieve the pruritus, possibly inducing sties, blepharitis, or keratitis.[23]
- Allergic skinfolds or pleats extending from under the eye to the epicanthal folds, parallel to the lower eyelid margins, are another common ophthalmic problem, as shown in Figure 14.2. These are called Morgan's lines or Dennie's sign, as illustrated in Figure 14.3.[8,17]

HEADACHE

Allergic rhinitis may cause frontal or sinus headaches, resulting in chronic fatigue and causing poor performance at work or school. Patients may self-medicate this headache with nonprescription analgesics, not realizing that more effective therapies could prevent the problem.

ALLERGIC IRRITABILITY SYNDROME

Some allergic rhinitis patients exhibit a constellation of psychosocial effects termed the "allergic irritability syndrome."[11] This syndrome includes mood swings, irritability, disruptive behavior, and a short attention span, which can cause poor performance and work at school.[3]

Differentiation from the Common Cold

The pharmacist should make an earnest attempt to help the patient discover whether the cause of the patient's symptoms is allergic rhinitis or the common cold, since they are often confused.(See Chapter 15, The Common Cold and Related Conditions.) Further, treatments and counseling points for these conditions vary.

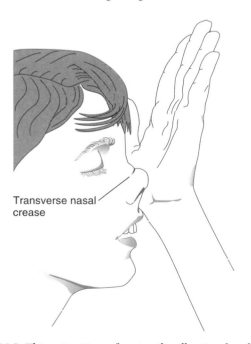

Figure 14.2. This patient is performing the allergic salute by pushing upward on the nose with the heel of the hand in an attempt to alleviate nasal pruritus. This produces the transverse nasal crease.

In regard to the four cardinal symptoms of allergic rhinitis (rhinorrhea, nasal congestion, sneezing, nasal pruritus), patients with the common cold also suffer rhinorrhea, but the initially clear discharge becomes purulent within a few days. Almost all patients with a common cold also experience nasal blockage, as allergic rhinitis sufferers do. Some sneezing may be evident; however, the sneezing of the common cold does not occur in repeated paroxysms as with allergic rhinitis. Nasal itching is an uncommon symptom of the common cold.

There are other characteristics of allergic rhinitis that are useful in differential recognition[24]:

- Symptoms of allergic rhinitis are usually of sudden onset, while the common cold often begins with a scratchy throat, progressing gradually to nasal congestion and other symptoms.
- Symptoms of the common cold last for 4 to 7 days. On the other hand, symptoms of allergic rhinitis continue as long as the individual is affected by the allergen.
- The common cold may only occur once or twice yearly in response to infection with different seasonal rhinoviruses. However, with perennial allergic rhinitis, symptoms occur whenever the patient is in contact with the allergen. With the seasonal variant, symptoms begin and end at the same time each year, probably coinciding with a certain pollen season.
- Other family members are often concurrently infected with the rhinovirus because of its highly contagious nature, but only one person in the house may be suffering from symptoms if allergic rhinitis is the cause.

Should these points fail to pin down the recognition of allergic rhinitis, the pharmacist should refer the patient for allergist screening. Components of the diagnosis include history, physical exam, skin testing, and radioallergosorbent testing.[17,27]

SPECIFIC CONSIDERATIONS OF ALLERGIC RHINITIS: SEASONAL VERSUS PERENNIAL ALLERGIC RHINITIS

After talking with the patient to determine whether he or she may have allergic rhinitis, the pharmacist may help determine the cause(s). The many possible triggers of allergic rhinitis have been grouped into two broad categories:

- Seasonal allergic rhinitis
- Perennial allergic rhinitis

The common thread in allergic rhinitis is the inhalation of a 5- to 50-micrometer **aeroallergen** (airborne allergenic substance) that the nose has failed to filter from inspired air.[8]

Seasonal allergic rhinitis has an incidence ten times that of perennial allergic rhinitis.[22] The two types of allergic rhinitis are not mutually exclusive, however.[17] A particular individual may suffer chronic, year-round, perennial allergies that worsen at certain times of the year because of a seasonal pollen.

Of course, should this discussion fail to pinpoint a possible allergen, the patient should be advised to visit an allergy clinic to determine the exact causes and potentially to undergo desensitization involving injections of allergen.

Seasonal Allergic Rhinitis

Seasonal allergic rhinitis is known as "rose fever" when caused by grass exposure in June and "hay fever" when caused by ragweed in August.[8] The problem is light, windborne pollen. Seasonal allergic rhinitis may cause symptoms from February through October in temperate climates where plants have a longer growing season.

The timing of seasonal allergic rhinitis depends on geographic location and plant ecology. For instance, from the northeast United States across the Midwest to the Rocky Mountains, the early spring heralds the arrival of tree pollens.[8] Grass pollens appear in April through June. Ragweed follows from July until the first hard frost. The timing of these three major antigens can be correlated with the times of peak symptoms to predict which allergen is responsible.[10,11,28]

If the individual experiences a worsening of symptoms after a rain, the probable cause is mold and fungi spores.[8] This allergen is worse in October, when the carpet of fallen leaves serves as an ideal substrate for the organisms. Mold and fungi allergens become less severe at the beginning of spring.[9,10]

Perennial Allergic Rhinitis

Those with chronic, perennial, allergic rhinitis often cannot pinpoint a specific aeroallergen. They may notice that symptoms are worse in the early morning from congestion in the venous lakes resulting from the nocturnal recumbent position and worse in the late evening from increased exposure to the allergens during the day.[8] Sneezing paroxysms tend not to be as severe as in patients with seasonal allergic rhinitis.[29]

Polluted air certainly plays a role with perennial allergic rhinitis sufferers.[8,30] Several studies confirm that allergic sensitization is more common in smokers and in children passively exposed to secondhand smoke.[1]

Some people notice that vacuuming or dusting worsens problems, ascribing the allergy to house dust.[31] Actually, the problem is usually the house dust mite, which is ubiquitous in the environment of the household. The mites live on human skin scales, and thus colonize stuffed toys, upholstered furniture (chairs, sofas), beds (especially mattresses, pillows, and bedding), and the carpeting surrounding these objects. Dust mite allergen tends to worsen in the early fall, when both temperatures and humidity rise, producing optimal conditions for their replication.[8,31] This allergy tends to be quite severe in the night and early morning when the individual is undergoing heavier exposure. Symptoms regress during the day for individuals who are out of the house.[17] Other allergenic components of house dust include cat dander, dog residues (saliva, hair), cockroaches, and indoor fungi. Interestingly, although nasal pruritus is very common in pollen allergy, it is quite rare in dust allergy.[10]

Pets are also a possible cause of perennial allergic rhinitis.[32] People may develop symptoms after entering a house where any animal had been several hours before, especially if they come into contact with their urine, dander, or saliva.[11,33]

Aerosol sprays and cosmetic preparations may cause symptoms, as may feather pillows.[18,32,34] When molds and mildew (causes of seasonal allergic rhinitis) actively grow inside the house in damp or humid areas, they can cause perennial allergic rhinitis.

Food allergies cause allergic rhinitis symptoms, and patients with allergic rhinitis are at higher risk for severe reactions such as anaphylaxis when eating foods contaminated with mites.[35] However, food allergies usually produce other symptoms, such as itching of the hard palate and oropharynx, diarrhea, or vomiting.[11]

TREATMENT OF ALLERGIC RHINITIS

Treatment Guidelines

The first step in treating allergic rhinitis may be to advise elimination of the cause(s). (See "Prevention of Allergic Rhinitis" and "A Pharmacist's Journal: Can You Stop My Child's Runny Nose?") Symptoms may persist despite the best efforts to eliminate or avoid the causes. In these cases medications are the next alternative (Patient Assessment Algorithm 14.1). The pharmacist is able to recommend ingredients from several groups of OTC products; eventually, if these avenues are exhausted, prescription medications may also be tried. Alternatively, the pharmacist may advise the patient to see an allergist for possible immunotherapy.

Nonprescription Medications

CROMOLYN SODIUM

Cromolyn sodium stabilizes mast cells, preventing their degranulation. Thus it is effective in prevention of allergic rhinitis symptoms and also acts to provide a measure of relief when symptoms are present through halting further release of chemical mediators. The nonprescription product, Nasalcrom Nasal Spray, is a 0.88–fluid ounce nasal solution administered with a pump spray bottle.[36] The patient may notice a brief stinging or sneezing directly following administration.

The nasal solution of cromolyn sodium provides prophylaxis against and treatment of rhinorrhea, nasal pruritus, and sneezing. For optimal prevention, Nasalcrom should be used for 1 week before allergen contact. The patient may not notice a maximal effect for 1 to 2 weeks.

If the individual has seasonal allergic rhinitis, Nasalcrom is used throughout the allergy season. The patient sprays once into each nostril, repeating this procedure three to four times daily—every 4 to 6 hours. It should not be used more than six times daily.

Nasalcrom should not be used in those younger than 6 years of age. The patient experiencing fever, discolored nasal discharge, sinus pain, or wheezing should ask a physician before using Nasalcrom. It should not be used to treat asthma, sinus infection, or cold symptoms. Should the patient's symptoms worsen or fail to improve after 2 weeks, or should new symptoms develop, the patient should cease use of Nasalcrom.

ANTIHISTAMINES

Single-entity antihistamines provide relief of sneezing; runny nose; itching of the nose, throat, and eyes; and watering of the eyes caused by allergic rhinitis or other upper respiratory allergies (Table 14.1).[37]

A Pharmacist's Journal

"Can You Stop My Child's Runny Nose?"

A woman in her late 20s asked if I could stop her child's nose from running. I discovered that this 4-year-old had typical symptoms of allergic rhinitis, but was most troubled by severe rhinorrhea. As I began to describe the role of allergens, the mother volunteered, "I know the cause perfectly well. My ex-husband gets to see him on weekends. He and his whole family smoke. Whenever I pick my son up, he stinks to high heaven and his nose is completely plugged or running because he's allergic to cigarettes." I asked if those extended family members were aware of the harm to the child. She replied, "They don't even care. It takes all week for me to get him normal again, and they mess him up every weekend. He's doing poorly in preschool because of this." Seeing that avoidance and environmental control appeared to be useless, I advised her that nonprescription antihistamines are contraindicated under the age of 6. I further urged her to seek professional advice about the detrimental effects of the allergens on her son's health, in light of the joint custody ruling, and to see a physician for medical advice regarding an appropriate antihistamine for her son.

Patient Assessment Algorithm 14.1. Suspected Allergic Rhinitis

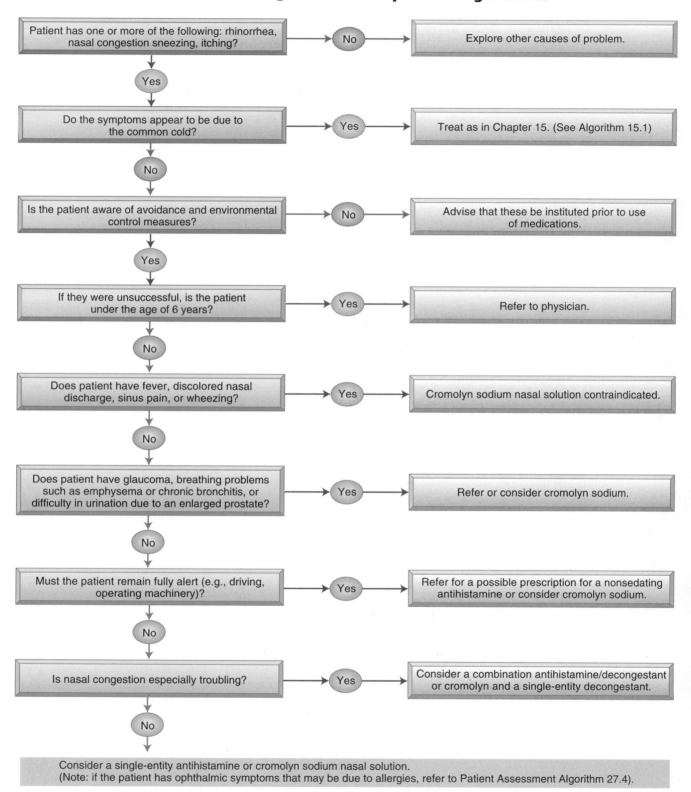

Patient has one or more of the following: rhinorrhea, nasal congestion sneezing, itching? — **No** → Explore other causes of problem.

↓ **Yes**

Do the symptoms appear to be due to the common cold? — **Yes** → Treat as in Chapter 15. (See Algorithm 15.1)

↓ **No**

Is the patient aware of avoidance and environmental control measures? — **No** → Advise that these be instituted prior to use of medications.

↓ **Yes**

If they were unsuccessful, is the patient under the age of 6 years? — **Yes** → Refer to physician.

↓ **No**

Does patient have fever, discolored nasal discharge, sinus pain, or wheezing? — **Yes** → Cromolyn sodium nasal solution contraindicated.

↓ **No**

Does patient have glaucoma, breathing problems such as emphysema or chronic bronchitis, or difficulty in urination due to an enlarged prostate? — **Yes** → Refer or consider cromolyn sodium.

↓ **No**

Must the patient remain fully alert (e.g., driving, operating machinery)? — **Yes** → Refer for a possible prescription for a nonsedating antihistamine or consider cromolyn sodium.

↓ **No**

Is nasal congestion especially troubling? — **Yes** → Consider a combination antihistamine/decongestant or cromolyn and a single-entity decongestant.

↓ **No**

Consider a single-entity antihistamine or cromolyn sodium nasal solution.
(Note: if the patient has ophthalmic symptoms that may be due to allergies, refer to Patient Assessment Algorithm 27.4).

Antihistamine Contraindications and Warnings

tip *Antihistamines are contraindicated with any breathing problem such as emphysema or chronic bronchitis, or difficulty in urination* caused by enlargement of the prostate gland. Antihistamines also carry a warning against glaucoma, but this precaution applies to narrow (acute)–angle glaucoma rather than open (wide)–angle glaucoma. However, should the patient be unaware of the type of glau-

Table 14.1. Representative Single-Entity Antihistamines for Allergic Rhinitis

PRODUCT	SELECTED INGREDIENTS/COMMENTS
Benadryl Allergy Capsule	Diphenhydramine HCl 25 mg
Benadryl Dye-Free Allergy Softgels	Diphenhydramine HCl 25 mg
Benadryl Allergy Liquid	Per 5 mL: diphenhydramine 12.5 mg
Benadryl Dye-Free Allergy Liquid	Per 5 mL: diphenhydramine 12.5 mg
Chlor-Trimeton Allergy Tablets	Chlorpheniramine maleate 4 mg (8 and 12 mg sustained-release)
Efidac 24 Chlorpheniramine Tablets	Chlorpheniramine maleate 16 mg (4 mg immediate release; 12 mg controlled release)
Nolahist Tablets	Phenindamine tartrate 25 mg
Tavist Allergy Tablets	Clemastine fumarate 1.34 mg

coma that they have, they should be asked to confirm a diagnosis of open angle before using antihistamines. *Antihistamines are contraindicated in children under 6*; excitability may occur.[37]

All approved antihistamine labels will carry a warning regarding the possible occurrence of drowsiness, and that the patient must exercise caution in driving and operating machinery. The label will also state that alcohol, sedatives, and tranquilizers may increase the drowsiness effect. *With diphenhydramine, the label must state "marked drowsiness."* Some work situations require extra vigilance; these patients may be advised to visit the physician for a trial of a nonsedating prescription antihistamine (terfenadine, astemizole).[38]

Labels of products containing phenindamine must also caution the patient that some individuals experience nervousness and insomnia.[37]

For many years FDA-approved OTC labeling for antihistamine dosing for allergies and the common cold has read, "Children under 6 years of age: Consult a doctor."[39] Antihistamines can have a stimulating effect on children instead of the usual sedative effect that occurs in adults.[37,40] Because antihistamines as a group cause the problem, and the effect cannot be predicted for an individual or for a specific antihistamine, the FDA concluded that the warning must apply to all antihistamines. (See "Pediatric Dosing Charts.")

Approved Antihistamines
Approved antihistamines include the following:
- Brompheniramine
- Chlorcyclizine
- Chlorpheniramine
- Dexbrompheniramine
- Dexchlorpheniramine
- Diphenhydramine
- Phenindamine
- Pheniramine
- Pyrilamine
- Thonzylamine
- Triprolidine

Doxylamine was added to the list of approved antihistamines somewhat later than the originally approved ingredients.[43] It was not placed on the original list because it had been implicated in birth defects and carcinogenicity reports.[37,44] However, in the 1994 report the FDA advised that the ingredient is safe and effective. A study of overdoses of doxylamine led authors to question nonprescription availability for doxylamine.[45]

Clemastine gained approval for OTC status in 1992. The products containing it are not timed-release, but the duration of clemastine is such that products containing it are effective for 12 hours.

Antihistamines for Skin Allergies
Allergic rhinitis remains the sole allergy-related nonprescription use of antihistamines. One comment to the FDA requested approval for oral diphenhydramine for "Temporary relief of itching associated with hives, minor skin irritations, or rashes due to food or animal allergies, insect bites, inhaled allergens (dust, mold, spores), poison ivy, oak, or sumac, soaps, detergents, cosmetics, and jewelry."[37] Another comment requested antihistamine labeling for pruritus, angioedema, and other manifestations of skin allergies. The FDA responded that hives and pruritic rashes secondary to foods, animal allergies, and insect stings and bites can be one component of a systemic anaphylaxis, and that the use of an OTC antihistamine in these cases could potentially delay more appropriate treatment that might be needed.[37] The agency was unaware of any data to demonstrate that the average person can distinguish between a mild allergic reaction and one that may be life-threatening that begins with itching only. Further, histamine is only one of the mediators released during mast-cell degranulation. Therefore, the use of an antihistamine alone may not be sufficient.

ORAL NASAL DECONGESTANTS
Oral nasal decongestants (e.g., pseudoephedrine, phenylephrine) used as sole therapy for allergic rhinitis have little effect on most of the hallmark symptoms of allergic rhinitis (e.g., sneezing, rhinorrhea, nasal pruritus) (See Table 15.3

for representative, single-entity, topical, nasal-decongestant products; Table 15.4 for representative, oral, nasal-decongestant products; and Table 14.2 for selected, combination products containing oral nasal-decongestants and antihistamines.) Their role in allergic rhinitis lies in the fact that they temporarily relieve nasal congestion.[46] (Antihistamines only partially relieve nasal congestion).[22] For this reason many allergic rhinitis products have an added decongestant to ensure an open airway.[18,19,24] Such combinations would only be needed when the patient complains of residual stuffiness after a single-entity antihistamine trial. Even then, the wide availability of single-entity decongestants allows the consumer to purchase one of these rather than a fixed combination. Subsequently, the patient can tailor his or her own therapy to the symptoms that are troublesome, rather than medicating with both ingredients of a fixed combination. Also, when a product includes a decongestant, it broadens the contraindications and lengthens the list of possible adverse effects. Decongestants may cause excitation and insomnia, thereby partially counteracting the drowsiness of antihistamines when the two are used concurrently.[25] The pharmacist must judge whether these limited benefits outweigh the risk of adverse effects. Packages containing them

FOCUS ON...

PEDIATRIC DOSING CHARTS

Several companies have provided dosing charts that purport to allow the pharmacist to dose antihistamine-containing products to children under the age of 6 years. The ages on these charts go down as low as 3 months. At least one company even provides stickers on which the pharmacist can fill in the dose from the appropriate table and place it on the bottle. It is true that most Federal Register OTC monographs include a section concerning "professional labeling," which includes information that is not to appear on the OTC labels. One of these sections is pediatric dosing information. The companies have evidently interpreted this to mean that they may not put it on the label, but may provide it to pharmacists, who will then, acting as the company's agent, verbally provide instructions that contravene approved labeling or repackage the box with the stickers provided.

In regard to antihistamines, the FDA has specifically stated, "The agency believes that evaluation of information concerning the safety of antihistamine use in children from 2 to under 6 years of age without the supervision of a physician is necessary before the agency can make a decision concerning the switch of dosage labeling for this age group for antihistamines from professional use only to OTC labeling for consumer use."[41] The question centers around the ability of the pharmacist to substitute for a physician and rely on the company-provided doses as safe and effective for children without physician approval.

A 1995 FDA summary-information document revealed that manufacturers have requested OTC labeling for antihistamines for children from 2 to under 6 years of age.[42] The FDA responded that more information concerning safety under the age of 6 is needed before such labeling can be moved from the professional section to the OTC labeling for consumer use.

highlight a number of cautions when patients are not supervised by a physician.[46] *The pharmacist must caution patients against the following situations:*

- *Exceeding recommended dosages to prevent nervousness, dizziness, or insomnia*
- *Dosing with oral decongestants for more than 7 days*
- *Use when the patient has fever*

Table 14.2. Representative Combination Products for Allergic Rhinitis

PRODUCT	SELECTED INGREDIENTS/COMMENTS
Actifed Cold & Allergy Tablets	Triprolidine HCl 2.5 mg, pseudoephedrine HCl 60 mg
Contac 12-Hour Cold Capsules	Chlorpheniramine maleate 8 mg, phenylpropanolamine HCl 75 mg
Dimetapp 12-Hour Extentabs	Brompheniramine maleate 12 mg, phenylpropanolamine HCl 75 mg
Dimetapp Elixir	Per 5 mL: brompheniramine maleate 12 mg; phenylpropanolamine HCl 12.5 mg
Dristan Nasal Spray	Pheniramine maleate 0.2% (not approved for topical use), phenylephrine HCl 0.5%
Drixoral Cold & Allergy 12-Hour Relief Tablets	Dexbrompheniramine maleate 6 mg, pseudoephedrine sulfate 120 mg
Vicks Nyquil Multi-Symptom Cold/Flu Relief Liquid	Per 30 mL: doxylamine succinate 12.5 mg, acetaminophen 1000 mg, pseudoephedrine HCl 60 mg, dextromethorphan hydrobromide 30 mg
Tavist-D Tablets	Clemastine fumarate 1.34 mg, phenylpropanolamine HCl 75 mg

Patients with heart disease, high blood pressure, thyroid disease, diabetes, or difficulty in urination caused by an enlarged prostate must not use them without physician approval. They may increase the severity of symptoms in hyperthyroid patients and can alter blood glucose regulation in the diabetic patient. Also, *patients taking monoamine oxidase inhibitors must first obtain physician approval for concomitant use.*

Phenylpropanolamine, often included in sinus, cold, and diet products, was not included in the final monograph because of unresolved safety questions. Phenylpropanolamine was one of several ingredients investigated for safety and effectiveness by the Select Committee on Aging of the House of Representatives.[42]

TOPICAL DECONGESTANTS

Topical nasal sprays, drops, and inhalers containing oxymetazoline, xylometazoline, phenylephrine, or other decongestants only alleviate nasal congestion associated with allergic rhinitis; like oral decongestants, they have little effect on the other three hallmark symptoms of allergic rhinitis. They cannot be used longer than 3 days since they may cause rebound congestion of the nasal mucosa (rhinitis medicamentosa).[19,24,46]

ANTITUSSIVES

While patients with allergic rhinitis may select combination products containing antitussives, cough is not one of the hallmark symptoms of allergic rhinitis, which limits the usefulness of both centrally and peripherally acting antitussives.

PREVENTION OF ALLERGIC RHINITIS: AVOIDANCE AND ENVIRONMENTAL CONTROL

The first lines of defense against allergic rhinitis are avoidance and environmental control.[32] These interventions both ameliorate symptoms and remove the cause of allergic rhinitis.[33] They may be the only treatment that is needed in some allergies such as those caused by pets and foods. (See "Parental Smoking Aggravates Allergic Rhinitis.") However, avoidance and environmental control may not be implemented because of either resistance (e.g., children of a smoker who is unable to quit) or impracticality (the cost of removing all carpeting and tiling the entire house).

Seasonal Allergic Rhinitis

For those with seasonal allergic rhinitis, influx of pollen-laden outside air into the household and workplace should be prevented. Keeping the windows shut at all times reduces pollen exposure by up to a factor of 10,000.[3,8] Air conditioners (with the vent closed) help in this regard, although they do not filter pollen from outside air.[3,33] The family should consider the purchase of high-efficiency particulate air (HEPA) filters, which are available as portable units for one or more rooms or for forced-air furnaces.[8] They do not generate ozone which worsens asthma and allergic rhinitis in a significant number of patients, as do electrostatic filters.[33]

Outdoor activities such as camping or hiking should be avoided during heavy pollen seasons.[33] Furthermore, allergic rhinitis sufferers should wear felted fiber masks for activities such as raking leaves, mowing grass, and baling hay.[3] Those whose jobs (and finances) permit may simply move away from the area during pollen seasons.

Perennial Allergic Rhinitis

Family allergies to the house dust mite may be controlled with chemical acaricides or fungicides, but attempting to eradicate the insects is an ongoing process, as they recolonize within a few months.[31] Acarosan, a product that contains benzyl benzoate, kills dust mites and larvae in carpets, but the treatment only lasts for 6 months.[47] Allergy Control Solution, which contains 3% tannic acid, inactivates dust-mite allergens when sprayed on carpets and upholstery, but its efficacy lasts for just 2 to 3 months.[48]

When attempting to control the dust mite, the family must pay special attention to bedrooms since a child may spend 12 to 13 hours of each day there and an adult may spend 8 to 9 hours there.[24] Allergenic items such as feather or down pillows should be exchanged for nonallergenic foam pillows.[22,32] The pillows, mattresses, and box springs should be covered with plastic casings, which in turn should be vacuumed weekly.[24,31,32] Bedding should be washed weekly (water must be 160 degrees to kill the mites) and dried thoroughly.[24]

All dust collectors such as venetian blinds, heavy drapes, overstuffed furniture, books, and assorted souvenirs and collectibles should be removed from the bedroom or moved to closets, drawers, or bookcases with doors.[3,8,32] The bedroom should be dusted and vacuumed thoroughly twice weekly, preferably by a member of the family who is not bothered when carrying out these activities. Dusting should be accomplished with sprays rather than dry cloths. During this cleaning activity, allergic family members should be away at work or school.[17]

FOCUS ON...

PARENTAL SMOKING AGGRAVATES ALLERGIC RHINITIS

The association of parental smoking with upper-airway symptoms in their children (e.g., wheezing, coughing, and bronchitis) mandates that smokers not smoke in the house or automobile, in consideration of their children's health.[25,32] However, for those children whose environments cannot be made healthier, the parents must accept that the tobacco smoke will act as a direct irritant on upper and lower respiratory airways, initiating and aggravating respiratory symptoms in children with allergic rhinitis.[24]

Dust mites are found in large concentrations in the rugs. Vacuuming with standard household units does not remove them.[31] While commercial carpet cleaning kills mites, they recolonize rapidly. For this reason removal of all rugs is the best defense. Floors should be an easily washable material such as tile.[33] Although these measures are critical for the bedrooms, they could also be applied to the entire house if finances permit.

Hot-air vents should be covered with dust filters.[33] Filters on heating/air conditioning systems should be replaced or cleaned every 2 to 4 weeks.[17,25] The ability of HEPA filters to reduce dust-mite symptoms is debatable.[17,31]

Control of molds and mildew can be enhanced by eradication of all areas in the house where they could conceivably grow.[24] Molds and mildew grow well in damp conditions, so moldy areas (bathroom walls, shower stalls, shower curtains, window sills, sinks, evaporative coolers, drip pans under refrigerators, plumbing fixtures, window moldings, and basement surfaces) should be wiped with diluted household bleach (3/4 cup of bleach per gallon of water).[8,24,31] A dehumidifier installed in humid areas also may help.[33] Cool-mist humidifiers should be cleaned with bleach (according to the manufacturer's directions) to prevent molds from growing in the reservoir. The trash must be emptied promptly as old food can serve as a focus of mold growth.[31] The possibility that a household pet is the cause of symptoms is often denied by the family because they had the pet for several months before the child or adult began to experience symptoms.[24] They must be informed that many months of exposure may be necessary prior to the development of an allergy. Rather than immediately getting rid of the pet, it may be boarded out for at least 5 to 6 weeks to see if symptoms improve.[31] (It takes that long for levels of cat allergen to be reduced.) If the pet is proven to be the culprit, it should be given away or kept out of bedrooms and seldom permitted to enter the house.[17,32] Pets may also carry pollen into the home.[8]

Exposure to such allergens as fresh paint, room deodorants, cosmetic sprays, insecticides, and formaldehyde from foam insulation must also be avoided whenever possible.[24]

SUMMARY

Allergic rhinitis is an uncomfortable condition that can be successfully controlled in the majority of patients through avoidance of allergens and control of the environment.

Accordingly, the pharmacist should attempt to discover the nature and frequency of the patient's symptoms. Should avoidance and environmental control not be implemented or should they fail to provide the degree of control desired, the pharmacist may recommend several nonprescription products. Nasal cromolyn sodium solution is a mast cell–stabilizing agent that prevents nasal symptoms of allergic rhinitis

AT THE COUNTER

 A woman in her late 30s asks the pharmacist about products for her allergies.

Interview/Patient Assessment

Her symptoms include watery eyes, nasal congestion and rhinorrhea, and sneezing. She denies use of any medication except "diet pills" and states that she has no medical conditions. In response to a question about the diet pills, she names a nonprescription product. The pharmacist knows that this particular product contains phenylpropanolamine. She asks if an antihistamine/decongestant combination might be helpful for her. She does not mind using a product that may cause drowsiness.

Pharmacist's Analysis

1. Are this woman's symptoms indicative of allergic rhinitis?
2. Does her use of diet pills influence therapy?
3. Should she use an antihistamine/decongestant combination?

This patient's symptoms indicate allergic rhinitis for which the first-line therapy is avoidance and environmental con-

trol. (Treatment options are summarized in Patient Assessment Algorithm 14.1.)

Patient Counseling

The patient should be questioned more fully about the nature of the allergen to determine if she has properly attempted avoidance and environmental control. Since she is an adult with no contraindications to the use of antihistamines, these agents should be considered. Her use of diet pills containing phenylpropanolamine is critical, however, since the concomitant use of an additional sympathomimetic amine (e.g., pseudoephedrine, phenylephrine, or any other product also containing phenylpropanolamine) could increase the risk of adverse reactions. For this reason she should be advised that a single-entity antihistamine would be a safer alternative than the combination. She may then be shown the various products, so she can choose one on the basis of such factors as price, duration of action, degree of drowsiness expected, and familiarity with a certain brand. Alternatively, she may use cromolyn sodium nasal solution, which will prevent symptoms in many patients and also relieve existing symptoms.

and relieves symptoms that are present. Single-entity anti-histamines can also provide relief for most patients. However, should nasal stuffiness be troublesome following the use of single-entity antihistamines, topical and oral nasal decongestants may also be necessary.

References

1. Zetterstrom O. The increased prevalence of allergic airway disease. Allergy 43(Suppl 8):10, 1988.
2. Meltzer EO. The use of antihistamines for the treatment of airway disease. Cutis 42(4A):22, 1988.
3. Dushay ME, Johnson CE. Management of allergic rhinitis: Focus on intranasal agents. Pharmacotherapy 9:338, 1989.
4. Nightingale CH. Treating allergic rhinitis with second-generation antihistamines. Pharmacotherapy 16:905, 1996.
5. Malone, et al. A cost of illness study of allergic rhinitis in the United States. J Allergy Clin Immunol 99 (1 Pt 1):22, 1997.
6. Fireman P. Treatment of allergic rhinitis: Effect on occupation productivity and work force costs. Allergy Asthma Proc 18:63, 1997.
7. Fireman P. Treatment strategies designed to minimize medical complications of allergic rhinitis. Am J Rhinol 11:95, 1997.
8. Demichiei ME, Nelson L. Allergic rhinitis. Am Fam Physician 37:251, 1988.
9. Tarnasky PR, Van Arsdel Jr PP. Antihistamine therapy in allergic rhinitis. J Fam Pract 30:71, 1990.
10. McDonald TJ. Nasal disorders in children. Postgrad Med 81:65, 1987(8).
11. Druce HM, Kaliner MA. Allergic rhinitis. JAMA 259:260, 1988.
12. Kelso JM. Skin test results in related and unrelated persons with allergic rhinitis. Ann Allergy Asthma Immunol 77:43, 1996.
13. Corren J. Allergic rhinitis and asthma: How important is the link? J Allergy Clin Immunol 99:S781, 1997.
14. Malo JL, et al. Prevalence and intensity of rhinoconjunctivitis in subjects with occupational asthma. Eur Respir J 10:1513, 1997.
15. Danielsson J, Jessen M. The natural course of allergic rhinitis during 12 years of follow-up. Allergy 52:331, 1997.
16. Ophir D, et al. Effects of inhaled humidified warm air on nasal patency and nasal symptoms in allergic rhinitis. Ann Allergy 60:239, 1988.
17. Conner BL, Georgitis JW. Practical diagnosis and treatment of allergic and nonallergic rhinitis. Prim Care 14:457, 1987.
18. Langer HM. Allergic rhinitis: A medical insight. J Otolaryngol 18:158, 1989.
19. Katelaris CH. Management of allergic rhinitis. Aust Fam Physician 18:769, 1989.
20. Djukanovic R, Wilson SJ, Howarth PH. Pathology of rhinitis and bronchial asthma. Clin Exp Allergy 26(Suppl 3):44, 1996.
21. Baraniuk JN. Pathogenesis of allergic rhinitis. J Allergy Clin Immunol 99:S763, 1997.
22. Pepper G. OTC vs. Rx for allergic rhinitis. Nurse Pract 12:58, 1987.
23. Ziering RW. Immediate and late side effects of hay fever. Postgrad Med 85:183, 1989(6).
24. Welch MJ, Kemp JP. Allergy in children. Prim Care 14:575, 1987.
25. Stafford CT. Allergic rhinitis. Postgrad Med 81:147, 1987.
26. Kaslow JE, Novey HS. When hay fever doesn't quit. Postgrad Med 85:164, 1989(6).
27. Thurmond M, Amedee R. Allergic diagnosis: Skin testing and RAST. J La State Med Soc 149:141, 1997.
28. Grant DF. Allergic and nonallergic rhinitis. Directing medical therapy at specific symptoms. Postgrad Med 100:64, 1996.
29. Lieberman P. Rhinitis, Allergic and Nonallergic. Hosp Pract 23:117, 1988(6).
30. Samir M, Magdy S, el Fetoh AA. Air pollution in relation to allergic and nonallergic rhinitis. Arch Otolaryngol Head Neck Surg 123:746, 1997.
31. Pollart SM, et al. House dust sensitivity and environmental control. Prim Care 14:591, 1987.
32. Klein GL. Persistent allergic rhinitis in older patients: Therapies worth trying. Geriatrics 42:91, 1987.
33. Kaliner M, et al. Rhinitis and Asthma. JAMA 258:2851, 1987.
34. Schwartz HJ, et al. Occupational allergic rhinitis in the hair care industry: Reactions to permanent wave solutions. J Occup Med 32:473, 1990.
35. Sanchez-Borges M, et al. A new triad: Sensitivity to aspirin, allergic rhinitis, and severe allergic reaction to ingested aeroallergens. Cutis 59:311, 1997.
36. Trade Package, Nasalcrom Nasal Spray: 1997.
37. Fed Reg 57:58355, 1992.
38. Storms WW. Treatment of allergic rhinitis: Effects of allergic rhinitis and antihistamines on performance. Allergy Asthma Proc 18:59, 1997.
39. Fed Reg 50:2219, 1985.
40. Simons FE, et al. Adverse central nervous system effects of older antihistamines in children. Pediatr Allergy Immunol 7:22, 1996.
41. Fed Reg 53:118, 1988.
42. Summary Information for January 13, 1995 Meeting of the Nonprescription Drugs Advisory Committee. Food and Drug Administration Docket # 88N-0004.
43. Fed Reg 59:4215, 1994.
44. Fed Reg 52:31891, 1987.
45. Koppel C, et al. Poisoning with over-the-counter doxylamine preparations: An evaluation of 109 cases. Hum Toxicol 6:355, 1987.
46. Fed Reg 59:43385, 1994.
47. Anon. Dust mite treatment. Am Drugg 203:34, 1991(3).
48. Anon. Allergy control. Am Drugg 201:26, 1990(7).

The Common Cold and Related Conditions

A female patient who appears to be in her 50s says she has been "stopped up" for several days and needs to be able to breathe through her nose again.

2. What is the significance of her scratchy throat and cough?
3. Should her cough also be treated?
4. Is a combination product appropriate for this patient?

Interview/Patient Assessment

The patient denies use of any medications and denies any health problems. She states that she began to have a runny nose about 3 days before, and she also had a scratchy throat. She has begun to cough, bringing up thick mucus from her lungs.

Pharmacist's Analysis

1. Are the patient's symptoms consistent with nasal problems associated with the common cold?

Patient Counseling

The symptoms indicate that this patient has a common cold. Since she has no medical conditions and is not using any medications, either oral or topical nasal decongestants could be recommended for her nasal obstruction. The cough appears to be productive, so an expectorant might be beneficial. A combination product containing guaifenesin and pseudoephedrine would treat both symptoms simultaneously, although with a combination product she will not be able to treat either symptom singly should the other abate at a later point. A topical anesthetic lozenge could provide relief from scratchy throat.

The common cold is the most frequent acute condition to which man is subjected.[1,2] Pharmacists receive more questions related to the common cold and its therapy than all other medical conditions combined. For this reason, an in-depth knowledge of the condition is essential for practicing pharmacists. Because it is advisable to limit sore throat product recommendations to patients with sore throat related to the common cold, discussion of sore throat has been included in this chapter.

THE COMMON COLD

PREVALENCE OF THE COMMON COLD

The common cold is so prevalent that a discussion of its incidence is not gauged in the usual epidemiologic measurements (e.g., incidence per 10,000 persons yearly), but in terms of number of colds per individual per year. On average, everyone has 3 to 12 colds yearly, depending on the age of the patient.[3] The common cold and its related conditions cause 250 million days of restricted activity in the United States each year and 30 million lost work or school days, which drains the resources of society and compromises recreation time.[4,5] A common cold during the first trimester of pregnancy may increase the risk of birth defects.[6]

EPIDEMIOLOGY OF THE COMMON COLD

Age

Children of kindergarten age, who are most likely to contract this viral infection, suffer an average of 12 colds yearly.[7] In-

cidence drops as age increases, and children aged 5 to 9 suffer only four to seven colds yearly.[1,7] Accordingly, adults experience even fewer episodes of the common cold, averaging only 3 colds yearly.[7] Once adults have children in daycare or preschool, however, the number of common colds rises as their children bring the virus home with them. Likewise, infants with older siblings are also more prone to catch the common cold than young singlets living at home.

Environmental Exposure

Contrary to popular myth, being in a cold or wet environment does not increase susceptibility to the common cold.[7] A solitary walk outside in the winter is preferable to sharing a warm room with people who are currently affected with the common cold.

Smoking

Smokers have an increased risk of the common cold.[8] Furthermore, smokers' symptoms are more severe than those of nonsmokers. The authors of one study confirming this link hypothesized that smoking may cause these problems either by hampering mucokinesis or by affecting the immune response.

ETIOLOGY OF THE COMMON COLD

The common cold can be produced by a number of viruses:[1,5]

- Rhinoviruses
- Influenza viruses
- Parainfluenza viruses

- Respiratory syncytial viruses
- Coronaviruses
- Adenoviruses
- Enteric cytopathic human orphan (ECHO) viruses
- Coxsackieviruses

Knowledge of the specific virus is not critical. Therefore, the physician will seldom attempt to discover exactly which virus is responsible for a common cold case.[5]

The rhinovirus is one of the more common causes, being responsible for 40 to 50% of all colds.[1,9] At least 100 specific types of rhinovirus have been identified, with many more remaining.[3] The virus antigen varies, so the protection afforded by the human immune system is erratic and uncertain.[5] Human antibodies do not resist the invaders vigorously.[4,5] The large number of rhinovirus types also makes immunization unfeasible.

The rhinoviruses begin the pathogenic process by first penetrating the mucous blanket of the nasal or bronchial mucociliary epithelium, attaching to a specific receptor. The next step in the viral assault is damage to the ciliated cells, which results in the release of bradykinin, prostaglandin, histamine, and cytokines.[10] These chemicals inflame the tissues lining the nose, and ciliated cells are sloughed, destroying the integrity of the epithelium.[10,11] As a result, the patient experiences sneezing, rhinorrhea, and nasal stuffiness. The chemicals are also responsible for sore throat.

As described in the previous chapter on allergic rhinitis, the pharmacist must ask the right types of questions to ensure that the patient does not have allergic rhinitis. A clinical allergist warned his colleagues to be wary of the patient who reports two colds a year, with one cold lasting for the duration of the spring pollen season and the second cold lasting for the duration of the fall pollen season, most likely because the cause is allergic rhinitis.[12]

TRANSMISSION OF THE COMMON COLD

Although time-honored wisdom holds that the common cold is contracted through coughing and sneezing, research has confirmed that indirect droplet spread is a secondary transmission method.[13] Kissing is also an uncommon method of transmission since cold viruses are not found in large numbers in the oral reservoir. The primary method is direct spread through contact with an inoculum of virus deposited by an infected patient, followed by self-inoculation through touching one's mucous membranes (e.g., the nose or eye).[5,14] These self-touching behaviors are extremely common. In fact, secret observers have recorded finger-to-nose or finger-to-eye contact of physicians during a conference, with each attendee logging at least one incident per hour.[5] Individuals with rhinovirus colds have been found to have virus on their fingers; objects in their homes also carry the virus.[15]

At least 75% of viral infections are transmitted by children. The major point of dissemination for the common cold virus is any location where children are concentrated such as the classroom or day care.[13] The children then return home to introduce the colds to the adults living there.

MANIFESTATIONS OF THE COMMON COLD

Symptoms of the common cold follow a characteristic progression.[16] About 2 to 4 days after viral contact, the patient feels a sore or scratchy throat.[17] Sneezing is next, followed by **rhinorrhea** (nasal discharge). The initially clear secretions become **purulent** (containing pus), and nasal obstruction alternates with rhinorrhea. Fever may occur in children, while older children and adults generally experience **malaise** (general sensation of discomfort) and muscular aches and pains. A nonproductive cough begins on day 3 or 4, but becomes loose and productive, gradually fading over the next several days. Possible constitutional symptoms include tiredness, shivering, and fever.[3]

Symptoms and their severity vary with the viral agent.[9] Rhinovirus colds usually result in involvement of adenoidal, nasal, and nasopharyngeal mucosa.[13,16] Some patients only experience a transient episode with minor symptoms lasting about 1 week.[7,17] The median duration of symptoms is 7 to 13 days.[1] Some patients, however, suffer extreme discomfort for a sustained period, with 20% of patients having symptoms for 2 weeks or more.[5,7] In one survey, 30% of patients still suffered from cough and runny nose by day 8.

The virus is able to involve other mucous membranes, including the lower airway, paranasal sinuses, the eustachian tube, and the middle ear.[9] Eustachian tube dysfunction and middle ear pressure abnormalities are frequent sequelae, with patients reporting earache or a feeling of pressure.[18] The frequent sinus involvement is caused by obstruction of normal sinus drainage.[19]

SPECIFIC CONSIDERATIONS OF THE COMMON COLD

Temporal Occurrence

Incidences of the common cold peak at three times of the year: September, October, and early spring. In temperate areas, the rhinovirus causes colds during early fall and late spring.[11] The September peak is likely the result of the reopening of schools.[17] Each time period represents a different causative agent. Rhinoviruses decline in importance during late fall to early spring. During the winter and early spring, the common cold is more likely to be caused by parainfluenza viruses, influenza viruses, respiratory syncytial virus, and the coronoaviruses.

Influenza

Many patients are confused about the nature of their disease condition, especially when a common cold occurs during flu season.[6]

The season for influenza, or flu, is from late December to early March, although it may continue into April. While influenza does mimic the common cold in some respects, important differences can be recognized. Like the common cold, flu does cause headache, sore throat, cough, runny nose, and sneezing.[20-22] However, the cough of flu is nonproductive. Further, whereas the common cold sufferer can usually continue his daily routine of work and school, influenza compromises one's ability to carry on. The disabling impact of influenza is partly caused by the additional symptoms not seen in the common cold, including chills, **myalgia** (aching of the muscles), malaise, backache, sweating, a sudden fever (as high as 104°), and sensitivity to light. Malaise may persist as long as 1 to 2 weeks. Influenza may be accompanied by such sequelae as bronchitis, pneumonia, and ear infections. While numerous nonprescription products are sold for influenza, they are typically mixtures of three to four ingredients such as dextromethorphan, guaifenesin, an analgesic, and a decongestant. No FDA Review panel has specifically examined influenza relief products, but individual ingredients may provide some relief.

Antihistamines may produce relief from runny nose of influenza. Likewise, antitussives may alleviate cough. Acetaminophen products are allowed to carry an indication for influenza, thereby helping alleviate body aches and pains and

headache. The pharmacist must recall that salicylates are absolutely contraindicated in influenza because of the risk of Reye's syndrome (See "Reye's Syndrome" in Chapter 18). Inclusion of antihistamines in flu products is questionable, since the syndrome is brought on by infective rather than allergic causes.

Sinus Involvement

The patient often complains of sinus trouble, sometimes as a sequela to the common cold. The inner wall of the sinus contains **cilia** (small, independently moving, hairlike projections attached to cell surfaces), which cleanse the sinus just as the ciliary system of the lungs cleans the lower respiratory passages.[23] As shown in Figure 15.1, each of the four pairs of sinuses (ethmoid, sphenoid, frontal, maxillary) is connected to the nasal cavity, which makes them susceptible to infection during a common cold or other upper respiratory infection. Should bacteria colonize the sinuses and the mucociliary defense system be impaired, a sinus infection results.

Symptoms of acute sinusitis include rhinorrhea with production of pus-filled mucus, headache, and discomfort. The typical cough and sore throat of the common cold are absent. Sinusitis can be further differentiated from the common cold by the presence of impaired taste and smell and a localized

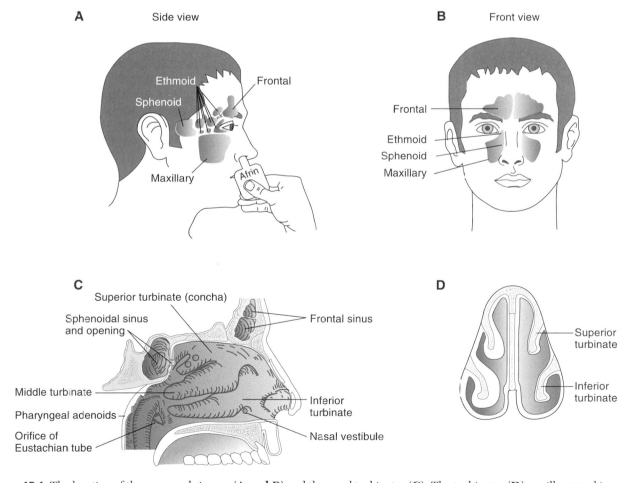

Figure 15.1. The location of the paranasal sinuses **(A and B)** and the nasal turbinates **(C)**. The turbinates **(D)** are illustrated in a congested state (*left*), and decongested state following use of the nasal decongestant (*right*).

pain and tenderness. The location of the pain depends on the specific sinus affected; for instance, infection of the maxillary sinus causes pain in the cheek and toothache. Sinus infection requires systemic antibiotic/antibacterial therapy, with such agents as amoxicillin, cotrimoxazole, or amoxicillin/clavulanate potassium.[24] The physician may also recommend intranasal steroids, topical decongestants, systemic decongestants, mucolytics, and normal saline nasal lavage.[24,25]

The FDA affirmed that antihistamines added to sinus products are not rational, as they do not reduce nasal congestion to aid in sinus drainage.[26] Further, the drying (anticholinergic) effect of antihistamines increases the viscosity of mucus and hinders sinus drainage. A possible use of antihistamines in sinus problems might be allergic **rhinosinusitis** (simultaneous inflammation of the nasal passages and sinus cavities), although the FDA has not specifically addressed treatment of this condition with antihistamines.[25]

Should the patient be taking an antibiotic/antibacterial, a rational combination sinus product would be one containing a decongestant and analgesic. (See Table 15.1 for examples.) It is improper, however, for the pharmacist to sell the patient any of the various nonprescription products for symptomatic relief without also stressing the need to see a physician.

TREATMENT OF THE COMMON COLD

Treatment Guidelines

The pharmacist fields numerous questions regarding the common cold and its associated problems. Since each patient is bothered by one or more possible symptoms, the pharmacist should first ascertain exactly which symptoms are troublesome, then recommend a product to relieve those symptoms.

Nonprescription Medications

Cough-cold items occupy a great deal of space on the shelves of the typical pharmacy, with manufacturers offering endless permutations on a common theme. Combination products are the rule; single-entity products the exception. (Table 15.2 presents examples of combination products.) Both types of products have specific advantages.

SINGLE-ENTITY PRODUCTS

Single-entity products are preferable for certain patients for several reasons. First, combination products assume that the patient is actually troubled with all of the symptoms that the product is marketed to alleviate. This may not be true, since common cold symptoms progress, so one symptom often fades as another is reaching its apex. Even if a patient does need all of those ingredients during a common cold episode, what happens in the future? Should a patient need relief from a single common cold symptom at another time, the combination product does not allow him or her to tailor therapy to their problem. Thus the prudent pharmacist may recommend two or three single-entity products for the common cold, carefully explaining to the patient why each is necessary.[27]

Secondly, a patient ingesting unneeded ingredients is prey to the adverse reactions caused by those ingredients. Thirdly, each ingredient carries certain contraindications. A

Table 15.1. Representative Sinus Products	
PRODUCT	SELECTED INGREDIENTS/COMMENTS
Advil Cold & Sinus Tablets	Ibuprofen 200 mg; pseudoephedrine HCl 30 mg
Contac Sinus Tablets	Acetaminophen 500 mg; pseudoephedrine HCl 30 mg
Dristan Sinus Tablets	Ibuprofen 200 mg, pseudoephedrine HCl 30 mg
Motrin Sinus Headache	Ibuprofen 200 mg, pseudoephedrine HCl 30 mg
Sine-Off Tablets	Acetaminophen 500 mg, pseudoephedrine HCl 30 mg, chlorpheniramine maleate 2 mg (antihistamine not likely to be necessary)
Sinutab Sinus Allergy Tablets	Acetaminophen 500 mg, pseudoephedrine HCl 30 mg, chlorpheniramine maleate 2 mg (antihistamine not likely to be necessary)
Sinutab Sinus No Drowsiness Maximum Strength Tablets	Acetaminophen 500 mg; pseudoephedrine HCl 30 mg
Sudafed Sinus Non-Drowsy Maximum Strength Tablets	Acetaminophen 500 mg; pseudoephedrine HCl 30 mg
Tavist Sinus Tablets	Acetaminophen 500 mg, pseudoephedrine HCl 30 mg
Tylenol Allergy Sinus Maximum Strength Tablets	Acetaminophen 500 mg, pseudoephedrine HCl 30 mg, chlorpheniramine maleate 2 mg (antihistamine not likely to be necessary)
Tylenol Sinus Maximum Strength Tablets	Acetaminophen 500 mg; pseudoephedrine HCl 30 mg

Table 15.2. Representative Combination Cough-Cold Products

PRODUCT	SELECTIVE INGREDIENTS/COMMENTS
Actifed Cold & Allergy Tablets	Pseudoephedrine HCl 60 mg, triprolidine HCl 2.5 mg
Benylin Cough Suppressant Expectorant Syrup	Per 5 mL: guaifenesin 100 mg, dextromethorphan 5 mg
Comtrex Day & Night Maximum Strength Cold & Flu Relief Tablets	Daytime products contain acetaminophen 500 mg, dextromethorphan hydrobromide 15 mg, pseudoephedrine HCl 30 mg; nighttime tablets add chlorpheniramine maleate 2 mg
Contac 12-Hour Cold Capsules	Phenylpropanolamine HCl 75 mg, chlorpheniramine maleate 8 mg
Contac Severe Cold & Flu Maximum Strength Caplets	Acetaminophen 500 mg, phenylpropanolamine HCl 12.5 mg, dextromethorphan hydrobromide 15 mg, chlorpheniramine maleate 2 mg
Dimetapp 12-Hour Extentabs	Phenylpropanolamine HCl 75 mg, brompheniramine maleate 12 mg
Drixoral Cold & Allergy 12-Hour Relief Tablets	Pseudoephedrine sulfate 120 mg, dexbrompheniramine maleate 6 mg
Robitussin CF Syrup	Per 5 mL: phenylpropanolamine HCl 12.5 mg, guaifenesin 100 mg, dextromethorphan hydrobromide 10 mg
Robitussin DM Syrup	Per 5 mL: guaifenesin 100 mg, dextromethorphan hydrobromide 10 mg
Robitussin PE Syrup	Per 5 mL: pseudoephedrine HCl 30 mg, guaifenesin 100 mg
Tavist-D Tablets	Phenylpropanolamine HCl 75 mg, clemastine fumarate 1.34 mg
Vicks Nyquil Multi-Symptom Cold/Flu Relief Liquid	Per 30 mL: doxylamine succinate 12.5 mg, acetaminophen 1000 mg, pseudoephedrine HCl 60 mg, dextromethorphan hydrobromide 30 mg

product containing four different ingredients (e.g., central antitussive, antihistamine, nasal decongestant, expectorant) may have so many contraindications that a significant number of patients may be unable to take it.

COMBINATION PRODUCTS

While single-entity products have advantages, patients often exhibit resistance when the pharmacist recommends as many as three or four different products. This resistance has several sources:

- Patients begin to see use of several products as too complicated.
- Different products carry different dosing intervals, requiring the patient to be more vigilant in remembering to take subsequent doses of three or four products.
- The cost may be prohibitive.
- The patient may not accept the burden of reading separate labels, each with its own set of directions, precautions, and contraindications.

Thus, if a patient actually has all of the symptoms that the ingredients of the combination product are able to treat, such a product carries several advantages:

- The patient only has to read one label, with the contraindications and precautions collected under a single heading.

- The patient is able to obtain relief from several ingredients by taking one dose of medication at a single dosing interval.
- The cost of one product is generally less than that of four products.

See "Unproven Therapies and the Common Cold."

PREVENTION OF THE COMMON COLD

Prevention of the common cold consists of preventing the invasion of the body by viral particles. Since the primary method of viral transfer is touching one's mucous membranes with contaminated hands, patients should be cautioned to wash the hands frequently and to avoid rubbing the eyes with the fingers, and avoid placing the fingers in the nose or mouth.

NASAL SYMPTOMS ASSOCIATED WITH THE COMMON COLD

PREVALENCE OF NASAL SYMPTOMS

The prevalence of patients exhibiting nasal symptoms associated with the common cold varies with the specific infective agent. In one study, the frequency of nasal discharge ranged from 82 to 100% for five different viruses, including three strains of rhinovirus, a respiratory syncytial virus, and a coronavirus.[14] In the same study, the frequency of nasal obstruction ranged from 64 to 100%. Nasal symptoms caused by allergic rhinitis, also quite common, are discussed in Chapter 14.

EPIDEMIOLOGY OF NASAL SYMPTOMS

The epidemiology of nasal symptoms associated with the common cold reflects the epidemiology of the common cold itself.

ETIOLOGY OF NASAL SYMPTOMS

Inhaled cold viruses attach to mucous membranes, producing cellular injury through a combination of physical pressure and pathologic damage.[31] The tissue injury activates cellular defense and plasma protein systems, which in turn releases chemical mediators of inflammation (e.g., prostaglandins, kinins, leukotrienes). Kinins and prostaglandins both produce vasodilation and increase vascular permeability. Vasodilation coupled with increased vascular permeability produces nasal obstruction and nasal discharge.

MANIFESTATIONS OF NASAL SYMPTOMS

Common cold viruses produce edema and hyperemia of the nasal mucous membranes.[27] Increased mucous gland activity causes clear and watery rhinorrhea. Inflammation of the mucous membranes and thickening of the turbinates eventually narrows the airways so that the individual cannot breathe through the nose. The patient then experiences alternating discharge and obstruction.[15]

TREATMENT OF NASAL SYMPTOMS ASSOCIATED WITH THE COMMON COLD

Treatment Guidelines

The patient can only treat nasal congestion caused by the common cold, or caused by allergic rhinitis, or associated with sinusitis.[26] *(Patient Assessment Algorithm 15.1)* Other medical conditions that cause stuffy nose are not amenable to self-treatment. (One condition is vasomotor rhinitis, alternating congestion and rhinorrhea caused by an inherent imbalance within the patient's autonomic nervous

---

FOCUS ON...

UNPROVEN THERAPIES AND THE COMMON COLD

Unproven therapies carry great implications for pharmacists and patients. An entire chapter is devoted to unproven therapies in this text. Unproven therapies associated with the common cold are included here since they are pervasive and firmly believed. Several examples of highly publicized but unproven therapies include the following:

- Vitamin C. Popular belief to the contrary, vitamin C has never been shown to prevent the common cold.[17,28] The myth began as a result of a book by Nobel-prize-winner Linus Pauling.[5] His Nobel was not in medicine, however. Studies demonstrating any effect of ascorbic acid on the course of the cold are contradictory. Vitamin C may produce a slight reduction in severity and duration, although further studies are needed to confirm this effect and clarify the exact doses that would be beneficial.[28]
- Zinc Gluconate Lozenges. Zinc gluconate lozenges are alleged to abort or relieve symptoms of the common cold. Many studies are equivocal, showing no effect or a minor effect.[29,30] Although another controlled medical study was positive, the full weight of scientific evidence has not conclusively proven their efficacy.[2] The metallic taste is unacceptable to many patients and the long-term consequences of zinc gluconate taken in this form are unknown.[5]

---

system.[32]) A major cause of vasomotor rhinitis is pregnancy, during which elevated levels of estrogen inhibit acetylcholinesterase, producing swelling and edema of the nasal mucosa. The phenomenon is more common at the end of the first trimester and may persist until delivery, and also for several weeks following delivery.[33] The same mechanism is responsible for rhinitis during menarche, puberty in both sexes, and with administration of estrogens and oral contraceptives. Elevated estrogen also causes vasomotor rhinitis in the late menstrual cycle, in hypothyroidism with myxedema, and in severe liver disease.

During pregnancy, patients with nasal congestion should be urged to consult their obstetricians. Nasal decongestants are not indicated for pregnant patients and may endanger the fetus. In one case a pregnant female was given large doses of an oxymetazoline nasal mist prior to two nonstress tests.[34] She was administered five doses over a 12.5-hour period rather than one dose every 12 hours as ordered. Systemic vasoconstriction resulted in a decline in uterine perfusion, which produced late decelerations in the fetal heart rate. Fortunately, the child was delivered spontaneously 14 hours after the final dose of topical nasal decongestant.

The pharmacist must be aware of the ages below which self-treatment is not indicated for nasal symptoms. Some companies market charts that purport to allow treatment below the ages at which the products are safe. (See "Pediatric Dosing Information.")

Nonprescription Medications

TOPICAL NASAL DECONGESTANTS
Dosage Forms
Topical nasal decongestants are sympathomimetic amines that stimulate adrenergic receptors of blood vessels (Table

Patient Assessment Algorithm 15.1. Nasal Congestion/Rhinorrhea

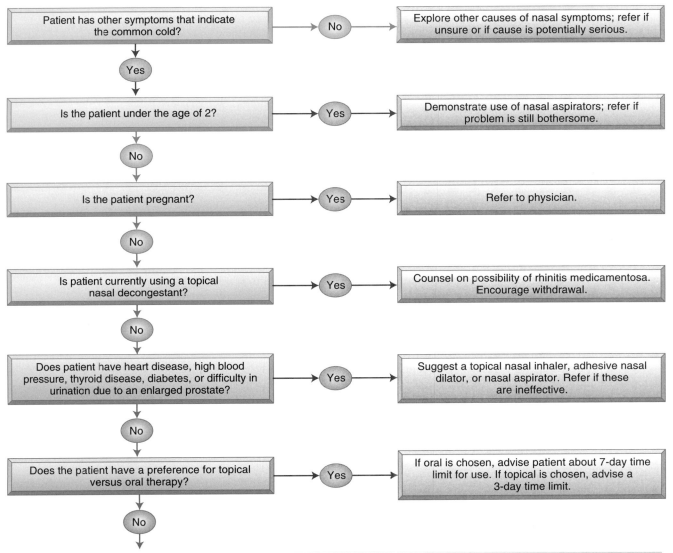

Recommend an age-appropriate, Category I ingredient, keeping in mind the 3-day time limit for topicals and the 7-day time limit for oral nasal decongestants. If runny nose and sneezing are still bothersome, consider recommending chlorpheniramine or doxylamine.

15.3).[39] They constrict dilated nasal blood vessels.[39,40] Available dosage forms include the following:

- Nasal drops, placed into the nose with the use of a dropper supplied by the manufacturer
- Nasal sprays, applied by placing the blunt end of the dropper bottle into the affected nostril(s) and spraying once or twice as indicated on the package (Fig. 15.1)
- A nasal jelly, placed into the affected nostril(s) with the fingers, then inhaled well back into the nasal passages[24] (no longer available)
- Inhalers, small tubes with a tapered end designed for nasal insertion. The decongestant is impregnated in a cotton plug inside the container. The patient blocks one nostril, inserts the inhaler into the other nostril, and inhales deeply. The volatilized ingredients contact the mucosa.

The medication in inhalers may be superior to topical drops or sprays, which only reach limited areas of the nasal mucosa.[41]

Required Labeling

The FDA requires several labels on all topical nasal decongestants.[26] *Patients should be advised that the topical products can cause temporary discomfort* such as burning, stinging, sneezing, or an increase in nasal discharge. *Patients should also be warned that use of the product by more than one person may spread the infection,* if the dropper tip contacts the nasal mucosa during administration.[40] *A sentence in bold-face type must warn the patient not to exceed the recommended dosage of topical nasal decongestants.* In one case a 61-year-old engineer with multiple sclerosis applied one full dropper of phenylephrine (instead of the recommended two to three drops) to each nostril several times daily.[42] This practice was suspected as the cause of a leukemoid reaction, which resolved 48 hours after cessation of phenylephrine.

tip *Topical products should state, "Do not use this product for more than 3 days. Use only as directed. Frequent or prolonged use may cause nasal congestion to recur or worsen. If symptoms persist, consult a doctor."* This warning is meant to reduce the occurrence of rhinitis medicamentosa, described below. It is also meant to prevent long-term adverse effects of nasal decongestants such as the occurrence of cerebral infarction that may have been caused by 20-year usage of oxymetazoline.[43]

tip *All topical nasal decongestants except those in inhalers should warn against use if the patient has heart disease, high blood pressure, thyroid disease, diabetes, or difficulty in urination caused by an enlarged prostate, unless directed by a doctor.* The topical ingredients listed below are fully approved except where specifically noted otherwise.

Naphazoline Hydrochloride

The 0.025% concentration of naphazoline can be recommended for patients as young as 6 years, but not younger. The stronger 0.05% concentration must not be used for patients younger than 12 and **tip** *must carry the warning: "Do not use this product in children under 12 because it may cause sedation if swallowed."*[26] (In an earlier document, the FDA stated that infants and young children suffer sedation, nervousness, increased systolic blood pressure and bradycardia with both nasal instillation and accidental oral ingestion.[40]) All of the imidazolines (naphazoline, oxymetazoline, xylometazoline) can sedate young children, and have been responsi-

FOCUS ON...

PEDIATRIC DOSING INFORMATION

The FDA guidelines on dosage for allowed ages are clearly stated in the references provided. The companies that market cough-cold products are usually quite careful to label their trade packages in conformance with approved FDA dosing guidelines. However, various manufacturers have provided pharmacists with charts, stickers, and pads that purport to allow safe dosing of their nonprescription products to children as young as 0 months of age and weighing as little as 6 pounds. Product lines for which these charts have been offered include Naldecon products, Triaminic products, Pedia-Care, Sudafed products, and Robitussin products. The intent is for the pharmacist to provide the tear-off pads and stickers to parents and guardians of those who are too young to be treated with the approved FDA labeling. Thus a mother with a 1-day-old baby with slight nasal congestion could be given 1/2 dropper of PediaCare (or of Tylenol Drops), according to a chart provided by McNeil.

Usage at ages younger than those listed is restricted to physician recommendation because of the lack of controlled clinical trials at those ages.[35] Generally, the safety of cough-cold products in patients younger than two has not been conclusively demonstrated. Antihistamines are not given for patients younger than 6 (with the exception of dimenhydrinate for motion sickness). This text provides many examples of instances in which infants and children were badly harmed by such improper administration. Pediatricians are also concerned, and have cited several instances in which prescription medications are prescribed by physicians for children who are too young to receive them.[36] The authors listed reasons why infants suffer greater toxicity: greater sensitivity to the effects of these medications and altered clearance and metabolism caused by age or the presence of diseases such as phenylketonuria or liver abnormalities. The authors stated "Given the lack of data on efficacy, and the increasing reports of toxicity in infants and children, rational therapeutics should not include combination cough and cold medication treatment of upper respiratory tract infections in infants."

Thus there are valid reasons to respect the age cutoffs provided by the FDA. In response to pharmacist queries about the legitimacy of these dosing charts, the companies respond that they will stand behind them. However, pharmacists are still uncomfortable, as placing a sticker on a bottle with handwritten note about a non-labeled dose in an infant is a clear example of relabeling, repackaging, and possible misbranding.

Attempts to involve the FDA in regulating this gray area have met with little success. A communication from the FDA discussed this "professional labeling," noting that some monographs include underage dosing as an aid to the physician.[37] This communication further noted that lay persons cannot safely use such products in pediatric patients without consultation with a physician, dentist, or other practitioner in which a doctor-patient relationship exists. The FDA further discussed the age cutoffs in a Nonprescription Drugs Advisory Committee meeting. During this meeting, the agency stressed that evaluation of additional information is mandatory before antihistamine dosing can be extended below age 6, for instance.[38]

Until the FDA either disciplines offending companies or approves these pediatric doses, the pharmacist is caught in a regulatory quagmire. An FDA official states that the pharmacist could be subject to civil liability in providing these doses. Yet the companies that promote these products state that they will protect the pharmacist should a lawsuit arise as a result of using these pediatric dosing charts. The prudent pharmacist should hold the welfare of the patient as the primary concern. The fact that these doses were not arrived at through legitimate double-blind placebo controlled trials should be sufficient to negate their use.

Table 15.3. Representative Topical Nasal Decongestant Products

PRODUCT	SELECTED INGREDIENTS/COMMENTS
Afrin Original 12-Hour Spray	Oxymetazoline HCl 0.05% drops or spray
Afrin Mentholated Spray	Oxymetazoline HCl 0.05%, menthol (menthol not approved as a decongestant)
Benzedrex Inhalers	Propylhexedrine 250 mg, lavender oil, menthol
Dristan 12-Hour Nasal Spray	Oxymetazoline HCl 0.05%
Neo-Synephrine 12-Hour Spray	Oxymetazoline HCl 0.05%
Neo-Synephrine	Phenylephrine HCl 0.125% drops; 0.25%, 0.5%, and 1% drops or spray
Nostrilla 12-Hour Spray	Oxymetazoline HCl 0.05%
Otrivin	Xylometazoline HCl 0.1% drops or spray
Privine	Naphazoline HCl 0.05% drops or spray
Vicks Sinex Nasal Spray	Phenylephrine HCl 0.5%
Vicks Vapor Inhalers	l-Desoxyephedrine 50 mg (an unapproved ingredient; see text)

ble for coma and hypothermia in neonates.[44] Naphazoline is applied in a dose of one to two drops or sprays no more than every 6 hours.

Oxymetazoline Hydrochloride
The 0.025% drop or spray can be given in a dose of two to three drops or sprays per nostril no more often than every 10 to 12 hours to patients 2 years old and older. *The product should have a calibrated dropper or be in a metered-dose spray that limits the dose for children.* The 0.05% concentration is given in the same dose to patients 6 years old and older.[26]

Propylhexedrine
This ingredient, only available as an inhaler, is not recommended for patients younger than 6 years. For patients 6 and older, the dosage is two inhalations in each nostril no more often than every 2 hours. *The inhaler must carry the statement, "This inhaler is effective for a maximum of 3 months after first use."*

Propylhexedrine possesses 10% of the power of amphetamines to stimulate the central nervous system.[45] It is known to drug abusers as "peanut butter meth" or "stove top speed" after its active ingredient is extracted or cooked.[45] Abusers ingest the cotton plug orally or inject its contents intravenously. Intravenous injection causes severe toxicity because of the active ingredient, along with menthol and other aromatics contained in the cotton plug. Because of this potential for abuse it must be sold cautiously.[45,46] The FDA issued a request for individuals to provide data regarding its abuse.[47,48] The pharmacist should store the products behind the pharmacy counter so potential buyers can be questioned. It is advisable to be wary of sale to individuals who request propylhexedrine products, offering nothing more than an unsupported refusal to consider alternative oral or topical

decongestants. These individuals are often abusers who should be denied the product.

Phenylephrine Hydrochloride
Phenylephrine is applied in a dose of two to three drops or sprays no more often than every 4 hours. *The 0.125% concentration is not to be used for patients younger than two; the 0.25% solution can be used for patients as young as 6, while the 0.5 and 1% concentrations should not be used for patients younger than 12.* The product should have a calibrated dropper or be in a metered-dose spray that limits the dose for children.

Xylometazoline Hydrochloride
Xylometazoline 0.05% solution or drops can be given to patients as young as 2 in a dose of two to three drops or sprays in each nostril, no more often than every 8 to 10 hours. The product should have a calibrated dropper or be in a metered-dose spray that limits the dose for children. The 0.1% concentration is not to be recommended in children younger than 12.

In one case a father followed the advice of a family friend and administered 0.1% xylometazoline to his 15-day-old daughter for slight nasal stuffiness to facilitate her feeding.[49] Within 2 hours, she was gray in color, hypotonic, and breathing irregularly. She became comatose after several hours, but eventually recovered. It is noteworthy that in this case it was not until "several hours after admission and many interviews with the parents" that the possibility of the nasal drop as a causative agent emerged. The physicians who reported the incident suggested that imidazolines be recognized as toxic products leading to coma in children.

In another case xylometazoline was used as a postsurgical nasal spray following submucous resection of the nose.[50] The patient's preexisting porphyria was worsened by the product, prompting the physicians who reported the case to suggest its avoidance in porphyric patients.

l-Desoxyephedrine

This ingredient (also known as l-methamphetamine) has had a checkered history.[45] It was given Category III status for lack of efficacy in the initial panel review process.[40] The Phase 2 document evaluated more recent studies, and assigned it to Category I, also finding that it does not cause nasal rebound within a 7-day period. For this reason, the agency recommended that it be used for 7 days, rather than the 3 days to which other topical nasal decongestants are limited.[46] The Phase 3 document explored the issue of l-desoxyephedrine being scheduled in the United States, with the inhaler being marketed through an exclusion.[26] Further, in this final document, the FDA revealed that l-desoxyephedrine is not currently standardized for quality and purity, and did not include it at that time as an approved topical nasal decongestant. A place for it was reserved, however, pending the development of compendial standards.

Systemic Adverse Reactions of Topical
Nasal Decongestants

Local vasoconstriction occurs fairly rapidly following application of topical nasal decongestants, thereby limiting the amount of active ingredient that reaches the systemic circulation.[40,51] However, nasal drops are difficult to administer and are often given incorrectly (e.g., excess quantities), which produces systemic absorption. Excess product drains into the stomach, with absorption causing systemic adverse reactions.[46] This eventuality can be prevented by proper administration of nasal drops. The patient should lie on the back across a bed, hanging the head over the edge of the bed and hyperextending the neck so that the patient is looking at a point behind him where the wall and floor meet.[52] The patient should remain in that position for 2 minutes or longer to allow absorption into the nasal mucosa.

tip *Imidazolines can produce arrhythmias—possibly as a result of coronary vasoconstriction—and should not be used by patients with heart disease.[46]*

tip *Topical nasal decongestants produce generalized vasoconstriction and also alter the balance of insulin and glucose in a diabetic, causing these medications to be contraindicated in the patient with diabetes mellitus.[46]*

Rhinitis Medicamentosa

The dramatic and rapid degree of relief afforded by topical nasal decongestants fosters abuse.[40] Patients tend to use them too frequently and for too prolonged a period.[46] Coupled with this is the problem of tachyphylaxis, in which repeated use lessens their effectiveness, which also makes patients tend to overuse the product.[32] Usage more frequently or longer than recommended causes a phenomenon known as rhinitis medicamentosa, in which the nasal mucosa rebounds to a more congested and edematous state as the product's effects subside.[53] Thus the patient tends to use more product to relieve the condition that the ingredient is

causing, perpetuating the condition.[46,54,55] Physician inspection of the patient with rhinitis medicamentosa shows nasal mucosa that is vasodilated, obstructed, reddened, and inflamed, producing watery rhinorrhea.[32] The optimal treatment is intervention to stop the vicious cycle through abrupt cessation of all topical vasoconstrictors.[32] Intense patient education is also needed to prevent recurrences.[33]

Rhinitis medicamentosa may be a form of **reactive hyperemia** (a phenomenon wherein excess blood rushes into an area when a temporary interruption of flow ceases, allowing free flow to resume), similar to the reaction commonly seen when one uncrosses one's legs. The leg that has borne the weight of the opposing leg reacts to the mechanical hypoxia with a reddened flush that signals a heightened blood flow into the area. Vasoconstriction via topical agents may also result in a reflexive hyperemia that is interpreted by the patient as stuffiness requiring additional topical nasal decongestant.[53] A worst-case scenario was seen when a 34-year-old patient presenting to the emergency room was found to be using three to four bottles of oxymetazoline and phenylephrine each day.[56] The medications were partly responsible for severe hypertension, cardiomegaly, and CHF. Craving his withheld nasal drops, the patient signed out against medical advice and was still abusing the products at the time of the report.

The neonate is particularly susceptible to the dangers of rhinitis medicamentosa, being an obligate nasal breather until 2 months of age.[32,41] Use of topical nasal decongestants in these infants can cause life-threatening cyanosis, apnea, respiratory distress, and cor pulmonale.[32,44]

ORAL NASAL DECONGESTANTS
Dosage Forms

Oral nasal decongestants are sympathomimetics that activate alpha-adrenergic receptors in nasal blood vessels to cause contraction of the smooth muscle of the nasal blood vessels (Table 15.4).[51,53] Pseudoephedrine is also a beta stimulant.[27] The resulting vasoconstriction facilitates breathing. Single-entity oral nasal decongestants, available as solutions, tablets, and capsules, are combined with other ingredients in these dosage forms and also in powder packets that are mixed in a hot or cold fluid prior to ingestion. While the onset of action of oral nasal decongestants is slower than that of topicals, they do reach all areas of the mucosa, unlike topicals.[41]

Required Labeling

The label of an oral nasal decongestant should warn the patient not to exceed the recommended dosage.[26] It will also caution patients that, if nervousness, dizziness, or sleeplessness occur, that the product should be discontinued and a

tip physician should be consulted. *Should patients also have fever, or should the symptoms fail to improve in 7 days, patients should also consult a physician. The label should warn that usage is prohibited unless recommended by a physician for patients with heart disease, high blood pressure, thyroid disease, diabetes, or difficulty in urination caused by enlargement of the prostate gland.*

Table 15.4. Representative Oral Nasal Decongestant Products

PRODUCT	SELECTED INGREDIENTS/COMMENTS
Drixoral Non-Drowsy Tablets	Pseudoephedrine sulfate 120 mg
PediaCare Infant Drops Decongestant	Pseudoephedrine HCl 7.5 mg/0.8 mL (Be cautious of infant dosing charts provided by the company)
Sudafed Children's Non-Drowsy Syrup	Pseudoephedrine HCl 15 mg/5 mL
Sudafed Tablets	Pseudoephedrine HCl 30 mg
Sudafed 12-Hour Tablets	Pseudoephedrine HCl 120 mg

(tip) *Products containing oral nasal decongestants will carry the following drug interaction warning: "Do not take this product if you are now taking a prescription monoamine oxidase inhibitor (MAOI) (certain drugs for depression, psychiatric or emotional conditions, or Parkinson's disease), or for 2 weeks after stopping the MAOI drug. If you are uncertain whether your prescription drug contains an MAOI, consult a health professional before taking this product."*[26]

See "Adverse Reactions of Oral Nasal Decongestants."

Phenylephrine Hydrochloride

Phenylephrine hydrochloride can be given orally every 4 hours a maximum of six times in 24 hours in the following dosages:

- 2.5 mg per dose (2 years and older)
- 5 mg per dose (6 years and older)
- 10 mg per dose (12 years and older).

There is no approved dose for patients younger than 2. No leading nonprescription oral product contains phenylephrine at this time.

Pseudoephedrine Hydrochloride/Sulfate

(tip) *Pseudoephedrine hydrochloride/sulfate is given orally every 4 to 6 hours a maximum of four times in 24 hours in the following doses:*

- *15 mg per dose (2 years and older)*
- *30 mg per dose (6 years and older)*
- *60 mg per dose (12 years and older).*

There is no approved dose for patients younger than 2. Pseudoephedrine is a popular ingredient in nonprescription cold products. The pharmacist must be wary of customers who attempt to purchase large quantities of pseudoephedrine tablets repeatedly. Because it is used in the illegal manufacture of methamphetamine and methcathinone (a so-called "designer drug"), the DEA proposed requiring pharmacies that sell more than a 120-day supply of pseudoephedrine to a single customer to keep records of such sales and to report them to the DEA.[57]

Phenylpropanolamine Hydrochloride

Phenylpropanolamine hydrochloride (popularly referred to as PPA) was recommended for Category I placement by the Review Panel in the original cough-cold monograph.[40] However, in the Phase 2 document, the FDA stated that it became aware of reports of blood pressure elevation with PPA.[46] Because of that, the FDA revoked the Category I designation for PPA and declined to discuss it further, stating that a future Federal Register publication would address the issue. PPA remained in limbo when the final monograph on oral nasal decongestants appeared in 1994.[26] The FDA repeated that the safety issues were still unresolved, and again deferred action on PPA, not assigning it a category designation. In the long-awaited 1996 Federal Register publication, the agency asked for information regarding hypertension, stroke, seizure, and the risk factors (e.g., hypertension, age, use of other medications, disease conditions) that increase the dangers of PPA.[58] The risk of hemorrhagic stroke was suggested by reports of intracranial bleeding in young females who use PPA for weight control. The FDA cautioned the public that the studies and their assessment would not be completed until 1998, but allowed marketing during this time since the agency did not feel that PPA presented a substantial health risk. While the studies were being carried out and evaluated, additional voluntary warnings proposed by industry appeared on product packages, with capitalization and bold printing proposed by the FDA in certain locations for increased emphasis. (See "Components of Voluntary Phenylpropanolamine Labeling.") This voluntary labeling was in some cases expanded on the warnings and precautions previously required for PPA and still required for other oral nasal decongestants.

Until these safety issues are fully resolved and the ingredient exonerated, pharmacists should be extremely cautious in recommending self-therapy with PPA.[27,51] Although it is found in many top-selling nonprescription products, some physicians have suggested that PPA's status as a nonprescription ingredient may not be appropriate, and that the FDA should carefully examine its safety.[59,60] PPA is also sold as a street substitute for amphetamines.[61–63]

ANTIHISTAMINES

The FDA OTC Review Panel originally assigned to cold products concluded that antihistamines could not be labeled as providing relief from rhinorrhea and sneezing of the common cold because of insufficient evidence.[40] However, industry studies submitted to the FDA prior to publication of the Phase 2 document provided evidence that chlorpheniramine effectively relieved runny nose and sneezing associated with the common cold.[90] In an unusual move, the agency concluded that, "Because the pharmacologic actions of the various Category I antihistamines are similar," that Category I status would be extended to all antihistamines. The FDA later reversed this decision, citing concerns that the pharmacologic effects of newer antihistamines might not reflect those of the older agents.[91] There was also concern that histamine is not the cause of common cold symptoms.[10,92] Because of these problems, the FDA announced that it would reconsider more recent studies of other antihistamines for the common cold, and deferred a final decision.[91] Two FDA committees voted in 1995 to continue approval for chlorpheniramine and doxylamine for relief of rhinorrhea and sneezing associated with the cold.[93] They also voted

---

FOCUS ON...

COMPONENTS OF VOLUNTARY PHENYLPROPANOLAMINE LABELING

(a) **DO NOT TAKE MORE THAN** 75 milligrams per day (24 hours). Taking more can be harmful.

(b) **DO NOT TAKE if you have the following:**

- Heart or thyroid disease
- High blood pressure
- An enlarged prostate gland

Unless directed by a doctor.

(c) **STOP USING IF you develop the following:**

- Nervousness
- Dizziness
- Sleeplessness
- Headache
- Palpitations

If symptoms continue, ask a doctor.

(d) **DO NOT USE WITH**

- A monoamine oxidase inhibitor (MAOI) (certain drugs for depression, psychiatric or emotional conditions, or Parkinson's disease), or for 2 weeks after stopping the MAOI drug. If unsure, ask a health professional.
- Any allergy, asthma, cough-cold, nasal decongestant, or weight control product (containing phenylpropanolamine, phenylephrine, pseudoephedrine, or ephedrine), or any prescription drug, unless directed by a doctor.

---

approval of this labeling for clemastine fumarate. Other antihistamines are of unknown worth for the common cold at present. Further, combination decongestant-antihistamine products that include unapproved ingredients simply add potential adverse reactions and contraindications without providing any proven benefit.

See "A Pharmacist's Journal: What Is in PediaCare That My Son's Cardiologist Doesn't Like?"

HYPOTONIC SODIUM CHLORIDE SOLUTIONS
During dry seasons, patients complain of dry nasal crusting that inhibits breathing and cannot be easily removed. Several manufacturers market 0.65% sodium chloride drops and sprays such as those listed in Table 15.5. Being hypotonic, they rehydrate nasal mucosa and liquefy dry secretions for easier removal.

Other Therapies: Devices to Reduce Nasal Congestion

Several devices may provide relief of nasal congestion. The older of the two is the simple nasal aspirator, a rubber bulb with a blunt plastic tip. Small nasal aspirators are often part of the "baby kit" that new mothers are given during the perinatal hospitalization period. The parent squeezes the bulb, inserting the tip of the aspirator into the plugged nostril. When the bulb is released, negative pressure may suck nasal secretions into the bulb. The procedure may be repeated on that nostril or the opposing nostril. The nasal aspirator must

be cleaned and dried thoroughly between uses to prevent cross-contamination.

A new device, the Breathe Right Nasal Dilator, is being aggressively marketed as an alternative therapy for nasal congestion. Consisting of a slender adhesive-backed plastic strip, the dilator is used by bending the plastic strip over the nose (between the bridge and the tip), pressing the strip into place, then releasing it. As the plastic strip attempts to resume its original flattened state, the adhesive pulls the nostrils into a more open state. The strip has received FDA approval as a medical device for relief of nasal congestion and snoring.[94–97] The product is available in Junior/Small, Small/Medium, and Medium/Large sizes. A transparent option is also available.

SORE THROAT ASSOCIATED WITH THE COMMON COLD

PREVALENCE OF SORE THROAT

Within any 2-week period, approximately 12% of adults suffer a sore throat.[98,99] The average adult experiences two to three sore throats per year.

EPIDEMIOLOGY OF SORE THROAT

Age studies of sore throat show that the distribution is bimodal, at the ages of 7 and 20.[98] In the majority of cases, the common cold is viral in origin, so that the epidemiology is similar to that of the common cold and other viral diseases.[100,101] Figure 15.2 shows a normal throat; Figure 15.3 compares the throat affected by viral pharyngitis to a throat affected with streptococcal pharyngitis.

ETIOLOGY OF SORE THROAT

As discussed earlier, a sore throat is often the initial symptom of the common cold. However, the pharmacist must not fall into the trap of assuming that all sore throat is related to the common cold. Sore throat is a symptom with many possible causes, some fatal if not seen by a physician. For instance, the sore throat may signal the presence of the following serious disorders and causes:

- Aplastic anemia
- Agranulocytosis
- Acute leukemia
- Viral diseases (e.g., measles, chickenpox, poliomyelitis, adenoviruses, influenza, herpes virus)
- Bacterial infections (e.g., diphtheria, scarlet fever, oral gonorrhea, streptococcal infection)
- Fungal infections (e.g., following use of oral antibiotics or as a result of an immunocompromised state)[98,102,103]
- Irritating foods or drinks
- **Postnasal drip** (purulent and thick nasal or pharyngeal secretions)
- Allergic rhinitis
- Gastroesophageal reflux
- Mouth breathing
- Inhalation of irritating fumes (e.g., smoke from fires or cigarettes) or noxious gases (e.g., chlorine)[98,101–104]

Trauma may induce sore throat such as from ingestion of foreign bodies (glass, fish bones, sharp pieces of bone) that scratch the

FOCUS ON...

ADVERSE REACTIONS OF ORAL NASAL DECONGESTANTS

Oral nasal decongestants potentially affect many body systems through activating extranasal alpha-receptors:[39]

- CNS reactions include anorexia, insomnia, excitation, headache, and irritability.
- The systemic vasculature is altered, elevating blood pressure.
- Urinary tract dysfunction may result in dysuria.[64]
- Oral (and topical) decongestants may produce impotence.[65]
- Cardiac symptoms include palpitations and tachycardia.

Unlike the topical agents, they do not cause rhinitis medicamentosa.[39]

While there have been scattered reports of the dangers of oral phenylephrine and pseudoephedrine, these dangers are dwarfed in both number and severity by the vast body of literature pertaining to phenylpropanolamine.

In some of the reports, severe danger resulted from doses just above those recommended by the manufacturer, illustrating the narrow margin of safety of PPA. As an example, a 25-year-old woman who wished to obtain relief from persistent symptoms of upper respiratory infection took four capsules of cold product, for a total dose of 600 mg of PPA and 48 mg of chlorpheniramine maleate.[60] She suffered hypertensive crisis, which necessitated several emergency interventions and admission to an intensive care unit. The authors cited an earlier study that listed eight deaths caused by PPA (caused by intracranial hemorrhage, cardiopulmonary arrest, and arrhythmia). A later correspondent referred to this patient, stressing that the cause of the patient's toxicity was more likely extreme sympathetic stimulation.[66]

As the above report indicated, PPA affects blood pressure.[58,67–69] One source states that single doses are probably safe in normotensive individuals, but are unsafe in those with preexisting hypertension.[70] However, the individual cited above did not have a previous problem with blood pressure. Further, other research demonstrated that conventional doses of a commercially available nonprescription product containing PPA caused significant increases in blood pressure in healthy young volunteers.[71] Some of the increases were startling: one patient's pressures rose from 106/69 to 168/96. In one case a 13-year-old girl ingested a capsule containing 75 mg of PPA, suffering hypertensive seizures as a result.[72] Hypertension may be accompanied by severe, throbbing bilateral headache.[61] PPA has also been implicated as a causal factor in stroke, intracranial hemorrhage, and sudden massive hemorrhage.[73–76] Cardiac arrhythmias may occur with normal dosing or with intentional overdosing.[77–79]

PPA is associated with many psychiatric reactions, but the most common is paranoid psychosis, which may persist after the medication is discontinued.[61,80,81] In one case a 55-year-old man took ten capsules containing 50 mg each of PPA daily for several months. On hospital admission, pathology included a 6-week history of withdrawal and abnormal behavior, including paranoid delusions that passersby were undercover "hit men" who were involved in a plot to kill him.[82] He had attempted to blow himself up so that he might elude his prosecutors. Complete recovery took 2 months. A report of seven patients documented amphetamine-like CNS effects attributed to PPA, including stimulation of the medullary respiratory center, tremor, restlessness, increased motor activity, agitation, and hallucinations.[83] Other psychiatric reactions reported with PPA include persecutory delusions, maniclike states, and déjà vu experiences.[61] In one case PPA was implicated so clearly in a mental disturbance that included aural hallucinations that the primary diagnosis was "Phenylpropanolamine Affective Disorder."[84] A 29-year-old student ingested 180 to 480 mL of PPA-containing cough syrup to combat depression and induce mania.[85] During one PPA-induced episode, he engaged in expensive shopping sprees, believing himself to be an undiscovered musical genius who had divine revelations. On discontinuation of PPA, all symptoms resolved rapidly.

Continued

mucosa or from damage to the external neck, perhaps as a result of child abuse.[100] All of these serious causes of sore throat mandate immediate physician referral for full evaluation.

Occasionally, the pharmacist may encounter the patient with a sore throat who also complains of painful dysphagia, respiratory distress, and fever.[105] The patient may have acute **epiglottitis** (inflammation of the epiglottis), a cause of sore throat that can be fatal by causing sudden lethal airway obstruction.[100] (Indirect laryngoscopy confirms the diagnosis.) Antibiotics and epinephrine (parenteral or via nebulizer) may be necessary.[106] In no case can nonprescription products be recommended. The FDA became aware of reports of 4 incidents of life-threatening laryngeal spasm (including one death) in the U.K. that occurred when individuals who may have had acute epiglottitis were given phenol-containing sore throat products.[107] On further investigation, the FDA discovered additional reports of this adverse reaction associated with use of phenol (24 cases), dyclonine (38 cases), benzocaine (4 cases), and 3 cases each involving benzyl alcohol, menthol, and hexylresorcinol.

Other adverse reactions attributed to PPA, in descending order of frequency, are nausea and emesis, anxiety, palpitations, **paresthesias** (strange sensations such as stinging or burning), tremor, tachycardia, myalgias, reversible renal failure, increased intracerebral pressure verified by lumbar puncture, disorientation to person, place, or time, bizarre behavior (e.g., disrobing in public), and suicidal behavior.[61,86,87] PPA also causes rare reactions such as acute renal failure and **rhabdomyolysis** (loss of muscle tissue through dissolving or disintegrating).[88,89]

Special mention should also be made of streptococcal pharyngitis ("strep throat"), a sore throat caused by streptococcal infection, because it is relatively more common than the other serious etiologies.[101] (About 30% of sore throats are streptococcal.[98,108]) Strep throat is usually caused by beta-hemolytic streptococcus, group A.[98,109] The infection is usually contracted through person-to-person transmission, although infected food may also be the causative agent.[110] The age-associated epidemiology exhibits a bimodal distribution, with peaks at 5 to 9 and 30 to 39 years of age.[111]

Streptococcal sore throat is usually extremely red and painful, of sudden onset, accompanied by halitosis, fever, headache, enlarged tender cervical lymph nodes, and tonsillar exudate.[98,110,112–114] Children are more likely than adults

A Pharmacist's Journal

"What Is in PediaCare That My Son's Cardiologist Doesn't Like?"

A young woman in her early 20s approached holding a box of PediaCare (containing 7.5 mg pseudoephedrine and 2.5 mg dextromethorphan per 0.8 mL) and Dimetapp Decongestant Drops (a single-entity product containing 7.5 mg pseudoephedrine per 0.8 mL). She asked, "What is in PediaCare that my son's cardiologist doesn't like? I wanted to give him PediaCare for his allergies, but his cardiologist said he'd prefer Dimetapp." I first asked the age of her son. She replied that he was four months old. I asked what his condition was. She said, "He's had aortic stenosis since birth." She said the cardiologist was worried about the effect of PediaCare on the child's heart and wanted him to use Dimetapp instead. I showed her the warning on the box of PediaCare against use in heart disease, and then pointed out that the same warning is on the box of Dimetapp Decongestant Drops, since pseudoephedrine is in both products. I then discussed the confusion in Dimetapp. "You know, the Dimetapp Decongestant is fairly new. I'll bet that

the cardiologist was referring to the regular Dimetapp. But that product contains phenylpropanolamine, which also causes problems with heart disease." She then replied, "But aortic stenosis isn't really a heart disease, is it?" I explained that any of the nasal decongestants could potentially increase the workload of the heart, and her son's heart is perhaps already stressed, depending on the severity of aortic narrowing. Further, I discussed the issue of the products being contraindicated under the age of 2 (decongestants) or 6 (antihistamines). The cardiologist had not given her a dose to use. I ventured the opinion, "It's difficult for physicians to keep up with these products. The cardiologist may not know that Dimetapp has a decongestant. If you are really going to use one of them, please have it in hand and call the cardiologist's office to let them know it contains an ingredient that can increase the workload of the heart and ask them what dose to give." After hearing this, she replied, "I'm taking my son to his pediatrician this afternoon. Maybe I'll ask him first." I told her that would be helpful, but urged that she stay in contact with the cardiologist also.

Table 15.5. Representative Hypotonic Sodium Chloride Nasal Products

PRODUCT	SELECTED INGREDIENTS
Afrin Saline Mist	Sodium chloride 0.65%
Ayr Nasal Mist	Sodium chloride 0.65%
Ocean Nasal Spray	Sodium chloride 0.65%

A. Viral pharyngitis

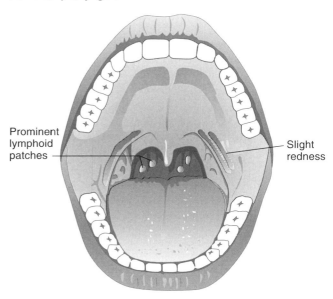

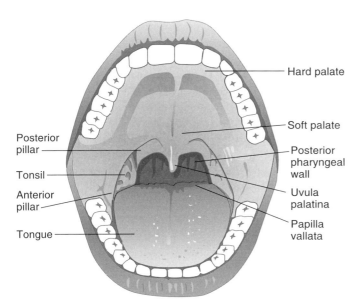

Figure 15.2. A normal throat as seen on superficial examination.

B. Streptococcal pharyngitis

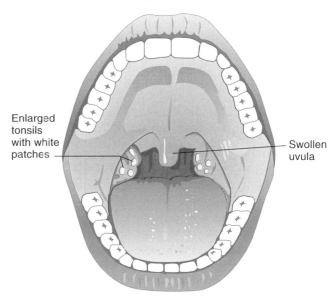

to experience pain, nausea, and vomiting as concurrent symptoms.[108] Concurrent cough and rhinorrhea are not as likely in strep throat as in the common cold.[108,109] As many as 20% of patients do not exhibit any symptoms.[113]

Streptococcal pharyngitis may result in rheumatic fever, glomerulonephritis, **erythema nodosum** (acute skin disease with erythematous nodules, itching, and burning), otitis media, sinusitis, mastoiditis, and peritonsillar abscess.[98,102] While most patients with strep throat spontaneously recover, it is not possible to predict exactly who will do so.[115] Appropriate therapy is systemic antibiotics (e.g., penicillin V, cephalosporins, erythromycin).[98,101,109,116]

MANIFESTATIONS OF SORE THROAT

The patient with sore throat caused by common cold viruses is usually troubled by a mild, scratchy feeling of discomfort, especially on swallowing.[102] The discomfort may proceed to an overt burning or painful feeling. However, severity of sore throat depends on the individual's unique response to pain. Some would describe strep throat as a minor discomfort, while others would describe sore throat of the common cold as a major problem.

Figure 15.3. A. Viral pharyngitis exhibits few visible signs. Mild redness, slight inflammation, and prominent lymphoid patches on the posterior pharyngeal wall may all be present. **B.** Streptococcal pharyngitis produces erythema, inflammation, and white patches on the tonsils.

TREATMENT OF SORE THROAT ASSOCIATED WITH THE COMMON COLD

Treatment Guidelines

 As noted above, *pharmacists would be well advised to limit sore throat product recommendations to patients*

with the common cold. Asking patients about concurrent nasal involvement and cough may be the optimal method to ensure that the patient has a common cold. It may be helpful to ascertain whether family members also have common cold symptoms.[100]

It is also useful to ask about severity, although the picture is clouded by the subjective responses described above. The common cold peaks of September, October, and early spring should aid in recognition of viral sore throat. (Strep throat occurs evenly throughout the year.[98]) (Patient Assessment Algorithm 15.2)

Nonprescription Products

While sore throat of the common cold is virally induced, no antiseptics exist that would be useful when applied topically to the throat.[117] This limits the pharmacist intervention to providing relief of discomfort, either topically or systemically with products such as those listed in Table 15.6. Topical sore throat products carry numerous FDA-mandated warnings

tip and precautions. *The first set of precautions is implied in the indications section for topical agents: "For the temporary relief of occasional minor irritation, pain, sore mouth and sore throat."*[107] Therefore, if the patient has a sore

Patient Assessment Algorithm 15.2. Sore Throat

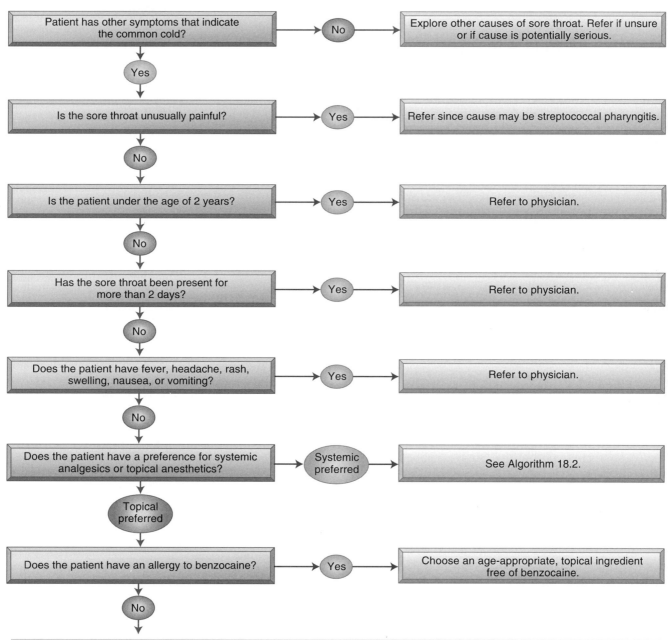

Patient has other symptoms that indicate the common cold? — No → Explore other causes of sore throat. Refer if unsure or if cause is potentially serious.

Yes ↓

Is the sore throat unusually painful? — Yes → Refer since cause may be streptococcal pharyngitis.

No ↓

Is the patient under the age of 2 years? — Yes → Refer to physician.

No ↓

Has the sore throat been present for more than 2 days? — Yes → Refer to physician.

No ↓

Does the patient have fever, headache, rash, swelling, nausea, or vomiting? — Yes → Refer to physician.

No ↓

Does the patient have a preference for systemic analgesics or topical anesthetics? — Systemic preferred → See Algorithm 18.2.

Topical preferred ↓

Does the patient have an allergy to benzocaine? — Yes → Choose an age-appropriate, topical ingredient free of benzocaine.

No ↓

Suggest product containing benzyl alcohol, butacaine, phenol, sodium phenolate, dyclonine, hexylresorcinol, or menthol, as appropriate for the patient's age (patient may take a systemic analgesic concurrently if desired).

Table 15.6. Representative Sore Throat Products

PRODUCT	SELECTED INGREDIENTS/COMMENTS
Aspergum	Aspirin 227 mg (not proven effective in this dosage form as a topical anesthetic for sore throat)
Cepastat Cherry Lozenges	Phenol 14.5 mg
Cepastat Extra Strength Lozenges	Phenol 29 mg
Halls Juniors Grape Lozenges	Menthol 2.5 mg
Halls Mentho-Lyptus Lozenges	Menthol 5–8.4 mg (concentration depends on flavor chosen)
Halls Plus Lozenges	Menthol 10 mg
Luden's Honey-Lemon Throat Drops	Menthol (amount not labeled)
Luden's Original Menthol Throat Drops	Menthol (amount not labeled)
Luden's Wild Cherry Throat Drops	Pectin, sugar
N'Ice Lozenges	Menthol 5 mg
Ricola Natural Honey-Herb Lozenges	Menthol (amount not labeled)
Robitussin Cough Drops	Menthol 7.4–10 mg (concentration depends on flavor chosen)
Sucrets Original Mint Lozenges	Hexylresorcinol 2.4 mg
Sucrets Wild Cherry Lozenges	Dyclonine HCl 2 mg
Sucrets Wintergreen Lozenges	Dyclonine HCl 3 mg
Vicks Chloraseptic Lozenges	Benzocaine 6 mg, menthol 10 mg; menthol or cherry
Vicks Chloraseptic Sprays	Phenol 1.4%; menthol or cherry

throat that is not occasional or minor, the products are clearly contraindicated. Further, *the products should warn, "If sore throat is severe, persists for more than 2 days, is accompanied or followed by fever, headache, rash, swelling, nausea, or vomiting, consult a doctor promptly."* All of these symptoms indicate a possible serious pathologic process (for instance, a rash with sore throat may be diagnostic for scarlet fever).[98] *The youngest age for which self-treatment is allowed is 2 years, for both oral and systemic products.*

TOPICAL NONPRESCRIPTION INGREDIENTS FOR SORE THROAT

The optimal dosage forms for sore throat are lozenges or sprays.[102] Both reach pharyngeal structures adequately. Lozenges are hard molded candies whose local anesthetics are released as they dissolve slowly in the mouth. The time limit for self-medication must be observed. One physician has noted several cases of patients who had used phenol sprays excessively.[118] Both suffered continual pharyngitis, which the author hypothesized was caused by product overuse. He christened this syndrome "pharyngitis medicamentosa."

In general, the patient is advised to use nonprescription throat lozenges every 2 hours.[107] Lozenges are limited to patients older than 2 (or older than 6 in the case of phenol/sodium phenolate). Liquid dosage forms are used by applying to the affected area (for example, by spraying),

swishing or gargling for 1 minute (or 15 seconds in the case of phenol/phenolate sodium), then expectorating, then repeating up to 4 times daily. Parents are directed to supervise use of liquid dosage forms for patients younger than 12.

Mouth rinses and gargles do not work as well as many people think. Research with colored solutions demonstrates that contact is limited to the oral cavity; the posterior pharyngeal wall is not affected by mouth rinses and gargles.[102] Perhaps the FDA includes gargle directions to allow treatment for the permissible labeled indication of sore mouth.

Permitted ingredients in topical sore throat anesthetics include benzyl alcohol, butacaine, phenol and sodium phenolate, dyclonine, hexylresorcinol, and menthol.

Benzocaine is also approved, but products containing benzocaine must carry the warning, "Do not use this product if you have a history of allergy to local anesthetics such as procaine, butacaine, benzocaine, or other "caine" anesthetics."[107]

SYSTEMIC NONPRESCRIPTION INGREDIENTS FOR SORE THROAT

Oral analgesics are also labeled as providing relief of sore throat, but they are covered extensively in Chapter 18. The labeling will be for "temporary relief of minor aches and pains associated with sore throat".[107] The sore throat labeling of systemic analgesics is essentially the same as that for topical analgesics, with one minor exception. Should an internal analgesic product carry a sore throat indication, it must carry the warning regarding concurrent symptoms, minus the caution against use with swelling.[119]

TOPICAL ASPIRIN FOR SORE THROAT

A topical aspirin gum has been sold for many years for sore throat. The panel assigned to these products disagreed on its efficacy when used topically.[102] The FDA agreed with the minority of the panel that the ingredient lacked sufficient data to allow final classification to be made, stating that the issue would be published under the auspices of the OTC internal analgesic review.[103] That panel confirmed that topical aspirin is devoid of local anesthetic effects, and that aspirin in a chewing gum would only be acceptable as a systemic product if it provided the minimum effective dose of 325 to 650 mg of aspirin per dose.[119]

COUGH ASSOCIATED WITH THE COMMON COLD

PREVALENCE OF COUGH

Cough is one of the most frequent reasons that patients seek medical help, and is a frequent symptom of the common cold.[120]

EPIDEMIOLOGY OF COUGH

The majority of coughs are associated with the common cold, thus their epidemiology is that of the common cold. However, chronic cough is common in young children, caused by consecutive upper respiratory tract infections.[24]

ETIOLOGY OF COUGH

Cough receptors located in the pharynx, stomach, external auditory canal, diaphragm, nose, and bifurcations of the large airways of the tracheobronchial tree initiate the cough reflex (Fig. 15.4).[120,121] Stimulation of these receptors causes neural activity that terminates in the central cough center in the upper brainstem and pons area of the brain.[122] Completion of the reflex arc results in an inspiratory gasp, a forceful contraction of the respiratory muscles against the closed glottis, which then suddenly opens.[24]

In many cases cough is protective, facilitating the removal of inhaled foreign particles and excessive secretions.[24,121] Most persons cough once or twice an hour when awake to clear the airways.[121]

The abrupt airway vibrations and high airflow velocity that cough produces are highly effective in mobilizing secretions; they also cause the characteristic sound of cough.[24] Suppressing the beneficial cough may delay pulmonary recovery from infection.[24] Cough is a symptom of underlying pathology, rather than a disease entity in itself.[120] When cough is

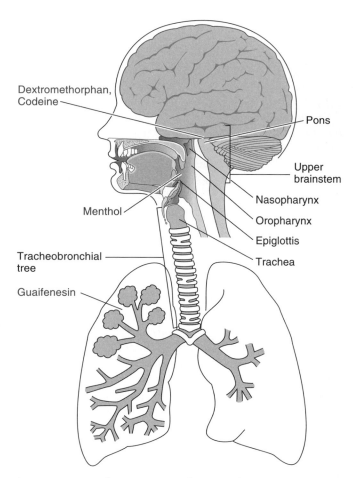

Figure 15.4. Cough originates in the upper brainstem and pons, which results in a cough reflex in the tracheobronchial tree. The sites of action of codeine, dextromethorphan, guaifenesin, and menthol are illustrated.

clearly the result of minor medical conditions such as the common cold, the pharmacist can allow self-treatment. However, if the pharmacist is not convinced that the cough etiology is the common cold, the patient must be referred for a full medical workup. Differential diagnosis of cough is difficult and extensive, including such etiologies as asthma, congenital heart defects, congestive heart failure, gastroesophageal reflux disease, cystic fibrosis, cigarette or wood fire exposure, inhalation of chlorine gas from swimming pool products, foreign body aspiration, immunodeficiency, pneumonia, mental aberration, glaucoma, and sinusitis.[24,121,123–135] Suppressing cough that is caused by a serious underlying disorder will mask the symptoms of the underlying disease.[24] Thus a minor symptom will abate while the medical condition continues unchecked.

The pharmacist must vigorously resist selling a cough suppressant to the smoker. Smoking of cigarettes, pipes, and cigars irritates the airways and produces chronic respiratory disease.[136,137] It also reduces the efficiency of the ciliated cells that move particle-laden mucus upwards for expectoration. Thus the traditional hacking smoker's cough actually aids the patient in mucokinesis, and morbidity may increase if this cough is suppressed. An expectorant may aid the smoker somewhat, but cessation of smoking reduces the incidence of cough by 50% and should be suggested as the best alternative for the coughing smoker. Eventually, the cough may abate in most patients following cessation.

tip Medications may induce cough. *About 15% of patients taking ACE inhibitors will experience a dry, hacking cough.[121,138–142]* These medications include benzapril hydrochloride (Lotensin), captopril (Capoten; also combined with hydrochlorothiazide in Capozide), enalapril maleate (Vasotec; also combined with hydrochlorothiazide in Vaseretic), fosinopril sodium (Monopril), lisinopril (Prinivil, Zestril; also combined with hydrochlorothiazide in Prinizide and Zestoretic), quinapril hydrochloride (Accupril), and ramipril (Altace). Beta-blockers may cause cough through narrowing the bronchioles.[121]

PROGNOSIS OF COUGH

The duration of the cough is a vital clue to etiology. Some single, upper-respiratory infections (influenza, adenovirus, *Bordetella pertussis*) produce ciliary defects that endure for as long as 10 weeks after the infection.[24] The patient suffers cough until normal ciliary activity is regained. Those with chronic persistent cough make up 10% of patients visiting outpatient pulmonary departments; it is the fifth most common symptom seen by primary care physicians.[142,143]

Some patients with chronic cough irritate the airways as they cough, which causes additional coughing. This irritant cough is nonproductive and may be helped with antitussive agents, if the patient has not yet exceeded the time cutoff for self-therapy. The most common causes of chronic cough are (in descending order) post nasal drip, bronchial asthma, GERD, chronic bronchitis, and **bronchiectasis** (chronic bronchial or bronchiolar dilation).[142,144]

COMPLICATIONS OF COUGH

Cough affects the musculoskeletal, pulmonary, cardiovascular, and central nervous systems.[120] It causes chest-wall pain,

muscle strain, dyspnea, fatigue, nausea and sleep disturbances.[121] Less common sequelae include rib fractures, **pneumothorax** (air or gas in the pleural cavity), syncope, urinary incontinence, and abdominal hernia.[142,145] Cough also plays a role in the transmission of disease.[146]

TREATMENT OF COUGH ASSOCIATED WITH THE COMMON COLD

Treatment Guidelines

When a patient with common cold requests medication for cough, the pharmacist must ascertain how long the cough has **tip** been present. *FDA-approved labeling for cough products cautions the patient that persistent cough may indicate a serious condition, and that a cough that persists for more than 1 week or tends to recur must not be self-treated.[147]*

The pharmacist must also ensure that the patient has a *minor* condition causing the cough. FDA-approved labeling will indicate that the product is useful for cough caused by minor bronchial irritation or minor throat irritation associated with the common cold or inhaled irritants.[147] *Labeling also will caution against use if the patient has* **tip** *fever, rash, or persistent headache. The label, too, will caution patients not to take the products if the patient has persistent or chronic cough such as that occurring with smoking, asthma, or emphysema, or if the cough is accompanied by excessive phlegm (sputum) unless directed by a physician.[147]* Assuming that the patient does not meet any of the FDA-mandated exclusions, the pharmacist must next discover the nature of the cough. A useful question is, "When you cough, do you feel loose secretions in your lungs?" Although couched in lay language, the question is designed to tailor therapy to the nature of cough. If the patient answers in the affirmative, the pharmacist may assume the presence of a productive cough that allows the patient to bring up accumulated mucus, preventing pneumonia (See Fig. 15.5). The productive cough must be allowed to continue to fully perform its cleansing function. It is difficult to make parents understand this. The parent simply wants all coughing to cease. A survey revealed that the reason for this fear of cough

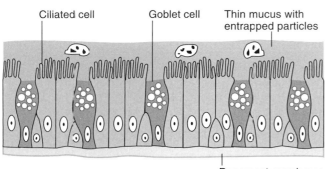

Ciliated cell   Goblet cell   Thin mucus with entrapped particles   Thick mucus that resists mucokinesis

Basement membrane

Figure 15.5. Mucus expectorated by the goblet cells, which entraps particles and pollution, can be easily moved upward by ciliated cells (*left*), unless it is excessively dried and thick (*right*).

is that parents fear that their children will die from choking on phlegm or vomit, will die from an attack of asthma, or will expire during their sleep.[148] Nevertheless, selling a child with productive cough a product that suppresses reflexive cough is counterproductive and could result in pneumonia because of retained secretions. However, the adult may be able to safely use these products if they are cautioned to periodically engage in voluntary coughing to help facilitate mukokinesis.

If the patient states that he or she does not feel secretions in the lungs, the pharmacist might next ask if the cough feels like a tight, dry hacking cough. If so, the pharmacist may assume the presence of a nonproductive cough, also known as the nuisance cough. This cough serves no purpose, and may be safely suppressed, as long as the pharmacist does not suspect that it is caused by any of the serious conditions previously mentioned.

The pharmacist must be aware of the ages below which self-treatment is not indicated for cough. Some companies market charts that purport to allow treatment below the ages at which the products are safe. (See "Pediatric Dosing Information.")

Nonprescription Medications

The FDA has approved numerous agents for relief of cough. They relieve cough through several mechanisms. Centrally acting agents (e.g., codeine, dextromethorphan, diphenhydramine) suppress the central cough center and others (e.g., camphor, menthol, guaifenesin) exert peripheral effects (Patient Assessment Algorithm 15.3).

CODEINE

Although codeine and its derivatives are usually prescription products, over 30 states allow nonprescription sales of certain properly labeled cough medications containing codeine, codeine sulfate, or codeine phosphate (Table 15.7).[149] These Schedule V narcotic nonprescription products have restrictions on their sale such as keeping a record of sales, verifying identity, and limiting sales to the same individual over a specified time. (The licenses of two Oklahoma pharmacists were suspended for 2 years for exceeding the sales limit of 48 hours to the same individual.[150])

Because of its abuse potential, the pharmacist should be suspicious of the patient who requests a codeine-containing product without trying the nonaddictive products. It may be most prudent to refuse to sell the products unless there is a justifiable reason to do so. Further, since codeine suppresses cough, it is not the preferred agent for a productive cough.

The labels of codeine-containing products must warn the patient that they may cause or aggravate constipation.[147] *Labels should caution against use if the patient has a chronic pulmonary disease or shortness of breath unless directed by a physician. Products labeled for children will caution against use if the child is taking other medications unless directed by a physician. Codeine is not to be recommended for children younger than 6.* The label should state that a special measuring device must be used to ensure accurate dosing if a physician recommends a dose

for a child younger than 6 and must clearly state that giving a higher dose than recommended by a doctor could result in serious side effects.

Codeine is given orally every 4 to 6 hours in the following doses:

- 5 to 10 mg with a daily maximum of 60 mg (6 years and older)
- 10 to 20 mg per dose with a daily maximum of 120 mg (12 years and older).

DEXTROMETHORPHAN

Dextromethorphan and its hydrobromide salt are alternative central agents that have little addictive potential and few adverse reactions (Table 15.8). Dextromethorphan hydrobromide is given orally as follows:

- Patients 2 and older may take 2.5 to 5 mg every 4 hours or 7.5 mg every 6 to 8 hours (not exceeding 30 mg/24 hours)
- Patients 6 and older may take 5 to 10 mg every 4 hours or 15 mg every 6 to 8 hours (not exceeding 60 mg/24 hours)
- Patients 12 and older may take 10 to 20 mg every 4 hours or 30 mg every 6 to 8 hours (not exceeding 120 mg/24 hours).

The ingredient's safety has not yet been demonstrated for children younger than 2. Dextromethorphan caused an unusual series of severe reactions in patients taking MAOI medications.[151] Concomitant use with phenelzine (Nardil) was responsible for two deaths and two hypertensive reactions, one that resulted in intracerebral bleeding. Concurrent isocarboxazid (Marplan) use caused persistent myoclonic jerking of the legs as long as 2 months after ingestion. Concomitant use with tranylcypromine (Parnate) resulted in psychotic reactions and hallucinations. *As a result of these problems, the FDA-mandated warning will read: "Do not use this product if you are now taking a prescription monoamine oxidase inhibitor (MAOI) (certain drugs for depression, psychiatric or emotional conditions, or Parkinson's disease), or for 2 weeks after stopping the MAOI drug. If you are uncertain whether your prescription drug contains an MAOI, consult a health professional before taking this product."*[152]

DIPHENHYDRAMINE

Diphenhydramine was approved for cough at one time, but the FDA expressed concern about the anticholinergic action of the ingredient drying secretions, which would hamper expectoration of mucus.[151,153,154] All diphenhydramine-containing combinations were given either Category II or III status. As an antihistamine, diphenhydramine is not approved for those aged under 6, limiting its utility greatly. It carries many FDA-required warnings. *Diphenhydramine may cause excitability, especially in children. It should not be given to patients who have breathing problems (such as emphysema or chronic bronchitis), glaucoma, or difficulty in urination caused by an enlarged prostate gland.* Patients are warned that *it causes marked drowsiness* and that the effect is increased with concomitant use of

Patient Assessment Algorithm 15.3. Cough

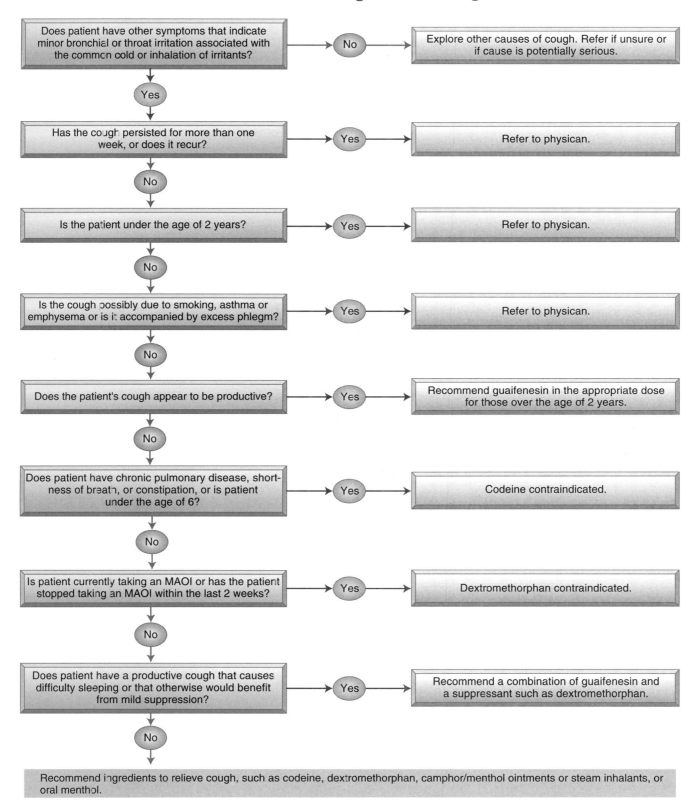

tip alcohol, sedatives, and tranquilizers. *The patient should exercise caution when driving or operating heavy machinery.* The manufacturer marketing the major diphenhydramine-containing cough syrup eliminated this in- gredient in a reformulation of the entire product line. As a result, it dramatically decreased in importance as an antitussive. In light of its many precautions and contraindications, diphenhydramine has been superseded by safer agents.

Table 15.7. Representative Cough Products Containing Codeine

PRODUCT	SELECTED INGREDIENTS/COMMENTS
Cheracol Syrup	Per 5 mL: codeine phosphate 10 mg; guaifenesin 100 mg
Naldecon-CX Syrup	Per 5 mL: codeine phosphate 10 mg; guaifenesin 200 mg, phenylpropanolamine HCl 12.5 mg (an unapproved decongestant)
Novahistine-DH Syrup	Per 5 mL: codeine phosphate 10 mg; pseudoephedrine HCl 30 mg; chlorpheniramine maleate 2 mg
Robitussin AC Syrup	Per 5 mL: codeine phosphate 10 mg; guaifenesin 100 mg

Table 15.8. Representative Cough Products Containing Dextromethorphan

PRODUCT	SELECTED INGREDIENTS/COMMENTS
Benylin Pediatric Syrup	Per 5 mL: dextromethorphan hydrobromide 7.5 mg
Delsym Cough Formula Suspension	Per 5 mL: dextromethorphan polistirex equivalent to dextromethorphan hydrobromide 30 mg
Hold DM Lozenges	Dextromethorphan hydrobromide 5 mg (not approved in this dosage form)
Robitussin Maximum Strength Cough Syrup	Per 5 mL: dextromethorphan hydrobromide 15 mg
Robitussin Pediatric Syrup	Per 5 mL: dextromethorphan hydrobromide 7.5 mg

CAMPHOR OR MENTHOL OINTMENTS

Several ointments are sold for the alleviation of cough (Table 15.9). Ointments containing 4.7 to 5.3% camphor or 2.6 to 2.8% menthol are approved for cough.[155] *Patients older than 2 apply the product by rubbing on the throat and chest in a thick layer no more than three times daily.* If desired, the patient may cover the site of application with a warm, dry cloth. The clothing is left loose around the throat and chest, and the vapors rise to the nose and mouth. *Labels of these products must caution the patient that they are for external use only and must not be taken by mouth or placed into the nostrils.*

CAMPHOR OR MENTHOL STEAM INHALANTS

Steam inhalants containing 6.2% camphor or 3.2% menthol are also approved for cough (Table 15.10). *For patients aged 2 and over add 5 mL of solution to a quart of hot water in the reservoir of a steam vaporizer, in a bowl, or in a wash basin.* (See the discussion of vaporizers in Chapter 16.) Alternatively, the Federal Register advises that 7.5 mL may be added to a pint of water in a boiling open container. The patient then breathes in the medicated vapors up to three times daily. *The containers of these products will caution patients that they are for steam inhalation only and must not be taken by mouth.* As noted in Chapter 16, manufacturers of vaporizers contradict the FDA-approved labeling, cautioning patients against adding medication directly to the reservoir, as the oils could coat the electrodes,

compromising the vaporizer's efficacy. The manufacturers suggest that they use the medication cup instead, which is the method pharmacists should recommend. Although some might be concerned about inhalation of volatile oils causing inhalation pneumonia, this potential risk has not been reported.

The safety of placing volatile oils in open containers of boiling water is hazardous. Hazards include steam burns and contact burns from accidental spills, so that this latter method should not be recommended by pharmacists.

ORAL MENTHOL

Lozenges or compressed tablets containing 5 to 10 mg of menthol per unit can be effective for cough through acting on nerve receptors within the respiratory tract to produce a local anesthetic effect (Table 15.11).[147,155] *Patients aged over 2 allow the product to dissolve slowly in the mouth once hourly or as directed by a physician.*

GUAIFENESIN

Guaifenesin is the only antitussive agent that acts as an expectorant. Expectorants are mucokinetic agents that loosen sputum and thin bronchial secretions to make the cough more productive.[156] They may accomplish this by irritating the gastric mucosa, which produces a reflex increase in respiratory tract secretions. Guaifenesin is therefore best suited for the productive cough, and is irrational for the dry, hack-

Table 15.9. Representative Cough Products Containing Camphor/Menthol in Cream/Ointment Form

PRODUCT	SELECTED INGREDIENTS/COMMENTS
Mentholatum Ointment	Camphor 9%, menthol 1.3% (subtherapeutic concentration of menthol for cough; supertherapeutic concentration of camphor: see text)
Vicks VapoRub Cream	Camphor 5.2%, menthol 2.8%, eucalyptus oil 1.2%
Vicks VapoRub Ointment	Camphor 4.8%, menthol 2.6%, eucalyptus oil 1.2%

Table 15.10. Representative Cough Products Containing Camphor/Menthol in Steam Inhalant Form

PRODUCT	SELECTED INGREDIENTS
DeVilbiss Hankscraft Vaporizer Inhalant	Vaporizer inhalant containing menthol 0.67%, methyl salicylate 2.34%, eucalyptus oil 1.8%
Kaz Inhalant	Vaporizer inhalant containing menthol, camphor 0.8%, methyl salicylate 0.4%, eucalyptus oil, peppermint oil
Vicks Vapo Steam	Vaporizer inhalant containing camphor 6.2%, menthol, eucalyptus oil

Table 15.11. Representative Cough Products Containing Menthol

PRODUCT	SELECTED INGREDIENTS/COMMENTS
Halls Juniors Grape Lozenges	Menthol 2.5 mg
Halls Mentho-Lyptus Lozenges	Menthol 5–8.4 mg (concentration depends on flavor chosen)
Halls-Plus Lozenges	Menthol 10 mg
N'Ice Lozenges	Menthol 5 mg
Robitussin Cough Drops	Menthol 7.4–10 mg (concentration depends on flavor chosen)

ing nonproductive cough (in which the patient does not feel loose secretions in the lungs). *In addition to the standard labeling for cough products, the label will also caution against use if the patient has chronic bronchitis.* The pharmacist must note that the label will carry the warning against use in a cough accompanied by excessive mucus.

The FDA intended to ensure that the patient with a morbid condition such as cystic fibrosis would not use the product. The pharmacist should note for the patient that the typical productive cough seems to involve a certain amount of loose mucus, but that any volume greater than previously encountered may be a sign of a more serious condition.

Guaifenesin is given orally every 4 hours in the following doses:

- *50 to 100 mg with a daily maximum of 600 mg (2 years and older)*
- *100 to 200 mg with a daily maximum of 1200 mg (6 years and older)*

- *200 to 400 mg per dose with a maximum of 2400 mg per 24 hours (12 years and older).*

The leading product, Robitussin Syrup, contains 100 mg per 5 mL.

A popular combination product containing guaifenesin and dextromethorphan (Robitussin-DM) deserves discussion. It would seem irrational to make a cough more productive with guaifenesin while simultaneously stopping the cough with a central suppressant. Yet this product is annually ranked as a major pharmacist-recommended cough product. It should most properly be reserved for the rare patient whose cough is productive, but who also has the ancillary complaint that cough interrupts sleep. Perhaps nighttime use of this combination will allow sleep by reducing the number of coughing episodes while keeping the cough productive. In other words, when the patient has bronchial congestion, the more aggressive productive cough might "break through" to help mucokinesis with the help of guaifenesin, while the minor nonproductive cough is usefully suppressed by the dextromethorphan.

SUMMARY

The patient who complains of the common cold may take several minutes of dedicated counseling by a pharmacist. To determine the cause of the symptoms and then recommend the appropriate medications, pharmacists need to keep in mind the symptoms indicative of the common cold and conditions related to the common cold:

- The common cold. Pharmacists must ask sufficient questions to ensure that symptoms are actually caused by a virus rather than a common imitator such as allergic rhinitis. Once this has been achieved, the pharmacist should recommend specific products for troublesome symptoms, while ensuring that the patient does not take ingredients that have no potential

benefit. This can be accomplished by recommending several single-entity products, or an appropriate combination product. Each ingredient should be recommended after the patient is questioned closely to ensure that there are no contraindications such as diabetes mellitus with oral nasal decongestants.

- Nasal symptoms. Oral pseudoephedrine or a short-term topical decongestant can effectively reduce nasal congestion.

FOCUS ON...

CHILDREN AND COLDS

The common cold is more frequent in the child and declines in frequency with age. There are several reasons for this. Children are in closer contact with each other than adults. They engage in close-contact play and sit in closely spaced desks. This allows the viral particles from an infected child to more easily contact other children. Adults more typically work in separate work areas. Children are also less likely to observe social mores that prohibit placing one's fingers in the nose and fingers or thumbs in the mouth. The child who picks the nose, sucks a thumb or fingers, or bites the nails stands a good chance of contracting the common cold. If the child is below the age of 2 years, a physician referral is the best advice. Above this age, nasal congestion can be treated with the nasal aspirator and pseudoephedrine. (The rebound phenomenon is a problem with topical products.) A sore throat can be treated with the appropriate dose of internal analgesic product, or with a topical ingredient such as dyclonine or menthol. The productive cough can be helped with guaifenesin, and the nonproductive cough with dextromethorphan or alternative antitussive agents. Codeine is not recommended for use under the age of 6 years. See "Pediatric Dosing Information."

AT THE COUNTER

 A mother requests a cold product for her child.

Interview/Patient Assessment

The mother says her child is three and a half. She says that his throat is sore, his nose is runny, and he is coughing. As the pharmacist asks about the quality of his cough, the mother says, "It is kind of loose, like there's something rattling around in his lungs." The sore throat has been present for 1 day, and is minor in severity. The runny nose and cough also began yesterday. He has no other symptoms and is currently taking a cotrimoxazole combination for chronic ear infections pending the implantation of tubes in both ears next month.

Pharmacist's Analysis

1. What is the significance of the quality of cough?
2. Is this child too young to be given nonprescription cough-cold products?
3. Have any of the child's symptoms been present too long to allow self-therapy?

4. Is the cotrimoxazole possibly contributory?
5. What product(s) could the pharmacist recommend?

Patient Counseling

This child has typical symptoms of the common cold. The cotrimoxazole is probably not contributory. The quality of cough is vital to determine since it will shape therapy. A loose cough such as this one requires the expectorant guaifenesin to facilitate removal of the secretions. It would be counterproductive to suggest a suppressant. The child could also be given a decongestant such as oral pseudoephedrine. A combination product such as Robitussin PE contains both guaifenesin and pseudoephedrine, but the mother should be cautioned to follow the dosing guidelines of the label carefully. In regard to the sore throat, he is too young to receive phenol/phenolate sodium products and some oral analgesics. However, he could be given oral ibuprofen suspension or acetaminophen, as well as any of the lozenges containing benzocaine, benzyl alcohol, menthol, hexylresorcinol, or dyclonine.

AT THE COUNTER

A male of college age asks the pharmacist which product would help his cough.

Interview/Patient Assessment

The patient says that it has been present for about 3 days and is loose and productive. He denies use of any tobacco products, but is taking oral tetracycline and applying topical clindamycin for acne. He has no other diagnosed medical problems and is not using any other medications. He also wants a product to help a "low-grade" fever that he has had for 4 days. He has not had nasal symptoms or a sore throat.

Pharmacist's Analysis

1. Has this patient's cough been present too long to allow self-therapy?

2. Do this patient's medications seem implicated in the cough?
3. Is the patient's fever significant?
4. Should the pharmacist recommend a nonprescription product or referral?

This patient's cough has only been present for 3 days, so the duration does not contraindicate self-therapy. His facial medications are not a likely source of problems. His fever, however, is troublesome. Patients are not to self-treat cough when they also have fever, rash, or persistent headache, as these symptoms indicate the presence of a disease process that must be seen by a physician.

Patient Counseling

The patient should be urged to make an appointment with a physician.

Oral pseudoephedrine is preferable to oral phenylpropanolamine, the safety of which is currently questionable. Topical products can cause rhinitis medicamentosa and should be recommended carefully to prevent the condition.

- Sore throat. Either topical or systemic analgesics can combat sore throat, assuming the patient does not have any of the contraindications and is of sufficient age. However, sore throat can indicate a serious condition and should only be self-medicated with caution.
- Cough. Any one of several antitussives (e.g, menthol, dextromethorphan) can be recommended for nonproductive cough, while guaifenesin is effective for productive cough. Keeping these principles in mind will allow the pharmacist to effectively recommend products for the common cold when required.

References

1. Monto AS. The common cold. JAMA 271:1122, 1994.
2. Mossad SB, et al. Zinc gluconate lozenges for treating the common cold. A randomized, double-blind, placebo-controlled study. Ann Intern Med 125:81, 1996.
3. Tyrell DAJ. Hot news on the common cold. Ann Rev Microb 42:35, 1988.
4. Raymond CA. Cold virus spurs range of remedies. JAMA 255:302, 1986.
5. Del Mar C. Managing viral upper respiratory infections. Aust Fam Physician 20:557, 1991.
6. Zhang J, Wen-wei C. Association of the common cold in the first trimester of pregnancy with birth defects. Pediatrics 92:559, 1993.
7. Saroea HG. Common colds. Can Fam Physician 39:2215, 1993.
8. Cohen S, et al. Smoking, alcohol consumption, and susceptibility to the common cold. Am J Public Health 83:1277, 1993.
9. Doyle WJ, et al. Therapeutic effect of an anticholinergic-sympathomimetic combination in induced rhinovirus colds. Ann Otol Rhinol Laryngol 102:521, 1993.
10. Hendeles L. Efficacy and safety of antihistamines and expectorants in nonprescription cough and cold remedies. Pharmacotherapy 13:154, 1993.
11. Winther B, et al. Pathology of naturally occurring colds. Eur J Respir Dis 64(Suppl 128):345, 1983.
12. Bookman R. Physician visits for 'colds'. JAMA 251:2793, 1984.
13. Gwaltney JM, Jr. Rhinovirus colds: epidemiology, clinical characteristics and transmission. Eur J Respir Dis 64(Suppl 128):336, 1983.
14. Raymond CA. 'Catching cold' may not be as easy as it seems. JAMA 255:305, 1986.
15. Dick EC, et al. Aerosol transmission of rhinovirus colds. J Infect Dis 156:442, 1987.
16. Tyrell DAJ, Cohen S, Schlarb JE. Signs and symptoms in common colds. Epidemiol Infect 111:143, 1993.
17. Stickler GB, Smith TF, Broughton DD. The common cold. Eur J Pediatr 144:4, 1985.
18. Elkhatieb A, et al. Middle ear abnormalities during natural rhinovirus colds in adults. J Infect Dis 168:618, 1993.
19. Gwaltney JM, Jr, et al. Computed tomographic study of the common cold. N Engl J Med 330:25, 1994.
20. Zamula E. How to avoid the flu. FDA Consumer 28(9):16, 1994.
21. Wiselka M. Influenza: diagnosis, management, and prophylaxis. BMJ 308:1341, 1994.
22. Anon. Prevention and control of influenza: part I, vaccines. MMWR 42(RR-6):1, 1993.
23. Hecht A. The sinuses are obsolete troublemakers. FDA Consumer 18(10):20, 1985.
24. Hatch RT, Carpenter GB, Smith LJ. Treatment options in the child with a chronic cough. Drugs 45:367, 1993.
25. Mabry RL. Therapeutic agents in the medical management of sinusitis. Otolaryngol Clin North Am 26:561, 1993.

26. Fed Reg 59:43386, 1994.

27. Lowenstein SR, Parrino TA. Management of the common cold. Adv Intern Med 32:207, 1987.

28. Hemilä H. Does vitamin C alleviate the symptoms of the common cold?—A review of current evidence. Scand J Infect Dis 26:1, 1994.

29. Godfrey JC, et al. Zinc gluconate and the common cold: a controlled clinical study. J Intern Med Res 20:234, 1992.

30. Farr BM, et al. Two randomized controlled trials of zinc gluconate lozenge therapy of experimentally induced rhinovirus colds. Antimicrob Agents Chemother 31:1183, 1987.

31. Braga PC. Inflammatory mediators in common colds. Int Pharm J 6 (Suppl 6):4, 1995.

32. Lekas MD. Rhinitis during pregnancy and rhinitis medicamentosa. Otolaryngol Head Neck Surg 106(6 Pt 2):845, 1992.

33. Mabry RL. The management of nasal obstruction during pregnancy. Ear Nose Throat J 62:28, 1983.

34. Baxi LV, et al. Fetal heart rate changes following maternal administration of a nasal decongestant. Am J Obstet Gynecol 153:799, 1985.

35. Fed Reg 53:23180, 1988.

36. Gadomski A, Horton L. The need for rational therapeutics in the use of cough and cold medicine in infants. Pediatrics 89(4 Pt 2):774, 1992.

37. Anon. Labeling for OTCs. Rx Ipsa Loquitur 14(1):1, 1987.

38. Anon. Summary information for January 13, 1995 meeting of the nonprescription drugs advisory committee. FDA Publication Docket # 88N-0004.

39. Krause HF. Antihistamines and decongestants. Otolaryngol Head Neck Surg 107(6 Pt 2):835, 1992.

40. Fed Reg 41:38312, 1976.

41. Pruitt AW. Rational use of cold and cough preparations. Pediatr Ann 14:289, 1985.

42. Huycke MM, et al. A leukemoid reaction caused by a nasal sympathomimetic. Clin Infect Dis 15:885, 1992.

43. Montalban J, et al. Cerebral infarction after excessive use of nasal decongestants. J Neurol Neurosurg Psychiatry 52:541, 1989.

44. Osguthorpe JD, Shirley R. Neonatal respiratory distress from rhinitis medicamentosa. Laryngoscope 97:829, 1987.

45. Wesson DR, Smith DE, Morgan JP. The international scheduling of OTC inhaler ingredients: an abuse perspective. J Psychoactive Drugs 18:151, 1986.

46. Fed Reg 50:2220, 1985.

47. Fed Reg 52:8970, 1987.

48. Fed Reg 52:24344, 1987.

49. Dunn C, Gauthier M, Gaudreault P. Coma in a neonate following single intranasal dose of xylometazoline. Eur J Pediatr 152:541, 1993.

50. Platt ND. Xylometazoline and porphyria. Br J Anaesth 70:491, 1993.

51. Johnson DA, Hricik JG. The pharmacology of alpha-adrenergic decongestants. Pharmacotherapy 13(6 Pt 2):110S, 1993.

52. Pracy R. What use are nose drops? Arch Dis Child 58:946, 1983.

53. Jackson RT. Mechanism of action of some commonly used nasal drugs. Otolaryngol Head Neck Surg 104:433, 1991.

54. Capel LH, Swanston AR. Beware congesting nasal decongestants. Br Med J 293:1258, 1986.

55. Graf P, Juto JE. Decongestion effect and rebound swelling of the nasal mucosa during four-week use of oxymetazoline. ORL J Otorhinolaryngol Related Spec 56;157, 1994.

56. Heyman SN, Mevorach D, Ghanem J. Hypertensive crisis from chronic intoxication with nasal decongestants and cough medications. Drug Intell Clin Pharm 25:1068, 1991.

57. Conlan MF. DEA targeting illegal diversion of some OTCs. Drug Topics 139(22):32, 1995.

58. Fed Reg 61:5916, 1996.

59. Horowitz JD, et al. Hypertensive responses induced by phenylpropanolamine in anorectic and decongestant preparations. Lancet 1:60, 1980.

60. Mueller SM. Phenylpropanolamine, a nonprescription drug with potentially fatal side effects. N Engl J Med 308:653, 1983.

61. Backlin SA. Decongestant-induced hypertensive crisis. Can Fam Physician 39:375, 1993.

62. Dilsaver SC, Votolato NA, Alessi NE. Complications of phenylpropanolamine. Am Fam Physician 39:201, 1989.

63. Blum A. Phenylpropanolamine: an over-the-counter amphetamine? JAMA 245:1346, 1981.

64. Napolez A, Lauth W. Drug-induced acute urinary retention. Ann Emerg Med 17:1367, 1988.

65. Zorgniotti AW, Rossman B. Possible role of chronic use of nasal vasoconstrictors in impotence. Urology 30:594, 1987.

66. Rubenzahl SE. Is it a hypertensive crisis? Can Fam Physician 39:1024, 1993.

67. McEwen J. Phenylpropanolamine-associated hypertension after the use of "over-the-counter" appetite-suppressant products. Med J Aust 2:71, 1983.

68. Finton CK, Barton M, Chernow B. Possible adverse effects of phenylpropanolamine (diet pills) on sympathetic nervous system function—caveat emptor! Mil Med 147:1072, 1982.

69. Pruitt AW, et al. "Look-alikes." Pediatrics 72:256, 1983.

70. Bradley JG. Nonprescription drugs and hypertension. Postgrad Med 89:195, 1991.

71. Thomas SHL, et al. A comparison of the cardiovascular effects of phenylpropanolamine and phenylephrine containing proprietary cold remedies. Br J Clin Pharmacol 32:705, 1991.

72. Howrie DL, Wolfson JH. Phenylpropanolamine-induced hypertensive seizures. J Pediatr 102:143, 1983.

73. Weintraub MI. Intracranial hemorrhage: cerebral amyloid angiopathy or nasal decongestants? JAMA 264:2213, 1990.

74. Johnson DA, Etter HS, Reeves DM. Stroke and phenylpropanolamine use. Lancet 2:970, 1983.

75. Mirsen T. Intracranial hemorrhage: cerebral amyloid angiopathy or nasal decongestants? JAMA 264:2113, 1990.

76. Kase CS, et al. Intracerebral hemorrhage and phenylpropanolamine use. Neurology 37:399, 1987.

77. Weesner KM, Denison M, Roberts RJ. Cardiac arrhythmias in an adolescent following ingestion of an over-the-counter stimulant. Clin Pediatr 21:700, 1982.

78. Clark JE, Simon WA. Cardiac arrhythmias after phenylpropanolamine ingestion. Drug Intell Clin Pharm 17:737, 1983.

79. Peterson RB. Phenylpropanolamine-induced arrhythmias. JAMA 223:324, 1973.

80. Gardner ER, Hall RCW. Psychiatric symptoms produced by over-the-counter drugs. Psychosomatics 23:186, 1982.

81. Hall RCW, et al. Psychiatric reactions produced by respiratory drugs. Psychosomatics 26:605, 1985.

82. Lambert MT. Paranoid psychoses after abuse of proprietary cold medicines. Br J Psychiatry 151:548, 1987.

83. Dietz AJ, Jr. Amphetamine-like reactions to phenylpropanolamine. JAMA 245:601, 1981.
84. Grigg JR, Goyer PF. Phenylpropanolamine anorexiants and affective disorders. Mil Med 151:387, 1986.
85. Mendez MF. Mania self-induced with cough syrup. J Clin Psychiatry 53:173, 1992.
86. Bennett WM. Hazards of the appetite suppressant phenylpropanolamine. Lancet 2:42, 1979.
87. Norvenius G, Widerlöv E, Lönnerholm G. Phenylpropanolamine and mental disturbances. Lancet 2:1367, 1979.
88. Swenson RD, Golper TA, Bennett WM. Acute renal failure and rhabdomyolysis after ingestion of phenylpropanolamine-containing diet pills. JAMA 248:1216, 1982.
89. Rumpf KW, et al. Rhabdomyolysis after ingestion of an appetite suppressant. JAMA 250:2112, 1983.
90. Fed Reg 50:2200, 1985.
91. Fed Reg 57:58356, 1992.
92. Gaffey MJ, et al. Intanasally and orally administered antihistamine treatment of experimental rhinovirus colds. Am Rev Respir Dis 136:556, 1987.
93. Anon. Three antihistamines okay for colds: NDAC. NDMA Executive Newsletter 24–95:2, 1995.
94. Anon. New Indication. Drug Topics 140(7):34, 1996.
95. Snyder K. Cinderella story. Drug Topics 139(7):34, 1995.
96. Griffin JW, et al. Physiologic effects of an external nasal dilator. Laryngoscope 107:1235, 1997.
97. Scharf MB, et al. Effects of an external nasal dilator on sleep and breathing patterns in newborn infants with and without congestion. J Pediatr 129:804, 1996.
98. Burke P. Sore throat. Practitioner 237:854, 1993.
99. Dagnelie CF, et al. Bacterial flora in patients presenting with sore throat in Dutch general practice. Fam Pract 10:371, 1993.
100. Goldstein MN. Office evaluation and management of the sore throat. Otorhinolaryngol Clin North Am 25:837, 1992.
101. Feldman WE. Pharyngitis in children. Postgrad Med 93:141, 1993.
102. Fed Reg 47:22712, 1982.
103. Fed Reg 53:2436, 1988.
104. Willatt DJ. Children's sore throats related to parental smoking. Clin Otolaryngol 11:317, 1986.
105. Denholm S, Rivron RP. Acute epiglottitis in adults: a potentially lethal cause of sore throat. J R Coll Surg Edinb 37:333, 1992.
106. Solomons N, Rowe-Jones J. Acute epiglottitis in children: a potentially lethal cause of sore throat. J R Coll Surg Edinb 38:265, 1993.
107. Fed Reg 56:48302, 1991.
108. Kiselica D. Group A beta-hemolytic-streptococcal pharyngitis: current clinical concepts. Am Fam Physician 49:1147, 1994.
109. Begovac J, et al. Asymptomatic pharyngeal carriage of beta-haemolytic streptococci and streptococcal pharyngitis among patients at an urban hospital in Croatia. Eur J Epidemiol 9:405, 1993.
110. Farley TA, et al. Direct inoculation of food as the cause of an outbreak of Group A streptococcal pharyngitis. J Infect Dis 167:1232, 1993.
111. Higgins PM. Streptococcal pharyngitis in general practice. 1. some unusual features of the epidemiology. Epidemiol Infect 109:181, 1992.
112. Nakar S, Kahan E, Weingarten M. Can you smell the strep? Lancet 343:729, 1994.
113. Patlak M. 'Strep' demands immediate care. FDA Consumer 25(8):25, 1991.
114. Steinbrook R. Pharyngitis. West J Med 143:534, 1985.
115. Shulman ST. Complications of streptococcal pharyngitis. Pediatr Infect Dis J 13(1 Suppl 1):S70, 1994.
116. Denny FW. Current management of streptococcal pharyngitis. J Fam Pract 35:619, 1992.
117. Fed Reg 59:6084, 1994.
118. Halwell R. Pharyngitis medicamentosa. Arch Otolaryngol Head Neck Surg 115:995, 1989.
119. Fed Reg 53:46204, 1988.
120. Irwin RS, Curley FJ, Bennett FM. Appropriate use of antitussives and protussives. Drugs 46:80, 1993.
121. Zervanos NJ, Shute KM. Acute, disruptive cough. Postgrad Med 95:153, 1994.
122. Leung AKC, Robson WLM, Tay-Uyboco J. Chronic cough in children. Can Fam Physician 40:531, 1994.
123. McKenzie S. Cough—but is it asthma? Arch Dis Child 70:1, 1994.
124. Katz PO. Is the chronic cougher a refluxer? Am J Gastroenterol 87:1520, 1992.
125. Putnam PE, Orenstein SR. Hoarseness in a child with gastroesophageal reflux. Acta Pediatr 81:635, 1992.
126. Mrvos R, Dean BS, Krenzelok EP. Home exposures to chlorine/chloramine gas: review of 216 cases. South Med J 86:654, 1993.
127. Ing AJ, Ngu MC, Breslin ABX. Pathogenesis of chronic persistent cough associated with gastroesophageal reflux. Am J Respir Crit Care Med 149:160, 1994.
128. Irwin RS, et al. Chronic cough due to gastroesophageal reflux. Chest 104:1511, 1993.
129. Koufman JA. Aerodigestive manifestations of gastroesophageal reflux. Chest 104:1321, 1993.
130. Ing AJ, Ngu MC, Breslin ABX. Chronic persistent cough and clearance of esophageal acid. Chest 102:1668, 1992.
131. Walcott DW, et al. Failure to thrive, diarrhea, cough, and oral candidiasis in a three-month-old boy. Ann Allergy 72:408, 1994.
132. Clough JB, Holgate ST. Episodes of respiratory morbidity in children with cough and wheeze. Am J Respir Crit Care Med 150:48, 1994.
133. Lenzo NP, Kendall PA. Cough and glaucoma: a possible association. Aust NZ J Med 24:67, 1994.
134. Boulet L-P, et al. Airway inflammation in nonasthmatic subjects with chronic cough. Am J Respir Crit Care Med 149(2 Pt 1):482, 1994.
135. Richards W, What's causing that child's chronic cough? Compr Ther 19:256, 1993.
136. Krzyzanowski M, Robbins DR, Lebowitz MD. Smoking cessation and changes in respiratory symptoms in two populations followed for 13 years. Int J Epidemiol 22:666, 1993.
137. Brown CA, Woodward M, Tunstall-Pedoe H. Prevalence of chronic cough and phlegm among male cigar and pipe smokers: results of the Scottish Home Health Study. Thorax 48:1163, 1993.
138. Punzi HA. Safety update: focus on cough. Am J Cardiol 72:45H, 1993.
139. Overlack A, et al. Cough induced by ACE-inhibitors. A kinin related phenomenon? Agents Actions Suppl 38(Pt 3):482, 1992.
140. Aggarwal P, Wali JP. Enalapril-induced cough in the emergency department. J Emerg Med 10:689, 1992.

141. Thornhill FLH. Clinical pharmacy without a net. Am J Hosp Pharm 47:2238, 1990.

142. Shuttari MF, Braun SR. Contemporary management of chronic persistent cough. Mo Med 89:795, 1992.

143. Hjalmarsson S, et al. Major hemorrhage as a complication of cough fracture. Chest 104:1310, 1993.

144. Irwin RS, Curley FJ, French CL. Chronic cough. Am Rev Respir Dis 141:640, 1990.

145. Pratter MR, et al. An algorithmic approach to chronic cough. Ann Intern Med 119:977, 1993.

146. Croughan-Minihane MS, et al. Clinical trial examining effectiveness of three cough syrups. J Am Board Fam Pract 6:109, 1993.

147. Fed Reg 52:30042, 1987.

148. Cornford CS, Morgan M, Ridsdale L. Why do mothers consult when their children cough? Fam Pract 10:193, 1993.

149. Survey of Pharmacy Law, 62: 1993, National Association of Boards of Pharmacy, Chicago.

150. Anon. Disciplinary hearings. Oklahoma State Board of Pharmacy 4(2):4, 1990.

151. Fed Reg 57:27666, 1992.

152. Fed Reg 58:54232, 1993.

153. Fed Reg 57:58378, 1992.

154. Fed Reg 60:10286, 1995.

155. Fed Reg 48:48576, 1983.

156. Fed Reg 54:8494, 1989.

CHAPTER 16

Humidity Deficit

OUTLINE

At the Counter. A young couple holding a bottle of vaporizer inhalant solution asks the pharmacist, "Does this stuff really work? Our 2-year-old son is kind of croupy. What kind of machine do we use it in?"

At the Counter. A couple in their late 60s are looking at vaporizers and humidifiers on a winter day. When the pharmacist asks if they require assistance, they say they want to know if one would help their dry skin and sore throats. They also can't seem to remove the secretions from their lungs.

References

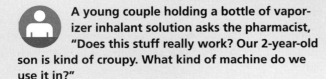

A young couple holding a bottle of vaporizer inhalant solution asks the pharmacist, "Does this stuff really work? Our 2-year-old son is kind of croupy. What kind of machine do we use it in?"

Interview/Patient Assessment

The pharmacist asks for more information about the child. The boy is not taking any medications and has no medical conditions. The main parental concerns are a runny nose and cough.

Pharmacist's Analysis

1. Is a vaporizer inhalant indicated for a child of this age?
2. Can a vaporizer inhalant solution alleviate rhinorrhea and cough?
3. How is a vaporizer inhalant used?
4. What is the possible utility of vapor therapy alone?

Vaporizer inhalant solutions do help cough, but are ineffective for rhinorrhea. They are placed into the medication cup of a vaporizer and volatilize to be breathed in by the patient.

Patient Counseling

A humidifier or vaporizer is safe for a child of this age, but is not likely to provide relief of either rhinorrhea or cough, unless the cough is caused by humidity deficit. This child's parents may use a vaporizer inhalant solution, which is proven to be safe and effective for the relief of cough and is safe for children as young as 2. The solution is added to the medication cup found on the top of the vaporizer, next to the steam outlet. The vaporizer may be allowed to run in the child's room, but must not be located less than 4 feet from his bed, and the vaporizer and cord should be out of reach. The vaporizer should be periodically cleansed, according to the manufacturer's directions.

Humans consume many nutrients during a typical day. Although the body is readily able to undergo short periods of starvation when denied access to most of these nutrients, humans cannot survive long if water is denied to them. (This need for water is not unique to humans, of course; all forms of life require water for survival.[1]) The weight of an average adult is 50 to 60% water. This water plays a role in virtually all of the bodily processes (e.g., circulation, digestion, excretion, metabolism, and temperature regulation). Humidity deficit, or insufficient moisture in the air, is critically important in respiration, which is why this topic is included in the section on respiratory problems.

PREVALENCE OF HUMIDITY DEFICIT

The prevalence of humidity deficit is unknown. It is thought to be quite common in the winter, although it often goes unrecognized. It can also appear in the summer, when it is also often unrecognized.

EPIDEMIOLOGY OF HUMIDITY DEFICIT

Several situations cause humans to suffer from less than optimal hydration. Diarrhea and vomiting can cause loss of fluid and electrolytes, and dehydration dangers multiply rapidly when the patient suffers from both. Less dramatic but equally important causes of water deficit must also be recognized. For instance, older patients often have a decreased thirst response and drink less fluids than they should, even-

tually becoming dehydrated.[2] Patients also suffer from a seasonally related fluid deficit. This seasonally related fluid deficit exists whenever the ambient air contains insufficient humidity and the individual does not take steps to replace water losses.

ETIOLOGY OF HUMIDITY DEFICIT

Humidity deficit can be caused by a combination of factors. The season of the year is a major variable, but climate control systems in buildings (heating and air conditioning systems) also play a role. The amount of time the climate control system runs is in turn influenced by the temperature extremes the geographic area normally experiences.

Relative Versus Absolute Humidity

Absolute humidity is the weight of water vapor in a given volume of gas, expressed as milligrams of water per liter of gas-vapor mixture.[3] The amount of water vapor that a gas can hold is directly related to the temperature of the gas: As the temperature of a gas (or the air) increases, the amount of water vapor that the gas (or the air) can hold increases. At a given temperature, a gas (or the air) is saturated when it contains the maximum amount of water vapor possible at that temperature.

Relative humidity (a percent) is the actual amount of water vapor in the air (the absolute humidity) divided by the amount of water vapor that the air is capable of holding at a given temperature, multiplied by 100:

$$\frac{\text{Actual water-vapor content of gas}}{\begin{array}{c}\text{Potential water-holding}\\\text{capacity of gas}\end{array}} \times 100 = \text{Relative humidity (\%)}$$

Thus, if cool outside (winter) air is warmed to room temperature, it is capable of holding more water vapor. Consequently, although the absolute humidity of the air has not changed, the relative humidity drops because warmer air can hold more water vapor.[4] In effect, the air has become drier, as explained below.

Impact of Low Relative Humidity

WINTERTIME IN COLD REGIONS

During hot summer weather, the relative humidity is often 90 to 95%. Since warm air is capable of holding a great deal of water, the high relative humidity of summer air represents a corresponding high weight of water vapor (absolute humidity). Colder winter air—which cannot hold as much moisture as its summer counterpart—generally also has a lower relative humidity, thus considerably less absolute humidity. As a consequence, when cool, low-moisture winter air is drawn inside and warmed, the relative humidity plummets.

When cool air is warmed in the winter—and its relative humidity drops—it in effect becomes much drier. Because it has such a low relative humidity, it becomes "water hungry." To meet its moisture deficit, the warm dry air draws moisture from sources in the house.[5,6] Woodwork shrinks, plaster cracks, furniture warps, plants require more frequent watering, static electricity increases, and we suffer the health effects of humidity deficit.

SUMMERTIME IN WARM REGIONS

Although the effects of desiccation are especially noticeable in colder climates where heaters run almost continuously all winter, air drying is a problem in warmer climates, too. In states with a high average temperature, such as Arizona or Texas, the air is usually quite dry. In the summer, homes and workplaces have recirculated, air-conditioned air that also has a low relative humidity.

"SICK" BUILDINGS

There is a trend to make modern buildings highly energy efficient. In the process, they are made tight with insulated seals and closed ventilation systems. The purpose is to keep outside air out. Up to 95% of the air is recirculated, becoming drier and drier as it does so. Buildings that become excessively dry as a result produce symptoms that are collectively known as "sick building syndrome," "tight building syndrome," "building illness," and "stuffy office illness."[7,8] The systems may also become contaminated with various bacteria, fungi, yeasts, and molds.[9]

OTHER LOW-RELATIVE-HUMIDITY SITUATIONS

The climate can also become quite dry in other enclosed compartments with air conditioning systems. People traveling cross-country in an automobile and those on a long airplane flight may notice that the air becomes progressively drier as the trip proceeds.

MANIFESTATIONS OF HUMIDITY DEFICIT

Health Effects of Dryness

Humidity deficit causes a number of common complaints besides those involving breathing, which will be discussed separately.

OPHTHALMIC SYMPTOMS

In a study of humidified versus dry air, office employees working in the dry air section complained of dryness, irritation, and itching of the eyes significantly more than those working in humidified air. All of these problems were significantly lessened by proper humidification.[6] Excessive dryness of the eye can result from dry indoor heating, which causes the sclera of the eye to lose its turgor.[10]

DERMATOLOGIC SYMPTOMS

Office employees working in dry air also found that itching, dryness, and irritation of the skin were reduced when proper humidification was introduced.[6] Most physicians agree that skin dryness can be relieved by proper humidification.[11] Low bodily hydration causes the skin to appear dry and wrinkled.[5,10]

OTIC SYMPTOMS

Earache can be caused by low humidity. The swollen eustachian tube prevents equalization of pressure. The patient may complain that swallowing fails to relieve the otic pressure.[10]

SORE THROAT

The patient who breathes dry air may complain of dysphagia caused by a perceived obstruction when attempting to swallow.[10] Inhalation of dry air also dries the laryngopharyngeal area to produce a feeling of sore throat.[5]

SUBSTERNAL PAIN

Breathing dry air causes a burning substernal sensation when the patient attempts a deep breath. While this mimics gastroesophageal reflux disease, it is not the result of acid reflux, but rather the result of airway tissue inflammation caused by breathing dry air.[10]

RESPIRATORY SYMPTOMS

People who breathe dry cold air often complain of rhinorrhea, nasal congestion, and irritation.[12] Cold air may also worsen allergic rhinitis.

In one study a device designed to deliver humidified warm air to the nasal mucosa relieved allergic rhinitis symptoms.[13] Further, general humidification relieved symptoms of allergic rhinitis in a group of office workers (e.g., eye symptoms, nasal congestion, nasal rhinorrhea, and sneezing).[6]

EXERCISE-INDUCED ASTHMA

The incidence of exercise-induced bronchospasm is greatly increased in cold dry air.[4,14] On the other hand, bronchoconstriction following exercise is minimal if the exercise is carried out in a facility with humidified air.[15,16]

Mucokinesis

The human body has a number of very effective specific and nonspecific defenses against infection. Specific defenses, which protect us against certain organisms only, include antibodies and other aspects of the immune system. Nonspecific defenses, which protect us against any pathogenic organism, include the skin (an excellent barrier to infection), inflammation, fever, phagocytosis, and the mucous membranes. Mucous membranes line body cavities that are open to the exterior environment such as the entire digestive tract, the eyelids, and the urinary and reproductive systems (the vagina). Mucous membranes prevent the tissues from drying out and prevent infection.

A good example of the role of mucous membranes is the respiratory tract. These membranes are the first barrier to viral penetration of the upper respiratory tract.[17] They also prevent further damage caused by inhalation of noxious substances (e.g., cigarette smoke, pollutants, and pollens).[18]

THE EFFECT OF DRYNESS ON MUCOKINESIS

Low humidity in the ambient air compromises the function of the mucous membranes of the respiratory tract by disrupting its surface epithelial cells, especially those of the **goblet cells** (cells that secrete mucus) and **ciliated cells** (cells with an upper surface covered with constantly beating hairlike projections) (Fig. 16.1).[19]

Goblet Cells

Goblet cells are scattered among ciliated cells in a 1:5 ratio. Their major function is the production of mucus.[3,10] The amount of mucus secreted from the goblet cells and other sites is approximately 65 to 90 mL/24 hours.[3] This mucus accumulates to form a "blanket" that lines the respiratory tree.[20] This mucus blanket consists of two layers:

- The lower layer (or sol layer), next to the cells, is a more fluid substance.
- The outermost layer (or gel layer), is less fluid and sticky, so that it will collect and hold inhaled foreign materials.

Ciliated Cells

Each ciliated cell has 200 to 250 cilia on its surface.[19–21] The tips of the cilia are embedded in the mucus blanket's upper gel layer, moving with a ciliary beat frequency (CBF) of 2000 beats per minute. Their wavelike motion propels the mucus blanket upward at an estimated rate of 10 to 15 mm/minute.[3,10] This waving action is similar to the wave cheer in a stadium, except that the ciliary movement more closely resembles a whipping motion. The mucus eventually reaches the lower pharyngeal area, where it is either expectorated or subconsciously swallowed, along with the viruses, bacteria, and pollutants entrapped within it. This process has been variously referred to as the mucociliary elevator, the tracheobronchial toilet, or mucokinesis.[10,14]

CONSEQUENCES OF IMPAIRED MUCOKINESIS

When mucokinesis is impaired or stopped completely so inhaled particles cannot be cleared, several adverse health consequences result[20]:

- Failure to clear inhaled microorganisms increases the risk of infections that are primarily transmitted through aerosol means such as the common cold and influenza.[22]
- The risk of bronchial cancer may be increased because of impaired clearance of inhaled carcinogens and prolonged contact time with the pulmonary mucosa.
- Accumulated airway lumen secretions obstruct airflow.

CONDITIONS KNOWN TO IMPAIR MUCOKINESIS

Several conditions impair mucokinesis, perhaps by reducing the numbers of ciliated cells or increasing the viscosity of the mucus blanket.

Infectious Agents

Rhinovirus infections reduce mucokinesis by inducing several types of damage.[17,23,24] They produce direct sloughing of epithelial cells, destruction of the epithelial layer, reduction in ciliary beat frequency, and they change the volume and rheologic properties of mucus.[16,23,25,26] Nasal secretions from patients with rhinovirus infection show expelled epithelial cells.[24,26] It is well known that influenza A virus can destroy ciliated cells, causing impaired tracheobronchial clearance.[27,28]

Dry Ambient Air

Low humidity levels desiccate airway secretions, resulting in reduced mucus layer adhesiveness and slowing of CBF

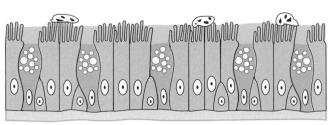

Figure 16.1. Mucus expectorated by the goblet cells, which entrap particles and pollution, can be easily moved upward by ciliated cells (*left*), unless it is excessively dried and thick (*right*).

frequency.[29] Even a short period of dry air breathing causes excessive nasal mucosal water loss, resulting in reduced nasal mucociliary clearance rate.[18] Ciliary action is impaired when relative humidity falls below 70% and ceases when relative humidity falls below 30%.[10] However, cilia are still capable of full activity within a few minutes when reheated and re-moisturized.[30]

Dry air breathing also hampers mucokinesis through damage to mucous glands, disorganization of the basement membrane, cytoplasmic and nuclear degeneration, desquamation of cells, mucosal ulceration, and flattening of the pulmonary epithelium.[14] Repair of ciliary damage takes only 2 to 3 days, but repair of full-thickness epithelial damage (should basement membrane damage occur) requires 2 to 3 weeks. During this time, the patient often suffers a dry, nonproductive hacking cough.[10] The patient frequently feels secretions present in the airways, but cannot loosen them through coughing.

TREATMENT OF HUMIDITY DEFICIT

Treatment Guidelines

Patients must ensure proper mucokinesis by keeping the body at a proper hydration level. Adequate hydration liquefies mucus viscosity for optimal, prompt removal through ciliary movements.

ADEQUATE WATER INGESTION

Patients must drink six to eight 8-ounce glasses of water daily to meet their needs for water.[1] Many people find it inconvenient or impossible to follow this simple recommendation, however.

AMBIENT AIR HYDRATION THROUGH EVAPORATION
Some people place a pan of water over floor air vents to add moisture to the air.[5] Air passively evaporates until the pan is empty. However, the efficacy of this method is uncertain.[1]

BOILING WATER
Some patients boil water in open containers, an intervention that is also of unknown efficacy.[5] **Holding one's head over boiling water could be hazardous**, in addition to being unpleasant.[31] Children have been severely scalded as parents attempt to hold them over a boiling pot. A sick, upset child struggling against being tightly held, can fall into the boiling water.[32,33] (A study of 11 scalds attained in this manner

showed that children required mean hospital stays of 14.7 days and had a mean complete healing time of 21.1 days, given the volume of water to which the child was exposed.[33]) For the same reasons, parents should never run hot water in the bathroom to humidify the air. A 10-month-old child was scalded when he fell into a tub half filled with boiling water.[33,34]

Nonprescription Medications

Nonprescription medications are often used in conjunction with devices to treat humidity deficit; however, their approved uses are to alleviate cough, and they are not used to treat humidity deficit per se. For this reason these medications are discussed in "Use of Medications with Vaporizers."

Nonpharmacologic Therapies

HUMIDITY INHALATION VIA VAPORIZERS AND HUMIDIFIERS
Overview of Vaporizers and Humidifiers
Given the unknown effectiveness of passive evaporation methods and the dangers of boiling pots and hot baths, alternate methods are preferable. Vaporizers and humidifiers are simple, inexpensive devices that can humidify air in the household or workplace. The term "vaporizer" applies to a device that produces steam to increase humidity; the term "humidifier" applies to a device that produces a nonheated mist to increase humidity. The devices also are referred to as "steam vaporizers" and "cool-mist humidifiers." Several manufacturers produce these items, and they differ in several important parameters, as highlighted in Table 16.1.

Manufacturer's directions for care of these units are printed in a brochure that is placed in the box of each humidifier or vaporizer. The consumer should contact the manufacturer for a replacement brochure if theirs was accidentally discarded or seems to be missing for any reason. *Also, patients must be reminded to keep the box to store the unit until the next season.* Figure 16.2 illustrates various appropriate locations for vaporizers and humidifiers in a typical household.

Pharmacists are often asked the fundamental question in home vapor therapy: Is a vaporizer or humidifier better? (Patient Assessment Algorithm 16.1). Both units add water vapor to the air.[5] However, they use different technologies to accomplish this goal. See Table 16.2 for a summary of the similarities and differences in vaporizers and humidifiers.

Table 16.1. Comparison of Representative Vaporizers

MANUFACTURER	COMPOSITION OF VAPORIZER ELECTRODES	CAN BOILING WATER BE EJECTED FROM VAPORIZER?	ELECTROLYTE TO ADD TO VAPORIZER WATER
DeVilbiss	Steel	Yes	Baking soda
Hankscraft	Steel	Yes	Baking soda
Kaz	Carbon	No	Salt
Sunbeam	Steel	No	Baking soda

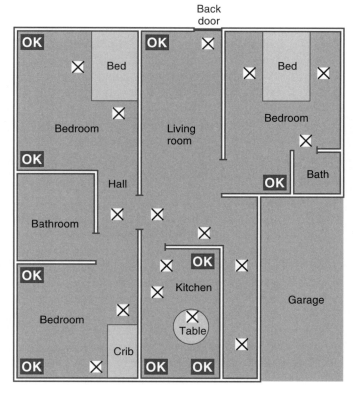

Figure 16.2. The various appropriate locations for vaporizers and humidifiers in a typical household (as noted). Note the spots a vaporizer should NOT be placed (as noted by an X): in traffic flow patterns (in halls, at entrances to rooms), next to a baby's crib, on top of a table, or next to a bedridden patient.

Despite their advantages, only 1% of elderly adults in one study used them to help relieve the symptoms of cold or influenza.[35] This is doubly disappointing when, in the same group of survey respondents, 7% incorrectly used vitamins to prevent colds and 3% incorrectly used vitamins to prevent influenza. These data suggest that much work remains to be done in the area of patient education regarding effective self-care interventions.

Table 16.2. Comparison of Vaporizer and Humidifier Characteristics

FEATURES/CHARACTERISTICS	VAPORIZERS	HUMIDIFIERS
Effective for humidity deficit?	Yes	Yes
Used with medication?	Yes	No
Cleaning requires disassembly?	Yes	No
Water may require electrolyte adjustment?	Yes	No
Device presents a burn hazard?	Yes	No
Potential hypersensitivity pneumonitis?	No	Yes
Device produces white dust?	No	Yes

The Effectiveness of Vaporizers and Humidifiers in Airway Conditions

The FDA does not require testing of vaporizers and humidifiers for efficacy in the manner that internal and topical nonprescription products must be tested. Thus research findings must be consulted to discover their efficacy.

Reportedly, physicians are divided in their assessments of these devices. However, in an unpublished national survey, a majority of pediatricians, family practitioners, and otorhinolaryngologists stated that the individual suffering from cold or flu should eliminate dryness by adding moisture to the indoor air to help relieve symptoms. In addition, they agreed that many people are simply unaware that the air in their homes is too dry, that people who already own vaporizers and humidifiers do not use them enough, and that vapor therapy is appropriate all of the time, not just when one has the cold or influenza.[11]

Objective studies proving the effectiveness of vaporizers and humidifiers are rare for several reasons. The gold standard in scientific investigation is the double-blind, placebo-controlled study with sample sizes sufficient to achieve statistical significance. But a double-blind, placebo-controlled trial using humidified air versus nonhumidified air may be impossible, if not highly difficult.[36] Choosing a variable to measure is also problematic, as is the fact that many patients in the trial will inevitably improve with or without therapy.[28]

Despite these potential problems in research design, investigators have attempted to document the efficacy of supplemental inhaled vapor. For instance, the previously mentioned study of office workers demonstrated that central humidification was highly effective in relieving many dry air symptoms.[6] As a justification for the research, the investigators stressed that indoor relative humidity often decreases to 10 to 20% in the winter. During the winter, they humidified one wing of an office building to 30 to 40% relative humidity, and did not humidify the other wing. After 1 week, they reversed the humidification. They repeated this so that each individual was exposed to three 1-week humidified phases and three 1-week dry phases. Subjects kept a diary of symptoms. As previously mentioned, humidification significantly reduced skin symptoms, and eye symptoms. Humidification also reduced pharyngeal dryness, nasal congestion, nasal excretion, and cough.

Another study examined 800 army recruits placed in humidified versus nonhumidified barracks, finding that those living in the humidified atmosphere suffered 18% fewer infections.[5] School children attending a humidified school suffered fewer respiratory infections than those in a nonhumidified school, and those whose homes were also humidified had an infection rate that was the lowest of all.[5]

Researchers investigated the design of barracks in a different military study, using 4000 trainees at four Army training centers. Recruits in barracks that were tightly closed suffered 50% more infections than those living in barracks that allowed fresh humid outside air in.[7] A device designed to deliver steam to the nose alleviated cold symptoms and increased nasal patency in a group of common-cold sufferers.[37]

An editorial in the *Journal of the Royal Society of Medicine* described a controlled clinical trial by a German physician.[38] The physician decided to study the health effects of saunas. He discovered that those who visited saunas two times weekly had half the colds of those who did not visit saunas, which may reflect the vapor that would be breathed in during a sauna visit. A group of physicians studied children with bronchitis. The children were randomly assigned to the steam group or a nonhumidified group. Those who breathed steam had a greater decrease in respiratory distress and recovered in a shorter period.[39]

A leading respiratory therapy textbook suggested several subjective observations that may be made to determine if a humidifier is effective[10]:

- Are the patient's secretions sufficiently thin and mobile to be easily evacuated?
- Has the patient stopped complaining of dryness?
- Is the patient able to loosen large amounts of previously immobile secretions?

Another benefit to humidification is in reduction of dry mouth associated with irradiation of the salivary glands. A humidifier should be used in the bedroom to promote comfort and sleep, according to a clinical oncology nurse specialist.[40] Further, the author of the report stressed that an increase in the moisture in the air reduces the mucosal dryness that caused patients to awaken frequently during the night.

Although numerous studies of the effectiveness of vapor therapy are not yet available, those that have been carried out point to effectiveness of vapor therapy in general. Further, anecdotal reports seem to show effectiveness for specific problems such as dry mouth.

Overhumidification

Overhumidification can promote the growth of dust mites, fungi, and molds in the house, so that humidification should be avoided when the environment is already above 50% humidity.[3,5] Allergies can result from overhumidification. Children with asthma or lower respiratory tract disease may experience worsening of symptoms since humidification increases airway resistance and can induce bronchospasm; they should only use humidification following a physician recommendation.[36,41]

VAPORIZERS
Method of Action

The vaporizer consists of a reservoir (filled as indicated by the manufacturer), and a boiling chamber that is placed into the reservoir (Fig. 16.3). Two electrodes inside the vaporizer's boiling chamber are connected to wall electricity. When the vaporizer is plugged in (and turned on if there is a separate switch), the electrical current attempts to bridge the electrodes. As this happens, it produces heat as a by-product, heating the water inside the chamber to boiling. Steam exits the vaporizer, humidifying the air. As the vaporizer produces steam the water level in the reservoir slowly falls, exposing more and more of the electrodes. When the water level is just touching the lower bit of the electrodes, the vaporizer no longer emits steam or uses electricity since the electrodes are not immersed in water.

At this point, the typical vaporizer still has about 3/4 inch of water in the reservoir. *The user must empty this water out before refilling the vaporizer, since the remaining water will contain a higher concentration of mineral than the tap water.* The electrolyte in the tank undergoes serial

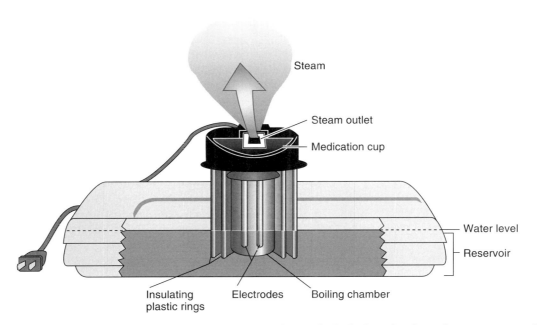

Figure 16.3. The steam vaporizer. Note the position of the electrodes inside the boiling chamber, where steam is produced.

concentration if the person fills the vaporizer numerous times by simply refilling to the fill line without ever emptying out the tank.

Cleaning the Vaporizer

tip *Vaporizer reservoirs must be rinsed with clean water and wiped dry (with a clean dry cloth) prior to each use.* Any accumulated minerals or residue around the edges of the reservoir should be removed. Since active boiling does not occur in the reservoir, this procedure is usually sufficient to cleanse it adequately.

Active boiling does occur within the boiling chamber surrounding the electrodes, so scale deposits readily within the

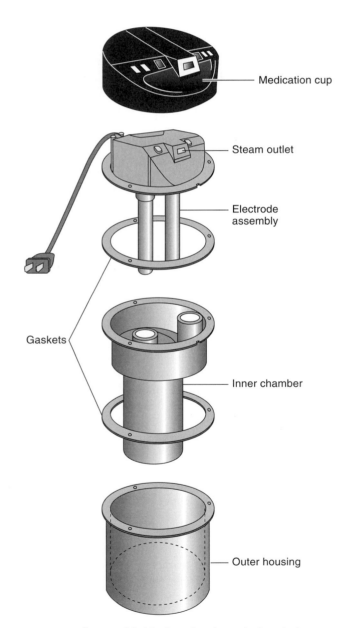

Figure 16.4. A disassembled boiling chamber, which includes outer housing, gaskets, electrode assembly, and inner chamber.

entire boiling chamber (Fig. 16.4). The vaporizer must be unplugged before cleaning the boiling chamber or taking it apart. ***Use extreme caution to prevent a curious toddler or unknowing adult from plugging in the vaporizer while it is being cleaned.***

If a vaporizer is used continually, about once a week, the user should soak the boiling chamber in a mixture of 50% water and 50% white vinegar for 10 minutes. The user then covers the bottom holes of the boiling chamber and adds water to the steam outlet. After placing the finger of the other hand over the steam outlet, the customer shakes the boiling chamber vigorously. The water is drained out of the chamber and the process repeated several times. If the hole in the bottom of the boiling chamber is plugged, the consumer should follow the manufacturer's instructions for unplugging the hole. (If there are no manufacturer's instructions, the user can unplug the vaporizer and use a toothpick or other nonmetallic object to try to clear the hole.) Periodically, the vaporizer's electrodes will require cleaning. How often depends on two variables:

- Type of electrode
- Hardness of water

tip *Stainless steel electrodes require cleaning every 50 hours (2 days). Carbon electrodes, which collect mineral less rapidly, only require cleaning about every 150 hours (1 week).*

Water is hard when it contains a large amount of dissolved substances—mainly calcium, but also iron, magnesium, and **tip** other metals. *If the water is quite hard, the consumer will need to clean the electrodes more often than recommended by the manufacturer.* Failing to clean the electrodes when necessary can compromise the function of the unit. ***Should scale span the electrodes completely, the unit will not heat water at all, or may spark.*** (See "A Pharmacist's Journal: My Vaporizer Doesn't Work.") The electrodes also may erode.

The consumer should follow manufacturer's directions to disassemble the boiling chamber surrounding the electrodes. (Disassembly may consist of removing a few screws and gaskets.) Scale buildup must be removed from the inside of the boiling chamber, and the electrodes must be scraped with a butter knife or other hard object to remove the scale. **tip** *The consumer may find it useful to use a pair of pliers or Vice Grips to break the scale from the electrodes. If the electrodes have very heavy scale accumulation, overnight soaking in vinegar may be helpful.* Cleaning tablets that contain citric acid may also help dissolve lime scale around the electrodes. Clean-Start Vaporizer Tablets are placed in the reservoir of a running vaporizer. Scale is more easily removed following their use.

Eventually steel electrodes that have been not been cleaned often enough will begin to erode (which reduces the output of the vaporizer). One electrode will usually begin to erode before the other. Since it is a little shorter than the other, scale will then precipitate more heavily onto the section of the electrode that is not yet eroded, causing more erosion. As the eroding

A Pharmacist's Journal

"My Vaporizer Doesn't Work."

I had given a continuing education program on humidification. One of the attendees said that a patient asked him to look at a vaporizer because it didn't work. He unscrewed the boiling chamber to examine the electrodes and found the inside of the boiling chamber completely blocked by accumulated scale. He asked her to return, and spent more than one-half hour cleaning the boiling chamber, electrodes, and tank. The customer thanked him as she took the unit back. The next day, she entered the pharmacy in a highly agitated state. Her household fuses had blown out, and the only cause she could think of was the clean vaporizer. The pharmacist explained that a properly running vaporizer should not blow out fuses, but she insisted that the pharmacy pay for new fuses.

steel electrode shortens more and more, the process of erosion speeds up. When this electrode is markedly shorter than the other, the vaporizer will not run as long as it should. At this point, the consumer should consider replacing the vaporizer. Vaporizers using carbon electrodes, which do not erode, last longer on the average than vaporizers using steel electrodes.

If the electrodes are bent during cleaning, they should be respaced to about the same distance that they were when the boiling chamber was opened. If they cannot be straightened or break during cleaning, a new unit should be purchased.

In normal conditions, steam should be visible within several minutes after the unit is plugged in, with a steady flow in 15 minutes or so. Some consumers become confused with the vaporizer when they do not hear moving parts and do not immediately see steam. The user should be patient in waiting for steam.

Adjustment of Electrolyte Content of Water

In order for vaporizers to work properly, the water must have the correct amount of minerals in it. Mineral content can be easily adjusted by the consumer if it is not ideal. *If the water is extremely soft (either naturally or because of a water softener), the vaporizer may fail to produce steam or may only do so slowly.* The consumer should adjust the electrolyte content by adding baking soda or salt to the reservoir as recommended by the manufacturer. (As an example, one company advises adding 4 to 5 pinches of salt to the reservoir if the vaporizer does not put out adequate steam.)

On the other hand, if the water is too hard, the vaporizer may blow fuses or trip electrical breakers (lights may flicker) as it draws excessive electrical power. Some brands of vaporizers may spit out boiling water if the water contains excessive electrolyte. (See "A Pharmacist's Journal: My Cat Doesn't Like This Vaporizer.") *Dilution of the tap water with distilled water will remedy this problem.*

Precautions in Use of Vaporizers

Vaporizer Safety. Modern vaporizers are extremely safe. Because of the steam outlet at the top of the unit, when the boiling chamber is placed into the vaporizer, the water level rises within the chamber. The steam that exits the steam outlet is sterile and free of minerals and bacteria.[5] Vaporizers are constructed to have a high tipover index (or low center of gravity), meaning that they can be tilted almost to vertical without the contents spilling out. Only the water in the boiling chamber is heated to boiling. The rest of the water in the reservoir is cool. Despite their overall safety when used as directed, improper or careless use of vaporizers can cause patient injury, especially involving young children, who are too young to appreciate the dangers of boiling water.

Burn Prevention

A few simple precautions can be communicated to patients to prevent burns. ***Never place the vaporizer on a table or other surface from which it could be overturned, and always keep the cord out of the reach of children and pets.*** In one case a mother placed a vaporizer on two blankets on a dresser next to the crib of a 7-month-old child.[42] He pulled the blankets and the vaporizer overturned, burning him. ***Parents must not leave children unattended around vaporizers.*** The steam that is coming out might be attractive to a baby. Also, parents must never place the units in a location where the child could accidentally fall on them.

To avoid being burned, the patient must not check to see if a vaporizer is working by placing the hand or finger over the steam outlet. Further, the vaporizer must be located at least 4 feet from people, and the steam must be directed away from patients.[43] Vaporizers should be located on the floor away from household traffic, with the cord out of reach of children and pets. A night light found on some vaporizers is an added safety feature.

Children must never be forced or allowed to breathe the steam directly. In one case a mother directed a 2-year-old to hold his face near the steam outlet to treat symptoms of upper respiratory infection.[44] When he cried, she noticed redness of the face and neck. He entered

A Pharmacist's Journal

"My Cat Doesn't Like This Vaporizer."

A female customer to whom I had sold a vaporizer wanted to return it several weeks later for a refund. When I asked what the problem was, she replied, "The cat doesn't like it." I asked her to clarify. "When the cat walks by the vaporizer, it hisses at her, then she hisses back at it. Now the cat won't go into the same room with the vaporizer." I asked if the vaporizer also spit out water. She assured me that it did. I ascertained that she was adding too much electrolyte to the water, which indeed causes some vaporizers to spit out boiling water, accompanied by hissing sounds. I advised her to reduce the amount of electrolyte, which evidently worked, since she did not return.

the emergency room with second-degree and third-degree burns and required 7 days of hospitalization.

Use of Medication with Vaporizers

Patients often request medications to help relieve coughs (Table 16.3). Medications used in conjunction with vaporizers and humidifiers were found to be safe and effective for cough in patients over 2, in the ongoing review of OTC products being undertaken by the FDA.[45] Camphor and menthol/peppermint oil were given Category I status (safe and effective).[46] Kaz Inhalant and DeVilbiss•Hankscraft Vaporizer Inhalant contain these ingredients, along with others. The products are poured into a medication cup located just below the steam outlet. The volatile oils slowly vaporize and infiltrate the room. Although the manufacturer of one such product advises the patient to pour it into the reservoir, manufacturers of vaporizers caution against this practice as the oils will interfere with the vaporizer's action and will void the warranty. The pharmacist should advise against adding any medication to the reservoir. Vaporizers were designed to properly deliver medication that is only added to the medication cup.

Medication is never used with any type of humidifier since they lack heat to volatilize the oils. Further, adding the medications to the tank will also void the warranty of humidifiers.

HUMIDIFIERS

Types of Humidifiers: Methods of Action and Cleaning

All humidifiers should be unplugged during filling and cleaning and should not be plugged in with wet hands. However, other information regarding cleaning varies according to the type of humidifier.

Impeller Humidifiers. The spinning disk or impeller humidifier is the most common type of home humidifier (Fig. 16.5). A motor rapidly rotates a hollow tube—the spindle—which is immersed in the reservoir. Water is drawn upward through the center of the spindle onto the upper part of a spinning disk and thrown by centrifugal force against a baffle or screen. The impact against the screen breaks the water droplets into a mist.

As the impeller rotates, it also draws room air into the humidifier through the air inlet. The room air is mixed with the mist around the impeller, and the fan action of the rotary impeller blows the humidified air out of the spout into the room. Thus the humidifier does not heat water like the vaporizer does, but produces humidification as the suspended droplets of water interact with the drier gas molecules of the room air.

The vaporizer ceases to function when the water level falls to the lowest level of the electrodes, but the impeller humidifier will continue to run, even when the reservoir is fully empty. Although the humidifier does not put out cool mist when empty, the noise of the impeller makes it appear to be functioning.

 The humidifier should be cleaned at least once weekly.[5] In the absence of manufacturer's directions, the user should follow these steps:

1. Unplug the motor unit and remove it from the reservoir.
2. Empty all water from the reservoir.
3. Partially fill the container with a solution of 1 teaspoonful of bleach per gallon of water. Cover the mist outlet.
4. Let stand for 20 minutes, shaking vigorously every few minutes.
5. Drain and rinse with clean water until the bleach smell is gone. Empty the reservoir and wipe the inside with a clean, dry cloth.
6. If scale is seen in the reservoir, place undiluted white vinegar into it and soak. Rinse thoroughly to remove the scale and vinegar with warm tap water.
7. Pry off and remove the pickup plug from the end of the impeller shaft.
8. Clean inside the impeller tube with a pipe cleaner.
9. Wash the tube with a bleach/water solution as described previously. Never submerge the motor or allow solution to enter the motor compartment. Clean the screen with a sponge.

To prevent bacterial growth, humidifiers should not be allowed to sit with water in the reservoir.

Table 16.3. Representative Medications for Use with Vaporizers

PRODUCT	SELECTED INGREDIENTS/COMMENTS
DeVilbiss•Hankscraft Vaporizer Inhalant	Methyl salicylate 2.34%, eucalyptus oil 1.8%, menthol 0.67%
Kaz Inhalant	Camphor 0.8%, methyl salicylate 0.4%, eucalyptus oil, peppermint oil, lavender oil (concentrations unlabeled)
Vicks Vapo Steam	Camphor 6.2%, menthol, eucalyptus oil (concentrations unlabeled); the manufacturer advises adding the product to the water in a steam vaporizer reservoir

Some humidifiers include a dust-trap covering over the air intake to filter room air. This filter should be cleaned periodically to ensure free flow of air into the humidifier. Warm soapy water is usually sufficient for cleaning the dust-trap filter, followed by rinsing; however, always advise consumers to follow the manufacturer's instructions.

Some humidifiers have air-cleaning filter cartridges. The air cleaning cartridge is placed over the air intake. The cartridge can remove 93% of small particles (such as pollen), as well as odors, tobacco smoke, and dust. The air filter should be changed as directed (about every 2 months or so).

Patients may object to the slight noise of the impeller in the humidifier. However, this constant motor whir masks other annoying noises. Its constant sound could be called "white noise." As droplets from the impeller humidifier evaporate on various spots around the room, they may leave a white dust. This is calcium carbonate, a harmless mineral found in tap water. It is harmless when inhaled, but may cause a problem in sophisticated electrical equipment such as computers and VCRs. White dust can be prevented by using distilled water in the reservoir rather than tap water.

Occasionally, people discover that water droplets fall out around the unit. Should this occur, it indicates one of three things. Either the room is already fully saturated with vapor, or the humidifier needs cleansing, or medication has been added to the water, which should never be done. (See "Use of Medication with Humidifiers.")

Evaporative Humidifiers. The evaporative humidifier employs another technology for household humidification. The typical evaporative humidifier has a reservoir of about 1.2 gallons. An absorbent paper wicking filter causes water in the reservoir to evaporate, and a fan circulates moist air into the room.[5]

Moisture is not actively forced into the air, but passively evaporates, thus the unit is self-regulating. Humidity output will increase when the air is drier, and decrease as the air becomes more saturated. Because the evaporative humidifier is a passive humidifier, the mineral in water does not enter the room, eliminating the problem of white dust.

The evaporative humidifier must be cleaned like the impeller humidifier. (Always follow the manufacturer's direc-

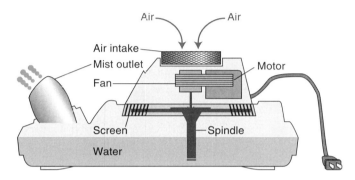

Figure 16.5. The impeller humidifier. Note the position of the spindle and motor.

tions.) Generally, the base should be cleaned and dried each day the humidifier is used. Each week, the wicking filter must be removed from its support ribs. Then, 8 ounces of white vinegar are poured into the reservoir. The solution should stand in the reservoir for 20 minutes. A cloth dampened with the vinegar should be used to wipe out the reservoir. The base is rinsed with warm water. To prevent electrical shock, the top housing containing the motor should never be immersed in water. The wicking filter can be removed from the housing and rinsed in warm water to remove mineral content (Fig. 16.6). Four conditions indicate that the wicking filter should be replaced:

- The wicking filter becomes discolored because of buildup of mineral and impurities from the water.
- The humidifier output decreases.
- The top of the wick becomes dry to the touch, indicating that water is not wicking up as it should.
- The wick has large holes or tears in it, perhaps as a result of forcing a support rib through it accidentally.

tip *If a family uses a humidifier seasonally (such as in the drier winter months in their particular climate), the wicking filter should be discarded at the end of the season, when the humidifier season is over. It should never be left in the humidifier while being stored.* In the pharmacy, replacement wicking filters should be stocked next to the evaporative units themselves.

A Pharmacist's Journal

"This Humidifier Isn't Very Good."

Store personnel once asked me if I would help a customer in the front of the store who needed help with a humidifier. I approached a woman holding one of the less expensive humidifiers. She asked me, "This isn't very good, is it?" I assured her that the unit was a good product, if used as directed. She replied, "But it only lasts for 24 hours." I agreed, and pointed out that we sold larger units that lasted a longer time, but they cost a little more. She listened politely, and responded, "But why would a person buy this?" I then explained the rationale for added humid-

ity and the benefits of proper humidification. After this explanation, she repeated, "But that's still not very good." As English was not her first language, I attempted again to explain the virtues of the unit. She repeated, "But it only lasts 24 hours." Finally, it dawned on me why she was puzzled. I then explained, "Although it only runs for 24 hours, you refill it and it runs another 24 hours." The light went on in her head, and she bought the unit. She had thought the humidifier was used once and then discarded. In that light, her questions were sensible and realistic.

tip *The base should be disinfected at the end of any seasonal use or when the unit is to stand for long periods. Follow the manufacturer's instructions or place 1 teaspoonful of household bleach in 1 gallon of water, and then allow the solution to remain in the reservoir for 20 minutes.*[5] Before use, the reservoir must be rinsed until the bleach smell is gone.

Ultrasonic Humidifiers. Ultrasonic humidifiers are another option for adding humidity to room air. The ultrasonic unit has no motor, but operates by means of a transducer, which vibrates 1.7 million times each second. High-frequency vibrations break the water droplets into an extremely fine mist.[5] A humidity control (the humidistat) sets the desired humidity level. The mist output control is a second control that regulates the fan and the amount of mist that the unit creates. When the unit reaches the level set with the humidistat, the ultrasonic humidifier cycles off automatically. As the humidity drops below the preset level, the unit cycles back on again. It operates quietly, comparable to the evaporative humidifier.

The ultrasonic humidifier with a tank holding 1.5 gallons will run for 14 to 16 hours. The customer should not allow the nozzle to be obstructed while it is operating. To prevent damage to the transducer, ultrasonic humidifiers should not be run while dry. While it is operating, the ultrasonic humidifier should not be tilted, emptied or filled.

tip *Whenever ultrasonic humidifiers are to sit for more than 48 hours, they should be emptied.* If they are not emptied, deposits may form in the base, impairing the transducer's action. The base should never be immersed in water.

tip *The ultrasonic should be cleaned weekly by following the manufacturer's instructions.* Clean the tank by placing some hydrogen peroxide 3% in it, shaking it vigor-

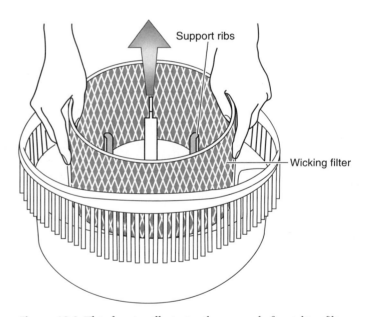

Figure 16.6. This drawing illustrates the removal of a wicking filter from an evaporative humidifier.

ously every few minutes for 20 minutes, and then draining and rinsing it.

Hydrogen peroxide is also poured into the humidifier base reservoir and allowed to stand for 20 minutes. If mineral deposits are in the base, white vinegar can be applied with a soft brush or cloth. The area also should be rinsed with clean water before using it.

White dust may also appear on surfaces around the ultrasonic humidifier.[5] The ultrasonic was quite popular in the mid to late 1980's, but the superfine mist produced carries the white dust to surrounding surfaces more easily than other humidifiers, causing them to diminish in popularity.[47] White dust is easily prevented through using distilled water in the reservoir.

Central Household Humidifiers.   Patients may ask about the efficiency of central household humidifiers. They may be built into the house or added on later.[5] However, they are not portable and are more expensive than the simpler units. Further, they can only be installed if you have forced-air heating. If you have hot-water, steam, or electrical-resistance heating, you cannot use a built-in humidifier.

Console Humidifiers.   Some companies market large console humidifiers with slowly rotating belts. They are not traditionally sold in pharmacies.

Precautions in the Use of Humidifiers:
Hypersensitivity Pneumonitis

The steam generated by vaporizers is sterile, but the droplets put out by humidifiers can carry organisms or their by-products to which the user may be allergic. Several case studies have reported a humidifier-related phenomenon variously known as hypersensitivity pneumonitis, humidifier fever, or allergic alveolitis.[48,49] Patients typically experience dyspnea, fever, cough, and headache that resolves on removal from the source and recurs on rechallenge with humidified air.[50–52] Other symptoms recently added to the syndrome include generalized malaise, myalgia, fever and chills, chest tightness, and weight loss.[53,54] Current theory subscribes to an allergic rather than infectious etiology.[53,55]

Often, the problem is seen with forced office humidification systems rather than simple home humidifiers, although a few scattered reports implicate home humidifiers in the problem.[49,56–61] The Consumer Product Safety Commission had no record of humidifiers causing allergies of this type.[62] Humidifier fever is easily prevented via cleansing of the unit as directed by the manufacturer. In light of the millions of humidifiers used every winter and the relatively small number of reported cases, the risk of allergic alveolitis occurring with a properly cleaned home humidifier appears to be negligible.

Use of Medication with Humidifiers

All nonprescription products used in conjunction with devices for humidity deficit require heat to volatilize them. Since humidifiers do not work by producing heat, adding any ingredient to the reservoir is irrational. Further, the manufacturers generally warn that this action will void the warranty of the item. Residue from the oily liquids could accumulate on the fan, impairing its action.

Patients should take care that only water is added to a humidifier. The accidental addition of 70% isopropyl alcohol to the humidifier allowed a newborn male infant to breathe the chemical for 2 hours, which resulted in death.[63]

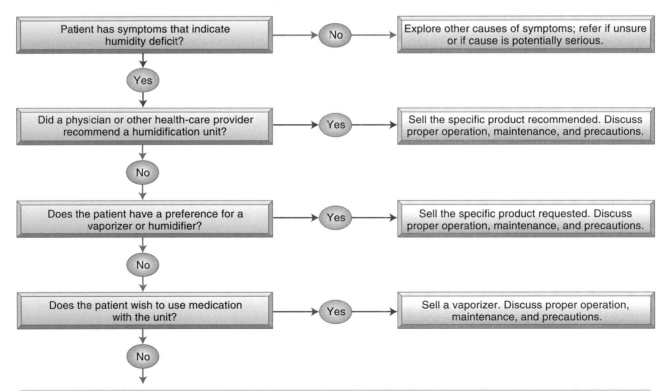

Patient Assessment Algorithm 16.1. Humidifiers and Vaporizers

PREVENTION OF HUMIDITY DEFICIT

The typical patient goes through a yearly cycle of gradually decreasing humidity in the home. When the problem becomes noticeable, humidifiers or vaporizers are purchased or brought out of storage and plugged in. Eventually, the symptoms of dryness resolve as humidity becomes optimal. However, those who tire of treating the problem may choose instead to prevent it by beginning the devices before winter dryness is intolerable. For instance, the patient would be well-advised to begin use of vaporizers and/or humidifiers in late fall (before humidity drops below the comfortable level). Their use could be continued as long as needed. These dates are approximate and wholly depend on the prevailing seasons in the particular geographic location. Using the products in this manner might also help prevent colds and flu by promoting mucokinesis.

SUMMARY

Humidity deficit is a common seasonal problem that often goes unrecognized. However, it may become the evident etiology as the pharmacist listens to the patient's complaints of sore throat, cough, dry skin, itching eyes, and the feeling of dried secretions in the airways. The pharmacist who suspects humidity deficit should discuss the need for adequate humidity and then demonstrate the various devices for providing humidity. To help the customer make a judgment on these products, the pharmacist should point out their relative advantages and disadvantages such as the use of medications to alleviate cough with vaporizers. Also, the pharmacist should note that while vaporizers require regular cleansing, the steam that exits from them does not cause health problems; humidifiers carry a small risk of allergic reactions unless the products are properly disinfected.

Used properly, according to manufacturers' directions, vaporizers and humidifiers are inexpensive, safe devices to prevent and treat health problems that arise from humidity deficit.

References

1. Lecos C. Water, the number one nutrient. FDA Consumer 17:28, 1983..
2. Phillips PA, et al. Disturbed fluid and electrolyte homeostasis following dehydration in elderly people. Age Aging 22:S26, 1993.
3. Burton GG, Hodgkin JE, Ward JJ, eds. Respiratory care: A guide to clinical practice. Philadelphia: JB Lippincott, 1991; p. 355.
4. Miyao H, et al. Relative humidity, not absolute humidity is of great importance when using a humidifier with a heating wire. Crit Care Med 20:674, 1992.
5. Cramer T. Humidifiers. FDA Consumer 26:33, 1992.
6. Reinikainen LM, et al. The effect of air humidification on symptoms and perception of indoor air quality in office workers: A six-period cross-over trial. Arch Environ Health 47:8, 1992.
7. Energy-tight buildings heighten disease risk. The Daily Oklahoman 4/27/88:3.
8. Sherin KM. Building-related illnesses and sick building syndrome. J Fla Med Assoc 80:472, 1993.
9. de Hoog GS, Beguin H, Batenburg-van de Vagte WH. Phaeotheca triangularis, a new meristematic black yeast from a humidifier. Antonie Van Leeuwenhoek 71:289, 1997.

AT THE COUNTER

A couple in their late 60s are looking at vaporizers and humidifiers on a winter day. When the pharmacist asks if they require assistance, they say they want to know if one would help their dry skin and sore throats. They also can't seem to remove the secretions from their lungs.

Interview/Patient Assessment

The wife has recently undergone chemotherapy for breast cancer. The husband has problems with irritable bowel syndrome.

Pharmacist's Analysis

1. Are the patients' symptoms possibly caused by humidity deficit?
2. Do their medical conditions contraindicate vapor therapy?
3. Which product should the pharmacist recommend?

The couple's symptoms are consistent with humidity deficit, especially since this occurs in the winter. Their medical conditions do not contraindicate vapor therapy with either a vaporizer or a humidifier.

Patient Counseling

The pharmacist could recommend either a vaporizer or humidifier to relieve the symptoms mentioned, as shown in Patient Assessment Algorithm 16.1. If the couple would like to try a vaporizer inhalant solution that is proven effective for cough, a vaporizer is required. At the point of sale, the pharmacist should point out the steps that must be taken to adjust water quality and to clean the vaporizer, boiling chamber, and electrodes. If the couple feel unable to undertake the more demanding cleaning steps required with vaporizers, the humidifier would be the best option, although they cannot use vaporizer inhalants with the humidifier.

10. Eubanks DH, Bone RC. Comprehensive respiratory care. 2nd ed. St. Louis: CV Mosby, 1990; p. 161.

11. Pray S. Humidifiers help skin (Letter). The New York Times, March 16, 1993.

12. Philip G, et al. Reflex activation of nasal secretion by unilateral inhalation of cold dry air. Am Rev Respir Dis 148:1616, 1993.

13. Ophir D, et al. Effects of elevated intranasal temperature on subjective and objective findings in perennial rhinitis. Ann Otol Rhinol Laryngol 97(3 pt 1):259, 1988.

14. Shelly MP, et al. A review of the mechanisms and methods of humidification of inspired gases. Intensive Care Med 14:1, 1988.

15. Boulet L-P, Turcotte H. Influence of water content of inspired air during and after exercise on induced bronchoconstriction. Eur Respir J 4:979, 1991.

16. Tyrrell DAJ. Rhinoviruses and coronaviruses—virologic aspects of their role in causing colds in man. Eur J Respir Dis 64(Suppl 128):332, 1983.

17. Sakakura Y. Changes of mucociliary function during colds. Eur J Respir Dis 64(Suppl 128):348, 1983.

18. Salah B, et al. Nasal mucociliary transport in healthy subjects is slower when breathing dry air. Eur Respir J 1:852, 1988.

19. Basbaum CB. Regulation of airway secretory cells. Clin Chest Med 7:231, 1986.

20. Wanner A. Mucociliary clearance in the trachea. Clin Chest Med 7:247, 1986.

21. Guus SM, et al. Correlation between nasal ciliary beat frequency and mucus transport rate in volunteers. Laryngoscope 95:854, 1985.

22. Dick EC, et al. Aerosol transmission of rhinovirus colds. J Infect Dis 156:442, 1987.

23. Wilson R, et al. Upper respiratory tract viral infection and mucociliary clearance. Eur J Respir Dis 70:272, 1987.

24. Pederson M, et al. Nasal mucociliary transport, number of ciliated cells, and beating pattern in naturally acquired common colds. Eur J Respir Dis 64(Suppl 128):355, 1983.

25. Winther B, et al. Pathology of naturally occurring colds. Eur J Respir Dis 64(Suppl 128):345, 1983.

26. Hendley JO. Rhinovirus colds: Immunology and pathogenesis. Eur J Respir Dis 64(Suppl 128):340, 1983.

27. Camner P, et al. Tracheobronchial clearance in patients with influenza. Am Rev Respir Dis 108: 131, 1973.

28. Parks CR. Mist therapy: Rationale and practice. J Pediatr 76:305, 1970.

29. Kuo C-D, et al. Aerosol, humidity and oxygenation. Chest 99:1352, 1991.

30. Mercke U. The influence of varying air humidity on mucociliary activity. Acta Otolaryngol 79:133, 1975.

31. Brown GW. Mucosal humidification (Letter). Lancet 338(8765):522, 1991.

32. Ebrahim MKH, et al. Scald accidents during water aerosol inhalation in infants. Burns 16:291, 1990.

33. Greally P, et al. Children with croup presenting with scalds. BMJ 301(6743):113, 1990.

34. Henry R. Moist air in the treatment of laryngotracheitis. Arch Dis Child 58:577, 1983.

35. Conn V. Self-care actions taken by older adults for influenza and colds. Nurs Res 40:176, 1991.

36. Szilagyi PG. Humidifiers and other symptomatic therapy for children with respiratory tract infections. Pediatr Infect Dis J 10:478, 1991.

37. DelMar C. Managing viral upper respiratory infections. Aust Fam Physician 20:557, 1991.

38. Ernst E. Saunas—A hobby or for health? J R Soc Med 11:639, 1989.

39. Singh M, et al. Evaluation of steam therapy in acute lower respiratory tract infections: a pilot study. Indian Pediatr 27:945, 1990.

40. Dunne CF. The dry mouth dilemma. Oncol Nurse Forum 18:785, 1991.

41. Infante-Rivard C. Childhood asthma and indoor environmental risk factors. Am J Epidemiol 137:834, 1993.

42. Barich DP. Steam vaporizers—Therapy or tragedy? Pediatrics 49:131, 1972.

43. Aggarwal A, Edlich RF, Himel HN. Steam vaporizer burn injuries. J Emerg Med 13:55, 1995.

44. Colombo JL, et al. Steam vaporizer injuries. Pediatrics 67:661, 1981.

45. Fed Reg 52:30041, 1987.

46. Fed Reg 48:48576, 1983.

47. Reese KM. Ultrasonic humidifiers said to threaten health. Chem Eng News 66:60, 1988..

48. Hodges GR, et al. Hypersensitivity pneumonitis caused by a contaminated cool-mist vaporizer. Ann Intern Med 80:501, 1974.

49. Burke GW, et al. Allergic alveolitis caused by home humidifiers. JAMA 238:2705, 1977.

50. Kane GC, et al. Hypersensitivity pneumonitis secondary to *Klebsiella oxytoca*. Chest 104:627, 1993.

51. Pal TM, et al. The clinical spectrum of humidifier disease in synthetic fiber plants. Am J Ind Med 31:682, 1997.

52. Mamolen M, et al. Investigation of an outbreak of "humidifier fever" in a print shop. Am J Ind Med 23:483, 1993.

53. Stankus RP. Hypersensitivity pneumonitis. NY St J Med 90:232, 1990.

54. Lewis C. Quantifying serum antibody class and subclass responses by enzyme immunoassay in humidifier-related disease. Clin Exp Allergy 21:601, 1991.

55. Embil J, et al. Pulmonary illness associated with exposure to Mycobacterium-avium complex in hot tub water. Hypersensitivity pneumonitis or infection? Chest 111:813, 1997.

56. McSharry C, et al. Serological and clinical investigation of humidifier fever. Clin Allergy 17:15, 1987.

57. Finnegan MJ. Amoebae and humidifier fever. Clin Allergy 17 235, 1987.

58. Anderson K, et al. Climate, intermittent humidification, and humidifier fever. Br J Ind Med 46:671, 1989.

59. Shiue S-T, et al. Hypersensitivity pneumonitis associated with the use of ultrasonic humidifiers. NY St J Med 90:263, 1990.

60. Volpe BT, et al. Hypersensitivity pneumonitis associated with a portable home humidifier. Conn Med 55:571, 1991.

61. Suda T, et al. Hypersensitivity pneumonitis associated with home ultrasonic humidifiers. Chest 107:711, 1995.

62. Duvall, DP. Personal communication. Washington, DC: U.S. Consumer Product Safety Commission, October 7, 1992.

63. Vicas IM, Beck R. Fatal inhalational isopropyl alcohol poisoning in a neonate. J Toxicol Clin Toxicol 31:473, 1993.

Asthma

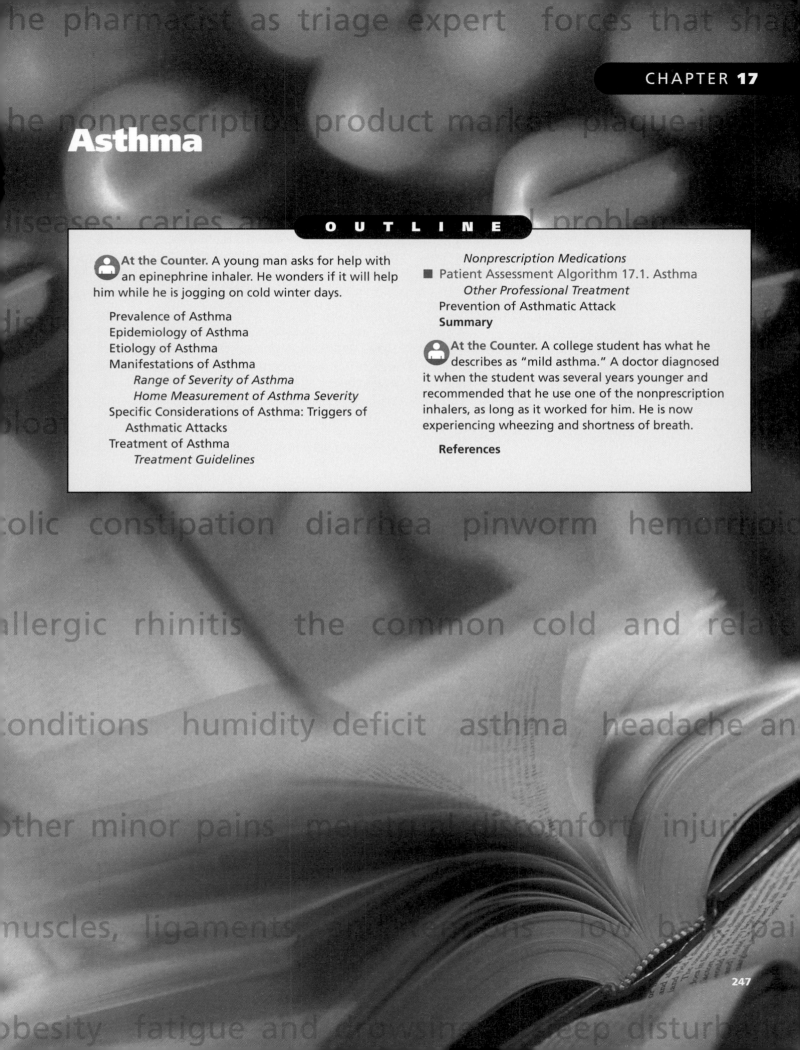

A young man asks for help with an epinephrine inhaler. He wonders if it will help him while he is jogging on cold winter days.

Interview/Patient Assessment

He has noticed for the past month or so that he cannot jog as much as he used to. He is affected with wheezing and shortness of breath after 1 mile and must rest before walking home. The pharmacist ascertains that he is taking no prescription medications and has no diagnosed medical conditions. However, he was diagnosed as an asthmatic when he was younger and used prescription medication for several years. His condition was never sufficiently serious to require hospitalization. He was symptom-free until this latest episode.

Pharmacist's Analysis

1. Are this man's symptoms consistent with asthma?
2. What is the importance of the type of activity and the season?
3. Can this patient use a nonprescription product?

The patient's symptoms are consistent with exercise-induced asthma (EIA), which is more common during a vigorous activity such as jogging in cold, dry air.

Patient Counseling

This patient once had a diagnosis of asthma, although his condition was not sufficiently serious to require hospitalization; currently, he is not using any medication. There are no potential drug interactions, and he has no contraindications to nonprescription asthma metered-dose inhalers.

Should the pharmacist choose to recommend an epinephrine inhaler, the patient should be warned not to exceed the recommended dose in either quantity or frequency of administration. Should his symptoms continue after 20 minutes, he should see a physician. He should be advised that physician monitoring might be preferable to self-treatment in this case, since asthma can be life-threatening. Finally, the pharmacist might point out the proven efficacy of prescription products (e.g., albuterol inhalation) in treatment of exercise-induced bronchospasm.

Asthma is a multifactorial condition that ranges in severity from mildly troubling to life-threatening. There are many prescription products available. However, the nonprescription market is limited to devices and a few oral or inhalation products. In most instances the retail pharmacist should refer the patient who wishes to self-treat asthma to a physician for diagnosis and care. Once the patient has been diagnosed, the pharmacist should undertake the elements of pharmaceutical care for all prescription asthma products.

PREVALENCE OF ASTHMA

The prevalence of asthma varies according to such population variables as age and geographic location. Asthma affects as many as 4% of the United States population.[1] This figure was found to be markedly higher in research that examined the incidence of asthma in well-educated, white adults whose ages were in the late 20s and early 30s.[2] At least 7.5% of females and 6.9% of males had a previous physician diagnosis of asthma. At least 2 to 3 million children are affected, although researchers estimate that as many as 14.3% of those in grades 3 to 5 suffer from undiagnosed asthma.[3,4]

Asthma increases the risk of death, which skews prevalence rates for certain ages. For instance, researchers followed a group of 1075 asthmatics that experienced over twice the number of deaths in an 8.6-year period when compared with a matched group of controls.[5]

EPIDEMIOLOGY OF ASTHMA

Symptoms of asthma can begin in any decade of life, although most people are diagnosed prior to the age of 25.[1] In a study of well-educated patients, asthma was more common in females, although other studies show a greater frequency in males.[2,6] Racial differences exist with asthma. One study revealed a lifetime prevalence of 12% for blacks and 6% for whites.[6]

ETIOLOGY OF ASTHMA

The cause of asthma is unknown, although various triggering factors have been identified.[1] Asthma's hallmark symptom is bronchospasm, with increased responsiveness of the smooth muscles of the airways, a condition known as bronchial hyperresponsiveness (BHR).[7–9] Figure 17.1 illustrates the normal airway contrasted to the situation in asthma. Many triggers may induce BHR. In exercise-induced asthma (EIA) the trigger is not antigenic, but is caused by airway cooling and drying.[10] In other cases the trigger is antigenic, involving inflammation and infiltration of the airways with eosinophils, neutrophils, and monocytes.[7,11,12] Further, asthma is charac-

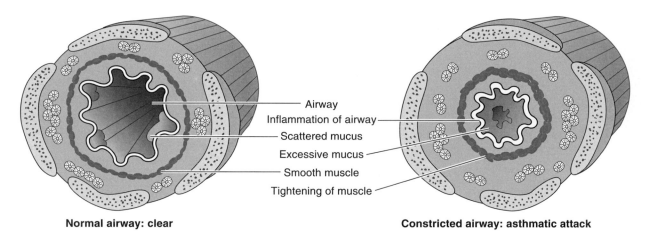

Normal airway: clear   **Constricted airway: asthmatic attack**

Figure 17.1. Although the asthma trigger varies with the type of asthma, the normal airway (*left*) becomes more constricted in all types of asthma. This airway constriction, along with other changes, causes the breathing problems of asthmatics.

terized by reversibility, either spontaneously or through pharmacologic interventions.[13]

MANIFESTATIONS OF ASTHMA

Range of Severity of Asthma

Asthma symptoms and signs may be classified as mild, moderate, or severe (see "Rating Asthma Severity"):

- With *mild* asthma, the patient may be asymptomatic or may experience minimal chest tightness with a slight increase in wheezing and perhaps a mild cough.[14]
- The patient with a *moderate* attack complains of moderate dyspnea or feeling of chest tightness; the patient is fully aware of airway obstruction.[14] In addition, inspiratory and expiratory wheezing, moderate coughing, and tachycardia develop.
- The patient in the throes of a *severe* attack suffers severe dyspnea; evident anxiety; **stridor** (a high-pitched, noisy respiration); coughing; rapid, shallow breathing; irritability; withdrawn behavior; cyanosis; fatigue; and stomach pain.

▲ *Asthma can be fatal with improper treatment.*
Asthma deaths often occur at night, prior to a trip to the hospital. In some cases night death occurs even though the patient uses a bronchodilator before bedtime, because the bronchodilator effect (about 4 hours after application) coincides with a natural nocturnal drop in airway function. A study of pediatric asthma deaths by an authority on pediatric psychiatry revealed that in all deaths the children had a history of stressful experiences prior to asthma episodes.[15] Further, 90% of children demonstrated a history of emotions or stress as a trigger. He also pinpointed a number of factors more common in children who die of asthma, including the following:

- Physiological factors (e.g., a history of seizures associated with asthma attacks)

- Large reductions in prednisone doses (by more than 50% of the initial dose)
- Wheezing with stress of discharge from a hospital

Psychological factors associated with pediatric asthma deaths included patient disregard of asthma symptoms, poor self-care when in a hospital, patient conflict with parents and hospital staff, manipulative use of asthma, emotional disturbances, symptoms of depression, and family dysfunction.

Overall, deaths from asthma almost doubled from 1978 to 1989.[16] Nonwhites experience death rates four times higher than those for whites. Many asthma deaths are caused by chronic obstructive pulmonary disease.[17]

Home Measurement of Asthma Severity

Peak-flow meters were primarily physician devices and seldom used at home until publication of a 1991 National Institutes of Health/National Heart, Lung and Blood Institute (NIH/NHLBI) report, which encouraged clinicians to recommend peak-flow meters for home use to monitor patients over age 5 with moderate-to-severe asthma (Fig. 17.2).[18] These handheld nonprescription devices, which measure the amount of air the individual can force from the airways in a rapid exhalation, allow the patient to obtain a number that correlates with lung function.[19] Although peak-flow meters primarily measure ease of exhalation from the large airways, they also measure the severity of asthma, a disease of the small airways.

To properly use a peak-flow meter, patients should follow these steps[19]:

1. Blow with all the force possible into the device.
2. Record the number.
3. Reset the pointer to zero and repeat steps 1 through 3.
4. Repeat steps 1 through 3 again.

The peak flow is the best of the three tries. The asthmatic is taught to track performance by learning a color zone system.

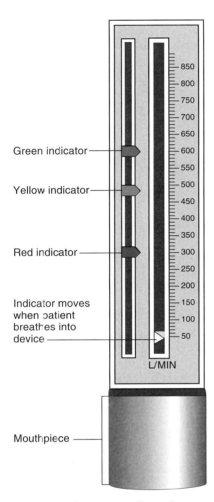

Figure 17.2. The peak-flow meter allows the patient to monitor lung function changes at home. This peak-flow meter is set for the patient with a peak flow of 600.

The medical professional will instruct the patient in setting three adjustable colored indicators on the scale of the peak-flow meter. For example, the top (green) marker is usually set at the patient's personal-best peak expiratory flow rate (PEFR). The middle (yellow) indicator may be set at 80 to 90% of the best PEFR, and the bottom (red) indicator set at 50 to 60% of the patient's best PEFR.

Since peak flow is affected by age, height, weight, sex, race, and strength, each patient is taught to use his or her own past personal best as their 100% level. Over a lifetime, the personal best peaks at age 30, diminishing thereafter. Patients may then use their best peak flow from the previous year as a 100% benchmark. The asthmatic is better able to manage asthma by correlating the symptoms or feelings they have about the severity of the episode with the peak flow rates on their own charts.[15]

Some physicians advocate using the peak-flow meter only when symptoms begin. Typically, however, when patients detect wheezing, small airways are usually 50 to 80% obstructed. At that time obstruction is so great that medication

needs are greatly increased. Instead, the devices should be used daily to detect drops in airway caliber that often occur 24 hours before symptoms develop. Current medical opinion is moving toward a minimum of two readings daily, morning (8:00 AM) and evening (4:00 PM), thus maximizing the preventive capability of the devices.[18] A patient who has trouble recognizing symptoms of an attack may be better able to pay more attention to those symptoms when his or her diary indicates that he or she is in airflow difficulty. If a specific PEFR reading on the peak-flow meter falls in the yellow zone, the patient's response is somewhat impaired. The patient should follow instructions given by the physician.

⚠️ *If the reading falls in the red zone, breathing is dangerously impaired, and the patient should call for medical assistance without delay.*

SPECIFIC CONSIDERATIONS OF ASTHMA: TRIGGERS OF ASTHMATIC ATTACKS

Many factors have been identified as triggers for asthmatic attacks. They include allergens, occupational exposures, exercise, stress, viral infections, and pollutants (Fig. 17.3).[19,20] Control of allergens, as described in Chapter 14 (Allergic Rhinitis), is also helpful for allergen-induced asthma. Occupational exposures include psyllium, as described in Chapter 10 (Constipation).

Inhalation of airborne particulates can induce asthma, depending on the size and nature of the particulates. Climatic conditions that result in the concentration of such pollutants as sulfur dioxide and ozone cause respiratory problems in the general population.[21] Individuals affected are often otherwise asymptomatic, but are later found to have hyperirritable airways. These conditions also initiate or aggravate wheezing and dyspnea in asthmatics. Similarly, irritants such as aerosol cosmetic sprays, fresh paint, room deodorants, and insecticides worsen breathing ability.[3]

EIA causes problems for some asthmatics.[22,23] Symptoms may begin as soon as 6 to 10 minutes after beginning exercise or not until after the exercise is over.[14] Usually, the condition is worse after exercise, reaching a peak in children at 4 to 8 minutes (6 to 10 minutes in adults) after stopping the exercise.[24] Symptoms gradually fade over a period of 30 to 60 minutes without medication.[14,25] Under most circumstances EIA is associated with moderate obstruction and is not life-threatening. Consequently, continued airway narrowing, which could necessitate hospitalization or emergency therapy, is extremely rare.[3]

TREATMENT OF ASTHMA

Treatment Guidelines

In 1991 the NIH/NHLBI established the National Asthma Education Program, which in turn developed consensus guidelines for diagnosis and treatment of asthma.[18] This well-received program described ideal treatment for chronic

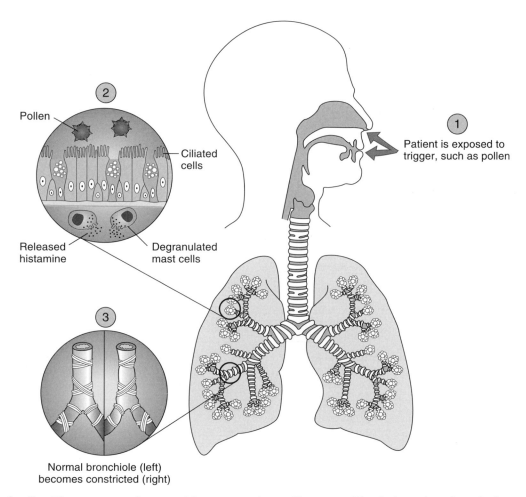

Figure 17.3. Inhaled pollen (*1*) triggers an asthma attack by causing release of histamine (*2*), which results in bronchiolar constriction (*3*).

and acute asthma, delineating roles for theophylline, inhaled beta-2 agonists, cromolyn, and corticosteroids.

In the original FDA OTC Review report on bronchodilators, the panel provided Category I classification for oral ephedrine, inhaled epinephrine, and oral theophylline, among other medications that are not currently marketed.[26] The FDA disagreed with the theophylline ranking and placed it in Category II status in its tentative final monograph.[27] The final monograph reaffirmed that judgment, making theophylline a nonmonograph ingredient for asthma.[28] In the same publications oral ephedrine and inhaled epinephrine eventually attained monograph status.

(tip) *The patient cannot use nonprescription products unless asthma has been diagnosed by a physician, because airway obstruction also occurs in widespread bronchial infection and in acute or chronic bronchitis.*[28] (*See Patient Assessment Algorithm 17.1.*) Oral beta agonists such as ephedrine were not accorded any role in treatment of asthma in the 1991 NIH/NHLBI report, with the experts stating that inhaled products are preferred.[18] Further, according to the report, more selective beta-2 agonists that have little beta-1 activity (e.g., albuterol or metaproterenol) are less likely to produce adverse cardiac effects. Because of

its mixed action on beta-2 and beta-1 receptors, epinephrine is a poor choice for asthma therapy. Thus, in the view of the expert NIH/NHLBI group assigned to delineate proper therapy for asthma, nonprescription products have little role, if any. (See "Rating Asthma Severity.")

Nonprescription Medications

INDICATIONS AND USE LIMITATIONS FOR NONPRESCRIPTION ASTHMA PRODUCTS

Nonprescription asthma products are indicated for temporary relief of shortness of breath, tightness of chest, and wheezing resulting from bronchial asthma.[28] However, *many* **(tip)** *patients should not use them.* See "Precautions with Nonprescription Asthma Products." The pharmacist should endeavor to stress the need for professional care for most asthmatics. Once the patient is under the guidance of a physician, pharmacist interventions include such activities as patient education, patient monitoring, and ensuring communication with the physician about such matters as noncompliance.[29–32]

EPINEPHRINE

When patients choose nonprescription asthma products, some understand that inhalers have a more rapid onset than

Patient Assessment Algorithm 17.1. Asthma

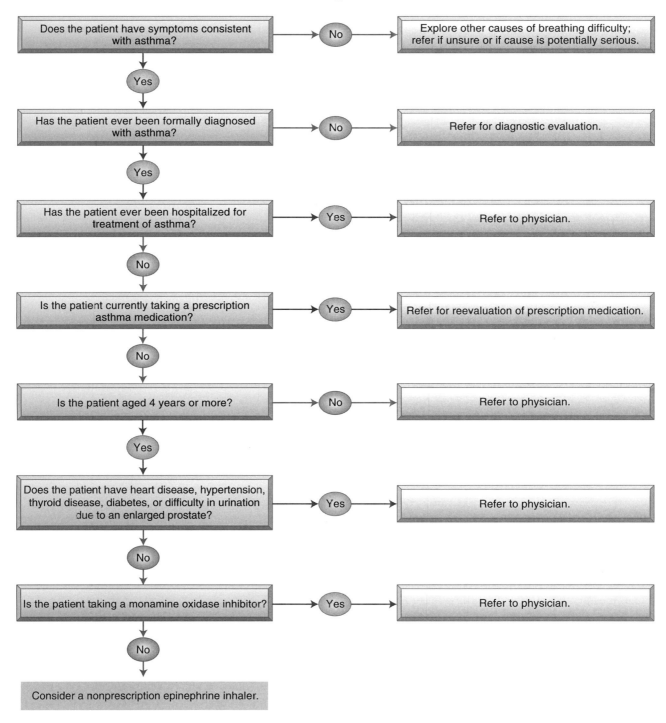

oral tablets. Epinephrine inhalers as listed in Table 17.1 have been the subject of debate in the Federal Register for some time.[27,28] (See "Correct Use of Metered-Dose Inhalers [MDIs].) Comments to the FDA mentioned their threat to the public health when marketed as nonprescription products. Some comments stressed that asthmatic patients rely too heavily on inhalers and overmedicate themselves in the mistaken belief that if the regular dose fails to achieve the desired results, a more frequent dose will work—a practice that can cause tolerance and dependency. Another comment

mentioned that some patients overmedicate to the point of tachyphylaxis (i.e., decreasing response following consecutive doses at short intervals). Comments submitted by physicians stressed that ***epinephrine causes serious adverse reactions and death and that it causes rebound congestion in the bronchial airways identical to the rebound congestion caused by epinephrine on the nasal mucosa.*** Despite all of these concerns, the FDA found none of the comments persuasive enough to limit the products to prescription-only status.

In one example of the dangers of epinephrine, a 19-year-old man obtained an epinephrine inhaler, sprayed the contents into a cup, and injected approximately 0.2 mL intravenously.[36] Within seconds he experienced palpitations, precordial chest tightness, pallor, diaphoresis, numbness, tingling of the hands and feet, and headache. He was hypotensive; 2000 mL of Lactated Ringer's solution maintained his systolic at 80 to 90 mm Hg. He remained asymptomatic during a 19-hour stay in the ICU and was discharged to inpatient psychiatric care.

A joint FDA advisory panel agreed that epinephrine should remain as a nonprescription drug product after hearing testimony. Nevertheless, the panel remained concerned about asthmatics who would not visit a physician, using nonprescription products instead.[37] In the most recent actions, the FDA has proposed the removal of all nonprescription, metered-dose inhalers.[38,39] This is a response to the reformulation of the products to remove ozone-depleting chlorofluorocarbon propellants. The agency proposed requiring premarket approval to ensure that the new inhaler system would be safe and effective. Epinephrine solutions for use in handheld nebulizers retained Category I status.

EPHEDRINE

Ephedrine-containing products with asthma labeling such as those in Table 17.2 are mostly combination products that include one or more other unapproved ingredients. ⚠ *Single-entity nonprescription products containing ephedrine are highly abused.*

Unfortunately, ephedrine is incorporated into numerous non–FDA-approved diet products under the name Ma huang and included in unapproved nonprescription stimulants found in gas stations, truck stops, and convenience stores.[40] Such packaging is in blatant disregard of the FDA labeling requirements for ephedrine. The FDA has seized many products that make these illegal stimulant claims.[41] In similar action, Texas has banned a diet product known as Formula One and has prohibited the sale to minors of any product containing ephedrine.[42] Adverse reactions to ephedrine products have included chest pain, myocardial infarction, hepatitis, stroke, seizures, psychosis, and death.[43]

Ephedrine is a key ingredient in the production of methamphetamine and of methcathinone ("cat"), a new "designer drug" that is more potent and addictive than crack cocaine. Emergency-room treatments of "cat" overdoses have been brisk in the upper Midwest. Unfortunately, ephedrine tablets can be purchased in bottles of 1000 for as little as $18 from mail-order magazines, who promote them in ads as diet and

---

FOCUS ON...

RATING ASTHMA SEVERITY

In addition to the NIH/NHLBI parameters for rating asthma[18] shown in the table, mild, moderate, and severe asthma exhibit the following characteristics:

- With *mild* asthma, exacerbations respond to bronchodilator medications more than 15% of the time, usually without steroids and usually in 12 to 24 hours.
- With *moderate* asthma, exacerbations respond to bronchodilators more than 15% of the time, but concomitant steroids are usually required. In addition, continuous daily drug treatment is required for maintenance plus aerosol steroids and cromolyn.
- With *severe* asthma, the patient has incomplete reversibility with aerosol bronchodilators, and high-dose steroids are required; continuous daily drug therapy is required for maintenance plus aerosolized and/or oral corticosteroids.[18]

NIH/NHLBI Ratings for Asthma

PARAMETER	DEGREE OF SEVERITY		
	MILD	MODERATE	SEVERE
Cough/wheeze	Less than 1–2 times weekly	More than 1–2 times weekly	
Emergency care?	None	Less than 3 times yearly	More than 2–3 times yearly
Description	Few clinical signs between episodes	Cough/low-grade wheezing between episodes	History of cough, syncope, hypoxic seizures, intubation, or respiratory failure
Exercise tolerance	Good	Diminished	Poor; limited activities
Nocturnal asthma	Less than 1–2 times monthly	2–3 nights/weekly	Nightly
School/work attendance	Good	May be affected	Poor
PEFR[a]	More than 80%	60–80%	Less than 60%
Am-Pm variability in PEFR	Less than 20%	20–30%	More than 30%
FEV_1[b] as % of predicted value	60–79%	41–59%	Less than 40%

[a]Peak expiratory flow rate.

[b]Forced expiratory volume in 1 second.

pep pills. As a result of the abuse, the DEA has sought authority to control these sales through legislation.[44] A 1994 bill signed by President Clinton subjected ephedrine tablets to stiffer controls to allow conviction of illegal drug traffickers.[45]

Rather than await federal action, many states have restricted the sale of products containing ephedrine only such as by making it a legend drug or a Schedule III, IV, or V drug.[46] Other states have restricted ephedrine combination products for asthma to legend status or to Schedule IV or V status.[47]

An FDA joint advisory panel has heard testimony from parents whose children suffered adverse effects from abused ephedrine products, with all speakers urging removal of OTC status for all ephedrine products. The panel agreed to removal after hearing all testimony.[48,49] As a result, the FDA proposed removal of ephedrine from asthma products, citing three recent developments[50,51]:

- The large-scale diversion of ephedrine for illicit use in the manufacture of methamphetamine and methcathinone.
- More recent information about ephedrine's harm with misuse and abuse when available as a nonprescription medication.
- The consensus from two FDA committees that the potential for illicit use outweighs any benefit to its use as a nonprescription bronchodilator.

Despite the threat of federal action, asthma products containing ephedrine are still widely available as of this writing.

UNAPPROVED INGREDIENTS IN ORAL COMBINATION ASTHMA PRODUCTS

Theophylline

The FDA does not allow the nonprescription sale of theophylline OTC as a single-entity product.[26] Thus theophylline

FOCUS ON...

PRECAUTIONS WITH NONPRESCRIPTION ASTHMA PRODUCTS

Patients must not use nonprescription asthma products if they have heart disease, high blood pressure, thyroid disease, diabetes, or difficulty in urination caused by enlargement of the prostate gland unless directed to do so by a physician. Furthermore, all packages must carry this FDA-mandated warning: "Do not use this product if you have ever been hospitalized for asthma or if you are taking any prescription drug for asthma unless directed by a doctor." Epinephrine and ephedrine must carry the following drug interaction warning: "Do not use this product if you are now taking a prescription monoamine oxidase inhibitor (MAOI) (certain drugs for depression, psychiatric or emotional conditions, or Parkinson's disease), or for 2 weeks after stopping the MAOI drug. If you are uncertain whether your prescription drug contains an MAOI, consult a health professional before taking this product."[33–35]

Products containing epinephrine must carry these warnings:

- Do not use this product more frequently or at higher doses than recommended unless directed by a doctor. (The preceding sentence must be in boldface type.) Excessive use may cause nervousness, rapid heart beat, and, possibly, adverse effects on the heart.
- Do not continue to use this product, but seek medical assistance immediately if symptoms are not relieved within 20 minutes or become worse.
- If the epinephrine is in solution form for nebulization, it must state: "Do not use this product if it is brown in color or cloudy."

Epinephrine-containing products may be administered to children 4 and older, with a dosage of one inhalation. After waiting 1 minute, the patient may use one additional inhalation. The product cannot be used for another 3 hours.

Products containing ephedrine must carry these warnings:

- Do not continue to use this product, but seek medical assistance immediately if symptoms are not relieved within 1 hour or become worse.
- Some users of this product may experience nervousness, tremor, sleeplessness, nausea, and loss of appetite. If these symptoms persist or become worse, consult your doctor.

Ephedrine-containing products must not be administered to children under the age of 12. Those over 12 may take 12.5 to 25 mg every 4 hours.

Table 17.1. Representative Inhalation Products for Asthma

PRODUCT	SELECTED INGREDIENTS/COMMENTS
AsthmaNefrin	Epinephrine solution for inhalation via nebulizer
Broncho-Saline	Aerosolized sterile normal saline for dilution of bronchodilator medications and other respiratory care applications
Primatene Mist	Per mL: 5.5 mg epinephrine in an MDI

was only found in combinations with ephedrine, possibly with other ingredients. Theophylline has well-known adverse reactions. In some cases nausea and vomiting occur when the doses are excessive, but frequently toxic effects associated with elevated serum levels of theophylline are not preceded by minor adverse effects. In addition, there is the question of synergistic toxicity of ingredients.[52,53]

Combination products containing ephedrine and theophylline were placed in Category II in 1988, a status that was finalized in 1995.[52–56] Virtually all products containing theophylline had been reformulated to exclude it by the mid 1990s.

Phenobarbital

Phenobarbital in asthma products was not examined by the FDA panel, and thus it is an unapproved ingredient. It was also removed from virtually all nonprescription asthma products by the mid 1990s.

Guaifenesin

Guaifenesin was not examined by the FDA panel and also must be considered an unapproved ingredient when included in asthma products.

Other Professional Treatment

Most asthmatics are monitored and treated by physicians, which is preferable to the unsupervised use of nonprescription medications. Asthma may be treated with the use of numerous protocols and algorithms, reflecting its multiple causes, various degrees of severity, and such demographic variables as the age of the patient.

PREVENTION OF ASTHMATIC ATTACK

Patients with allergen-induced asthma must limit their exposure to these allergens, as described in Chapter 14.

FOCUS ON...

CORRECT USE OF METERED-DOSE INHALERS (MDIs)

Prescription MDIs are often a component of the patient's asthma program. Nonprescription MDIs containing epinephrine are also available. For the patient to obtain the full benefits from using these products, all usage steps must be followed. While exact directions vary depending on the construction of the inhaler, the following steps may be used with modifications for most MDIs:

1. Remove the plastic dust cover from the mouthpiece.
2. Assemble the inhaler—for example, by placing the correct end of the mouthpiece over the top of the MDI.
3. Invert the assembled MDI.
4. If a spacer is recommended, place it on the MDI.
5. Shake the MDI-spacer assembly vigorously.
6. Place the assembled MDI close to the mouth.
7. Empty the lungs as completely as possible by exhaling deeply.
8. Place the mouthpiece (of either the spacer or the MDI) in the mouth, closing the lips tightly around the open end of the mouthpiece.
9. Inhale deeply while activating the MDI.
10. Remove the MDI from the mouth immediately after the activation.
11. Finish the deep inhalation and hold this breath as long as comfortable.
12. Exhale slowly, keeping the lips barely open.
13. Clean the MDI (and spacer) as recommended.
14. Keep a record of the number of activations of the device. Subtract one more activation from the total listed on the MDI to determine the remaining contents.

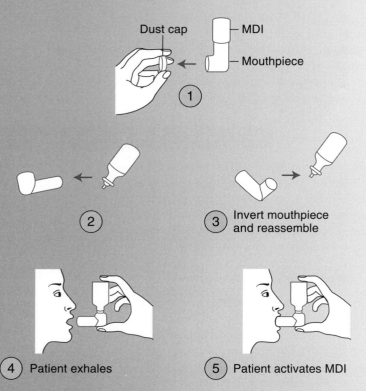

This sequence illustrates the typical use of a nonprescription inhaler (manufacturer's instructions may be more specific). *MDI*, Metered-dose inhaler.

Table 17.2. Representative Oral Products for Asthma

PRODUCT	SELECTED INGREDIENTS/COMMENTS
Bronkaid Caplets	Ephedrine sulfate 25 mg, guaifenesin 400 mg; an unapproved combination
Primatene Tablets	Ephedrine HCl 12.5 mg, guaifenesin 200 mg; an unapproved combination

tip Patients with EIA can reduce the possibility of an attack by undergoing a warm-up 15 to 60 minutes prior to the main event.[19] The warm-up should not be strenuous enough to trigger bronchoconstriction. EIA is often associated with exercise in cold, dry air.[57] Exercises more prone to trigger EIA include high-intensity sports of intermediate duration performed in a cold, dry, or dusty environment such as basketball, cycling, soccer, or track.[6,7] These sports result in high ventilation rates. Asthmatics who experience severe symptoms with outdoor sports may try swimming in an indoor pool; indoor jogging; or alternating outdoor sports such as football, baseball, isometric exercises, downhill skiing, sprinting, and walking. The intermittent nature of these exercises gradually releases mast-cell mediators. Avoidance of stress—particularly when suffering from a viral illness—may also prevent attacks.

SUMMARY

Asthma is a condition of unknown etiology, although several triggering factors have been pinpointed. ***Because asthma ranges in severity from mild to deadly, patients should not use nonprescription asthma products unless asthma has been diagnosed by a physician.*** Thus nonprescription products have a very limited role in self-treatment of asthma. A physician diagnosis invariably leads to one or more prescriptions for any of the numerous prescription products. *Patients using prescription asthma products must not use the nonprescription products.* Therefore, the legitimate market for these products is of necessity quite small, limited solely to patients with diagnosed asthma whose physician-prescribed regimen includes these products.

Various aspects of the pharmacist's role in asthma care when patients request nonprescription products include the following:

- Questioning the patient to determine if a diagnosis of asthma has been made by a physician
- Asking the patient if he or she has ever been hospitalized with asthma
- Asking the patient if he or she is currently taking any prescription medication for asthma (if so, the pharmacist must stress the importance of compliance with a prescribed regimen and must determine the reason for the proposed purchase of a nonprescription product)
- Asking whether the patient has used nonprescription products at any previous time (if so, what were the results?)
- Discovering if the patient has other medical conditions or is taking other medications that would contraindicate nonprescription asthma products

AT THE COUNTER

A college student has what he describes as "mild asthma." A doctor diagnosed it when the student was several years younger and recommended that he use one of the nonprescription inhalers, as long as it worked for him. He is now experiencing wheezing and shortness of breath.

Interview/Patient Assessment

He does not especially want to use an inhaler and asks whether one of the asthma tablets would be just as good. He is taking no medication for asthma or any other condition and has no other diagnosed medical conditions.

Pharmacist's Analysis

1. Are the patient's symptoms consistent with asthma?

2. Should this patient use a nonprescription product?
3. Should he use an oral product or an inhalation product?

This patient's symptoms are consistent with asthma. His prior physician diagnosis allows him to use nonprescription products when appropriate. However, tablets are not approved for asthma since they contain ingredients not proven safe and/or effective.

Patient Counseling

Since he is not currently taking any asthma medication, he could try an epinephrine metered-dose inhaler or inhalation solution with a nebulizer. If the patient chooses self-therapy, the pharmacist should point out the various precautions associated with the use of epinephrine.

- Pointing out the numerous precautions associated with the use of nonprescription products
- Recommending that the patient visit a physician to allow the asthma triggers to be identified
- Pointing out the usefulness of peak-flow meters

References

1. Darzen JM. Asthma. In: Wyngaarden JB, Smith LH, Bennett JC, eds. Cecil Textbook of Medicine. 19th ed. Philadelphia: WB Saunders, 1992; p. 381.
2. Ownby DR, Johnson CC, Peterson EL. Incidence and prevalence of physician-diagnosed asthma in a suburban population of young adults. Ann Allergy Asthma Immunol 77:304, 1996.
3. Rados B. Asthma is all in the chest. FDA Consumer 18:22, 1985.
4. Joseph CL, et al. Prevalence of possible undiagnosed asthma and associated morbidity among urban schoolchildren. J Pediatr 129:735, 1996.
5. Ulrik CD, Frederiksen J. Mortality and markers of risk of asthma death among 1,075 outpatients with asthma. Chest 108:10, 1995.
6. Nelson DA, et al. Ethnic differences in the prevalence of asthma in middle class children. Ann Allergy Asthma Immunol 78:21, 1997.
7. Bone RC. Step care for asthma. JAMA 260:543, 1988.
8. Armour C, et al. Mediators on human airway smooth muscle. Clin Exp Pharmacol Physiol 24:269, 1997.
9. Spahn JD, Szefler SJ. The etiology and control of bronchial hyperresponsiveness in children. Curr Opin Pediatr 8:591, 1996.
10. Giesbrecht GG, Younes M. Exercise- and cold-induced asthma. Can J Appl Physiol 20:300, 1995.
11. Howarth PH, et al. Influence of albuterol, cromolyn sodium and ipratropium bromide on the airway and circulating mediator responses to allergen bronchial provocation in asthma. Am Rev Respir Dis 132:986, 1985.
12. Blyth DI, et al. Lung inflammation and epithelial changes in a murine model of atopic asthma. Am J Respir Cell Mol Biol 14:425, 1996.
13. Ciprandi G, et al. Allergen-specific conjunctival challenge in children with allergic asthma: a clinical tool. Allergy 49:489, 1994.
14. McFadden ER Jr. Exercise and asthma (Editorial). N Engl J Med 317:502, 1987.
15. Anon. Pediatric asthma deaths continue to increase. Am Fam Physician 38:372, 1988.
16. Arrighi HM. US asthma mortality: 1941 to 1989. Ann Allergy Asthma Immunol 74:321, 1995.
17. Huovinen E, et al. Mortality of adults with asthma: a prospective cohort study. Thorax 52:49, 1997.
18. Guidelines for the diagnosis and management of asthma. Expert Panel Report, National Heart, Lung and Blood Institute, 1991.
19. Papazian R. Being a sport with exercise-induced asthma. FDA Consumer 28:30, 1994.
20. Tessier P, et al. Bronchoconstriction due to exercise combined with cold air inhalation does not generally influence bronchial responsiveness to inhaled histamine in asthmatic subjects. Eur Respir J 1:133, 1988.
21. Zawadski DK, et al. Effect of exercise on nonspecific airway reactivity in asthmatics. J Appl Physiol 64:812, 1988.
22. Rohr AS, et al. A comparison of inhaled albuterol and cromolyn in the prophylaxis of exercise-induced bronchospasm. Ann Allergy 59:107, 1987.
23. Mayol PM, et al. Exercise-induced asthma: preliminary report. Bol Assoc Med P R 78:535, 1986.
24. Gilbert IA, et al. Heat and water flux in the intrathoracic airways and exercise-induced asthma. J Appl Physiol 63:1681, 1987.
25. Hunt CH. Exercise induced asthma (Editorial). Del Med J 59:690, 1987.
26. Fed Reg 41:38311, 1976.
27. Fed Reg 47:47519, 1982.
28. Fed Reg 51, 35326, 1986.
29. Anon. Role of the pharmacist in improving asthma care. National Asthma Education and Prevention Program. Am J Health Syst Pharm 52:1411, 1995.
30. Pauley TR, Magee MJ, Cury JD. Pharmacist-managed, physician-directed asthma management program reduces emergency department visits. Ann Pharmacother 29:5, 1995.
31. Gupchup GV, Wolfgang AP, Thomas J 3rd. Development of a scale to measure directive guidance by pharmacists. Ann Pharmacother 30:1369, 1996.
32. Munroe WP, et al. Economic evaluation of pharmacist involvement in disease management in a community pharmacy setting. Clin Ther 19:113, 1997.
33. Fed Reg 57:27662, 1992.
34. Fed Reg 57:34733, 1992.
35. Fed Reg 58:54238, 1993.
36. Hall AH, et al. Intravenous epinephrine abuse. Am J Emerg Med 5:65, 1987.
37. Epinephrine OTC inhaled products draw divided response. Weekly Pharmacy Reports 43:3, 1994.
38. Fed Reg 60:13014, 1995.
39. Fed Reg 61:25142, 1996.
40. Federal and state actions against ephedrine abuse. National Pharm Compliance News 10/94.
41. FDA Consumer 27:39, 1993.
42. Diet Supplement Banned. The Saturday Oklahoman and Times 5/14/94:9.
43. Adverse effects with ephedra and other botanical dietary supplements. FDA Medical Bulletin 24:3, 1994.
44. Skat cat. Drug Topics 137:100, 1993.
45. Clinton signs ephedrine curb. NDMA Exec Newsletter 1–94:4, 1994.
46. State Actions. NDMA Exec Newsletter 1–94:4, 1994.
47. States act on ephedrine abuse. NABP Newsletter 23:81, 1994.
48. Panel questions OTC status of ephedrine. NDMA Newsletter 41–94:2, 1994.
49. Ephedrine status opposed by FDA advisory committee. Weekly Pharmacy Reports 43:3, 1994.
50. Fed Reg 60:38643, 1995.
51. Fed Reg 60:44787, 1995.
52. Fed Reg 53:30521, 1988.
53. Drugs for asthma. Med Lett Drugs Ther 29:11, 1987.
54. Theophylline brouhaha. US Pharm 15:14, 1990.
55. Fed Reg 60:38636, 1995.
56. OTC theophylline cough/cold combinations: FDA will decide this year. Weekly Pharmacy Reports 40:3, 1991.
57. Malo J-L, et al. Kinetics of the recovery from bronchial obstruction due to hyperventilation of cold air in asthmatic subjects. Eur Respir J 1:384, 1988.

Pain Conditions

Headache and Other Minor Pains

Headache—a symptom, not a disease entity—is one of the most common complaints for which patients seek help from the pharmacist. This chapter focuses on headache and the nonprescription products used for headache treatment. In addition, the chapter briefly discusses the utility of nonprescription internal analgesics in alleviating other causes of pain that are not covered elsewhere in this text. The chapter also describes the emerging uses of aspirin in prevention of infarction and stroke.

Nonprescription internal analgesics are a wide variety of ingredients sold for an equally wide variety of pain conditions. The approved indications for adult products include the following[1]:

- Temporary relief of minor aches and pains associated with the common cold
- Sore throat
- Headache
- Toothache
- Muscular aches
- Backache
- Menstrual and premenstrual periods
- Minor pain of arthritis
- Reduction of fever

Internal analgesics intended for use in patients under the age of 12 cannot be labeled for relief of muscular aches, backache, or arthritis, however. When these problems are seen in children, etiologies and treatment should be directed by a physician.[1] Also, labeling pediatric products for treatment of menstrually related claims is considered inappropriate by the FDA.

Acetaminophen may also be labeled for the minor aches and pains of influenza. Internal analgesics may also be labeled for relief of low back pain or sinusitis, as long as these more specific warnings do not intermix with the more strict labeling established by the FDA.[1] Internal analgesic products are advertised for uses for which no ingredient is proven to be safe and effective (e.g., urinary tract infections, nocturnal leg cramps).

See Chapter 26, Fever, for information on the use of internal analgesics with that condition.

HEADACHE

PREVALENCE OF HEADACHE

There are many different types of headaches (see "Benign Headaches That May Be Treatable With Nonprescription Internal Analgesics"), including the following:

- Chronic daily headache
- Migraine
- Tension
- Cluster

In an average year, 70 to 90% of people in the United States report one or more headaches.[2] Over 5% will seek medical care for headache; more than 1% of all physicians' office visits and emergency room visits are primarily for treatment of headache.[2] One-half of headache sufferers reported that their activity was limited to more than 50% of normal by headache.[3] Up to 75% of children under the age of 15 experience headache of some type.[4] Chronic headache is by far the most common chronic pain syndrome (with most of the chronic headaches being caused by tension).[5]

EPIDEMIOLOGY OF HEADACHE

The epidemiology of headache is as diverse as its many causes. Different patients suffer from different headache. The patients most prone to each type of headache are described below as each subtype of headache is discussed. (See "Benign Headaches That May Be Treatable with Nonprescription Internal Analgesics.")

ETIOLOGY OF HEADACHE

Headache has neither a specific physiologic marker nor a physical sign, making it difficult to study (Fig. 18.1).[6] As it is a wholly subjective phenomenon, distinguishing between the different types of headache is difficult.

A carefully elicited family and personal history is the most important tool for the physician in arriving at a correct headache diagnosis.[7] The history should include the first occurrence of headache, whether the presenting headache is a new *type* of headache, and the course of all of the patient's past headaches. Possible triggers (shown below) should be identified so avoidance strategies may be instituted[8]:

- Dietary triggers reportedly include such foods and drinks as those containing caffeine, aspartame, monosodium glutamate, nitrates and nitrites, ice cream, and chocolate
- Sexual activity[9]
- Stressful situations such as divorce, marital strife, job conflicts, death of a close relative or friend, or impending deadlines
- Changes from normal routines or patterns such as dieting or traveling; even alterations in altitude, seasons, or sleeping patterns can induce headache

Variables of pain such as location of the pain, its frequency and character (e.g., throbbing versus penetrating), presence of a prodrome or aura, and associated signs and symptoms are all potentially helpful in identification of cause.[2,10,11]

Unfortunately, headache directly affects the ability to concentrate, so a detailed interview may worsen the condition.[6] The pharmacist should attempt to discover whether

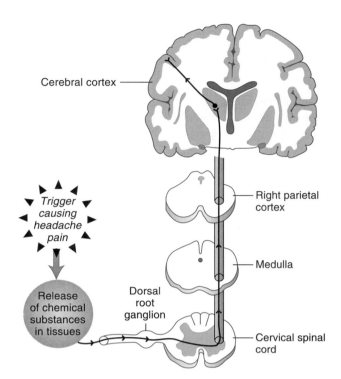

Figure 18.1. The pain stimulus begins with damage or injury to cells, triggering release of neurotransmitters.

the patient has previously been through a diagnostic workup and, if so, from which headache variant the patient suffers.

Benign (Primary) Versus Organic (Secondary) Headache

The International Headache Society has developed a comprehensive and rigid classification taxonomy for all types of headache, including primary benign disorders such as migraine, tension, and cluster headaches and the more dangerous headaches that are secondary to some underlying organic pathology.[12] Only 1% of patients present with headache caused by organic pathology such as headache caused by subarachnoid hemorrhage or ruptured **aneurysm** (dilation of an artery); the other 99% are benign.[3]

This chapter will focus on the benign headache, but the pharmacist must always be alert for serious causes of headache.

Possible Causes of Secondary (Organic) Headache

POSTTRAUMATIC HEADACHE

A headache that follows head injury or a hyperextension/flexion injury to the neck is known as posttraumatic headache.[13,14] This headache may be migraine, but more often displays a symptom mix suggesting several types of headache. For instance, patients may suffer from a dull pain in the cervical area, coupled with throbbing temporal and/or frontal pain. Concomitant symptoms include dizziness, irritability, fatigability, anxiety, insomnia, and impaired concentration and/or memory.[15] The pharmacist should refer patients with a recent history of trauma to a physician to rule out any serious intracranial damage.

TMJ-INDUCED HEADACHE

Temporomandibular joint (TMJ) disorders may produce headache.[16,17] Theories of causation have focused on spasm of the muscles of mastication.[18] Surgery may be required for **myofascial** (limited to the fascia surrounding and separating the muscle tissue) TMJ pain that is resistant to medication or physical therapy.

SPHENOID SINUSITIS HEADACHE

Acute sphenoid sinusitis causes a headache that is curable if the infection is diagnosed early and treated appropriately.[19] Headache may also be related to visual problems, especially if the patient states that reading or watching television for 20 to 30 minutes seems to cause the headache.

CO-INDUCED HEADACHE

Headache is one of the earliest symptoms seen in those suffering from carbon monoxide (CO) poisoning. If they present with headache, suspect toxic inhalation of CO for patients working in the vicinity of gas-powered engines or propane-fueled forklifts; exposed to fumes from pool heaters, vehicles (e.g., a leaky exhaust in the family automobile), wood stoves, water heaters, Sterno fuel, or paint removers containing methylene oxide; or in contact with tobacco smoke.[20,21] Note that ice resurfacing machinery in indoor ice rinks produces CO, which accumulates nearest the surface of the ice, endangering small children.[22]

MISCELLANEOUS SECONDARY HEADACHE

Many less serious etiologies have also been documented in the literature. Certain patients only suffer headache as they eat cold food, experience menstrual flow, or engage in sexual activity.[23–27] Of course, their occurrence can be extremely unpleasant for the sufferer, nonetheless.

MANIFESTATIONS OF HEADACHE

Symptoms That Necessitate Physician Referral

There are several clues that serious pathology underlies a headache. If any of these are present, immediate physician referral is mandatory. The sudden appearance of the first headache of one's life may indicate a neurologic etiology.[2] If the headache was brought on by exertion or exercise, it could indicate an aneurysm.[2] If the patient also becomes less aware of his surroundings or if his mental functioning is not as good as normal, these are dangerous signs.[11]

The same caution applies if a headache is the "worst one of my life."[2] If a headache is similar to those previously suffered, it is less dangerous, but, if it is unusually severe, an emergency room visit is indicated.[3,28] Pain of acute onset (known as the "thunderclap headache") may indicate subarachnoid hemorrhage.[2,3]

If a headache occurs along with a stiff neck, sensitivity to light, nausea, vomiting, and loss of consciousness or coma, it may indicate intracranial hemorrhage and must be checked immediately.[2]

A headache that begins gradually but worsens over a period of days or weeks is also cause for concern, especially when accompanied by fever. This type of headache may indicate an infection such as sinusitis.[2]

Patients with glaucoma must be aware that pain around the eye may indicate an acute attack that must be immediately checked.[2]

Headache in children younger than 7 is troubling because posterior brain tumors are most common at that age, and serious etiologies such as viral meningitis predominate.[4,29] Thus they should be referred for physician evaluation.

Benign Headaches That May Be Treatable with Nonprescription Internal Analgesics

CHRONIC DAILY HEADACHE

Many patients have a headache almost every day.[30] It may be dull to moderate the majority of the time, but several days of each month it may be so serious that it limits the amount and type of activities that can be engaged in. Symptoms such as nausea or vomiting and sensitivity to light may occur with the headache.[31] This type of headache is medically termed the chronic daily headache. The chronic daily headache is usually not serious, but the prudent person should still visit the physician to see if any further care is needed. The chronic daily headache is usually a combined tension-migraine etiology.[3,32]

MIGRAINE HEADACHE

About 15 to 30% of women and 3 to 13% of men suffer from migraine.[3,33,34] Onset may occur at any age. The patient is typically well between episodes and may be in complete remission for 10 to 20 years.[2,3] The frequency ranges from less than one per year to daily.[35] A migraineur is an individual who has suffered five migraine headaches.[3]

Migraine is a moderate to severe unilateral/bilateral headache with aching or throbbing pain that worsens with such normal movements as bending over or climbing stairs. Each episode can last for 4 to 24 hours in the most intense form.[2,3] Anorexia, **photophobia** (abnormal sensitivity to light), **phonophobia** (abnormal sensitivity to sound), nausea, and vomiting often accompany the headache.[36] Some patients experience a less intense headache persisting for an additional 4 to 24 hours in some cases, often accompanied by a drained, tired, or exhausted feeling.

An aura may precede the attack, typically manifesting as visual disturbances (e.g., movement of geometric figures or spots across the field of vision).[37] The visual aspects of the aura usually begin 15 to 30 minutes prior to the headache and cease with its onset.[38] The aura may also include unilateral paresthesia such as a pins-and-needles sensation moving along one side of the face or body, a sense of numbness or weakness, and inability to speak or other speech difficulty.[3,39]

TENSION HEADACHE

The tension headache (also known as muscle contraction headaches) is the most common headache and affects patients of all ages.[2,3,31] The headache consists of bandlike tightness, pressure, or constriction around the forehead and temples that often radiates to or from the neck. The pain is steady, dull, deep, and usually bilateral, lasting for 30 minutes to as long as 7 days.[2] It varies from mild to moderate in severity as the day progresses and is not aggravated by exertion. It is thought to be associated with sustained skeletal muscle contraction as a reaction to life stresses. The patient may suffer from chronic tension headache for months to years.[40]

Ancillary symptoms include anorexia, photophobia, phonophobia, and **pericranial** (surrounding the skull) muscle tenderness.[2] Tension headache is not preceded by an aura and does not produce gastrointestinal (GI) or neurologic symptoms. However, the patient often has a history of psychosocial problems such as marital or job stress.[41,42] The chronic daily headache is usually a combined tension-migraine etiology.[3,32]

CLUSTER HEADACHE

Cluster headache, which is uncommon, has a male:female ratio as high as 9:1.[3] Onset is usually the late 20s, but infants and children may also experience them.[43] While each attack is typically brief, lasting only 30 to 90 minutes, they recur in a "cluster" two to six times daily for 1 to 2 weeks to as long as 4 to 5 months.[3] Cluster periods typically recur about once yearly, nocturnally in about 50% of patients.[16,43]

The patient complains of severe, excruciating unilateral pain that is deep and boring, behind the eye or in the **periorbital** (surrounding the orbit of the eyeball) region.[2,3] The ophthalmic location produces the feeling that a hot poker is being pushed into the eyeball itself. Pain may also center in the maxillary area, shoulder, or anterior neck.

The patient may experience coexisting symptoms such as unilateral nasal congestion or unilateral ophthalmic tearing, both occurring on the side of the head affected with the headache.[2,3,44] Unlike the migraineur, there is a negative family history with cluster headache. It exhibits no aura and is only rarely accompanied by gastrointestinal (GI) symptoms.[3] Lying down often increases the discomfort level.

TREATMENT OF HEADACHE

Headache that is self-treatable may respond to any safe and effective nonprescription analgesic. However, in late 1997 a nonprescription product was given specific approval for migraine headache.[45–47] The product, Excedrin Extra Strength, contains acetaminophen, aspirin, and caffeine and is newly positioned as Excedrin Migraine. This approval is the first time that an internal analgesic has been proven safe and effective for any specific subtype of headache. Patient Assessment Algorithm 18.1 illustrates the steps used in determining if a headache is self-treatable.

Treatment Guidelines

🛈 *The time limitation for unsupervised self-usage of internal analgesics is 10 days for pain in an adult, but only 5 days for pain in a child.*

🛈 *An alcohol warning has been proposed for all OTC analgesics. "If you generally consume three or more alcohol-containing drinks per day, you should consult your physician for advice on when and how you should take this product."[48,49]*

Nonprescription Medications: Internal Analgesics

Patient Assessment Algorithm 18.2 illustrates the steps in choosing an appropriate internal analgesic product for headache.

SALICYLATES

Although several salicylates are approved for use as internal analgesics, the best known and most widely used of these is aspirin. Magnesium salicylate, sodium salicylate, choline salicylate, and calcium carbaspirin are the additional approved salicylates, as seen in the products listed in Table 18.1.[1] *Use* ⚠ *extreme caution when recommending products containing salicylates for children* because of the risk of Reye syndrome (discussed below). For uses of aspirin in the prevention of stroke and myocardial infarction, see "Aspirin in Stroke Prevention" and "Aspirin in Myocardial Infarction."

Salicylate Dosage Forms

The adult dosage for aspirin and sodium salicylate is 325 to 500 mg every 3 hours, or 325 to 650 mg every 4 hours, or 650 to 1000 mg every 6 hours.[1]

A pediatric dosing schedule may be followed every 4 hours with 81 mg tablets. The number of tablets taken varies with age:

- Age 2 to 3: two 81 mg tablets
- Age 4 to 5: three 81 mg tablets
- Age 6 to 8: four 81 mg tablets
- Age 9 to 10: four to five 81 mg tablets
- Age 11: five to six 81 mg tablets
- Age 12 and up: adult dose

Doses may be repeated every 4 hours while symptoms persist, up to 5 times daily, or as directed by a physician. However, the danger of Reye syndrome in pediatric patients argues against the use of aspirin and other implicated ingredients in pediatric patients at any time.

🛈 *Aspirin in tablet or capsule form must carry an FDA-mandated warning to drink a full glass of water with each dose.[1]* Enteric-coated aspirin tablets may reduce GI blood loss. Endoscopic study has shown lower incidence of GI erosion and ulceration than with buffered or plain tablets; however, their bioavailability may be decreased.[50] More recent evidence demonstrates that enteric-coated aspirin tablets may carry an increased risk of upper GI bleeding when compared with plain aspirin.[51]

Patient Assessment Algorithm 18.1. Headache

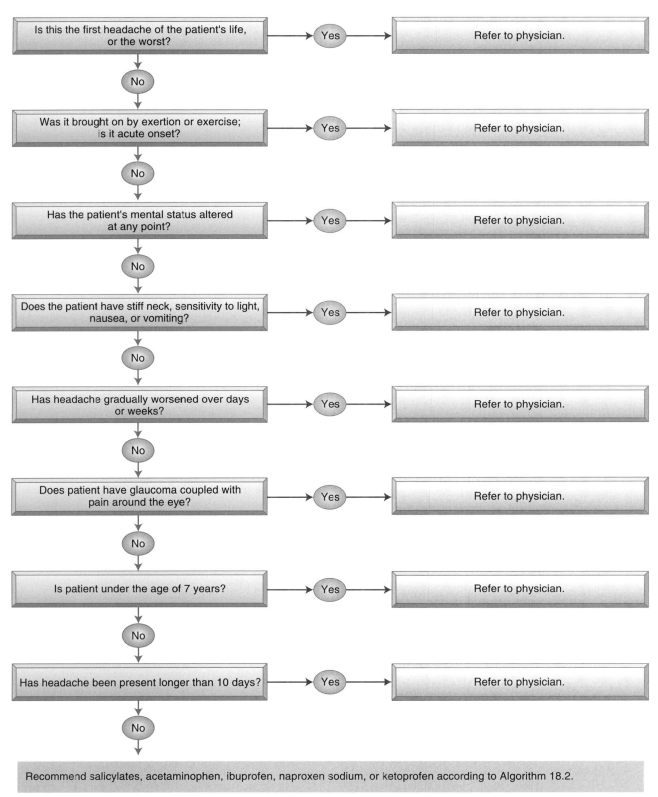

Is this the first headache of the patient's life, or the worst? — Yes → Refer to physician.
No ↓
Was it brought on by exertion or exercise; is it acute onset? — Yes → Refer to physician.
No ↓
Has the patient's mental status altered at any point? — Yes → Refer to physician.
No ↓
Does the patient have stiff neck, sensitivity to light, nausea, or vomiting? — Yes → Refer to physician.
No ↓
Has headache gradually worsened over days or weeks? — Yes → Refer to physician.
No ↓
Does patient have glaucoma coupled with pain around the eye? — Yes → Refer to physician.
No ↓
Is patient under the age of 7 years? — Yes → Refer to physician.
No ↓
Has headache been present longer than 10 days? — Yes → Refer to physician.
No ↓
Recommend salicylates, acetaminophen, ibuprofen, naproxen sodium, or ketoprofen according to Algorithm 18.2.

Aspirin powder dosage forms are absorbed faster than tablets, reaching effective blood levels faster. However, the FDA was not provided with clinical data to prove that this advantage results in any difference in onset, intensity, or incidence of relief of pain.[1] Powders may be easier to give to children than tablets or capsules. Prior to ingestion, they must be dissolved in a full glass of water.

Aspirin suppositories yield unpredictable therapeutic lev-

Patient Assessment Algorithm 18.2. Part 1 Internal Analgesics

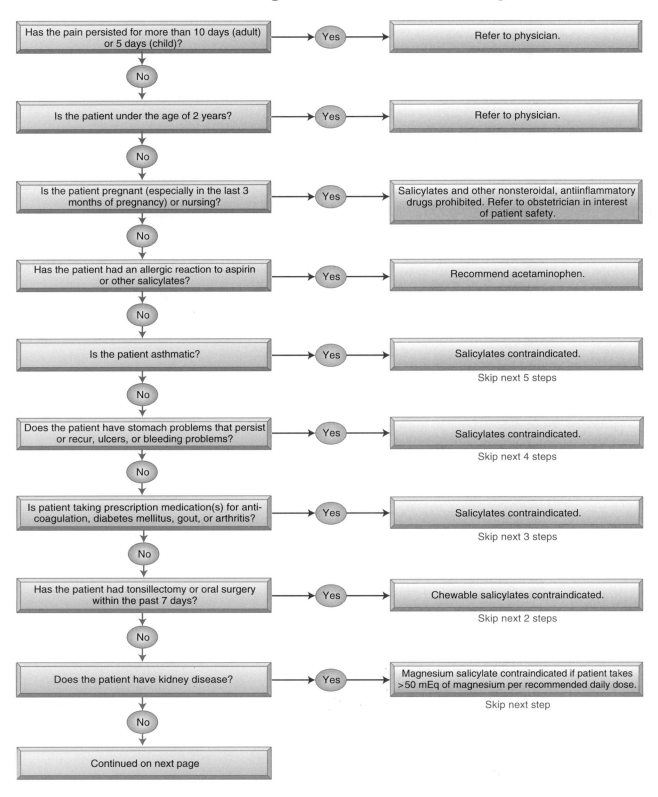

els as a result of erratic absorption.[1] They may be of value in patients who are vomiting, unconscious, or otherwise unable to ingest oral medications. The FDA has assigned them a Category III rating because of these problems.[1]

Timed-release aspirin may provide a limited benefit by preventing the need for multiple daily doses. However, the FDA is concerned about the labeling of one such product in regard to the recommended dose.[1] (It advises two 650 mg

Patient Assessment Algorithm 18.2. Part 2 Internal Analgesics

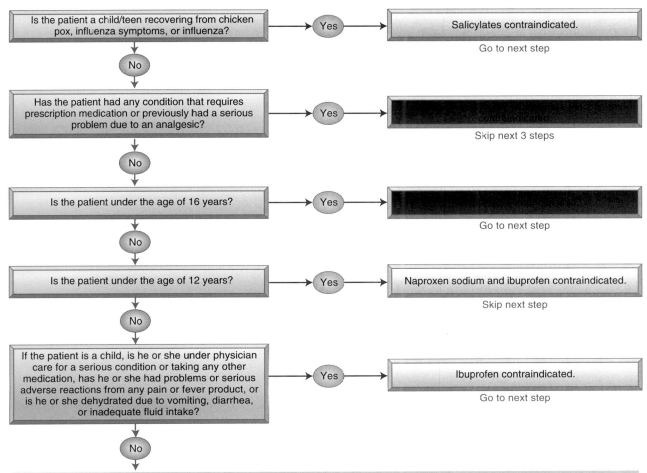

Is the patient a child/teen recovering from chicken pox, influenza symptoms, or influenza?	→ Yes →	Salicylates contraindicated.
		Go to next step

↓ No

Has the patient had any condition that requires prescription medication or previously had a serious problem due to an analgesic?	→ Yes →	Contraindicated.
		Skip next 3 steps

↓ No

Is the patient under the age of 16 years?	→ Yes →	
		Go to next step

↓ No

Is the patient under the age of 12 years?	→ Yes →	Naproxen sodium and ibuprofen contraindicated.
		Skip next step

↓ No

If the patient is a child, is he or she under physician care for a serious condition or taking any other medication, has he or she had problems or serious adverse reactions from any pain or fever product, or is he or she dehydrated due to vomiting, diarrhea, or inadequate fluid intake?	→ Yes →	Ibuprofen contraindicated.
		Go to next step

↓ No

Recommend salicylates, acetaminophen, ibuprofen, naproxen sodium, or ketoprofen in an age-appropriate dosage form, unless contraindicated. If the headache appears to be migraine, consider Excedrin Migraine™.

Table 18.1. Representative Single-Entity Salicylate Internal Analgesic Products

PRODUCT	SELECTED INGREDIENTS/COMMENTS
Aspirin Regimen Bayer Adult Low Strength	Aspirin 81 mg
Aspirin Regimen Bayer Adult Low Strength with Calcium	Aspirin 81 mg, calcium carbonate 250 mg
Bayer Aspirin	Aspirin 325 mg
Aspirin Regimen Bayer Children's	Aspirin 81 mg (orange or cherry)
Bayer Extra Strength	Aspirin 500 mg
Bufferin Low Dose Adult Regimen Strength	Aspirin 81 mg
Doan's Pills	Magnesium salicylate 303.7 mg
Ecotrin	Enteric-coated aspirin 325 or 500 mg
Ecotrin Adult Low Strength	Enteric-coated aspirin 81 mg
Halfprin	Aspirin 81 or 162 mg
Momentum	Magnesium salicylate 467 mg
Nuprin Backache	Magnesium salicylate 467 mg
St. Joseph Adult Chewable	Aspirin 81 mg

tablets, followed by one to two tablets every 8 hours. Should the product release 1300 mg of aspirin too quickly, it would exceed the safe single dose.) Therefore, the FDA has stated that products such as this must undergo the New Drug Application process to prove safety.

The efficacy of aspirin in chewing gum form is unproven, as aspirin has no topical effect. Such products as Aspergum, sold for sore throat pain, may cause oral mucosal damage.[1]

Salicylate Use Limitations

(tip) *Age Recommendation. Salicylates must not be given below age 2.[1]* Further, their administration to any child or teenager is dangerous because of Reye's syndrome. (See "Reye's Syndrome.")

(tip) *Contraindications. Patients should not take salicylates if they have stomach problems that persist or recur (such as heartburn, upset stomach, or stomach pain), ulcers, or bleeding problems, unless directed by a doctor.[1]*

(tip) *Patients also should not take salicylates (especially aspirin or calcium carbaspirin) if they are allergic to salicylates (including aspirin) or if they are asthmatic, unless directed by a physician.[1]*

(tip) Like virtually all other nonprescription products, *aspirin must carry the general warning against use when pregnant or nursing unless directed by a physician.*[52] Aspirin use during earlier stages of pregnancy is associated with congenital heart defects and closure of the ductus arteriosus.[50] Animal research suggests that aspirin may cause skeletal and central nervous system malformations.[53] Aspirin also increases the incidence of stillbirths and neonatal deaths.

(tip) In addition, a special warning cautions that *patients must not use aspirin during the last 3 months of pregnancy unless specifically directed to do so by a doctor* because it may cause problems in the unborn child or complications during delivery. Aspirin taken during the third trimester can affect fetal circulation and uterine contractions.[54] The mother can suffer antepartum and postpartum bleeding disorders, as well as prolonged labor and/or gestation. The fetus can suffer from bleeding disorders and intraventricular hemorrhage.

(tip) *Products in a chewable dosage form (e.g., chewable tablet, chewing gum) should not be taken for 7 days after tonsillectomy or oral surgery* because of a possible effect on blood clotting.[1]

(tip) *Products containing magnesium salicylate at a concentration that would allow a patient to take more than 50 mEq of magnesium in the recommended daily dose must warn patients with kidney disease not to take them unless directed by a physician.[1]*

(tip) *The label of salicylates must warn patients not to take the product if they are taking a prescription drug for anticoagulation (thinning blood), diabetes, gout, or arthritis, except under a physician's supervision.[1]*

A study in JAMA reported that aspirin, when taken by men drinking alcohol on a full stomach, causes unexpected increases in blood alcohol concentrations (approximately 26% higher than expected).[55] This information is important because many people believe that they can drink more if they also eat with alcohol. The mechanism may be noncompetitive inhibition of gastric alcohol dehydrogenase activity. An alcohol warning has been proposed with aspirin, ibuprofen, and naproxen because of gastritis.

Reye's Syndrome

Reye's syndrome is a rare, acute, life-threatening condition that occurs primarily in children or teenagers in the course of or while recovering from a mild respiratory tract infection, (⚠) flu, chicken pox, or other viral illness.[56] **Because it confers a 35% higher risk of Reye's syndrome, children and teenagers should not use aspirin for chicken pox or flu symptoms.**

Early symptoms of Reye's syndrome are excessive, repeated vomiting.[57] Other symptoms are cold, clammy hands and feet and a negative, irritable, or belligerent attitude. A period of disorientation leads to inability to recognize family members and then deep coma and death. Death can occur as early as the first day of the disease to several weeks later (average time from vomiting to death is 3 to 5 days).

The label warning for oral and rectal aspirin and (tip) nonaspirin salicylates is as follows: *"Children and teenagers who have or are recovering from chicken pox, flu symptoms, or flu should NOT use this product. If nausea, vomiting, or fever occur, consult a doctor because these symptoms could be an early sign of Reye's syndrome, a rare but serious illness."*[58]

Because of concern about Reye's syndrome, children have been given aspirin much less in recent years. The number of Reye's syndrome cases has decreased during this time, also helping provide evidence for the salicylate connection.[57]

Salicylate Allergies

Allergic reactions to aspirin occur in 0.3 to 0.9% of healthy individuals and in 1.9 to 2.8% of asthmatics. Also, 30% of patients with sinusitis or nasal polyps, in addition to asthma, are allergic to aspirin.[1] Those with aspirin allergies may also react to nonsteroidal antiinflammatory drugs (NSAIDs), tartrazine, sodium benzoate, and acetaminophen.[59] Symptoms usually appear within 20 minutes and include generalized urticaria, angioedema, rhinitis, and bronchial asthma.[60]

Allergic-reaction cases include the following:

- A female with a history of asthma, aspirin sensitivity, and nasal polyps after undergoing a nasal polypectomy took a capsule containing 270 mg of aspirin and died of respiratory distress within 10 minutes.[61]
- In a well-publicized lawsuit, a patient's wife alleged that she told a pharmacist that her husband was aspirin-allergic.[62] He later died from a reaction (acute bronchospasm) to Indocin. The patient settled out of court for $900,000, alleging that the pharmacist should have known about the possibility of cross-allergenicity.

Miscellaneous Warnings with Salicylates

Publicity about the newer uses of aspirin has caused the FDA to require this warning on all aspirin products:

tip "IMPORTANT: See your doctor before taking this product for your heart or for other new uses of aspirin, because serious side effects could occur with self-treatment."[57]

tip Patients must also be notified that, *should ringing in the ears or a loss of hearing occur, consult a doctor before taking any more of the product.*[1]

Adverse Reactions of Aspirin

As age increases, the risk of adverse effects from aspirin also increases. Unfortunately, older patients are likely to use aspirin for cardiac and circulatory problems.

Gastrointestinal (GI). Studies indicate a significant relationship between the dose of aspirin given and the severity and extent of GI discomfort and bleeding.[63,64] Doses of 1200 mg daily produce increased symptoms when compared with a placebo. A study of 100 mg aspirin doses per day in elderly patients produced GI symptoms in 18% of patients.[65] Diarrhea and nausea were the GI symptoms for which aspirin caused the greatest relative risk. Aspirin produced clinically evident GI bleeding symptoms in 3% of patients, while the placebo produced symptoms in no subject. One subject required hospitalization and transfusion.

A study examined 14 patients who had taken 100 to 325 mg of aspirin daily.[64] All had been admitted to the hospital for acute-onset, major upper-GI bleeding. Twelve presented with **melena** (stools that appear black, discolored, or tarry because of the presence of blood that has been affected by intestinal contents), one with melena coupled with hematemesis, and one with coffee-ground vomiting. Two had only used aspirin for 7 days. Erosive gastritis was found in eight of these patients, gastric ulcer in four, and duodenal ulcer in five. The potential of even low-dose as-

FOCUS ON...

ASPIRIN IN STROKE PREVENTION

Stroke is defined as a rapid onset of a neurologic deficit lasting longer than 24 hours and having either a transient or permanent effect on the brain.[68,69] As the third leading cause of death in the United States, stroke causes 150,000 deaths yearly, with an incidence of about 500,000 yearly.[70,71] Twenty percent of the deaths occur within 1 month; another 10% die within 1 year.

Stroke is the leading cause of disability in adults.[72] Each year, at least 35,000 stroke survivors must begin institutional care as a result of severe stroke-induced disability.[69] Another 100,000 can remain at home since their injury is less severe. Unfortunately, the individuals at greatest risk of stroke are those over age 50, an expanding subpopulation.[73]

Preventive interventions have helped reduce the incidence of stroke over the past 40 years.[74] The first step is primary stroke prevention, prevention of stroke in an individual who has not yet suffered one.[74] Examining an individual's risk factors for stroke is the key to advance identification of potential targets. The risk of stroke can be reduced by cessation of cigarettes and alcohol, loss of weight, tight control of blood glucose (if diabetic), and reduction of elevated serum cholesterol and lipid levels and blood pressures.[68,72,75] Although aspirin has possible utility in stroke, other known risk factors for stroke include advancing age, atrial fibrillation, cardiovascular disease, and sickle cell disease. The person who fails to reduce these risk factors and takes aspirin to compensate is ignoring some very vital protective steps and assuming a false sense of security.[76,77]

Secondary stroke prevention refers to intervention in individuals for whom the primary preventive measures have failed or were not tried, with the patient having a past history of stroke or stroke-related symptoms. These patients may have experienced cerebral or retinal ischemic events that serve as harbingers of stroke such as transient ischemic attacks (TIAs) or transient monocular blindness.[78] Previous TIAs increase the risk of stroke by a factor of five. Stroke itself is a risk factor for further stroke, so that patients with a history of minor stroke are at risk for a major incident.[78] Stroke has a recurrence rate of 13 to 20% for the following 24 months and a 16 to 42% rate for the next 5-year period.[76,79] Most major clinical stroke prevention trials target patients with prior or existing ischemic symptoms in an attempt at secondary prevention.

A family physician first noted in 1956 that use of aspirin might confer some protection against stroke, but the findings were published in an obscure medical journal.[71,80] However, in the 1970s controlled clinical trials of aspirin in stroke and TIA began to appear, confirming the physician's preliminary suggestion.

THE MECHANISM OF ASPIRIN IN STROKE PREVENTION

In human platelets, a substance known as cyclooxygenase converts arachidonic acid to prostaglandin endoperoxides and then to thromboxane A2.[63,78] Thromboxane stimulates a change in shape of the platelet and augments secretion of aggregatory and coagulation factors. Both actions result in clumping of platelets, which is the first step in the formation of a blood clot.

Aspirin acetylates cyclooxygenase in platelets, inhibiting its action.[71,78,81] Thus inhibition of the thromboxane pathway reduces blood clotting. The action of aspirin on cyclooxygenase inhibition is irreversible, even though it rapidly disappears from the circulation. Therefore, the platelets it affects do not return to normal.[82] Normal platelet activity only resumes when unaffected platelets are released into the circulation.[63] Each platelet has an average life of 10 days, corresponding to a replacement of 10% each day. Thus within 5 to 6 days of one dose of aspirin about 50% of the platelets exhibit normal cyclooxygenase activity. Aspirin also affects megakaryocytes prior to their release into the circulation, which extends its effects somewhat.[63]

Continued

pirin to cause GI bleeding underlines the importance of the FDA-mandated labeling precautions.

Stroke. Although aspirin is used in secondary prevention of ischemic stroke, it may actually induce hemorrhagic stroke.[63,66] This possibility was raised as a result of the studies carried out by the American Steering Committee of the Physicians' Health Study Research Group and also the British Physicians' Primary Prevention Studies.[63] In these studies, men chosen to receive aspirin experienced an increased risk of stroke. Although the reason is unknown, some hypothesize that aspirin may increase the risk of cerebral hemorrhage because of its antihemostatic effect.

EFFICACY OF ASPIRIN FOR STROKE PREVENTION

In a tentative final monograph, the FDA reviewed several pre-1981 studies of aspirin in TIA and stroke prevention.[1] The Peripheral and Central Nervous System Drugs Advisory Committee concluded that aspirin and buffered aspirin both reduce the risk of recurrent TIAs or stroke in males who have experienced transient ischemia of the brain caused by fibrin platelet emboli. The FDA proposed addition of wording to that effect to the professional labeling section of aspirin products. Recent studies also seem to extend the protective effect to females, although others are contradictory. This conjecture is difficult to substantiate, since at one point, only 25 to 33% of subjects in all studies were females, making it difficult to generalize to all females.[71,73]

Subsequent to that FDA report, numerous additional studies have appeared, many of which directly conflict with other results. However, at this time, aspirin does not seem to be helpful in primary prevention of stroke.

ASPIRIN DOSAGE FOR STROKE PREVENTION

The FDA originally recommended a dose of 1300 mg of aspirin per day in divided doses of 650 mg twice daily or 325 mg four times daily, based on its extensive literature review.[1] However, in an attempt to minimize adverse effects, investigators found that lower doses may be sufficient.[65,74,83]

Neonatal Hemorrhage. Although the relatively young pregnant female is not the typical patient to request aspirin for prophylaxis of stroke and myocardial infarction (MI), she may request it for headache or other more traditional uses. However, pharmacists must recall that aspirin is absolutely contraindicated in pregnancy. In an incident described in *Clinical Pediatrics,* a female ingested six Alka-Seltzer Effervescent Antacid and Pain Reliever tablets daily for 2 weeks prior to delivery to treat heartburn and hangover.[67] (Her aspirin intake was 1950 to 3000 mg daily.) The infant, delivered at term, suffered severe intracranial hemorrhage, which required 23 days hospitalization after birth. (The pregnancy was also complicated by chronic alcohol abuse.)

ACETAMINOPHEN
Acetaminophen Dosage Forms

The adult dosage for acetaminophen (APAP) is 325 to 500 mg every 3 hours, 325 to 650 mg every 4 hours, or 650 to 1000 mg every 6 hours.[1] Doses may be repeated every 4 hours while symptoms persist, up to 5 times daily, or as directed by a physician. APAP is available in a wide range of dosage forms, as listed in Table 18.2. Solid dosage forms include tablets and/or caplets in typical adult strengths of 325 or 500 mg.

Dosing of pediatric 80-mg tablets varies with age:

- Age 2 to 3: two 80 mg tablets
- Age 4 to 5: three 80 mg tablets
- Age 6 to 8: four 80 mg tablets
- Age 9 to 10: four to five 80 mg tablets
- Age 11: five to six 80 mg tablets
- Age 12 and up: adult dose

Doses may be repeated every 4 hours while symptoms persist, up to 5 times daily, or as directed by a physician. A cap-

sule containing 80 mg in powder form is marketed to allow the caregiver to sprinkle the powder in water or another liquid for easier ingestion.

Liquid dosage forms include pediatric drops (containing 80 mg per 0.8 mL or per 1.66 mL), a pediatric elixir or suspension (containing 160 mg/5 mL), and an adult elixir (containing 500 mg/15 mL). (See "A Pharmacist's Journal: What Dose Should I Use?")

APAP may also be combined with antacids for such problems as overindulgence in food and alcohol and hangover (see Chapter 5). APAP suppositories were placed in Category III by the FDA because of unpredictable therapeutic levels.[1]

Acetaminophen Use Limitations

Age Recommendation. The youngest age that can be safely treated with nonprescription APAP without a physician recommendation is 2 years.[1] One company has published a dosing chart for its brand of APAP that purports to allow the pharmacist to dose the drop dosage form down to 0 months of age (6 pounds). There is already confusion about Tylenol, which can be worsened when pharmacists fail to refer the parent to the pediatrician. For instance, elixirs for older children contain 160 mg/5 mL. But the infant drops contain 500 mg/5 mL, a much stronger concentration.

Using the infant dropper with the elixir will result in underdosing. Using the directions on the elixir bottle to measure a dose of drops will result in overdosing. (See Figure 18.2 for examples of the dosing instructions and dosing devices available for use with various acetaminophen products.)

In one case the mother of a 6-year-old with measles was told in an emergency room to give APAP 325 mg every 6 hours.[90] She believed that it was nontoxic since it was advertised to children, so she increased the dose to 500 mg every 4 hours for a 48-hour period. When the child suffered fever and abdominal pain, she further increased the dose to 500 mg every 2 to 3 hours for the next 12 hours. Despite administration of dopamine and acetylcysteine, the child developed hepatic and renal failure, followed by seizures. Brain death occurred on the eleventh hospital day. Autopsy findings were consistent with APAP toxicity (centrilobar hepatic and renal tubular necrosis). The authors of the study concluded, "There is no defined treatment for APAP toxicity resulting from long-term overdosage. The lethal outcome in this case illustrates the need to educate the public about the potential toxicity of nonprescription medications."

In another case a 10-year-old was given repeated acetaminophen doses for the fever of influenza B.[91] The child experienced abdominal pain, nausea, and vomiting, all signs of acetaminophen toxicity. Medical personnel administered additional acetaminophen with resulting lethal hepatotoxicity.

In recognition of its toxicity when not dosed as directed, the FDA-mandated warning on all APAP packages will state the fol-

(tip) lowing: "*Do not exceed recommended dosage; in an overdose situation, prompt medical attention is critical for adults as well as for children, even if you do not notice any signs or symptoms.*"[1]

FOCUS ON . . .

ASPIRIN IN MYOCARDIAL INFARCTION (MI)

MI is the leading cause of death in the United States.[78] Any particular patient's post-MI prognosis depends on the size of the infarction, the presence of ventricular arrhythmias, and the degree of underlying coronary artery disease.[84] Like stroke, MI prevention efforts are categorized into primary and secondary aspects.[85] While some patients are genetically predisposed to MI, primary prevention consists of control of known risk factors in all patients. These risk factors include cigarette smoking, high serum cholesterol, hypertension, and diabetes mellitus. Secondary prevention, on the other hand, consists of attempts to prevent a second MI, when primary methods of prevention failed or were not instituted and an MI occurred.

THE MECHANISM OF ASPIRIN IN MYOCARDIAL INFARCTION PREVENTION

The mechanism of action of aspirin in prevention of MI is probably the same as its action against stroke.[86] The FDA also summarized the literature concerning the utility of aspirin in MI.[1] Six large, randomized, multicenter, placebo-controlled studies of post-MI males and one of males with unstable angina demonstrated that use of aspirin reduced the risk of subsequent death and/or nonfatal reinfarction by 20%. In patients with unstable angina aspirin reduced the risk by 50%.

NONPRESCRIPTION ASPIRIN LABELING FOR CARDIAC/CIRCULATORY PATHOLOGY

The FDA will allow professional labeling for aspirin to carry this MI-associated statement: "Aspirin is indicated to reduce the risk of death and/or nonfatal myocardial infarction in patients with a previous infarction or unstable angina pectoris."[1] In 1996 the FDA expanded this labeling to include the statement, "Aspirin is indicated to reduce the risk of vascular mortality in patients with a suspected acute MI."[87]

In an issue of the *Federal Register* the FDA recognized the role of newspapers, magazines, television, and radio in communicating these findings about aspirin to the lay public and discussed the issue of consumer labeling.[1] A major FDA concern was that patients would ingest aspirin on a long-term basis without consulting a physician and that the average patient lacks the necessary training to determine whether benefits are likely. The following warning statement developed by the agency reflects these concerns: "IMPORTANT: See your doctor before taking this product for your heart or for other new uses of aspirin, because serious side effects could occur with self treatment." The warning does not apply to aspirin in combination products for cough-cold, or when it is combined with acetaminophen or any diuretic.[88,89]

(tip) *Use by Heavy Drinkers.* An FDA advisory panel recommended in July 1993 that *heavy drinkers should not take more than the 4 gram daily maximum dose of APAP because of the risk of serious liver damage.*[92]

APAP was a factor in three cases of liver injury in alcoholics.[93,94] Both had used Nyquil, which contains 1 gram of APAP per 30 mL. One patient used an entire 14-ounce bottle of Nyquil over one 24-hour period. Another drank 12 ounces over a 12-hour period. The latter patient suffered massive hepatic necrosis. The third took eight to ten Tylenol Extra Strength each day for 2 weeks before admission and drank a 14-ounce bottle of Nyquil during the 72 hours before admission. All survived despite massive hepatic necrosis and/or jaundice. A later study demonstrated that the risk of APAP toxicity is increased when the alcoholic is fasting.[95]

Use in Renal Patients. Daily users of analgesic mixtures may have a greater risk of renal damage. In one article, after the researchers adjusted for other analgesics, APAP was tentatively suggested as the culprit in renal toxicity.[96] There had been previous anecdotal reports. Analgesic abuse produces a characteristic lesion of renal papillary necrosis, possibly associated with chronic interstitial nephritis and chronic renal failure.[97–99] Patient symptoms included chronic pain syndromes and somatic conditions such as malaise, weight loss, anemia, peptic ulcer, recurrent urinary infections, renal colic, or nephrolithiasis. Physicians often did not link these conditions to the underlying renal papillary necrosis that caused them. Further, the symptoms such as peptic ulcer and low loin pain often triggered further use, which caused the patients to enter a vicious cycle in which they used more

PRODUCT	SELECTED INGREDIENTS/COMMENTS
Anacin Aspirin Free	Acetaminophen 500 mg
Feverall Children's Sprinkle Caps	Acetaminophen 80 mg or 160 mg
Feverall Infant Suppositories	Acetaminophen 80 mg
Feverall Suppositories	Acetaminophen 120 mg, 325 mg, or 650 mg
Panadol Adult Tablet	Acetaminophen 500 mg
Tempra Quicklets	Acetaminophen 80 mg or 160 mg (quick dissolving)
Tylenol Caplets, Geltabs, Tablets, Gelcaps	Acetaminophen 325 mg
Tylenol Children's Chewable Tablets	Acetaminophen 80 mg (grape, bubble gum, or fruit burst)
Tylenol Children's Elixir and Suspension Liquid	Acetaminophen 160 mg/5 mL
Tylenol Arthritis	Acetaminophen 650 mg; up to 8 hours duration
Tylenol Extra-Strength Adult Liquid	Acetaminophen 500/15 mL
Tylenol Extra-Strength Caplets, Geltabs	Acetaminophen 500 mg
Tylenol Infant Drops and Suspension Drops	Acetaminophen 80 mg/0.8 mL (cherry, grape)
Tylenol Junior Strength Chewable Tablets or Swallow Caplets	Acetaminophen 160 mg

Table 18.2. Representative Single-Entity Acetaminophen Internal Analgesic Products

A Pharmacist's Journal

"What Dose Should I Use?"

I was filling a prescription when the student pharmacist on duty answered the phone. I noticed him listening intently, after which he put the caller on hold and went to the nonprescription product shelves. He returned and began to explain a dose to the caller. After listening for another short period, he turned to me looking thoroughly confused. "I'm not sure what she is asking for." The caller explained to me that she had purchased a Tylenol combination product for her 11-month-old and wanted to know what dose to give him. I took several minutes to explain that 11 months was too young to allow therapy without calling her physician. However, she was insistent that I get the box from the shelf and bring it to the phone so she could ask me several questions about the product she had purchased. The intern had apparently brought the wrong box, so I asked her carefully what product she had purchased. I wrote down the product, and attempted to locate it on our shelves. I could not find it, and told her that we must not have it at this time. She then admitted that she had bought it at another store and, hung up, frustrated, convinced that the real reason the pharmacist would not create a dose for her 11-month-old was that she did not make the purchase from our store.

of the product that was causing the problem. The authors suggested that the diagnosis could be made more easily if a history of regular analgesic intake was taken, leading to further confirmation through radiographic studies. An editorial in the same issue of that journal cautioned, "Some patients frequently underestimate their analgesic intake, and others are unaware that medications bought without prescription may have serious side effects. Many of these patients also behave addictively with respect to analgesic mixtures."[97]

In other research, investigators examined the average

Various liquid acetaminophen dosing devices and the product concentration with which they are supplied

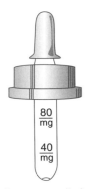

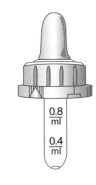

The dropper supplied with a pediatric drop with a concentration of 80 mg/1.66 mL

The dropper supplied with a pediatric drop with a concentration of 80 mg/0.8 mL

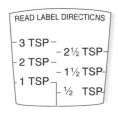

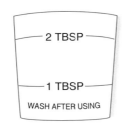

The dose cup supplied with a children's liquid with a concentration of 80 mg/5 mL

The dose cup supplied with an adult's liquid with a concentration of 500 mg/15 mL

Figure 18.2. Acetaminophen products are available as pediatric drops, a pediatric elixir, and an adult elixir. Concentrations differ, so that the caregiver must be sure to measure the correct dose of the correct liquid.

number of tablets taken yearly in relation to end-stage renal disease (ESRD).[100] They discovered that frequent use of acetaminophen and other NSAIDs (e.g., taking more than 364 pills yearly) increased risk of ESRD, whereas frequent use of aspirin did not. Further, total lifetime ingestion of as many as 1000 to over 5000 acetaminophen tablets also increased the risk of ESRD.

The FDA is concerned about evidence that combinations of antipyretic analgesics taken over a sustained time period cause a specific form of kidney failure and chronic renal failure, as well as an increased risk of uroepithelial tumors. The agency invited specific comments on the issue of limiting nonprescription drug products to single antipyretic-analgesic agents, and later extended the comment date to 1990.[1,101] Despite the long interval between this publication and the present, no further decision has been published in the *Federal Register*.

IBUPROFEN

Approved for nonprescription sale in 1984, ibuprofen is available as 200-mg tablets/caplets, a suspension containing 100 mg/5 mL, 50-mg children's tablets, and 100-mg junior tablets or swallow caplets, as listed in Table 18.3. The nonprescription dosage is one caplet or tablet every 4 to 6 hours, to a maximum of six tablets in 24 hours. While the patient may take two tablets at once if pain or fever does not respond **tip** to one tablet, *the label cautions the patient to take the smallest effective dose.* Further, *if occasional mild* **tip** *heartburn, upset stomach, or stomach pain occurs with use, the label advises the patient to take the product with food or milk.*

Ibuprofen Use Limitations

Age Recommendation. The age cutoff for nonprescription ibuprofen use was 12 years until the Rx-to-OTC switch of a pediatric ibuprofen suspension in September of 1995.[102–104] **tip** *The introduction of Children's Motrin Oral Suspension extended the age for self-therapy with ibuprofen down to the age of 2 years.* Children's Motrin is also available in drops, children's tablets, and junior-strength tablets (for ages 6 to 11). However, when the product is administered to children, it should not be given for pain longer than 3 days.[104] Children's Advil appeared as another pediatric ibuprofen suspension for nonprescription sale in July 1996.

tip *Contraindications. Patients who have had a severe allergic reaction to aspirin (asthma, inflammation, hives, anaphylaxis) should not take ibuprofen* because of the possibility of cross-allergenicity.[105] **tip** *Ibuprofen is contraindicated in pregnancy* and carries the same warning as aspirin regarding an absolute prohibition against use in the last 3 months of pregnancy.[105] **tip** *If the patient has any condition that requires the use of prescription drugs, or has previously had a serious problem from taking a nonprescription pain reliever, self-medication with ibuprofen is contraindicated. Furthermore, ibuprofen should not be combined with other nonprescription internal analgesics.*[105]

In addition to the other ibuprofen and general analgesic **tip** precautions, *pediatric ibuprofen products should not be given if the child is under a physician's care for any serious condition or is taking any other medication, has problems or serious adverse reactions from products used for fever or pain, does not obtain relief in the first 24 hours, if the pain or fever worsens, if any new symptoms appear, or if the child is dehydrated because of vomiting, diarrhea, or lack of fluid intake.*[104]

Adverse Reactions to Ibuprofen

Ibuprofen and Renal Problems. With the nonprescription availability of ibuprofen, several physicians have expressed concern about possible renal toxicity.[106–107] In 1990 headlines appeared that linked ibuprofen with kidney damage. Articles reported the results of a study showing that ibuprofen caused renal failure in people with mild kidney dis-

Table 18.3. Representative Internal Analgesic Products Containing Ibuprofen

PRODUCT	SELECTED INGREDIENTS/COMMENTS
Advil	Ibuprofen 200 mg
Children's Advil	Ibuprofen 100 mg/5 mL
Children's Motrin Oral Suspension	Ibuprofen 100 mg/5 mL
Children's Motrin Tablets	Ibuprofen 50 mg
Junior Strength Motrin Tablets	Ibuprofen 100 mg (orange chewable or swallow caplets)
Motrin IB	Ibuprofen 200 mg
Nuprin	Ibuprofen 200 mg

ease.[108] The 3-year study included 12 women. Within a short period of time, one manufacturer of nonprescription ibuprofen products sent a letter to pharmacists and physicians detailing some valid criticisms of the study. For instance, some patients had more than mild renal failure, and all suffered from concurrent diseases such as diabetes mellitus, hypertension, and gout. Further, the doses given were prescription doses rather than OTC doses.

Another review article described various nephrotoxicity syndromes associated with NSAIDs. It provided the following risk factors for NSAID nephrotoxicity:

- Age over 60, atherosclerotic cardiovascular disease, receiving a concurrent diuretic
- Renal insufficiency, usually serum creatinine level > 180 micromol/L (2.0 mg/dL)
- States of renal hypoperfusion (sodium depletion, diuretic use, hypotension, sodium avid states such as hepatic cirrhosis, nephrotic syndrome, and congestive heart failure)[97]

An ad hoc panel of the National Kidney Foundation recommended that these risk factors be included in the labeling of nonprescription ibuprofen products. However, at this time the manufacturers have not done so, and the FDA has not required these warnings.[97]

A physician responding to the controversy stressed that an NIH conference found that chronic analgesic nephropathy causes 2 to 10% of end-stage renal disease.[109] The author further pointed out the inhibition of cyclooxygenase and hydroperoxidase system caused by ibuprofen and noted that these systems are responsible for APAP metabolism. In light of the fact that consumers frequently combine various nonprescription products, he terms a combination of ibuprofen (or any other NSAID) and APAP as "the nephrolethal combination of the 1990s.

Aseptic Meningitis. Aseptic meningitis can occur in NSAID users, especially those with a connective-tissue disorder such as systemic lupus erythematosus (SLE). A 52-year-old woman with a past history of SLE had a previous history of aseptic meningitis in conjunction with ingestion of prescription Motrin.[110] She had avoided use of ibuprofen since that time. However, on the day in question she purchased Nuprin, unaware that it was a nonprescription form of Motrin. She took one tablet for leg pain caused by superficial thrombophlebitis and subsequently developed symptoms consistent with drug-induced aseptic meningitis. They resolved shortly thereafter.

GI Hemorrhage. NSAID-associated gastric problems result in 200,000 hospitalizations each year and perhaps 20,000 deaths.[111] While the lower doses of nonprescription ibuprofen are undoubtedly safer in this regard, they may still cause gastric pathology. An elderly British woman with a history of gastric ulceration associated with NSAID usage took nonprescription ibuprofen for 3 days for backache.[112] She developed melena and was admitted to the hospital, where her hemoglobin was 4.5 (normal=14). Despite transfusion, she developed irreversible cardiac failure and died. Her physician brought the case to the attention of the British Pharmaceutical Society to emphasize that *pharmacists should ask patients whether they have a history of stomach problems prior to selling nonprescription ibuprofen.*

Visual Disturbances. Ibuprofen has been associated with visual disturbances.[113] Patients experienced fluctuating and generalized blurring of near and distance vision, as though they were "looking through a film" or "seeing shadows at night when there was nothing there." One patient had taken two to six ibuprofen 200-mg tablets 5 days of each week for 8 months. Another had taken 10 tablets weekly for 2 months. The authors of the report cautioned, "It is striking that, despite chronic use of this drug, none of these patients included ibuprofen as part of their initial drug history. It was only after more selective and direct questioning that the discovery was made."

NAPROXEN SODIUM

Naproxen was given OTC status in early 1994. It is available as Aleve tablets or caplets containing 220 mg of naproxen sodium. The dosage is one tablet every 8 to 12 hours while symptoms persist. The manufacturer suggests that greater relief can be obtained by an initial dose of two tablets, fol-

(tip) lowed by a single tablet 12 hours later. *The daily maximum of three tablets per 24 hours should not be exceeded (a full glass of water should be ingested with each dose), but the smallest effective dose should be used.*[114] Patients over 65 should not exceed one tablet every 12 hours.

Naproxen Sodium Age Recommendation

(tip) *The age cutoff for nonprescription naproxen sodium use is 12 years.*[114]

Naproxen Sodium Contraindications

(tip) *Patients who have had a severe allergic reaction to aspirin (asthma, inflammation, hives, anaphylaxis) should not take naproxen sodium because of the possibility of cross-allergenicity.*[114]

(tip) *Naproxen sodium is contraindicated in pregnancy and carries the same warning as aspirin regarding an absolute prohibition against use in the last 3 months of pregnancy.*

(tip) *If the patient has any condition that requires the use of prescription drugs, or has previously had a serious problem from taking a nonprescription pain reliever, self-medication with naproxen sodium is contraindicated. Naproxen sodium should not be combined with other nonprescription internal analgesics.*

KETOPROFEN

Ketoprofen became a nonprescription product in December of 1995. It may be purchased as Orudis KT tablets or caplets, each containing 12.5 mg of ketoprofen, given to adults in a dosage of one tablet every 4 to 6 hours. If the patient does not experience relief in 1 hour, the dose may be repeated. The patient who has experience with the product may find that two tablets initially are necessary, although the smallest effective dose should be used.

(tip) *Patients must not exceed two tablets each 4- to 6-hour period, with a daily maximum of six tablets. A full glass of water or other liquid must be ingested with each dose.*

Ketoprofen Age Recommendation

(tip) *The age cutoff for nonprescription ketoprofen use is 16 years.*[115,116]

Ketoprofen Contraindications

(tip) *Patients who have had a severe allergic reaction to aspirin (asthma, inflammation, hives, anaphylaxis) should not take ketoprofen because of the possibility of cross-allergenicity.*

(tip) *Ketoprofen is contraindicated in pregnancy and carries the same warning as aspirin regarding an absolute prohibition against use in the last 3 months of pregnancy.*

(tip) *If the patient has any continuing medical condition for which he or she is under the care of a physician, or has previously had problems or side effects with any pain reliever or fever reducer, self-medication with ketoprofen is contraindicated. Ketoprofen should not be combined with other nonprescription internal analgesics/fever reducers.*

A Pharmacist's Journal

"What's the Dose of Tonic Water?"

For many years, quinine was available in nonprescription products for nocturnal leg cramps. People used it in an indiscriminate manner, and its unapproved use for this condition caused many adverse reactions such as hypersensitivity, thrombocytopenia, renal and hepatic dysfunction, hemorrhage, cerebrovascular accident, anaphylaxis, and death. Thus its removal from the market in the early 1990s was an appropriate move by the FDA. However, once it was removed, patients began to ask where it was and when the product would be coming in. Thus for the first time pharmacists began to find out who had been buying it and what they had been using it for. I had people tell me that they had been using it for the muscle aches of dehydration as they carried out football exercises in the hot summer sun and for leg cramps caused by sitting for long stretches in wheat combines. One of my students counseled a patient at the pharmacy about the nonavailability of quinine. This patient returned to ask another question. "What's the dose of tonic water?" A well-meaning friend told him that tonic water contains quinine. This patient decided to dose himself, but wanted to know what quantity of tonic water would be needed to equal his previous self-administered dose of quinine capsules. Tonic water does contain quinine. Occasional use as a mixer for mixed drinks would be safe for most patients, but could cause hypersensitivity reactions. For this reason its use should be avoided altogether. The student attempted to dissuade the patient from indiscriminate use of tonic water as a medication, but the patient became resistant and left the store.

OTHER INGREDIENTS IN INTERNAL ANALGESIC PRODUCTS

Caffeine

Studies confirmed that caffeine safely and effectively synergizes aspirin or aspirin-APAP combinations but does not do so with APAP alone.[101,117–119] The mechanism may be that of mood elevation.[120] Various caffeine combinations are listed in Table 18.4. The suggested ratio of ingredients is a 10:1 milligram ratio of aspirin to caffeine. Caffeine/APAP combinations remain on the market until the final FDA monograph is issued. Caffeine may contribute to the nephrotoxicity of analgesics, perhaps through its action as an adenosine antagonist.[97]

Buffering Agents

Various buffers are often added to aspirin or aspirin/APAP products, as listed in Table 18.5. By raising the pH of the microenvironment of the stomach lining surrounding the dissolving aspirin particles, they supposedly reduce the risk of stomach irritation. However, the FDA did not discover sufficient clinical studies to prove this claim and placed all such claims in Category III.[1]

Salicylamide

Salicylamide is not a salicylate, but is the amide derivative of salicylic acid. It is of unproven efficacy and can cause severe reactions such as tinnitus, ecchymoses, hemorrhagic lesions, leukopenia, or thrombocytopenia.[1] All other salicylate precautions should be observed. Salicylamide is found in the products listed in Table 18.6.

Antihistamines

Antihistamines are combined with internal analgesics both to synergize analgesics and to induce sleep, as listed in Table 18.7. Phenyltoloxamine is usually chosen as a synergizing agent, but this combination has not been proven to be more efficacious than the internal analgesic alone and has been given Category III status.[1] *Since it has no proven efficacy, the patient is needlessly exposed to adverse reactions from the antihistamine.*

Diphenhydramine is added as a sleep aid.[50] (See Chapter 24, which discusses sleep aids, for information on the efficacy of this combination.)

Potassium Nitrate (Saltpeter)

This ingredient was not submitted to the FDA for review, making it unapproved. Saltpeter can cause gastroenteritis, muscle weakness, and seizures.[121] It is found in a product known as DeWitt's Pills, along with salicylamide and caffeine.

Nonpharmacologic Therapies

Some people find it helpful to rest in a quiet, dark room when headache begins, with an ice pack on the head.[122]

Table 18.4. Representative Internal Analgesic Products Containing Caffeine in Approved Combinations

PRODUCT	SELECTED INGREDIENTS
Anacin	Aspirin 400 mg, caffeine 32 mg
Excedrin Aspirin Free	Acetaminophen 500 mg, caffeine 65 mg
Excedrin Migraine	Aspirin 250 mg, acetaminophen 250 mg, caffeine 65 mg
Goody's Powders	Aspirin 520 mg, acetaminophen 260 mg, caffeine 32.5 mg
Vanquish	Aspirin 227 mg, acetaminophen 194 mg, caffeine 33 mg, aluminum hydroxide, magnesium hydroxide

---

Table 18.5. Representative Internal Analgesic Products Containing Only Aspirin and/or Acetaminophen and Buffers

PRODUCT	SELECTED INGREDIENTS/COMMENTS
Alka-Seltzer Original	Aspirin 325 mg, sodium bicarbonate 1916 mg, citric acid (in effervescent tablets which form sodium citrate)
Arthritis Strength Bufferin	Aspirin 500 mg, calcium carbonate, magnesium oxide, magnesium carbonate
Ascriptin Maximum Strength	Aspirin 500 mg, alumina-magnesia, calcium carbonate
Ascriptin	Aspirin 325 mg, alumina-magnesia, calcium carbonate
Extra Strength Bayer Plus	Aspirin 500 mg, calcium carbonate
Bufferin	Aspirin 325 mg, calcium carbonate, magnesium oxide, magnesium carbonate

Table 18.6. Representative Internal Analgesic Products Containing Salicylamide

PRODUCT	SELECTED INGREDIENTS/COMMENTS
BC Powder	Aspirin 650 mg, salicylamide 195 mg, caffeine 32 mg; an unapproved combination
DeWitt's Pills	Salicylamide, caffeine, potassium nitrate (an unapproved combination; unlabeled amounts)

Table 18.7. Representative Internal Analgesic Products Containing Antihistamines

PRODUCT	SELECTED INGREDIENTS/COMMENTS
Bayer Extra Strength PM	Aspirin 500 mg, diphenhydramine HCl 25 mg (an unapproved combination)
Doan's P.M.	Magnesium salicylate 467.2 mg, diphenhydramine HCl 25 mg (an unapproved combination)
Excedrin P.M.	Acetaminophen 500 mg, diphenhydramine citrate 38 mg (an unapproved combination)
Percogesic	Acetaminophen 325 mg, phenyltoloxamine citrate 30 mg (an unapproved combination)
Tylenol PM	Acetaminophen 500 mg, diphenhydramine HCl 25 mg (an unapproved combination)

PREVENTION OF HEADACHE

For some patients, investigation identifies certain factors that trigger benign headache. Triggering factors for migraine include heat, bright lights, too little or too much sleep, odors, physical fatigue, emotional stress, alcohol, chocolate, skipping meals, schedule changes, and certain food additives (such as MSG).[4] Their avoidance may prevent triggering headache.

ARTHRITIS

In regard to self-treatment of arthritis pain, the FDA has described several comments that had been received in response to an earlier document (Fig. 18.3).[1] The agency agreed with comments that the patient must not attempt to self-diagnose arthritis, since nonprescription treatment could delay proper diagnosis and treatment, as in the case of rheumatoid arthritis. The FDA has allowed labeling of internal analgesics for minor pain of arthritis, in light of the required warning against use for more than 10 days and the required caution to see a physician if the pain persists or worsens, if new symptoms occur, or if either redness or swelling is present. To prevent use in children, internal analgesic products should be labeled, "Do not give this product to children for the pain of arthritis unless directed by a physician." For information on internal analgesics used for the treatment of arthritis, see "Nonprescription Medications: Internal Analgesics."

SORE THROAT

Treatment of sore throat with topical anesthetics is described in Chapter 18. Internal analgesics are also effective for mi-

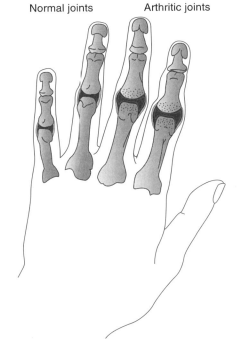

Figure 18.3. Arthritis produces inflammation of the joints, with accompanying pain and stiffness.

nor sore throat. The FDA has noted that sore throat may indicate a more serious condition such as streptococcal infection ("strep throat"), which left untreated can progress to rheumatic fever or glomerulonephritis.[1] Additionally, sore throat accompanied by rash may indicate rheumatic fever or measles. Serious illness could compromise the patient's life if treatment delay were to occur with use of nonprescription internal analgesics. Therefore, the FDA requires a warning on products labeled for sore throat: "If sore throat is severe,

Table 18.8. Representative Products Marketed for Urinary Tract Pain

PRODUCT	SELECTED INGREDIENTS/COMMENTS
Azo-Standard	Phenazopyridine 95 mg (an unapproved ingredient)
Cystex	Methenamine 162 mg, sodium salicylate 162.5 mg (an unapproved combination)
Prodium	Phenazopyridine 95 mg (an unapproved ingredient)
Uristat	Phenazopyridine 95 mg (an unapproved ingredient)

persists for more than 2 days, is accompanied or followed by fever, headache, rash, nausea, or vomiting, consult a doctor promptly."[1] For information on internal analgesics used for the treatment of sore throat, see "Nonprescription Medications: Internal Analgesics."

URINARY TRACT PAIN

Although some products have been marketed for relief of urinary tract problems, the FDA has not approved this labeling, *nor has the FDA approved any ingredient as* *safe or effective for urinary tract pain. Patients requesting help for this problem should be referred to a physician for diagnosis and treatment with an appropriate antibacterial/antibiotic if necessary.*

Phenazopyridine, methenamine, and benzoic acid, found in the products listed in Table 18.8, were not submitted to the FDA for review of any condition. Many patients (especially females) purchase these products for self-treatment of the pain arising from urinary tract infections. As noted, this is not a recommended practice.

Phenazopyridine can cause methemoglobinemia, hemolytic anemia, skin pigmentation, and transient acute renal failure. Jaundice and hepatitis occur, probably resulting from hypersensitivity. It may precipitate in the urine to form stones and can also stain contact lenses. It is a potential carcinogen. Use of phenazopyridine as sole therapy to treat the pain of urinary tract infection is irrational in any case, since the patient should obtain an antibiotic/antibacterial prescription to eradicate the source of the urinary tract infection.

SUMMARY

Headache is a common symptom that can be the result of benign or organic causes. The patient may safely self-treat such benign symptoms as chronic daily headache, migraine, tension headache, and cluster headache. However, the following indicate a possibly serious etiology that should be referred for medical investigation:

- The sudden appearance of the first headache of one's life
- The worst headache one has ever had

AT THE COUNTER

A 58-year-old male patient asks about the efficacy of aspirin in stroke prevention. He also hopes it may help stop his occasional headaches. He wants to know if one baby aspirin a day is sufficient.

Interview/Patient Assessment

The patient's computer profile shows that he is currently taking imipramine, probenecid, Accupril, and Lanoxin.

Pharmacist's Analysis

1. Is aspirin effective in stroke prevention?
2. Would a pediatric aspirin tablet daily be effective for stroke prevention?
3. Can this patient take aspirin without a physician recommendation?

A great deal of evidence has accumulated to indicate that aspirin is effective in prevention of stroke, even in doses as small as those equivalent to one baby aspirin daily. However, this patient has gout, as evidenced by his use of probenecid. Therefore, although aspirin may be of benefit to the patient, the risks of unsupervised use outweigh the potential benefits.

Patient Counseling

The patient should be told that unsupervised use of aspirin is unwise because of a drug interaction with his gout medication. The dangers of an acute attack of gout should be stressed. The patient should be urged to discuss the situation with his physician.

AT THE COUNTER

 A college-aged female asks for a product to help with her headache.

Interview/Patient Assessment

Her headaches began her first year of college and seem to intensify around the time of final examinations. The pain is steady and becomes worse in the night as she tries to study. Her present headache has persisted for 4 days. She is taking ranitidine for treatment of active ulcer and birth control tablets. She has no other diagnosed medical conditions.

Pharmacist's Analysis

1. Does this patient's headache appear to be self-treatable?
2. Since her headache has been present for 4 days, should she self-treat?

3. What is the significance of her medication regimen?

This patient's condition appears to be consistent with tension headache, an etiology that is amenable to self-treatment. Since the limit for treatment of pain in adults is 10 days, she may self-treat for 6 more days before seeing a physician.

Patient Counseling

The patient's ranitidine usage and history of active ulcer contraindicate aspirin. However, neither APAP, naproxen, nor ketoprofen are contraindicated with stomach problems, and any could be recommended for this patient. Since the NSAIDs could cause gastric problems, APAP might be the best choice.

- Acute onset headache pain
- Headache that begins gradually but worsens over a period of days or weeks
- Headache along with loss of awareness of the surroundings, compromised mental function, stiff neck, sensitivity to light, nausea, vomiting, loss of consciousness or coma, fever
- Pain around the eye in the glaucoma patient
- Headache in children

Assuming the headache is not caused by serious underlying pathology, the pharmacist may advise self-treatment with such products as salicylates, APAP, ibuprofen, naproxen sodium, or ketoprofen. Each ingredient must be recommended carefully, however, with full knowledge of its contraindications, warnings, and other use precautions.

Internal analgesics are also useful for aches and pains when caused by such problems as the common cold, sore throat, toothache, muscle problems, back pain, menstrual and premenstrual etiologies, and arthritis. However, pain caused by the urinary tract must be referred to a physician for care.

References

1. Fed Reg 53:46203, 1988.
2. Silberstein SD. Evaluation and emergency treatment of headache. Headache 32:396, 1992.
3. Couch JR. Headache to worry about. Med Clin North Am 77:141, 1993.
4. Chu ML, Shinnar S. Headaches in children younger than 7 years of age. Arch Neurol 49:79, 1992.
5. Forgays DG, et al. Headache in college students: A comparison of four populations. Headache 33:182, 1993.
6. Schachtel BP, et al. Headache pain model for assessing and comparing the efficacy of over-the-counter analgesic agents. Clin Pharmacol Ther 50:322, 1991.
7. Silberstein SD. Office management of benign headache. Postgrad Med 93:223, 1993.
8. Schulman EA, Silberstein SD. Symptomatic and prophylactic treatment of migraine and tension-type headache. Neurology 42(3 Suppl 2):16, 1992.
9. Coutin IB, Glass SF. Recognizing uncommon headache syndromes. Am Fam Physician 54:2247, 1996.
10. Silberstein SD. Advances in understanding the pathophysiology of headache. Neurology 43(3 Suppl 2):6, 1992.
11. Rapoport AM, Silberstein SD. Emergency treatment of headache. Neurology 42(3 Suppl 2):43, 1992.
12. Anon. Classification and diagnostic criteria for headache disorders, cranial neuralgia, and facial pain. Cephalagia 8(Suppl 7):1, 1988.
13. Gawel MJ, et al. Subcutaneous sumatriptan in the treatment of acute episodes of posttraumatic headache. Headache 33:96, 1993.
14. Yamaguchi M. Incidence of headache and severity of head injury. Headache 32:427, 1992.
15. Packard RC. Posttraumatic headache: Permanency and relationship to legal settlement. Headache 32:496, 1992.
16. Kowal L. Headaches and the ophthalmologist. Aust Fam Physician 20:1326, 1991.
17. Haley D, et al. The comparison of patients suffering from temporomandibular disorders and a general headache population. Headache 33:210, 1993.
18. Kirk WS Jr. Chronic temporomandibular joint disease and head pain. NC Med J 54:30, 1993.
19. Anon. Sinusitis: More than a headache (Editorial). JSC Med Assoc 87:514, 1991.
20. Sadovnikoff N, et al. Carbon monoxide poisoning. Postgrad Med 92:86, 1992.

21. Wilson MS. Headaches caused by exhaust fumes (Letter). Br J Gen Pract 41:522, 1991.

22. Fawcett TA, et al. Warehouse worker's headache. J Occup Med 34:12, 1991.

23. Keenan PA, Lindamer LA. Non-migraine headache across the menstrual cycle in women with and without premenstrual syndrome. Cephalagia 12:356, 1992.

24. Bird N, et al. Ice cream headache—Site, duration, and relationship to migraine. Headache 32:35, 1992.

25. Silberstein SD. The role of sex hormones in headache. Neurology 42(Suppl 2):37, 1992.

26. Lance JW. Solved and unsolved headache problems. Headache 31:439, 1991.

27. Østergaard JR, Kraft M. Natural course of benign coital headache. BMJ 305:1129, 1992.

28. Rubino FA. Initial evaluation of headache. J Fla Med Assoc 84:20, 1997.

29. Burton LJ, et al. Headache etiology in a pediatric emergency department. Pediatr Emerg Care 13:1, 1997.

30. Solomon S, et al. Evaluation of chronic daily headache—Comparison to criteria for chronic tension-type headache. Cephalagia 12:365, 1992.

31. Sheftell FD. Chronic daily headache. Neurology 42(3 Suppl 2):32, 1992.

32. Diamond S. Coexisting migraine and tension-type headache (Letter). Arch Neurol 50:795, 1993.

33. Pryse-Phillips W, et al. A Canadian population survey on the clinical, epidemiological and societal impact of migraine and tension-type headache. Can J Neurol Sci 19:333, 1992.

34. Laughey WF, et al. How many different headaches do you have? Cephalagia 13:136, 1993.

35. Skaer TL. Clinical presentation and treatment of migraine. Clin Ther 18:229, 1996.

36. Mathew NT. Dosing and administration of ergotamine tartrate and dihydroergotamine. Headache 37(Suppl 1):S26, 1997.

37. Saper JR. Diagnosis and treatment of migraine. Headache 37(Suppl 1):S1, 1997.

38. Linet MS, et al. Headaches preceded by visual aura among adolescents and young adults. Arch Neurol 49:512, 1992.

39. Leone M, et al. A review of the treatment of primary headaches. I. Migraine. Ital J Neurol Sci 16:577, 1995.

40. Olesen J, Rasmussen BK. The International Headache Society classification of chronic daily and near-daily headaches: A critique of the criticism. Cephalagia 16:407, 1996.

41. De Benedittis G, Lorenzetti A. The role of stressful life events in the persistence of primary headache: Major events vs. daily hassles. Pain 51:35, 1992.

42. Martin PR, Theunissen C. The role of life event stress, coping and social support in chronic headaches. Headache 33:301, 1993.

43. Mathew NT. Cluster headache. Neurology 42(3 Suppl 2):22, 1992.

44. D'Amico D, et al. Coexistence of migraine and cluster headache: Report of 10 cases and possible pathogenetic implications. Headache 37:21, 1997.

45. Portyansky E. Separate directions. Drug Topics 141(16):22, 1997.

46. Vogel MR. Excedrin Extra Strength recommended for migraine relief. Pharm Today 3(8):15, 1997.

47. Anon. Advisory panel okays OTC Excedrin Extra Strength for migraine pain. NDMA Exec Newsletter 16–97:1, 1997.

48. Anon. Tylenol relabeled. Drug Topics 138:22, 1994(22).

49. Anon. FDA promises alcohol warning on all analgesics. NDMA Exec Newsletter 1/20/95.

50. Federal Register 42:35345, 1977.

51. Kelly JP, et al. Risk of aspirin-associated major upper-gastrointestinal bleeding with enteric-coated or buffered product. Lancet 348:1413, 1996.

52. Fed Reg 55:27776, 1990.

53. Collins E. Maternal and fetal effects of acetaminophen and salicylates in pregnancy. Obstet Gynecol 58(Suppl):57S, 1981.

54. Anon. Aspirin warning strengthened. The Daily Oklahoman 7/3/90:2.

55. Roine R, et al. Aspirin increases blood alcohol concentrations in humans after ingestion of ethanol. JAMA 264:2406, 1990.

56. Zamula E. Reye syndrome. FDA Consumer 24:21, 1990(9).

57. Anon. Reye syndrome cases. FDA Consumer 23:3, 1989(8).

58. Fed Reg 58:545227, 1993.

59. Savitsky ME, Wiens JA, Miwa LJ. Cross-reactivity in aspirin-sensitive patients. Drug Intell Clin Pharm 21:338, 1987.

60. Bowen CA. Drug forum. US Pharmacist 12:24, 1987(2).

61. Aaron TH, Muttitt ELC. Reactions to acetylsalicylic acid. Can Med Assoc J 126:609, 1982.

62. O'Donnell J. Drug chain reaches settlement in aspirin allergy case. Drug Topics 136:72, 1992(22).

63. Hirsh, et al. Aspirin and other platelet-active drugs. Chest 102(4 Suppl):327S, 1992.

64. Oren R, et al. Gastro-duodenal injury associated with intake of 100–325 mg aspirin daily. Postgrad Med J 69:712, 1993.

65. Silagy CA, et al. Adverse effects of low-dose aspirin in a healthy elderly population. Clin Pharmacol Ther 54:84, 1993.

66. Kelly R. Selection from current literature: Using aspirin for primary or secondary prevention. Fam Pract 10:88, 1993.

67. Karlowicz MG, White LE. Severe intracranial hemorrhage in a term neonate associated with maternal acetylsalicylic acid ingestion. Clin Pediatr 32:740, 1993.

68. Sila CA. Prophylaxis and treatment of stroke. Drugs 45:329, 1993.

69. Besdine RW. Stroke prevention in the elderly. Conn Med 57:287, 1993.

70. Matchar DB, et al. The stroke prevention patient outcomes research team. Stroke 24:2135, 1993.

71. Unwin DH, Greenlee RG. Prophylactic drug therapy in cerebrovascular disease. Am Fam Physician 48:85, 1993.

72. Brass LM, et al. Transient ischemic attacks in the elderly: Diagnosis and treatment. Geriatrics 47:36, 1992.

73. Sivenius J, et al. European stroke prevention study (ESPS): Antithrombotic therapy is also effective in the elderly. Acta Neurol Scand 87:111, 1993.

74. Tortorice KL, Carter BL. Stroke prophylaxis: Hypertension management and antithrombotic therapy. Ann Pharmacother 27:471, 1993.

75. Yusuf S, et al. Primary and secondary prevention of myocardial infarction and strokes: An update of randomly allocated, controlled trials. J Hypertens Suppl 11:S61, 1993.

76. Bornstein NM, et al. Failure of aspirin treatment after stroke. Stroke 25:275, 1994.

77. Segal M. Should you take aspirin to help prevent a heart attack? FDA Consumer 22:19, 1988(5).

78. Couch JR. Antiplatelet therapy in the treatment of cerebrovascular disease. Clin Cardiol 16:703, 1993.

79. Kelley RE, Berger JR. TIA and minor stroke. Postgrad Med 91:197, 1992.

80. Craven LL. Prevention of coronary and cerebral thrombosis. Miss Vall Med J 78:213, 1956.

81. Grotemeyer KH, et al. Two-year follow-up of aspirin responder and aspirin non responder. A pilot study including 180 post-stroke patients. Thromb Res 71:397, 1993.

82. Antiplatelet Trialists' Collaboration. Collaborative overview of randomised trials of antiplatelet therapy. I. Prevention of death, myocardial infarction, and stroke by prolonged antiplatelet therapy in various categories of patients. BMJ 308: 81, 1994.

83. Dalen JE, Hirsh J. Introduction. Chest 102(4 Suppl):303S, 1992.

84. Flaker GC, Singh VN. Prevention of myocardial reinfarction. Postgrad Med 94:94, 1993.

85. Prentice CRM. Antithrombotic therapy in the secondary prevention of myocardial infarction. Am J Cardiol 72:175G, 1993.

86. Byers JF. The use of aspirin in cardiovascular disease. J Cardiovasc Nursing 8:1, 1993.

87. Fed Reg 61:30002, 1996.

88. Fed Reg 58:54223, 1993.

89. Nightingale SL. From the Food and Drug Administration. JAMA 270:2669, 1993.

90. Blake KV, et al. Death of a child associated with multiple overdoses of acetaminophen. Am J Hosp Pharm 45:1438, 1988.

91. Nadir A, et al. Parental and medical over-administration of acetaminophen causing lethal hepatotoxicity in a 10-year-old. J Okla State Med Assoc 87:261, 1994.

92. Anon. OTC Warnings. Drug Topics 137:64, 1993(14).

93. Fleckenstein JL. Nyquil and acute hepatic necrosis (Letter). N Engl J Med 313:48, 1985.

94. Foust RT, et al. Nyquil-associated liver injury. Am J Gastroenterol 84 422, 1989.

95. Whitcomb DC, Block HD. Association of acetaminophen hepatotoxicity with fasting and ethanol use. JAMA 272:1845, 1994.

96. Sandler DP, et al. Analgesic use and chronic renal disease. N Engl J Med 320 1238, 1989.

97. Bennett WM, DeBroe ME. Analgesic nephropathy—A preventable renal disease. N Engl J Med 320:1269, 1989.

98. Nanra RS, et al. Analgesic nephropathy induced by common proprietary mixtures. Med J Aust 1:486, 1980(10).

99. Stewart JH. Analgesic abuse and renal failure in Australasia. Kidney Int 13:72, 1978.

100. Perneger TV. Whelton PK, Klag MJ. Risk of kidney failure associated with the use of acetaminophen, aspirin, and nonsteroidal antiinflammatory drugs. N Engl J Med 331:1675, 1994.

101. Sawynok J. Pharmacological rationale for the clinical use of caffeine. Drugs 49:37, 1995.

102. Walson PD, et al. Comparison of multidose ibuprofen and acetaminophen therapy in febrile children. AJDC 146:626, 1992.

103. Anon. McNeil consumer products. Weekly Pharmacy Rep 44:1, 1995(16).

104. Trade package. Children's Motrin: 1995.

105. Gossel TA. OTC ibuprofen: The track record today. US Pharmacist 12:77,1987(11).

106. Nashel DJ, et al. Labeling of ibuprofen for over-the-counter use. (Letter). N Engl J Med 312:377, 1985.

107. Stillman MT, Schlesinger PA. Nonsteroidal anti-inflammatory drug nephrotoxicity. Arch Intern Med 150:268, 1990.

108. Whelton A, et al. Renal effects of ibuprofen, piroxicam, and sulindac in patients with asymptomatic renal failure. Ann Intern Med 112:568, 1990.

109. Mitchell SR. Tell your kidneys to take a powder (Letter). Arch Intern Med 151:617, 1991.

110. Grimm AM, Wolf JE. Aseptic meningitis associated with nonprescription ibuprofen use (Letter). DICP 23:712, 1989.

111. Agrawal N. NSAIDs: Is over-the-counter the best? (Letter). J Am Geriatr Soc 38:956, 1990.

112. Anon. Ibuprofen fatality. Pharm J 239:299, 1987.

113. Nicastro NJ. Visual disturbances associated with over-the-counter ibuprofen in three patients. Ann Ophthalmol 21:447, 1989.

114. Newton GD, et al. New OTC drugs and devices: A selected review. Am Pharm NS35:35, 1995(2).

115. Trade package. Orudis KT: (undated).

116. Trade package. Actron: (undated).

117. Schachtel BP, et al. Caffeine as an analgesic adjuvant. A double-blind study comparing aspirin with caffeine to aspirin and placebo in patients with sore throat. Arch Intern Med 151:733, 1991.

118. Migliardi JR, et al. Caffeine as an analgesic adjuvant in tension headache. Clin Pharmacol Ther 56:576, 1994.

119. Ward N, et al. The analgesic effects of caffeine in headache. Pain 44:151, 1991.

120. Papazian R. Pain, pain go away. FDA Consumer 29(1):11, 1995.

121. Cunningham EE. Early patent and proprietary medicines and the treatment of kidney and urinary tract diseases. Am J Nephrol 7:45, 1987.

122. Spierings ELH. Practical aspects of the pharmacotherapy of headache. Compr Ther 18:36, 1992.

Menstrual Discomfort

A woman in her late 40s requests help with the menstrual products.

Interview/Patient Assessment

She is experiencing increased discomfort at onset of her menstrual flow, which began today. She has painful abdominal cramping with bloating, fatigue, and a faint feeling. The symptoms of dysmenorrhea have worsened gradually since she was diagnosed as having uterine fibroids several months ago. She wonders if a combination product containing pamabrom and acetaminophen would be helpful.

Pharmacist's Analysis

1. Would a product containing pamabrom and acetaminophen be likely to provide relief from her symptoms?
2. Does this patient have primary dysmenorrhea?
3. Should this patient be allowed to self-treat her menstrual complaints?

The product the patient wishes to use is suitable for most patients with primary dysmenorrhea or premenstrual syndrome. Her symptoms are not premenstrual in time of onset, so the pharmacist must suspect some condition other than PMS. The presence of uterine fibroids suggests that she does not have primary dysmenorrhea, but secondary dysmenorrhea, which must be treated by a physician. Alleviating the symptoms produced by uterine fibroids may cause her to neglect medical care.

Patient Counseling

This patient should be urged to speak with her physician so that an informed decision may be made about treatment of the fibroids themselves, since the symptoms they produce are worsening. Her physician may suggest treatment that would allow symptoms to resolve completely.

While menstrual problems directly affect females, they can have a much wider impact, affecting family, friends, and coworkers. Fortunately, nonprescription products can provide relief from certain symptoms related to menstrual periods.

The average menstrual cycle lasts for 28 days.[1] The events that occur in the cycle may be earlier or later in certain females and may even occur at different times during different cycles in the same patient. However, the menstrual phase occurs roughly on days 1 through 4, and the proliferative phase on days 5 to 14 (Fig. 19.1). During the proliferative phase the uterine lining prepares to nurture a fertilized ovum, under the influence of rising estrogen levels. The secretory phase begins at day 14 (on the average) and continues through day 28, dominated by progesterone. If the ovum remains unfertilized, it atrophies on days 24 to 25 and estrogen/progesterone levels decline rapidly. At this point endometrial development halts, and the uterine lining is shed as menses commences. Days 1 to 14 (approximately) are also known as the follicular phase, and the remainder of the cycle is known as the luteal phase.

The pharmacist can suggest self-treatment for two conditions related to the menstrual period, premenstrual syndrome (PMS), which occurs prior to the onset of flow, and dysmenorrhea, a syndrome that usually begins with the onset of flow. Other menstrual disorders such as precocious onset of first menses, delayed onset of first menses, disappearance of menstrual flow after a series of normal periods, excessive bleeding during menses, and breakthrough bleeding between menses may indicate a serious underlying condition and should be referred.

PREMENSTRUAL SYNDROME

There is no universally accepted definition of PMS, partly because symptoms are inconsistent from female to female and from cycle to cycle in the same person.[2–6] As a result it is more easily described than defined. PMS begins around the time of ovulation (usually midcycle, or on day 14) in the late luteal phase, up to a week prior to the onset of flow.[7,8]

PREVALENCE OF PREMENSTRUAL SYNDROME

The prevalence of PMS depends on criteria used to define the disorder.[9,10] About 3 to 5% of females are free of PMS symptoms.[1,11] Of the remaining 95 to 97% most have only mild symptomatology, although as many as 20 to 40% of females may be moderately to severely affected.[1,12] Only 5% of females have PMS that is so severe as to completely disrupt their lives. While the disruption is usually minor (e.g., absence from school or work), in extreme cases it can lead to suicide gestures, suicide, and violent behavior directed at others.[4,11] (French officials recognize PMS as a legitimate criminal defense, asserting that it is a form of insanity.[13] Similar defenses have been used in England, Canada, and the United States.[14,15])

EPIDEMIOLOGY OF PREMENSTRUAL SYNDROME

Age affects PMS. Over one-half of females with PMS reported that their symptoms began in adolescence, while one-

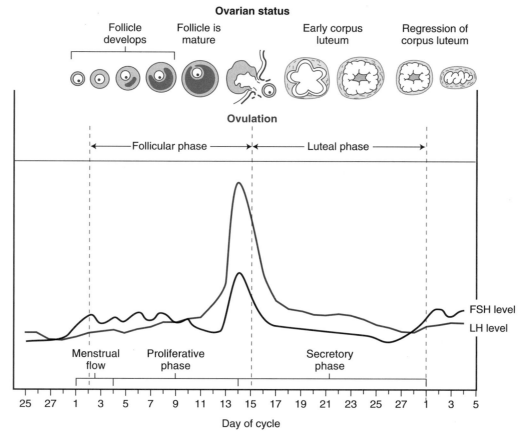

Figure 19.1. The female ovulatory/menstrual cycle, showing ovarian status in relation to levels of follicle-stimulating hormone (FSH) and luteinizing hormone (LH). Times are approximate.

fourth stated that the symptoms began with the first period.[16] During the late 20s symptoms become less common, and they may disappear in the late 30s to early 40s.[17–20] Genetics also play a role in PMS. Monozygous (identical) twins both suffer from PMS more often than both dizygous (fraternal) twins.[21]

Symptoms worsen with increased parity.[22] Other predisposing factors for PMS include past history or family history of mental illness or PMS, or past history of sexual abuse, working outside of the home (but not by choice), and toxemia during a past pregnancy.[22–26] PMS is more common in females who have a past history of oral contraceptive use, alcohol consumption, and use of drugs.[27]

PMS cannot occur in patients with chemical or surgical **oophorectomy** (removal of the ovaries).[13,28] Patients with hysterectomies, however, may still experience symptoms as long as ovaries are intact.

ETIOLOGY OF PREMENSTRUAL SYNDROME

The greatest controversy in PMS is the clash over etiology. There are those who assert that the problem is psychological, and others who assert strongly that the problem is physiologic.[2]

Physiological Etiology

The cyclical nature of PMS points to the natural conclusion that its etiology is tied to monthly hormonal fluctuations (Fig. 19.2). At one time a monthly hormonal imbalance was suspected as causal for PMS, but most researchers now feel that the cause is normal ovarian function, which triggers biochemical events in the central nervous system (CNS) and other target tissues.[11]

Progesterone has been linked to PMS symptoms in research.[29] Patients with oophorectomy and hysterectomy are free of symptoms, as noted, and do not develop them again when given supplemental estrogen therapy.[11] However, symptoms recur when the patient is given progesterone or related chemicals.

The role of other hormones has been investigated, including estrogen, prolactin, growth hormone, thyroid hormones, follicle-stimulating hormone, antidiuretic hormone, insulin, prostaglandins, and cortisol.[29–31] Preliminary studies of these hormones are rarely replicated, and none is thought to be primarily causal at this time.[13,32]

Investigation of the role of neurotransmitters may be more fruitful, since these are thought to be altered by progesterone and estrogen.[13] Bodily changes are induced by

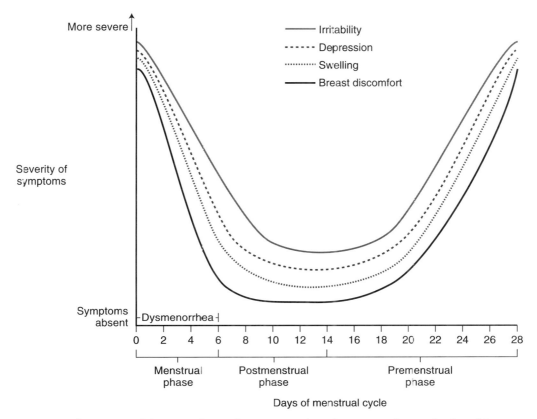

Figure 19.2. Severity of symptoms of dysmenorrhea and premenstrual syndrome according to the day of the menstrual cycle.

serotonin, endorphins, and monoamines. Serotonin, for instance, modulates mood and behavior; mood changes may be linked to cyclic alterations in serotonergic activity.[33,34]

Vitamin B$_6$ is a cofactor in neurotransmitter synthesis. For this reason it has been included in numerous nonprescription products used to alleviate PMS symptoms. However, it has not been shown to help PMS in controlled trials.[35] Further, it is doubtful that pyridoxine deficiency exists in large numbers of American females. Females who have taken as little as 50 mg of pyridoxine daily have experienced neurotoxicity. The risk of adverse effects when combined with lack of proven merit argues against self-administration with pyridoxine.

Psychiatric Etiology

Many physicians do not believe that PMS is an actual entity.[36] In a proposed revision of the American Psychological Association's authoritative manual, *Diagnostic and Statistical Manual of Mental Disorders* (DSM-III-R), PMS was placed in a controversial appendix and given the name "Late Luteal Phase Dysphoric Disorder (LLPDD)."[2,37,38] The DSM-IV Work Group considered renaming the condition (e.g., Premenstrual Dysphoric Disorder, Periodic Mood Disorder, Cyclic Mood Disorder).[39]

Several research studies point to a psychiatric causation for PMS. In one study patients who were convinced by researchers that they were in the premenstrual phase reported

a higher index of physical symptoms (e.g., water retention, pain, and/or sexual arousal) than others who were convinced by researchers that they were intermenstrual.[21,40]

Medication-Related PMS

In one instance a medication induced PMS. Phenobarbital produced symptoms indistinguishable from PMS, all of which ceased immediately on cessation of phenobarbital.[41] However, this was the only report discovered of a reaction of this type.

MANIFESTATIONS OF PREMENSTRUAL SYNDROME

Symptoms of premenstrual syndrome include water retention and bloating, abdominal pain, cramping, breast tenderness, headache, fatigue, irritability, feelings of depression, abnormal eating patterns, increased libido, excitement, feelings of inadequacy, tension, and anxiety (see Fig. 19.2).[7, 42–50] "Suggested Criteria for a Patient Diagnosis of Premenstrual Dysphoric Disorder" below included these and additional diagnostic criteria for the condition. More severe symptoms include seemingly psychotic behavior and acts of violence. Some researchers assert that true PMS symptoms cease at onset of flow and are absent in the postmenstrual period.[2]

SPECIFIC CONSIDERATIONS OF PREMENSTRUAL SYNDROME

See "Specific Considerations of Menstrual Discomfort: Treating Patients with Tact and Sensitivity."

PROGNOSIS OF PREMENSTRUAL SYNDROME

When treated with nonprescription medications or other interventions, PMS symptoms may be greatly ameliorated. However, if PMS remains untreated, researchers allege that the patient may suffer an entire set of adverse life consequences, including loss of self-confidence, decreased self-esteem, altered body image, feelings of inadequacy, low assertiveness, broken engagements, marital distress, divorce, alterations in mother/child relationships, and an inability to maintain a job or pursue educational goals.[16] Regardless of the validity of these perceptions, the patient should be encouraged to seek treatment rather than to endure the problem month after month.

TREATMENT OF PREMENSTRUAL SYNDROME

FOCUS ON...

SUGGESTED CRITERIA FOR A PATIENT DIAGNOSIS OF PREMENSTRUAL DYSPHORIC DISORDER[51]

(These criteria were suggested for inclusion in the Appendix of DSM-IV by a Task Force of the American Psychological Association.)

A. In the majority of cycles over the past 12 months, the symptoms listed in part C occurred during the last week of the luteal phase, began to remit within a few days after the onset of the follicular phase, and were absent in the week following menses. (In menstruating females the luteal phase corresponds to the period between ovulation and the onset of the menses, and the follicular phase begins with menses.)

B. The disturbance markedly interferes with work or school or with usual social activities and relationships with others (e.g., causes avoidance of social activities, decreased productivity, and inefficiency at home, at work, and/or at school).

C. At least five of the following symptoms were present most of the time during the late luteal phase, with at least one of the symptoms being one of the first four:

1. Markedly depressed mood, feelings of hopelessness, or self-deprecating thoughts
2. Marked anxiety, tension, feelings of being "keyed up," or "on edge"
3. Marked affective lability (e.g., feeling suddenly sad or tearful or with an increased sensitivity to rejection)
4. Persistent and marked anger or irritability or increased interpersonal conflicts
5. Decreased interest in usual activities (e.g., work, school, friends, or hobbies)
6. Subjective sense of difficulty in concentrating
7. Lethargy, easy fatigability, or marked lack of energy
8. Marked change in appetite, overeating, or specific food cravings
9. Hypersomnia or insomnia
10. A subjective sense of being overwhelmed or out-of-control
11. Other physical symptoms such as breast tenderness or swelling, headaches, joint or muscle pain, a sensation of "bloating," or weight gain

D. The disturbance is not merely an exacerbation of the symptoms of another disorder such as major depressive disorder, panic disorder, dysthymic disorder, or a personality disorder, although it may be superimposed on any of these disorders.

E. Criteria A, B, C, and D must be confirmed by prospective daily ratings during at least two symptomatic cycles. (A diagnosis may be made provisionally prior to this confirmation.)

A number of studies indicate that PMS might be worsened by some foods and beverages[13]:

- High sodium foods and simple sugars (can lead to water retention)[13,29]
- Protein (e.g., red meat) and dairy products[22]
- Chocolate, fruit juices, and beer[52]
- Alcoholic beverages, especially during the postmenstrual period[53]
- Recreational drugs (promote emotional instability)[13]
- Nicotine (a vasoconstrictor, it can reduce ovarian blood flow)[1]
- Caffeine, which produces tension and irritability and contributes to sleep disorders, also should be avoided.[13,29,54] It may also contribute to breast-related symptoms.[1] In surveys it is strongly associated with prevalence of PMS.[55] *If the patient cannot cease her consumption of caffeine altogether, she should at least halt or moderate her intake on days 3 to 4 prior to the onset of menses and during menses.[56]*

Rest also may be helpful in alleviating PMS symptoms, perhaps by relieving stress.[57,58] *Patients with sleep disorders are predisposed to fatigue and irritability, which add to PMS symptoms.*

Exercise also reduces PMS severity.[13,19] Exercise is thought to raise levels of beta endorphins, which elevates the mood.[59] See "Treatment of Menstrual Discomfort."

DYSMENORRHEA

Dysmenorrhea is pain or discomfort occurring during menstruation.[60] It usually begins the first day of menses.[61]

PREVALENCE OF DYSMENORRHEA

Dysmenorrhea is the major cause of short-term school absenteeism and of work-related absences.[16,28,62] As many as 91% of high-school females experience dysmenorrhea, and the problem is severe for 23%.[16] As many as 26% of students miss class, and 55% of students report that cramps interfere with their school work.

EPIDEMIOLOGY OF DYSMENORRHEA

The patient with dysmenorrhea is more likely to also have PMS, with severity of symptoms of one condition mirroring that of the other (see Fig. 19.2).[2] When patients suffer from both syndromes, onset of pain is usually premenstrual. Incidence of dysmenorrhea does not vary according to most sociodemographic variables, although one study demonstrated increased incidence in those of low income.[63,64] Users of cigarettes and alcohol may have more severe cramps, although other studies show no difference.[61,65] Excess weight is also a risk factor for the cramping pain of dysmenorrhea.[61]

ETIOLOGY OF DYSMENORRHEA

Primary Dysmenorrhea

Primary dysmenorrhea is thought to result from prostaglandin 2 alpha released from sloughed uterine lining.[16,66] Prostaglandins induce strong uterine contractions, causing the familiar cramping pain.[59] In this sense the cramps are actually a signal that uterine contractions are functioning normally to help expel menstrual discharge. Dysmenorrhea usually begins within 3 years of **menarche** (the time that the patient first has menstrual flow, approximately at age 12 to 14) and may cease with aging or childbirth (as the cervical os enlarges), facilitating expulsion of menstrual discharge.[67] However, dysmenorrhea may continue until menopause.

Secondary Dysmenorrhea

The more dangerous subtype of dysmenorrhea, secondary dysmenorrhea, is secondary to some underlying pathologic process (e.g., pelvic inflammatory disease, uterine fibroids, endometriosis, ovarian cyst, neoplasm, uterine polyps, ectopic pregnancy, an abnormally positioned uterus, or appendicitis).[28,59]

Dysmenorrheic pain is more likely to be the result of secondary dysmenorrhea if it occurs at other times of the cycle or during intercourse.[59] Since the patient cannot know the cause of her dysmenorrhea, she should visit a physician when she first experiences pain during the period. Should she be found free of secondary pathology, she has primary dysmenorrhea, a diagnosis of exclusion.[28]

MANIFESTATIONS OF DYSMENORRHEA

In addition to pain and/or cramping, the syndrome of dysmenorrhea also includes headache, nausea, bloating, dizziness, fatigue, vomiting, lower backache, diarrhea, and syncope in more than 50% of patients.[7,28,60,68] The spasms or cramping may begin a few hours prior to onset of flow or begin at onset of flow. Pain often stops after 48 hours, but may last as long as 72 hours or continue through the entire period.[61] Pain is mainly confined to the pelvic region and lower abdomen, but may also occur in other areas of the body. The pain is mild in 49% of patients, moderate in another 37%, and severe in 14% of patients.[16]

SPECIFIC CONSIDERATIONS OF DYSMENORRHEA

See "Specific Considerations of Menstrual Discomfort: Treating Patients with Tact and Sensitivity."

TREATMENT OF DYSMENORRHEA

See "Treatment of Menstrual Discomfort."

MENSTRUAL DISCOMFORT

For prevalence, epidemiology, etiology, manifestations, prognosis, and treatment of premenstrual syndrome, see discussion above. For prevalence, epidemiology, etiology, and manifestations of dysmenorrhea, see discussion above.

SPECIFIC CONSIDERATIONS OF MENSTRUAL DISCOMFORT: TREATING PATIENTS WITH TACT AND SENSITIVITY

It is unfortunate that menstrual complaints are often not seen as real illnesses.[69] Too often, school nurses, physical education teachers, parents, health educators, physicians, and other health professionals "wonder if a girl's complaint is an excuse to shirk responsibility or to gain sympathy or attention" when young women report these discomforts to them.[16] More sympathetic—and enlightened—professionals allow the patient to miss school or sit out athletic activities.

The lack of tact and sensitivity is deep-seated, however. Even a leading researcher on menstrual problems states that cyclic mood swings "transform a happy school girl into a lazy, bad-tempered, selfish individual whose academic work and behavior deteriorate."[16]

Because females have experienced a variety of attitudes toward complaints of menstrual discomfort, the pharmacist must be acutely aware that a caring, empathetic approach is appreciated when discussing these problems.[70]

TREATMENT OF MENSTRUAL DISCOMFORT

Treatment Guidelines

Only 14.5% of patients with dysmenorrhea and 2% of patients with severe dysmenorrhea in one study sought help from a physician; as many as 66% of those who do seek physician care remain dissatisfied with their treatment.[16,63] Many daughters do not inform their parents that they have reached menarche, and only 30% of parents understand their daugh-

ter's pain. Thus a majority of patients who wish to treat symptoms of dysmenorrhea will choose self-treatment (see Patient Assessment Algorithm 19.1). The same may be true of PMS. As an important note, *a young female seeking relief from PMS or dysmenorrhea may not be accompanied by an adult who might help her understand directions and precautions associated with the nonprescription ingredients.* In one study adolescents reported that they began to self-administer medications for menstrual pain without

Patient Assessment Algorithm 19.1. Menstrually Related Discomfort

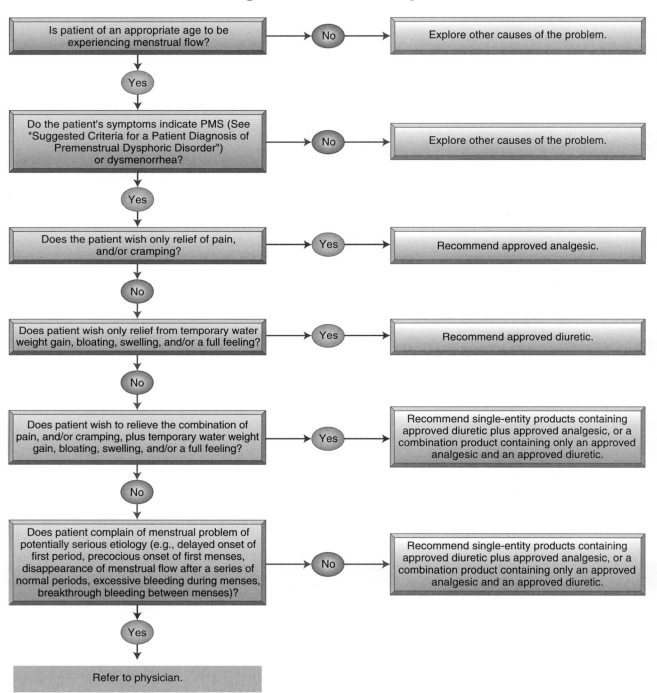

checking with an adult at ages 11 to 12 (this study also included treatment of pain of the head, stomach, throat, and back).[71]

Nonprescription Medications

While PMS and dysmenorrhea are distinct clinical entities, symptoms overlap somewhat.[68] Thus nonprescription products for menstrual problems such as those shown in Table 19.1 are usually combinations of ingredients from several categories indicated for the symptoms of PMS and primary dysmenorrhea (labeled as "menstrual symptoms" for ease of consumer understanding). These ingredient categories include analgesics, diuretics, and antihistamines.[68] Permitted combinations include a diuretic combined with an approved analgesic, or ammonium chloride combined with either caffeine or pamabrom.[72] If the antihistamine pyrilamine is eventually found to be safe and effective, it will also be permitted in combination products.

Nonprescription menstrual products provide relief for mild-to-moderate symptoms, but will probably not help those with severe symptoms.[4] The lower age cutoff for self-treatment is the highest age cutoff of the product's various ingredients, if it is a combination. Of course, there are no legitimate requests for their use prior to the age of menarche.

The products are not indicated for treatment of either amenorrhea or menopause. Menopause was specifically excluded from the discussion of nonprescription products in the original panel report.[68] Menopause occurs between the ages of 48 and 51 on the average.[67]

ANALGESICS

All Category I analgesics are approved for the treatment of pain and/or cramping of the premenstrual and menstrual periods.[68] *Since prostaglandins are responsible for the cramping of dysmenorrhea, it would be logical to recommend nonsteroidal anti-inflammatory agents (NSAIDs), as they inhibit synthesis of prostaglandins.*[59] Aspirin is not as potent in this use as the other NSAIDs (e.g., ibuprofen, ketoprofen, naproxen sodium). Acetaminophen is not thought to prevent prostaglandin production, but it is helpful for treating the headache and backache that may occur with menstrual cramping or PMS.[59]

DIURETICS

 Diuretics are effective for the temporary water weight gain, bloating, swelling, and/or full feeling of PMS and

the menstrual period.[59,68,72] The original panel report found three diuretics to be effective.

Ammonium Chloride

Ammonium chloride is an acidifying diuretic that may cause progressive hyperchloremic acidosis if used in patients with impaired kidney function.[68] ***If it is taken by patients with liver disease, a hepatic coma may occur.*** *For this reason products containing it must be labeled against use if the patient has kidney or liver disease.*[68] Ammonium chloride is approved for use in dosages of 1 gram three times daily for no longer than 6 days. *At those doses ammonium chloride causes adverse reactions that also must be listed on the label: nausea, vomiting, and gastrointestinal distress.*

Caffeine

Caffeine was found to be effective as a diuretic in dosages of 100 to 200 mg every 3 to 4 hours. It is also labeled "For the relief of fatigue associated with the premenstrual and menstrual periods."[68,72] *However, research indicates that caffeine worsens symptoms of PMS.* For this reason another diuretic may be preferable. Further, caffeine products must be labeled, "The recommended dose of this product contains about as much caffeine as a cup of coffee. Limit the use of caffeine-containing medications, foods, or beverages while taking this product because too much caffeine may cause nervousness, irritability, sleeplessness, and occasionally rapid heart beat."[72]

Pamabrom

Pamabrom is a xanthine derivative approved as a diuretic in doses of 50 mg four times daily to a maximum of 200 mg daily.[68]

PYRILAMINE

Pyrilamine has been the subject of considerable controversy for use in menstrual problems. In the Phase I report the panel rated it as Category I for providing relief from a variety of symptoms:

- Emotional changes or mood changes related to the premenstrual period such as anxiety, nervous tension, and irritability
- Water-retention symptoms such as temporary weight gain and swelling occurring during the menstrual or premenstrual periods

Table 19.1. Representative Approved Combination Products for Menstrual Problems	
PRODUCT	SELECTED INGREDIENTS
Diurex 2 Tablets	Magnesium salicylate tetrahydrate 404 mg, pamabrom 50 mg
Midol Teen	Acetaminophen 400 mg, pamabrom 25 mg
Pamprin Maximum Pain Relief	Acetaminophen 500 mg, magnesium salicylate 250 mg, pamabrom 25 mg

A Pharmacist's Journal

"I Need to Get the Water Off."

A young girl who appeared to be in her late teens or early 20s asked where our water pills were. I showed them to her and asked if the swelling was related to the menstrual period. She said it was not. I asked where the swelling was. "My feet and hands. My hands are so swollen now that I can hardly get my wedding ring off." I explained that she should see a physician since her heart or kidneys might be damaged. She replied, "I've had this for two years. My kidneys work just fine, they just don't get enough fluid off." I repeated that she really needed to see her physician. However, she began to turn her body away from me as she looked at the products and would no longer speak to me or acknowledge my presence in any way. I never saw her again. The pharmacist is often left with only half of the story, wondering what the outcome was.

- Cramps and backache of the premenstrual or menstrual period[68]

However, in the same report the FDA made editorial comments regarding its effectiveness, stating that it should not be marketed as an ingredient in single-entity products. The recommended dosage is 25 to 30 mg every 3 to 4 hours or 60 mg every 12 hours, not to exceed 200 mg in any 24-hour period.

In the Phase II document the FDA reviewed data and concluded that pyrilamine did not have sufficient evidence of effectiveness to warrant Category I designation (alone or in combination) and relegated it to Category III.[72] Pursuant to this decision, the Nonprescription Drug Manufacturers Association submitted new data to prove effectiveness.[73] The FDA concluded that these data did not support efficacy, but supplied recommendation for reanalysis of the data, which it suggested would then support a claim for relief of menstrual cramps.

UNPROVEN PRODUCTS FOR MENSTRUAL PROBLEMS
Botanical/Vegetable Herbs
The original panel assigned to review menstrual products examined various herbs and botanical agents such as those in some of the products in Table 19.2. The panel stated that Category II labeling should be assigned to all herbs, including Jamaica dogwood, pleurisy root, black cohosh, life root, dandelion root, blessed thistle, corn silk, couch grass, dog grass extract, buchu, uva ursi, golden seal, oil of juniper, pipsissewa, and triticum.[68,72]

Vitamins/Minerals
Ferrous sulfate has been included in menstrual products. The original review panel concluded that treatment of iron deficiency anemia was not within its purview.[68] The decision was reaffirmed by the FDA, which stated that adding iron to menstrual products would be unwarranted.[72] All vitamins were placed in Category II except for pyridoxine, which was given Category III status.

Evening Primrose Oil
Primrose oil has been the subject of numerous consumer ads and health-food-store products.[29] However, convincing clinical research demonstrating its efficacy in either PMS or dysmenorrhea has not been carried out.[74,75] The purported active ingredient is gamma-linoleic acid.[22]

Antifungal Agents
For several years lay publications have touted a theory that hypothesizes that numerous medical problems (e.g., PMS, ulcer, diarrhea, etc.) are the result of yeast overgrowth in the bowel.[4] Supposedly, this overgrowth is caused by oral contraceptives and the use of oral antibiotics. This theory has no scientific support, and the patient who asks about it should be urged not to take health-food-store products that claim to treat this problem.

Nonpharmacologic Therapies

Lay therapies abound for both PMS and dysmenorrhea, but pharmacists may recommend local heat to relieve the problem. Such thermotherapy products as heating pads are widely perceived to provide menstrual relief.[76] (See Chapter 20 for an in-depth discussion of products that deliver thermotherapy).

SUMMARY

Menstrual disorders have the potential to disrupt life immeasurably. While the patient may suffer from several menstrually related problems, she may only self-treat PMS and primary dysmenorrhea. Nonprescription products containing approved analgesics and diuretics may provide relief if the problem is not severe. However, should the problem continue or fail to lessen in severity after a trial of these products, a physician visit is indicated to rule out severe underlying pathology.

Table 19.2. Representative Unapproved Combination Products for Menstrual Problems

PRODUCT	SELECTED INGREDIENTS/COMMENTS
Diurex Water Capsules	Potassium salicylate, caffeine, APAP (unlabeled amounts; an unapproved combination)
Diurex Water Pills	Potassium salicylate, caffeine, salicylamide (unlabeled amounts)
Lydia E. Pinkham Tablets	Jamaica dogwood, pleurisy root, licorice, ferrous sulfate (an unapproved combination)
Midol Maximum Strength Menstrual Formula	Acetaminophen 500 mg, caffeine 60 mg, pyrilamine maleate 15 mg (pyrilamine not yet fully approved)
Midol Maximum Strength PMS Formula	Acetaminophen 500 mg, pamabrom 25 mg, pyrilamine maleate 15 mg (pyrilamine not yet fully approved)
Pamprin Multi-Symptom Maximum Strength	Acetaminophen 500 mg, pamabrom 25 mg, pyrilamine maleate 15 mg (pyrilamine not yet fully approved)
Premsyn PMS	Acetaminophen 500 mg, pamabrom 25 mg, pyrilamine maleate 15 mg (pyrilamine not yet fully approved)
Rejuvex	Bovine glandular powders (mammary 25 mg, ovary 19 mg, uterus 10 mg, adrenal 10 mg, pituitary 5 mg), dong quai 200 mg, boron 3 mg, vitamins, minerals, trace elements (an unapproved combination labeled as "the natural way to ease the symptoms of menopause")
Sundown Natural Water Pills	Potassium gluconate 20 mg, dextrate, uva ursi, alfalfa, parsley, couchgrass, juniper berry extract, asparagus, buchu (an unapproved combination)

AT THE COUNTER

 A female patient appearing to be 17 or 18 asks for help with the menstrual products.

Interview/Patient Assessment

The pharmacist questions the patient about the type of pain she is experiencing. "During school, it hurts pretty bad some days." About a week before her flow begins, she experiences cramping abdominal pain, a swollen feeling, and her head feels stuffy and painful. Symptoms virtually disappear once flow begins. She denies use of any medication and says that she has no medical conditions.

Pharmacist's Analysis

1. Are this patient's symptoms consistent with premenstrual syndrome?
2. Which ingredients would provide relief from her symptoms?
3. Is there a combination product that would be suitable for her?

This patient's symptoms appear to be caused by premenstrual syndrome. An analgesic would relieve cramping and head pain. A diuretic may alleviate the swollen feeling. However, some ingredients are not the best choices, even though they are approved by the FDA as diuretics. For instance, caffeine may worsen PMS symptoms and ammonium chloride may cause gastrointestinal upset. Pamabrom is an approved diuretic that produces less adverse reactions than either caffeine or ammonium chloride.

Patient Counseling

Normally, an NSAID (e.g., ibuprofen, ketoprofen, naproxen sodium) is an excellent choice for the discomfort of PMS. Since this patient would also benefit from a diuretic, a single-entity product containing pamabrom taken concomitantly would be appropriate. Should the patient not wish to purchase two separate products, a combination product containing an approved analgesic (acetaminophen, magnesium salicylate, or ibuprofen) and pamabrom would be suitable. Several products contain this combination (e.g., Midol Teen, Pamprin Maximum Pain Relief).

Products containing pyrilamine should not be recommended at this time. Further, a large number of products with possibly dangerous or ineffective ingredients such as herbs and plants should be avoided altogether.

References

1. Smith MA, Youngkin EQ. Managing the premenstrual syndrome. Clin Pharm 5:788, 1986.
2. Bancroft J. The premenstrual syndrome. Psychol Med 93(Suppl 24):1, 1993.
3. York R, et al. Characteristics of premenstrual syndrome. Obstet Gynecol 73:601, 1989.
4. Keye WR Jr. Premenstrual symptoms: Evaluation and treatment. Compr Ther 14:19, 1988.
5. Anderson M, et al. Premenstrual syndrome research: Using the NIMH guidelines. J Clin Psychiatry 49:484, 1988.
6. Richardson JT. The premenstrual syndrome: A brief history. Soc Sci Med 41:761, 1995.
7. Willis J. Doing something about 'the curse'. FDA Consumer 17(5):11, 1983.
8. Severino SK, Moline ML. Premenstrual syndrome. Identification and management. Drugs 49:71, 1995.
9. Fisher M, Trieller K, Napolitano B. Premenstrual symptoms in adolescents. J Adolesc Health Care 10:369, 1989.
10. Sherry S, et al. Anxiety, depression, and menstrual symptoms among freshman medical students. J Clin Psychiatry 49:490, 1988.
11. O'Brien PMS. Helping women with premenstrual syndrome. BMJ 307:1471, 1993.
12. Busch CM, et al. Severe perimenstrual symptoms: Prevalence and effects on absenteeism and health care seeking in a nonclinical sample. Women Health 14:59, 1988.
13. Parker PD. Premenstrual syndrome. Am Fam Physician 50:1309, 1994.
14. Benedek EP. Premenstrual syndrome: A view from the bench. J Clin Psychiatry 49:498, 1988.
15. Spiegel AD. Temporary insanity and premenstrual syndrome: Medical testimony in an 1865 murder trial. NY St J Med 88:482, 1988.
16. Wilson CA, Keye WR Jr. A survey of adolescent dysmenorrhea and premenstrual symptom frequency. J Adolesc Health Care 10:317, 1989.
17. Osofsky HJ, Keppel W, Kuczmierczyk AR. Evaluation and management of premenstrual syndrome in clinical psychiatric practice. J Clin Psychiatry 49:494, 1988.
18. Hamilton JA, Parry BL, Blumenthal SJ. The menstrual cycle in context. I. Affective syndromes associated with reproductive hormonal changes. J Clin Psychiatry 49:474, 1988.
19. Devalon ML, Bachman JW. Premenstrual syndrome. Postgrad Med 86:51, 1989.
20. Ainscough CE. Premenstrual emotional changes a prospective study of symptomatology in normal women (sic). J Psychosom Res 34:35, 1990.
21. Lurie S, Borenstein R. The premenstrual syndrome. Obstet Gynecol Surv 45:220, 1990.
22. Robinson GE. Premenstrual syndrome: Current knowledge and management. Can Med Assoc J 140:605, 1989.
23. Gise LH, et al. Issues in the identification of premenstrual syndromes. J Nerv Ment Dis 178:228, 1990.
24. Coughlin PC. Premenstrual syndrome: How marital satisfaction and role choice affect symptom severity. Soc Work 35:351, 1990.
25. Paddison PL, et al. Sexual abuse and premenstrual syndrome: Comparison between a lower and higher socioeconomic group. Psychosomatics 31:265, 1990.
26. Pearlstein TB. Hormones and depression: What are the facts about premenstrual syndrome menopause, and hormone replacement therapy? Am J Obstet Gynecol 173:646, 1995.
27. Chuong CJ, Burgos DM. Medical history in women with premenstrual syndrome. J Psychosom Obstet Gynecol 16:21, 1995.
28. Yankauskas E. Primary female syndromes: An update. NY St J Med 90:295, 1990.
29. Smith S, Schiff I. The premenstrual syndrome—Diagnosis and management. Fertil Steril 52:527, 1989.
30. Hamilton JA, Parry BL, Blumenthal SJ. The menstrual cycle in context. II. Human gonadal steroid hormone variability. J Clin Psychiatry 49:480, 1988.
31. Spellacy WN, et al. Plasma glucose and insulin levels during the menstrual cycles of normal women and premenstrual syndrome patients. J Reprod Med 35:508, 1990.
32. Trunnell EP, Turner CW, Keye WR. A comparison of the psychological and hormonal factors in women with and without premenstrual syndrome. J Abnorm Psychol 97:429, 1988.
33. Bancroft J. The menstrual cycle and the well being of women. Soc Sci Med 41:785, 1995.
34. Ozeren S, et al. Fluoxetine in the treatment of premenstrual syndrome. Eur J Obstet Gynecol Reprod Biol 73:167, 1997.
35. Corney RH, Clare AW. The treatment of premenstrual syndrome. Practitioner 233:233, 1989.
36. Trott A, Trott A, Trott E. Premenstrual syndrome: Diagnosis and treatment. Del Med J 68:357, 1996.
37. Blumenthal SJ, Nadelson CC. Late luteal phase dysphoric disorder (premenstrual syndromes): Clinical implications. J Clin Psychiatry 49:469, 1988.
38. Fitz-Gerald M. Premenstrual syndromes. J La State Med Soc 142:37, 1990.
39. Severino SK. Late luteal phase dysphoric disorder: A scientific puzzle. Med Hypotheses 41:229, 1993.
40. Gitlin MJ, Pasnau RO. Psychiatric syndromes linked to reproductive function in women: A review of current knowledge. Am J Psychiatry 146:1413, 1989.
41. Campbell JJ, McNamara ME. A case of phenobarbital behavioral toxicity presenting as a menstrually related mood disorder (Letter). J Clin Psychiatry 54:441, 1993.
42. Rapkin AJ, Chang LC, Reading AE. Mood and cognitive style in premenstrual syndrome. Obstet Gynecol 74:644, 1989.
43. Pazy A, Yedlin N, Lomranz J. The measurement of perimenstrual distress. J Psychol 123:571, 1989.
44. Keye WR Jr. Premenstrual syndrome. West J Med 149:765, 1988.
45. Endicott J, Halbreich U. Clinical significance of premenstrual dysphoric changes. J Clin Psychiatry 49:486, 1988.
46. Wurtman JJ, et al. Effect of nutrient intake on premenstrual depression. Am J Obstet Gynecol 161:1228, 1989.
47. Stewart DE. Positive changes in the premenstrual period. Acta Psychiatr Scand 79:400, 1989.
48. Kornstein SG, Parker AJ. Menstrual migraines: Etiology, treatment, and relationship to premenstrual syndrome. Curr Opin Obstet Gynecol 9:154, 1997.
49. Morgan M, et al. Cognitive functioning in premenstrual syndrome. Obstet Gynecol 88:961, 1996.

50. Fontana AM, Badawy S. Perceptual and coping processes across the menstrual cycle: An investigation in a premenstrual syndrome clinic and a community sample. Behav Med 22:152, 1997.

51. Endicott J. The menstrual cycle and mood disorders. J Affect Disord 29:193, 1993.

52. Rossignol AM, Bonnlander H. Prevalence and severity of the premenstrual syndrome. J Reprod Med 36:131, 1991.

53. Caan B, et al. Association between alcoholic and caffeinated beverages and premenstrual syndrome. J Reprod Med 38:630, 1993.

54. Rossignol AM, et al. Tea and premenstrual syndrome in the People's Republic of China. Am J Public Health 79:67, 1989.

55. Rossignol AM, Bonnlander H. Caffeine-containing beverages, total fluid consumption, and premenstrual syndrome. Am J Public Health 80:1106, 1990.

56. Phillis JW. Caffeine and premenstrual syndrome (Letter). Am J Public Health 79:1680, 1989.

57. Heilbrun AB Jr, Frank ME. Self-preoccupation and general stress level as sensitizing factors in premenstrual and menstrual distress. J Psychosom Res 33:571, 1989.

58. Rosen LN, Moghdam LZ, Endicott J. Relationship between premenstrual symptoms and general well-being. Psychosomatics 31:47, 1990.

59. Hale E. Taming menstrual cramps. FDA Consumer 25(5):27, 1991.

60. Carmichael JM, Thornley SM. Treatment options for dysmenorrhea. US Pharmacist Women's Health Issues Suppl 18 (2):35, 1993.

61. Harlow SD, Park M. A longitudinal study of risk factors for the occurrence, duration and severity of menstrual cramps in a cohort of college women. Br J Obstet Gynaecol 103:1134, 1996.

62. Segal M. A balanced look at the menstrual cycle. FDA Consumer 27(10):32, 1993.

63. Hewison A, van den Akker OB. Dysmenorrhea, menstrual attitude and GP consultation. Br J Nurs 5:480, 1996.

64. Jamieson DJ, Steege JF. The prevalence of dysmenorrhea, dyspareunia, pelvic pain, and irritable bowel syndrome in primary care practices. Obstet Gynecol 87:55, 1996.

65. Jarrett M, Heitkemper MM, Shaver JF. Symptoms and self-care strategies in women with and without dysmenorrhea. Health Care Women Int 16:167, 1995.

66. Apgar BS. Dysmenorrhea and dysfunctional uterine bleeding. Prim Care 24:161, 1997.

67. Jarvis C. Physical Examination and Health Assessment. Philadelphia: WB Saunders, 1992; p. 834.

68. Fed Reg 47:55076, 1982.

69. Halbreich U. Premenstrual changes, the gentle Ms. Jekyll and the hideous Ms. Hyde: The saga of catchy titles, myths and facts. Psychol Rep 65(3 Pt 2):1209, 1989.

70. Chrisler JC, Levy KB. The media construct a menstrual monster: A content analysis of PMS articles in the popular press. Women Health 16:89, 1990.

71. Chambers CT, et al. Self-administration of over-the-counter medication for pain among adolescents. Arch Pediatr Adolesc Med 151:449, 1997.

72. Fed Reg 53:46194, 1988.

73. Anon. FDA asks to re-look at pyrilamine data. NDMA Executive Newsletter 3–95:3, 1995.

74. McMurchie M, Hindmarsh E. Premenstrual syndrome. Aust Fam Physician 18:105, 1989.

75. Budeiri D, Li Wan Po A, Dornan JC. Is evening primrose oil of value in the treatment of premenstrual syndrome? Control Clin Trials 17:60, 1996.

76. Vance AR, Hayes SH, Spielholz NI. Microwave diathermy treatment for primary dysmenorrhea. Phys Ther 76:1003, 1996.

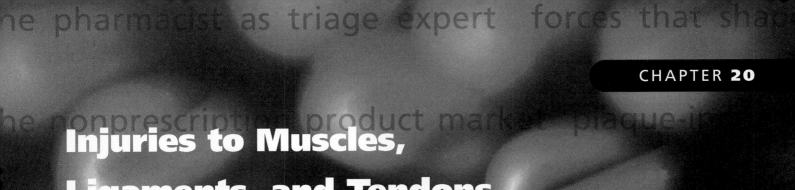

Injuries to Muscles, Ligaments, and Tendons

A 29-year-old female with two young children in her shopping cart wants to know which arm splint and external analgesic ointment will best help her.

Interview/Patient Assessment

The patient awakened this morning with a stiff wrist. When she lifted her child from the car seat the previous day, her wrist felt as though it had been "pulled too far." In response to the pharmacist's questions, she denies any medical condition and said she was not taking any prescription or nonprescription medications other than multivitamins and oral contraceptives.

Pharmacist's Analysis

1. What are the possible causes of this patient's arm pain?
2. Could her medications be contributing to the condition?
3. Should she use an arm splint and an external analgesic ointment?

This patient appears to have a minor strain caused by the repetitive actions involved with lifting her children. Her use of oral contraceptives and multivitamins is unlikely to be important. The fact that her injury only occurred the previous day suggests that self-treatment with cryotherapy may be helpful in the short term in preventing inflammation. However, in another day thermotherapy may be helpful. Alternatively, various external analgesics may also provide symptomatic relief.

Patient Counseling

The pharmacist may recommend a device to produce cooling on the wrist to reduce inflammation during the next 24-hour period. She could choose cryogel packs or use an ice bag. Once 48 to 72 hours have passed since the time of the injury, she may choose to use a heating pad or other modality for producing thermotherapy. As an alternative, various external analgesics provide relief of symptoms, although they cannot be used in conjunction with a thermotherapy device. If the pain persists for more than 7 days or if the symptoms seem to clear up but recur, she should see a physician.

People suffer many injuries to muscles, ligaments, and tendons during the typical year. While some are sports-related or work-related, others occur simply when walking or climbing steps. This chapter describes some of the injuries people experience and the possible interventions the pharmacist may suggest to help alleviate the patient's symptoms. Aside from back pain (discussed in Chapter 21), most of the common injuries to muscles, ligaments, and tendons initially seen by a pharmacist are ankle injuries, knee injuries, tendon injuries, bursitis, repetitive-strain injury, strains and sprains, and contusions.

Ankle injuries, the most frequent injury seen by pharmacists, are discussed in greater detail than other injuries because of their high prevalence. Although knee injuries are also common, they are usually related to sports activity and a coach or athletic trainer usually offers advice and monitoring for them, including a physician referral if needed. Tendon injuries, strains and sprains—general conditions that affect various parts of the body (including the ankles and knees)—are discussed in a general sense to allow the pharmacist to understand the meaning of these terms. Repetitive-strain injury, which can affect any part of the body subjected to repeated, stereotyped activity, also is discussed briefly.

ANKLE INJURIES

PREVALENCE OF ANKLE INJURIES

Acute ankle injury (usually ankle sprain) is one of the most common reasons for emergency room and general practi-

tioner visits and the most common acute sports injury.[1,2] The incidence of ankle injury is estimated to be 1 per 10,000 population each day.[1]

EPIDEMIOLOGY OF ANKLE INJURIES

Males aged 20 to 30 and females aged 10 to 20 suffer the greatest number of injuries.[3] Injuries occur most often in the afternoon or early evening and more frequently in the spring.[3] Ankle injuries in adolescents are more severe than in children because of their relatively greater body mass and strength.[4] In one study 45% of ankle injuries were sports related, while 20% arose during play and 16% at work.[3]

ETIOLOGY OF ANKLE INJURIES

Ankle sprain, the most common ankle injury, occurs when fibers or collagen of the ankle ligaments are stretched sufficiently to result in total disruption (Fig. 20.1).[5,6] (See "Strains and Sprains.") On X-ray, there is no fracture.[3] The injury is usually a result of inward motion of the sole of the foot, which damages the anterior **talofibular** (relating to the talus and fibula) ligament, although 20% of injuries also show involvement of the **calcaneoifibular** (relating to the calcaneus and fibula) ligament.[7]

In the majority of cases the ankle injury is caused by stumbling or sliding on ground level.[3] Ankle injury also often results from a bad step from a curb or underestimating the number of steps remaining when walking down a flight of

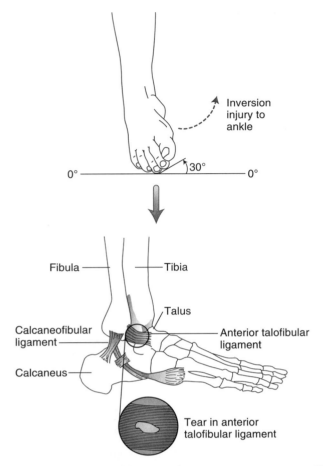

Figure 20.1. The inward (inversion) movement, a common ankle injury, often tears the anterior talofibular or calcaneofibular ligament.

stairs, causing the patient to land on the lateral part of the foot.[8] Less commonly, the patient jumps from a height, landing poorly.

Sports is a major cause of ankle injuries, especially those whose activities include running, jumping, and turning.[5] Football and basketball are particularly high-risk sports with as many as 67% of football players and 80% of basketball players having sprained one or both ankles.[5] Other high-risk sports include volleyball and soccer.[1] Injury to the dominant ankle is more common than to the nondominant ankle, probably because the dominant leg is more often subjected to force **inversion** (turning contrary to the existing position such as inward) when jumping or kicking.[1]

MANIFESTATIONS OF ANKLE INJURIES

Patients with a typical ankle sprain (such as an inversion sprain) often report that they heard a loud popping sound coming from the joint, followed by sudden onset of severe pain.[1] Further, they were usually unable to bear weight and noticed marked bleeding under the skin.

PROGNOSIS OF ANKLE INJURIES

While the time needed for complete rehabilitation from ankle sprain ranges from 36 to 72 days, as many as 40% of patients with a past history of ankle sprain experience long-term problems such as chronic pain, **crepitus** (a noise or vibration produced when irregular cartilage surfaces or bone are rubbed together), stiffness, swelling, muscular weakness, and residual ligament laxity.[1,5] These problems may persist as long as 6.5 years after the initial insult.[9] Instability caused by ligament laxity produces ease of giving way.[2,5,7] Ankle sprain is also highly predictive for future sprain caused by residual proprioceptive inadequacy, with as many as 31% of patients complaining of recurrent, chronic sprains.[2,8]

The pharmacist should refer the patient with ankle sprain to a physician for initial evaluation (although the pharmacist can also advise interim cryotherapy). The severity of the sprain must be assessed, and the possibility of fracture eliminated, as indicated by tenderness over bony structures.[6] In addition, the patient should be urged to make an appointment as soon as possible, via emergency room if the primary care physician's office is closed. Bleeding into the ankle joint and soft tissues obscures diagnosis.[1]

Past medical history is a predictor of future complications.[1] The patient with diabetes mellitus may not experience pain that would normally limit activity during the rehabilitation phase. Engaging in activity may thus cause total destruction of the foot and ankle joints in the diabetic. Similarly, the patient with a history of deep-vein thrombosis may develop thrombosis during recovery. Patients with either of these conditions should be referred for physician consultation, as should patients with either foot insensitivity or neuropathic abnormalities.

TREATMENT OF ANKLE INJURIES

See "Treatment of Injuries to Muscles, Ligaments, and Tendons." In particular, note "Ankle Injuries" under "Cryotherapy" and "Strains and Sprains" under "Thermotherapy."

KNEE INJURIES

While the pharmacist may be asked to counsel patients with knee injury, the majority of knee injuries result from sports-related activities such as basketball and football. Thus pharmacists are not often involved in the selection of products for the immediate care of knee injury. Further, the coach or athletic trainer usually provides advice to the patient about which treatment to follow.

Racquetball and squash produce a condition known as patellar pain syndrome, which the patient experiences as dull, aching, poorly localized pain that radiates to the sides and back of the knee.[10] The trend to play racquetball and squash on bare, unvarnished floors has increased the number of anterior cruciate ligamentous knee injuries (Fig. 20.2). Typically, when injury occurs, the patient hears an audible "snap" or "pop" followed by deep knee pain and a fall to the ground.

For treatment of knee injuries, see "Treatment of Injuries to Muscles, Ligaments, and Tendons." In particular, note "Knee Injuries" under "Cryotherapy" and "Strains and Sprains" under "Thermotherapy."

TENDON INJURIES

Tendinitis is the term used for inflammation of a tendon; tenosynovitis also includes inflammation of the associated connective tissue sheath of the tendon.[11]

A number of tendons are targets for injury, especially those that connect highly active muscle to bone. The most common sites are the shoulder, elbow, hip, wrist, hand, thigh, and foot.[11] As with many other injuries the pharmacist counsels, many acute tendon injuries are related to sports. (The more chronic injuries are discussed in the "Repetitive Strain Injury" section.)

Bursitis is a condition that is closely related to tendinitis. A bursa (plural = bursae) is a fluid-filled capsule found in areas where the body experiences friction. For instance, exposed or prominent protrusions may have an overlying bursa. Bursae are also located in areas where a tendon passes over a bone. The bursa functions to provide a fluid resistance against friction. The etiology, manifestations, and treatment are similar to those produced by tendinitis.

ETIOLOGY OF TENDON INJURIES

Usually, tendon injury is caused by overuse of an associated muscle either during sports activity or work.

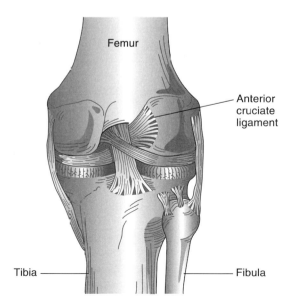

Figure 20.2. The anterior cruciate ligament is a common site for sports-related injury of the knee.

MANIFESTATIONS OF TENDON INJURIES

When a tendon suffers injury, the patient experiences pain and inflammation. The symptoms may be sufficiently severe to inhibit movement of the affected area.

Tennis elbow (lateral epicondylitis), a tendinitis resulting from repetitive motion, is the most common upper-extremity injury seen in racquetball and squash athletes[10] (Fig. 20.3).

Patellar tendinitis is most often a result of engaging in running or jumping sports (e.g., soccer, basketball, and volleyball).[10] The activity, when combined with personal contact during play and hard playing surfaces, results in inflammation of the patellar tendon, which the patient experiences as a tenderness over the tendon.

Swimmer's shoulder is a tendinitis that affects young competitive swimmers.[10] This inflammation of the rotator cuff produces imbalances in flexibility and strength and limited mobility.

TREATMENT OF TENDON INJURIES

For treatment of tendon injuries, see "Treatment of Injuries to Muscles, Ligaments, and Tendons." In particular, note "Tendon Injuries" under "Cryotherapy."

STRAINS AND SPRAINS

A strain is a "blunt injury resulting from overextension of the articular capsular ligamentous apparatus of a joint."[12] Single, violent forces cause acute strains, while overuse and fatigue produce chronic strain.[13] A first-degree strain (little damage to muscle fibers and an intact muscle sheath) produces pain, mild spasm, tenderness, and edema, with mild compromise of function (Fig. 20.4). A second-degree strain exhibits many torn muscle fibers, with an intact muscle sheath, which produces bleeding, pain, and functional disability. Heavy bleeding, disabling pain, and muscle spasms

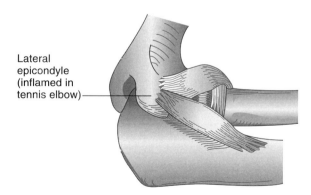

Figure 20.3. The lateral epicondyle of the elbow is a common site for tendinitis of the elbow.

A Pharmacist's Journal

"Where's Your Medicine for Muscle Cramps?"

A patient in his 60s asked me where medication for his muscle cramps was located. I asked what type of cramp and how long they had been present. He stated that his leg, arm, and hand had been cramping for several weeks. He said, "I may need potassium. Where's the potassium?" I tried to let him know that nonprescription potassium supplements are dangerous and asked what medications he was taking. He became evasive, and said, "I can't remember, but I got some of them here. They should be on your computer." A look at the computer profile showed prescriptions for glipizide and glyburide, both over 1 year old. I questioned him about them, and he reluctantly said he receives them through mail-order. I asked what else he gets through mail-order, and he said, "They give me Prinivil, Lasix, Lanoxin, glipizide, and glyburide. My doctor told me to take K-Dur, but I stopped taking it." I explained that his cramps may be caused by low potassium for which he must not take any type of nonprescription product. I urged him to see his physician to have a potassium level drawn instead. (I can only hope that he appreciated the fact that a local pharmacist was willing to provide a free consultation for products bought elsewhere. One wonders whether the pharmacists at the mail-order facility would be as willing to counsel on medications bought at the patient's neighborhood pharmacy.)

characterize the third-degree sprain, in which many muscle fibers have been crushed, and the muscle sheath is partially torn.

Sprains occur when the patient's ligaments have been overstretched by direct or indirect joint trauma.[13] Common features include varying degrees of pain, tenderness, edema, and restricted functional capability. The first-degree acute sprain shows few damaged fibers and no muscle disability, while the second-degree sprain exhibits muscle disability, edema, pain, and hemorrhage. The third-degree sprain is characterized by complete tears, with severe pain, rapid bruising, muscle instability, and sudden and complete loss of muscle function.[13] Symptoms of sprain include reddening, rise in temperature, restriction of movement, inflammation, and hematoma.[12]

Shoulder sprains, often the result of falling or hitting a wall, are common with racquet sports such as racquetball and squash.[10]

For treatment of strains and sprains, see "Treatment of Injuries to Muscles, Ligaments, and Tendons." In particular, note "Strains and Sprains" under "Cryotherapy" and "Strains and Sprains" under "Thermotherapy."

REPETITIVE STRAIN INJURY

This problem is also referred to as cumulative trauma disorder, repetitive motion disorder, or overuse syndrome.[14] Repetitive strain injury occurs when an individual subjects the same part of the body to repetitive motions, perhaps during work-related or sports-related activities that require

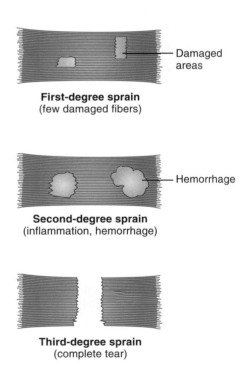

Figure 20.4. Ligament with different degrees of damage. The first-degree sprain has few damaged fibers, the second-degree sprain produces inflammation and hemorrhage, and the third-degree sprain is a complete ligamental tear.

highly stereotyped movements and static postures (e.g., musicians, packers, butchers, postal workers, assembly workers, small parts assemblers and, of course, computer users).[15,16] According to the National Institute for Occupational Safety and Health, this problem could occur in 15 to 20% of the work force in the United States because of the nature of their jobs.[14]

Abnormal postures are thought to contribute to cumulative trauma disorder.[15] They lead to overuse of certain muscle groups, with a resultant underuse and weakness of the opposing musculature. Certain extremity positions also produce nerve compression.

An example of repetitive strain injury familiar to college students is writer's cramp caused by writing for long periods without adequate rest.[15] The upper extremities and hands are also subjected to these strains when engaging in data entry and word processing.[14] A well-known example of repetitive strain injury is carpal tunnel syndrome, sometimes seen in pharmacists and pharmacy technicians because of the need to remove and replace childproof caps on prescription bottles when dispensing medications. Symptoms of repetitive strain injury of the upper extremities include pain, weakness, numbness, and tingling in the shoulders, neck, and arms.[15]

For treatment of repetitive strain injuries, see "Treatment of Injuries to Muscles, Ligaments, and Tendons." In particular, note "Strains and Sprains" under "Cryotherapy" and "Strains and Sprains" under "Thermotherapy."

CONTUSIONS

Contusions (bruises) occur when a patient suffers a direct blow to the body.[13] Tissue damage manifests as edema and inflammation. Infiltration of blood produces the hematoma that the lay person recognizes as the typical bruise. The bruised area is painful, tender to touch, and stiff. The patient may not be able to continue to participate in sports, depending on the severity and site of the contusion.

For treatment of contusions, see "Treatment of Injuries to Muscles, Ligaments, and Tendons."

INJURIES TO MUSCLES, LIGAMENTS, AND TENDONS

For prevalence, epidemiology, etiology, manifestations, and prognosis of ankle injuries, see above. For information on knee injuries, see above. For information on tendon injuries, strains and sprains, repetitive strain injury, and contusions, see above.

TREATMENT OF INJURIES TO MUSCLES, LIGAMENTS, AND TENDONS

Treatment Guidelines

Acute injuries are best treated with a combination approach known as PRICE (protection, rest, ice, compression, and elevation) or RICE (rest, ice, compression, and elevation). Cryotherapy, whether in the form of ice or other cold modalities, has beneficial effects when applied soon after the in-

jury. After 48 to 72 hours, the injury is rehabilitated by continuing the above modalities (e.g., PRICE), except some form of thermotherapy should be substituted for the cryotherapy devices. Further, gradual institution of monitored exercise will help preserve the functional capacity of the affected area. A group of products known as external analgesics may also provide relief, especially during the subacute phase. Oral analgesics may also be beneficial. (See Patient Assessment Algorithm 20.1.)

Nonprescription Medications

EXTERNAL ANALGESICS

External analgesics are defined as topically applied substances that exert topical analgesic, anesthetic, antipruritic, or counterirritant effects.[17] Topical analgesics relieve pain without causing numbness by raising the threshold for the pain response at subcutaneous terminal nerve endings. Topical anesthetics completely block pain receptors to numb the area, so that responses to painful stimuli are abolished while the product is active. Antipruritics simply relieve itching. Counterirritants cause irritation or mild inflammation of the skin to relieve pain in muscles, joints, or viscera beneath the site of application.[17] This chapter is mainly concerned with the counterirritant group of external analgesics, since they are the agents used for strains, sprains, and related complaints.[17]

Usefulness of Counterirritants

While counterirritants are applied topically to intact skin to relieve pain similar to the other external analgesics, their method of producing analgesia is radically different. The other analgesics act by depressing cutaneous sensory receptors, but counterirritants act by stimulating these receptors in skin, affecting deeper structures of the body. Counterirritants produce reversible, transient inflammation or irritation of the skin. While their mechanism is still obscure, experts theorize that the sensation they produce at the skin surface (e.g., itching, burning, warmth, or cooling) masks the pain that is occurring more deeply in the body. Thus counterirritants do not produce a cure, but simply make underlying pain more bearable. Their action is comparable with other physical coping methods such as scratching an itch, applying a heat lamp, or rubbing a bumped elbow.

The specific labeled indications of counterirritants are, "For the temporary relief of minor aches and pains of muscles and joints such as simple backache, lumbago, arthritis, neuralgia, strains, bruises, and sprains."[17]

Categories of Counterirritants

Counterirritants are not a discrete group of chemicals.[17] Rather, chemicals that produce counterirritation are a diverse group of substances, mostly of plant origin. The actions of counterirritants depend on several factors such as concentration, solvent, period of contact, and amount of friction used in application.

Some counterirritants are known as **rubefacients** (chemicals that in a certain concentration redden the skin to pro-

Patient Assessment Algorithm 20.1. Suspected Injury to Muscle, Ligament, or Tendon

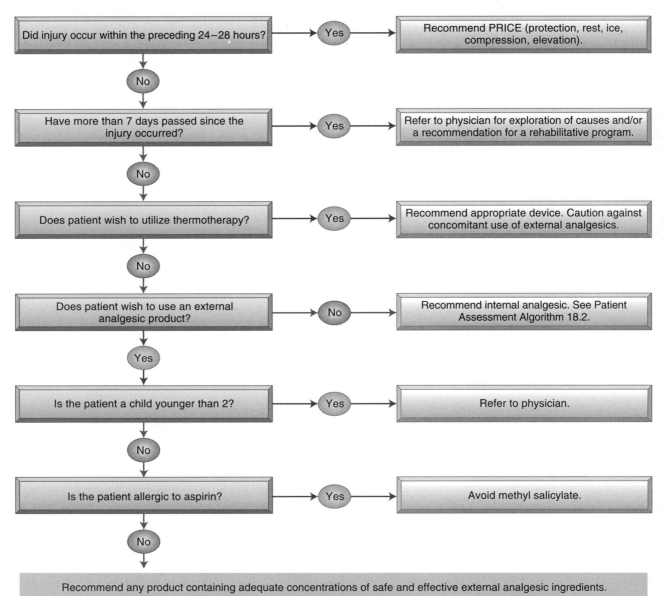

Recommend any product containing adequate concentrations of safe and effective external analgesic ingredients.

duce a feeling of warmth, but do not cause inflammation). However, at higher concentrations, rubefacients may induce inflammation and have a vesicant action. ***Inflammation is not desirable with these products since it produces blistering.*** At lower concentrations some of the ingredients might even produce a feeling of coolness (e.g., menthol, camphor).

The FDA has categorized counterirritants into four distinct groups[18]:

1. Irritants that produce redness: allyl isothiocyanate, strong ammonia solution, methyl salicylate, and turpentine oil
2. Irritants that produce a cooling sensation: camphor and menthol
3. Irritants that produce vasodilation: histamine and methyl nicotinate

4. Irritants that do not produce redness: capsicum and capsaicin

Cautions in Self-Use of Counterirritants

Some people react badly to counterirritants, developing rash and blisters with even modest amounts. For this reason counterirritants are all labeled: *"If condition worsens, or if symptoms persist for more than 7 days or clear up and occur again within a few days, discontinue use of this product and consult a physician."*[18] Other guidelines for safely using counterirritants include the following[17]:

*   Do not apply to wounds or damaged skin.
*   Do not bandage.
*   Do not use in the eyes.
*   The products are for external use only.

- The products are not to be used in children below the age of 2 years.
- The products are not to be used more than three to four times daily.

While it is not part of the FDA-required official labeling, the pharmacist must caution patients who purchase counterirritants not to use heating pads or any other thermotherapy device concurrently (see "Precautions and Contraindications to Thermotherapy"). ***The severe burns that this dangerous combination produces can be disfiguring.***

Specific Counterirritants

Allyl Isothiocyanate. This ingredient is also known as volatile oil of mustard. First used as poultices of powdered mustard seed and as plasters, it is considered to be safe in concentrations of 0.5 to 5%. *Patients should be cautioned against homemade compresses using mustard seeds.* In one case a 34-year-old woman used such a product on her back and experienced severe burning that healed slowly over several days.[19] The incident also produced a sensitivity reaction to orally ingested mustard.

Stronger Ammonia Water. Seldom found in nonprescription products, this ingredient is approved for use in concentrations of 1 to 2.5%, applied not more than three to four times daily.

Camphor. Camphor, a common ingredient in counterirritants, was found to be safe in concentrations of 3 to 11% in the original 1979 panel document.[17] Shortly thereafter, however, another FDA panel concluded that any camphor product containing more than 2.5% camphor should be placed in Category II because of toxicity.[17,20] Further, the FDA acted to remove camphorated oil from the nonprescription market because of numerous incidents of poisoning following its misidentification as castor oil.[20–22] (*Pharmacists who discover old bottles of this product, also known as cam-*

phor liniment, should immediately discard them.) Despite this controversy, the FDA panel responsible for external analgesics chose to allow camphor products in excess of 2.5% to remain on the market, with the justification that there are few adverse-reaction reports from ingestion of solid dosage forms of camphor.[20] Somewhat later, another publication limited camphor products to concentrations of 11% or lower.[18]

The FDA strongly recommended that manufacturers adopt child-proof packaging to prevent ingestion, and further urged that the caution, "For external use only" be in larger size print and/or different color print. Unfortunately, this latter approach may not halt the ingestions such as those of ointments by children too young to read.[23]

Capsicum Preparations. Capsicum is the fruit of African chile, Tabasco pepper, or several other peppers.[17] Its active ingredient is capsaicin, which produces erythema and burning without blistering the skin. It was found safe for use in concentrations yielding the equivalent of 0.025 to 0.25% capsaicin (Table 20.1). Capsaicin has recently been recommended for postherpetic neuralgia (PHN), a painful condition that persists beyond an attack of shingles, and is reported to be the leading cause of suicide in chronic pain sufferers over the age of 70.[24] It may reduce pain of PHN through depleting substance P, a chemical that allows transmission of pain impulses. Patients contemplating use of capsaicin for PHN should first consult with a physician and must not apply the products until lesions are completely healed.

Histamine. Histamine dilates blood vessels in concentrations of 0.025 to 0.1%. It is seldom included in nonprescription external analgesic products.

Menthol. Menthol produces coolness when initially applied to the skin, but shortly after begins to produce warmth. In concentrations of 1% or less menthol is a cutaneous sen-

A Pharmacist's Journal

"How Much Soltice Can I Eat?"

A former student who had taken a job with a chain in West Virginia returned to interview students. He visited me in my office and related this story: "I was probably like most students in your class. I listened to your practice experiences and thought, 'That stuff doesn't really happen!' Well, I found out the truth when I began to work. The things that happened to me are as bad and worse than your stories. Just the other day a man came in the store and said, 'How much Soltice can I eat?' I remembered that you spoke about the dangers of camphor ingestion and that Soltice has 5% camphor. I asked, 'Why do you eat Soltice?' He replied, 'It keeps my nasal congestion away.' I asked him how much he was eating, and he replied, 'I eat a jar of it every 2 days.' Needless to say, I was careful to tell him that it could kill him, but he didn't seem to think it was any big deal."

Table 20.1. Representative Single-Entity External Analgesic Products Containing Capsaicin

PRODUCT	SELECTED INGREDIENTS
Capzasin-P	Capsaicin 0.025% (cream and lotion)
Capzasin•HP Cream	Capsaicin 0.075%
Zostrix Cream	Capsaicin 0.025%
Zostrix-HP Cream	Capsaicin 0.075%

sory depressant, producing topical analgesia. However, in concentrations of 1.25% up to the maximum allowed concentration of 16%, menthol is a stimulant counterirritant (Table 20.2). When applied topically, it causes sensitization, producing symptoms of urticaria, erythema, and additional cutaneous lesions. ***Should excess menthol be ingested, the patient experiences nausea, abdominal pain, vomiting, and symptoms of central-nervous-system depression (e.g., dizziness, staggering gait, flushed face, sleepiness, slow respirations, coma).***[20]

Methyl Nicotinate. Seldom found in counterirritants, methyl nicotinate produces direct vasodilation. ***If methyl nicotinate is applied to large areas of the body, it could produce generalized vascular dilation, manifested by fall in blood pressure, change in pulse rate, and syncope.***[17] It is applied in concentrations limited to 0.25 to 1%.

Methyl Salicylate. This ingredient may also be referred to as wintergreen oil or teaberry oil.[17] Its use as a pleasant flavor/aroma for candy and other foods can lead to ingestion of toxic quantities by children. ***As little as 4 mL of wintergreen oil is fatal for children.*** Methyl salicylate produces toxicity typical of other salicylates, although metabolic acidosis may be more common with it than with the other salicylates.[17] *Pharmacists selling small bottles of wintergreen oil must caution parents or caregivers to dispose of any remaining amounts after cooking or food preparation to prevent a toxic ingestion.* The author advises against dumpster disposal, advocating the method of pouring any remaining chemical onto soil in a backyard. Wintergreen does not present any environmental toxicity, so this method of disposal is acceptable (as opposed to the disposal of gasoline, used oil, etc.).

Use of methyl salicylate as an internal home remedy for various stomach complaints is potentially deadly. In one such case a 46-year-old man ingested 30 mL of wintergreen oil to suppress persistent hiccups.[25] He entered the emergency department with confusion, agitation, and acidosis. His salicylate level of 102 mg/dL far exceeded the level considered toxic (above 40 mg/dL). Despite aggressive care, he expired 17 hours after ingestion.

Aside from the toxicity of methyl salicylate at high doses,

Table 20.2. Representative Single-Entity External Analgesic Products Containing Menthol

PRODUCT	SELECTED INGREDIENTS
Absorbine jr Liniment	Menthol 1.27%
Mineral Ice Gel	Menthol 2%

the products are widely used and usually safe. Toxic ingestions of ointments and other topicals containing methyl salicylate are rare, although they occasionally cause local irritation. Products containing 10 to 60% may be used safely by the patient. Few products contain methyl salicylate as a single active ingredient. One, however, is Theragesic Cream, which contains 15% methyl salicylate.

Patients allergic to aspirin may be allergic to methyl salicylate and should avoid it.[26] Although the potential for cross-reactivity is rare, there are other products that can be recommended that are free of methyl salicylate.

Turpentine Oil. While the ingredient is potentially toxic, no fatalities have been reported from topical medications.[17] Turpentine oil is, however, a primary skin irritant and a sensitizer. The irritant effect stems from defatting of the skin, which produces dryness and fissuring. Painters and those in similar occupations experience hand eczema as a result of cleaning paintbrushes in the chemical.

In its role as a sensitizer, turpentine oil produces cross-sensitivity with ragweed, chrysanthemum, and pyrethrum. In one case a man known to be allergic to turpentine applied Sloan's Liniment (a product still available that contained turpentine at that time).[27] Within 24 hours he developed an acute, weeping, eczematous reaction with eventual purpuric annular lesions. A diagnosis of erythema multiforme was made.

Turpentine oil is used in concentrations of 6 to 50% in nonprescription products.

Combinations. The FDA allows combinations of external analgesics, as shown in Table 20.3. However, only one ingredient from the four categories mentioned earlier (products that produce redness, coolants, vasodilators, and irritants

Table 20.3. Representative Combination External Analgesic Products

PRODUCT	SELECTED INGREDIENTS/COMMENTS
Absorbine Arthritis Strength Liquid	Menthol 4%, capsaicin 0.025%
Arthritis Hot Cream	Methyl salicylate 15%, menthol 10%
ArthriCare Rub	Menthol 1.25%, methyl nicotinate 0.25%, capsaicin 0.025%, aloe vera gel
ArthriCare Ultra	Menthol 2%, capsaicin 0.075%
Ben Gay Cream	Methyl salicylate 15%, menthol 10%
Ben Gay Gel	Menthol 2.5%, camphor (no concentration provided, listed as an active ingredient)
Ben Gay Ointment	Methyl salicyate 18.3%, menthol 16%
Ben Gay Ultra Strength Cream	Methyl salicylate 30%, menthol 10%, camphor 4%
Flex-all 454 Gel	Menthol 7%, methyl salicylate (no concentration provided, listed under "Also Contains"), aloe vera gel
Hospital Strength Banalg Lotion	Methyl salicylate 14%, menthol 3%
Icy Hot Ointment	Methyl salicylate 29%, menthol 7.6%
Menthacin	Menthol 4%, capsaicin 0.025%
Mentholatum Deep Heating Lotion Extra Strength	Methyl salicylate 20%, menthol 6%
Mentholatum Ointment	Menthol 1.3%, camphor 9%
Mentholatum Deep Heating Rub	Methyl salicylate 30%, menthol 8%
Soltice Rub	Menthol 5.1%, camphor 5.1% (methyl salicylate and eucalyptus oil, but no concentrations provided; listed as "Other Ingredients")

that do not produce redness) may be included in each product. Thus an approved combination product might contain *(tip)* methyl salicylate, menthol, histamine, and capsaicin. *It is irrational to combine a counterirritant with a topical analgesic, anesthetic, or antipruritic since these would numb the skin, nullifying the effect of the counterirritant.*

Unapproved Ingredients

Two ingredients widely found in counterirritants have not yet gained FDA approval:

- Eucalyptus oil
- Trolamine

Eucalyptus oil, while traditionally used in concentrations of 0.5 to 3%, has not yet been found to have effectiveness as a counterirritant.

Trolamine (triethanolamine salicylate) has been advertised with the unique claim that it is absorbed into the skin, passing directly into affected deeper structures. However, the FDA has not yet been furnished with proof of this claim.[17,20] The ingredient also does not function as a typical counterirritant. At this time there is no justification for recommending it. One firm marketing a trolamine salicylate product (Aspercreme) was barred by the Federal Trade Commission from claiming effectiveness for arthritis without

support from scientific studies.[28] The firm was also forbidden to use the brand name unless labels clearly indicated that the product did not contain aspirin. The company declined to comply, choosing to appeal. Representative products containing trolamine are listed in Table 20.4.

INTERNAL ANALGESICS

Internal analgesics are safe and effective for providing temporary relief of minor aches and pains associated with muscular aches and the minor pain of arthritis. For a full discussion of these agents, see Chapter 18, Headache and Other Minor Pains.

Nonpharmacologic Therapies

CRYOTHERAPY

Cold is widely advocated as a critical component of the immediate care of sprains, strains, fractures, and other inflammatory conditions.[29–33] As such, it is referred to as "the treatment of *(tip)* choice for all acute musculoskeletal injuries."[34] *Used during the first 24 to 48 hours of acute injury, cryotherapy decreases inflammation within injured ligaments through inhibiting histamine, neutrophil activation, collagenase activity, and synovial leukocytes.*[29,35] Limiting inflammation in this manner speeds the return to normal func-

Table 20.4. Representative External Analgesics Containing Trolamine

PRODUCT	SELECTED INGREDIENTS/COMMENTS
Aspercreme Lotion, Cream	Trolamine 10% (trade-named "Salycin," but not approved), aloe vera gel
Myoflex Cream	Trolamine 10% (not approved)
Sportscreme Lotion	Trolamine 10% (trade-named "Salycin," but not approved)

tion.[34] Cryotherapy also limits secondary tissue damage that might result from hypoxia by lowering tissue metabolism.[29] Thus marginally viable cells may survive the injury, whereas they would not without cryotherapy.[34]

When used for acute injuries, cold is combined with compression, rest, and elevation in an attempt to limit inflammation.[29] If inflammation is not a concern, compression is unnecessary.

Effects of Cryotherapy

Cryotherapy, or local cooling, results in vasoconstriction, which decreases the temperature of the skin and underlying subcutaneous tissues.[5,29] Variables that affect the extent of cooling include the following[29,30]:

- Modality employed (e.g., ice pack versus cryogel)
- Lengths of exposure
- Temperature of the modality used

The temperature of muscular tissue falls somewhat but less than the temperature of the more superficial layers of skin above the muscles. Because of the insulation provided by the upper layers, any temperature decrease in the muscles lasts longer than that in upper layers.[29] Cold applications also decrease temperature within the joints.[36]

Cryotherapy reduces edema caused by acute injury, especially when used in conjunction with compression.[30] Application of a cold gel pack can decrease resting ankle volume significantly.[5,10]

Cryotherapy vasoconstricts regional vessels, which reduces the extent of hematoma following injury.[29,30] However, because of the body's compensatory mechanisms, cold interrupts vascular sympathetic nerve conduction, which produces vasodilation, resulting in a paradoxical rewarming, a phenomenon known as the hunting reaction.[30] Thus during cryotherapy vessels alternate between vasodilation and vasoconstriction.

Cryotherapy decreases muscular spindle activity, which reduces muscle spasticity. Cryotherapy also reduces postinjury pain, perhaps by decreasing or blocking conduction velocity in peripheral nerves by interrupting a "pain → spasm → pain" cycle.[5,29] During cryotherapy application, the patient reports an uncomfortable cold feeling, followed by burning, aching, and numbness.[29]

Cryotherapy's effects in reducing circulatory flow, bleeding, edema, and tissue damage minimize the requirement for removal of debris (e.g., phagocytosis, waste product buildup) during the healing process.[37]

Applications of Cryotherapy

(tip) *Ankle Injuries. While the pharmacist should refer ankle injuries to a physician for initial evaluation, he or she should also recommend that the patient institute immediate (up to 48 hours after injury) cryotherapy until the appointment time.*[5,38]

Most ankle sprains are treated with functional management, also known as early controlled movement.[3,4] The goal of this therapy is to allow ankle utilization in a protected manner as permitted by the severity of injury, which speeds the rate and quality of ligament healing. Cryotherapy is combined with rest, compression, and elevation to control pain and edema, thereby aiding in weightbearing. A typical regimen is one to two daily applications, each lasting 20 to 30 minutes, or four treatments of 10 to 15 minutes each.[4,8] Application is coupled with elevation, which aids in controlling (tip) postinjury edema.[5] *If a bag of ice is used, the patient may add some water to optimize its conformance to the shape of the ankle.*[39]

Knee Injuries. Cryotherapy is a component of therapy for patellar pain syndrome and anterior-cruciate ligament injury.[10] Others recommend cryotherapy for patellar tendinitis at the conclusion of an activity that might aggravate the condition.[40]

Tendon Injuries. Cryotherapy affects superficial tendons and is helpful during the immobilization phase of tendon injuries.[41,42] When a resting splint is indicated, cryotherapy acts to reduce pain and inflammation. Tennis elbow is helped by flexible gel packs that may be wrapped around the elbow.[43] Shin splints also respond to cryotherapy treatments of 10 to 15 minutes two to three times daily.[44]

Strains and Sprains. Cryotherapy is also useful for all degrees of strains and sprains, as described above. Cryotherapy benefits sports-related shoulder sprains and is helpful in treating chronic muscle strain that is a result of overuse.[4,13,16]

Cryotherapy also controls bleeding from contusions that did not cause an overt sprain.[13] Used immediately, it limits the size of the hematoma by reducing the amount of blood that infiltrates into the tissues. The cryotherapy should be continued for 10 minutes for minor contusions that do not limit the function of the area.

Rehabilitation. Rehabilitation encompasses all postinjury procedures that are instituted to allow maximal function.[29,45]

Its objective is to minimize risk of reinjury while instituting exercises that allow a return to preinjury status.[45] Cryotherapy aids rehabilitation by allowing immediate mobilization and facilitating therapeutic exercise.[5,30] In ankle injuries, for instance, a three-phase rehabilitation program may be followed:

- Phase I consists of PRICE (protection, rest, ice, compression, elevation). In this phase cryotherapy is applied three times daily to decrease the degree of edema.
- Phase II incorporates stretching exercises.
- Phase III includes conditioning with proprioception boards.

Cryotherapy is used during the latter phases to limit pain and inflammation.[3,5]

Arthritis. Cryotherapy is generally considered to help arthritic joints. In one study, local cooling was beneficial in reducing the temperature in the knee joint cavity of healthy subjects and was recommended by the authors for inflammatory joint disease.[46] (See Chapter 18.)

Methods of Applying Cryotherapy

Cryotherapy includes methods not available for pharmacists to recommend such as cold whirlpools and ice massage.[35] Patients at home may opt to apply ice in chipped, flaked, cubed, or crushed form to the injury. A pack of frozen peas or beans in a plastic bag will also cool tissue.[2] Pharmacists may select among such cryotherapy devices as ice packs, single-use chemical packs, and flexible cryogel packs.[5,29]

Gel packs produce maximal vasoconstriction within 13 to 14 minutes after application.[8] Placed in the nonfreezer section of the refrigerator, they retain their flexibility and are easily fitted to different anatomical areas.[13]

Single-use packs contain two chemicals in a dual-compartment, flexible, plastic container. When the container is squeezed, the inner membrane ruptures, allowing the two chemicals to mix in an endothermic reaction.[30] Because they can only be used once, chemical packs are relatively more expensive than cryogel packs, but they can be a useful addition to a first aid kit for use when a refrigerator is not available (e.g., hiking, an overnight camping trip). Their cooling power is not as good as other modalities.[13]

tip The pharmacist might advise that *a wet towel or cloth placed between the skin and the cryotherapy device can facilitate transfer of cold to the skin and lengthen the time of application by reducing patient discomfort* (Fig. 20.5).[29] In addition, a towel placed between the cryotherapy device and the skin helps avoid nerve damage and frostbite.[34]

Precautions and Contraindications to Cryotherapy

Cold must not be applied so long that it causes tissue damage. **tip** *A rule of thumb is to remove the cryotherapy device when the skin feels numb or when 20 minutes have passed, whichever is shorter.*[34] After 20 minutes, the dose-response curve flattens, so that there is little added benefit, but the risks of tissue freezing increase.

Cryotherapy must be avoided in patients with Raynaud's disease, since these patients already suffer from restricted

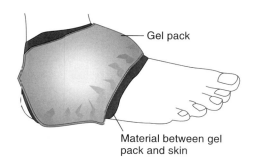

Gel pack should be cooled in lower refrigerator, not in freezer.

Figure 20.5. A cryotherapy device (a gel pack) properly placed on an ankle, with a cloth material between the gel pack and the skin.

blood flow.[47] It also must not be applied to the patient with cold-induced allergy.[13,30]

tip *Cryogel packs must be cooled in the lower refrigerator.*[29] If they are frozen, their application to the skin can cause frostbite and deeper injury. A 47-year-old male placed a frozen, reusable, cold compress on the thigh.[48] He sat on the product on and off for a total 25-minute application time. When seen, he had sustained a frostbite injury with erythema, hyperpigmentation, and bulla formation that required over a month to heal. The authors of the report also reported that the patient secured the compress to the skin with an elastic bandage and cautioned against applying such a product with firm pressure.

Cryotherapy must be applied cautiously to superficial nerves.[29] Unless the devices are well padded, they may cause nerve palsy when applied over superficial nerves. One report listed several cases where college athletes were given cryotherapy ranging from 15 minutes to 2 hours.[49] Nerve damage consisted of motor and sensory deficit and lasted from 1 hour to 6 months. The authors concluded that cryotherapy on areas with little subcutaneous fat (e.g., knee, dorsum of the foot, shoulder) does not allow fat insulation of nerves and increases the risk of nerve injury. They suggested that cryotherapy be limited to 20 minutes' duration to reduce risk of cryogenic injury.

Cryotherapy reduces the flexibility of muscles and tendons, making it of little use in warming activities carried out before activity.[30,37] Since the inflexible collagen is also anesthetized, the risk of injury is enhanced.

THERMOTHERAPY

Local heat, known as thermotherapy, is not useful during an acute injury, but is invaluable during the follow-up care of injuries to muscles, ligaments, and tendons.

- **tip** Heat During Acute Injury. *Local heat increases inflammation and worsens tissue hypoxia, and this is contraindicated during the acute phase of injury.*[29] The application of heat should be postponed until all signs and symptoms of inflammation have fully abated.[34] According to some authors, heat also increases pain associated with an acute injury by allowing increased blood flow to place pressure on free nerve endings.[29] Other authors, however, allege that heat decreases pain by increasing the pain threshold.[50] This difference of opinion highlights the subjective nature of pain.

- Heat During the Subacute Phase of Injury. Heat has value during subacute stages of inflammation by neutralizing noxious stimuli and increasing removal of cellular waste products and debris (e.g., metabolites and lactic acid).[29] Local heat also reduces pain, soreness, and stiffness in the subacute phase. Heat and cold may be alternated during rehabilitation by using a 4-minute heat cycle and a 2-minute cold cycle, repeating both treatments three times.[51] Combined with stretching techniques, heat prepares injured ligaments for range-of-motion exercises by allowing the tissue to stretch more easily.[41]

Effects of Thermotherapy

Thermotherapy exerts optimal effects when tissue temperatures reach 104 to 113.9°F. *The optimal exposure time is 3 to 30 minutes, but some authorities suggest a maximal exposure time of 20 minutes.*[34] These parameters are critical; excessive heat is dangerous, producing severe burns in patients who do not follow guidelines for its safe use.[35] Burns begin at 114.8°F, depending on the duration of exposure.

Thermotherapy and Blood Flow. Thermotherapy increases temperature in the skin and subcutaneous tissues. The initial steady temperature increase slows as regional vasodilation acts to diffuse the heat.[29,37] This vasodilation-induced heat redistribution is vital in preventing tissue damage caused by burns. The skin becomes reddened as vasodilation proceeds. Blood flow through skeletal muscle is only minimally affected by heat unless the individual also exercises. In this case thermotherapy augments the effect of exercise to prolong the improved muscular perfusion.[29]

Thermotherapy and Inflammation. Thermotherapy also releases chemicals that cause inflammation such as histamine and prostaglandins.[29] Thus an acute inflammation results, which in turn causes vasodilation. The vasodilation increases edema and hemorrhage, thereby increasing the extent of injury and time required to regain normal function. ***Thermotherapy applied to an acute injury worsens inflammation and extends the time of return to normal function.***

Thermotherapy and Tissue Metabolism. Thermotherapy increases regional tissue metabolism. The tissues demand increased oxygen and nutrients, which enhances the risk of secondary postinjury tissue hypoxia in healthy tissues.

Thermotherapy and Collagen. Thermotherapy makes muscles and tendons more flexible by allowing collagen to become more elastic, thereby relieving stiffness in the joints.[29,35,37] Simultaneous strengthening exercises maximize the potential benefit of enhanced elasticity.[29,50] Heat acts optimally when applied to superficial joints (e.g., the knee or ankle), which have minimal overlying soft tissue.[29] Rheuma-

toid arthritis, which results in impaired joint mobility, is helped by heat. The mechanism of thermotherapy in relieving joint stiffness may be that it allows greater stretch of the joint capsule.[50] Preheating the elbow 5 minutes before playing can reduce the discomfort of tennis elbow.[52]

Strains and Sprains. Heat is recommended for various strains and sprains, as well as tendinitis.[53,54] For instance, it is helpful in the subacute phase of calf strain.[55] Heat is also recommended for painful neck and shin splints.[44,56]

Methods of Applying Thermotherapy

While many methods are available for producing heat, they differ mainly in the depth to which they penetrate.[29] Ultrasound is a deep heating modality that causes heat to penetrate for up to 5 cm. Other physician-recommended modalities include hydrotherapy, contrast baths, hydrocollator packs, radiant heat, and the paraffin wax bath.[35] The pharmacist is limited to recommending superficial heating treatments, which only penetrate for 1 to 5 mm.[35]

Hot Water Bottles. These rubber items are inexpensive and simple to use, but their temperature cannot be regulated once they are filled with water of a certain temperature.[35,57] As they cool, they must be reheated by adding warmer water.

Heating Pads. Heating pads operate through the principle of electrical resistance.[58] When attached to electrical current, they allow electricity to flow through a set of resistance wires embedded in insulating material inside the pad. The natural resistance of the wire to electrical passage produces heat as a by-product, delivering a constant supply of regulated heat.[35] The devices are controlled by a thermostat, which controls the wattage.[58] *Heating pads must always be used with the covers in place.*

Clay/Gel Packs. Consumers may purchase various nonelectrical alternatives to heating pads. Some require microwave heating to warm a clay or gel substance, after which the patient places a cover over the pack and uses it as a heating pad. Others require heating with the use of boiling water, which presents the hazard of potential burns.

Exothermic Chemicals. Another type of thermotherapy device consists of a fluid-filled, flexible, plastic bag containing a chemical solution and a small metal button. Clicking the metal button triggers a cascade of chemical precipitation that causes an exothermic reaction. The patient readies the device for reuse by boiling or microwave heating to redissolve the crystals and then allows it to cool to room temperature.

Precautions and Contraindications to Thermotherapy

The heating pad—common in most homes, as well as in institutional and clinical settings—is generally considered to be a safe method of producing local heat.[59] A survey of nursing home patients revealed that 15% had a heating pad in their room.[60] Unfortunately, widespread misconceptions about their safety combined with their ubiquitous distribution mean that the average patient has ready access to heating pads and often does not take precautions to prevent heat damage to skin.[59]

(tip) *Heat increases active bleeding and should not be placed on a hemorrhaging area or fresh hematoma such as a contusion.*[29,35,47] Heat is contraindicated in malignancies as it may increase the rate and/or extent of metastasis and may enhance the rate of cell growth.[29,30] Application to patients with fever is avoided since any additional rise in core temperature may overstress the cardiopulmonary system.

(tip) *Heat should not be applied to insensitive skin, since the patient cannot gauge the extent of heat, therefore promoting the risk of burns.*[35] In one case a 35-year-old quadriplegic with a demyelinating disorder used a heating pad over the left shoulder and upper arm for a short period to treat pain.[61] He developed a third-degree burn. Another patient suffered burns when she applied a heating pad to a post–breast reconstruction site that was partially anesthetized.[62] A spina bifida patient with reduced foot sensation used a heating pad for 20 minutes on the medium setting, resulting in burns requiring debridement and grafting.[58] One lesion only healed after 10 months of intensive care.

Patients with diabetes mellitus have insensitive skin because of peripheral neuropathy.[63] The feet also feel cold because of impaired circulation, prompting some diabetics to resort to foot-warming techniques such as application of local heat. **⚠ *Thermotherapy devices and even hot water can cause burns in the diabetic.*** The diabetic has an impaired healing ability, requiring a great deal more care for a burn than the nondiabetic. Amputation may result. A 39-year-old male with Type I diabetes rested his foot on top of a heating pad for one night.[58] He suffered a full-thickness burn that required excision and grafting, further debridement, and several additional attempts to graft tissue to the wound.

Skin that is poorly perfused or ischemic may not be able to redistribute the heat through blood flow, also promoting the risk of burn injury.[29] Inadequate arterial flow is also seen in pressure sores, which may be worsened by local heat application.[37]

Heat increases metabolism, and thereby also increases the accumulation rate of metabolic wastes.[37] In patients recovering from crushing amputation or replantation, local heat could be dangerous if venous or lymphatic drainage were to be impaired.

(tip) *Heat should be used cautiously in patients with rheumatoid osteoarthritis.*[36,46] The activity of enzymes that produce damage to cartilage is increased as temperature in the joint is increased. Therefore, application of heat to arthritic joints could worsen debility. **(tip)** *Heat should never be applied to the abdomen of pregnant patients, and it should be avoided over the eyes or the genital area of all patients.*[34]

(tip) *Patients must never lie or sit on a local heat product.* The weight of the body reduces blood flow to the area, which allows heat to build to harmful levels.[58] Two patients with anesthetic skin caused by flap muscle reconstructions slept on heating pads.[62] Both suffered burns as a result. In another case a 3-month-old child was placed on a heating pad for the duration of a surgical hernia repair.[64] He suffered third-degree burns that required grafting. This case illustrates violation of the dual warnings against pediatric use and also against lying or sitting on a heating pad.

(tip) *Patients must never go to sleep on a heating pad or be allowed to use a heating pad if not fully conscious.*[35] An elderly, institutionalized patient was left lying on a heating pad for 40 hours.[59] Although it was on the lowest setting, the patient suffered an extensive second-degree burn. This incident prompted the author of the paper to undertake a study that revealed that a heating pad on the low setting could produce a second-degree burn in 12 to 20 hours. In another case the physician for a postsurgical patient who had undergone abdominoplasty ordered a "heating pad to abdomen PRN."[65] Stainless-steel staples, which acted as heat conductors, facilitated a burn that significantly delayed healing. The damage was augmented since the patient was asleep when the pad was applied initially and had received five Demerol injections to minimize postsurgical pain.

(tip) *Heating devices must be used carefully in children.* A 3-year-old developmentally delayed child was given a microwave-heated cryogel pack to improve an extravasated IV site.[66] Because of combativeness, she was restrained, which hampered her ability to remove the device. Later checking revealed a burn that required debridement and skin grafting.

Heating devices are contraindicated with bites of the spider *Loxosceles reclusa* (fiddleback spider, brown recluse).[67] Although it may be recommended as adjunctive therapy, **(tip)** *thermotherapy increases the risk and extent of blisters, ulceration, and necrosis.* Cryotherapy, conversely, produces a more favorable outcome. This recommendation is based on anecdotal evidence rather than controlled trials; recommendations for the bites of other dermonecrotic spiders may differ; therapy for the bites of nondermonecrotic spiders is also quite variable.

(tip) *Thermotherapy devices must never be used with counterirritant external analgesic ingredients such as camphor, menthol, and methyl salicylate.* Many of these products carry a warning not to use them with heating pads, heat lamps, or other heat sources, and some heating devices carry a warning against use with external analgesics. These external analgesics increase superficial blood flow. Locally applied heat (e.g., via heating pad) cannot be redistributed via peripheral circulation and remains in the area, increasing the risk of local burns. In one such case a 62-year-old male applied an external ointment containing 18.3% methyl salicylate and 16% menthol.[68] Despite the manufacturer's warning against it, he applied a heating pad for 15 to 20 minutes. He developed necrosis that extended into the deep fascia and underlying muscles. One year of hospitalization was required, including debridement and grafting. He also experienced renal sequelae. The pharmacist selling either external analgesics or thermotherapy devices must warn the patient against concomitant use with the other product.

SUMMARY

Patients suffer many injuries of muscles, tendons, and ligaments. The majority of these are related to normal daily ac-

AT THE COUNTER

 A high-school girl's basketball team member injured her ankle the previous night when an opposing team member accidentally ran into her. The physician found no evidence of fracture and confirmed a sprain, suggesting that she rent crutches and buy an ankle brace. She also asks whether there is anything else she should be doing.

Interview/Patient Assessment

The patient is wearing a sandal and an elastic wrap, allowing the pharmacist to see that the ankle is grossly swollen and purple. She states that it is exquisitely painful, not allowing her to bear weight.

Pharmacist's Analysis

1. Should this patient be allowed to self-treat her ankle sprain?

2. What is the role of cryotherapy for this patient?
3. What is the role of thermotherapy for this patient?
4. What is the role of external analgesics for this patient?

This patient's physician diagnosis allows self-therapy for her ankle sprain.

Patient Counseling

In accord with the principles of PRICE (protection, rest, ice, compression, elevation), she should be urged to give the injured ankle protection, rest (crutches will help), compression (the wrap and ankle brace will help here), and elevation when possible. Cryotherapy should have begun immediately and must continue for at least 24 to 48 hours after the injury. At that point thermotherapy can speed recovery. External analgesics may help relieve pain, but they must not be used during the same period as thermotherapy, since concurrent use of these modalities can cause burning of the skin.

---

tivities or to sports and are minor in nature. The pharmacist often counsels patients on ankle injuries, knee injuries, tendon injuries, bursitis, repetitive strain injuries, miscellaneous strains and sprains, and contusions. The pharmacist can help the patient limit the extent of injury by judicious and rapid application of cryotherapy. Later application of thermotherapy can reduce symptoms and speed recovery. Cryotherapy and thermotherapy may also be components of a physician-directed rehabilitation program.

External and internal analgesics also play a role in pain relief. External analgesics, also known as counterirritants, work to relieve pain by inducing a feeling of warmth, cooling, or burning over the site of injury, or by directly dilating the vessels in the area to produce a regional warmth. Should the condition persist for more than 7 days, or clear up but then worsen, the patient should see a physician. However, the pharmacist must not hesitate to refer patients who are clearly beyond the scope of self-therapy to a physician for care.

References

1. Trevino SG, Davis P, Hecht PJ. Management of acute and chronic lateral ligament injuries of the ankle. Orthop Clin North Am 25:1, 1994.
2. Mascaro TB, Swanson LE. Rehabilitation of the foot and ankle. Orthop Clin North Am 25:147, 1994.
3. Hølmer P, et al. Epidemiology of sprains in the lateral ankle and foot. Foot Ankle Int 15:72, 1994.
4. Griffin LY. Common sports injuries of the foot and ankle seen in children and adolescents. Orthop Clin North Am 25:83, 1994.
5. Yeung MS, Chan K-M, So CH. An epidemiologic survey on ankle sprain. Br J Sports Med 28:112, 1994.
6. Murtagh J. Sprained ankle. Aust Fam Physician 24:434, 1995.
7. Wilkerson GB, Horn-Kingery HM. Treatment of the inver-

sion ankle sprain: Comparison of different modes of compression and cryotherapy. J Orthop Sports Phys Ther 17:240, 1993.
8. McDowell LD, Seymour SF. Diagnosis and treatment of ankle sprains. Nurse Pract 19:36, 1994.
9. Verhagen RAW, DeKeizer G, vanDijk CN. Long-term follow-up of inversion trauma of the ankle. Arch Orthop Trauma Surg 114:92, 1995.
10. Silko GJ, Cullen PT. Indoor racquet sports injuries. Am Fam Physician 50:374, 1994.
11. Hole JW Jr, Koos KA. Human Anatomy. 2nd ed. Wm. C. Brown, 1994; p. 215.
12. Frahm E, Elsasser U, Kämmereit A. Topical treatment of acute sprains. Br J Clin Pract 47:321, 1993.
13. Meeroff JC. Cryotherapy for minor athletic injuries. Hosp Pract 29:97, 1985.
14. Harris NR II, Gianacakes N. Repetitive motion disorders of the upper extremity. J Fla Med Assoc 81:831, 1994.
15. Higgs PE, Mackinnon SL. Repetitive motion injuries. Annu Rev Med 46:1, 1995.
16. Rempel DM, Harrison RJ, Barnhart S. Work-related cumulative trauma disorders of the upper extremity. JAMA 267:838, 1992.
17. Fed Reg 44:69768, 1979.
18. Fed Reg 48:5852, 1983.
19. Kohl PK, Frosch PJ. Irritant contact dermatitis induced by a mustard compress. Contact Derm 23:189, 1990.
20. Fed Reg 45:63878, 1980.
21. Fed Reg 45:63869, 1980.
22. Fed Reg 47:41716, 1982.
23. Phelan WJ III. Camphor poisoning: Over-the-counter dangers. Pediatrics 57:428, 1976.
24. Flieger K. Shingles—or chickenpox, part two. FDA Consumer 25(6):37, 1991.
25. Fleet WM III, Morgan HJ, Morello PJ. A fatal case of hiccups. J Tenn Med Assoc 83:79, 1990.
26. Generali JA. Should a patient who cannot tolerate or is

allergic to aspirin avoid using products that contain methyl salicylate? US Pharm 12(1):29, 1987.

27. Fisher AA. Erythema multiforme-like eruptions due to exotic woods and ordinary plants: Part I. Cutis 38:101, 1986.
28. Anon. The notebook. FDA Consumer 19(3):30, 1985.
29. Irrgang JJ, et al. Rehabilitation of the injured athlete. Orthop Clin North Am 26:561, 1995.
30. Grana WA. Physical agents in musculoskeletal problems: Heat and cold therapy modalities. Am Acad Orthop Surg 43:439, 1993.
31. Reider B, et al. Treatment of isolated medial collateral ligament injuries in athletes with early functional rehabilitation. Am J Sports Med 22:470, 1994.
32. McCoy RL II, Dec KL, McKeag DB. Caring for the school-aged athlete. Prim Care 21:781, 1994.
33. Risser WL. The acute management of minor soft tissue injuries. Pediatr Ann 21:170, 1992.
34. Baumert PW Jr. Acute inflammation after injury. Postgrad Med 97:35, 1995.
35. Delisa JA. Practical use of therapeutic physical modalities. Am Fam Physician 27:129, 1983.
36. Oosterveld FGJ, Rasker JJ. Effects of local heat and cold treatment on surface and articular temperature of arthritic knees. Arthritis Rheum 37:1578, 1994.
37. Nanneman D. Thermal modalities: Heat and cold. AAOHN J 39:70, 1991.
38. Litt JCB. The sprained ankle. Aust Fam Physician 21:447, 1992.
39. Hergenroeder AC. Diagnosis and treatment of ankle sprains. Am J Dis Child 144:809, 1990.
40. Mulherin WB. Treating injuries in tennis. J Med Assoc Ga 81:317, 1992.
41. Sailer SM, Lewis SB. Rehabilitation and splinting of common upper extremity injuries in athletes. Clin Sports Med 14:411, 1995.
42. Stanish WD, Curwin S, Rubinovich M. Tendinitis: The analysis and treatment for running. Clin Sports Med 4:593, 1985.
43. Chop WM Jr. Tennis elbow. Postgrad Med 86:301, 1989.
44. Moore MP. Shin splints. Postgrad Med 83:199, 1988.
45. Lephart SM, Henry TJ. Functional rehabilitation for the upper and lower extremity. Orthop Clin North Am 26:579, 1995.
46. Oosterveld FGJ, et al. The effect of local heat and cold therapy on the intraarticular and skin surface temperature of the knee. Arthritis Rheum 35:146, 1992.
47. Tepperman PS, Devlin M. The therapeutic use of local heat and cold. Can Fam Physician 32:1110, 1986.
48. Cipollaro VA. Cryogenic injury due to local application of a reusable cold compress. Cutis 50:111, 1992.
49. Bassett FH III, et al. Cryotherapy-induced nerve injury. Am J Sports Med 20:516, 1992.
50. Rivenburgh DW. Physical modalities in the treatment of tendon injuries. Clin Sports Med 11:645, 1992.
51. Seto JL, Brewster CE. Treatment approaches following foot and ankle injury. Clin Sports Med 13:695, 1994.
52. Kohn HS. Current status and treatment of tennis elbow. Wis Med J 83:18, 1984.
53. Guidotti TL. Occupational repetitive strain injury. Am Fam Physician 45:585, 1992.
54. Sayer GR, et al. The management of sprains and strains in general practice. Aust Fam Physician 23:1763, 1994.
55. Sando B. Calf strain. Aust Fam Physician 17:1060, 1988.
56. Spicer GL. Treatment of painful neck (Letter). Aust Fam Physician 19:600, 1990.
57. Tepperman PS, Devlin M. Therapeutic heat and cold. Postgrad Med 73:69, 1983.
58. Bill TJ, Edlich RF, Himel HN. Electric heating pad burns. J Emerg Med 12:819, 1994.
59. Diller KR. Analysis of burns caused by long-term exposure to a heating pad. J Burn Care Rehab 12:214, 1991.
60. Ferrell BA, Ferrell BR, Osterweil D. Pain in the nursing home. J Am Geriatr Soc 38:409, 1990.
61. Sandanam J. Burns caused by heating pads (Letter). Med J Aust 1:369, 1982.
62. Stevenson TR, et al. Heating pad burns in anesthetic skin. Ann Plast Surg 15:73, 1985.
63. Katcher ML, Shapiro MM. Lower extremity burns related to sensory loss in diabetes mellitus. J Fam Pract 24:149, 1987.
64. Anon. Infant severely burned by heating pad. Regan Report on Nursing Law 28:2, 1987.
65. Anon. "Heating pad PRN-Patient burned: Dr. accuses nurses." Regan Report on Nursing Law 33:4, 1993.
66. Dave AL. Third-degree burn following use of microwave-heated cryogel pack. Clin Pediatr 32:191, 1993.
67. King LE Jr. Brown recluse spider bites: Stay cool (Letter). JAMA 254:2895, 1985.
68. Heng MCY. Local necrosis and interstitial nephritis due to topical methyl salicylate and menthol. Cutis 39:442, 1987.

Low Back Pain

AT THE COUNTER

 A male in his mid 30s asks the pharmacist if there is something he can take for his back pain.

Interview/Patient Assessment

The pharmacist asks the patient to describe his back pain, where it is located, and when it occurs. The patient, who works in construction, relates a 3-day history of pain in the lower back. He feels better at night, but his back begins to bother him before noon and aches until soon after bedtime. He denies any use of prescription medication, denies use of alcohol or IV drugs, and denies any medical conditions or concomitant symptoms. He had no trauma. He wonders if a heating pad would be helpful.

Pharmacist's Analysis

1. Should this patient be referred to a physician?
2. Would thermotherapy delivered by a heating pad be beneficial for this patient?

3. What is the role of internal analgesics in this patient?

Patient Counseling

The patient appears to have typical, nonspecific, low back pain. He has not revealed any danger signals that warrant physician referral. Treatment may encompass one or more of several options:

- Thermotherapy, using a heating pad or other device
- **Cryotherapy** (therapy employing devices that are cold), using a cryogel pack or other device
- Internal analgesics, which can be used with physical modalities

The pharmacist should advise the patient that if the pain persists for longer than 10 days from the time of onset, he should see a physician.

Back pain may originate in any part of the spine, from the lumbosacral area up to the neck or upper back. The degree of discomfort ranges from a minor irritation to disabling pain.

Patients complaining of back pain are usually referring to low back pain, which can be generalized as acute and/or chronic pain that tends to be localized to the lumbar region (the anatomic area below the posterior ribs and above the lower margins of the buttock).[1]

Pain in the neck or upper back, a separate entity, is more often caused by some form of repetitive strain injury, as described in Chapter 20, "Injuries to Muscles, Ligaments, and Tendons."[2,3]

PREVALENCE OF LOW BACK PAIN

Overall, low back pain is the fifth most common reason that patients see physicians, with Americans spending $50 billion on this complaint yearly.[4] More patients see orthopedists and neurosurgeons for low back pain than any other condition for which those specialties are consulted.[5] As many as 1 to 2% of the population is considered totally disabled from low back pain, with another 5% partially disabled.[6,7] Low back pain, which is thought to be the first or second (behind the common cold) most frequent cause of lost work time, affects perhaps 80% of the population at some time.[7,8] An estimated 7 to 10% of patients suffer from chronic low back pain.[9]

At least 2% of employees experience a work-related back injury, resulting in 175 million occupational lost days.[7,9]

The reasons for the high incidence of back pain are nu-

merous, ranging from a general lack of fitness of the population to the stresses induced by the switch from quadrupedal to bipedal locomotion.[10] The costs of low back pain are staggering. Direct costs (diagnosing, treatment) are estimated at $24 billion yearly, and indirect costs (e.g., lost earnings) are another $35 billion per year.[11]

EPIDEMIOLOGY OF LOW BACK PAIN

Occupational Factors

Occupational factors that cause low back pain may be sudden injuries or more gradual, long-term damage. As noted above, as many as 2% of all employees injure their backs yearly.[7,9] Predisposing factors for low back pain include many occupationally related factors such as long-distance driving, prolonged standing, prolonged sitting without position changes, lifting heavy objects, performing intense physical effort on short notice, and working with vibrating tools.[6] High-risk occupations include jobs involving heavy manual labor such as construction, mining, transportation, and garbage collection; warehouse work; truck, auto, and equipment repair; nursing (particularly nurse's aides); and repetitive tasks in manufacturing.[6,7,12,13]

Age

Back pain is rare in children.[14] Peak incidence of back pain occurs in the 30 to 50 age group.[7] Back pain is the leading cause of disability in patients under 45 years of age in the United States.[15,16]

Gender

Low back pain is more common in females, partly because of the fact that 50% of pregnant females experience it.[17,18] However, males and females in industry experience back pain at the same rate.[7]

Sports

Certain sports such as gymnastics, figure skating, and dance cause a high incidence of low back pain because of the stresses they place on the back.[19] Golf can cause back problems as a result of improper swing mechanics and/or practice patterns.[20] Bicycling can cause neck and lower back pain because of the posture required to maintain balance.[21]

Physical Fitness

Patients who are not physically fit experience ten times the rate of back injuries as those who are fit.[22] Physicians hypothesize that exercises increase the strength and flexibility of the lower back.

Other Factors

Additional risk factors for low back pain include cigarette smoking, coughing, and twisting or bending, although the reasons are not always clear.[23,24] A recent poor evaluation on the job is also predictive of low back pain, attesting to the psychologic or intentionally deceptive nature of the problem.[7,25] Obesity and tall stature are associated with back pain, as are legs of differing lengths.[9,26,27] In the case of the tall person, some stoop over to ease interactions with others. Also, the tall individual has a greater spinal length and upper body weight, both of which place increased stress on the lower back.[27]

White residents of the western United States and individuals with psychological stress are all more prone to have back pain.[11] Once again, however, these epidemiological studies cannot identify causation.

ETIOLOGY OF LOW BACK PAIN

Most back pain (as much as 85 to 97%) is not the result of any demonstrable medical cause and thus is known as nonspecific back pain.[22,28] For patients with diagnosable abnormalities, low back pain is most commonly caused by malignancy and infection.[5] Less common causes include structural abnormalities (e.g., herniated disc, spinal stenosis), neurologic deficits, arthritis, minor strains, overexertion, trauma, and spondylarthropathies.[29,30]

MANIFESTATIONS OF LOW BACK PAIN

The onset of low back pain—the most common and most easily treated back pain—generally occurs between ages 30 and 50. The pain, which is described as aching, stiffness,

---

FOCUS ON...

SCIATICA

Many patients with back pain also experience sciatica, a pain in the lower back or hip that radiates down the back of the thigh to the leg.[31] Sciatica is a common problem, affecting as many as 40% of Americans at some time.[32] Sciatica may be caused by lumbar disk herniation with compression of nerve roots, but the exact causes are not known.[33]

The prognosis of sciatica is good, although a minority of patients require surgical intervention, especially when lumbar herniation is the cause.[32,34] Patients with sciatica must be referred to a physician for evaluation of possible herniation. Nonprescription products should not be recommended for this condition.

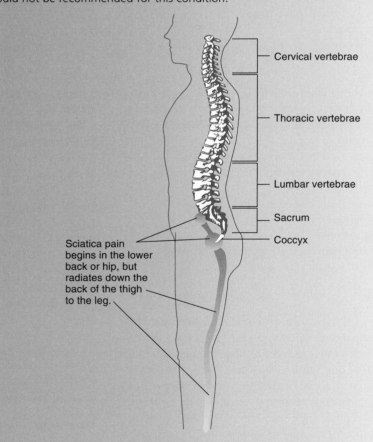

Sections of the spinal column and sites of sciatica pain.

and/or burning, begins suddenly in the case of an acute injury, but gradually increases in intensity with overuse syndromes.[9] Low back pain occurs normally in the lumbosacral region and perhaps in the buttocks and/or thighs and/or legs (sciatica) (see "Sciatica").[15,26] Pain varies with the nature and extent of physical activity and often wanes with the passage of time, particularly if treated. It eases during the night, only to worsen during the day. The patient is otherwise well.

SPECIFIC CONSIDERATIONS OF LOW BACK PAIN

Danger Signs

Pharmacists should recognize various "danger signs" that indicate a serious cause of the back pain, necessitating immediate referral to a physician.[14,29,35] These danger signs include the following:

- Age at onset of younger than 20 or older than 55 years
- Pain in the lower back or hip that radiates down the back of the thigh to the leg
- Weakness, numbness, or tingling associated with the back pain
- Bowel and/or bladder incontinence
- Gait abnormalities
- Pain associated with a traumatic event (e.g., a fall, motor vehicle accident, or contact sport injury)
- Persistent, progressive pain unrelieved by medication, rest, or immobilization
- Systemic weight loss (e.g., 10 pounds in 90 days) or systemic illness
- Fever or chills
- Back pain in young children who have previous fractures as part of the history, which is a possible sign of child abuse (see Chapter 1, The Pharmacist as Triage Expert)
- History of cancer
- Back pain worsens at night or when lying down
- Use/abuse of intravenous drugs
- Frequent ingestion of alcohol
- Chronic disease (e.g., diabetes, HIV, or hepatitis)
- Urethral discharge/burning on urination
- Immunosuppression
- High risk for fracture (e.g., advanced age or history of osteoporosis)

The Sick Role

Some patients with back pain do not understand that they should strive to maintain activity, despite the back pain. Instead, they become convinced that the back pain is disabling and may decide to quit work and reduce or cease extracurricular activities (e.g., social organizations) and normal family activities (e.g., driving children to school). These patients may further take on a "sick role" behavior, assuming the identity of a victim.[36] Pharmacists with patients who continually seek self-care devices and medications for chronic backache should refer the patients.

Back pain patients in the sick role may resist any attempt

to address their behaviors. Successful treatment of this patient may necessitate psychotherapy.

PROGNOSIS OF LOW BACK PAIN

The prognosis for back pain in general is quite good. About 80 to 90% of patients with low back pain will be able to return to work within 8 to 10 weeks.[37,38] Once an individual has had an episode of low back pain, however, the rate of recurrence is fairly high.[22] Surgery is necessary in only 0.25 to 2% of all patients with low back pain.[9]

Taking time off work increases the risk of chronic low back pain.[26] Studies show that patients who take 1 year off work have only a 25% chance of ever regaining productive employment. The chances plummet to 10% for patients who take 2 years off, partly because of the sick role (see "The Sick Role").[26] For this reason patients should be encouraged to undergo early rehabilitation.[39,40]

Low back pain in young athletes is generally self-limited, but should be checked by a physician if it lasts longer than 2 to 3 weeks to ensure that serious damage has not occurred.[41]

TREATMENT OF LOW BACK PAIN

tip *Patients with low back pain that has persisted for too long a period (10 days in adults) should be referred for physician evaluation, since differential diagnosis of low back pain consists of ruling out such pernicious possibilities as neoplasms, infection, metabolic bone diseases, spondylarthropathies, and neurologic deficits.[42]* Most physicians suggest nonsteroidal antiinflammatories or muscle relaxants initially, coupled with bed rest (typically no longer than 2 days in bed).[43]

Importantly, bed rest alone is counterproductive if it goes on for too long a period (more than 1 day).[7,8] Bed rest deconditions the patient's body and leads to depression toward life in general and an increasing unwillingness to resume normal household and personal activities.[44] Patients should be encouraged to engage in exercise, as it reduces recurrences, reduces time off work, and lessens usage of health-care resources.[26] In addition to general beneficial exercises, patients should be taught specific exercises for the treatment and prevention of lumbar back pain. However, these specific exercises should be prescribed by a physician and monitored by a physical therapist to ensure that they do not worsen the pain.[7]

Other components of conservative management of chronic low back pain include traction, manipulation, the use of corsets and braces, exercises, TENS (transcutaneous electrical nerve stimulation), spinal manipulation, and physical modalities.[45]

Treatment Guidelines

When patients complain of back pain, pharmacists should first ask about the duration of pain; if it is more than 10 days, the patient should be referred. Other danger signs also re-

Patient Assessment Algorithm 21.1. **Low Back Pain**

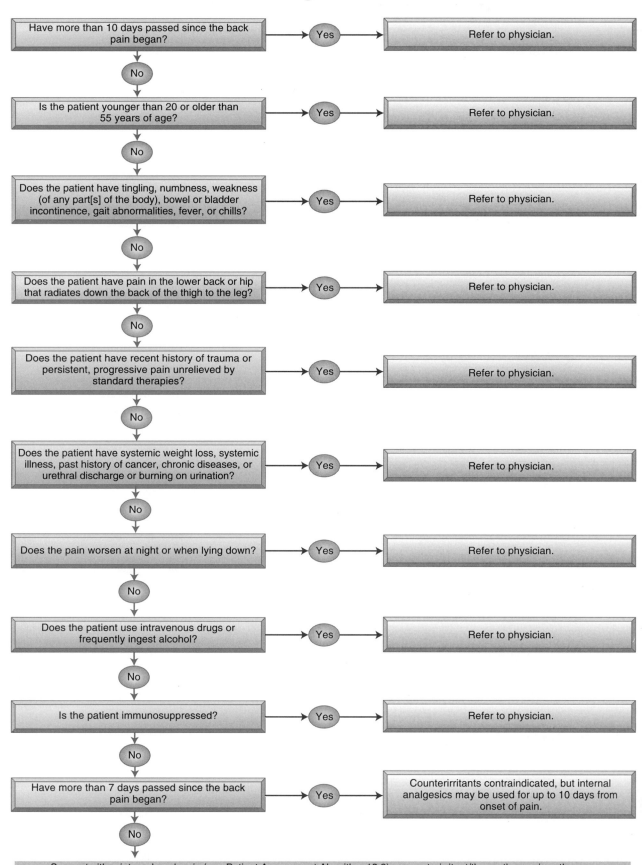

Table 21.1. Representative Products Marketed for Back Pain	
PRODUCT	SELECTED INGREDIENTS
Backaid Maximum Strength	Acetaminophen 500 mg, pamabrom 25 mg
Doan's Regular Strength Caplets	Magnesium salicylate tetrahydrate 377 mg (equivalent to 303.7 mg of magnesium salicylate)
Doan's Extra Strength Caplets	Magnesium salicylate tetrahydrate 580 mg (equivalent to 467.2 mg of magnesium salicylate)
Doan's P.M. Extra Strength Caplets	Magnesium salicylate tetrahydrate 580 mg (equivalent to 467.2 mg of magnesium salicylate), diphenhydramine HCl 25 mg
Momentum	Magnesium salicylate tetrahydrate 580 mg (equivalent to 467 mg of magnesium salicylate anhydrous), diphenhydramine HCl 25 mg

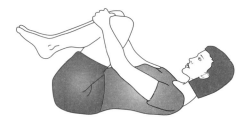

Figure 21.1. Position for passive flexion of the lumbar spine.

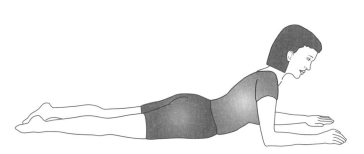

Figure 21.2. Position for passive extension of the lumbar spine.

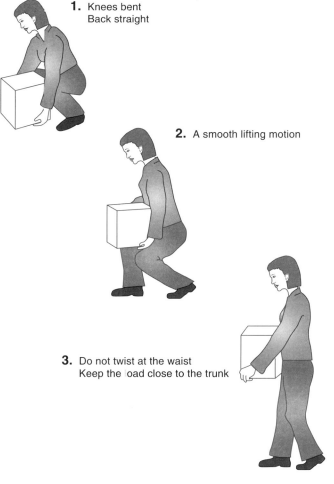

1. Knees bent
Back straight

2. A smooth lifting motion

3. Do not twist at the waist
Keep the load close to the trunk

Figure 21.3. The proper steps used in lifting.

quire referral to a physician. (See Patient Assessment Algorithm 21.1 for the steps used in recommending nonprescription medications.) Patients who have experienced back pain less than 10 days and who are free of the warning signals may be self-treated.

Nonprescription Medications

Internal analgesics (e.g., acetaminophen, ibuprofen, ketoprofen, naproxen) are safe and effective for acute back pain.[46] *The time limit for unsupervised self-usage of internal analgesics in back pain is 10 days in adults.* For a full discussion of these medications, see Chapter 18, Headache and Other Minor Pains. Some manufacturers have targeted back pain in their advertising. For a list of these medications see Table 21.1.

Back pain also may be relieved by the application of counterirritant products, as long as it has not been present for longer than 7 days. For a full discussion of these medications, see Chapter 20, Injuries to Muscles, Ligaments, and Tendons.

Nonpharmacologic Therapies

Back pain may respond to such interventions as thermotherapy and cryotherapy.[46] For a full discussion of these modalities, see Chapter 20, Injuries to Muscles, Ligaments, and Tendons.

PREVENTION OF LOW BACK PAIN

Useful steps to prevent back pain include back flexion and extension exercises and general fitness interventions.[47] Figures 21.1 and 21.2 show passive exercise positions for a series of back strengthening exercises that have been proven beneficial for many patients.

Patients can also avoid back pain of mechanical origin (e.g., sprains and strains) by following the proper steps in lifting and carrying a load (Fig. 21.3)[26]:

1. Place the feet apart when lifting to give a firm, stable, lifting base. Bend the knees and lower the trunk so the hands are as level with the waist as possible. Do not kneel or overflex the knees. Keep the back straight and the shoulders level and face in the same direction as the hips.
2. Lift smoothly, without jerking.
3. Carry the load, holding it close to the trunk. (Holding a load at arm's length can increase the stress by a factor of five.)

SUMMARY

Back pain is a term used by patients to refer to pain anywhere along the spine, from the lumbosacral area to the neck and upper back. Low back pain, one of the most common medical complaints, resolves without sequelae in the majority of patients. However, in some patients low back pain can be a chromic—even disabling—condition, while in other patients it can be a sign of serious underlying pathology such as malignancy or infection. The following back pain patients should be referred to a physician:

- Those who are younger than 20 or older than 55 years
- Those who are immunosuppressed
- Those who habitually use alcohol or intravenous drugs
- Those who also exhibit a number of signs, including weakness, numbness, or tingling, or who have a history of trauma, persistent or progressive pain, systemic weight loss, fever or chills, pain that worsens at night or when lying down, urethral discharge, or pain on urination (among others)
- Those who have pain in the lower back or hip that radiates down the back of the thigh to the leg, which may be sciatica

Lower back pain can be self-treated using several nonprescription medications and some nonpharmacologic therapies. Internal analgesics (e.g., ibuprofen, acetaminophen, naproxen) provide relief from back pain, but must not be used longer than 10 days. Topical medications such as counterirritants may provide symptomatic relief, but must not be used for longer than 7 days. Physical modalities such as thermotherapy and cryotherapy may also be useful.

AT THE COUNTER

 A female patient appearing to be in her late 60s to early 70s asks the pharmacist whether a nonprescription product containing phenazopyridine will help her back pain by "cleaning out her kidneys."

Interview/Patient Assessment

The pharmacist asks the patient's age and the nature of her back pain. The patient states that she is 74 years of age and has not had back pain before. The problem began after a plane trip to visit her grandchildren the previous week. She has no weight loss, fever, or other danger signal that would indicate a physician referral is necessary.

Pharmacist's Analysis

1. What is a possible cause of this patient's back pain?
2. What is the role of phenazopyridine nonprescription products in back pain?

3. Should this patient use internal analgesics, external analgesics, or physical modalities?

Patient Counseling

This patient has several problems that necessitate a physician visit. Her first onset of back pain past the age of 55 indicates a potentially serious etiology such as fracture caused by osteoporosis (although the patient might not remember any trauma, even a minor event such as sneezing can cause a fracture in the osteoporotic spine). She also should not use internal analgesics, external analgesics, or physical modalities without a physician recommendation. They may alleviate the pain, giving her a false sense of security that may prevent her from actually making a physician appointment. Phenazopyridine is not approved by the FDA for any use, especially back pain of unknown origin. She should be urged to make an immediate appointment with her physician.

References

1. Borenstein DG. Chronic low back pain. Rheum Dis Clin North Am 22:439, 1996.
2. Miller DLG. Nintendo neck (Letter). Can Med Assoc J 145:1202, 1991.
3. Wheeler AH. Diagnosis and management of low back pain and sciatica. Am Fam Physician 52:1333, 1995.
4. Borenstein DG. Epidemiology, etiology, diagnostic evaluation, and treatment of low back pain. Curr Opin Rheumatol 8:124, 1996.
5. Wipf JE, Deyo RA. Low back pain. Med Clin North Am 79:231, 1995.
6. Fast A. Low back disorders: Conservative management. Arch Phys Med Rehab 69:880, 1988.
7. Dorsher PT. Evaluation and treatment of low back pain. J Fla Med Assoc 84:24, 1997.
8. Lewis C. What to do when your back is in pain. FDA Consumer 32(2):26, 1998.
9. Teasell RW, White K. Clinical approaches to low back pain. Part 1. Epidemiology, diagnosis, and prevention. Can Fam Physician 40:481, 1994.
10. Dreisinger TE, Nelson B. Management of back pain in athletes. Sports Med 21:313, 1996.
11. Mazanec DJ. Back pain: Medical evaluation and therapy. Cleve Clin J Med 62:163, 1995.
12. Hignett S. Work-related back pain in nurses. J Adv Nursing 23:1238, 1996.
13. Smedley J, et al. Prospective cohort study of predictors of incident low back pain in nurses. BMJ 314:1225, 1997.
14. Payne WK III, Ogilvie JW. Back pain in children and adolescents. Pediatr Clin North Am 43:899, 1996.
15. Phillips JA, Forrester B, Brown KC. Low back pain. AAOHN 44:40, 1996.
16. Wheeler AH, Hanley EN Jr. Spine update. Nonoperative treatment for low back pain. Spine 20:375, 1995.
17. Ostgaard HC. Assessment and treatment of low back pain in working pregnant women. Semin Perinatol 20:61, 1996.
18. Harreby M, et al. Epidemiologic aspects and risk factors for low back pain in 38-year-old men and women: A 25-year prospective cohort study of 640 school children. Eur Spine J 5:312, 1996.
19. Micheli LJ, Wood R. Back pain in young adults. Arch Pediatr Adolesc Med 149:15, 1995.
20. Hosea TM, Gatt CJ Jr. Back pain in golf. Clin Sports Med 15:37, 1996.
21. Mellion MB. Neck and back pain in bicycling. Clin Sports Med 13:137, 1994.
22. Margo K. Diagnosis, treatment and prognosis in patients with low back pain. Am Fam Physician 49:171, 1994.
23. MacEvilly M, Buggy D. Back pain and pregnancy: A review. Pain 64:405, 1996.
24. Hainline B. Low-back pain in pregnancy. Adv Neurol 64:65, 1994.
25. Kummel BM. Nonorganic signs of significance in low back pain. Spine 21:1077, 1996.
26. Jayson MIV. Back pain. BMJ 313:355, 1996.
27. Kuritzky L, Brunton SA. Steps in the management of low back pain. Hosp Pract 31:109, 1996.
28. Bueff HU, Van Der Reis W. Low back pain. Prim Care 23:345, 1996.
29. Connelly C. Patients with low back pain. Postgrad Med 100:143, 1996.
30. Kraemer J. Natural course and prognosis of intervertebral disc diseases. Spine 20:635, 1995.
31. Douglas S. Sciatic pain and piriformis syndrome. Nurse Pract 22:166, 1997.
32. Frymoyer JW. Lumbar disk disease epidemiology. Instr Course Lect 41:217, 1992.
33. Olmarker K, Rydevik B. Pathophysiology of sciatica. Orthop Clin North Am 22:223, 1991.
34. Nachemson AL. Newest knowledge of low back pain: A critical look. Clin Orthop 279:8, 1992.
35. Porter RW, Ralston SH. Pharmacological management of back pain syndromes. Drugs 48:189, 1994.
36. Gillette RD. Behavioral factors in the management of back pain. Am Fam Physician 53:1313, 1996.
37. Daniels JM II. Treatment of occupationally acquired low back pain. Am Fam Physician 55:587, 1997.
38. Brody M. Low back pain. Ann Emerg Med 27:454, 1996.
39. Manniche C. Assessment and exercise in low back pain. With special reference to the management of pain and disability following first time lumbar disc surgery. Dan Med Bull 42:301, 1995.
40. Borenstein DG. A clinician's approach to acute low back pain. Am J Med 102:16S, 1997.
41. McCoy RL, et al. Common injuries in the child or adolescent athlete. Prim Care 22:117, 1995.
42. Martinelli TA, Wiesel SW. Low back pain: The algorithmic approach. Compr Ther 67:22, 1991.
43. Lazaro L IV, Quinet RJ. Low back pain: How to make the diagnosis in the older patient. Geriatrics 49:48, 1994.
44. Teasell RW, White K. Clinical approaches to low back pain. Part 2. Management, sequelae, and disability and compensation. Can Fam Physician 40:490, 1994.
45. Assendelft WJJ, et al. The relationship between methodological quality and conclusions in review of spinal manipulation. JAMA 274:1942, 1995.
46. Gillette RD. A practical approach to the patient with back pain. Am Fam Physician 53:670, 1996.
47. Lahad A, et al. The effectiveness of four interventions for the prevention of low back pain. JAMA 272:1286, 1994.

Miscellaneous Internal Conditions

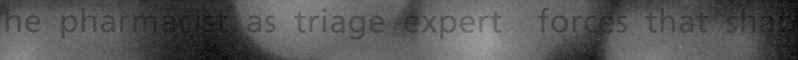

Obesity

AT THE COUNTER

 A female patient appearing to be in her early 20s requests help with the diet products. She appears perhaps 50 pounds overweight.

Interview/Patient Assessment

She has not used these products before, but wants to lose weight prior to her fifth high-school reunion in 2 months. She denies any medical condition other than nasal allergies for which her physician has suggested the use of Tavist-D. She also takes birth-control tablets.

Pharmacist's Analysis

1. What is the significance of the pharmacist making a rough estimate of the patient's weight?
2. Is short-term weight loss a legitimate use of these products?
3. Is her medication regimen of concern?

It is critical to refuse to recommend these products to patients with normal or below-average body weight, as they may be suffering from anorexia nervosa. However, this pa-

tient appears to be overweight, so anorexia is probably not an issue. Use of these products for weight loss in her situation is rational, but the pharmacist should stress the role of exercise and caloric reduction. A problem arises in her use of Tavist-D, which contains phenylpropanolamine.

Patient Counseling

She must be advised against use of any weight-control product containing phenylpropanolamine as long as she is taking any other product containing phenylpropanolamine or any product containing phenylephrine, pseudoephedrine, or ephedrine. The only other safe and effective weight-loss product is benzocaine, but it is not marketed in any widely available nonprescription product at this time. Therefore, this patient should be advised to refrain from using any weight-control product. Should she eventually choose to use phenylpropanolamine, she must be made aware of the many precautions to be observed in its use. The pharmacist should stress the safety and long-term benefits of incorporating an exercise regimen into her lifestyle, along with overall portion reduction.

Weight control is an elusive goal for most Americans.[1] Because of this, quack diet schemes and deceptive, ineffective, and sometimes dangerous products have proliferated wildly in the past 2 decades. All promise what they cannot deliver: easy weight loss.[2] The discrepancy between what people expect and what the few FDA-approved diet products can do is wider than with any other group of legitimate nonprescription drug products. The problem is further compounded by the vast number of quack weight-loss schemes, gimmicks, and products.

The definition of obesity is body fat (adipose tissue) present in excess amounts.[2] However, obesity is further quantified by measures of weight and height. The American Heart Association (AHA) uses criterion for obesity derived from the Metropolitan Life weight tables first published in 1959, as seen in Table 22.1.[3] Although these tables were revised in 1983 to allow an extra 10% body weight, the AHA has continued to use the 1959 version, feeling it more accurately reflects the relationship between weight and health. These tables for males and females have been accepted for decades as valid predictors of health-related problems with excess body weight.

One of the most useful obesity indicators is the body mass index (BMI) (also known as the Quetelet index), defined as the weight in kilograms divided by the height in meters squared.[4,5] To use nonmetric figures, the pharmacist may use this formula:

$$\text{weight (lbs)} \times 705/(\text{height in inches})^2 = \text{BMI}$$

This figure provides a good correlation with percentage of body fat. Experts differ, but most sources define obesity as a BMI of 28 to 30 or above.[2,6] As an example, a 5'10" male weighing 160 pounds would have a BMI of 23. However, a 5'10" male weighing 207 pounds would have a BMI of 30. A 5' female weighing 118 has a BMI of 23, but should she weigh 153 pounds, her BMI would be 30.[7]

The BMI is widely accepted because it is easily obtained and it allows a comparison of different people. However, researchers have also focused on less easily obtained measures such as body-region fat-distribution patterns.[8–10] Some people tend to become obese in the trunk or central upper body (known as male, abdominal, upper-body, or android obesity)—referred to as "apples" in the popular press.[11] Others gain preferentially in the limbs, hips, and legs, while remaining relatively small in the stomach and upper body (known as female, gluteal, femoral, lower-body, or gynoid obesity)—referred to as "pears."[5] These differences are quantified through such ratios as waist-to-hip circumference and subcapsular-to-triceps skinfold thickness. BMI correlates with the waist-to-hip ratio, so that consideration of both may provide important predictive clinical data.[12] These patterns predict such complications of obesity as gallstones, lipid metabolism disorders, hypertension, and type 2 diabetes mellitus.[13] Also, a waist-to-hip ratio of 1 or more (an android pattern) predicts cardiovascular problems in males and females more than a waist-to-hip ratio of less than 1 (the gynoid pattern).[5,14,15]

Table 22.1. The American Heart Association Desirable Weight Tables[a]

MEN HEIGHT (FEET/INCHES)	SMALL FRAME (LBS)	MEDIUM FRAME (LBS)	LARGE FRAME (LBS)
5'2"	112–120	118–129	124–141
5'3"	115–123	121–133	129–144
5'4"	118–126	124–136	132–148
5'5"	121–129	127–139	135–142
5'6"	124–133	130–143	138–156
5'7"	128–137	134–147	142–161
5'8"	132–141	138–152	147–162
5'9"	136–145	142–156	151–170
5'10"	140–150	146–160	155–174
5'11"	144–154	150–165	159–179
6'0"	148–158	154–170	164–184
6'1"	152–162	158–175	168–189
6'2"	156–167	162–180	173–194
6'3"	160–171	167–185	178–199
6'4"	164–175	172–190	182–204

WOMEN[b] HEIGHT (FEET/INCHES)	SMALL FRAME (LBS)	MEDIUM FRAME (LBS)	LARGE FRAME (LBS)
4'10"	92–98	96–107	104–119
4'11"	94–101	98–110	106–122
5'0"	96–104	101–113	109–125
5'1"	99–107	104–116	112–128
5'2"	102–110	107–119	115–131
5'3"	105–113	110–122	118–134
5'4"	108–116	113–126	121–138
5'5"	111–119	116–130	125–142
5'6"	114–123	120–135	129–146
5'7"	118–127	124–139	133–150
5'8"	122–131	128–143	137–154
5'9"	126–135	132–147	141–158
5'10"	130–140	136–151	145–163
5'11"	134–144	140–155	149–168
6'0"	138–148	144–159	153–173

Adapted from http://www.amhrt.org/Heart_and_Stroke_A_Z_Guide/dweight.html. 1998.

[a]The height in feet and inches includes shoes; the weight includes indoor clothing. This assumes that male indoor clothing has a weight of 7 pounds and female clothing a weight of 4 pounds, both including shoes.

[b]Women between 18 and 25 years of age should subtract 1 pound for each year under 25.

Another definition of obesity is morbid obesity. An individual is considered to be morbidly obese if he or she weighs double their ideal body weight or more.[16] The term is also used to indicate an individual who is 100 pounds or more above ideal body weight.

PREVALENCE OF OBESITY

What is the incidence of obesity in the United States? The numbers depend on the definition and BMI cutpoint used, but it is variously stated to affect 25 to 33% of all Americans —at a cost of more than 70 billion dollars yearly.[7,17–19] Louisiana, for example, has reported that 30% of its population exceeds ideal body weight by 20%, which is that state's definition of obesity.[20] These figures increase each year.[21,22]

EPIDEMIOLOGY OF OBESITY

Obesity increases with age, with the highest numbers of obese individuals aged 45 and over.[18] As many as 37% of those aged 65 or older are obese.[4] However, obesity also affects 25% of all United States children.[23]

The prevalence of obesity is higher in females than males and higher in pubertal females than prepubertal females.[7,24] At puberty the percentage of fat in females rises, while that of males plummets.[25,26]

Certain ethnic groups have greater obesity, although the underlying cause may be a mixture of environmental and genetic factors.[7,25] For example, Black-American and Hispanic females are more likely to be obese than white women, according to epidemiologic studies.[7,18,27,28]

In developing countries, the wealthy tend to be obese and

the poor are more likely to be undernourished and thus experience protein-calorie malnutrition. However, in heterogeneous, affluent societies such as the United States, social class and obesity are inversely related in all patients.[29,30] The female link in the United States is age dependent, so that prepubertal upper-to-middle-class children are more overweight than prepubertal lower-class females.[31] However, at puberty and beyond, lower-class females are 7 to 12 times more likely to be overweight than middle-class and upper-class women.[25] Social class and obesity are not well correlated in males.

Thus the distribution of obesity in the human population is marked by several trends that can be examined in attempting to understand the etiology of obesity.[29]

ETIOLOGY OF OBESITY

All else aside, the simple explanation for obesity is too little exercise coupled with excess caloric intake.[32] However, this is much too facile to provide meaningful clues to the prevention or treatment of obesity because it implies that willpower is at the heart of the problem.

A National Institutes of Health conference stated, "the underlying causes of overweight are unknown."[7] Although there is an obvious imbalance between energy intake and energy expenditure, the reason for the imbalance is not so obvious and may be multifactorial. In any individual obesity may be caused by a mixture of inherited, environmental, cultural, socioeconomic, and physiologic factors.

Evidence suggests that certain genetically determined physiologic processes cause obesity and prevent successful weight loss in 25% of cases.[2] One genetic theory that attempts to explain the high incidence of obesity in developed countries points out that humans were hunter-gatherers for 95 to 99% of our history.[29,33] During this time there were alternating periods of excess and starvation as game became scarce and gathering was unsuccessful. Natural selection dictated that only certain individuals would survive in times of widespread tribal starvation; notably, those whose ability to store calories in times of excess were most efficient. These primitive societies did not experience obesity because starvation cycles occurred every 2 to 3 years. During starvation those who had been able to store fat efficiently survived, while those unable to do so perished. Thus a genetic predisposition to store fat efficiently became dominant. Furthermore, since obesity probably did not occur in these semistarvation societies, it was not selected against in an evolutionary sense.

About 12,000 years ago, during the Neolithic revolution, humans converted to an agricultural society in which both plants and animals were domesticated. Now, in modern societies such as the United States food is so plentiful that even the poor can become obese.[2] Periods of starvation such as those experienced by prehistoric man simply do not exist in these modern societies. Those with a tendency to store fat efficiently do so as a result of genetic background.

Thus genetics is thought to play an important role in obesity. Research has tentatively identified obesity genes that help determine body fat mass and the proportion of fat that enters either central or peripheral stores.[34–37] Having obese parents more than doubles the risk of obesity in adults.[38]

Other research into the etiology of obesity has focused on the body-weight set point.[39] According to this theory, each person has an internal "best weight," known as the body-weight set point.[40] In obese individuals the set point is too high and the individual cannot easily balance intake and expenditure. For instance, a reduction in calories may be compensated for by an involuntary lowering of basal metabolism. Defects in thermogenesis or changes in physical activity may also be responsible for the body's defense of the set point.[41]

Other research refutes the genetic and set-point theories. Both of those theories begin with the assumption that the obese patient eats as little or less than the person of normal body weight. These assumptions are based on such interventions as the use of self-reports and food diaries. However, when obese people are actually observed, their self-studies often are found to be unreliable.[42] Obese persons consistently choose and eat larger meals than lean persons and eat more rapidly.[25] They also tend to be less active than lean people: they choose an escalator instead of stairs, for example.[25] If these observations can be generalized to the population at large, it follows that behavioral interventions to control weight are more likely to be successful.

Finally, researchers have advanced numerous other theories for obesity such as reduced sympathetic activity in obese patients, thermogenesis and its effects on brown adipose tissues, and differences in the size versus the number of fat cells.[25] Some show promise in developing novel approaches to the treatment of obesity.

COMPLICATIONS OF OBESITY

Obesity, which predisposes people to numerous health risks, is a primary factor in early death (along with other known factors such as cigarette smoking). Since the degree of obesity is critically important, the BMI has been used to assign probabilities of medical complications. Those with a BMI of 20 to 25 are at very low risk, those with a BMI of 25 to 30 are at low risk, 30 to 35 denotes moderate risk, 35 to 40 indicates high risk, and over 40 are at very high risk (Fig. 22.1).[25]

Obesity is a major factor in the development of severe medical problems that cause premature mortality, primarily cardiovascular disease, diabetes, and gallbladder disease, and it increases the risk of many other medical conditions (Fig. 22.2).[17,25] For instance, obese adolescent males exhibited increased mortality for as long as 50 years after adolescence, a finding independent of their adult weight.[12] Mortality is 5 to 12 times higher for obese men than lean men, a difference that is even more pronounced in the morbidly obese.[20] Modest weight loss improves survival by reducing the risk factors for cardiac disease—more so when the weight loss is accompanied by permanent lifestyle changes.[5] Even a 5% reduction in body weight reduces the risk of death.[43]

Ironically, weight loss also has been associated with an in-

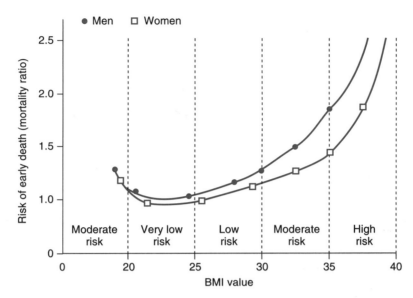

Figure 22.1. The risk of early death in terms of mortality ratio at different body mass index (BMI) values (e.g., a BMI of 35 approximately doubles the risk of early death). (Adapted from Bray GA, Gray DS. Obesity. I. Pathogenesis. West J Med 149:429, 1988.)

creased risk of death, even when studies target voluntary weight loss, controlling for involuntary weight loss caused by illnesses such as cancer.[44,45] Weight cycling ("yo-yo dieting")—the process of gaining and losing weight repeatedly over time—has been shown to increase the risk of early death.[46] In the face of conflicting data and known risks of obesity, it is prudent to attempt to prevent obesity in the first place.

Hypertension

Obese individuals face a 3 to 5.6 times greater risk for hypertension.[20] Likewise, obese patients with hypertension can often reduce blood pressure with weight loss.[47]

Coronary Heart Disease

Central **adiposity** (excessive accumulation of fat) is a risk factor for coronary artery disease, principally because of obesity-related hypertension.[8,17,48] (Perhaps central adiposity is more dangerous because abdominal body fat is more easily mobilized.[5]) Obesity increases the work of the heart, even in normotensive patients.[25] However, obesity also causes cardiovascular disease through its role in the development of diabetes mellitus, hypercholesterolemia, and left ventricular hypertrophy.[4,49] Weight loss lowers lipid levels and allows atherosclerotic plaques to resolve.[20]

Non–Insulin Dependent (Type 2) Diabetes Mellitus (NIDDM)

Central adiposity is also a risk factor for NIDDM.[8,50] Even moderate obesity increases the risk of developing NIDDM tenfold, while morbid obesity confers a risk that is 30 times greater.[20] Overweight type 2 diabetics who lose weight may

be able to improve glycemic control to the point where they no longer require oral hypoglycemics or insulin to reach euglycemia.[7,51] Since not all obese individuals develop diabetes, it is possible that those who become symptomatic had a preexisting tendency for its development.[41,52]

Gallstones/Gall Bladder Problems

Obesity is one of the cardinal risk factors for gallstones. Overweight women with a BMI of 30 or more double their risk of gallstones.[8] By the age of 60, gallbladder disease will have occurred in over 30% of obese females.[25] The incidence of gallbladder disease in men and women is tied to central obesity. Obese individuals tend to hypersecrete cholesterol so bile becomes supersaturated, contributing to the formation of cholesterol gallstones. In addition, obese individuals who consider weight reduction through the use of very low calorie diets are also at increased risk of developing gallstones, perhaps because the diets do not contain sufficient fat and protein to stimulate gallbladder contraction.[8]

Cancer

Obesity is a risk factor for certain types of cancer.[12,45] These include cancers of the breast, gallbladder, biliary passages, cervix, ovaries, and endometrium in females.[41,53] Obese males experience a heightened risk of colon, rectal, and prostate cancers.[41,54]

Work-Related Accidents and Disability

Obesity contributes to work-related injuries such as accidental falls and increases the number of work disability days.[20] The Social Security Disability laws recognize obesity as a cause of disability when an individual's weight exceeds tabled

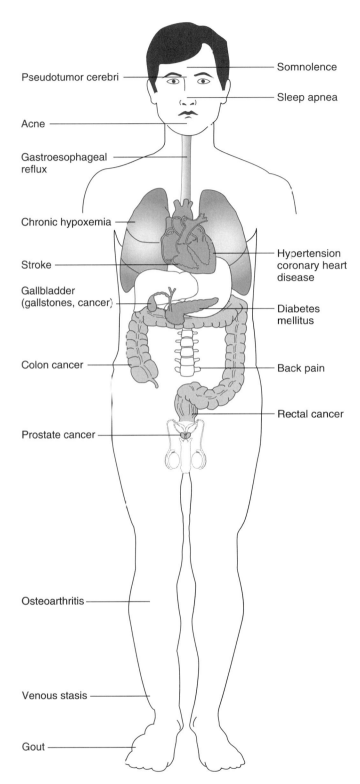

Pseudotumor cerebri — Somnolence

Sleep apnea

Acne —

Gastroesophageal reflux

Chronic hypoxemia —

Stroke —

Hypertension coronary heart disease

Gallbladder (gallstones, cancer)

Diabetes mellitus

Colon cancer —

Back pain

Rectal cancer

Prostate cancer —

Osteoarthritis —

Venous stasis —

Gout —

Figure 22.2. Obesity increases the risk of many serious medical conditions.

Joint Disease

Degenerative joint disease (osteoarthritis) is common in weight-bearing joints of obese individuals.[7,55] However, osteoarthritis also occurs in non–weight-bearing joints, suggesting that obesity aggravates joint symptoms.[41] Obesity is also a risk factor for low back pain.[56]

Respiratory Problems

Obesity hypoventilation syndrome (also known as Pickwickian syndrome from Joe, the overweight boy in Dickens' *Pickwick Papers*) is a combination of the following:

- Obesity
- Somnolence
- Sleep apnea
- Chronic **hypoxemia** (arterial blood low in oxygenation but not yet anoxic)
- **Hypercapnia** (carbon dioxide retention)
- Secondary **polycythemia** (a higher than normal number of erythrocytes in the blood)[41,57]

These problems increase obese individuals' risk of congestive heart failure and pulmonary hypertension.[20] Sleep apnea and the entire hypoventilation syndrome is reduced in prevalence and severity with weight loss.[7]

Self-Esteem

Weight loss is a difficult goal; many people wish to lose weight in order to improve the overall appearance, feel better, and enhance self-esteem.[19,58] However, many patients are unsuccessful in this attempt, and those who do lose weight often regain it within 5 years, causing a sense of failure and further lowering the self-esteem. Unfortunately, some people react to inability to lose weight with a depression that is alleviated somewhat by eating. This vicious cycle of eating to relieve the depression caused by low self-esteem defeats many patients seen by the pharmacist. Thus extreme tact must be exercised by the pharmacist in counseling patients with weight problems, so that a poor body image will not be exacerbated.

Other Conditions

Gout, shortness of breath, gastroesophageal reflux disease, stroke, polycystic ovary syndrome, **pseudotumor cerebri** (vascular tumor, brain swelling, or other conditions that mimic an intracranial tumor), and venous stasis are more common with obesity.[11,12,20] Obesity also causes or contributes to such dermatologic abnormalities as hirsutism, acne, abdominal striae, and **benign acanthosis nigricans** (darkening of the skin in the creases of the neck, axillary region, and over the knuckles).[57]

TREATMENT OF OBESITY

Treatment Guidelines

Weight gain occurs gradually; it is not realistic for most people to expect a simple and rapid weight loss.[59] Weight loss

figures by 10% or more.[20] For instance, a man is considered disabled if he is 5'10" and weighs 10% or more above 318 pounds; a female of 5' would be disabled if she weighed 10% or more above 230 pounds.

can greatly reduce or prevent the complications arising from obesity. In addition, weight loss also allows greater functional capacity, reduces work absenteeism, decreases pain, and increases the quality and quantity of social interactions.[7]

As a consequence, it is no surprise that many people attempt weight loss. As many as 61% of adults have dieted at some time.[27] In a national survey 45% of Americans reported that they were overweight (37% of males and 52% of females).[18] Almost two-thirds of those surveyed were attempting to lose weight. Significantly, 4% of self-reported, underweight persons and 11% of self-reported, normal-weight persons were also trying to lose weight. A survey of high-school students revealed that 44% of females and 15% of males were trying to lose weight.[60]

Dietary alterations are the most common weight-loss intervention. Patients reduce meal portions, manipulate their ratios of fat-carbohydrate-protein, and/or substitute lower-calorie foods and drinks.[61] The average duration of a weight-loss regimen was found to be 6.4 months for females and 5.8 months for males for those who had dieted in the past year.[7] Patients reported in a survey that they had made two to two and a half attempts to lose weight in the past 24 months, which highlights the tendency for weight regain with these low-effectiveness methods. For an historical perspective, it is interesting to compare the late Paleolithic diet with the average American diet and with today's dietary recommendations (Table 22.2). The most striking difference is the high amount of fat ingested by the average American.

Exercise is another vital component of healthy weight loss, but it is chosen less frequently as a weight-loss method, perhaps because it involves instituting lifelong lifestyle changes.[7,62] (Studies have demonstrated that males exhibit a direct correlation between weight and hours spent watching television.[5]) Exercise must be accompanied by reduced caloric intake to gain maximal benefits, which include increased cardiovascular fitness and a more favorable choles-

Patient Assessment Algorithm 22.1. Weight Loss

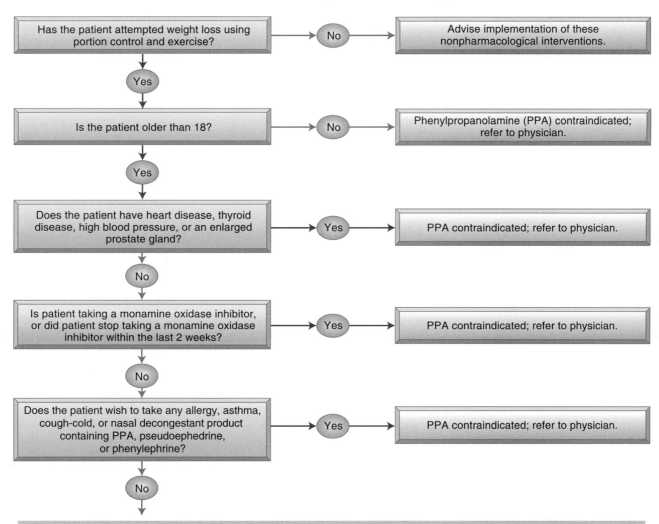

terol profile.[63] Patient Assessment Algorithm 22.1 illustrates the steps used in guiding the patient who seeks weight loss.

Nonprescription Medications

The original FDA review panel assigned to review weight-control products agreed in 1982 that it would be rational to market products for appetite control in the treatment of obesity.[64] Although many products that lack evidence of safety and effectiveness have been marketed for weight loss, the original report found only two ingredients to be safe and effective: phenylpropanolamine and benzocaine. (See "Dangerous, Ineffective, and/or Deceptive Weight-Loss Interventions.") The panel also recommended that these ingredients not be used by individuals younger than 12. Further, the FDA recommended that products containing these ingredients include the following advice, *"This product's effectiveness is directly related to the degree to which you reduce your usual daily food intake. Attempts at weight reduction that involve the use of this product should be limited to periods not exceeding 3 months, because that should be enough time to establish new eating habits."*

PHENYLPROPANOLAMINE (PPA)

Various diet products containing PPA are listed in Table 22.3. In 1982 the FDA OTC Review panel recommended an initial dose and precautions for PPA. However, in 1991 the FDA reopened the administrative record to discuss PPA.[65] Following a Congressional hearing concerned with diet pills, PPA, and their abuses, Congressman Ron Wyden, chair of the meeting, notified the FDA that PPA led all other OTC remedies in serious problems such as the following:

- Number of serious and fatal adverse effects
- The degree of seriousness of these adverse effects
- The number of calls to poison control centers

The hearing also revealed other problems with PPA diet products:

- Significant increases in blood pressure
- Ineffective for the majority of users
- Misuse by the majority of users (who do not follow label instructions or indications)
- A primary pathologic pathway in the deterioration of patients with anorexia nervosa
- Caused weight loss that was temporary and quickly regained as fat, predisposing the user to further diet failure
- Suspected of wasting lean-muscle mass

In response to these concerns the FDA held an open public meeting to discuss the safety and efficacy of PPA.

A proposed rule summarized the results of the PPA data-

Table 22.2. The Late Paleolithic Diet Compared with the Current Recommendations and the Diet Consumed by the Average American

DIETARY COMPONENT	LATE PALEOLITHIC DIET	CURRENT RECOMMENDATIONS	AVERAGE AMERICAN DIET
% Protein	34	10–15	12
% Carbohydrate	45	50–70	46
% Fat	21	15–30	42
Cholesterol (mg)	591	0–300	600
Fiber (g)	45.7	30–60	19.7
Sodium (mg)	690	1100–3300	2300–6900
Calcium (mg)	1580	800–1200	740

Modified from Brown PJ, Konner M. An anthropological perspective on obesity. Ann NY Acad Sci 499:29, 1987.

Table 22.3. Representative Single-Entity Weight-Control Products Containing Phenylpropanolamine

PRODUCT	SELECTED INGREDIENTS
Acutrim 16 Hour Steady Control	Phenylpropanolamine 75 mg
Acutrim Maximum Strength	Phenylpropanolamine 75 mg
Acutrim Late Day Strength	Phenylpropanolamine 75 mg
Control	Phenylpropanolamine 75 mg
Dexatrim Extended Duration	Phenylpropanolamine 75 mg
Dexatrim Maximum Strength	Phenylpropanolamine 75 mg
Permathene-12 Maximum Strength	Phenylpropanolamine 75 mg

gathering processes.[66] The agency did document that PPA raises blood pressure and became concerned about the risk of hemorrhagic stroke. Young female patients were more likely to suffer intracranial bleeding, a risk that increased if the patient inadvertently (or intentionally) exceeded the recommended dose, as in taking two different PPA-containing products labeled for different uses. The FDA suggested relabeling PPA-containing products to reduce risk—boldfaced type and capital letters for certain key phrases. The FDA-proposed warning would read as follows:

tip *"For use by people 18 years of age and older. Do not take more than 75 mg per day (24 hours). Taking more* **WILL NOT** *increase weight loss and can be harmful.* **DO NOT TAKE IF** *you have heart or thyroid disease, high blood pressure, or an enlarged prostate gland, unless directed by a doctor.* **STOP USING IF** *you develop nervousness, dizziness, sleeplessness, headache, or palpitations. If symptoms continue, ask a doctor.* **DO NOT USE WITH:** *(a) A monoamine oxidase inhibitor (MAOI) (certain drugs for depression, psychiatric, or emotional conditions, or Parkinson's disease), or for 2 weeks after stopping the MAOI drug. If unsure, ask a health professional. (b) Any allergy, asthma, cough-cold, nasal decongestant, or weight-control product (containing phenylpropanolamine, phenylephrine, pseudoephedrine, or ephedrine), or any prescription drug, unless directed by a doctor."*

At present this proposal remains a suggestion. Some products contain older FDA-approved labeling. If the new labeling is approved, these newer warnings would nullify and supersede the older warnings.

BENZOCAINE

The only other nonprescription diet aid recommended for Cate-

---

DANGEROUS, INEFFECTIVE, AND/OR DECEPTIVE WEIGHT-LOSS INTERVENTIONS

The great number of people attempting weight loss make it a lucrative market. Prescription medications are effective when used properly, but for a variety of reasons, many patients prefer to self-treat. Unfortunately, self-treatment opens the door for dangerous and/or ineffective methods and ineffective and/or unsafe products.

Representative Products Advertised for Weight Control That Contain Ingredients Lacking Proof of Safety and/or Efficacy[a]

PRODUCT	SELECTED INGREDIENTS/COMMENTS
CitraLean	Hydroxycitric acid, gymnema sylvestre, vanadyl sulfate, chromium picolinate, chromium polynicotinate (an unapproved combination)
Dexatrim Maximum Strength Plus Vitamins	Phenylpropanolamine 75 mg, vitamins, minerals, trace elements
Dexatrim Maximum Strength With Vitamin C	Phenylpropanolamine 75 mg, Vitamin C 180 mg
Diet Now!	B_6, potassium, kola nut, Ma huang, siberian ginseng, ginger, dulse, spirulina, fenugreek, dandelion, parsley, cranberry, fennel, chia seed, grapefruit pectin, hawthorne berry, lemon grass (an unapproved combination)
Fat Burner Sustained Release	Kola nut, chromium picolinate, carnitine, cinnamon powder, mustard seed powder, grapefruit extract
Fat Burner	Hydroxycitric acid, chromium picolinate, carnitine, uva ursi, kola nut, B_6, cayenne
Fat Burners	Choline, methionine, chromium picolinate, carnitine, lysine, inositol, betaine, lecithin
Fat Burner Thermogenic Diet Drink	l-carnitine, chromium picolinate, inositol, ginseng, guarana, vanadyl sulfate, creatine monohydrate (an unapproved combination)
Health Brands Dieters Tea	Locust plant, wymote, sagekhomi, ginseng, honeysuckle, chrysanthemum, papaya, chapparal, orange peel (an unapproved combination)
High Energy Maximum Strength	Kola nut, panax ginseng
KLB6 Grapefruit Diet Plan	Grapefruit extract, glucomannan, vitamin B_6, lecithin, kelp, cider vinegar, uva ursi, l-phenylalanine (an unapproved combination)
Laci Le Beau Super Dieter's Tea	Senna, orange peel, licorice root, althaea, siberian ginseng, papaya, honeysuckle, German chamomile (an unapproved combination)
Maximum Strength Chromium Picolinate	Chromium picolinate 200 mg/tablet (an unapproved ingredient)
Nature's Bounty Water Pill	Buchu, uva ursi, parsley, juniper berries, potassium gluconate (an unapproved combination)

Continued

gory I status, benzocaine has been overlooked in the FDA rush to deal with water-soluble gums and PPA. However, the agency has not revoked its recommended Category I status, nor has its age limit been changed from 12 years of age. It is effective in doses of 3 to 15 mg when used in the form of gum, lozenges, or candy just prior to eating. It works as an anorexiant by decreasing the ability to detect sweetness. At this time no leading weight-control product contains benzocaine. The reason may be lack of perceived marketing potential, since several older products were discontinued because of poor sales.

Nonpharmacologic Therapies: Nonnutritive Sweeteners and Fat Substitutes

The potential health hazards of PPA and unavailability of benzocaine restrict the ability of the pharmacist to counsel patients mainly to dietary manipulation and exercise. In this regard, patients may ask about various nonnutritive sweeteners that are available in most pharmacies, as well as about the recently approved fat substitute, olestra. (These products are considered food additives rather than nonprescription products.)

ASPARTAME

Aspartame is a chemical composed of phenylalanine and aspartic acid.[67] Heating (e.g., cooking) or exposing the molecule to an alkaline pH allows the formation of breakdown products (methanol, diketopiperazine, and aspartyl-phenylalanine), which lack sweetness.

Marketed as NutraSweet, aspartame is 180 to 200 times sweeter than table sugar (sucrose) and is devoid of any bitter aftertaste.[67] Aspartame may be purchased as packets containing NutraSweet in combination with additives such as dextrose and cellulose, in a product trade-named

The Perfect Solution	Ma huang, guarana, bladderwrack, yerba mute, ginseng, guaranine, bissey nut, ginger, fo-ti, licorice root, chromium picolinate, chromium chelavite, B_{12}
SeQuester	Barley-rice fiber, sodium choleate complex, cellulose, acacia, croscarmellose sodium, lemon pectin, carrot, etc.
Sleeper's Diet	l-arginine, l-ornithine, l-lysine (an unapproved combination)
T-Lite	Kola nut, plantain, wood betony, eleuthro, bladderwrack, guarana, garlic, cascara sagrada, senna, beet fiber, gymnema, almond, grapefruit, hydrangea, vitamins, minerals, trace elements
Ultra Lean	Brindall berry, dandelion, horsetail, juniper berries, cayenne, betaine, iodine, potassium, magnesium, vanadyl sulfate, chromium polynicotinate (an unapproved combination)
Under-Eat	Glucomannan (an unapproved ingredient)
Weider Dynamic Fat Burners	Choline bitartrate, inositol, dl-methionine, vitamin B_6, betaine (an unapproved combination)

aVitamins and minerals are not rational in weight-loss combinations; they have no proven benefit in reducing weight. Further, if the weight-loss product induces a vitamin/mineral deficiency, it is unsafe for self-use.

DANGEROUS DIETARY INTERVENTIONS

Skipping meals and starvation are common interventions for patients who have difficulty reducing portions.[61] Some dieters also vomit to reduce weight, with 14% of high-school students in one survey reporting that they had done so.[60] **Bulimia** (a chronic psychiatric disorder characterized by episodes of eating large quantities of food, followed by guilt, depression, and self-disgust that lead to self-induced vomiting, use of laxatives, and anorexia), engaged in by over 50% of patients with anorexia nervosa, may follow binge eating or guilt over regular meal ingestion.[73] (Bulimia and anorexia nervosa are most often seen in young females.)

USE OF EMETICS AND/OR LAXATIVES

Most patients purchasing syrup of ipecac undoubtedly do so for use following ingestion of poison (or to keep for future use in a poisoning episode), its FDA-approved use. However, the pharmacist should ask to ensure that these are actually the reasons for purchase. The patient should be strongly suspected of bulimia unless a convincing reason is given. Even then, repeated sales of this emetic to the same individual suggest self-induced vomiting. *The pharmacist who notes high shoplifting of syrup of ipecac should suspect theft by bulimics and consider placing the product behind the counter to thwart its unwarranted use. Bulimia is extremely dangerous in its own right, but much more so when the individual uses syrup of ipecac as an emesis tool.[14]* Similarly, some bulimics purchase laxatives (e.g., those containing stimulants such as bisacodyl or senna) repeatedly to reduce weight. Some pharmacies have already removed them from self-serve areas, with a sign directing patients to consult with the pharmacist if they wish to purchase the products. (In addition to purchases of laxatives and emetics, some anorexics and bulimics may be identified through noticing young, underweight female patients who appear extremely anxious about weight gain and proper nutrition.)

Quack products often include laxatives, while not labeling them as such. Some dieter's teas include such laxatives as Cassia (containing senna) and Rhamnus purshiana (containing cascara sagrada).[74] The FDA has cautioned that these products have caused laxative-abuse syndromes, including such complications as severe electrolyte imbalances,

Continued

which can lead to cardiac arrhythmias and death. The FDA stresses that the marketing of these products as dietary supplements allows the manufacturers to evade FDA premarketing review of safety, effectiveness, dosing information, and monitoring advice. Anorexics and bulimics also purchase such products as dieter's teas.

INTENTIONAL DEHYDRATION

Patients have the mistaken idea that diuresis is a safe and effective method for weight loss. Diuresis is undoubtedly effective, as the person loses water weight. However, this practice must be discouraged for several reasons:

- Most people are already poorly hydrated, and the use of a diuretic further endangers their functional capability.
- Diuresis does not cause loss of water alone, but also loss of the electrolytes that accompany the water such as potassium, sodium, calcium, and magnesium. The individual who diureses at home with a diuretic will not have the potassium status evaluated.
- When diuretic use is halted, the body will regain their normal hydration status, so that any weight loss is short-term, as well as dangerous.

Nonprescription products containing reputed diuretics for weight loss have been sold for many years. These products usually contain such herbs as buchu, uva ursi, parsley, and juniper berries. None of these ingredients have been proven safe or effective as diuretics, and all purported diuretics were placed in Category II in the original FDA OTC Review Panel document.[64] A later document from the FDA also listed these diuretics in the group of ingredients not recognized as safe and effective for weight control.[75] One such product even adds potassium gluconate to each tablet, which could cause hyperkalemia in light of the ineffectiveness of the herbal diuretics. The pharmacist selling such products must alert the patients to the dangers of hyperkalemia with their use, in case the products do not diurese as advertised.

Athletes commonly use dehydration to reach and maintain a lower-weight classification in an attempt to increase their competitive edge. One author has noted that with regard to wrestling, "Many coaches consider rapid weight loss to be an essential part of the sport . . . "[76] There is no approved indication for diuretic use in males. *All males attempting to purchase such products should be strongly questioned, since the only approved use for nonprescription diuretics is menstrually related swelling.*

DANGEROUS STIMULANTS

Many diet products and combinations contain ephedrine and/or caffeine, both of which lack proof of safety and efficacy for weight loss.[77] Caffeine was listed in the original FDA OTC Panel Review document as an ingredient devoid of anorexiant effect.[64] A later document from the FDA listed caffeine in the group of ingredients not recognized as safe and effective for weight control.[76]

Manufacturers may market ephedrine/caffeine combinations as "fat burners" that will enhance metabolism.[74] Some manufacturers also use deceptive techniques to mask the presence of these unapproved weight-loss ingredients such as labeling the product with the sources used to obtain ephedrine (the oriental herb Ma huang, also known as *Ephedra sinica,* or Chinese ephedra) or caffeine (guarana or kola nut).

Continued

AT THE COUNTER

A male patient aged approximately 35 is intently reading the boxes of the nonprescription diuretics. His weight appears to be in excess of 200 pounds on a 5 foot, 5 inch frame. He asks whether the diuretics are helpful for weight loss since he's concerned about a heart attack.

Interview/Patient Assessment

The pharmacist determines that the patient's concerns stems from the fact that his father suffered a heart attack in his mid 30s and was also overweight. This patient denies the use of any medications and states that he has no medical condition.

Pharmacist's Analysis

1. Is this patient justifiably concerned about a link between excess weight and heart attack?

2. Are diuretics effective for a patient such as this?
3. What should the pharmacist recommend?

The link between obesity and hypertension is well established, as is that between obesity and coronary heart disease.

Patient Counseling

This patient should be advised that the only safe and effective use for nonprescription diuretics is menstrually related swelling. Further, any weight loss caused by a diuretic would be transient and potentially dangerous. The patient might be shown a phenylpropanolamine-containing weight-loss product, while being advised that he should also eat less and exercise more. The pharmacist should also communicate to him the other risk factors for myocardial infarction (e.g., cholesterol), so that he might institute other lifestyle changes as well.

Equal. The use of aspartame has been linked with numerous adverse health reactions in the popular press, but legitimate scientific research has failed to confirm these associations.[68–70] However, patients with phenylketonuria, a rare genetic disorder, should not use aspartame as they cannot metabolize phenylalanine.[68]

SACCHARIN

Saccharin is 300 times sweeter than table sugar.[68] Its availability in liquid, tablets, bulk powder, and unit-of-use packets has ensured its widespread acceptance. (Sweet 'N Low is one major trade name.) The major consumer question about saccharin concerns a link with cancer of the bladder in rats, first reported in the 1970s.[71] However, intensive research has failed to verify a link in humans.

ACESULFAME POTASSIUM

Acesulfame is a permitted sweetener for certain foods.[68] Also approved by the FDA for use as packets or tablets, acesulfame potassium is 130 times sweeter than sucrose. It does not break down during cooking.

OLESTRA

Olestra (trade-named Olean) is a fat substitute used in food that is free of fat and calories.[72] Olestra is of interest to pharmacists because of its adverse reactions, which are mainly gastrointestinal. It can cause abdominal cramping, increased frequency of bowel movements, and loose stools. These problems are not of medical significance, according to the FDA. However, olestra inhibits absorption of fat-soluble vitamins A, D, E, and K if foods are eaten at the same time. Therefore, labels will warn that *consumers may need to supplement with vitamins A, D, E, and K while using olestra.* It also reduces the amount of carotenoids available from carrots, sweet potatoes, leafy green vegetables, and animal tissues, although the effects of reduced carotenoid absorption are unknown.

Use of these ingredients is unsafe. They have caused nervousness, dizziness, tremor, altered blood pressure and heart rate, gastrointestinal distress, chest pain, myocardial infarction, hepatitis, stroke, seizures, psychosis, and death.[74] The adverse reactions can occur in young, healthy individuals. In children and teenagers who use them, a stimulant overdose syndrome is increasingly seen.

An example of the ephedrine/caffeine combination is a product known as Nature's Nutrition Formula One.[78] (This product is also an example of nutritional products sold through multilevel marketing techniques.) The promotional brochure promises opportunities in "this community and throughout the United States for persons interested in marketing our growing line of products." Independent distributors need not have medical or pharmaceutical training (or any education at all, for that matter) and may not be cognizant of the hazards of unapproved weight-loss products. Sales of this particular product were banned in Texas because it was suspected of causing at least one death and numerous illnesses.[79] The FDA informed the manufacturer that the product was in violation of federal law, but the company refused to institute a recall, prompting the FDA to issue a national warning against its use.[78,80] At that time the agency noted that reports of several deaths and more than 100 injuries caused by ephedrine/caffeine combinations had been received.[81]

TOPICAL AMINOPHYLLINE

In the mid 1990s word spread about the weight-loss properties of aminophylline creams. (These products were also sold through multilevel marketing schemes, with sales projected to top 200 million dollars in 1994.[82]) Supposedly, these creams allow the user to target weight loss to the thighs, hence the names such as Thigh Cream and Beautiful Thighs. Like most diet fads, they were sold widely before any substantial and legitimate medical evidence was offered to prove them both safe and effective. Users risked absorption of aminophylline with the product's use, with its eventual conversion to theophylline. The dangers of excessive theophylline blood levels are well known, yet manufacturers did not place any warnings regarding this ingredient on the labels. A 1998 Internet search revealed numerous locations where the unwary consumer could purchase these products.

DIET PROGRAMS

Even diet programs are not exempt from scrutiny. The Federal Trade Commission (FTC) charged five of the nation's leading weight-loss programs with making false claims and using deceptive testimonials.[83] The agency discovered that none of the five could back up claims that customers are successful in reaching weight goals or maintaining weight loss.[84] Three of the commercial programs agreed to settle the charges through consent agreements (e.g., Nutri/System, Inc.), and two others (e.g., Jenny Craig, Inc. and Weight Watchers International, Inc.) challenged the charges.[83]

LIQUID DIET PRODUCTS

Liquid diet products usually consist of canned vitamin/mineral/calorie mixtures. Those wishing to lose weight are instructed to replace one or two meals a day with the canned product. Supposedly, the meal being replaced would have been higher in calorie/fat content than the canned product. Some products include instructions regarding dietary restriction and activity that should be adhered to while they are used. Should an individual be sufficiently motivated to follow these instructions, weight loss is more probable, but not assured.

The FTC examined several liquid diet products and found that they used "unsubstantiated hype" in promotions. The FTC cautioned the manufacturers of Optifast, Medifast, and Ultrafast to cease misleading advertising.[85] The companies agreed to stop misrepresenting the possibility of weight regain and further agreed to include a warning about the need for monitoring by a physician while using the products.[86]

FIBERS/BULK FORMERS

Products containing fiber and bulk formers were classified as Category III in the original FDA panel monograph.[64] Their purported action involved swelling in the gastrointestinal tract, producing a nonnutritive bulk that would inhibit hunger.[64] These products include

Continued

the laxative ingredients methylcellulose and psyllium, chondrus, guar gum, carrageenan, karaya gum, sea kelp, and xanthan gum. They also included alginic acid/sodium bicarbonate, which forms a combination of sodium alginate and carbon dioxide on ingestion, which was alleged to produce a bulking foam, to inhibit hunger. At the time of the original document, the safety of these ingredients was not in question.

Following the original panel report, a product known as Cal-Ban 3000 began to be sold in pharmacies. Cal-Ban 3000 was promoted as a "new medical breakthrough" and
a "powerful new weight-loss formula that causes rapid weight loss without conventional dieting or exercise."[87] The FDA eventually discovered that the so-called medical breakthrough was guar gum (listed on the label as "specially prepared ground endosperm of *Cyamopsis tetragonolobus*," the genus and species of guar gum, and sold without an approved marketing application, it was not subject to mandatory reporting requirements for adverse reactions) and that the directions for the product advised consumers to take up to ten of the 500-mg tablets at a time.[88] (Seventeen patients developed esophageal obstruction, and ten were hospitalized as a result of guar gum blockages of the esophagus or intestinal tract when the product expanded after coming in contact with mucosal moisture; one died.[89,90]) When the FDA instituted a full-scale investigation of the product and its hazards, the manufacturer attempted to evade the FDA by hiding its inventory, which was eventually destroyed.[87,91] The manufacturer was also issued a fine of $1.3 million. *This incident highlights the need for pharmacists to be especially careful when selling products that have not yet been fully evaluated for safety.* The Cal-Ban 3000 incident caused the FDA to issue a warning for water-soluble gums.[89] (See the warning under "Ingestion of Adequate Water with Bulk Laxatives" in Chapter 10, Constipation.) Further, it was reclassified into Category II as a weight-control product.[92] All other such ingredients were also designated as not generally recognized as safe and effective for weight loss (e.g., alginic acid, carboxymethylcellulose, carrageenan, etc.).[75]

VITAMINS/MINERALS

No vitamin or mineral has been found by the FDA to have an anorexiant effect; all were placed in Category II in the original FDA Panel document.[64] A comment questioned whether the FDA would allow their combination with active weight-control medications, and the agency agreed that it might be reasonable to do so.[75] The issue of combining vitamins and minerals with an active anorexiant is pending at the present time.

OTHER INGREDIENTS/METHODS

A full review of additional weight-loss methods would fill an entire textbook of quackery. Nevertheless, a few should be mentioned because pharmacists sometimes receive questions about them, and they are often included in unapproved diet products.

Spirulina

Spirulina, an extract of blue-green algae, is alleged to have diet properties. Although it is a protein, it has an incomplete amino-acid profile. Thus it lacks value as a nutritional supplement and is useless as a diet aid.

Grapefruit

Numerous products contain grapefruit, which is alleged to burn away fat through its inherent acidity. Of course, the tablets are taken orally, so grapefruit's acidity is dwarfed by the greater acidity of the gastric contents. Thus these tablets are also worthless as a diet aid.

The Sleeper's Diet

Occasionally, a product appears that is so absurd that it would be laughable were it not for the fact that it dupes unwary consumers. One such product is the "Sleeper's Diet," which alleges to allow weight loss while one sleeps. (Supposedly, one does not even need to alter eating or exercise habits.) The Sleeper's Diet contains arginine, ornithine, and lysine, a "special combination of amino acids based on a popular weight-loss program."

Glucomannan

Glucomannan is another water-soluble gum, but it was not covered specifically under the FDA guidelines mentioned earlier. However, the FDA did report seven cases of glucomannan-induced esophageal obstruction from Australia.[90] Five of the patients suffered complete esophageal obstruction. In all but one case the obstruction resulted from a single tablet. The obstruction required esophagoscopy for removal in five cases. One subject experienced an esophageal perforation that required 2 months of hospitalization. Apparently, the FDA intended to control this ingredient with the other bulking agents by including the phrase, "These ingredients include, but are not limited to . . . ." when providing an illustrative list of water-soluble gums.

Chromium Picolinate

This ingredient has taken over as the fad diet aid for the late 1990s. Several studies show no effect in weight loss, and one actually illustrated weight gain in young, obese women.[93–95] Its reputation is apparently based on word-of-mouth endorsements from users, although testimonials are meaningless to science regardless of their quantity or sincerity. Nevertheless, chromium picolinate continues to be incorporated into products sold through multilevel marketing schemes, independent distributorships, and pharmacies. The long-term effects of chromium supplementation are unknown at present. It may worsen behavioral disorders as a result of its effect on neurochemicals.[96]

SUMMARY

Obesity is a medical condition of uncertain etiology but with tremendous medical consequences such as increased risk of the following:

- Hypertension
- Coronary heart disease
- Type 2 diabetes mellitus
- Gallstones and gallbladder problems
- Cancer
- Work-related accidents and disability
- Joint disease
- Respiratory problems

Left untreated, obesity can be deadly. Unfortunately, there is little the pharmacist can offer in the way of nonprescription products for obesity. Nonprescription products containing phenylpropanolamine have not yet been proven free of substantial risk, yet there are no safe and effective pharmacologic alternatives (until benzocaine is widely marketed). The patient should be made aware of nonnutritive sweeteners, fat substitutes, and liquid diet products, which seem to be relatively safe when used as directed. Should they fail to result in a safe and gradual weight loss, the patient who wishes assistance should be referred to a physician for initial evaluation and professional medical care.

The pharmacist should also stress the long-term effectiveness of instituting lifestyle changes such as portion control, lowering the fat content of the diet, and increasing the exercise regimen. Further, the patient should be warned against the use of the many dangerous and/or ineffective diet products that are available.

References

1. Clark MM, Guise BJ, Niaura RS. Obesity level and attrition: Support for patient-treatment matching in obesity treatment. Obes Res 3:63, 1995.
2. Robison, et al. Obesity, weight loss, and health. J Am Diet Assoc 93:445, 1993.
3. http://www.amhrt.org/Heart_and_Stroke_A_Z_Guide/dweight.html.1998.
4. Harris TB, et al. Overweight, weight loss, and risk of coronary heart disease in older women. Am J Epidemiol 137:1318, 1993.
5. Phillips WG. Obesity and weight cycling. J Med Assoc Ga 82:537, 1993.
6. Seidell JC, Flegal KM. Assessing obesity: Classification and epidemiology. Br Med Bull 53:238, 1997.
7. Fletcher SW, et al. National Institutes of Health Technology Assessment Conference Statement: Methods for voluntary weight loss and control, March 30–April 1, 1992. Nutr Rev 50:340, 1992.
8. Everhart JE. Contributions of obesity and weight loss to gallstone disease. Ann Intern Med 119:1029, 1993.
9. Bjorntorp P. Regional patterns of fat distribution. Ann Intern Med 103:994, 1985.
10. Logue E, Smucker WD, Bourget CC. Identification of obesity: Waistlines or weight? Nutrition, Exercise and Obesity Research Group. J Fam Pract 41:357, 1995.
11. Lerman RH, Cave DR. Medical and surgical management of obesity. Adv Intern Med 34:127, 1989.
12. National Task Force on the Prevention and Treatment of Obesity. Weight cycling. JAMA 272:1196, 1994.
13. Zamboni M, et al. Effect of weight loss on regional body fat distribution in premenopausal women. Am J Clin Nutr 58:29, 1993.
14. Kirkland L, Anderson R. Achieving healthy weights. Can Family Physician 39:157, 1993.
15. Bouchard C. Genetic factors in obesity. Med Clin North Am 73:67, 1989.
16. Kral JG. Morbid obesity and related health risks. Ann Intern Med 103:1043, 1985.
17. Kern PA, et al. Combined use of behavior modification and very low-calorie diet in weight loss and weight maintenance. Am J Med Sci 307:325, 1994.
18. Horm J, Anderson K. Who in America is trying to lose weight? Ann Intern Med 119:672, 1993.
19. Stern JS, et al. Weighing the options: Criteria for evaluating weight-management programs. The Committee to Develop Criteria for Evaluating the Outcomes of Approaches to Prevent and Treat Obesity. Obes Res 3:591, 1995.
20. Martin LF, Hunter SM. Are there effective treatments for the severely obese? J La State Med Soc 146:348, 1994.
21. Goodrick GK, Poston WS II, Foreyt JP. Methods for voluntary weight loss and control: Update 1996. Nutrition 12:672, 1996.
22. Cheah JS. Current management of obesity. Singapore Med J 37:299, 1996.
23. Nuutinen O, Knip M. Predictors of weight reduction in obese children. Eur J Clin Nutr 46:785, 1992.
24. Legato MJ. Gender-specific aspects of obesity. Int J Fertil Womens Med 42:184, 1997.
25. Bray GA, Gray DS. Obesity. I. Pathogenesis. West J Med 149:429, 1988.
26. Gray DS. Diagnosis and prevalence of obesity. Med Clin North Am 73:1, 1989.
27. French SA, Jeffery RW. Consequences of dieting to lose weight: Effects on physical and mental health. Health Psychol 13:195, 1994.
28. Van Itallie TB. Health implications of overweight and obesity in the United States. Ann Intern Med 103:983, 1985.
29. Brown PJ, Konner M. An anthropological perspective on obesity. Ann NY Acad Sci 499:29, 1987.
30. Sorensen TI. Socio-economic aspects of obesity: Causes or effects? Int J Obes Relat Metab Disord 19(Suppl 6):S6, 1995.
31. Patterson ML, et al. Sociodemographic factors and obesity in preadolescent black and white girls: NHLBI's Growth and Health Study. J Natl Med Assoc 89:594, 1997.
32. Weiser M, et al. The pharmacologic approach to the treatment of obesity. J Clin Pharmacol 37:453, 1997.
33. Ferro-Luzzi A, Martino L. Obesity and physical activity. CIBA Found Symp 201:207, 1996.
34. Roberts SB, Greenberg AS. The new obesity genes. Nutr Rev 54(2 Pt 1):41, 1996.
35. Bray GA. Progress in understanding the genetics of obesity. J Nutr 127(5 Suppl):940S, 1997.
36. Leibel RL. Single gene obesities in rodents: Possible relevance to human obesity. J Nutr 127:1908S, 1997.

37. Hansen BC. Obesity, diabetes, and insulin resistance: Implications from molecular biology, epidemiology, and experimental studies in humans and animals. Diabetes Care 18:A2, 1995.

38. Whitaker RC, et al. Predicting obesity in young adulthood from childhood and parental obesity. N Engl J Med 337:869, 1997.

39. Porter S. How to treat the overweight patient. Ohio St Med J 81:859, 1985.

40. Keesey RE. The body-weight set point. Postgrad Med 83:114, 1988.

41. Weinsier RL. Etiology, complications, and treatment of obesity. Ala J Med Sci 24:435, 1987.

42. Price GM, et al. Characteristics of the low-energy reporters in a longitudinal national dietary survey. Br J Nutr 77:833, 1997.

43. Goldstein DJ, Potvin JH. Long-term weight loss: The effect of pharmacologic agents. Am J Clin Nutr 60:647, 1994.

44. Pamuk ER, et al. Weight loss and subsequent death in a cohort of U.S. adults. Ann Intern Med 119:744, 1993.

45. Pamuk ER, et al. Weight loss and mortality in a national cohort of adults, 1971–1987. Am J Epidemiol 136:686, 1992.

46. Kuller L, Wing R. Weight loss and mortality. Ann Intern Med 119:630, 1993.

47. Stevens VJ, et al. Weight loss intervention in phase I of the trials of hypertension prevention. Arch Intern Med 153, 849, 1993.

48. Peiris AN, et al. Adiposity, fat distribution, and cardiovascular risk. Ann Intern Med 110:867, 1989.

49. Rexrode KM, Manson JE, Hennekens CH. Obesity and cardiovascular disease. Curr Opin Cardiol 11:490, 1996.

50. James WP. The epidemiology of obesity. CIBA Found Symp 201:1, 1996.

51. Pontiroli AE, et al. Weight loss reverses secondary failure of oral hypoglycaemic agents in obese non–insulin-dependent diabetic patients independently of the duration of the disease. Diabete Metab 19:30, 1993.

52. Bjorntorp P. Neuroendocrine abnormalities in human obesity. Metabolism 44(2 Suppl 2):38, 1995.

53. Brancati FL, et al. Patient characteristics related to intensity of weight reduction care in a university medical clinic. J Gen Intern Med 7:609, 1992.

54. Kissebah AH, Freedman DS, Peiris AN. Health risks of obesity. Med Clin North Am 73:111, 1989.

55. Seidell JC. Time trends in obesity: An epidemiological perspective. Horm Metab Res 29:155, 1997.

56. Deyo RA, Bass JE. Lifestyle and low-back pain. Spine 14:501, 1989.

57. Bray GA. Complications of obesity. Ann Intern Med 103:1052, 1985.

58. Atkinson RL. Use of drugs in the treatment of obesity. Annu Rev Nutr 17:383, 1997.

59. Gill TP. Key issues in the prevention of obesity. Br Med Bull 53:359, 1997.

60. Serdula MK, et al. Weight control practices of U.S. adolescents and adults. Ann Intern Med 119:667, 1993.

61. Levy AS, Heaton AW. Weight control practices of U.S. adults trying to lose weight. Ann Intern Med 119:661, 1993.

62. Blocker WP Jr, Ostermann HJ. Obesity: Evaluation and treatment. Dis Mon 42:829, 1996.

63. Bray GA, DeLany J. Opinions of obesity experts on the causes and treatment of obesity—A new survey. Obes Res 3(Suppl 4):419S, 1995.

64. Fed Reg 47:8466, 1982.

65. Fed Reg 56:13295, 1991.

66. Fed Reg 61:5912, 1996.

67. Garriga MM, Metcalfe DD. Aspartame intolerance. Ann Allergy 61:63, 1988.

68. Greeley A. Not only sugar is sweet. FDA Consumer 26(3):17, 1992.

69. Lapierre KA, et al. The neuropsychiatric effects of aspartame in normal volunteers. J Clin Pharmacol 30:454, 1990.

70. Yost DA. Clinical safety of aspartame. Am Fam Physician 39:201, 1989.

71. Grenby TH. Update on low-calorie sweeteners to benefit dental health. Int Dent J 41:217, 1991.

72. Papazian R. Healthful snacks for the chip & dip crowd. FDA Consumer 30(3):8, 1996.

73. Wilson GT. Relation of dieting and voluntary weight loss to psychological functioning and binge eating. Ann Intern Med 119:727, 1993.

74. Anon. Adverse events with ephedra and other botanical dietary supplements. FDA Med Bull 24(2):3, 1994.

75. Fed Reg 56:37792, 1991.

76. Woodworth M, Sitler M. Iowa wrestlers continue detrimental weight loss practices. Iowa Med 83:375, 1993.

77. Ryan DH. Medicating the obese patient. Endocrinol Metab Clin North Am 25:989, 1996.

78. Anon. FDA warns against using Nature's Nutrition Formula One. Pharm Today 1(8):3, 1995.

79. Stanley D. Popular pep pill banned by state. Austin American-Statesman A1, 1994 (May 13).

80. Anon. Ma huang and kola nut combination can be deadly. FDA Consumer 29(4):3, 1995.

81. Klinka K. Product dangerous, health official warns. The Daily Oklahoman 10, 1995(March 1).

82. Doheny K. Thigh high. Am Drugg 211(1):39, 1994.

83. Anon. FTC accuses five diet programs of deceptive advertising. FDA Consumer 27(10):3, 1993.

84. Schwartz R. Skinning the slimmers. Am Drugg 209(1):12, 1993.

85. Anon. FTC cautions on liquid protein diets. Am Drugg 205(1):1, 1991.

86. Anon. Weighty claims. Drug Topics 135(20):5, 1991.

87. Cramer T. Cal-Ban banned. FDA Consumer 26(5):39, 1992.

88. Fed Reg 55:45788, 1990.

89. Anon. Guar gum diet products under investigation. FDA Consumer 24(8):3, 1990.

90. Fed Reg 55:45782, 1990.

91. Anon. Drugs/Human Use Recalls: Cal-Ban 3000 guar gum tablets and capsules. FDA Consumer 27(7):45, 1993.

92. Fed Reg 58:45194, 1993.

93. Grant KE, et al. Chromium and exercise training: Effect on obese women. Med Sci Sports Exerc 29:992, 1997.

94. Lukaski HC, et al. Chromium supplementation and resistance training: Effects on body composition, strength, and trace element status of men. Am J Clin Nutr 63:954, 1996.

95. Trent LK, Thieding D. Effects of chromium picolinate on body composition. J Sports Med Phys Fitness 35:273, 1995.

96. Reading SA. Chromium picolinate. J Fla Med Assoc 83:29, 1996.

97. http://www.amhrt.org/Heart_and_Stroke_A_Z_Guide/dweight.html. 1998.

Fatigue and Drowsiness

AT THE COUNTER

A college student asks the pharmacist which product is best to keep him awake all night so he can study for an exam.

Interview/Patient Assessment

The student has a final the next day and must pass it to graduate. He also says he plans to eat all night and drink a caffeinated soft drink to stay awake. He has asthma for which he uses Serevent and albuterol inhalers.

Pharmacist's Analysis

1. Is caffeine indicated for this type of problem?
2. Is his asthma a contraindication for caffeine?
3. Do his medications present any contraindication with caffeine?

Neither this patient's medications nor his disease state contraindicates use of nonprescription caffeine. However, non-

prescription products containing caffeine are only suitable for maintaining alertness when performing boring or repetitive activities and when the patient would normally be awake. Therefore, this proposed use, during a time when the patient would normally be asleep, is not suitable for these products. They are not indicated in those who wish to stay awake all night, and they do not substitute for sleep.

Patient Counseling

It would be best to advise the patient that lack of sleep likely will hamper his performance on the examination. Further, the adverse reactions of caffeine (e.g., urination and anxiety) also could have a negative impact on his performance. He should be encouraged to get a good night's rest and take his final with a clear head.

Fatigue and drowsiness affect a large percentage of the population.[1,2] Both problems are likely to affect people performing tasks they perceive as boring or routine. Unfortunately, some people find their jobs or automobile driving to be boring. Potentially fatal consequences may result from fatigue or drowsiness while driving or with certain jobs.

FATIGUE

Fatigue is synonymous with lethargy, tiredness, lassitude, being run down, or lack of energy. It has no standard definition shared by the lay public and the medical establishment, so many patients use it to denote related conditions such as simply a need for sleep.[3] Fatigue may be related to underlying medical diagnoses or treatment, but also may exist independent of any of these.[4,5] Fatigue is different from drowsiness, which is discussed below.

PREVALENCE OF FATIGUE

Fatigue may be the most common symptom of illness that manifests in both acute and chronic forms.[2] One-half of the subjects noticed fatigue when they first awakened in the morning, while one-fifth of subjects had experienced fatigue for 5 to 10 years and another fifth for greater than 10 years. Only 28% of patients are likely to improve, meaning that for them fatigue is a chronic problem.

EPIDEMIOLOGY OF FATIGUE

The incidence of fatigue varies by gender, with more females in one study being fatigued.[3] Patients who complain of fatigue do not exercise as much as patients who do not experience fatigue. Smokers tend to experience fatigue more than nonsmokers, and patients with a high body mass index also experience more fatigue.[3] Fatigue is the most common symptom reported by cancer patients.[6,7]

ETIOLOGY OF FATIGUE

Fatigue is a component of numerous conditions such as psychiatric illnesses, which account for many cases.[8–10] Other fatigue-related diagnoses include depression, stress, and anxiety.[8,11–13] Organic causes of fatigue include infection (e.g., mononucleosis, HIV), influenza-like illnesses, hypoglycemia, anemia, Parkinson's disease, systemic lupus erythematosus, circulatory disorders, pregnancy, hypertension, multiple sclerosis, fibromyalgia, and ischemic heart disease.[14–22] Several possible reasons for fatigue related to underlying conditions have been advanced such as disruption of the sleep-wake cycle or the hypothalamic-pituitary-adrenal axis.[23,24]

Caffeine produces central nervous system (CNS) stimulation with short-term use. However, continued use can result in fatigue, which may cause an increase in caffeine intake, further worsening the fatigue. The remedy for caffeine-induced fatigue is to discontinue the use of caffeine. (See "Hazards of Caffeine.")

Some patients suffer from a chronic fatigue, which reduces employability and increases use of health care services.[25] One version of this is a viral condition. (see "Chronic Fatigue Syndrome.")

TREATMENT OF FATIGUE

See "Treatment of Fatigue and Drowsiness."

PREVENTION OF FATIGUE

See "Prevention of Fatigue and Drowsiness."

DROWSINESS

As opposed to fatigue, drowsiness (or sleepiness) is the feeling that one has a need to sleep. Drowsiness may be seen as a continuum between full wakefulness and being fully asleep.[28] Drowsiness is normal and expected when individuals approach usual sleep times (as determined by each individual's 24-hour circadian cycle). This discussion concerns drowsiness that occurs at inappropriate times such as late morning or mid afternoon.

PREVALENCE OF DROWSINESS

Daytime drowsiness is not confined to insomniacs. Many people tend to become drowsy at certain times during the

FOCUS ON...

CHRONIC FATIGUE SYNDROME

Chronic fatigue syndrome (CFS) is a chronic mononucleosis in which patients exhibit several nonspecific complaints such as severe fatigue, weakness, malaise, subjective fever, sore throat, painful lymph nodes, decreased memory, confusion, depression, decreased ability to concentrate on tasks, and/or absence of objective physical or laboratory findings.[26,27] Complete recovery is rare.[26] In any case caffeine is not suggested; a physician visit should be suggested if the pharmacist suspects the presence of CFS.

day, from awakening (e.g., perhaps 6:00 or 7:00 AM) to about 10:00 AM and again from noon to 6:00 PM (Fig. 23.1).[29]

EPIDEMIOLOGY OF DROWSINESS

No data are available on the epidemiology of drowsiness, but it is assumed to be a widespread phenomenon that affects every person at some time. Elderly patients are known to complain of daytime drowsiness more than younger patients, probably related to sleep difficulties.[28]

ETIOLOGY OF DROWSINESS

A major cause of drowsiness is insufficient sleep[30] (see Chapter 24, "Sleep Disturbances"), since insomniacs exhibit impaired performance on tasks performed during daytime.[31] The greater the sleep debt incurred by an individual, the greater the likelihood that the individual will inadvertently fall asleep.[29] In addition, unintended

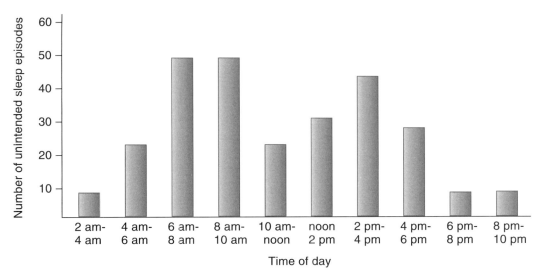

Figure 23.1. Unintentional sleep episodes during the day (summarized from several studies). Note that the sleepiness increases steadily from noon to 4:00 PM and then decreases. (Modified from Mitler MM, et al. Catastrophes, sleep, and public policy: Consensus report. Sleep 11:100, 1988.)

A Pharmacist's Journal

"My Wife Is Weaving on the Road."

A couple approached me at about 10:00 AM to ask about nonprescription stimulants. The husband said, "My wife is weaving on the road. What can she take to stay awake?" I discovered that they were moving from Chicago to Albuquerque, both driving rental moving trucks. They had left Chicago at 9:00 AM the day before, had slept no more than 3 to 4 hours, and now, she was becoming drowsy in western Oklahoma. I asked, "Do you mean the stretch of interstate just east of here?" The husband replied affirmatively, and I cringed. Because of construction, westbound traffic had been narrowed to one small lane. The narrow lane was a challenge even for a seasoned driver. I could well imagine the husband's concern if his wife was weaving back and forth, but particularly in a rental truck in that narrow lane.

I suggested NoDoz, telling him it was a caffeine-containing product that may help. "Do you really think it will help?" he asked. "My wife already drinks three pots of coffee a day." I agreed that this small additional amount might not provide any benefit. I suggested they stop for a nap, but they said they had to arrive that night. I gave them my best wishes and urged extreme caution.

sleeping is more likely if the person is required to be immobile.[29]

Drowsiness is also a side effect of many medications, both prescription and nonprescription. Further, it may be a symptom of 20 or more underlying medical disorders, including sleep apnea and narcolepsy.[32]

SPECIAL CONSIDERATIONS OF DROWSINESS

Drowsiness is potentially lethal, since unintentionally falling asleep prevents a person from performing critical activities such as driving.[33] (See "A Pharmacist's Journal: My Wife Is Weaving on the Road.") Falling asleep at the wheel is the second most common cause of fatal auto accidents, exceeded only by alcohol-related fatalities.[33,34] Accidents caused by drowsiness often are more severe because the sleeping driver does not attempt corrective maneuvers to lessen the severity of impact. Drowsiness-related auto accidents most commonly occur between 1:00 AM and 4:00 AM and between 1:00 PM and 4:00 PM.[29]

Errors in job performance also occur more commonly at these times. Drowsiness (perhaps occurring as a result of impaired or inadequate sleep) has been cited as partly or wholly to blame for the Three Mile Island and Chernobyl nuclear power plant disasters, the *Challenger* explosion, and the *Exxon Valdez* oil spill.[35]

TREATMENT OF DROWSINESS

See "Treatment of Fatigue and Drowsiness."

PREVENTION OF DROWSINESS

See "Prevention of Fatigue and Drowsiness."

FATIGUE AND DROWSINESS

For prevalence, epidemiology, and etiology of fatigue, see "Fatigue." For prevalence, epidemiology, etiology, and specific considerations of drowsiness, see "Drowsiness" above.

TREATMENT OF FATIGUE AND DROWSINESS

Treatment Guidelines

Caffeine, the only FDA-approved stimulant ingredient for treating fatigue and drowsiness, occurs naturally in some foods and beverages and is added to others.[36] It may produce its therapeutic effect through blockade of methylxanthine-sensitive adenosine receptors.[37] Before recommending caffeine, however, the pharmacist should attempt to discover the amount of caffeine the patient currently ingests. (Table 23.1, which gives average amounts of caffeine in various foods and beverages, can be used to estimate intake.) At least 20 to 30% of the population ingest 500 to 600 mg of caffeine daily.[38] The pharmacist should not recommend nonprescription products to patients who consume more than the FDA-recommended dosage, which is 100 to 200 mg not more often than every 3 to 4 hours. See Patient Assessment Algorithm 23.1 for the steps used to determine whether a nonprescription product is appropriate for the patient with a complaint of fatigue or drowsiness.

Table 23.1. Sources of Caffeine

CAFFEINE SOURCE	MILLIGRAMS OF CAFFEINE
Coffees[a]	
Espresso (7 ounces)	100
Decaffeinated (6 ounces)	2–8
Instant, regular (6 ounces)	35–169
Flavored instant (e.g., Cafe Vienna) (6 ounces)	40
Freeze-dried (5 ounces)	66
Percolated (5 ounces)	110
Drip (6 ounces)	70–215
Soft Drinks (12-ounce can)	
Pepsi Lite, Pepsi Free	0
7-Up, Diet 7-Up	0
Diet Sunkist Orange, Fanta Orange	0
Sprite, Fresca	0
Hires Root Beer	0
Diet Rite Cola	34
Pepsi-Cola, Diet Pepsi-Cola	35
Royal Crown Cola	36
Diet Dr. Pepper	37
Dr. Pepper	41
Shasta Cola, Sunkist Orange	42
Tab	44
Coca-Cola, Diet Coca-Cola	46
Mellow Yello	51
Diet Mr. Pibb	52
Mountain Dew	54
Josta (labeled as guarana)	58
Jolt	100
Teas	
Brewed (Most U.S. brands) (8 ounces)	20–90
Brewed (Imported) (8 ounces)	25–110
Iced (8 ounce glass)	9–50
Instant (8 ounces)	25–50
Foods	
Cocoa beverage (water mix; 6 ounce)	3–32
Milk chocolate (1 ounce)	1–15
Sweet/dark chocolate (1 ounce)	5–35
Baking chocolate (1 ounce)	26
Chocolate syrup (1 ounce)	13
Chocolate milk (8 ounces)	2–7

Adapted from references 81 through 84.

[a]Amounts of caffeine in cappuccino and latte may vary from coffee because of the addition of steamed milk and/or frothed milk.

Table 23.2. Representative Products for Fatigue and Drowsiness

PRODUCT	SELECTED INGREDIENTS
Caffedrine Timed Release	Caffeine, 200 mg
Maximum Strength NoDoz	Caffeine, 200 mg
NoDoz	Caffeine, 100 mg
Vivarin	Caffeine, 200 mg

Nonprescription Medications

INDICATIONS FOR CAFFEINE USE

Nonprescription stimulants are indicated for restoring mental alertness or wakefulness to patients suffering from fatigue or drowsiness[39] (Table 23.2). With the use of caffeine products, patients generally experience a clearer and more rapid flow of thought and feel reversal of drowsiness and fatigue.[34,40,41] It enhances the ability of patients to engage in physical activities such as swimming.[42,43]

A common reason for use of caffeine-containing nonprescription products is to help students to stay awake all night studying for examinations. *Pharmacists must strongly advise such purchasers that this is not an approved indication, that caffeine products are not a substitute for normal sleep in those who wish to stay awake rather than sleeping.*

The individual who lacks mental alertness because of insufficient sleep the previous night might benefit from caffeine, but this should be a short-term solution for an occasional problem.[44]

PRECAUTIONS IN CAFFEINE USE

Caffeine-containing stimulants must be labeled with the following precautions: "The recommended dose of this product contains about as much caffeine as a cup of coffee. Limit the use of caffeine-containing medications, foods, or beverages while taking this product because *too much caffeine may cause nervousness, irritability, sleeplessness, and, occasionally, rapid heart beat.*"[39] Labels must further caution potential users that *caffeine products are for occasional use only and will not substitute for sleep.* Should fatigue or drowsiness persist or continue to recur, patients should be advised to see a physician. Because of side effects and the potential for misuse, caffeine is a potentially hazardous ingredient in nonprescription products. For possible risks in the use of caffeine, see "Hazards of Caffeine."

DOSAGE OF CAFFEINE

Caffeine-containing stimulants are only to be used in patients age 12 and older. Recommended doses are 100 to 200 mg, not more often than every 3 to 4 hours.[39]

CAFFEINE WITHDRAWAL

Caffeine is an addictive drug.[45–47] This is perhaps the reason that moderate and heavy coffee drinkers do not reduce intake, even when confronted with clear evidence about its health risks.[48] Caffeine withdrawal presents a well-known set of symptoms, including headache and anxiety.[49,50] Other withdrawal symptoms include jitters, upset stomach, tiredness, lassitude, rhinorrhea, leg pains, diaphoresis, and general muscle pain.[51]

PREVENTION OF FATIGUE AND DROWSINESS

Fatigue and drowsiness may be prevented in many cases simply by obtaining sufficient rest and sleep.[52,53] While the amount of sleep is variable among individuals, the patient

Patient Assessment Algorithm 23.1. Fatigue and Drowsiness

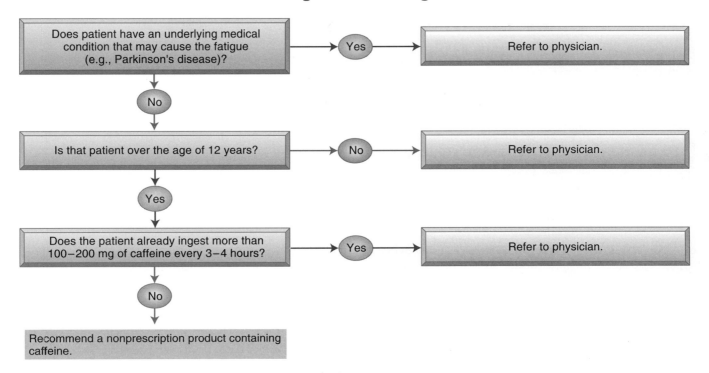

FOCUS ON...

HAZARDS OF CAFFEINE

Because caffeine is so widely used throughout the world, it has accumulated perhaps more reports of adverse reactions than any other nonprescription ingredient. Its widespread use also ensures that each new report is met with widespread consumer concern. While many reports implicate coffee or other caffeine-containing beverages, remember that caffeine is the major pharmacologic ingredient of these beverages. Its presence must be assumed to be causal unless a study with decaffeinated beverages as a control exonerates caffeine. Further, even though coffee and teas also contain other xanthines (e.g., theophylline and theobromine), caffeine is the most potent of these.[54]

Many of the reported associations (e.g., cancers) are preliminary, and some are contradicted by other research.

EPIDEMIOLOGY OF RECREATIONAL CAFFEINE INGESTION

Caffeine is the most widely consumed drug in the United States and Europe, making it *de facto* the most widely used stimulant.[54] At least 80% of Americans drink caffeinated beverages. American adults consume an average of 4 mg/kg of caffeine daily (1 mg/kg for those younger than 18 years of age).[55] Women generally drink more than men of the same age. However, men aged 40 to 49 are the exception, since they consume more caffeine than any other age group, male or female. People living on the West Coast drink more than those on the East Coast. Those drinking coffee tend to have less active leisure pursuits.[56]

CENTRAL NERVOUS SYSTEM EFFECTS

Of course, the primary reason caffeine is used is to stimulate the CNS.[57] Caffeine-naive subjects (those who do not regularly ingest caffeine) experience stimulation as caffeine approaches peak plasma levels, normally about 15 to 45 minutes after ingestion.[54,58] The effect is adrenal medullary stimulation, which releases epinephrine and norepinephrine. The catecholamine release is similar to that produced during the "fight or flight" reaction. However, with continued use the effect becomes less pronounced through the pharmacologic phenomenon known as tolerance.

Continued

Coffee drinkers do not show marked increased catecholamine levels after a test dose of caffeine. Over time, coffee drinkers who desire stimulation from caffeine generally must increase intake to achieve the same degree of stimulation, but tolerance ensures that this amount will also eventually become ineffective.[59] Thus patients may consume several caffeinated beverages each day (e.g., one or more liters of diet colas), either in an effort to reexperience the "high" or simply to reach a normal level of functioning.

Other than stimulation, caffeine also may produce a number of short-term effects, popularly known as caffeinism or "coffee nerves."[60] The syndrome, which occurs at doses of 200 to 500 mg of caffeine, includes headaches, tremors, nervousness, insomnia, agitation, and irritability.[49] (Caffeinism effects other than those on the central nervous system include arrhythmias, diuresis, palpitations, and flushing.) (See "A Pharmacist's Journal: Is There Anything That Will Keep Me Awake Without Dehydrating Me?") At doses above these, caffeine produces delirium and sensory disturbances.

Habitual caffeine use is reported to produce increased hostility, irritability, depression, panic attacks, stress, and anxiety.[61] Particularly, it can increase anxiety in stressful tasks.[61] (Anxiety can be so severe that one physician cautioned fellow practitioners not to "fall into the trap of prescribing benzodiazepines for the treatment of anxiety when the appropriate management is reduction of caffeine intake."[62]) Ingestion of large quantities of NoDoz (a nonprescription product) has been reported to induce acute psychosis.[62]

In one study decaffeinated coffee was secretly substituted for regular coffee in a closed ward of psychiatric patients.[58] To exclude rater bias, neither patients nor staff were informed of the switch. Reduced caffeine ingestion decreased patients' hostility, suspicion, and tension. Each of the measures reversed when the regular coffee was reintroduced secretly.

Continued caffeine intake can produce paradoxical drowsiness. In one series of six patients, pathologic sleepiness was only relieved after cessation of caffeine.[63] One of the patients drank 10 cups of coffee and two liters of cola drinks daily in an attempt to remedy the sleepiness that the caffeine itself was causing. The patients in this series took frequent naps, awakened unrefreshed, and fell asleep while driving and eating. Needless to add, their work was affected.

PREGNANCY-RELATED PROBLEMS

Scattered data indicate that caffeine may be responsible for pregnancy-related problems. For instance, caffeine and smoking may reduce fetal growth.[64] Spontaneous abortion is another possible effect, although it does not appear to be teratogenic.[65] Consideration of these and similar reports has prompted the FDA to warn pregnant women to avoid or minimize caffeine intake.[66]

EFFECTS ON THE HEART

Caffeine can increase heart rate, cardiac output, and the force of cardiac contractions. Blood pressure is usually increased with its use.[67] In one study caffeine (in a dose of 3.3 mg/kg, equivalent to 2 to 3 cups of coffee) elevated systolic blood pressures in both normotensive and mild hypertensive patients, increasing the workload on the heart.[68] Caffeine is associated with increased risk of myocardial infarction, premature ventricular beats, and other arrhythmias.[64] Those who drink more than 5 cups of coffee per day (approximately 687 mg) experience a modestly elevated risk of cardiac arrest.[69] Coffee use is strongly correlated with cigarette smoking, an association that is frustrating for epidemiologists, who must endeavor to discover the independent cardiac risks of smoking and caffeine.[58]

CARCINOGENICITY

Coffee may be causal in bladder and renal carcinoma.[64] Evidence for causation in pancreatic carcinoma has accumulated. Breast, ovarian, and bowel cancer may also be caused by caffeine.

GASTROINTESTINAL PROBLEMS

Caffeine increases output of stomach acid, although it does not appear to increase the risk of duodenal ulcer.[64] Caffeine also worsens gastroesophageal reflux.

CAFFEINE-INDUCED MORTALITY

Caffeine is deadly in overdose—which can range from a suicide attempt to child abuse.[70–75] In one case, for instance, a 20-year-old bulimic female ingested 20 g of caffeine in a suicide attempt, which caused a myocardial infarction.[72]

MISCELLANEOUS PROBLEMS

Caffeine is implicated in the following:

- Anemia[64]
- Increased risk of fractures caused by osteoporosis in middle-aged women[76–78]
- Dental fluorosis[79]
- More severe premenstrual syndrome symptoms[80]

A Pharmacist's Journal

"Is There Anything That Will Keep Me Awake Without Dehydrating Me?"

A man in his 30s came to the pharmacy window and asked, "Is there anything that will keep me awake without dehydrating me?" I told him that the only nonprescription stimulant we had was caffeine, which has a side effect of increasing urinary output. He said he wanted black pills like he bought one time because they didn't dry him out. I asked where he bought them. He said

he got them "somewhere." I assumed he might have purchased illegal stimulants (e.g, amphetamines). I then asked what he used them for. He said he routinely drives a tractor-trailer rig cross country, and he needs to stay awake for long stretches. However, since he could not get his black pills he had to use caffeine, and he didn't want to stop all of the time to urinate. I advised obtaining proper rest instead because all we had was caffeine.

AT THE COUNTER

 A male patient in his late teens asks for help staying awake on the job.

Interview/Patient Assessment

The patient is required to enter customer data on a company computer system for long stretches. He states, "This work is incredibly boring, but I need the job for my college tuition next year. I'm getting at least 8 hours of sleep at night since I'm living at home with my parents." He is taking Claritin for allergies and Orudis KT for a minor knee injury. He denies the use of any other medications, prescribed or recreational. He does not use caffeine in any form at the present time.

Pharmacist's Analysis

1. Is his request an approved use for nonprescription stimulants?
2. Could his medications cause drowsiness?
3. Is caffeine contraindicated for him?

This patient's medication regimen is not likely to be a cause

of his drowsiness; Claritin is a nonsedating antihistamine, and drowsiness is not common with Orudis KT. His sleep habits appear to be adequate. This patient seems to have simple drowsiness related to the nature of the work he is required to perform. Alleviating drowsiness resulting from this etiology is an approved use of nonprescription stimulants. Any of the caffeine-containing nonprescription products could be recommended. Alternatively, he might ingest a caffeinated beverage.

If the caffeine products are chosen, the patient should be cautioned not to ingest other caffeine-containing foods or beverages while taking the products. He should be warned that the products could cause nervousness, irritability, sleeplessness, and rapid heart beat. He should be instructed not to exceed the maximum dose of 100 to 200 mg every 3 to 4 hours.

Patient Counseling

Caffeine does not appear to be contraindicated for him and could be recommended.

should be urged to gradually increase sleep times until fatigue or drowsiness are no longer a problem. If this simple remedy is ineffective, other causes may be responsible.

Fatigue caused by infective agents cannot be prevented. Fatigue or drowsiness caused by excessive caffeine ingestion, however, can be prevented through caffeine withdrawal. To prevent fatigue or drowsiness resulting from insomnia or other sleep problems, the underlying condition must be treated. (See Chapter 24, "Sleep Disturbances.") In some in-

stances medication-induced drowsiness can be prevented by substituting alternative agents with a lower index of drowsiness under the advice of the physician.

SUMMARY

Fatigue and drowsiness are common problems that affect virtually everyone at some time or another. They may be related to infections, medication usage, or inadequate sleep. Caffeine is the only FDA-approved stimulant to combat fatigue and drowsiness. Used properly, caffeine can help restore mental alertness or wakefulness. However, used improperly, caffeine can cause such problems as nervousness, irritability, sleeplessness, and tachycardia.

The pharmacist should determine the patient's current caffeine intake prior to recommending a caffeine product, considering such sources as foods and beverages. The maximum safe dose is 100 to 200 mg, no more than every 3 to 4 hours. Unfortunately, many patients exceed these guidelines, and the excess caffeine may be responsible for fatigue or drowsiness. The widespread dietary and recreational overuse of caffeine (such as coffee consumption) is best treated by reducing caffeine ingestion rather than adding a nonprescription product. Further, recreational/dietary use is responsible for numerous physical and mental problems that could be helped by judicious pharmacist counseling regarding complete caffeine withdrawal.

References

1. Nail LM, Winningham ML. Fatigue and weakness in cancer patients: The symptoms experience. Semin Oncol Nurs 11:272, 1995.
2. Ream E, Richardson A. Fatigue: A concept analysis. Int J Nurs Stud 33:519, 1996.
3. Lichstein KL, et al. Fatigue and sleep disorders. Behav Res Ther 35:733, 1997.
4. Tiesinga LJ, Dassen TW, Halfens RJ. Fatigue: A summary of the definitions, dimensions, and indicators. Nurs Diagn 7:51, 1996.
5. Cook NF, Boore JR. Managing patients suffering from acute and chronic fatigue. Br J Nurs 6:811, 1997.
6. Yarbro CH. Interventions in fatigue. Eur J Cancer Care 5(2 Suppl):35, 1996.
7. Smets EM, et al. Fatigue in cancer patients. Br J Cancer 68:220, 1993.
8. Epstein KR. The chronically fatigued patient. Med Clin North Am 79:315, 1995.
9. Katerndahl DA. Differentiation of physical and psychological fatigue. Fam Pract Res J 13:81, 1993.
10. Cathebras PJ, et al. Fatigue in primary care: Prevalence, psychiatric comorbidity, illness behavior, and outcome. J Gen Intern Med 7:276, 1992.
11. Llewelyn MB. Assessing the fatigued patient. Br J Hosp Med 55:125, 1996.
12. Ridsdale L, et al. Patients with fatigue in general practice: A prospective study. BMJ 307:103, 1993.
13. Gift AG, Pugh LC. Dyspnea and fatigue. Nurs Clin North Am 28:373, 1993.
14. Mengshoel AM, Vollestad NK, Forre O. Pain and fatigue induced by exercise in fibromyalgia patients and sedentary healthy subjects. Clin Exp Rheumatol 13:477, 1995.
15. Bates DW, et al. Prevalence of fatigue and chronic fatigue syndrome in a primary care practice. Arch Intern Med 153:2759, 1993.
16. Darko DF, et al. Fatigue, sleep disturbance, disability, and indices of progression of HIV infection. Am J Psychiatry 149:514, 1992.
17. van Lier D, et al. Nausea and fatigue during early pregnancy. Birth 20:193, 1993.
18. Friedman J, Friedman H. Fatigue in Parkinson's disease. Neurology 43:2016, 1993.
19. Wysenbeek AJ, et al. Fatigue in systemic lupus erythematosus. Prevalence and relation to disease expression. Br J Rheumatol 32:633, 1993.
20. Hubsky EP, Sears JH. Fatigue in multiple sclerosis: Guidelines for nursing care. Rehabil Nurs 17:176, 1992.
21. Sandroni P, Walker C, Starr A. 'Fatigue' in patients with multiple sclerosis. Motor pathway conduction and event-related potentials. Arch Neurol 49: 517, 1992.
22. van Hilten JJ, et al. Sleep, excessive daytime sleepiness and fatigue in Parkinson's disease. J Neural Transm Park Dis Dement Sect 5:235, 1993.
23. Hickie I, et al. Is there a postinfection fatigue syndrome? Aust Fam Physician 25:1847, 1996.
24. Rosekind MR, et al. Managing fatigue in operational settings. I. Physiological considerations and countermeasures. Behav Med 21:157, 1996.
25. Bombardier CH, Buchwald D. Chronic fatigue, chronic fatigue syndrome, and fibromyalgia. Disability and health-care use. Med Care 34:924, 1996.
26. Bombardier CH, Buchwald D. Outcome and prognosis of patients with chronic fatigue vs chronic fatigue syndrome. Arch Intern Med 155:2105, 1995.
27. Komaroff AL. Clinical presentation of chronic fatigue syndrome. CIBA Found Symp 173:43, 1993.
28. Haimov I, Lavie P. Circadian characteristics of sleep propensity function in healthy elderly: A comparison with young adults. Sleep 20:294, 1997.
29. Mitler MM, et al. Catastrophes, sleep, and public policy: Consensus report. Sleep 11:100, 1988.
30. Hirvonen K, et al. The detection of drowsiness and sleep onset periods from ambulatory recorded polygraphic data. Electronecephalogr Clin Neurophysiol 102:132, 1997.
31. Aldrich CK, et al. Asleep at the wheel. Postgrad Med 80:233, 1986.
32. Weck E. A bedtime story. FDA Consumer 23(8):13, 1989.
33. Hansotia P. Sleep, sleep disorders and motor vehicle crashes. Wis Med J 96:42, 1997.
34. Horne JA, Reyner LA. Counteracting driver sleepiness: Effects of napping, caffeine, and placebo. Psychophysiology 33: 306, 1996.
35. Brown LK. Update on sleep disorders. Mt Sinai J Med 61:95, 1994.
36. Fed Reg 52:18923, 1987.
37. Sawynok J. Pharmacological rationale for the clinical use of caffeine. Drugs 49:37, 1995.
38. Mathew RJ, Wilson WH. Caffeine induced changes in cerebral circulation. Stroke 16:814, 1985.
39. Fed Reg 53:6100, 1988.
40. Lorist MM, et al. Aging, caffeine, and information processing: An event-related potential analysis. Electroencephalogr Clin Neurophysiol 96:453, 1995.
41. Pasman WJ, et al. The effect of different dosages of caffeine on endurance performance time. Int J Sports Med 16:225, 1995.
42. MacIntosh BR, Wright BM. Caffeine ingestion and performance of a 1,500 metre swim. Can J Appl Physiol 20:168, 1995.
43. Spriet LL. Caffeine and performance. Int J Sport Nutr 5(Suppl):S84, 1995.

Chapter 23 / Fatigue and Drowsiness

345

44. Wright KP Jr, et al. Combination of bright light and caffeine as a countermeasure for impaired alertness and performance during extended sleep deprivation. J Sleep Res 6:26, 1997.

45. Liguori A, Hughes JR. Caffeine self-administration in humans: 2. A within-subjects comparison of coffee and tea vehicles. Exp Clin Psychopharmacol 5:295, 1997.

46. Liguori A, Hughes JR, Oliveto AH. Caffeine self-administration in humans: 1. Efficacy of cola vehicle. Exp Clin Psychopharmacol 5:286, 1997.

47. Mitchell SH, De Wit H, Zacny JP. Caffeine withdrawal symptoms and self-administration following caffeine deprivation. Pharmacol Biochem Behav 51:941, 1995.

48. Weinstein ND. Reactions to life-style warnings: Coffee and cancer. Health Educ Q 12:129, 1985.

49. Schuh KJ, Griffiths RR. Caffeine reinforcement: The role of withdrawal. Psychopharmacology 130:320, 1997.

50. Couturier EG, et al. Influence of caffeine and caffeine withdrawal on headache and cerebral blood flow velocities. Cephalalgia 17:188, 1997.

51. Rogers PJ, Richardson NJ, Dernoncourt C. Caffeine use: Is there a net benefit for mood and psychomotor performance? Neuropsychobiology 31:195, 1995.

52. Rosekind MR, et al. Managing fatigue in operational settings. 2: An integrated approach. Behav Med 21:166, 1996.

53. Bonnet MH, et al. The use of caffeine versus prophylactic naps in sustained performance. Sleep 18:97, 1995.

54. Schneider JR. Effects of caffeine ingestion on heart rate, blood pressure, myocardial oxygen consumption, and cardiac rhythm in acute myocardial infarction patients. Heart Lung 16:167, 1987.

55. Barone JJ, Roberts HR. Caffeine consumption. Food Chem Toxicol 34:119, 1996.

56. Jacobsen BK, Thelle DS. The Tromso heart study: Is coffee drinking an indicator of a life style with high risk for ischemic heart disease? Acta Med Scand 222;215, 1987.

57. Linde L. Mental effects of caffeine in fatigued and non-fatigued female and male subjects. Ergonomics 38:864, 1995.

58. Henry JP, Stephens PM. Caffeine, stress, and cardiomyopathy. J SC Med Assoc 79:545, 1983.

59. Rogers PJ, Richardson NJ, Elliman NA. Overnight caffeine abstinence and negative reinforcement of preference for caffeine-containing drinks. Psychopharmacology 120:457, 1995.

60. Richardson NJ, et al. Mood and performance effects of caffeine in relation to acute and chronic caffeine deprivation. Pharmacol Biochem Behav 52:313, 1995.

61. Iancu I, Dolberg OT, Zohar J. Is caffeine involved in the pathogenesis of combat-stress reaction? Mil Med 161:230, 1996.

62. Roberts JA. Caffeine and disease (Letter). Med J Aust 155:275, 1991.

63. Regestein QR. Pathologic sleepiness induced by caffeine. Am J Med 87:586, 1989.

64. Etherton GM, Kochar MS. Coffee. Facts and controversies. Arch Fam Med 2:317, 1993.

65. Hinds TS, et al. The effect of caffeine on pregnancy outcome variables. Nutr Rev 54:203, 1996.

66. Lecos CW. Caffeine jitters: Some safety questions remain. FDA Consumer 21(10):22, 1987/1988.

67. Lotshaw SC, Bradley JR, Brooks LR. Illustrating caffeine's pharmacological and expectancy effects utilizing a balanced placebo design. J Drug Educ 26:13, 1996.

68. Sung BH, et al. Caffeine elevates blood pressure response to exercise in mild hypertensive men. Am J Hypertens 8(12 Pt 1):1184, 1995.

69. Weinmann S, et al. Caffeine intake in relation to the risk of primary cardiac arrest. Epidemiology 8:505, 1997.

70. Shum S, et al. Acute caffeine ingestion fatalities: Management issues. Vet Hum Toxicol 39:228, 1997.

71. Mrvos RM, et al. Massive caffeine ingestion resulting in death. Vet Hum Toxicol 31:571, 1989.

72. Forman J, Aizer A, Young CR. Myocardial infarction resulting from caffeine overdose in an anorectic woman. Ann Emerg Med 29:178, 199.7

73. Dietrich AM, Mortensen ME. Presentation and management of an acute caffeine overdose. Pediatr Emerg Care 6:296, 1990.

74. Fligner CL, Opheim KE. Caffeine and its dimethylxanthine metabolites in two cases of caffeine overdose: A cause of falsely elevated theophylline concentrations in serum. J Anal Toxicol 12:339, 1988.

75. Leson CL, McGuigan MA, Bryson SM. Caffeine overdose in an adolescent male. J Toxicol Clin Toxicol 26:407, 1988.

76. Hernandez-Avila M, et al. Caffeine, moderate alcohol intake, and risk of fractures of the hip and forearm in middle-aged women. Am J Clin Nutr 54:157, 1991.

77. Kiel DP, et al. Caffeine and the risk of hip fracture: The Framingham study. Am J Epidemiol 132:675, 1990.

78. Lloyd T, et al. Dietary caffeine intake and bone status of postmenopausal women. Am J Clin Nutr 65:1826, 1997.

79. Chan JT, Yip TT, Jeske AH. The role of caffeinated beverages in dental fluorosis. Med Hypotheses 33:21, 1990.

80. Rossignol AM, Bonnlander H. Caffeine-containing beverages, total fluid consumption, and premenstrual syndrome. Am J Public Health 80:1106, 1990.

81. Brooten D, Jordan CH. Caffeine and pregnancy. JOGN Nursing 12:190, 1983.

82. Lecos C. The latest caffeine scorecard. FDA Consumer 18(2):14, 1984.

83. Anon. Instant coffee. Consumer Reports 59(10):646, 1994.

84. Caffeine safety and labeling of foods & beverages: International Food Information Council. http://ificinfo.health.org/qanda/caflabel.html. 1998.

Sleep Disturbances

AT THE COUNTER

 A male patient asks for help with sleep-aids.

Interview/Patient Assessment

The patient, who is 47, states that he has had trouble sleeping for the past 2 to 3 days because of an impending divorce. He has just moved into an apartment and is concerned about his ability to meet his financial obligations. In response to a question about medical conditions, he lists allergies, which he is not treating at the present time, and glaucoma. For the glaucoma he uses pilocarpine 4% drops four times daily and levobunolol 0.5% twice daily. He has undergone two argon laser trabeculoplasties for the glaucoma. His intraocular pressures are now stabilized, although he suffered a 5% visual loss in one eye 4 years ago, before beginning treatment.

Pharmacist's Analysis

1. Is this patient's insomnia the type that is amenable to nonprescription products?
2. What is the significance of this patient's glaucoma?

3. Can this patient be treated with nonprescription products?

This patient's insomnia appears to be of the short-term type. It has not lasted for 2 weeks, so it potentially could be treated with a nonprescription product. However, this patient has glaucoma, which is a contraindication to the use of nonprescription antihistamines. Some pharmacists argue that narrow-angle (angle-closure) glaucoma is the only true contraindication and that patients with open-angle glaucoma should be able to use these products. The problem with this reasoning is that the glaucoma patient may not be aware of the type of glaucoma and may guess incorrectly.

Patient Counseling

The pharmacist should advise the patient that all nonprescription products for insomnia are contraindicated with a diagnosis of glaucoma and should suggest that the patient speak with his eye-care practitioner prior to using these products. Alternatively, the pharmacist might call the patient's eye-care practitioner to obtain clarification prior to a product recommendation.

Sleep occupies approximately one-third of our lives.[1] Fortunately, most people sleep well most of the time. To obtain the full benefit from sleep and to prevent sleep deprivation, an individual must obtain adequate sleep and must cycle through the stages of sleep in a normal manner.[2,3]

For most people past the age of adolescence, 8 hours of sleep is adequate. During this time the person's normal sleep architecture should be divided into two phases: rapid eye movement (REM) sleep and non–rapid eye movement (NREM) sleep.[2,4] REM sleep is characterized by several features:

- Rapid eye movements beneath the eyelids
- Muscle twitching
- Changes in blood pressure and heart rate
- The majority of dream time

NREM sleep differs from REM sleep in the following manner:

- Physiologic activity is generally reduced.
- Brain activity, heart rate, blood pressure, and respiratory rates drop.
- There is comparatively little dream time.

NREM sleep is also subdivided into several stages, according to electroencephalographic patterns:

- Stage 1 is usually a brief period between wakefulness and sleep.

- Stage 2 bridges the gap between Stage 1 and the deeper sleep stages.
- Stages 3 and 4 give the body the greatest amount of rest.

Whenever the quality or quantity of either of these is affected (e.g., through the use of prescription hypnotics), the patient may experience symptoms.[5]

Several sleep disorders affect either the quality or quantity of sleep. They include insomnia, which may be amenable to self-treatment. All other sleep disorders such as narcolepsy, sleep apnea, and restless legs syndrome should be referred to a physician, who may recommend a sleep disorder clinic[6] (Fig. 24.1).

INSOMNIA

Insomnia is the most common sleep disorder and has several subtypes.[7] With the possible exception of daytime drowsiness (see Chapter 23), insomnia is the only sleep disturbance treatable with nonprescription products.

The term "insomnia" is often misunderstood, with the result that the stereotypical insomniac is a wide-awake individual who cannot sleep at all.[8,9] Arbitrary definitions may also include assessment information such as restricting the diagnosis to patients whose **sleep latency time** (the period from lying down to actually falling asleep) exceeds 30 minutes and

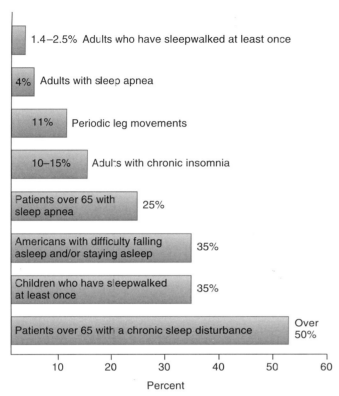

Figure 24.1. The percentage of patients with certain sleep disorders.

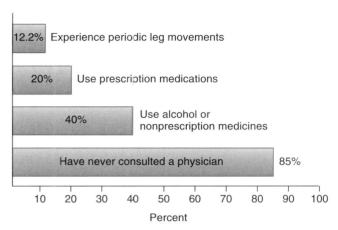

Figure 24.2. Qualities of patients with insomnia.

whose **sleep efficiency** (the percentage of time in bed that one is actually asleep) is less than 85%.[10] Medically, the term indicates unusual difficulty falling asleep and sleeping, sleep that is unusually disturbed, or sleep that causes the individual to suffer from residual daytime tiredness.[2,8] Insomnia is classified as severe when the problem occurs nearly every night.[11]

In diagnosing insomnia it is vital to rule out patients who may be worried because they cannot sleep a total of 8 hours, as the popular press often recommends. As long as these individuals feel rested and energetic the following day, the sleep they did get was sufficient for them. They are referred to as "short sleepers."[8]

PREVALENCE OF INSOMNIA

A 1991 Gallup Poll concluded that 36% of adults in the United States are affected with insomnia, mostly with intermittent episodes.[8,12] This figure is almost identical to those obtained in Europe and Australia.[13,14] Almost half of those who report insomnia state that they are bothered by it a great deal.[11,15] About 5% of all adults have chronic insomnia; the problem is so severe in 0.1% of the United States population that they require medication for insomnia frequently, if not nightly.[15]

Most people who suffer from insomnia do not seek medical care[6,8] (Fig. 24.2). (See "Historical Lack of Treatment for

Insomnia.") Thus estimates of the incidence of insomnia derived from such data are probably low.

EPIDEMIOLOGY OF INSOMNIA

At some time virtually everyone is affected with insomnia.[2] Insomnia affects both sexes and occurs in all ages, racial categories, and socioeconomic strata.[2] Some associations with certain demographic variables do exist, however. The disorder does occur with higher frequency in females.[2,14,16] In addition, females are more likely to see a physician and to use medications for insomnia.[11,17] The majority of insomnia sufferers are elderly women.[18] (In one survey of patients aged over 65, 8% of men as opposed to 18% of women used hypnotics regularly.[18])

Age is another variable strongly associated with insomnia.[1,11,19,20] Perhaps 50% of older patients experience some type of chronic sleep disturbance, often associated with poor physical health and pain.[21–23] As many as 66% of elderly people living in institutions have insomnia.[12] As a result of this age-related sleep disorder, elderly people take more medications for insomnia and correspondingly experience a greater number of adverse reactions because of them than the general population.[24,25] Insomnia in the aged patient is more often refractory to hypnotics.[24] The elderly not only wake more often during sleep, but take four times longer to fall asleep again.[21]

As many as 74 to 98% of patients with idiopathic Parkinson's disease experience insomnia because of difficulties associated with the condition such as limb or facial dystonia and other problems such as nocturia and painful leg cramps.[26]

ETIOLOGY OF INSOMNIA

During a typical year 80% of adults will suffer from insomnia of less than 2 weeks' duration.[27] Whether the pharmacist can advise self-treatment of insomnia with nonprescription products depends in part on the duration of the problem. Insomnia may occur on one night, causing nothing more than residual tiredness the following day and not interfering with a normal sleep the next night.[8] However, insomnia may persist for several days, weeks, months, or even years. Because of this wide time span, it is useful to divide insomnia into several categories[11,12]:

- Transient (lasting less than 7 days)
- Short term (lasting from 7 days to 3 weeks)
- Long term (lasting more than 3 weeks)

Transient Insomnia

With transient insomnia, patients usually have had no previous sleep complaints.[12] The causes include acute stress, environmental disturbances, and time zone changes.[8,15] Acute stress may be caused by such anxiety-producing events as an examination in school, upcoming surgical procedure, or marital strife.[28] Environmental disturbances include sleeping in an unfamiliar bed, excess noise or light, extremes in weather, or sleeping in a room that is too hot or cool.[29] Eating a large meal or drinking alcohol before bedtime are also possible causes of insomnia.[2,12] Circumstances such as these normally cause insomnia for no more than a few days. Transient insomnia usually responds well to the principles of sleep hygiene, discussed under "Prevention of Insomnia."[12] It may be helpful to recommend nonprescription sleep-aids or to refer patients to their physicians for a short course of prescription benzodiazepine therapy.[6,12]

Short-Term Insomnia

Short-term insomnia is caused by more severe stressors such as loss of a job, starting a new job, one's own illness, illness or death of a family member or friend, upcoming marriage or divorce, moving to a new area, severe financial difficulties, or guilt over sexual conflicts related to going to bed with one's sleep partner.[2,12] Since these problems do not resolve rapidly, they may cause insomnia for longer periods as the person continues to worry about them.[30] This type of insomnia also responds well to sleep hygiene measures (see "Prevention of Insomnia"), especially avoiding stimulants such as caffeine and nicotine.[12] The patient also may benefit from nonprescription sleep-aids or benzodiazepine therapy.[12]

FOCUS ON...

HISTORICAL LACK OF TREATMENT FOR INSOMNIA

Although insomnia is quite common, many patients do not see a physician because of it.[6] Only about 5% of patients with insomnia make an appointment with the physician to discuss that specific problem.[2,8] Another 26% of patients with insomnia visited the physician for another problem, but mentioned insomnia almost as an afterthought.[8,16] These figures lead one to the conclusion that the majority of insomniacs (the remaining 69%) do not feel that the problem should be handled by physicians or with the use of a prescription medication. Perhaps they consider insomnia a routine problem to be dealt with on one's own.[2] As alarming as these percentages are, the problem may be even worse. A United States Senate commission estimated that only one out of every 250 patients with insomnia discusses the issue with a physician.[6]

Research verifies that physicians rarely ask about insomnia or other sleep disturbances.[8] In fact, one geriatric physician was quoted as stating, "I never ask my patients about sleep difficulties for fear they may answer me."[16] Another physician noted that the reluctance of physicians to ask about sleep difficulties may be caused by scheduling demands that do not allow for time-intensive questioning, pessimism regarding treatment success, or lack of interest and/or training.[8,13] A random survey of physicians revealed that even when the complaint is brought to their attention, history taking is minimal, and the usual reaction is to prescribe hypnotics.[11] (These observations regarding insufficient patient contact time become more critical in light of the impact of managed care on physician-patient consultation time, which requires the physician to see more patients per hour to increase the profit margin.)

Long-Term Insomnia

Long-term insomnia may be caused by underlying medical pathology (e.g., sleep apnea, need to urinate, restless legs syndrome, nocturnal myoclonus, cluster headache, pain from rheumatic disease or dental problems, angina, or peptic ulcer), use or abuse of sedative-hypnotics or narcotics, illegal drugs, or alcohol.[2,12,13,27,31–37] Psychiatric/psychologic disorders such as depression, obsessive worrying, persistent hypochondria, panic disorder, obsessive-compulsive disorder, anorexia nervosa, dementia, and phobias can all produce chronic insomnia.[2,38–40] Chronic insomnia may be caused by an acute stressor, and then persist as a habit.[41,42]

Chronic psychophysiologic insomnia ("learned insomnia") is a variant of long-term insomnia.[10,12,15,43] In this behavioral condition the patient does not associate the bedroom with sleep, but with lack of sleep or rest.[12,41] As bedtime approaches, the typical patient begins to experience anxiety related to the amount of sleep they will lose during the sleep cycle. If sleep does not come on as rapidly as the patient thinks it should, a cascade of worries is triggered such as how they will look, feel, or act the next day; whether they will be able to work as they must; and what the quality and quantity of that work will be.[13] Thus this type of insomnia is a pernicious vicious cycle in which the more one worries about lack of sleep, the less likely one is to sleep.[6] A key that this process underlies the insomnia is the patient volunteering the information that he or she sleeps well when away from home or on vacation.[12] Patients may also fall asleep during class or when watching television, but be unable to sleep in bed a short time after the nap.[10,44]

(tip) *Nonprescription products are inappropriate for long-term insomnia because the etiology should be determined, perhaps through referral to a sleep laboratory.[11,41]* Then, depending on the etiology, treatment may consist of surgery (e.g., correction of a physiologic cause of sleep apnea), behavioral therapy, or prescription medications.

SPECIFIC CONSIDERATIONS OF INSOMNIA

The consequences of insomnia are dependent on its duration. Intermittent, transient insomnia usually causes little disturbance for most individuals. However, the effects of repeated episodes of short-term insomnia or long-term insomnia can be devastating.

Since the purpose of sleep is to prepare the patient for the next day, it is axiomatic that the first effects of insomnia will show up then.[45] Typically, the patient who has not slept well the previous night feels fatigued, tired, jittery, irritable, anxious, not refreshed, confused, and unable to concentrate.[1,8,44,46]

Chronic insomnia adversely affects an individual's psychosocial health by increasing psychologic distress, reducing the quality of family and social relationships, and producing a greater awareness of one's somatic problems.[47] It also decreases one's occupational viability by increasing the rates of job-related injuries and industrial errors.[6,27,48] Increased susceptibility to illness with chronic insomnia culminates in the finding that these individuals utilize more health-care resources and take more sick leave than people who sleep normally.[6,47] Chronic insomnia is also a predictor for major depression.[49]

Daytime sleepiness can be devastating.[50,51] Those with chronic insomnia report lowered daytime functioning.[47] Automobile collisions occur with greatest frequency when the circadian rhythm is at its peak for producing sleep (e.g., between 4:00 AM and 6:00 AM and between 2:00 PM and 4:00 PM), resulting in thousands of injuries and deaths and billions of dollars in damages.[2,44,48] A British study found that 30% of automobile accidents were caused by falling asleep while driving; 85% involved fatalities.[6] In the United States fatigue resulting from sleep deprivation is partly or wholly responsible for 57% of deadly truck accidents and 10% of fatal car accidents, costing 56 billion dollars yearly.[45] Drowsiness (perhaps occurring as a result of insomnia) was thought to be partly or wholly to blame for the Three Mile Island and Chernobyl nuclear power plant disasters, the *Challenger* explosion, and the Exxon *Valdez* oil spill[48,52] (Fig. 24.3).

TREATMENT OF INSOMNIA

Treatment Guidelines

Because of the general reticence to seek physician consultation, pharmacists questioned about insomnia should suggest physician evaluation if the guidelines for nonprescription products are exceeded (e.g., use in excess of 2 weeks).[53] Pharmacists also can help patients by discussing the principles of sleep hygiene (see "Prevention of Insomnia"). For an overview of the steps used in helping patients with insomnia, see Patient Assessment Algorithm 24.1.

Nonprescription Medications

SINGLE-ENTITY INSOMNIA PRODUCTS

In 1989 the FDA completed the review of nonprescription sleep-aids such as those products listed in Table 24.1. They are safe and effective when used for the following[31]:

- Reducing the time to fall asleep if the patient has difficulty doing so
- Relieving occasional sleeplessness
- Reducing difficulty falling asleep

Children with sleep disorders should be referred, since the most appropriate therapy is behavioral intervention and (tip) supportive treatment.[54,55] *Nonprescription sleep-aids should not be used by patients younger than 12.* In addition, these products are not appropriate if sleeplessness persists continuously for more than 2 weeks.[56] (See "A Pharmacist's Journal: What Do You Have for a Child Who Just Wants to Play?")

(tip)   The label on these products cautions that *insomnia may be a symptom of a serious underlying medical illness.* The label also warns against use in individuals who have a breathing problem (such as emphysema or chronic bronchitis), glaucoma, or difficulty in urination caused by enlargement of the prostate gland.[57] The label cautions against use of alcoholic beverages while using the products. It also states, "Do not take this product if you are taking sedatives or tranquilizers without first consulting your doctor." Finally, the label bears the general warning against use in pregnancy and by nursing females.[56]

Diphenhydramine in a dose of 50 mg at bedtime is the only ingredient approved as a sleep-aid through the FDA OTC Review process.[56] Doxylamine is also marketed as a sleep-aid through an approved new drug application. Both diphenhydramine and doxylamine are ethanolamine antihistamines with a pronounced tendency to sedate the patient. Unfortunately, they also possess atropine-like anticholinergic effects, although the incidence of gastrointestinal symptoms is low.

ANTIHISTAMINE/ANALGESIC COMBINATION PRODUCTS

Manufacturers are marketing a number of products that combine a sleep-aid with an analgesic (Table 24.2). The FDA has allowed these combinations to remain on the market pending a final decision regarding their efficacy.[56] The agency is concerned that an appropriate population for use of these products may not exist. The pharmacist should only recommend this combination to the patient who has sleeplessness combined with occasional minor aches, pains, and headaches.

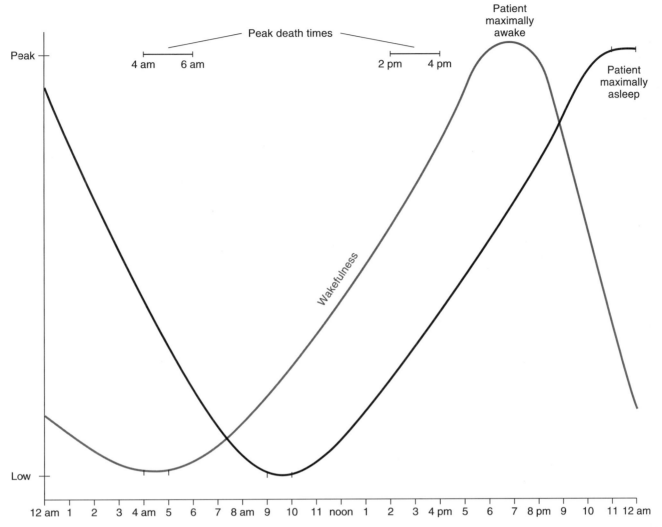

Figure 24.3. The circadian drives for sleep and wakefulness provide clues for the peak times for all causes of death. Death occurs most often in the midst of the sleep-wakefulness cycles.

ALTERNATIVE THERAPIES

Other supposed remedies for insomnia lack proof of safety and/or efficacy, although many are sold with the promise of helping alleviate insomnia.

Melatonin

Melatonin is a naturally occurring human hormone that is evidently linked to circadian cycles.[58] Sold as a nonprescription item, it is widely touted for insomnia but proof of safety and efficacy are lacking.[58-60] This hormone is widely available in pharmacies and health-food stores and through Internet sites. In one study 5 mg of melatonin was administered to patients with psychophysiologic insomnia for 1 week. It was of no value when compared with placebos and caused headache and an objectionable taste in the mouth.[61]

Valerian

Valerian is an herb widely promoted in health-food stores and on the Internet as a sleep-aid. However, a search of the American medical literature (Medline) reveals only four citations during the period from 1990 to 1998. One is a review of European plants.[62] Another is a German study of fourteen elderly patients who seemed to demonstrate an increase in slow-wave sleep with valerian 405 mg three times daily.[63] However, of the final two studies, one describes valerian as benign in overdose, but the other implicates it as a possible cause of hepatotoxicity, central nervous system depression, and anticholinergic reactions.[64,65] Since its safety and efficacy remain to be demonstrated, it should not be recommended for any use.

Miscellaneous Alternative Therapies

Accessing the Internet brings a host of information on supposed treatments for insomnia. They include chamomile, hops, passion flower, skullcap, germanium, and homeopathic arsenic and crude coffee. None of these have been proven safe and effective in preventing or treating insomnia.

Patient Assessment Algorithm 24.1. Insomnia

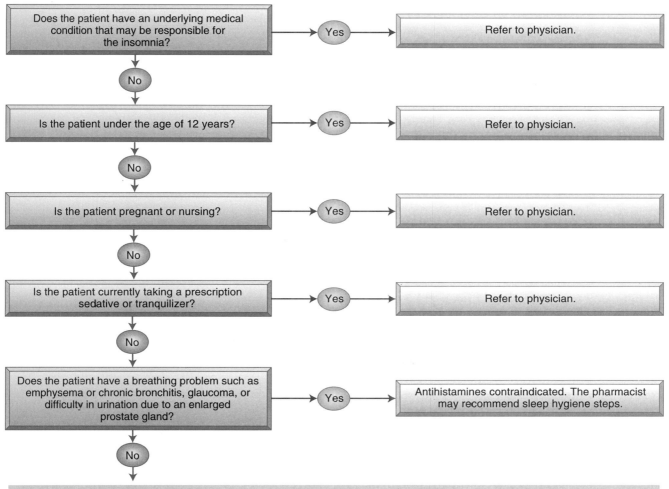

PREVENTION OF INSOMNIA: SLEEP HYGIENE

Sleep hygiene refers to patient behaviors and practices that affect sleep. Improper sleep hygiene can cause stimulation, preventing or delaying the onset of sleep, or disorganizing sleep.[15,66] Discussing sleep-inhibitive factors with a patient could help resolve the insomnia, obviating the need for prescription or nonprescription medications.[67]

The Role of Medications and Food

Many medications can cause insomnia, including propranolol, antiarrhythmics, oral contraceptives, methyldopa, theophylline, thyroid supplements, and fluoxetine.[15] However, patients should always check with their physician prior to discontinuing medications suspected of causing insomnia. *Patients may not be aware of nonprescription medications that stimulate the central nervous system* such as oral nasal decongestants, topical nasal decongestants, diet products containing phenylpropanolamine, certain antihistamines (e.g., phenindamine), and antiasthmatics. *The*

pharmacist selling any of these products (e.g., a nonprescription oral decongestant containing pseudoephedrine) should caution the patient not to take the product too close to bedtime, unless previous experience has demonstrated that it does not cause a problem for them.

Since hunger can inhibit sleep, patients should be advised not to go to bed hungry.[2] However, a heavy meal taken too close to bedtime can also inhibit sleep, perhaps through causing gastroesophageal reflux. The last meal should end by 6:00 to 7:00 PM if the bedtime is 10:30 to 11:00 PM.

Caffeine, Nicotine, Alcohol, and Drugs of Abuse

Caffeine is a major cause of insomnia.[10,15] For patients with insomnia, caffeine should be avoided completely after noon.[11] This includes chocolate, cola drinks, coffee, tea, and all other foods and drinks containing caffeine (e.g., certain root beer or orange drinks).[2] (See Table 23.1.)

Nicotine also causes CNS stimulation.[2,15] Patients should avoid cigarettes, cigars, chewing tobacco, snuff, and all other forms of nicotine.

Table 24.1. Representative Insomnia Products

PRODUCT	SELECTED INGREDIENTS/COMMENTS
Calms Forte Tablets	Per 4-grain tablet: Passion flower 1X triple strength, oat 1X double strength, hops 1X double strength, chamomile 2X, calcium phosphate 3X, iron phosphate 3X, potassium phosphate 3X, sodium phosphate 3X, magnesium phosphate 3X; a homeopathic product lacking proof of efficacy
Compoz	Diphenhydramine HCl 50 mg
Mile's Nervine	Diphenhydramine HCl 25 mg
Nytol	Diphenhydramine HCl 25 mg
Nytol Maximum Strength	Doxylamine succinate 25 mg
Nytol Natural	Equal parts ignatia ama (St. Ignatius' Bean) 3X, Aconitum radix (Aconite root) 6X; a homeopathic formula lacking proof of efficacy
Sleep-Eze 3	Diphenhydramine HCl 25 mg
Sleepinal Capsules	Diphenhydramine HCl 50 mg
Sleepinal Softgels	Diphenhydramine HCl 50 mg
Sominex	Diphenhydramine HCl 25 mg
Unisom	Doxylamine succinate 25 mg
Unisom SleepGels	Diphenhydramine HCl 50 mg

A Pharmacist's Journal

"What Do You Have for a Child Who Just Wants to Play?"

A man in his 20s asked me, "What do you have for a child who just wants to play?" I told him the toy section was in another part of the store. He said, "No, I mean my child won't go to sleep. He just wants to play." In response to my question regarding age, he told me the child was only 18 months old. I told him that this is a time of child curiosity and high energy in which the child will naturally want to play with his parents and learn about the world. He said, "I understand that, but can't we give him something to put him to sleep because we're losing out on our sleep. He would play all night if he could." I told him he should see a pediatrician since our sleep products are only for adult insomnia and are not to be used for patients younger than 12.

Alcohol is a common cause of insomnia, although it is often used to facilitate sleep.[68] About 12% of patients complaining of chronic insomnia are alcohol users.[15] While alcohol initially does induce sleep, during the second half of the night, heavy drinkers often are subjected to more awakenings than normal.[2,10,15] Withdrawal from alcohol addiction also causes insomnia.[35]

Drugs of abuse may also cause insomnia since many have stimulant properties such as the amphetamines. Illegal drugs such as marijuana reduce the efficiency of sleep and may induce insomnia.

Daytime Behaviors

Regardless of how sleepy patients are following a night of insomnia, they should not nap at all during the day.[11,69] Engaging in regular, moderate exercise around midday or in the early evening has been found to facilitate sleep.[1,11,70] Many people go to bed and arise at odd hours or whenever the mood strikes them, a lack of routine that plays havoc with the internal circadian rhythms. To foster proper sleep, it is desirable to go to sleep and arise at the same times each day, so the body will adjust to getting the same hours of sleep each night.[11,69]

Table 24.2. Representative Antihistamine/Analgesic Combination Products

PRODUCT	SELECTED INGREDIENTS/COMMENTS
Alka-Seltzer PM	Aspirin 325 mg, diphenhydramine citrate 38 mg (an unapproved combination in an effervescent tablet)
Bayer Extra Strength PM	Aspirin 500 mg, diphenhydramine HCl 25 mg (an unapproved combination)
Doan's P.M.	Magnesium salicylate 467.2 mg, diphenhydramine HCl 25 mg (an unapproved combination)
Doan's P.M. Extra Strength	Aspirin 500 mg, diphenhydramine HCl 25 mg (an unapproved combination)
Excedrin P.M.	Acetaminophen 500 mg, diphenhydramine citrate 38 mg; an unapproved combination
Sominex Pain Relief Formula	Acetaminophen 500 mg, diphenhydramine HCl 25 mg; an unapproved combination
Tylenol PM	Acetaminophen 500 mg, diphenhydramine HCl 25 mg; an unapproved combination
Unisom with Pain Relief	Acetaminophen 650 mg, diphenhydramine HCl 50 mg; an unapproved combination

In addition, an hour or so should be set aside before bedtime to wind down from the day and allow relaxation.[1,11,71] Working on stressful tasks up to the point of sleep does not allow the body to begin to rest.[10] The patient should go to bed only when truly sleepy.[69]

After several days of implementation of sleep hygiene, sleepiness at bedtime should become natural.[11]

The Role of the Bedroom

The bedroom should be comfortable and present a sense of security to the patient (with the use of locks on doors if necessary).[11] It should not be used for anything except sleep and sexual activity.[11,69] The patient should not read or watch television in the bedroom (unless these consistently make that particular patient sleepy).[1] It should not be used for marital squabbles. The bedroom temperature should avoid extremes and the room itself should be kept quiet.[2,10] Darken the room to minimize visual stimulation.[10]

After Lying Down

The patient should try not worry about the day behind or the day ahead.[1,69] *If the patient is unable to sleep within 10 minutes after going to bed, he or she should simply get up and engage in a nonstimulating activity such as reading or watching television.*[11] When the patient becomes sleepy again, he or she should attempt to sleep, but repeat the 10-minute rule as many times as needed.[11] If the patient cannot sleep after several hours, it should be remembered that most people usually cope fairly well after a night with no sleep (as opposed to excessively worrying about the coming day).[1]

NARCOLEPSY AND HYPERSOMNIA

Narcolepsy is traditionally thought of as sudden episodes of sleep, but the condition can be more involved than that simple perception.[72] As a syndrome, narcolepsy includes a tetrad of symptoms: sleepiness, cataplexy, hallucinations, and sleep paralysis.[73] The sleepiness may be most severe in a boring situation, or may suddenly appear in a dangerous situation such as when driving.[15] Cataplexy, considered pathognomonic for narcolepsy, is a condition in which strong emotion such as laughing causes a weakness of the musculature. The patient may feel it as a weakness of the knees when laughing. In the worst cases the patient may collapse and appear nonresponsive for a short period.

Hallucinations associated with narcolepsy occur either when falling asleep or awakening and may be accompanied by sleep paralysis in which the patient is unable to move.

Hypersomnia is different from narcolepsy in that it does not occur as part of the tetrad of narcoleptic symptoms. Further, episodes of sleep are not irresistible, but are nevertheless prolonged and excessive.[72]

OBSTRUCTIVE SLEEP APNEA

Sleep apnea is the most dangerous sleep-related problem, possibly causing cardiovascular morbidity and mortality, as well as persistent insomnia and drowsiness in the daytime in some cases.[13,72,74–75] It occurs in an many as 4% of adults.[76] The prototypical patient is a male adult whose sleeping partner complains that he snores extremely loudly. The patient has no trouble falling asleep at the beginning of the night, but is awakened many times during the night without knowing why. The cause is a narrowed upper airway that allows pharyngeal airway collapse during sleep.[76] There may be as many as 10 incidents lasting over 10 seconds each hour. The impeded breathing causes the patient to awaken. Treatment may involve surgery, tricyclic antidepressants, or benzodiazepines.

RESTLESS LEGS SYNDROME

Restless legs syndrome may result from genetic causes, pregnancy, or iron deficiency anemia, as well as various other factors.[43] On becoming relaxed and sleepy, this patient begins to experience an uncomfortable feeling in the lower legs, similar to ants crawling under the skin.[77] It is relieved only by moving the legs or walking, which inhibits sleep.[78] The condition can prevent the patient from falling asleep for a long period. About one-half of patients with restless legs syndrome also experience periodic limb movements during sleep, a related condition discussed below.

PERIODIC LIMB MOVEMENTS

In contrast to the patient with restless legs syndrome, the patient with periodic limb movements does not experience difficulty in falling asleep, but cannot maintain restful sleep because of limb movements that occur during sleep.[13,79] The bed partner describes a certain pattern of stereotyped repetitive movements of the limbs, most commonly the legs.[15] The legs may move so consistently in these patterns that they produce repeated periodic limb movements during sleep, disrupting sleep to the point of causing daytime sleepiness.[72] Short-acting benzodiazepines may be helpful.[13]

ADVANCED AND DELAYED SLEEP-PHASE SYNDROMES

With advanced sleep-phase syndrome, the patient falls asleep in the early evening, but awakens in the early morning, a common problem in the elderly.[13,80,81] Exposure to light at the end of the day may allow the patient to delay sleeping until a more appropriate time.[82]

The typical patient with delayed sleep-phase syndrome complains of inability to fall asleep until perhaps 2:00 to 3:00 AM, coupled with extreme difficulty awakening to attend school or work.[13] They may sleep uninterrupted on a weekend until noon. Younger adults and adolescents are the usual victims and may be helped with chronotherapy in which the sleep times are advanced by 3 hours daily, until the patient is able to sleep at the desirable time. The treatment is approximately 1 week in length and difficult for the family.

NOCTURNAL WANDERING

Episodes of nocturnal wandering ("sleepwalking," perhaps associated with "night terrors") usually begin in childhood.[83–85] The patient appears unresponsive, walking in a clumsy manner through the house, perhaps stumbling over objects, threatening those who are in their way, making decisive gestures such as trying to escape, and at times carrying out activities such as mistaking a closet door for the exit.[86] The patient may injure himself or others in the episode. When awakened, the patient usually relates a nightmare in which there is a threat to the subject or a loved one (such as a fire, earthquake, burglary, being buried alive). Treatment includes benzodiazepines, counseling, and measures to provide a safe sleeping environment.[87]

SUMMARY

Patients experience a wide variety of sleep disorders, the most common being insomnia. Insomnia is a common condition that refers to unusual difficulty in falling asleep, unusually disturbed sleep, or sleep that causes a residual daytime tiredness. The condition is more common in older patients and in females. Pharmacists should discuss the various sleep hygiene

AT THE COUNTER

A college-aged student is concerned about his sleeplessness.

Interview/Patient Assessment

This patient has an upcoming medical-school admissions examination for which he has been preparing strenuously. He has slept poorly for the previous week. He is taking stress vitamins and wants to know if they could be causing the problem. He is not taking any other medications and denies any medical problems.

Pharmacist's Analysis

1. Is this student's insomnia the type for which nonprescription sleep-aids are approved?
2. Could his vitamins be contributing to the problem?
3. Are nonprescription sleep-aids appropriate for him?

This student appears to have typical short-term (transient) insomnia for which nonprescription sleep-aids are approved. His insomnia is probably related to the upcoming examination. His stress-vitamin usage is irrational since no vitamin or mineral has been found effective in helping prevent or treat stress; however, the vitamin combination is probably not contributing to the problem.

Patient Counseling

The patient should be shown the single-entity nonprescription products since he has none of the conditions that contraindicate their use (e.g., emphysema, chronic bronchitis, glaucoma, difficulty in urination caused by an enlargement of the prostate gland). The products may only be used for insomnia of less than 2 weeks' duration; since the insomnia has persisted for 1 week, he may only self-treat for 1 additional week. If the insomnia continues beyond that point, he should see a physician.

steps that may alleviate insomnia with patients such as the roles of medications and food, caffeine, nicotine, alcohol, drugs of abuse, daytime behaviors, the role of the bedroom, and steps to institute when trying to go to sleep. Should interventions based on sleep hygiene fail to alleviate the insomnia, nonprescription products containing either doxylamine or diphenhydramine have been proven safe and effective for self-treatment of transient or short-term insomnia of less than 2 weeks' duration, although other ingredients such as herbs and melatonin have not been proven safe and effective. Patients with long-term insomnia (longer than 2 weeks) should be referred for evaluation by a physician.

Other sleep disorders such as narcolepsy, hypersomnia, obstructive sleep apnea, restless legs syndrome, periodic limb movements, advanced and delayed sleep phase syndromes, and nocturnal wandering should be referred to a physician for evaluation.

References

1. Espie C. Sleep disorders in adults. Practitioner 238:137, 1994.
2. Rakel RE. Insomnia: Concerns of the family physician. J Fam Pract 36:551, 1993.
3. Harrison Y, Horne JA. Should we be taking more sleep? Sleep 18:901, 1995.
4. Mahowald MW, Schenck CH. NREM sleep parasomnias. Neurol Clin 14:675, 1996.
5. Dotto L. Sleep stages, memory and learning. CMAJ 154:1193, 1996.
6. Lechky O. Questions about sleep should be routine part of patient visits, physician says. Can Med Assoc J 149:1296, 1993.
7. Edinger JD, et al. The empirical identification of insomnia subtypes: A cluster analytic approach. Sleep 19:398, 1996.
8. Dement WC. The proper use of sleeping pills in the primary care setting. J Clin Psychiatry 53(Suppl):50, 1992.
9. Spielman AJ, Nunes J, Glovinsky PB. Insomnia Neurol Clin 14:513, 1996.
10. Barthelen GM, Stacy C. Dyssomnias, parasomnias, and sleep disorders associated with medical and psychiatric diseases. Mt Sinai J Med 61:139, 1994.
11. Becker PM, Jamieson AO, Brown WD. Insomnia. Postgrad Med 93:66, 1993.
12. Maczaj M. Pharmacological treatment of insomnia. Drugs 45:44, 1993.
13. Nino-Murcia G. Diagnosis and treatment of insomnia and risks associated with lack of treatment. J Clin Psychiatry 53(Suppl):43, 1992.
14. Dodge R, Cline MG, Quan SF. The natural history of insomnia and its relationship to respiratory symptoms. Arch Intern Med 155:1797, 1995.
15. Hayes MJ, Grunstein RR. The nonrespiratory disorders of sleep. Aust NZ J Med 24:194, 1994.
16. Anderson EG. Night people: Avoiding the quick fix for insomnia. Geriatrics 47:65, 1992.
17. Walsh JK, Engelhardt CL. Trends in the pharmacological treatment of insomnia. J Clin Psychiatry 53(Suppl):10, 1992.
18. Pearse PAE. Use of the sleep diary in the management of patients with insomnia. Aust Fam Physician 22:744, 1993.
19. Prinz PN. Sleep and sleep disorders in older adults. J Clin Neurophysiol 12:139, 1995.
20. Ancoli IS. Sleep problems in older adults: Putting myths to bed. Geriatrics 52:20, 1997.
21. Campbell SS, Dawson D, Anderson MW. Alleviation of sleep maintenance insomnia with timed exposure to bright light. J Am Geriatr Soc 41:829, 1993.
22. Henderson S, et al. Insomnia in the elderly: Its prevalence and correlates in the general population. Med J Aust 162:22, 1995.
23. Myers BL, Badia P. Changes in circadian rhythms and sleep quality with aging: Mechanisms and interventions. Neurosci Biobehav Rev 19:553, 1995.
24. Lichstein KL, Johnson RS. Relaxation for insomnia and hypnotic medication use in older women. Psychol Aging 8:103, 1993.
25. Pollak CP, Perlick D, Linsner JP. Sleep and motor activity of community elderly who frequently use bedtime medications. Biol Psychiatry 35:73, 1994.
26. Patinen M. Sleep disorder related to Parkinson's disease. J Neurol 244(4 Suppl):S3, 1997.
27. Pagel JF. Treatment of insomnia. Am Fam Physician 49:1417, 1994.
28. Mahowald MW. Diagnostic testing: Sleep disorders. Neurol Clin 14:183, 1996.
29. Nivison ME, Endreson IM. An analysis of relationships among environmental noise, annoyance and sensitivity to noise, and the consequences for health and sleep. J Behav Med 16:257, 1993.
30. Watts FN, Coyle K, East MP. The contribution of worry to insomnia. Br J Clin Psychol 33(Pt 2):211, 1994.
31. Asplund R, Aberg HE. Micturition habits of older people. Scand J Urol Nephrol 26:345, 1992.
32. Calverly PMA, Shapiro CM. Medical problems during sleep. BMJ 306:1403, 1993.
33. Sahota PK, Dexter JD. Transient recurrent situational insomnia associated with cluster headache. Sleep 16:255, 1993.
34. Hardo PG, Wasti SA, Tennant A. Night pain in arthritis: Patients at risk from prescribed night sedation. Ann Rheum Dis 51:972, 1992.
35. Shinba T, Murashima YL, Yamamoto K-I. Alcohol consumption and insomnia in a sample of Japanese alcoholics. Addiction 89:587, 1994.
36. Novak M, Shapiro CM. Drug-induced sleep disturbances: Focus on nonpsychotropic medications. Drug Saf 16:133, 1997.
37. Bailey DR. Sleep disorders. Overview and relationship to orofacial pain. Dent Clin North Am 41:189, 1997.
38. Morgan K, Clarke D. Risk factors for late-life insomnia in a representative general practice sample. Br J Gen Pract 47:166, 1997.
39. Benca RM. Sleep in psychiatric disorders. Neurol Clin 14:739, 1996.
40. Neylan TC. Treatment of sleep disturbances in depressed patients. J Clin Psychiatry 56(Suppl)2:56, 1995.
41. Morawetz D. Helping patients to sleep better without drugs. Aust Fam Physician 22:329, 1993.
42. Mendelson WB, Jain B. An assessment of short-acting hypnotics. Drug Saf 13:257, 1995.
43. Johns M. Understanding insomnia. Aust Fam Physician 22:318, 1993.
44. Mendelson WB. Insomnia and related sleep disorders. Psychiatr Clin North Am 16:841, 1993.
45. Bonnet MH, Arand DL. We are chronically sleep deprived. Sleep 18:908, 1995.

46. Bonnet MH, Arand DL. The consequences of a week of insomnia. Sleep 19:453, 1996.
47. Morin CM, Culbert JP, Schwartz SM. Nonpharmacological interventions for insomnia: A meta-analysis of treatment efficacy. Am J Psychiatry 151:1172, 1994.
48. Brown LK. Update on sleep disorders. Mt Sinai J Med 61:95, 1994.
49. Breslau N, et al. Sleep disturbance and psychiatric disorders: A longitudinal epidemiological study of young adults. Biol Psychiatry 39:411, 1996.
50. Mahendran R. Management of insomnia. Singapore Med J 36:80, 1995.
51. Farney RJ, Walker JM. Office management of common sleep-wake disorders. Med Clin North Am 79:391, 1995.
52. Roth T, Roehrs TA. Etiologies and sequelae of excessive daytime sleepiness. Clin Ther 18:562, 1996.
53. Wincor MZ. The pharmacist's role in the recognition and management of insomnia. J Clin Psychiatry 53(Suppl):80, 1992.
54. Anders TF, Eiben LA. Pediatric sleep disorders: A review of the past 10 years. J Am Acad Child Adolesc Psychiatry 36:9, 1997.
55. Ferber R. Childhood sleep disorders. Neurol Clin 14:493, 1996.
56. Fed Reg 54:6814, 1989.
57. Fed Reg 59:16982, 1994.
58. Chase JE, Gidal BE. Melatonin: Therapeutic use in sleep disorders. Ann Pharmacother 31:1218, 1997.
59. Cupp MJ. Melatonin. Am Fam Physician 56:1421, 1997.
60. Arendt J, Deacon S. Treatment of circadian rhythm disorders—Melatonin. Chronobiol Int 14:185, 1997.
61. Ellis CM, Lemmens G, Parkes JD. Melatonin and insomnia. J Sleep Res 5:61, 1996.
62. Cott J. NCDEU update. Natural product formulations available in Europe for psychotropic indications. Psychopharmacol Bull 31:745, 1995.
63. Schulz H, Stolz C, Muller J. The effect of valerian extract on sleep polygraphy in poor sleepers: A pilot study. Pharmacopsychiatry 27:147, 1994.
64. Chan TY, Tang CH, Critchley JA. Poisoning due to an over-the-counter hypnotic, Sleep-Qik (hyoscine, cyproheptadine, valerian). Postgrad Med J 71:227, 1995.
65. Willey LB, et al. Valerian overdose: A case report. Vet Hum Toxicol 37:364, 1995.
66. Pary R, et al. Treatment of insomnia. Getting to the root of sleeping problems. Postgrad Med 100:195, 1996.
67. Flamer HE. Sleep problems. Med J Aust 162, 603, 1995.
68. Johnson JE. Insomnia, alcohol, and over-the-counter drug use in old-old urban women. J Community Health Nurs 14:181, 1997.
69. Morawetz D. Nine rules for better sleep. Aust Fam Physician 22:387, 1993.
70. O'Connor PJ, Youngstedt SD. Influence of exercise on human sleep. Exerc Sport Sci Rev 23:105, 1995.
71. Richards KC. Sleep promotion. Crit Care Nurs Clin North Am 8:39, 1996.
72. Aldrich MS. The clinical spectrum of narcolepsy and idiopathic hypersomnia. Neurology 46:393, 1996.
73. Bassetti C, Aldrich MS. Narcolepsy. Neurol Clin 14:545, 1996.
74. Stoohs RA. Picking up the pieces—The consequences of sleep fragmentation. Chest 109:1417, 1996.
75. Berry RB, et al. Sleep apnea impairs the arousal response to airway occlusion. Chest 109:1490, 1996.
76. Levy P, et al. Is sleep apnea syndrome in the elderly a specific entity? Sleep 19(3 Suppl):S29, 1996.
77. Walters AS. Toward a better definition of the restless legs syndrome. The International Restless Legs Syndrome Study Group. Mov Disord 10:634, 1995.
78. Wetter TC, Pollmacher T. Restless legs and periodic leg movements in sleep syndromes. J Neurol 244(4 Suppl 1), S37, 1997.
79. Trenkwalder C, Walters AS, Hening W. Periodic limb movements and restless legs syndrome. Neurol Clin 14:629, 1996.
80. Wagner DR. Disorders of the circadian sleep-wake cycle. Neurol Clin 14:651, 1996.
81. Richardson GS, Malin HV. Circadian rhythm sleep disorders: Pathophysiology and treatment. J Clin Neurophysiol 13:17, 1996.
82. Regestein QR, Pavolva M. Treatment of delayed sleep phase syndrome. Gen Hosp Psychiatry 17:335, 1995.
83. Gilleminault C, Moscovitch A, Leger D. Forensic sleep medicine: Nocturnal wandering and violence. Sleep 18:740, 1995.
84. Stores G. Practitioner review: Assessment and treatment of sleep disorders in children and adolescents. J Child Psychol Psychiatry 37:907, 1996.
85. King N, Ollendick TH, Tonge BJ. Children's nighttime fears. Clin Psychol Rev 17:431, 1997.
86. Schenck CH, Mahowald MW. REM sleep parasomnias. Neurol Clin 14:697, 1996.
87. Crisp AH. The sleepwalking/night terrors syndrome in adults. Postgrad Med J 72:599, 1996.

Poisoning Emergencies

AT THE COUNTER

 The pharmacist answers the phone and hears a woman ask, with obvious anxiety, "What should I do? My child took medicine."

Interview/Patient Assessment

On questioning by the pharmacist, the woman explains that her 3-year-old daughter was found by the medicine cabinet several minutes before with a bottle of imipramine 50 mg tablets that the woman takes for exogenous depression. The mother received 30 tablets from the pharmacy a week earlier, and has taken one a day since. The bottle only has four tablets left in it. She has ipecac but doesn't know whether she needs to give it to the child since she seems calm and it's her afternoon nap time.

Pharmacist's Analysis

1. How many tablets might the child have taken?

2. Is the child in imminent danger from imipramine ingestion?
3. Should the child be awakened to give syrup of ipecac?

The child could have taken as many as 19 tablets (the original 30 minus seven taken minus four remaining). Imipramine is one of the most dangerous agents in overdose situations, according to poison authorities. The child's calm demeanor may be deceptive, since the medication induces drowsiness. Syrup of ipecac is contraindicated in any patient who is not fully conscious because of the risk of aspiration.

Patient Counseling

The mother should be cautioned to call a Poison Control Center for emergency directions. The mother should also be advised to transport the child to the emergency room if a Poison Control Center cannot be contacted. A need for urgency must be conveyed to the mother.

Poisoning, whether intentional or accidental, is one of the few true medical emergencies for which the average pharmacist practicing in a retail situation might provide advice. Although poisoning is popularly associated with young children ingesting substances to which they should not have access, it also occurs when young adults attempt suicide and in accidents such as exposure to cleaners or solvents.

Pharmacy coursework usually includes toxicology. While few pharmacists go on to specialize in this area, those who do may work in poison control centers where they have access to up–to-date technologies with which they can provide competent advice in a poisoning emergency.[1,2] (See "Poison Control Centers.") The chapter does not provide the specialized knowledge base needed to substitute for these comprehensive sources of information; rather, this chapter reviews poisoning for pharmacists who typically receive urgent calls while working in the typical retail or hospital setting.

PREVALENCE OF POISONING

In 1995, poison control centers in the United States reported over 2 million incidents.[5]

EPIDEMIOLOGY OF POISONING

Common Age of Poisoning Patients

ACCIDENTAL POISONING
Accidental poisoning (as opposed to intentional administration to others or oneself) is an age-dependent phenomenon. About 40% of poisonings involve children younger than 3,

54% children younger than 6.[6] There are several reasons for such a powerful age association. Most young children who are able to crawl, toddle, or walk, are extremely curious about their environment and they exhibit the natural tendency to place all objects into the mouth.[7–9]

INTENTIONAL POISONING
Intentional poisoning (as opposed to accidental self-administration of a toxic agent) is a result of willful intent to do self-harm. This may be an attempt to gain attention (a suicide gesture) or a true suicide attempt. Those younger than 6 years are only involved in 0.4% of intentional poisonings, with those 6 to 12 being involved in another 3.2%.[6] Thus the majority of intentional poisonings involve those aged 13 to 19 (29.2%), and those over the age of 19 (65.3%), with 1.9% being of unknown age. Of 410 fatalities listed as intentional suicides reported in 1 year, none occurred in the ages below 6 years, one was in the age of 6 to 12, 19 were in the ages of 13 to 19, and 390 were over the age of 19.[6]

Gender of Poisoning Patients

Gender is also a predictor of self-poisoning. Males are more likely to ingest toxins up to the age of 13, which encompasses most of the accidental ingestions.[6] At all higher ages, females predominate because of their propensity to employ self-poisoning as a method for suicide (as opposed to suicide methods more commonly used by males such as the use of firearms). For example, for poisonings in the ages from 6 to 12, males are 56.2% of the total, with females being 42.9%; however, for the ages of 13 to 19 (the majority of which are intentional), only 41.8% were in males, with the balance being in females.[6]

Locations of Poisoning

It should be no surprise that the primary location for poisoning is a residence (whether one's own or another's home), where 80 to 90% of incidents take place.[7] The workplace and school account for 4% of incidents.[6]

Locations of Toxic Substances

Although the danger of placing hazardous substances into "non-hazardous" containers—such as filling a soft drink bottle with gasoline for the lawnmower—has been a focus of poison education for decades, many poisonings still result from this practice.[7] Removing medications from child-resistant containers to facilitate opening them, for example, defeats the intent of the closures.[10,11]

Poisoning statistics also show that many incidents occur because hazardous substances are not in a secure storage location.[7]

Family-Associated Factors

When not being given personal attention, children can become bored; often this is when young children choose to explore their environment. Thus peak times for poisoning include those when caregivers are inattentive or neglectful, and during family crises.[7] For example, in one survey, poison control centers reported receiving the greatest number of calls between 4:00 and 10:00 PM (as compared with other periods), which could be indicative of the stress associated with tired, harried parents attempting to make supper and supervise homework while young children clamor for attention.[6]

ETIOLOGY OF POISONING

Categories of Poisoning

There are many methods by which people are exposed to

FOCUS ON...

POISON CONTROL CENTERS

Poison control centers generally are located in medical centers, children's hospitals, or state-affiliated locations such as the health department of a university. These regional centers maintain comprehensive computerized databases and current antidote and treatment protocols on hundreds of thousands of potential poisons (including drugs, plants, and chemicals).[3] Poison control centers may be certified by the American Association of Poison Control Centers. To become certified, professional staff members must be nurses or pharmacists, must have at least a year's experience in a poison center, and must pass a written examination. The professional staff of poison control centers is trained to elicit the applicable data from stressed callers.

Poison Control Centers

Note: The information below was collected by the KidsHealth.org staff. If a number fails to connect properly, call your information directory to obtain the latest number for your area.

ALABAMA
Alabama Poison Center
408-A Paul Bryant Drive
Tuscaloosa, Al 35401
Emergency Phone: (800) 462-0800 [AL only]; (205) 345-0600

Regional Poison Control Center
The Children's Hospital of Alabama
1600-7th Avenue South
Birmingham, Al 35233-1711
Emergency Phone: (205) 939-9201; (205) 939-9202;
(800) 292-6678 [AL only]; (205) 933-4050

ALASKA
Anchorage Poison Control Center
Providence Hospital Pharmacy
PO Box 196604
Anchorage, AK 95516-6604
Emergency Phone: (800) 478-3193; (907) 261-3193

ARIZONA
Arizona Poison and Drug Information Center
Arizona Health Sciences Center
1501 N. Campbell Avenue, Rm #1156
Tucson, AZ 85724
Emergency Phone: (800) 362-0101 [AZ only]; (520) 626-6016

Samaritan Regional Poison Center
1111 E. McDowell Road, Ancillary-1
Phoenix, AZ 85006
Emergency Phone: (602) 253-3334; (800) 362-0101 [AZ only]

ARKANSAS
Arkansas Poison and Drug Information Center
University of Arkansas for Medical Sciences
4301 West Markham-Slot 522
Little Rock, AR 72205
Emergency Phone: (800) 376-4766

Continued

toxic substances. Most poisoning episodes (about 86%) are unintentional, but 11% are intentional (the balance are unknown or other minor categories).[6] Intentional episodes are more common with increasing age, and are more likely to be fatal than accidental episodes.

Occupational Exposures

People become exposed to dangerous substances as a result of activity in the workplace. As an example, vapors may be inhaled at a hazardous material spill.[6] Carcinogenic agents may be contacted by the pharmacist working with antineoplastic agents in a horizontal laminar flow hood or without proper protection.

Environmental Exposures

People are exposed to hazardous substances when contacting contaminated air or soil, or drinking contaminated water.[6]

Recreational Exposures

Some people expose themselves to a dangerous substance voluntarily to obtain a euphoric or psychotropic effect. Alternatively, the exposure may be a requirement to join a group such as fraternity hazing involving ingestion of dangerous or lethal quantities of alcohol.

Poisoning As Child Abuse

Unfortunately, child abuse sometimes takes the form of poisoning. The usual agents employed fall into the following three categories.[12]

- Common household agents (e.g., antifreeze, lye, hydrocarbons, sodium bicarbonate)
- Nonprescription medications (e.g., emetics, laxatives, antacids, acetaminophen, salicylates)

CALIFORNIA
Central California Regional Poison Control Center
Valley Children's Hospital
3151 N. Millbrook
Fresno, CA 93703
Emergency Phone: (800) 346-5922 [Central CA only];
(209) 445-1222

Los Angeles Regional Drug and Poison Information Center
LAC + USC Medical Center
GH Room 1107 A & B
1200 N. State Street
Los Angeles, CA 90033
Emergency Phone: (213) 222-3212; (800)777-6476

San Diego Regional Poison Center
UCSD Medical Center
200 West Arbor Drive
San Diego, CA 92103-8925
Emergency Phone: (619) 543-6000;
(800) 876-4766 [in 619 area code only]

San Francisco Bay Area Regional Poison Control Center
San Francisco General Hospital
1001 Potrero Avenue, Building 80, Room 230
San Francisco, CA 94110
Emergency Phone: (800) 523-2222

Santa Clara Valley Medical Center
Regional Poison Center
750 South Bescom Avenue, Suite 310
San Jose, CA 95128
Emergency Phone: (408) 885-6000; (800) 662-9886 [CA only]

Davis Medical Center Regional Poison Control Center
University of California
2315 Stockton Blvd., Room 1024
Sacramento, CA 95817
Emergency Phone: (916) 734-3692;
(800) 342-9293 [Northern CA]

COLORADO
Rocky Mountain Poison and Drug Center
8802 E. 9th Avenue
Denver, CO 80220-6800
Emergency Phone: (303) 629-1123

CONNECTICUT
Connecticut Poison Control Center
University of Connecticut Health Center
263 Farmington Avenue
Farmington, CT 06030
Emergency Phone: (800) 343-2722 [CT only]; (203) 679-3056

DELAWARE
The Poison Control Center
3600 Sciences Center, Ste. 220
Philadelphia, PA 19104-2641
Emergency Phone: (215) 386-2100; (800) 722-7112

Continued

- Prescription medications and drugs of abuse

In one instance, a 21-month-old child was given muriatic acid (a form of hydrochloric acid, sometimes used in construction) by a baby-sitter.[13] The 15-year-old sitter had a history of psychiatric treatment that neither the sitter nor her parents disclosed to the employers. (Abuse of an older sibling was also suspected.) The sitter admitted the abuse, stating that she thought the child was attacking her.

MANIFESTATIONS OF POISONING

The manifestations of poisoning are as varied as are the different products that can be ingested as poisons. The pharmacist must utilize knowledge of pharmacology to predict which symptoms would be expected. For instance, if the product's major pharmacologic effect is central nervous system sedation, lethargy should be expected.

SPECIFIC CONSIDERATIONS OF POISONING

The Most Commonly Ingested Poisons

A survey of seven poison control centers revealed that the most common medications ingested by children under the age of 6, in descending order, were as follows[14]:

- Analgesics
- Cold medications
- Topical products
- Multivitamins
- Antibiotics
- Antacid/gastrointestinal products
- Hormones

In another survey, which included all ingestants for all ages, the most common poisons were as follows[6]:

- Cleaning substances (10.6% of all calls)

DISTRICT OF COLUMBIA
National Capital Poison Center
3201 New Mexico Avenue, N.W., Suite 310
Washington, DC 20016
Emergency Phone: (202) 625-3333; (202) 362-8563 [TTY]

FLORIDA
Florida Poison Information Center
University Medical Center
University of Florida Health Science Center
655 West 8th Street
Jacksonville, FL 32209
Emergency Numbers: (904) 549-4465; (800) 282-3171 [FL only]

Florida Poison Information Center
University of Miami/Jackson Memorial Hospital
1611 NW 12th Avenue
Urgent Care Center Bldg., Rm. 219
Miami, FL 33136
Emergency Phone: (800) 282-3171 [FL Only]

The Florida Poison Information and Toxicology Resource Center
Tampa General Hospital
PO Box 1289
Tampa, FL 33601
Emergency Phone: (813) 256-4444 [Tampa only];
(800) 282-3171 [FL only]

GEORGIA
Georgia Poison Center
Hughes Spalding Children's Hospital
Grady Health Systems
80 Butler Street, S.E.
PO Box 26066
Atlanta, GA 30335-3801
Emergency Phone: (800) 282-5846; (404) 616-9000 [GA only]

HAWAII
Hawaii Poison Center
1500 S. Beretania Street, Rm. #113
Honolulu, HI 96826
Emergency Phone: (808) 941-4411

IDAHO
Idaho Poison Center
3092 Elder Street
Boise, ID 83720-0036
Emergency Phone: (208) 334-4570; (800) 632-8000 [ID Only]

ILLINOIS
BroMenn Poison Control Center
BroMenn Regional Medical Center
Franklin at Virginia
Normal, IL 61761
Emergency Phone: (309) 454-6666

Chicago and Northeastern Illinois Regional Poison Control Center
Rush-Presbyterian-St. Luke's Medical Center
1653 West Congress Parkway
Chicago, IL 60612
Emergency Phone: (312) 942-5969; (800) 942-5969

Continued

- Analgesics (9.4%)
- Cosmetics and other personal care products (8.5%)
- Plants (5.4%)
- Cough/cold preparations (5.2%)
- Pesticides
- Topicals
- Food products
- Hydrocarbons
- Antimicrobials
- Sedatives/hypnotics/antipsychotics
- Alcohols
- Antidepressants
- Chemicals and vitamins

The Most Dangerous Poisons

A survey of poison control centers found the greatest number of poisoning deaths associated with the following poisons, most of which are medications, in descending order[6]:

- Analgesics
- Antidepressants
- Sedatives/hypnotics/antipsychotics
- Stimulants
- Street drugs
- Cardiovascular drugs
- Alcohols
- Asthma medications
- Chemicals
- Hydrocarbons
- Antihistamines
- Cleaning substances

Another expert listed the following as the most toxic prescription medications[15]:

- Tricyclic antidepressants
- Antimalarials (chloroquine)
- Antidiarrheals (e.g., Lomotil)
- Hydrocodone-based cough syrups (e.g., Hycodan, Tussionex)
- Propoxyphene
- Ethchlorvynol
- Lindane
- Lithium carbonate
- Glyburide/glipizide
- Clonidine

Efforts have been made to identify medications that can cause

INDIANA
Indiana Poison Center
Methodist Hospital of Indiana
I-65 and 21st St.
PO Box 1367
Indianapolis, IN 46206-1367
Emergency Phone: (800) 382-9097 [IN only]; (317) 929-2323

IOWA
St. Luke's Poison Center
St. Luke's Regional Medical Center
2720 Stone Park Boulevard
Sioux City, IA 51104
Emergency Phone: (712) 277-2222; (800) 352-2222

Mid-Iowa Poison and Drug Information Center
Variety Club Poison and Drug Information Center
Iowa Methodist Medical Center
1200 Pleasant Street
Des Moines, IA 50309
Emergency Phone: (515) 241-6254; (800) 362-2327 [IA only]

Poison Control Center
The University of Iowa Hospitals and Clinics
Pharmacy Department
200 Hawkins Drive
Iowa City, IA 52242
Emergency Phone: (800) 272-6477

KANSAS
Mid-America Poison Control Center
University of Kansas Medical Center
3901 Rainbow Blvd., Room B-400
Kansas City, KS 66160-7231
Emergency Phone: (913) 588-6633;
(800) 332-6633 [KS only & KC metro area]

KENTUCKY
Kentucky Regional Poison Center of Kosair Children's Hospital
Medical Towers South, Suite 572
PO Box 35070
Louisville, KY 40232-5070
Emergency Phone: (502) 589-8222; (800) 722-5725 [KY only]

LOUISIANA
Louisiana Drug and Poison Information Center
Northeast Louisiana University
Sugar Hill
Monroe, LA 71209-6430
Emergency Phone: (800) 256-9822 [LA only]; (318) 362-5393

MAINE
Maine Poison Control Center
Maine Medical Center
Department of Emergency Medicine
22 Bramhall Street
Portland, ME 04102
Emergency Phone: (207) 871-2950; (800) 442-6305 [ME only]

Continued

the death of a 22-pound toddler if as little as one tablet or teaspoonful is ingested. The highly toxic medications include the following[8]:

- Camphor (in such nonprescription products as Campho-Phenique)
- Chloroquine
- Tricyclic antidepressants
- Phenothiazines
- Quinine (available as a nonprescription medication through the mid 1990s)
- Methyl salicylate (a leading ingredient in external analgesics sold for muscle strain; also sold as a flavoring agent in liquid form)
- Theophylline (once a major ingredient in nonprescription antiasthmatics, but should have been removed by the major manufacturers)

This group of medications produces nearly half of the deaths in children younger than 2 in the United States. The author of the report suggests that the extreme danger of the highly toxic medications is obscured by the large number of less toxic products (e.g., most nonprescription drugs) that routinely place the warning to "Keep out of reach of children" on the labels.[8] Pharmacists should take special care to point out the toxicity associated with the nonprescription products on the list above, since camphor and methyl salicylate can kill a child if as little as 1 teaspoonful is ingested. Nonprescription products not on the list that can be extremely dangerous include iron supplements, eucalyptus oil, and a dibucaine-containing local anesthetic ointment.[8,16]

Another aspect of poisoning concerns hazardous substances that do not cause early symptoms, but that may cause severe toxicity later. (See "A Pharmacist's Journal: Are You Still Open? Do You Have Ipecac?") Sometimes called "time bombs," these ingredients include acetaminophen,

MARYLAND
Maryland Poison Center
University of Maryland School of Pharmacy
20 N. Pine Street
Baltimore, MD 21201
Emergency Phone: (410) 528-7701; (800) 492-2414 [MD only]

MASSACHUSETTS
Massachusetts Poison Control System
300 Longwood Avenue
Boston, MA 02115
Emergency Phone: (617) 232-2120; (800) 682-9211

MICHIGAN
Blodgett Regional Poison Center
1840 Wealthy S.E.
Grand Rapids, MI 49506-2968
Emergency Phone: (800) POISON1; (800) 356-3232 [TTY]

Poison Control Center
Children's Hospital of Michigan
Harper Professional Office Bldg.
4160 John R., Suite 425
Detroit, MI 48201
Emergency Phone: (313) 745-5711; (800) 764-7661

Marquette General Hospital
420 W. Magnetic Street
Marquette, MI 49855
Emergency Phone: (906) 225-3497; (800) 562-9781

MINNESOTA
Hennepin Regional Poison Center
Hennepin County Medical Center
701 Park Avenue
Minneapolis, MN 55415
Emergency Phone: (612) 347-3141; (612) 337-7387 [Petline]; (612) 337-7474 [TDD]

Minnesota Regional Poison Center
8100 34th Avenue S.
P.O. Box 1309
Minneapolis, MN 55440-1309
Emergency Phone: (612) 221-2113

MISSISSIPPI
Mississippi Regional Poison Control Center
University of Mississippi Medical Center
2500 North State Street
Jackson, MS 39216-4505
Emergency Phone: (601) 354-7660

MISSOURI
Cardinal Glennon Children's Hospital Regional Poison Center
1465 S. Grand Blvd.
St. Louis, MO 63104
Emergency Phone: (314) 772-5200; (800) 366-8888; (800) 392-9111

Children's Mercy Hospital
2401 Gillham Road
Kansas City, MO 64108
Emergency Phone: (816) 234-3430

Continued

iron, lithium, monoamine oxidase inhibitors, ethanol and methanol, phenytoin, carbamazepine, and hepatotoxic mushrooms, as well as timed-release formulations.[2,17] Patients who have ingested these products may need extended observation, sometimes for as long as 12 to 24 hours, or perhaps even longer in the case of a hepatotoxic medication such as acetaminophen.

TREATMENT OF POISONING

Treatment Guidelines

When the parent, caregiver, or other person is advised to administer a nonprescription poisoning treatment medication, the product must be used correctly. If not, it may be ineffective or produce adverse reactions. (See "General Labeling for All Poison Treatment Products" and "Problems Regarding Syrup of Ipecac.") For steps that may be used in handling a poisoning incident, refer to Patient Assessment Algorithm 25.1.

Nonprescription Medications

Two nonprescription products are available for poisonings. One, syrup of ipecac (usually referred to as simply "ipecac"), is an emetic agent widely available in pharmacies. The other, activated charcoal, is an ingredient that adsorbs poisons, but it is not commonly sold in pharmacies. Some companies that sell activated-charcoal products prefer to target hospitals to ensure that the product is used properly (e.g., concomitant administration of cathartics to prevent obstruction and facilitate elimination). However, other products may be available to the retail pharmacy through the traditional wholesale channels for the use by informed patients. Cathartics may also be used as a component of poisoning treatment, and are available in the laxative sec-

MONTANA
Rocky Mountain Poison and Drug Center
8802 E. 9th Avenue
Denver, CO 80220-6800
Emergency Phone: (303) 629-1123

NEBRASKA
The Poison Center
8301 Dodge Street
Omaha, NE 68114
Emergency Phone: (402) 390-5555 [Omaha];
(800) 955-9119 [NE & WY]

NEVADA
Rocky Mountain Poison and Drug Center
8802 E. 9th Avenue
Denver, CO 80220-6800
Emergency Phone: (303) 629-1123; (800) 332-3073 [COLO WATTS]; (800) 525-5042 [MONT WATTS];
(800) 446-6179 [NEV WATTS]; (303) 739-1127 [TTY]

NEW HAMPSHIRE
New Hampshire Poison Information Center
Dartmouth-Hitchcock Medical Center
One Medical Center Drive
Lebanon, NH 03756
Emergency Phone: (603) 650-8000; (603) 650-5000 [11pm–8am];
(800) 562-8236 [NH only]

NEW JERSEY
New Jersey Poison Information and Education System
201 Lyons Avenue
Newark, NJ 07112
Emergency Phone: (800) POISON1 [(800) 764-7661]

NEW MEXICO
New Mexico Poison and Drug Information Center
University of New Mexico
Health Sciences Library, Room 125
Albuquerque, NM 87131-1076
Emergency Phone: (505) 843-2551; (800) 432-6866 [NM only]

NEW YORK
Central New York Poison Control Center
SUNY Health Science Center
750 E. Adams Street
Syracuse, NY 13210
Emergency Phone: (315) 476-4766; (800) 252-5655

Finger Lakes Regional Poison Center
Box 777
University of Rochester Medical Center
601 Elmwood Avenue, Box 321, Rm. G-3275
Rochester, NY 14642
Emergency Phone: (716) 275-5151;
(800) 333-0542

Hudson Valley Regional Poison Center
Phelps Memorial Hospital Center
701 North Broadway
North Tarrytown, NY 10591
Emergency Phone: (800) 336-6997; (914) 366-3030

Continued

tion of retail pharmacies when their use is considered medically necessary.

IPECAC

Ipecac is the only safe and effective nonprescription emetic. Although other emetics are sometimes used as home remedies, they are not proven to be safe or effective. (See "Additional Methods of Gastric Emptying.")

Content of Ipecac

Ipecac contains the alkaloids emetine and cephaeline.[24] Cephaeline serves to produce nausea and vomiting, whereas emetine is a less powerful emetic, and produces two major adverse effects of chronic ipecac administration: cardiomyopathy and skeletal myopathy.

Mechanism of Ipecac

Ipecac induces vomiting through a combination of local and central effects. It causes irritation of the gastrointestinal tract and activates the central vomiting center through stimulation of the chemoreceptor zone.[18,25] Ipecac is so effective that in one study, 99.6% of children vomited an average of 23 minutes after administration.[26]

Advantages of Ipecac

Ipecac is administered to tens of thousands of children younger than 6 each year.[6,26] Ipecac given at home can reduce the costs associated with ingestion of poisons without increasing the risk to the patient.[14] Allowing the patient to stay at home also reduces anxiety and stress. *The American Academy of Pediatrics has recommended that all homes with young children stock ipecac.*[26]

Problems with Ipecac

Questionable Benefit of Gastric Emptying. Although emesis seems beneficial in certain instances, physicians disagree about the value of gastric emptying in the treatment of poisoning, whether with ipecac or by gastric lavage.[2,20,27,28]

Long Island Regional Poison Control Center
Winthrop University Hospital
259 First Street
Mineola, NY 11501
Emergency Phone: (516) 542-2323

New York City Poison Control Center
N.Y.C. Department of Health
455 First Avenue, Room 123
New York, NY 10016
Emergency Phone: (212) 340-4494; (212) POISONS;
(212) 689-9014 [TDD]

Western New York Regional Poison Control Center
Children's Hospital of Buffalo
219 Bryant Street
Buffalo, NY 14222
Emergency Phone: (716) 878-7654; Also Extensions: 7655, 7856, 7857

NORTH CAROLINA
Carolinas Poison Center
1000 Blythe Boulevard
P.O. Box 32861
Charlotte, NC 28232-2861
Emergency Phone: (704) 355-4000;
(800) 84-TOXIN [(800) 848-6946]

Catawba Memorial Hospital Poison Control Center
Pharmacy Department
810 Fairgrove Church Road
Hickory, NC 28602
Emergency Phone: (704) 322-6649

Duke Poison Control Center
North Carolina Regional Center
Box 3007
Duke University
Durham, NC 27710
Emergency Phone: (919) 684-8111; (800) 672-1697 [NC only]

Triad Poison Center
1200 N. Elm Street
Greensboro, NC 27401-1020
Emergency Phone: (910) 574-8105; (800) 953-4001 [NC only]

NORTH DAKOTA
North Dakota Poison Information Center
MeritCare Medical Center
720 4th Street North
Fargo, ND 58122
Emergency Phone: (701) 234-5575;
(800) 732-2200 [ND, MN, SD only]

OHIO
Akron Regional Poison Center
1 Perkins Square
Akron, OH 44308
Emergency Phone: (216) 379-8562;
(800) 362-9922 [OH only]; (216) 379-8446 [TTY]

Continued

Ipecac, which produces emesis, is widely thought to reduce the quantity of toxin absorbed following a toxic ingestion.[14] However, few data are available to confirm that the reduction in the amount of drug absorbed is significant enough to favorably alter the patient's course. Some studies do show benefit, however. In one, serum concentrations of acetaminophen were lower for overdose patients given ipecac early in the episode.[29] If an ingested medication has an extremely rapid onset of action (e.g., zolpidem), especially with the production of sedative-hypnotic effects, emesis may not be an option because of the time elapsed before administration and the dangers in allowing emesis in a sedated patient.[30]

Adverse Effects of Ipecac. Ipecac is usually safe when used as directed, although minor side effects are common: lethargy in almost one-fourth of patients and diarrhea in one-tenth.[26] However, ⚠ *ipecac can be highly toxic when accidentally ingested.* A 15-month-old child ingested one or two bottles of ipecac syrup.[31] She underwent two hospitalizations and experienced protracted vomiting lasting for 1 week. In addition, she had such severe weakness that she was unable to support her head or bear weight, and deep tendon reflexes were absent.

Emetine produces direct toxic effects on muscle tissue, producing weakness that may proceed to paralysis.[31] The neuromuscular effects—which may not occur until 1 week after ipecac ingestion and may take up to 1 month to resolve—include skeletal muscle stiffness, tremors, weakness of the proximal rather than distal areas, tenderness, aching, and edema.[32] Effects generally resolve if ipecac is discontinued, although full recovery may not occur for 6 to 12 months.

Bethesda Poison Control Center
2951 Maple Avenue
Zanesville, OH 43701
Emergency Phone: (614) 454-4221

Central Ohio Poison Center
700 Children's Drive
Columbus, OH 43205-2696
Emergency Phone: (614) 228-1323; (800) 682-7625;
    (614) 228-2272 [TTY]; (614) 461-2012

Cincinnati Drug & Poison Information and Regional Poison Control System
P.O. Box 670144
Cincinnati, OH 45267-0144
Emergency Phone: (513) 558-5111; (800) 872-5111 [OH only]
(800) 253-7955 [TTY]

Greater Cleveland Poison Control Center
11100 Euclid Avenue
Cleveland, OH 44106
Emergency Phone: (216) 231-4455

Medical College of Ohio Poison and Drug Information Center
3000 Arlington Avenue
Toledo, OH 43614
Emergency Phone: (419) 381-3897; (800) 589-3897 [419 area code only]

Northeast Ohio Poison Education/Information Center
1320 Timken Mercy Drive N.W.
Canton, OH 44708
Emergency Phone: (800) 456-8662 [OH only]

OKLAHOMA
Oklahoma Poison Control Center
940 N.E. 13th Street, Rm. 3N118
Oklahoma, OK 73104
Emergency Phone: (405) 271-5454; (800) 522-4611 [OK only]

OREGON
Oregon Poison Center
Oregon Health Sciences University
3181 S.W. Sam Jackson Park Road, CB550
Portland, OR 97201
Emergency Phone: (503) 494-8968; (800) 452-7165 [OR only]

PENNSYLVANIA
Central Pennsylvania Poison Center
University Hospital
Milton S. Hershey Medical Center
Hershey, PA 17033-0850
Emergency Phone: (800) 521-6110; (717) 531-6111

Lehigh Valley Hospital Poison Prevention Program
17th & Chew Streets
P.O. Box 7017
Allentown, PA 18105-7017

The Poison Control Center
3600 Sciences Center, Suite 220
Philadelphia, PA 19104-2641
Emergency Phone: (215) 386-2100

Continued

Cardiomyopathy (disease of the myocardium) caused by emetine is a result of direct toxicity to heart muscle fibers, which reduces contractility.[32] Cardiomyopathy often manifests initially as tachycardia, progressing to inverted T waves, hypotension, chest pain, shortness of breath, prolonged QRS complex, premature atrial beats, and atrial tachycardia. Cardiac arrest results from asystole or ventricular fibrillation.

Questions about ipecac persist.[33–37] Research indicates that administration of ipecac delays the administration of activated charcoal (since the patient should have vomited prior to administration of charcoal), hinders the retention of the charcoal, and prolongs the time in the emergency room.[25,38–40] Perhaps because of these issues, administration of ipecac in poisonings decreased by 80% between 1983 and 1994.[6]

Abuse of Ipecac. Ipecac abuse falls into two categories:

- Child abuse: Administration to children when the caregiver knows it is not indicated
- Self abuse: Self-usage to induce vomiting such as with anorexia/bulimia

CHILD ABUSE USING IPECAC. Parents or other caregivers may give ipecac as part of a psychiatric disturbance known as **Munchausen syndrome by proxy** (simulating medical conditions in others for the purpose of gaining medical attention).[41] An indication of long-term abuse of ipecac is repeated hospital or emergency room visits for children suffering from protracted vomiting and diarrhea, and/or skeletal and cardiac myopathy. The diarrhea and vomiting may be sufficiently severe to cause dehydration.

In one such case, a 29-month-old boy was admitted to the hospital for dehydration, vomiting, and diarrhea.[41] The mother was

Pittsburgh Poison Center
3705 Fifth Avenue
Pittsburgh, PA 15213
Emergency Phone: (412) 681-6669; (800) 722-7112

Regional Poison Prevention Education Center
Mercy Regional Health System
2500 Seventh Avenue
Altoona, PA 16602

RHODE ISLAND
Rhode Island Poison Center
593 Eddy Street
Providence, RI 02903
Emergency Phone: (401) 444-5727

SOUTH CAROLINA
Palmetto Poison Center
College of Pharmacy
University of South Carolina
Columbia, SC 29208
Emergency Phone: (803) 765-7359; (800) 922-1117 [SC only];
(706) 724-5050; (803) 777-1117

SOUTH DAKOTA
McKennan Poison Control Center
Box 5045
800 E. 21st Street
Sioux Falls, SD 57117-5045
Emergency Phone: (605) 336-3894; (800) 952-0123; (800) 843-0505

TENNESSEE
Middle Tennessee Poison Center
The Center for Clinical Toxicology
Vanderbilt University Medical Center
1161 21st Avenue South
501 Oxford House
Nashville, TN 37232-4632
Emergency Phone: (615) 936-2034 [local];
(800) 288-9999 [regional]; (615) 322-0157 [TDD]

Southern Poison Center, Inc.
847 Monroe Avenue, Suite 230
Memphis, TN 38163
Emergency Phone: (901) 528-6048; (800) 228-9999 [TN only]

TEXAS
Central Texas Poison Center
Scott & White Memorial Clinic & Hospital
2401 S. 31st Street
Temple, TX 76508
Emergency Phone: (817) 774-2005; (800) POISON1; (800) 764-7661

North Texas Poison Center
Texas Poison Center Network at Parkland Memorial Hospital
5201 Harry Hines Blvd.
P.O. Box 35926
Dallas, TX 75235
Emergency Phone: (800) POISON1 [(800) 746-7661]

Continued

friendly, cooperative, and supportive. The boy's symptoms recurred every 2 to 4 months for an 18-month period. All diagnostic studies (e.g., stool parasites) were negative, but urine was positive for emetine and cephaeline. The boy also exhibited symptoms of significant right heart failure consistent with ipecac usage. He improved only after forcible removal from the mother and placement with grandparents.

In a second example, a 5-year-old boy was subjected to similar abuse by his mother, a drug abuser. His symptoms involved skeletal myopathy, manifested as weakness of the shoulder and hip muscles, in addition to cardiac abnormalities. The mother vehemently denied administering ipecac to her son, but several bottles were discovered in her belongings.

IPECAC ABUSE IN ANOREXIA/BULIMIA. Patients with severe eating disorders such as anorexia/bulimia often abuse ipecac, along with additional destructive behaviors (such as laxative abuse, binge eating, starvation, and the induction of vomiting using other methods).[42] Patients may drink ipecac several times a day for many months prior to discovery. Nationally, experts estimate that 35,000 of America's 1 million bulimics abuse ipecac.

Because ipecac is slowly excreted (more than one-third of the active ingredients is retained by the body more than 35 days after consumption), ingestion of just 30 mL daily (21 mg of emetine in 30 mL of ipecac) will eventually produce symptoms of skeletal and cardiac myopathy.[32,43] The clinical picture duplicates that of Munchausen syndrome by proxy.[24] Ipecac has been responsible for several deaths when abused in this manner. *Ipecac abuse is more common in young women than any other age/gender group.*

South Texas Poison Center
7703 Floyd Curl Drive
San Antonio, TX 78284-7834
Emergency Phone: (800) POISON1 [(800) 764-7661] [TX Only]

Texas Poison Control Network
PO Box 1110, 1501 S. Coulter
Amarillo, TX 79175
Emergency Phone: (800) 764-7661

Texas Poison Control Network
Southeast Texas Poison Center
The University of Texas Medical Branch
301 University Avenue
Galveston, TX 77555-1175
Emergency Phone: (409) 765-1420 [Galveston]; (713) 654-1701 [Houston]; (800) 764-7661 [TX only]

West Texas Regional Poison Center
4815 Alameda Avenue
Et Paso, TX 79905
Emergency Phone: (800) 764-7661 [TX only]

UTAH
Utah Poison Control Center
410 Chipeta Way, Suite 230
Salt Lake City, UT 84108
Emergency Phone: (801) 581-2151; (800) 456-7707 [UT only]

VERMONT
Vermont Poison Center
Fletcher Allen Health Care
111 Colchester Avenue
Burlington, VT 05401
Emergency Phone: (802) 658-3456

VIRGINIA
Blue Ridge Poison Center
University of Virginia
Blue Ridge Hospital
Box 67
Charlottesville, VA 22901
Emergency Phone: (804) 924-5543; (800) 451-1428

Virginia Poison Center
401 N. 12th Street
Virginia Commonwealth University
Richmond, VA 23298-0522
Emergency Phone: (804) 828-9123 [Richmond]; (800) 552-6337 [VA only]

WASHINGTON
Washington Poison Center
155 N.E. 100th Street, Suite #400
Seattle, WA 98125
Emergency Phone: (206) 526-2121; (800) 732-6985 [WA only]; (206) 517-2394 [TDD]; (206) 517-2394 [TDD; WA only]

WEST VIRGINIA
West Virginia Poison Center
3110 MacCorkle Avenue, S.E.
Charleston, WV 25304
Emergency Phone: (800) 642-3625 [WV only]; (304) 348-4211

Continued

The singer Karen Carpenter was a well-known victim of ipecac toxicity.[34] It is troubling that when her psychotherapist was asked on a nationally televised program why pharmacists continue to sell ipecac to individuals who are abusing the product, he said that he believes that pharmacists "would not refuse to sell ipecac to a bulimic individual because they would lose profit from the sale."[34] Pharmacists should be suspicious when a patient who may be anorexic/bulimic attempts to buy ipecac. Abnormally low body weight is a helpful tip-off, as are repeated sales to the same individual or the purchase of multiple bottles. (High-school students have reported that they buy bottles at different pharmacies to minimize the risks of detection.[32]) Pharmacists might place ipecac behind the counter, filling the space with a shelf notice asking prospective buyers to consult the pharmacist about poisoning incidents to ensure that ipecac is actually indicated.

FDA-Approved Labeling for Ipecac

Ipecac dosing depends on patient age, as illustrated in Table 25.1. To facilitate its action, the patient should drink water or another clear fluid after drinking ipecac. The amount of liquid taken concomitantly with ipecac also varies with patient age. ***Babies younger than 6 months are not usually ambulatory enough to self-ingest poisons; they also have immature airway defenses against aspiration; thus they should not be given ipecac.***[23] All ages may repeat the initial ipecac dose one time if vomiting does not occur in 30 minutes. The maximum bottle size that may be sold on a nonprescription basis is 30 mL.

While FDA-approved labeling for ipecac cautions against concomitant ingestion with milk,

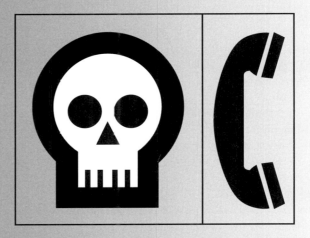

The official poisoning control symbol, which is the logo of the American Association of Poison Control Centers.

Each home should have the number of a certified poison control center posted prominently next to the telephone, alongside other emergency numbers.[4] Likewise, each pharmacy should keep the number of a certified poison control center for quick reference when a patient calls. *To obtain an updated list of certified centers, contact www.usmedicine.com/poison.html or http://Kidshealth.org/parent/community/ poison_control_center.a_k.html.*

There are several reasons why the pharmacist should refer calls to the poison control center. Most calls involve an ongoing incident that may require immediate and intensive counseling. The typical pharmacy is busy with routine duties such as prescription filling and counseling, nonprescription product counseling, and technician monitoring. It may

Continued

studies are equivocal.[18,26] Some studies show increased time to emesis with concomitant milk, but others show no effect. The issue is important since a poisoned child may be unwilling to drink large quantities of water and no other clear fluid may be available.

⚠️ *Ipecac must not be used for patients who risk aspiration during emesis.* For this reason, it is contraindicated when patients are not fully conscious, perhaps as a result of an ingested medication.[18] Commonly ingested medications altering mental status include antihistamines, opioids, benzodiazepines, ethanol, tricyclic antidepressants, beta-blockers, phenothiazines, theophylline, and barbiturates.[20] To illustrate this hazard, a patient being treated for tricyclic overdose aspirated after a rapid change in mental status.[20]

tip *The ipecac label cautions the person administering the ipecac not to give activated charcoal until the patient has vomited since the activated charcoal will adsorb ipecac.[18]*

be difficult to give a poisoning incident the attention it deserves. Furthermore, the pharmacy library is virtually useless when compared with an up-to-date poison control center database. Finally, a pharmacist who handles just one or two poisoning calls per month

tip cannot maintain the expertise of the poison control center personnel, who field many calls each day. *As a pharmacist, do not hesitate to refer all calls to the experts.*

When the pharmacist receives a phone call involving a poisoning incident, it is vital to immediately obtain the caller's phone number in case the call is interrupted on either end and communication needs to be reestablished. When referring callers or customers to a poison control center, the pharmacist should advise them to have the following information ready:

- The patient's age
- The patient's weight
- The patient's preexisting health conditions or problems, if any
- The current status of the patient
- The substance involved and whether it was inhaled, swallowed, absorbed through skin contact, or splashed into the eyes
- Any first aid or other treatment that may have been given
- Whether the victim has vomited
- The victim's location, and how long it would take to get to an emergency room

For more information on poison control centers, write Secretary, Poison Prevention Week Council, Box 1543, Washington, D.C. 20013.

Other Precautions to Observe With Ipecac

tip *When a patient requests ipecac, the pharmacist should ask whether it is for a possible poisoning or merely to stock the medicine cabinet for later use when needed. (See "A*

A Pharmacist's Journal

"Are You Still Open? Do You Have Ipecac?"

The discount store in which our pharmacy is located had just closed one evening when the phone rang. I was backing the computer and about ready to leave and I hesitated a moment before answering. When I did, a frantic voice asked, "Are you still open? Do you have ipecac?" I asked the caller to briefly tell me what had happened after assuring her that I would make sure that she could get ipecac if she needed it. She said that a 2-year-old visiting his grandparents had been found with a bottle of Tylenol tablets about 30 minutes earlier. They were afraid he had eaten 30 or more tablets. Someone had told them that all they needed to do was give him syrup of ipecac. I urged them to reconsider and take the child to the emergency room immediately because of the extreme danger posed by acetaminophen. They said they would, but

wanted to get the ipecac on the way to the hospital. I told the person manning the front door to expect the grandparents and to admit them without any argument. They arrived a few minutes later and said they were on the way to the emergency room. I sold them the ipecac and stressed that speed was of the essence.

I later saw the grandparents in town and asked what the outcome was. They said that the child was considered to be sufficiently serious that he was airlifted to a larger hospital. He regurgitated several times while in the helicopter and recovered uneventfully. Needless to say, that was one time I was glad I answered the phone, even though the pharmacy was closed.

In retrospect, I should have provided the phone number of the Poison Control Center, but I was so intent on getting the child to the emergency room that I neglected to think of this most basic advice.

Patient Assessment Algorithm 25.1. Part 1 Poisoning

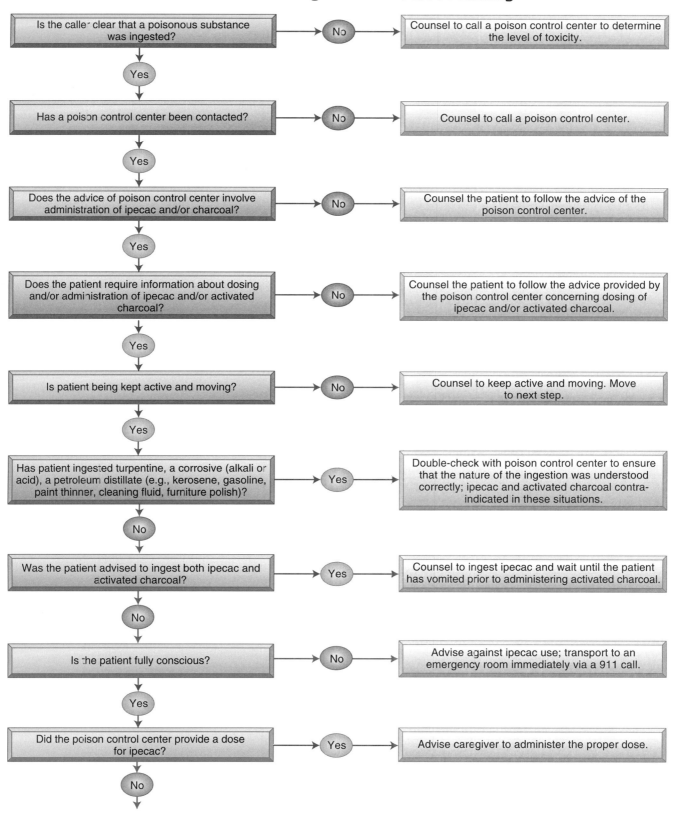

Pharmacist's Journal: Will Ipecac Work for This Problem?") When a customer wants to purchase ipecac to have ready in case of a poisoning emergency, the pharmacist should point out the expiration date and caution the customer to purchase a product prior to that date. The pharmacist should explain that it could be futile to use an expired bottle and could delay proper care.

If a toxic situation has occurred, the pharmacist should provide all of the directions, cautions, and warnings associated with ipecac. ***Ipecac is contraindicated when a***

Patient Assessment Algorithm 25.1. Part 2 Poisoning

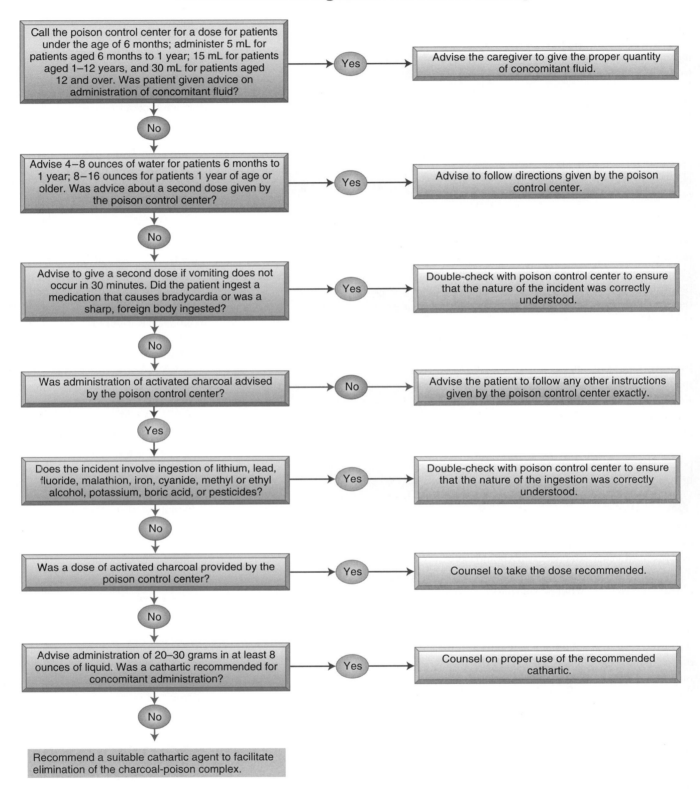

Call the poison control center for a dose for patients under the age of 6 months; administer 5 mL for patients aged 6 months to 1 year; 15 mL for patients aged 1–12 years, and 30 mL for patients aged 12 and over. Was patient given advice on administration of concomitant fluid?

Yes → Advise the caregiver to give the proper quantity of concomitant fluid.

No ↓

Advise 4–8 ounces of water for patients 6 months to 1 year; 8–16 ounces for patients 1 year of age or older. Was advice about a second dose given by the poison control center?

Yes → Advise to follow directions given by the poison control center.

No ↓

Advise to give a second dose if vomiting does not occur in 30 minutes. Did the patient ingest a medication that causes bradycardia or was a sharp, foreign body ingested?

Yes → Double-check with poison control center to ensure that the nature of the incident was correctly understood.

No ↓

Was administration of activated charcoal advised by the poison control center?

No → Advise the patient to follow any other instructions given by the poison control center exactly.

Yes ↓

Does the incident involve ingestion of lithium, lead, fluoride, malathion, iron, cyanide, methyl or ethyl alcohol, potassium, boric acid, or pesticides?

Yes → Double-check with poison control center to ensure that the nature of the ingestion was correctly understood.

No ↓

Was a dose of activated charcoal provided by the poison control center?

Yes → Counsel to take the dose recommended.

No ↓

Advise administration of 20–30 grams in at least 8 ounces of liquid. Was a cathartic recommended for concomitant administration?

Yes → Counsel on proper use of the recommended cathartic.

No ↓

Recommend a suitable cathartic agent to facilitate elimination of the charcoal-poison complex.

---

patient is experiencing seizures because of the risk of as- piration. (In one case, a patient who overdosed on isoniazid had unexpected convulsions and aspirated during ipecac- induced regurgitation.[20]) It is also contraindicated when the medication ingested produces seizures (e.g., lindane).[15]

If more than 1 hour has elapsed since the ingestion, the efficacy of ipecac is reduced.[20] Given within 1 hour of ingestion, ipecac removes an average of 30 to 60% of stom- ach contents; the figure drops to 15 to 30% if 1 hour has elapsed since the ingestion.[25] If the ingestant is a liquid, the time is shorter, since liquids do not require dissolution prior to absorption. Since studies confirm that the average parent takes more than 1 hour to get the child to the emergency room, ipecac is best used at home. While it is true that some medications slow gastrointestinal motility, perhaps allowing ipecac to retain effectiveness beyond 60 minutes, they may also alter mental status (e.g., anticholinergics, opioids) and are contraindicated with emesis.[20] Ipecac is of questionable usefulness if the patient has already vomited, so pharmacists should not recommend it.

Ipecac should not be used in nontoxic ingestions (e.g., a single berry or leaf from a plant, two or three tablets of non–iron-containing vitamin) because of the risk of adverse effects such as **prolonged hyperemesis** (an abnormally long period of vomiting). For instance, it was used in one situation to "teach the child a lesson" and another when a child ate only a small piece of toilet paper.[20] Hyperemesis may necessitate hospital admission.

⚠ *Ipecac should not be used if the ingested substance might cause bradycardia* (e.g., beta-blockers), since it may potentiate bradycardia as a result of vagal effects.[20,44] It should only be used under a physician's supervision if the patient is very young or very old and in instances where a sharp foreign body has been ingested.

ACTIVATED CHARCOAL

Activated charcoal is a nonspecific antidote for a wide range of poisoning emergencies.[46–48] It adsorbs many toxins, and may be followed with a cathartic to facilitate elimination of the adsorbed poison-charcoal complex and prevent obstruction. (See "Cathartics.")

Production and Mechanism of Activated Charcoal

Activated charcoal is produced when vegetable matter (e.g., wood pulp) is subjected to heat in excess of 1650°F, followed by acid or steam washing—a process known as destructive distillation.[22,49] This process produces an activated charcoal with an extremely intricate internal honeycomb-like pore structure that is able to adsorb many different substances.[25,50] The surface area of activated charcoal increases from 2 to 4 square meters per gram to over 1000 square meters (10,000 square feet) per gram, giving it tremendous ad-

GENERAL LABELING FOR ALL POISON-TREATMENT PRODUCTS

The FDA requires the labels of all poison control drug products to include several important precautions[18]:

- Those who plan to administer the product are directed to call a poison control center, emergency facility, or health professional before using the product.
- They are advised to follow directions as stated on the container if help cannot be contacted.
- They are advised to read the warnings and directions as soon as the product is purchased and insert an emergency phone number in a blank space on the label.
- Those administering the product are directed to keep the patient active and moving and to save the poison container.
- If previously unable to contact a poison control center, emergency medical facility, or health professional, they will be cautioned to continue trying.

The only products approved for treating poisoning in the United States at this time are syrup of ipecac as an emetic and activated charcoal as an adsorbent. *Neither ipecac nor activated charcoal should be administered to patients who are not fully conscious, since their ability to protect the airway during emesis is compromised.*[18] Both are required to carry additional labeling. The labels of both products will caution against use if the patient has ingested turpentine, corrosives (e.g., alkalies such as lye or strong acids), or petroleum distillates (e.g., kerosene, gasoline, paint thinner, cleaning fluid, or furniture polish), unless directed to do so by a health professional.[18,19] Ipecac-induced regurgitation of caustics or corrosives (e.g., drain cleaners, dishwasher detergents) would reexpose the esophagus to the chemicals. (Some authorities advise administration of large volumes of water or milk to dilute the toxin, although this may also produce a dangerous emesis.)[18,20–22] Aspiration could occur with emesis of hydrocarbons and petroleum distillates since their low viscosity allows them to enter the bronchial tree without detection by the patient, causing lipid pneumonia.[22,23] (Even though activated charcoal is not an emetic, these warnings are still required on its labels since its administration can produce vomiting, perhaps because of the taste.)

Table 25.1. Dose of Ipecac and Water Recommended for Various Ages

PATIENT AGE	IPECAC DOSE	AMOUNT OF WATER
Younger than 6 months	No dose; call physician immediately	
6 months–1 year	5 mL	4–8 ounces
1–12 years	15 mL	8–16 ounces
12 years and over	30 mL	8–16 ounces

Adapted from Fed Reg 50:2244, 1985.

sorptive capacity. Medications and other substances adsorb to the surface of activated charcoal, forming a poison-toxin complex (Fig. 25.1).[25,51]

Preparation of Activated Charcoal

Activated charcoal is available premixed in sorbitol or water, in squeeze tubes, or as a powder that must be suspended in liquid prior to administration (Table 25.2).[46] Premixed bot-

A Pharmacist's Journal

"Will Ipecac Work for This Problem?"

I teach the students to question ipecac purchasers about the nature of the ingestion. However, the things you hear may surprise you. A young mother came in to buy ipecac and asked if it would be appropriate in the following circumstance: "I just went in to the store for a few minutes," she said. "When I returned, the 1-year-old was chewing on something. It appeared to be a greenish material. I asked his 4-year-old sister what he was eating, since there wasn't anything in the car to eat. She pretended that she didn't know, but eventually she pointed under the front seat. I reached under the seat and pulled out a fast-food foil wrapper.

Then I remembered that I had not finished a fast-food hamburger several months earlier and threw it under the seat. I guess his big sister wanted to play carhop and delivered him the hamburger. Would he need to take syrup of ipecac?"

I explained that it might be helpful, since the old meat would probably be contaminated with bacteria and perhaps fungi. I suggested she observe him for any symptoms indicative of a GI infection and call his pediatrician if they developed. Of course, this incident also points out the dangers inherent in leaving young children alone in any situation, especially in a car in a parking lot.

---

tles should be agitated thoroughly before use to ensure uniform suspension of the activated charcoal. (Sorbitol is under FDA scrutiny since it was not approved as a vehicle in the tentative final monograph and may eventually be removed from these products because of lack of efficacy as an adjunctive agent.[52]) Squeezable tubes include tips that fit nasogastric tubes to allow passage directly into the stomach, reducing the risk of aspiration.

Advantages of Activated Charcoal

Because of its relative safety and efficacy, use of activated charcoal increased in emergency departments by 71% from 1986 to 1992, displacing ipecac syrup.[14]

Activated charcoal has demonstrated effectiveness in poisonings involving acetaminophen, aminophylline, amitriptyline, ampicillin, aspirin, barbiturates, carbamazepine, chlorpheniramine, chlorpromazine, colchicine, dextroamphetamine, digoxin, doxepin, ethchlorvynol, fluoxetine, phenobarbital, phenylpropanolamine, phenytoin, propoxyphene, strychnine, tetracycline, theophylline, and tricyclic antidepressants.[22,50,53,54]

Activated charcoal is most effective given soon after ingestion since medications that have already passed the pylorus may not be bound unless the charcoal moves rapidly enough to contact them.[22]

Usefulness of Activated Charcoal with Other Modalities

Activated charcoal does not reduce the effectiveness of most other poisoning interventions. For instance, the action of *N*-acetylcysteine in treatment of acetaminophen overdosage is not compromised if the patient also receives activated charcoal.[55]

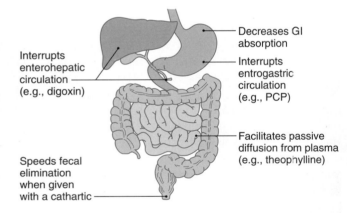

Figure 25.1. Multidose activated charcoal is thought to be helpful in poison ingestion through several mechanisms. *GI, gastrointestinal; PCP, phencyclidine.*

Multidose Activated Charcoal

Multiple doses of activated charcoal (e.g., 40 g initially in phenobarbital ingestion, followed by 40 g every 4 hours for five doses) seem beneficial for several reasons: unabsorbed poison may be adsorbed (Fig 25.1).[50,56,57] Also, medications that are secreted in bile are adsorbed, so that the cycle of enterohepatic circulation is halted. Finally, medications that diffuse passively back into the gastric lumen from the circulation are also adsorbed, interrupting the phenomenon of enterogastric recirculation.[46,50] In this sense, multiple-dose activated charcoal is an alternative to dialysis (by using the gut as a dialysis membrane) or hemoperfusion for such medications as phenobarbital, carbamazepine, theophylline, phenytoin, aspirin, dapsone, vancomycin, and quinine, although it does not appear to be helpful for sodium valproate.[2,56,58–61]

Superiority to the "Universal Antidote"

Occasionally, patients ask about the "universal antidote," which contained activated charcoal, tannic acid, and magnesium oxide. However, the added ingredients have no advantage over activated charcoal alone, and may interfere with its effectiveness.[22] The tannic acid also may be hepatotoxic.

Disadvantages of Activated Charcoal

Although activated charcoal is considered by most medical authorities to have desirable characteristics, its use is not without controversy and some research has failed to show benefits to its use.[28] It should be given as quickly as possible after ingestion, for instance, to maximize its effectiveness.[62]

Adverse Effects of Activated **tip** *Charcoal. Occasionally, activated charcoal may be aspirated into the pulmonary system,* the most serious complication arising from its use.[63] In one

---

FOCUS ON...

ADDITIONAL METHODS OF GASTRIC EMPTYING

GASTRIC LAVAGE

Gastric lavage is another option for gastric emptying for patients with a contraindication to emesis.[25,45] If the airway is protected, lavage is safe, although some adverse effects may occur such as epistaxis, hypothermia if the solution is too cool, and esophageal perforation. Gastric lavage is also a more rapid method than ipecac.

MANUAL PRODUCTION OF EMESIS

Many people believe that emesis stimulated by mechanical means is also effective. Usually an object such as the blunt end of a spoon or a finger is placed down the back of the throat to trigger gagging that should culminate in the vomiting reflex.[22] If the patient undertakes this procedure, s/he should keep her/his head lower than the hips to lessen the risk of aspiration. Also, drinking several glasses of water before the procedure helps ensure effectiveness.

Mechanical means are usually unsuccessful, and return of gastric contents is incomplete.

ZINC SULFATE

Zinc sulfate produces vomiting through a local effect on gastric mucosa.[18] However, its toxicity is such that the FDA did not consider it for nonprescription use. While the effective dose is 2 g in 200 mL of water, repeated once in 15 minutes, the zinc sulfate might not produce emesis. *If zinc sulfate does not result in emesis, it must be removed by suction tube, since its absorption produces hemolytic effects, renal toxicity, and death.* The lethal dose is 3 to 15 g. Patients considering its use must be strongly dissuaded.

OTHER METHODS

Copper sulfate, not available as a nonprescription product, can cause toxicity and should be avoided. Mustard powder in water, mustard in milk, salt water, and dishwashing detergent are old home remedies that are of unknown effectiveness. Relying on them instead of using an effective product or seeking professional help would be unwise. Further, salt water could produce sodium toxicity itself. At least one Internet site promotes cat's claw (uncaria tomentosa) for environmental toxin poisoning, but this herb lacks any scientific proof of effectiveness.

Table 25.2. Representative Activated Charcoal Products for Treatment of Poisoning

PRODUCT	SELECTED INGREDIENTS/COMMENTS
Actidose with Sorbitol	Activated charcoal 25 g per 120 mL or 50 g per 240 mL, with sorbitol 48 g per 120 mL or 96 g per 240 mL in bottles or tubes
Actidose-Aqua	Activated charcoal 25 g per 120 mL or 50 g per 240 mL in bottles or tubes
Charcoaid	Activated charcoal 30 g per 150 mL in sorbitol solution
Charcoaid G	Activated charcoal with a surface area of 2000 square meters/g, available in 15-g bottles of dry powder
CharcoAid 2000	Activated charcoal with a surface area of 2000 square meters/g, available in 240-mL bottles containing 50 g of activated charcoal
Insta-Char Aqueous	Activated charcoal 25 g per 120 mL or 50 g per 240 mL, unflavored or cherry flavored
Insta-Char/Sorbitol	Activated charcoal 25 g per 120 mL or 50 g per 240 mL with sorbitol 25 g per 120 mL or 50 g per 240 mL, cherry flavored
Liqui-Char Tubes	Activated charcoal alone or with sorbitol
Liqui-Char Bottles	Activated charcoal alone or with sorbitol

such case, a 30-year-old man being treated for overdose of amitriptyline was given gastric lavage through a nasogastric tube.[46] He removed his tube, and it was accidentally reinserted into the right mainstream bronchus, and activated charcoal/sorbitol was inadvertently introduced into his lungs. After the mistake was discovered, the material was suctioned from the lungs, although he continued to have charcoal-tinged sputum, as well as adult respiratory distress syndrome. He was discharged after 2 weeks. (The case highlights the dangers of aspiration in patients with depressed mental status, as well as the need to verify nasogastric tube placement via auscultation or x-ray prior to administration of any medication or feeding.)

tip *Activated charcoal may cause bowel obstruction in rare instances requiring surgical intervention*, especially when a cathartic is not given concurrently.[63,64] The risk is heightened in patients taking medications that slow intestinal motility (e.g., anticholinergics) and those with past surgical adhesions in the bowel.[65] A patient with adhesions from an earlier surgery was given multiple-dose activated charcoal (a total of 350 g) for theophylline toxicity. She experienced vomiting, constipation, periumbilical pain, abdominal distension, and dehydration. Subsequently, a 4.5 by 5 by 3 cm charcoal obstruction was found that required surgical removal. In another case, a patient taking methadone and amitriptyline was given 100 g of activated charcoal to treat abnormally high amitriptyline levels.[66] Pursuant to complaints of abdominal discomfort, she was found to have a **stercolith** (a fecal mass, composed of charcoal in this case) that weighed 120 g. The stercolith produced a 4 cm tear in the sigmoid colon that necessitated resection and construction of a diverting colostomy. No cathartics had been given to help ease elimination of the charcoal. The possibility of bowel obstruction argues for concomitant cathartic administration.

Activated charcoal should only be given cautiously to the combative or agitated patient. In two such cases, it was accidentally spilled onto the patient's face and into the eyes.[67] The product may have caused corneal abrasions suffered by both patients, which resolved without ophthalmic sequelae. The authors recommended irrigation and fluorescein examination in such cases.

Constipation, empyema, **bronchiolitis obliterans** (obstruction of the terminal bronchioles caused by aspiration of activated charcoal), perforation, and vomiting also may occur with use of activated charcoal.[65,67]

Desorption. The charcoal-poison complex may undergo a phenomenon known as **desorption** (a process in which the toxic substance loses its affinity for the charcoal and thus might be absorbed).[68] Patients may be given laxatives or cathartics to hasten removal of the complex prior to desorption, but the phenomenon of desorption may not occur as often as believed.[22]

Ineffectiveness for Certain Substances. Activated charcoal is not effective for lithium, lead, fluoride, malathion, iron, cyanide, methyl and ethyl alcohol, potassium, boric acid, and some pesticides.[19,25,50,69]

Pediatric Resistance. The black color of the activated charcoal slurry can cause apprehension in some children, who examine products visually with great care before ingestion.[22] Should a child swallow some and balk at another mouthful, they may spit or spew the remainder out, which could stain clothing and walls.[22]

FDA-Approved Labeling for Activated Charcoal

Experts recommend doses 8 to 10 times that of the toxic agent.[22,49] About 5 to 10 g of activated charcoal will adsorb 1 g of most substances.[22] However, the inability to estimate quantities of ingestant makes large doses (50 to 100 g) advisable. The FDA requested that activated charcoal products contain a minimum of 30 g of activated charcoal.[18,22] The labeled dose is 20 to 30 g in a minimum of 8 ounces of liquid, repeated immediately if possible.[18] For this reason, the patient may need to purchase several bottles.

tip *The label cautions against administering activated charcoal until the patient has vomited, unless directed to do so by a health professional.[18] Thus the patient may wish to purchase ipecac for initial administration.*

As noted above, activated charcoal is not a specific antidote for any substance but serves as an adjunctive agent while any specific antidotes that may exist are also being used.[22] This characteristic of activated charcoal is justification for the label instruction to continue trying to contact a poison control center, emergency medical facility, or health professional if unable to do so prior to administering charcoal. (See "General Labeling for All Poison Treatment Products.")

CATHARTICS

Catharsis is a final component of gastric decontamination.[68,70] Used in conjunction with activated charcoal, an oral cathartic helps remove the charcoal-substance complex and also may facilitate removal of remaining toxin that has neither been absorbed by the body nor adsorbed onto the activated charcoal.[66,71]

The use of cathartics is also controversial, however, since these agents present their own set of adverse reactions in all age groups, and their use is not conclusively proven to be beneficial.[2,56] In one study, magnesium citrate decreased the gastrointestinal transit times of activated charcoal, although the authors suggested further studies to determine the exact medical benefit one could expect.[68] Like many medical controversies, the issue has not been settled.

If rapid catharsis is indicated the oral saline laxatives (e.g., magnesium citrate, magnesium sulfate, magnesium hydroxide, sodium phosphate/biphosphate) are usually appropriate.

PREVENTION OF POISONING

Like many medical conditions prevention can reduce the need for treatment. When pharmacists sell ipecac for possible future use, a list of reminders could be provided to customers to help reduce the risk of accidental poisoning:

- Ensure that all medications, household chemicals, and pesticides are stored in containers with child-resistant caps.

- Keep all hazardous household products separate from foods and medicines, away from children, preferably in a locked cabinet or in a cabinet with a childproof latch.
- Store medicines separately from household chemicals and food, away from children, preferably in a locked cabinet or in a cabinet with a childproof latch.
- Keep all household chemical products and medicines out of sight and out of reach of children, preferably in a locked cabinet or in a cabinet with a childproof latch.
- Do not take medication in front of children. (They tend to imitate adults.)
- When using a household chemical or medicine, never leave it near a child. If necessary, take the child along when leaving the area—such as to answer the phone or doorbell.
- Store pesticides in a locked cabinet or household shed. Remove children and their toys from the area before using these products.
- Keep all products in original containers. Never transfer hazardous substances to food or beverage containers.
- Read labels before using any product. Never take any medications from an unlabeled bottle.
- Never give or take medicine in the dark.
- Never refer to medicine as "candy" when giving it to children.
- Ensure all medications remain in their childproof containers.
- Teach children not to eat berries, leaves, or other parts of plants.
- Remember: Many poisonings occur when children are under parental supervision. Having a parent in the house will not necessarily prevent poisonings.
- Discard medicines more than 2 years old or when expired. Do not throw old medicine in the trash—flush it and rinse the container before discarding.
- Before giving a medication that is packaged with a dose device (e.g., a dosing cup), read the directions and examine the device carefully to ensure that the correct dose is given.[72]

Prevention of intentional poisoning is more difficult since it involves an act of intentional will. Pharmacists who become aware of suicide threats such as potential poisonings should take immediate action (e.g., notify the patient's family, a physician, social services, law enforcement officials, etc.). If the patient receives mental help, serious injury or death may be prevented.

SUMMARY

Accidental and intentional poisoning present a challenge to the typical pharmacist since counseling must be immediate and accurate. A lack of specialized references in the typical pharmacy argues for referring calls to a poison control center. However, pharmacists must be capable of answering questions regarding the two safe and effective nonprescription products for poisonings: syrup of ipecac and activated charcoal.

Syrup of ipecac is the traditional agent of choice for first-line therapy of accidental poisoning in the home, although its

AT THE COUNTER

 A father phones the pharmacy at 6:00 PM to ask about a possible poisoning.

Interview/Patient Assessment

The caller's 4-year-old son opened his prescription bottle of Zantac and ingested some tablets about 30 minutes before. The bottle originally contained 60 tablets, and only 35 remain; however, the father doesn't know how many had been in the bottle since he only takes it when symptoms occur. The child is alert and playing. The father wants to know if he should give the child the ipecac he bought several months ago.

Pharmacist's Analysis

1. Is Zantac one of the most dangerous poisons?
2. Is syrup of ipecac indicated for Zantac ingestion?
3. What dose of syrup of ipecac is appropriate? What ancillary measures should be recommended?

Zantac is not one of the most dangerous agents in accidental ingestion episodes (as listed in this chapter). Its ingestion does not contraindicate use of ipecac or activated charcoal.

Patient Counseling

The father should first be given the phone number of a Poison Control Center for formal instruction. If this information is not available, the father should administer a 15-mL dosage of syrup of ipecac, then repeat once after 30 minutes if the boy has not vomited. The father should be advised to keep the child active to augment the efficacy of ipecac. The father should also be cautioned to consider a visit to the emergency room if the ipecac does not induce vomiting or if the child begins to exhibit any symptoms at all.

use should be considered part of a total therapeutic plan coordinated by a poison control center, emergency medical facility, or health professional. While activated charcoal is often chosen as treatment in the emergency room, it is not yet sold in many pharmacies nor is it stocked in the average home. Therefore, the pharmacist must be fully aware of the shortcomings and advantages of both agents, as well as the precautions associated with their use and abuse.

References

1. Wigder HN, et al. Emergency department poison advice telephone calls. Ann Emerg Med 25:349, 1995

2. Bond GR. The poisoned child. Emerg Med Clin North Am 13:343, 1995.

3. Kelly NR, et al. Effectiveness of a poison center: Impact on medical facility visits. Vet Hum Toxicol 39:44, 1997.

4. Bablouzian L, et al. Evaluation of a community based childhood injury prevention program. Inj Prev 3:14, 1997.

5. Bowden CA, Krenzelok EP. Clinical applications of commonly used contemporary antidotes. A US perspective. Drug Saf 16:9, 1997.

6. Litovitz TL, et al. 1994 annual report of the American Association of Poison Control Centers toxic exposure surveillance system. Am J Emerg Med 13:551, 1995.

7. Meredith TJ. Epidemiology of poisoning. Pharmacol Ther 59:251, 1993.

8. Koren G. Medications which can kill a toddler with one tablet or teaspoonful. J Toxicol Clin Toxicol 31:407, 1993.

9. Henretig FM. Special considerations in the poisoned pediatric patient. Emerg Med Clin North Am 12:549, 1994.

10. Armstrong DS. Childproof containers (Letter). Can Med Assoc J 148:1674, 1993.

11. Jackson RH, Craft AW. Poisoning and child resistant containers. BMJ 305:522, 1992.

12. Dees DN, Dees DJ. Child abuse by poisoning. SD J Med 46:91, 1993.

13. Gotschlich T, Beltran RS. Poisoning of a 21-month-old child by a baby-sitter. Clin Pediatr 34:52, 1995.

14. Bond GR. Home use of syrup of ipecac is associated with a reduction in pediatric emergency department visits. Ann Emerg Med 25:338, 1995.

15. Morelli J. Pediatric poisonings: The 10 most toxic prescription drugs. Am J Nurs 93:27, 1993.

16. Tibballs J. Clinical effects and management of eucalyptus oil ingestion in infants and young children. Med J Aust 163:177, 1995.

17. Buckley NA, Dawson AH, Reith DA. Controlled release drugs in overdose. Clinical considerations. Drug Saf 12:73, 1995.

18. Fed Reg 50:2244, 1985.

19. Lamminpaa A, Vilska J, Hoppu K. Medical charcoal for a child's poisoning at home: Availability and success of administration in Finland. Hum Exp Toxicol 12:29, 1993.

20. Wrenn K, Rodewald L, Dockstader L. Potential misuse of ipecac. Ann Emerg Med 22:1408, 1993.

21. Johannsen HG, Mikkelsen JB, Larsen CF. Poisoning with household chemicals in children. Acta Pediatr Scand 83:1317, 1994.

22. Fed Reg 47:444, 1982.

23. Holdsclaw VA, Nykamp D. Treating poisonings: Focus on syrup of ipecac. Am Pharm NS32:31, 1992

24. Dresser LP, et al. Ipecac myopathy and cardiomyopathy. J Neurol Neurosurg Psychiatry 56:560, 1993.

25. Gaar GG. Gastrointestinal decontamination for acute poisoning by ingestion. J Fla Med Assoc 81:747, 1994.

26. Klein-Schwartz W, et al. The effect of milk on ipecac-induced emesis. J Toxicol Clin Toxicol 29:505, 1991.

27. Saetta JP, Quinton DN. Residual gastric content after gastric lavage and ipecacuanha-induced emesis in self-poisoned patients: An endoscopic study. JR Soc Med 84:35, 1991.

28. Merigian KS, et al. Prospective evaluation of gastric emptying in the self-poisoned patient. Am J Emerg Med 8:479, 1990.

29. Garrettson LK. Ipecac home use: We need hope replaced with data. J Toxicol Clin Toxicol 29:515, 1991.

30. Kurta DL, Myers LB, Krenzelok EP. Zolpidem (Ambien): A pediatric case series. J Toxicol Clin Toxicol 35:453, 1997.

31. Carraccio C, Blotny K, Ringel R. Sudden onset of profound weakness in a toddler. J Pediatr 122:663, 1993.

32. Vanin JR. Ipecac abuse—Danger. J Am Coll Health 40:237, 1992.

33. Angle CR. Is ipecac obsolete? J Toxicol Clin Toxicol 29:513, 1991.

34. Brushwood DB, Tietze KJ. Regulatory controversy surrounding ipecac use and misuse. Am J Hosp Pharm 43:157, 1986.

35. Lovejoy FH, Shannon M, Woolf AD. Recent advances in clinical toxicology. Curr Probl Pediatr 22:119, 1992.

36. Greaves I, Goodacre S, Group P. Management of drug overdoses in accident and emergency departments in the United Kingdom. J Accid Emerg Med 13:46, 1996.

37. Minton NA, Glucksman E, Henry JA. Prevention of drug absorption in simulated theophylline overdose. Hum Exp Toxicol 14:170, 1995.

38. Kornberg AE, Dolgin J. Pediatric ingestions: Charcoal alone versus ipecac and charcoal. Ann Emerg Med 20:648, 1991.

39. Albertson TE, et al. Superiority of activated charcoal alone compared with ipecac and activated charcoal in the treatment of acute toxic ingestions. Ann Emerg Med 18:56, 1989.

40. Pond SM, et al. Gastric emptying in acute overdose: A prospective randomised controlled trial. Med J Aust 163:345, 1995.

41. Goebel J, Gremse DA, Artman M. Cardiomyopathy from ipecac administration in Munchausen syndrome by proxy. Pediatrics 92:601, 1993.

42. Greenfeld D, et al. Ipecac abuse in a sample of eating disordered outpatients. Int J Eat Disord 13:411, 1993.

43. Lacomis D. Case of the month. June 1996—Anorexia nervosa. Brain Pathol 6:535, 1996.

44. Reith DM, et al. Relative toxicity of beta blockers in overdose. J Toxicol Clin Toxicol 34:273, 1996.

45. Bayer MJ, McKay C. Advances in poison management. Clin Chem 42(8 Pt 2):1361, 1996.

46. Harris CR, Filandrinos D. Accidental aspiration of activated charcoal into the lung: Aspiration by proxy. Ann Emerg Med 22:1470, 1993.

47. Smilkstein MJ. Therapy for toxicologic emergencies. Acad Emerg Med 1:126, 1994.

48. Krenzelok EP, Leikin JB. Approach to the poisoned patient. Dis Mon 42:509, 1996.

49. Orisakwe OE. Activated charcoal: Is failure to use it negligence or ignorance? South Med J 87:165, 1994.

50. Vale JA, Proudfoot AT. How useful is activated charcoal? BMJ 306:78, 1993.

51. Roberts JR, Gracely EJ, Schoffstall JM. Advantage of high-surface-area charcoal for gastrointestinal decontamination in a human acetaminophen ingestion model. Acad Emerg Med 4:167, 1997.

52. Cooney DO. *In vitro* adsorption of phenobarbital, chlorpheniramine maleate, and theophylline by four commercially available activated charcoal suspensions. J Toxicol Clin Toxicol 33:213, 1995.

53. Laine K, et al. The effect of activated charcoal on the absorption of fluoxetine, with special reference to delayed charcoal administration. Pharmacol Toxicol 79:270, 1996.

54. Ibanez C, et al. Activated charcoal increases digoxin elimination in patients. Int J Cardiol 48:27, 1995.

55. Spiller HA, et al. A prospective evaluation of the effect of activated charcoal before oral *N*-acetylcysteine in acetaminophen overdose. Ann Emerg Med 23:519, 1994.

56. Bradberry SM, Vale JA. Multiple-dose activated charcoal: A review of relevant clinical studies. J Toxicol Clin Toxicol 33:407, 1995.

57. Chyka PA. Multiple-dose activated charcoal and enhancement of systemic drug clearance: Summary of studies in animals and human volunteers. J Toxicol Clin Toxicol 33:399, 1995.

58. Chyka PA, et al. Correlation of drug pharmacokinetics and effectiveness of multiple-dose activated charcoal therapy. Ann Emerg Med 25:356, 1995.

59. Frenia ML, et al. Multiple-dose activated charcoal compared to urinary alkalinization for the enhancement of phenobarbital elimination. J Toxicol Clin Toxicol 34:169, 1996.

60. Kucukguchu S, et al. Multiple-dose activated charcoal in an accidental vancomycin overdose. J Toxicol Clin Toxicol 34:83, 1996.

61. al-Shareef A, et al. The effect of repeated-dose activated charcoal on the pharmacokinetics of sodium valproate in healthy volunteers. Br J Clin Pharmacol 43:109, 1997.

62. Crockett R, et al. Prehospital use of activated charcoal: A pilot study. J Emerg Med 14:335, 1996.

63. Mauro LS, Nawarskas JJ, Mauro VF. Misadventures with activated charcoal and recommendations for safe use. Ann Pharmacother 28:915, 1994.

64. Atkinson SW, Young Y, Trotter GA. Treatment with activated charcoal complicated by gastrointestinal obstruction requiring surgery. BMJ 305:563, 1992.

65. Goulbourne KB, Cisek JE. Small-bowel obstruction secondary to activated charcoal and adhesions. Ann Emerg Med 24:108, 1994.

66. Gomez HF, et al. Charcoal stercolith with intestinal perforation in a patient treated for amitriptyline ingestion. J Emerg Med 12:57, 1994

67. McKinney PE, et al. Corneal abrasions secondary to activated charcoal. Am J Emerg Med 11:562, 1993

68. Sue Y-J, Woolf A, Shannon M. Efficacy of magnesium citrate cathartic in pediatric toxic ingestions. Ann Emerg Med 24:709, 1994

69. Graves HB, et al. Clinical policy for the initial approach to patients presenting with acute toxic ingestion or dermal or inhalation exposure. Ann Emerg Med 25:570, 1995

70. James LP, Nichols MH, King WD. A comparison of cathartics in pediatric ingestions. Pediatrics 96:235, 1995

71. McFarland AK III, Chyka PA. Selection of activated charcoal products for the treatment of poisonings. Ann Pharmacother 27:358, 1993.

72. Litovitz T, et al. Surveillance of loperamide ingestions: An analysis of 216 poison control center reports. J Toxicol Clin Toxicol 35:11, 1997.

Fever

AT THE COUNTER

A college-aged student asks the pharmacist how much Tylenol he can take for a fever.

Interview/Patient Assessment

The patient says he is not taking any medications and says that he does not have any medical conditions. He said he began to feel "achy" yesterday and he missed class today because he did not feel well. He reported a fever of 101 to 102°F, taken orally an hour or so before.

Pharmacist's Analysis

1. What is the probable cause of this patient's fever?
2. Is a fever of this magnitude dangerous?
3. Which antipyretics would be effective for this patient?

The patient may have any one of a number of minor conditions that produce fever, a protective response that aug-

ments the body's ability to fight infection. A temperature of 101 to 102°F is not dangerous but may add to the malaise caused by the infectious process itself.

Patient Counseling

The patient should be urged to consider the fever as a normal body process that can be helpful in fighting illness. He should also be urged to continue to monitor his temperature and see a physician if the fever exceeds 103°F, worsens, or lasts longer than 3 days total. Should he wish to treat the fever, he may use any of several antipyretics, although the risk of Reye syndrome argues against the use of aspirin. Acetaminophen, ibuprofen, naproxen, or ketoprofen could all be used by this patient for a total of 3 days from the onset of fever. If the fever is still present after 3 days total, he should see a physician.

Fever indicates body temperature above the "normal" value—traditionally cited as 98.6°F (37°C).[1–3] For purposes of this chapter, "normal" will refer to this well-accepted value. A range of measurements are presented as "normal" in the medical literature, however, from 96°F (35.6°C) to 99.9°F (37.7°C). The wide discrepancy in these figures only serves to stress the inadequacy of choosing a specific figure or range as "normal" because of the many variables that affect body temperature.[1,4–6] (See "Body Temperature Regulation.") The issue is further clouded by the use of such terms as "low-grade fever" (perhaps used by medical authors to refer to a body temperature of as low as 99.6 to 100°F, although the author's definition should be consulted), and "high-grade fever" (perhaps used to refer to temperatures of 102 to 104°F or more, although the specific author's definition should be consulted here also).[5]

Fever, like other symptoms, is not a medical condition in itself, but is a reflection of a pathologic process. Once considered an abnormal problem that must be corrected, fever is increasingly recognized as a critical mechanism in the body's disease defense, a mechanism associated with increased disease survival and more rapid recovery from disease.[2,8]

PREVALENCE OF FEVER

Good data on the prevalence of fever are lacking. In general screenings, only 5 to 10% of patients have temperatures exceeding 100.4°F.[9] In one study, fever was the primary presenting complaint in 20% of emergency room visits with children and 6% with adult patients.[10] In another study, 39% (87 of 224) of all children younger than 3 presenting to an emergency room were **febrile** (having an excessive body temper-

ature), defined as axillary temperatures in excess of 99.2 and tympanic membrane temperatures in excess of 100.4.[11]

EPIDEMIOLOGY OF FEVER

Since fever is a symptom that might result from many underlying conditions, the epidemiology mirrors the epidemiology of the conditions that produce fever (e.g., rhinovirus infection). Other epidemiologic variables offer useful information.

Gender, Race, and Age

Women may have slightly higher temperatures than men.[1] There is little if any difference in the races regarding normal temperatures.[1] Neonates do not have well-developed thermoregulatory mechanisms, and their temperatures may be higher than expected—a finding that can be incorrectly interpreted as fever.[5] On the other end of the age spectrum, the elderly may respond less predictably with fever when challenged by various pyrogenic stimuli.[12,13] Also, body temperature generally drops with aging (leading to the medical maxim, "the older, the colder"). In an elderly patient, a potentially lethal fever may be disregarded by medical caregivers simply because it would be considered to fall within the upper limits of "normal" (e.g., 99.9).[5]

Food Ingestion

Ingestion of a large, protein-rich meal often increases temperature by 1°F or more. Individuals who eat this type of meal and also drink alcoholic beverages may experience a warm feeling; if they take their temperature they may discover a "fever." The temperature usually returns to normal after 2 to 3 hours.[5]

Ovulation

The menstrual cycle is responsible for variations in body temperature. (See Chapter 43, Problems Related to Sexual Activity, for a description of temperature in relation to ovulation.)

Tobacco and Chewing Gum

Smoking pipes, cigars, and cigarettes can cause a sustained rise in the oral temperature, reportedly to greater than 100°F, perhaps as a result of vasodilation of buccal vessels.[5] Refraining from smoking for 3 to 4 hours will usually allow the intraoral temperature to return to a more normal value.

Chewing gum or tobacco can also raise the intraoral temperature, reportedly by as much as 1°F, perhaps by a friction-induced buccal vasodilation.[5] Patients should take their temperature when not chewing, or perhaps as long as an hour or two after ceasing.

Exercise

Studies of football players, long-distance runners and rowing crews reveal that exercise can raise temperature by as much as 1.5°F.

ETIOLOGY OF FEVER

Generally speaking, fever is produced by **pyrogens** (chemicals that produce fever), either of endogenous or exogenous origin.[14] Endogenous pyrogens are proteins that induce fever, including such chemicals as interleukin-1, tumor necrosis factor, interleukin-6 and interferon alpha. Exogenous pyrogens are chemicals produced by bacteria or by components of the organisms.

Bacterial Infection

Bacterial infections produce as many as 74% of fevers.[15] Bacterial pyrogens stimulate the hypothalamus to increase the temperature it normally attempts to maintain (i.e., the temperature set point).[4] In one study of **nosocomial** (transmitted to a patient while hospitalized) infections, the most common bacterial causes of fever (in descending order) were urinary tract infections, pneumonia, bloodstream infections, and vascular infections (e.g., phlebitis).[15]

FOCUS ON...

BODY TEMPERATURE REGULATION

The human body balances heat loss (via conduction, radiation, and evaporation) with heat production (through metabolic processes) to maintain an acceptable body temperature by a homeostatic process called thermoregulation.[4] The unclothed human has the ability to adapt to ambient temperature swings as wide as 55 to 140°F in dry air, with core temperatures varying no more than 1°F.[4] Because the process of thermoregulation begins when ambient temperatures rise above 91.4°F or dip below 80.6°F, the 80.6 to 91.4°F temperature range is known as the "thermoneutral zone."

To achieve temperature homeostasis in the body, thermosensitive neurons in the hypothalamus—the body's thermostat—collect and interpret information from temperature sensors and control thermoregulatory function.[4,7] Temperature sensors used by the hypothalamus include heat-sensitive cells in the preoptic anterior hypothalamus, heat-sensitive and cold-sensitive receptors in the skin, and cold-sensitive receptors in the hypothalamus, midbrain, and spinal cord. Based on input from these sensors, the hypothalamus decreases heat when the person is too warm by shunting blood to surface vessels, which allows loss of heat to the environment and initiates sweating (to more rapidly reduce heat). If the person is too cold, the hypothalamus initiates processes that conserve warmth such as peripheral vasoconstriction, increased cellular metabolism, and shivering.[4]

An individual's body temperature normally undergoes circadian variation, peaking between 4 pm and 9 pm each day, and reaching a low between 2 am and 8 am.[1,4] (The amplitude of the daily variation usually does not exceed 1°F.) There can be considerable body-temperature variations from person to person.[1]

As shown in the figure, body temperature is not only affected by circadian variation, but also by numerous other factors such as the temperature of the environment, recent exercise, menstrual status, and emotions.

Endogenous variables:

a. Circadian variation
   High: 4 pm–9 pm
   Low: 2 am–8 am

b. Gender
   Female: Higher ↑
   Male: Lower ↓

c. Age
   Neonatal: Higher ↑
   Elderly: Lower ↓

d. Ovulation ↑

e. Infections ↑

f. Cancer ↑

g. Multisystem
   diseases ↑
   (e.g., rheumatic
   diseases)

Exogenous variables:

a. Recent meal and alcohol: ↑↓

b. Tobacco, chewing gum ↑

c. Exercise ↑

d. Medications ↑
   (e.g., antibiotics)

e. Factitious fevers ↑

f. Exposure to cold ↓

g. Oral measurements
   • Mouth breathing ↓
   • Incorrect thermometer
     location ↓
   • Dentures ↑

Many variables affect the body temperature, some endogenous (not affected directly by the patient) and some exogenous (affected by patient activities), as described in the chapter.

Bacterial disease is strongly correlated with the severity of fever in infants and young children.[11] When the rectal temperature exceeds 103.1°F, at least 3 to 15% of young children are found to be bacteremic. In those with rectal temperatures above 105.8°F, as many as 10% are found to have meningitis.

Patients with cancer who are **neutropenic** (having an abnormally low number of neutrophils in the blood) are subject to life-threatening infection.[16] Fever is often the herald of such infection.

Elderly patients with infections may not produce a fever as consistently as younger patients because of a combination of factors.[2] For example, aging causes central and peripheral changes that blunt the fever response, as does chronic disease in the nervous, circulatory, and immune systems.

Viral Infection

Several viruses can produce fever, including influenza, rhinoviruses, varicella, cytomegalovirus, Epstein-Barr virus, and HIV.[17–19]

Cancer

Fever is an important clue to some tumors, especially colon cancer.[17] Non-Hodgkin's lymphomas and metastatic disease to the liver or central nervous system are also responsible for fevers.[20]

Multisystem Diseases

Multisystem diseases that often produce fever include rheumatic diseases, connective tissue disorders, vasculitis (e.g., temporal arteritis), polymyalgia rheumatica, or sarcoidosis.[17]

Medications

Drug-induced fever, which occurs in about 10% of hospital inpatients, can be low or high-grade (over 104°F).[21] Several clues help implicate the medication regimen as a source of fever:

- The patient with fever is given thorough diagnostic examinations to discover the source of the fever, but the diagnostic examinations are negative.[22]
- The patient is given antimicrobial therapy, but it has no effect.
- When a medication is suspected and is discontinued, the patient's **defervescence** (the falling of an elevated fever) generally correlates with the excretion of the drug.

With some reports, drug-induced fever is the only manifestation of medication hypersensitivity.[23] In other cases, patients experience additional symptoms such as generalized myalgia, chills, and headache.[24] Prescription medications that produce fever include antibiotics (e.g., penicillin, cephalosporins), antibacterials (e.g., sulfonamides, nitrofurantoin), barbiturates, iodides, azathioprine, mercaptopurine, procarbazine, hydroxyurea, quinidine, allopurinol, propylthiouracil, methyldopa, dobutamine, diltiazem, pro-

cainamide, atropine, and the tuberculostatics (e.g., isoniazid, ethambutol, para-aminosalicylic acid).[5,25–34]

Nonprescription medications can also induce fever. In one case, a 55-year-old man developed fever 5 days after cimetidine administration was commenced.[35] The temperatures exceeded 104°F, only stopping when cimetidine was discontinued. In this case, the mechanism was an IgE-mediated reaction.

A challenge test may be used to confirm the existence of drug-induced fever. If the fever abates following cessation of the medication, a challenge dose may be given, followed by scrupulous surveillance of temperatures.[24] Should the temperature rise once again, the medication can be circumstantially blamed for the fever. The medication should not be used in the patient again. In one such case, a patient with tuberculosis was given a medication regimen that included isoniazid, developing isoniazid-induced fever 2 weeks later.[34] Isoniazid was given three additional times, almost causing her death until it was finally identified as the cause of the reaction and discontinued.

Fever of Unknown Origin

Fever of unknown origin (FUO) is the term used for fevers (reaching at least 101°F on several occasions) that persist for a sustained period (3 weeks or longer), but for which no readily apparent cause can be found after 1 week in the hospital.[5,20,36,37] An intensive diagnostic workup often allows the physician to discover the underlying cause.[17]

Factitious Fever

Factitious fever is a false fever produced by a patient by tampering with a measuring device. When the fever is factitious, medical caregivers may be tipped off by the clue that elevated temperature is usually the only abnormal finding.[5] The most common patient is a young female medical professional, although reports cite factitious fevers with older patients such as one 79-year-old female who did not wish to be discharged from the hospital.[17] Patients may heat a glass thermometer over a light bulb or in hot water, may rub the thermometer until friction produces the desired "fever", or may bring a thermometer that already registers a high fever to the office or hospital, surreptitiously substituting it for the one provided. A carefully monitored rectal temperature will uncover a factitious fever.

Fever and Concomitant Rash

Fever along with rash is a potentially deadly combination of symptoms.[38] The most serious type of coexisting rash is petechial, which indicates bleeding into the skin. The lesions do not blanch with pressure via **diascopy** (placing pressure on an area with the fingers to see if blood can be forced from the area). Potential causes include bacterial endocarditis, meningococcemia, and Rocky Mountain Spotted Fever. The rash may also be maculopapular, indicating such causes as typhoid fever, Lyme disease, rubeola, or primary HIV. Fever with a vesicular or bullous rash may be caused by poison ivy dermatitis, allergies, herpes simplex virus, or staphylococcal skin infections.

MANIFESTATIONS OF FEVER

Common Symptoms

When an individual has a fever, thermoregulatory mechanisms initiate the processes necessary to allow homeostasis. When this occurs, peripheral vasodilation causes the individual's skin to feel hot; the individual also may perspire (a visible sign of higher than normal body temperature).

A slightly elevated body temperature (e.g., 99.4 to 100°F) may produce symptoms such as lassitude, fatigue, and generalized malaise.[5,39,40] Generally, however, a temperature of 102 to 103°F is necessary to produce symptoms.[41,42]

Fever is often thought to cause headache. In one study of children with headache, almost three times as many had fever as a control group of children without headache.[43] Fever-induced headache is described as steady, aching, producing pressure, or burning.

Febrile Seizures

Fever can induce convulsions in young children.[39] These febrile seizures are most common in male children between the ages of 18 months to 3 years, but those aged 3 months to 5 years are at higher risk than younger and older children. Generally, they do not begin until the patient's temperature exceeds 103°F.[44]

Febrile seizures occur so early in the course of the elevated temperature that they may be the first sign that the child's temperature has risen.[44] Fever-induced convulsions are usually less than 15 minutes in duration. Febrile seizures do not lead to morbidity or mortality as commonly as seizures from other causes. Administration of antipyretics is not proven to prevent the recurrence of febrile seizures after an initial episode.[39]

SPECIFIC CONSIDERATIONS OF FEVER

Temperature Measurement

Body temperature, one of the "vital signs," can reveal the presence of life-threatening medical conditions.[45] For temperature measurement to be useful, however, it must be an accurate reflection of **core temperature** (the general thermal status of the body tissues).[4] It is especially important to estimate the temperature of the deep brain structures and the location of the temperature regulation centers.

Numerous factors affect accuracy of measurement of temperature, including the environmental (ambient) temperature, exercise (exercise can cause a sustained rise in temperature), phase of the menstrual cycle, and emotional state.[4] (See "Body Temperature Regulation.")

When someone suspects the presence of a fever in another person, it is traditional to first test the subject's forehead or face with the hand. According to studies, however, this tactile assessment of fever is only accurate perhaps half of the time.[41,46] Nevertheless, when the hand seems to confirm that a fever is present, the next step is to use a temperature measurement device.

Numerous controversies are associated with the measurement of body temperature such as the optimal site for measurement and its correlation with core body temperature and the advantages and disadvantages of the various measuring devices.

SITES FOR TEMPERATURE MEASUREMENT

Since different body sites reflect core temperatures with different degrees of accuracy, measurements are site specific, and the site should be cited with each measurement.[1]

Oral Measurement

Oral (sublingual) temperatures are a good reflection of core temperatures, although their absolute values are consistently lower.[4] For this reason, many experts suggest adding approximately 1°F to the oral temperature to obtain a more accurate reflection of core temperature.[9] Temperature readings that are lower than core temperature can result from breathing through the mouth while taking the temperature, placing the thermometer incorrectly in the mouth (e.g., above the tongue or supralingual placement), eating or drinking before taking the temperature (although this can also raise the temperature), smoking, and the presence of dentures.[12]

The intraoral environment can register widely divergent temperature values. The highest values are obtained below the tongue, as far back as possible. These "heat pockets" best reflect core temperature (Fig 26.1). If a thermometer is placed in other sites such as those just inside the front teeth, it yields values as low as 96.8°F (the sites closest to the outside environment).

Rectal Measurement

Rectal temperatures—which are approximately 1°F above oral—are thought to be the most accurate measure of core temperature generally available to patients.[4,12] Nevertheless, rectal measurement has many disadvantages. Because of lag time, rectal measurements are not a good reflection of temperature at the thermoregulation centers of the deep brain. Should the patient undergo a rapid change in core temperature, rectal measurements will tend to lag behind somewhat.[11]

Rectal measurements also can cause discomfort, take time to perform correctly, and can cause rectal perforations, particularly in very young infants (Fig. 26.2).[11] Young children often fight, cry, and struggle while the rectal thermometer is being inserted, perhaps because they mistakenly think the thermometer is a needle or because of a natural fear of restraint for any reason.[41] Thermometers are sometimes broken when taking the temperature rectally, particularly when patients vigorously resist. The use of plastic

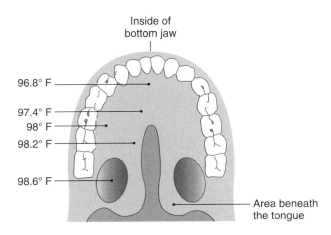

Inside of bottom jaw

96.8° F
97.4° F
98° F
98.2° F
98.6° F

Area beneath the tongue

Figure 26.1. The "heat pockets," locations that most closely approximate core temperature. Note that temperatures drop as the oral opening is approached.

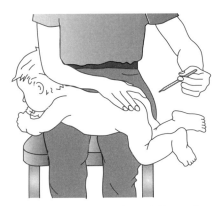

Figure 26.2. The baby must be held carefully to take a rectal temperature to prevent rectal perforation.

sheaths—usually stocked next to the thermometers—reduces the hazards associated with breakage (Fig 26.3).

Rectal measurement cannot be used for certain patients such as those with recent rectal surgery (because of the danger of reopening a sutured wound or causing pain), neutropenia, or acute myocardial infarction (because of potential changes in heart rate).[45]

Tympanic Measurement

Tympanic temperature measurement has gained in popularity in recent years. This site appears physiologically sound because blood flow to the tympanic membrane is the same vasculature as blood reaching the hypothalamus. Thus tympanic measurements should correlate closely with the central temperature receptors, although tympanic measurements are affected by changes in ambient temperature.[4,11]

Axillary Measurement

The greatest drawback in axillary (armpit) temperature measurement is its questionable validity.[11,47] The axillae are subject to inaccuracies arising from the temperature of the environment and physiologic factors. For instance, during

1. Patient tears upper outer wrap.

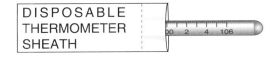

DISPOSABLE
THERMOMETER
SHEATH

2. Patient removes thermometer with sheath surrounding it.

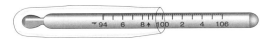

Figure 26.3. Following directions provided, the patient should cover the end of a glass or digital thermometer with a disposable plastic sheath prior to oral, rectal, or axillary use.

fever, blood is shunted from the skin and peripheral sites. Thus the axillary temperature might appear normal when fever is present. The axillary temperature is approximately 1°F below the oral measurement.[15]

Other Sites

Indwelling devices known as thermistors may be used to measure the temperature of the esophagus or pulmonary artery.[11,45] Although they most accurately measure core temperatures, these methods are reserved for critically ill patients.

Bladder and vaginal measurements reflect core temperature well also, but as with rectal measurement suffer from a prolonged lag time. Bladder and vaginal measurement generally is not used.

Skin temperatures other than axillary are easy to take, but reflect core temperatures poorly.[4]

DEVICES FOR TEMPERATURE MEASUREMENT

Several temperature measurement devices are listed in Table 26.1. The ideal device for measurement of body temperature has several desirable characteristics[7]:

- Accurate reflection of core temperature
- Rapid results
- Easy to use
- Comfortable for the patient
- Free of complications (e.g., rectal perforation)

Glass Thermometers

In use for over a century, the glass thermometer has a bulb of mercury at the insertion end and a measurement scale along the side.[1] Both oral and rectal glass instruments are available. The oral thermometer should be left in place for a minimum of 9 minutes to obtain an accurate reading.[12] Disposable plastic sheaths should be placed over the thermometer prior to placement to help prevent the spread of infection (see Fig. 26.3).[47] (See Figure 26.1 for placement locations.)

Oral Digital Thermometers

The digital oral thermometer reduces the time required to obtain an oral temperature reading from 9 minutes to less

Table 26.1. Representative Temperature Measurement Devices

DEVICE	COMMENTS
B-D Baby Fever Thermometer	Glass thermometer calibrated from 96°F to 106°F (the baby thermometer has a shorter bulb to help reduce the possibility of rectal perforation; may also be used for axillary temperatures)
B-D Oral Fever Thermometer	Glass thermometer calibrated from 96°F to 106°F (may be used to measure oral, rectal, or axillary temperatures)
B-D Digital Fever Thermometer	Measures temperatures from 96°F to 105°F (may be used to measure oral, rectal, or axillary temperatures)
Family Medical Aids Fever Reader	A chemical strip placed against the forehead and read after one minute
Thermoscan Instant Thermometer	Measures tympanic temperatures in one second; replacement lens filters available

than 1 minute in most cases. Plastic sheaths (probe covers) can also be used with them (see Fig. 26.3). (See Figure 26.1 for placement locations.)

Tympanic Thermometers

The tympanic thermometer uses infrared technology for temperature measurement[11] (Fig. 26.4). To use a tympanic thermometer, a disposable probe is placed in the external ear and aimed toward the tympanic membrane, while performing an "ear tug" to facilitate measurement (Fig.26.5).[7] Tympanic thermometers are quite comfortable for patients, provide rapid results, and are simple to use. In addition, patients are not required to disrobe, as with a rectal measurement.

The usefulness of tympanic thermometry has been debated, with some studies finding it inadequate.[48–61] In one, it did not reliably detect fever in children under the age of 3 years.[11] However, some of these studies compare tympanic measurements to rectal, oral, or axillary measurements rather than to the ideal: actual core temperature.[60]

Chemical Dots/Strips

Certain heat-sensitive chemicals are manufactured as dots or strips that are placed on the skin.[7] Although skin reflects core temperature poorly, some studies indicate that certain chemical measurement devices provide acceptable accuracy.[7]

Temperature Measurement Units

Medical articles often discuss temperature measurement in centigrade units. However, the American public is generally only familiar with Fahrenheit units. This chapter reports the temperature in Fahrenheit units to facilitate the pharmacist in counseling patients who are generally only familiar with this system. However, should the reader wish to convert one value in this chapter to another, Table 26.2 provides equivalent values, as well as other common values. For conversions not listed on the table, any of the following equivalent formulas may be used[62]:

$$9\,C° = 5\,F° - 160 \qquad F° = 9/5\,C° + 32 \qquad C° = 5/9\,(F° - 32)$$

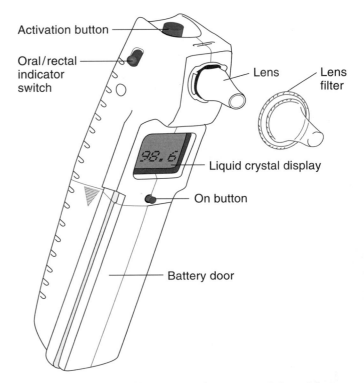

Figure 26.4. The parts of a tympanic thermometer (adapted from a brochure illustrating the Thermoscan Instant Thermometer).

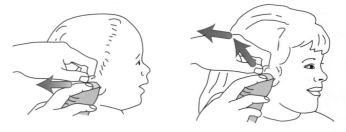

Figure 26.5. The "ear tug" is performed with tympanic thermometer measurements by either pulling the ear straight back (for a child under 1 year of age) or up and back (for those over the age of 1 year)

Table 26.2. Temperature Equivalencies: Fahrenheit and Centigrade

FAHRENHEIT TEMPERATURE	CENTIGRADE TEMPERATURE
55.4	13
80.6	27
91.4	33
95	35
95.5	35.3
96	35.6
96.5	35.8
97	36.1
97.5	36.4
98	36.7
98.6	37
99	37.2
99.4	37.4
99.5	37.5
99.9	37.7
100	37.8
100.4	38
100.5	38.1
101	38.3
101.5	38.6
102	38.9
102.2	39
102.5	39.2
103	39.4
103.1	39.5
103.5	39.7
104	40
104.5	40.3
105	40.6
105.8	41
106	41.1
107	41.7
140	60

TREATMENT OF FEVER

Treatment Guidelines

Fever treatment is controversial since research indicates that reduction of fever in some conditions (e.g., viral illnesses) prolongs the period of **viral shedding** (the period in which a carrier is yielding infective viral particles to the environment).[63] Specifically, fever increases the release of interferons, increases neutrophil release, and improves chemotaxis. Ideally, treatment of fever should be directed toward relieving discomfort, discovering the cause of fever, and treating it appropriately.[39] (See Patient Assessment Algorithm 26.1.)

Many patients suffer from "fever phobia," the irrational fear that body temperatures from 100 to 104°F will cause severe harm (e.g., brain damage) to their children, themselves, or loved ones.[41,64] Temperatures from 104 to 106°F cause undue worries about convulsions, stroke, coma, death, dehydration, and blindness. Parents and caregivers also worry that the temperature will continue to rise as high as 120°F. The patient may be told by the pharmacist that fevers help boost the activity of the immune system, helping the patient combat viral and bacterial infections.[41] Perhaps this advice would help those with fever phobia.

Age can help pharmacists determine the gravity of fever. Fever in a child 3 months of age or younger is more likely to be caused by a serious illness than fever in an older child; parents of these children should be warned more carefully to obtain medical advice.[7]

The current FDA proposed labeling for ingredients approved for fever warns patients as follows: "Do not take this product for fever for more than 3 days unless directed by a doctor. If fever persists or gets worse, consult a doctor."[65] No specific temperature is required on the label, although the

Patient Assessment Algorithm 26.1. Fever

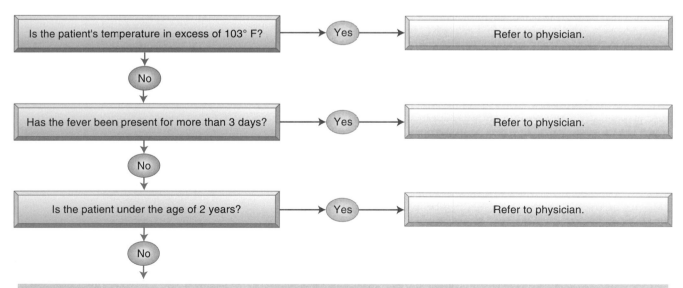

original panel assigned to review antipyretics recommended that patients not self-treat fevers of more than 103°F.

Caregivers must be advised not to awaken a child to treat a fever.[41] Sleeping will help the child recover from the conditions causing the fever. If the child becomes sufficiently uncomfortable, he or she will usually awaken and indicate discomfort.

See "Specific Considerations of Fever" for details on temperature measurement and temperature measurement devices.

Nonprescription Medications

Antipyretic agents reduce fever through inhibiting the synthesis of prostaglandins, which resets the hypothalamic set point.[39]

ASPIRIN

Aspirin is discussed in detail in Chapter 18, Headache and Other Minor Pains. *The major risk of taking aspirin for fever is Reye's syndrome, which most often occurs in children with influenza or chickenpox who are given aspirin.*[38] (See "Reye's Syndrome" in Chapter 18.)

ACETAMINOPHEN

 Acetaminophen is only necessary for fever if the patient is uncomfortable.[18] Patients or caregivers wishing to administer acetaminophen must understand that it only lowers a temperature by 2 to 3°F. It cannot return a fever of 103°F to normal. Pharmacists must advise patients and caregivers that administering more acetaminophen to "break the fever" is extremely dangerous because of the toxicity of acetaminophen. Acetaminophen is discussed in detail in Chapter 18, Headache and Other Minor Pains.

OTHER ANTIPYRETICS

Ibuprofen, naproxen, and ketoprofen are discussed in detail in Chapter 18, Headache and Other Minor Pains.

Nonpharmacologic Therapies

Several nonpharmacologic therapies may be instituted to reduce fever, augmenting heat dissipation through evaporation, radiation, convection, and conduction. Sponge baths may be useful, but patients and caregivers must be cautioned not to use water that is too cool, since patients may be plunged into hypothermia and experience such symptoms as shivering and frostbite. Ice packs carry the same precaution. Alcohol baths are also used, but patients may undergo cutaneous absorption of the alcohol or its denaturing agent, either of which can be dangerous. Patients may also be cooled with air conditioning or fans, although their effectiveness is limited by discomfort and shivering.[39]

SUMMARY

Thermoregulation via the hypothalamus is the process used by the body to maintain a stable temperature in health. Fever occurs when the body temperature exceeds a "normal" temperature level—although the specific temperature at which elevated temperature is considered to be fever is debated. Fever also has an adaptive value, allowing the body to better mobilize the defenses against infection.

Fever is not a medical condition in itself, but reflects some underlying pathology. In most cases, an infectious etiology is

AT THE COUNTER

A mother and father bring a 4-year-old child to the counter to ask the pharmacist for help treating the child's fever.

Interview/Patient Assessment

The mother asks the pharmacist to perform a tactile fever assessment. The forehead feels hot. The child appears well-oriented and fully alert. The parents state that they have been measuring the child's oral temperature during the past 2 days with a digital thermometer and it has been as high as 102.5°F. The child is taking no medications, has had no recent immunizations, and has no medical condition. Several children at the day care center the child attends have also been sick within the last week. The syndrome does not include any additional symptoms other than malaise (e.g., the patient does not have vomiting, diarrhea, or rhinorrhea).

Pharmacist's Analysis

1. What is the probable cause of this child's fever?

2. Are there dangers to overmedicating this fever?
3. Which antipyretics would be appropriate for this child?

The child's fever is not yet a cause for alarm. In all likelihood he has contracted a minor viral illness. The parents' concern about the fever may cause them to medicate aggressively in an attempt to bring it to "normal."

Patient Counseling

The parents must be informed that the child's fever is not yet at a dangerous stage. They should be cautioned that overmedicating the fever exposes the child to the hazards of medications, as well as possibly reducing the ability of the child to fight the infection. Should they wish to treat the fever anyway, the pharmacist may point out acetaminophen or ibuprofen liquids, urging them to pay close attention to all warnings, precautions, and dosing instructions. If the temperature persists beyond one additional day or worsens, the child should see a physician.

responsible. For these reasons, treatment of fever by any means is controversial.

Measurement of fever is also controversial. Common measurement sites include the mouth (oral), the rectum, the armpit (axilla), and the ear (tympanic membrane). Measurement devices include glass/mercury, digital, and tympanic thermometers, as well as various chemical strips or dots.

When a patient has fever, the pharmacist should first attempt to discover the specific temperature, how and where the temperature was taken, and any ancillary symptoms. If a fever lasts more than 3 days or worsens, a physician should be consulted.

Finally, although the FDA does not specify a specific temperature for referral, 103°F was mentioned by an early FDA panel as a lower danger point. For this reason, it is prudent for the pharmacist to refer patients with temperatures of 103° or more to ensure that proper care is received.

References

1. Mackowiak PA, Wasserman SS. Physicians' perceptions regarding body temperature in health and disease. South Med J 88:934, 1995.
2. Castle SC, et al. Fever response in elderly nursing home residents: Are the older truly colder? J Am Geriatr Soc 39:853, 1991.
3. Sarwari AR, Mackowiak PA. The pharmacologic consequences of fever. Inf Dis Clin North Am 10:21, 1996.
4. Schmidt KD, Chan CW. Thermoregulation and fever in normal persons and in those with spinal cord injuries. Mayo Clinic Proc 67:469, 1992.
5. Weinstein L. Clinically benign fever of unknown origin: A personal retrospective. Rev Infect Dis 7:692, 1985.
6. Donowitz GR. Fever in the compromised host. Inf Dis Clin North Am 10:129, 1996.
7. Pontious SL. Accuracy and reliability of temperature measurement in the emergency department by instrument and site in children. Pediatr Nurs 20:58, 1994.
8. Kluger MJ, et al. The adaptive value of fever. Inf Dis Clin North Am 10:1, 1996.
9. Jensen BN, et al. The superiority of rectal thermometry to oral thermometry with regard to accuracy. J Adv Nurs 20:660, 1994.
10. Kresovich-Wendler K, Levitt MA, Yearly L. An evaluation of clinical predictors to determine the need for rectal temperature measurement in the emergency department. Am J Emerg Med 7:391, 1989.
11. Muma BK, et al. Comparison of rectal, axillary, and tympanic membrane temperatures in infants and young children. Ann Emerg Med 20:41, 1991.
12. Marion GS, McGann KP, Camp DL. Core body temperature in the elderly and factors which influence its measurement. Gerontology 37:225, 1991.
13. Norman DC, Yoshikawa TT. Fever in the elderly. Inf Dis Clin North Am 10:93, 1996.
14. Whitby M. The febrile patient. Aust Fam Physician 10:1753, 1993.
15. Arbo MJ, et al. Fever of nosocomial origin: Etiology, risk factors, and outcomes. Am J Med 95:505, 1993.
16. Shenep JL, et al. Infrared, thermistor, and glass-mercury thermometry for measurement of body temperature in children with cancer. Clin Pediatr 30(4 Suppl):36, 1991.
17. Knockaert DC, Vanneste LJ, Bobbaers HJ. Fever of unknown origin in elderly patients. J Am Geriatr Soc 41:1187, 1993.
18. Carsons SE. Fever in rheumatic and autoimmune disease. Inf Dis Clin North Am 10:67, 1996.
19. Sullivan M, Feinberg J, Bartlett JG. Fever in patients with HIV infection. Inf Dis Clin North Am 10:149, 1996.
20. Cunha BA. Fever of unknown origin. Inf Dis Clin North Am 10:111, 1996.
21. Johnson DH, Cunha BA. Drug fever. Inf Dis Clin North Am 10:85, 1996.
22. Rehr EL, Swanson KA, Kern JA. Mercaptopurine-induced fever in a patient with Crohn's disease. Ann Pharmacother 26:907, 1992.
23. Dominguez EA, Hamill RJ. Drug-induced fever due to diltiazem. Arch Intern Med 151:1869, 1991.
24. Puyana J, et al. Drug-induced fever: A clinical report and challenge test with calcium dobesilate. Int Arch Allergy Appl Immunol 92:364, 1990.
25. Webster J, Koch HF. Aspects of tolerability of centrally acting antihypertensive agents. J Cardiovasc Pharmacol 27(Suppl 3):S49, 1996.
26. Lossos IS, Matzner Y. Hydroxyurea-induced fever: Case report and review of the literature. Ann Pharmacother 29:132, 1995.
27. O'Rourke DJ, et al. Propafenone-induced drug fever in the absence of agranulocytosis. Clin Cardiol 20:662, 1997.
28. Akyol H, et al. Cytotoxic drug-induced fever: A report on procarbazine-induced hyperpyrexia. Med Pediatr Oncol 18:173, 1990.
29. Robison-Strane SR, Bubik JS. Dobutamine-induced fever. Ann Pharmacother 26:1523, 1992.
30. Mevorach D, Lossos IS, Oren R. Cefuroxime-induced fever. Ann Pharmacother 27:881, 1993.
31. Pleasants RA, Walker TR, Samuelson WM. Allergic reactions to parenteral beta-lactam antibiotics in patients with cystic fibrosis. Chest 106:1124, 1994.
32. Arias J, Fernandez Rivas M, Panadero P. Selective fixed drug eruption to amoxycillin. Clin Exp Dermatol 20:339, 1995.
33. Jeurissen ME, et al. Azathioprine induced fever, chills, rash, and hepatotoxicity in rheumatoid arthritis. Am Rheum Dis 49:25, 1990.
34. Salomaa ER, et al. Pulmonary infiltrates and fever induced by isoniazid. Postgrad Med J 66:647, 1990.
35. Hiraide A, Yoshioka T, Ohshima S. IgE-mediated drug fever due to histamine H2-receptor blockers. Drug Saf 5:455, 1990.
36. Knockaert DC, et al. Fever of unknown origin in the 1980s. Arch Intern Med 152:51, 1992.
37. Petersdorf RG. Fever of unknown origin (Editorial). Arch Intern Med 152:21, 1992.
38. Schlossberg D. Fever and rash. Inf Dis Clin North Am 10:101, 1996.
39. Klein NC, Cunha BA. Treatment of fever. Inf Dis Clin North Am 10:211, 1996.
40. Styrt B, Mummaw N, Stein G. Symptoms and rate of temperature change in febrile outpatients. Am J Emerg Med 12:339, 1994.
41. Schmitt BD. Behavioral aspects of temperature-taking. Clin Pediatr 30(4 Suppl):8, 1991.

42. Cunha BA. The clinical significance of fever patterns. Inf Dis Clin North Am 10:33, 1996.
43. Kandt RS, Levine RM. Headache and acute illness in children. J Child Neurol 2:22, 1987.
44. Powers JH, Scheld WM. Fever in neurologic diseases. Inf Dis Clin North Am 10:45, 1996.
45. Milewski A, Ferguson KL, Terndrup TE. Comparison of pulmonary artery, rectal, and tympanic membrane temperatures in adult intensive care unit patients. Clin Pediatr 39(4 Suppl):13, 1991.
46. Singhi S, Sood V. Reliability of subjective assessment of fever by mothers. Indian Pediatr 27:811, 1990.
47. Ogren JM. The inaccuracy of axillary temperatures measured with an electronic thermometer. Am J Dis Child 144:109, 1990.
48. Hooker EA. Use of tympanic thermometers to screen for fever in patients in a pediatric emergency department. South Med J 86:855, 1993.
49. Terndrup TE. Tympanic thermometers (Letter). South Med J 87:1059, 1994.
50. Schuman AJ. The accuracy of infrared auditory canal thermometry in infants and children. Clin Pediatr 32:347, 1993.
51. Fraden J. The development of Thermoscan Instant Thermometer. Clin Pediatr 30(4 Suppl):11, 1991.
52. Beach PS, McCormick DP. Clinical applications of ear thermometry (Editorial). Clin Pediatr 30(4 Suppl):3, 1991.
53. Zehner WJ, Terndrup TE. The impact of moderate ambient temperature variance on the relationship between oral, rectal, and tympanic membrane temperatures. Clin Pediatr 30(4 Suppl):61, 1991.
54. Fraden J, Lackey RP. Estimation of body sites temperatures from tympanic measurements. Clin Pediatr 30(4 Suppl):65, 1991.
55. Talo H, Macknin ML, Medendorp SV. Tympanic membrane temperatures compared to rectal and oral temperatures. Clin Pediatr 30 4 Suppl):30, 1991.
56. Chamberlain JM, et al. Comparison of a tympanic thermometer to rectal and oral thermometers in a pediatric emergency department. Clin Pediatr 30(4 Suppl):24, 1991.
57. Terndrup TE, Milewski A. The performance of two tympanic thermometers in a pediatric emergency department. Clin Pediatr 30(4 Suppl):18, 1991.
58. Hooker EA, Houston H. Screening for fever in an adult emergency department: Oral vs. tympanic thermometry. South Med J 89:230, 1996.
59. Yaron M, Lowenstein SR, Koziol-McLain J. Measuring the accuracy of the infrared tympanic thermometer: Correlation does not signify agreement. J Emerg Med 13:617, 1995.
60. Erickson RS, Woo TM. Accuracy of infrared ear thermometry and traditional temperature methods in young children. Heart Lung 23:181, 1994.
61. Fed Reg 42:35346, 1977.
62. Stoklosa MJ, Ansel HC. Pharmaceutical calculations. 9th ed. Philadelphia: Lea & Febiger, 1991; p. 287.
63. Doran TF, et al. Acetaminophen: More harm than good for chickenpox? J Pediatr 114:1045, 1989.
64. Stein MJ. Historical perspective on fever and thermometry. Clin Pediatr 30(4 Suppl):5, 1991.
65. Fed Reg 53:46204, 1988.

Ophthalmic/Otic Conditions

Ophthalmic Conditions

Patients present to pharmacists with ophthalmic conditions that range from minor discomfort that is easily treatable with nonprescription products to serious conditions that can result in visual loss if not immediately treated by an ophthalmologist.

The FDA Review Panel assigned to review ophthalmic products considered the etiologies, severity, prognoses, and consequences of various ophthalmic conditions, with the initial publication appearing in 1980.[1,2] The panel decided that several conditions could potentially be treated without physician consultation:

- Dry eye
- Loose foreign material
- Redness caused by minor eye irritation
- Discomfort caused by minor eye irritation
- Corneal edema
- Ophthalmic allergic conjunctivitis (this was allowed as an indication in a later FDA decision)

Most FDA-mandated warnings regarding safe use of nonprescription eye-care products are ingredient specific and are described in the sections of the chapter for which the ingredients are approved. However, some warnings are required on all products:

- If patients experience eye pain, changes in vision, continued redness, or irritation of the eye, or if the condition worsens or persists ("for more than 72 hours" in the case of vasoconstrictors, emollients, demulcents, and astringents), patients must discontinue use and see a physician.
- Products containing mercury or a mercury-containing compound (e.g., thimerosal) as a preservative must be avoided by patients sensitive to mercury.[1]

- Patients should avoid contamination of ophthalmic drops by not touching the tip of the container to any surface and by replacing the cap after using. (See "Instructions for Use of Ophthalmic Drops.")
- Unit-dose products must be discarded after the single use.
- Patients using eye drops should discard the product if the solution changes color or becomes cloudy.

See Figure 27.1 to review eye anatomy. Also see "Miscellaneous Ophthalmic Issues."

PART 1: OPHTHALMIC CONDITIONS THAT CAN BE SELF-TREATED

DRY EYE

Patients often complain of having dry eyes.[3] "Dry eye" refers to a syndrome resulting from many conditions that produce abnormalities of tear film flow and/or stability rather than denoting a specific disease entity.[4] Broadly speaking, dry eye is a state of tear-film instability caused by a deficiency of any component of the tear film and by insufficient interaction between the mucin layer of tears and cell surface glycoprotein (Fig. 27.2). The recognition of early and mild cases is difficult for even trained professionals (e.g., optometrists, ophthalmologists). Symptoms include ocular discomfort, blurred vision, discharge, an awareness of the eyes, a desire to rub or itch the eyes, a feeling that sand or dirt is in the eyes, burning, or redness.[3]

The human cornea has no known nerve receptors for dryness or wetness and cannot interpret dry eye in this manner.[5] Rather, dry eye is thought to be perceived through stimula-

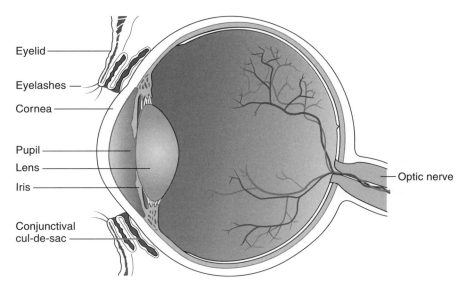

Figure 27.1. Cross-section of the eye.

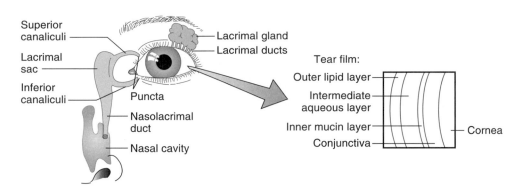

Figure 27.2. The lacrimal apparatus that produces tears, introduces them into the eye, and allows them to drain into the nasal cavity. The layers of the tear film are also illustrated.

tion of receptors for touch and possibly for cold, warmth, and pain. Further, some combination of receptor stimulus of the eyelids, cornea, or conjunctiva may interact to produce a message to the brain that results in a perception of dryness.

PREVALENCE OF DRY EYE

The prevalence of dry eye is unknown, although as many as 75% of soft contact-lens wearers experience it.[6] Further, 14% of patients aged 65 and older also report dry eye.[7]

EPIDEMIOLOGY OF DRY EYE

Dry eye can result from a number of conditions, including aqueous tear deficiency, exposure to dry air, keratoconjunctivitis sicca, primary Sjögren's syndrome, blepharitis, vitamin A deficiency, allergic conjunctivitis, certain medications, and contact lenses.[8–10] Many of the discussions concerning epi-

demiology of dry eye also encompass etiology, as underlying medical conditions that cause dry eye carry their own etiologic variables.

Aqueous Deficiency

The most common cause of dry eye is partial or absolute tear aqueous deficiency. Partial or total occlusion of lacrimal glands is often responsible for this tear deficiency.[11] This can result from ocular diseases such as trachoma, chemical burns, and erythema multiforme, as well as from other conditions such as lacrimal gland atrophy.[2]

Dry Air

Dry ambient air can cause the eyes to become dry. This effect is often seen in the winter with central heating systems.[12] (See Chapter 16, Humidity Deficit.) Dry eye from dry air can also occur in an air-conditioned environment such as in long automobile trips or on aircraft flights.[13]

Keratoconjunctivitis Sicca

Dry eye is usually the result of an abnormality in one or more tear stability–dependent factors.[14] There are six to eight different types of possible abnormal tear film conditions, but the most severe form is keratoconjunctivitis sicca (KCS), which causes approximately 80 to 90% of diagnosed cases of dry eye.[15] The typical patient afflicted with KCS produces less mucin than normal, so that filaments of corneal epithelium and mucus form on the eye, causing ocular pain.[16] The process can cause **keratinization** (development of a cornified or horny layer) of the cornea, producing burning, pain, discomfort, a feeling of fullness, and/or a gritty foreign body sensation, with possible loss of vision.[17] Hot ambient air and wind increase evaporation of tears and worsen the symptoms. KCS may be induced by ocular diseases that scar lacrimal ducts and block the secretion of fluid, by Sjögren's syndrome, by vitamin A deficiency, by HIV infection, and by lacrimal gland atrophy.[18] However, most patients with isolated dry-eye complaints have no major underlying systemic disease.[3] The condition is most commonly seen in menopausal or postmenopausal women, which has prompted a hypothesized but unproven estrogen-dependent mechanism.[3]

By the time an individual reaches the age of 40 to 45 years, approximately 50% of the ability to produce the aqueous layers of tear film is lost. Thus the prevalence of KCS in the elderly is a function of this age-associated decrease in aqueous production. While artificial tear products provide symptomatic relief, the patient may also require soft contact lenses, as well as surgery to close the inferior puncta and lessen tear drainage.[16]

Primary Sjögren's Syndrome

A possible cause of KCS-associated dry eye is the symptom complex known as primary Sjögren's syndrome. Characterized by minor exacerbations and remissions throughout the life of the patient, it occurs primarily in postmenopausal females and is caused by lymphocytic destruction of moisture-producing glands.[16] The patient generally complains of excessive dryness in several areas of the body, causing several conditions[3]:

- Dry eye
- **Xerostomia** (dry mouth)—results in complaints of difficulty chewing or ingesting dry foods
- Upper airway dryness—can cause a persistent cough or hoarseness
- Vaginal dryness—may lead to painful intercourse

Rheumatoid polyarthritis is another common component of Sjögren's.[19]

The syndrome develops after infectious mononucleosis, as well as infections with Epstein-Barr virus, cytomegalovirus, or adenovirus.[3] Other ophthalmic complaints seen with Sjögren's include chronic conjunctivitis and **keratitis** (inflammation of the cornea). While artificial tear substitutes provide symptomatic relief, prolonged use of the products should be monitored by a physician. Other medical or surgical intervention may be warranted.

Vitamin A Deficiency

Vitamin A deficiency is a major cause of childhood blindness in underdeveloped countries because vitamin A deficiency results in mucin deficiency.[3] The eye undergoes a loss of mucin-secreting goblet cells resulting in an unstable tear film that causes dry patches on the conjunctiva. If not corrected, mucin deficiency can cause corneal and conjunctival xerosis. Impaired **dark adaptation** (ability of the eyes to adapt to darkness, allowing the person only limited vision) is a sensitive test for vitamin A deficiency. Adequate dietary intake of green, leafy vegetables prevents vitamin A deficiency, but disorders of digestion, absorption, transport, storage, and metabolism can result in deficiency of Vitamin A despite an adequate diet. Vitamin A malabsorption is common in patients with chronic pancreatitis, chronic liver disease, alcoholism, and cystic fibrosis.[3]

Medication-Induced Dry Eye

Dry eye is a possible adverse reaction induced by a long list of medications, including the following:

- Certain diuretics (e.g., hydrochlorothiazide, chlorthalidone)
- Antihistamines (e.g., diphenhydramine, dexbrompheniramine, chlorpheniramine)
- Anticholinergics (e.g., atropine, scopolamine)
- Phenothiazines (e.g., trifluoperazine, thioridazine)
- Tricyclic antidepressants (e.g., amitriptyline, imipramine)
- Isotretinoin, indapamide, cimetidine, and clonidine
- Radiotherapy[20]

Contact Lenses

Contact lenses may produce a mild form of dry eye—both from exacerbating a previously unnoticed dry-eye condition or from causing discomfort that is perceived as dry eye.[6,21,22] In addition, additives such as preservatives in contact lens solutions may either induce tear film breakdown or result in toxicity or allergy that is interpreted as dry eye.[5]

ETIOLOGY OF DRY EYE

As noted, much of the etiology of dry eye was described in the section discussing epidemiology of dry eye. However, the production and functions of tears is germane to a discussion of etiology of dry eye.

Production and Functions of Tears

Tears are produced by ophthalmic lacrimal, sebaceous and mucous glands[2] (see Fig. 27.2). Tears flow over the corneal surface, collect in the conjunctival cul-de-sac, and then drain through the **puncta** (openings located in the inner corners of the upper and lower eyelids). Next, the lacrimal drainage system (consisting of the inferior and superior canaliculi, the lacrimal sac, and the nasolacrimal duct) directs tears into the nasal cavity. Tears provide nutrition for anterior surface cells;

aid in metabolism, secretion, waste removal, and maintenance of optical clarity; and exert an antibacterial action.[5,19]

Composition of Tears

Tears are 0.7% protein (e.g., mucin, albumin) with a total solids content of about 1.8%.[5] Tears are slightly alkaline with an osmotic concentration of 0.9% sodium chloride.

A discussion of dry eye must include a description of tear-film physiology. The preocular tear film is a three-layer system[19,23]:

- Mucin (innermost)
- Aqueous (intermediate)
- Lipid (outermost)

The innermost layer, the mucin layer, adheres to the corneal and conjunctival cell microvilli. Mucin, produced by goblet cells, changes the normally hydrophobic surface of the corneal epithelium to hydrophilic by a surfactant action, enabling it to become more wet.[3,24] Thus the intermediate aqueous layer of the precorneal tear film can spread more easily over the conjunctiva. This intermediate aqueous layer, which composes approximately 90% of the thickness of the tear film, contains chemicals responsible for corneal metabolism (e.g., glucose, inorganic ions) and the antimicrobial agent lysozyme.[15,19] The outermost lipid layer of tears, which is composed of wax monoesters, cholesterol esters, and diesters, retards evaporation and prevents instability or rupture of the tear film.[19,25] Aging and certain hormonal disorders may alter the composition of this lipid layer, resulting in dry eye.[25]

Factors Determining Tear Volume

Three separate processes determine the volume of tears[26,27]:

- Tear production by lacrimal glands
- Tear outflow via the lacrimal system
- Evaporation from the surface of the eye

Lacrimal gland tear production is influenced by body hydration. Aqueous peripheral secretions—such as tears and saliva—are compromised with insufficient body water as the body preferentially supplies the cells of more vital organs.

Some patients with qualitative changes in tear composition may complain of dry eye in the presence of normal tear volume.[19] Several tests allow clinical diagnosis of dry eye (e.g., tear film viscosity, tear lactoferrin levels, tear osmolarity, rose bengal staining, and Schirmer's test), confirming an absolute deficiency of tears.[21,28–31]

TREATMENT OF DRY EYE

Treatment Guidelines

Professional monitoring and the use of nonprescription tear substitutes usually proves sufficient treatment for dry eye, but some cases may require surgical correction (Patient Assessment Algorithm 27.1).

Nonprescription Medications

ARTIFICIAL TEARS

Tear-replacement products (tear substitutes, more commonly known as artificial tears) such as those in Table 27.1, contain **demulcents** (high molecular weight compounds, water-soluble polymers, or water-soluble polyols), which act like mucin to coat the surface of irritated mucous membranes and their abraded surfaces, thereby protecting underlying cells from external stimuli such as environmental irritants (e.g., wind or sun).[2] They also facilitate wetting of the cornea and prevent drying of the affected tissue through increasing the volume of fluid in the eye.[32] Their effects in preventing and alleviating irritation and dry eye makes them useful ophthalmic ingredients in products for dry eye and in products intended to relieve irritation and allergic conditions. FDA-approved self-care directions instruct the patient to use 1 to 2 drops as needed.[1] *Use twice daily is sufficient for most patients; instillation more than six times daily may wash away natural tears and cause a rippled appearance on the ocular surface not unlike "dishpan hands" caused by excessive immersion of the hands in water.*[21]

Artificial-tear products can temporarily relieve the burning and irritation caused by dryness of the eye. They should not be used longer than 72 hours unless directed to do so by an eye-care specialist. *Patients who experience eye pain, changes in vision (central or peripheral), continued redness, or irritation of the eye must discontinue use and obtain an appointment with an eye-care specialist at once.*

Cellulose derivatives (e.g., carboxymethylcellulose, hydroxyethyl cellulose, hydroxypropyl methylcellulose, methylcellulose), common ingredients in artificial tears, provide enhanced duration when compared with other ingredients. These water-soluble compounds form viscous, transparent solutions. Cellulose derivations are safe, and other than dry crusts that form on the lids during the use of cellulose derivatives, they are virtually free of adverse reactions. (The crusts do not adhere tightly and are easily wiped or washed away.)

Polyvinyl alcohol is another common component of tear substitutes. A nontoxic, long-chain, plastic polymer that lowers surface tension, it has a lower viscosity than the cellulose derivatives. Therefore, it does not form crusts, but its duration is shorter. Polyols used in dry-eye products include glycerin, propylene glycol, polyethylene glycols, and polysorbate 80.

Povidone and dextran 70 are also effective dry-eye ingredients, but dextran 70 can cause transient stinging and temporarily blur the patient's vision. Gelatin may not be used as a single ingredient, but can be added to another demulcent to raise the protein content of tears.

OCULAR EMOLLIENTS

Ocular emollients may also be used to treat dry eye (Table 27.2). These products are ophthalmic ointments containing lanolin, mineral oil, paraffin, petrolatum, white petrolatum, white ointment, white wax, or yellow wax. They soften tissue by forming an occlusive film on the surface of the eye. Just as with tear substitutes, emollients relieve burning and irritation of dry eye, relieve discomfort caused by minor irritations of the

Table 27.1. Representative Artificial Tears

PRODUCT	SELECTED INGREDIENTS/COMMENTS
AquaSite Preservative Free	Unit dose: dextran 70, 0.1%; polyethylene glycol 400, 0.2%
Bausch & Lomb Moisture Eyes	Propylene glycol 1%, glycerin 0.3%
Bion Tears	Unit dose: dextran 70, 0.1%; hydroxypropyl methylcellulose 2910, 0.3%
Celluvisc Preservative Free	Unit dose: carboxymethylcellulose sodium 1%
Clear Eyes CLR (Contact Lens Relief)	Hydroxypropyl methylcellulose, glycerin, sodium chloride, borate buffers (concentrations unlabeled)
Hypo Tears Eye Drops	Polyethylene glycol 400, 1%; polyvinyl alcohol 1%
Hypo Tears PF Eye Drops	Unit dose: polyethylene glycol 400, 1%; polyvinyl alcohol 1%
Murine Tears	Polyvinyl alcohol 0.5%, povidone 0.6%
OcuCoat PF Eye Drops	Unit dose: dextran 70, 0.1%; hydroxypropyl methylcellulose 2910, 0.8%
Refresh Plus Preservative Free	Unit dose: carboxymethylcellulose sodium 0.5%
Refresh Preservative Free	Unit dose: polyvinyl alcohol 1.4%, povidone 0.6%
Tears Naturale Eye Drops	Dextran 70, 0.1%; hydroxypropyl methylcellulose 0.3%
Tears Naturale II	Dextran 70, 0.1%; hydroxypropyl methylcellulose 2910, 0.3% (electrolyte content differs from Tears Naturale)
Tears Naturale Free Lubricated Eye Drops	Unit dose: dextran 70, 0.1%; hydroxypropyl methylcellulose 2910, 0.3%
Tears Plus	Polyvinyl alcohol, povidone

Table 27.2. Representative Ocular Emollients

PRODUCT	SELECTED INGREDIENTS/COMMENTS
Bausch & Lomb Moisture Eyes PM	Ointment; white petrolatum 80%, mineral oil 20%
Hypo Tears Lubricant Eye Ointment	Ointment: mineral oil; white petrolatum (concentrations unlabeled)
Lacri-Lube S.O.P.	Ointment: mineral oil 42.5%; white petrolatum 56.8%
Refresh P.M.	Ointment: mineral oil 41.5%; white petrolatum 56.8%
Stye	Ointment: mineral oil 31.9%; white petrolatum 57.7% (the product was sold for many years to treat styes until the FDA required that such labeling be removed); in spite of the trade name, it cannot cure or prevent styes—patients with styes should be referred to a physician

eye or wind/sun exposure, protect against further irritation, and lubricate.[1] *Because they may cause blurred vision, their optimal time of use is at bedtime.*[16] When using ointments, the patient should pull down the lower eyelid and apply a small ribbon (1/4 in) of ointment to the inside of the eyelid, while taking care not to touch the tip of the ointment tube to anything (e.g., the eye, eyelid, a finger, the counter, etc.). (See "Instructions for Use of Ophthalmic Ointments and Gels.")

Nonpharmacologic Therapies

Patients may notice that dry eye is caused or worsened by certain environmental factors such as smoke, chemical vapors, and cold drafts.[3] These irritants should be avoided whenever possible. *If the eye worsens when the patient reads, watches television, or stares closely and intently at a computer monitor, it may be caused by a depressed blink reflex induced by intense concentration.*[33] Blinking carries the liquid over the surfaces of the eye, preventing tear-film breakdown.[14,34] To bathe the tissues of the eye, the patient may need to consciously learn to blink fully and often.[35] *If the problem is worse in the winter, the patient may need to consider the use of a cool-mist humidifier or warm-steam vaporizer to combat the effects of the dry winter air (especially the heated air inside the house) on the eyes.*[3,36,37] (See Chapter 16, Humidity Deficit.)

Other Professional Treatment

Surgery to relieve dry eye traditionally consists of narrowing the puncta to restrict tear outflow or closing it entirely.[38] In another approach a team of researchers in Australia has transferred submandibular salivary glands to the temple region through microvascular anastomosis, suturing the duct orifice to an opening in the conjunctiva.[39] The transplanted gland secretes saliva in a continuous basal mode, thereby relieving ocular dryness.

LOOSE FOREIGN MATERIAL IN THE EYE

MANIFESTATIONS OF LOOSE FOREIGN MATERIAL IN THE EYE

Loose foreign material underneath the eyelids produces irritation and inflammation, often accompanied by redness, swelling, mucous discharge, and/or involuntary tearing.[2] The patient may blink uncontrollably. Typical complaints include foreign-body sensation, discomfort, burning, stinging, smart-

ing, and itching. The foreign material may be dirt, an eyelash, or particles that are solubilized in or suspended by the tears. (See "A Pharmacist's Journal: She Pulled This Ropy Stuff Out of Her Eye.")

TREATMENT OF LOOSE FOREIGN MATERIAL IN THE EYE

Treatment Guidelines

If it is not removed, loose foreign material in the eye may cause an ocular infection. However, if the eye is not damaged, symptoms usually resolve with removal of the object. An eye irrigating solution—also known as an eyewash or eye lotion—can help remove the object (Patient Assessment Algorithm 27.1).

Nonprescription Medications

The rational formulation for an eyewash is nothing more than an isotonic, buffered solution of sterile water, with agents to establish appropriate pH and preservatives (Table 27.3). An

A Pharmacist's Journal

"She Pulled This Ropy Stuff Out of Her Eye."

An older woman approached me to ask about products for minor eye irritation for her granddaughter. She said her granddaughter had been playing with her eyelid the day before. The granddaughter had some irritation and was trying to see if something was under her eyelid. The young girl apparently felt something protruding slightly from her eyelid. The grandmother said she pulled at it and "this thick, ropy

stuff came out from under the eyelid." The grandmother said she thought that the girl's eye cosmetics had collected under the eyelid over the last several months, until they accumulated into this strange crusty thing. I told her that, although the girl might be able to cleanse the eye with a sterile eyewash, she should see a general practitioner to ensure that no residual remained that could cause an infection at some point.

Table 27.3. Representative Eyewashes

PRODUCT	SELECTED INGREDIENTS/COMMENTS
Bausch & Lomb Eye Wash	Sterile isotonic solution; boric acid, sodium borate, sodium chloride, purified water; packaged with an eye cup (concentrations unlabeled)
Collyrium for Fresh Eyes Eye Wash	Sterile isotonic solution; boric acid, sodium borate, water; packaged with an eye cup

Patient Assessment Algorithm 27.1. Ophthalmic Problems

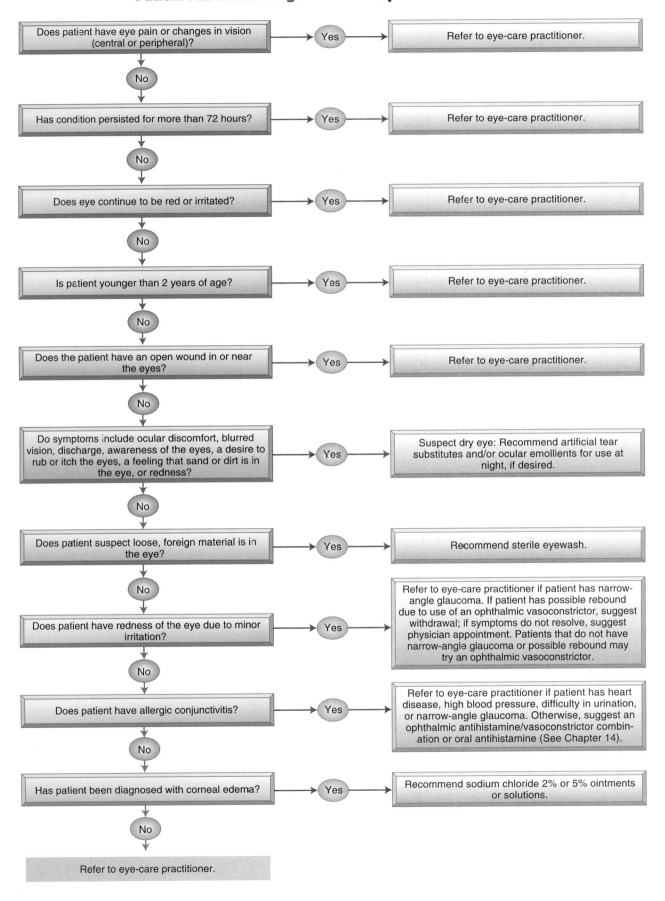

eyewash, which can help wash away foreign material and dilute irritating substances dissolved or suspended in tears, does not contain any active ingredients.

The labeled indications for eyewash products are as follows: flushing, irrigating, cleansing, washing, or bathing the eye to remove loose foreign material, air pollutants (smog or pollen), or chlorinated water, or to help relieve irritation, discomfort, burning, stinging, smarting, or itching caused by these problems.[1] *Eyewash labels must warn patients to obtain immediate medical attention for all open wounds in or near the eyes.*[1]

Some eyewashes are packaged with eyecups, archaic applicators that have been available for decades. The eyecup is a receptacle (usually made of plastic) wrapped in a plastic overwrap that maintains sterility until the overwrap is opened. The eyecup holds approximately 11 to 12 mL of eyewash. To use the eyecup in conjunction with an eyewash, the patient should rinse the eyecup with clean water (or the eyewash itself) before use.[1] Eyewash is placed in the cup until it is half filled. The patient bends over until the periorbital area is surrounded by the rim of the eyecup. The patient opens the eye and tilts the head back, hyperextending the neck, until the fluid in the eyecup bathes ocular tissues. The eyeball must be rotated to ensure thorough bathing. With gentle pressure, fluid in the eyecup should not leak out onto the clothing. The patient must rinse the eyecup with clean water (or the eyewash solution) after each use.

The eyecup is only sterile before the manufacturer's package is opened. Once the package has been opened, the eyecup is contaminated through contact with room air, which renders it nonsterile. Although the FDA cautions that the patient should avoid contaminating the rim and inside surface of the cup, the necessity of touching it to skin makes this admonition impossible. Further, if several individuals in the household use the eyecup, the eyes may become infected through cross-contamination. Finally, the plastic composition of most eyecups currently supplied with eyewashes does not permit sterilization through boiling. Attempted disinfection through application of alcohol or other substances is also unwise since trace amounts of these chemicals may contact the eye with subsequent use of the eyecup.

Because of the disadvantages of eyecups, the pharmacist should recommend that the patient not use them. A better alternative is to hold the head over a sink, holding the eyewash at an angle slightly away from the eyes, aimed in such a manner that when the bottle is squeezed, the solution will stream gently across the surface of the eye, flushing or irrigating it.

REDNESS OF THE EYE CAUSED BY MINOR IRRITATION

ETIOLOGY OF REDNESS OF THE EYE CAUSED BY MINOR IRRITATION

Irritation of the eye may result from exposure to numerous irritants, including noxious airborne pollutants (such as gases

or smoke) and chlorinated water. These chemicals, gases, or other microparticulates can become solubilized or suspended in tears, irritating the eye and resulting in inflammation and redness.[2,40]

Infectious diseases and glaucoma are two examples of serious conditions that could also cause irritation/inflammation. For this reason pharmacists must stress the 72-hour use limit when eye-care products are sold for redness and must counsel patients to discontinue use and see an eye-care specialist (e.g., physician, optometrist) if redness and irritation continue.[1]

TREATMENT OF REDNESS OF THE EYE CAUSED BY MINOR IRRITATION

Treatment Guidelines

Ophthalmic redness resulting from minor irritation can be safely and effectively treated with ophthalmic vasoconstrictors such as those found in the products listed in Table 27.4 (Patient Assessment Algorithm 27.1). Like nasal vasoconstrictors, these sympathomimetic amine ingredients shrink swollen blood vessels. The transient vasoconstriction reduces redness of the eye. The approved dosage is 1 to 2 drops in the affected eye(s) up to four times daily.

Ophthalmic vasoconstrictors are contraindicated in patients with glaucoma since they may produce **mydriasis** (dilation of the pupil), even in normal doses. The mydriasis can, in turn, trigger an attack of narrow-angle glaucoma, which may compromise the patient's vision.[1,2] Since most glaucoma patients do not know what type of glaucoma they have, pharmacists should caution all glaucoma patients against using ophthalmic vasoconstrictors unless they know for certain that they have open-angle glaucoma. (Alternatively, the pharmacist could contact the patient's eye-care specialist to ascertain the type of glaucoma.) Patients predisposed to mydriasis with normal dosing of vasoconstrictors include patients with contact lenses, lightly colored irises, and a corneal abrasion. The FDA has proposed a revision to the previous nonprescription decongestant ophthalmic warning, "Pupils may become dilated (enlarged). This is temporary and not serious. If you have narrow-angle glaucoma, do not use this product except under the advice and supervision of a doctor."[41]

Like nasal vasoconstrictors, ophthalmic ingredients can also cause a rebound **hyperemia** (presence of increased blood caused by cessation of circulation followed by restoration of circulation), especially when the products are used too often or for too long a period. As the product's effects abate, the eye returns to its former congested state, but appears worse than it was before the medication was used. This phenomenon, which has been referred to as "conjunctivitis medicamentosa," could prompt patients to use the product for longer periods and at shorter intervals than intended, long after the original cause of the redness is no longer present. Thus the product can cause the condition for which it is being used—another classical vicious cycle. Effects may persist even when the drops are discontinued, necessitating

Table 27.4. Representative Ophthalmic Products Containing Astringents and/or Vasoconstrictors

PRODUCT	SELECTED INGREDIENTS
Bausch & Lomb Sensitive Eyes	Naphazoline HCl 0.012%; polyethylene glycol 300, 0.2%
Bausch & Lomb Sensitive Eyes Maximum Strength	Naphazoline HCl 0.03%; hydroxypropyl methylcellulose 0.5%
Clear Eyes	Naphazoline HCl 0.012%, glycerin 0.2%
Clear Eyes ACR	Naphazoline HCl 0.012%, glycerin 0.2%, zinc sulfate 0.25%
Murine Tears Plus	Polyvinyl alcohol 0.5%, povidone 0.6%, tetrahydrozoline HCl 0.05%
OcuClear	Oxymetazoline HCl 0.025%
Visine	Tetrahydrozoline HCl 0.05%
Visine A.C.	Tetrahydrozoline HCl 0.05%, zinc sulfate 0.25%
Visine Advanced Relief	Dextran 70, 0.1%; polyethylene glycol 400, 1%; povidone 1%; tetrahydrozoline HCl 0.05%
Visine L.R.	Oxymetazoline HCl 0.025%

a physician visit.[42] For this reason all vasoconstrictors should be labeled, *"Overuse of this product may produce increased redness of the eye."*

Nonprescription Medications

Ingredients found in nonprescription products such as vasoconstrictors include naphazoline, tetrahydrozoline, phenylephrine, and oxymetazoline. Many products also have ingredients for dry eye (e.g., polyethylene glycol, glycerin) added to their formulation.

The FDA panel that reviewed ophthalmic vasoconstrictors in 1980 recognized that they are potentially toxic if ingested. Two cases of poisoning by tetrahydrozoline have been reported. In both pediatric cases (15 and 23 months of age), children were admitted to the emergency room with fatigue, lethargy, and limpness, followed by agitation, thrashing movements, irritability, poor balance, and ataxic movements.[43] In one case treatment with activated charcoal and sorbitol via nasogastric tube was effective. In a second case the patient, who was managed by observation, improved within 20 hours.[43]

DISCOMFORT CAUSED BY MINOR EYE IRRITATION

Eye irritation also causes discomfort, which can be relieved by the ophthalmic demulcents described in "Treatment of Dry Eye" above. In addition to their use in relieving dry eye, they also relieve discomfort caused by minor irritation of the eye or exposure to wind or sun.

Zinc sulfate 0.25% also relieves the discomfort of minor eye irritation by acting as an astringent, which precipitates the proteinaceous components of mucus. The precipitated protein is more easily removed from the eye.[2] The approved

dosage of zinc sulfate is 1 to 2 drops in the affected eye(s) up to four times daily.

ALLERGIC CONJUNCTIVITIS

EPIDEMIOLOGY OF ALLERGIC CONJUNCTIVITIS

Chapter 14 discusses the ophthalmic manifestations of allergic rhinitis. The pharmacist can recognize ophthalmic allergic conjunctivitis by discovering that the patient has a personal or family history of dermatitis, concurrent nasal involvement, asthma, or atopic disease.[44] Age of onset occurs before age 30 in 80% of patients.

MANIFESTATIONS OF ALLERGIC CONJUNCTIVITIS

Allergic conjunctivitis is usually bilateral, chronic, and recurring with prominent itching. The eyes are slightly red, tearing, and burning, but with little discharge.[45] The problem seems worse when the patient initially awakens.

ETIOLOGY OF ALLERGIC CONJUNCTIVITIS

Allergic conjunctivitis is caused by the same types of exposure that trigger allergic rhinitis. It may be caused by exposure to animal hair, pollen, ragweed, or other plants.

TREATMENT OF ALLERGIC CONJUNCTIVITIS

Treatment Guidelines

The FDA Review Panel originally appointed to examine nonprescription ophthalmics in 1980 explicitly opposed the use of single-entity vasoconstrictors for any indication relating to allergic rhinitis. However, in 1995 several prescription products were given approval for OTC marketing with allergic conjunctivitis their primary indication. (See Patient Assessment Algorithm 27.1.)

Nonprescription Medications

The combination products as shown in Table 27.5 contain a vasoconstrictor (naphazoline) and an antihistamine (pheniramine or antazoline). They are indicated for relieving ophthalmic redness and itching caused by exposure to animal hair, pollen, or ragweed at a dosage of 1 to 2 drops in the affected eye(s) up to four times daily.[46–48] *Warnings prohibit the use of nonprescription products for allergic conjunctivitis by patients with heart disease, high blood pressure, difficulty in urination, and narrow-angle glaucoma or by patients younger than 6.*

CORNEAL EDEMA

The water content of the cornea occasionally increases, causing the cornea to swell and lose transparency.[2]

ETIOLOGY OF CORNEAL EDEMA

Corneal edema may be caused by a number of conditions, including prolonged contact lens wearing, corneal inflammation, infection, glaucoma, iritis, or degeneration of cells lining the back of the cornea.[2] *Since corneal edema is potentially produced by a serious underlying problem, it must be checked by a physician.* Further, blurred vision and ophthalmic pain may indicate corneal ulceration or glaucoma, so that even the symptoms of corneal edema are difficult to differentiate.

MANIFESTATIONS OF CORNEAL EDEMA

Patients with corneal edema often complain of foggy vision and haloes around lights. If the condition worsens, blisters can form, causing photophobia and irritation. Should blisters rupture, patients may describe a foreign-body sensation with excruciating pain.

TREATMENT OF CORNEAL EDEMA: NONPRESCRIPTION MEDICATIONS

Hypertonic sodium chloride in a 2 to 5% concentration in a sterile solution or ointment creates an osmotic gradient that draws fluid from the cornea (Table 27.6).[2] To ensure safe use of nonprescription ophthalmics for corneal edema, the FDA requires a warning label, *"Do not use this product except under the advice and supervision of a doctor."* Other labeling warns the purchaser that the products may cause temporary burning and irritation when instilled into the eye. The patient is directed to use 1 to 2 drops in the affected eye(s) every 3 or 4 hours or as directed by a physician.[1] (See Patient Assessment Algorithm 27.1.) Although the FDA considered making these products prescription only (in light of a pre–physician diagnosis requirement), the agency felt that such a move would unduly restrict access to products that are safe and effective when self-administered.

PART 2: OPHTHALMIC CONDITIONS THAT MUST BE REFERRED TO A PHYSICIAN

Because of their prominent location on the face and the need for clear vision, the eyes are often uncovered and exposed to various types of damage that require evaluation by a physician.[49]

Table 27.5. Representative Products for Allergic Conjunctivitis

PRODUCT	SELECTED INGREDIENTS
Naphcon A	Naphazoline HCl 0.025%; pheniramine maleate 0.3%
Opcon-A	Naphazoline HCl 0.02675%; pheniramine maleate 0.315%
Vasocon-A	Naphazoline HCl 0.05%, antazoline phosphate 0.5%
Visine A	Naphazoline HCl 0.025%; pheniramine maleate 0.3%

Table 27.6. Representative Products for Corneal Edema

PRODUCT	SELECTED INGREDIENTS
Adsorbonac	Sodium chloride 2% or 5% solutions
Muro 128	Sodium chloride 2% or 5% ointments and solutions

A Pharmacist's Journal

"Where Are the Magnets?"

I was once approached by a patient who asked "Where are the magnets?" I told him that they would be in the toy section, unless he was using them for a purpose such as finding studs in walls. He replied, "No, I'm looking for a medical magnet." On further questioning, the patient revealed that he wanted a strong medical mag-net such as they use in emergency rooms. I told him that I had never seen one, and he would probably have to get one in a medical supply house. He expressed dissatisfaction and revealed that he wished to remove a metal shaving from his eye. I urged him to seek immediate emergency care instead.

FOREIGN BODY IN THE EYE

There are many circumstances that result in a foreign body entering the eye. For example, people engaged in metal working and wood working—particularly with power tools—occasionally feel a particle enter the eye (especially if they neglect protective eyewear).

Striking metal objects with other metal objects is a primary cause of foreign bodies in the eye, since small pieces of metal may be ejected at high speed, penetrating the eyes.[50–53] Keeping tarantulas as pets is popular, but when they are handled they may mount a defensive reaction that consists of rubbing the back legs to cause barbed hairs to fly at the attacker's face. These barbed hairs can penetrate the cornea and conjunctiva, causing eye redness and pain.[54] Ophthalmic corticosteroids may be helpful.

As discussed above, the only time a patient can self-treat a foreign body in the eye is for loose foreign material that is easily removed with an eyewash. Unfortunately, patients attempt to self-treat a wide range of more serious foreign bodies. (See "A Pharmacist's Journal: Where Are the Magnets?")

Particles embedded in the cornea usually cause some initial discomfort.[2] However, the cornea has a remarkable ability to adapt to continued stimulation so that the uncomfortable feeling fades rapidly.[55] (The cornea adapts in this manner with hard contact lenses.) Patients asking pharmacists for advice often suspect the presence of a foreign body, but might think it is gone since its presence does not cause discomfort any longer.

Patients may attempt to remove an embedded object themselves, but should not do so. Foreign bodies that are not promptly removed may cause cataracts within a matter of hours if the lens retains the object or is pierced by it. Toxic effects caused by the foreign body may cause glaucoma. Sclerosis of the trabecular meshwork may also result in glaucoma. Metallic foreign bodies that remain imbedded in the cornea for a sufficient period can produce a "rust ring," which requires a corneal curette or motorized device for removal.[56]

Objects may be removed from the eye by a physician or other qualified medical professional in the emergency room or a physician's office with the use of sterile needles, cycloplegics, and cobalt blue light; topical antibiotics are often prescribed.[57,58] At times, damage is so subtle that emergency room referral to an ophthalmologist is required. As an example, a patient hammering metal bearings produced a fragment of metal with a velocity sufficient to penetrate his cornea.[59] His symptoms were minor, which underscores the need for pharmacist referral for any suspected ocular foreign object.

OCULAR TRAUMA

Ocular trauma is a major cause of disability, and the second most common cause of visual impairment.[60] Patients suffer ophthalmic traumas that vary tremendously in etiology and severity. All patients with ocular trauma must be referred immediately for evaluation.[56,57,61]

Young men are especially at risk because of their tendency to take risks.[62] Injury can result from a range of causes:

- Elastic cords with hooks on the ends such as bungee cords[63]
- Sports (such baseball, basketball, lacrosse, bicycling, football, soccer, and hockey) [60,64–70]
- Pursuit games such as paint ball competitions[71]
- Close proximity to lawnmowers[72]
- Fireworks[73,74]
- Workplace-associated injuries[50,75–79]
- Dangerous toys (e.g., air guns, BB guns) [80–83]
- Merchandise display hooks[84]
- Airbags[85,86]
- Automobile collisions[87,88]

A Pharmacist's Journal

"Where's the Visine?"

When I was working in a store near a fairground many years ago, a man and his wife approached to ask where the Visine was. As I showed the product to him, he nonchalantly removed his sunglasses to show me his eyes. His eyes had no whites. They were completely black, as though he were an alien. I asked what had happened to his eyes. He said that he raced stock cars at the fairgrounds and that on the previous day a car overturned in front of him and he hit it with great force. The seat belt snapped, and his head ricocheted off of the dashboard. His racing goggles were pushed into his face hard and produced total bruising of the whites of his eyes. I told him that Visine is for minor redness and he needed to see an ophthalmologist for a problem of his magnitude.

A Pharmacist's Journal

"Is Visine Good for Red in the Eye?"

A woman asked if Visine would be appropriate to get the red out. I told her that it is for that kind of problem. I asked how long she had the problem. She replied, "It's my husband. He was playing soccer a week ago. His friend hit him in the eye with his elbow, and his eyeball is bruised and irritated." I told her that the eye products were for minor problems, not for eye trauma. I further urged that she caution her husband to see a physician for the trauma.

See "A Pharmacist's Journal: Where's the Visine?" and "A Pharmacist's Journal: Is Visine Good for Red in the Eye?"

Even seemingly minor trauma must be professionally evaluated to ensure that there is not a deeper injury. Forceful sneezing and eye rubbing may produce rupture of the fragile conjunctival blood vessels, which appears as a painless, bright-red accumulation of blood.[58] Patients may scratch the eye with a fingernail, causing a conjunctival laceration. See "A Pharmacist's Journal: What Do You Have for Bloody Spots in the Eye?"

CHEMICAL EXPOSURE

The eyes are exposed to many substances in a typical day. Some chemicals can irritate or damage the eyes. Aerosol sprays are a common source of chemical exposure. Perfume, polish, deodorant, capsicum sprays, and fire extinguisher chemicals, for example, can cause potentially serious injury and mandate referral.[89,90] In one unfortunate case, a 55-year-old woman undergoing facial reconstructive surgery was disinfected with Hibiclens. The product contacted her eye, causing severe visual loss that necessitated corneal transplantation.[91]

tip Exposure of the eye to strong acids or alkalis calls for immediate emergency treatment (irrigation with clean water for as long as 30 minutes) and then referral to an emergency room.[56–58,61] Delayed therapy will most likely result in visual loss. Alkali injuries (e.g., lye, lime, plaster, mortar, cement) may not show apparent damage at first, but the chemical continues to penetrate tissue, eventually resulting in severe scarring.[92] The FDA is considering the use of nonprescription eye irrigants intended for first aid for chemical burns of the eye and called for data in 1989 to allow evaluation of their safety and efficacy.[93] The evaluation has not appeared as of a decade later.

INFECTIONS OF THE EYE AND SURROUNDING SKIN

The FDA Panel appointed to examine nonprescription ophthalmics in 1980 considered that minor external ocular infec-

A Pharmacist's Journal

"What Do You Have for Bloody Spots in the Eye?"

A young woman asked me what I had for bloody spots in the eye. I showed her the ophthalmic vasoconstrictors and asked what her problem was. She said, "It's not me. It's my husband. He awakened this morning with bloody spots in his eye." I asked about possible causes. She stated that he had never had this problem before, had gone to sleep early the previous night, and did not smoke or use alcohol. She said that neither of them had any memory of his eye being hit the previous day and neither could recall her having accidentally elbowed him in their sleep. I asked if the eye looked like small vessels had swollen. She said, "No, it's got these bloody spots like someone took an icepick and stabbed it several times." She denied his use of drugs of abuse and said he did not wear contact lenses. I told her he should see a physician to rule out bacterial infection.

tions might be amenable to non-prescription products, including the hordeolum (stye), blepharitis (granulated eyelids), and bacterial conjunctivitis.[2] However, the panel argued against the use of local anesthetics in the eye, as they could mask symptoms of serious disorders. The panel also considered ocular antiinfectives marketed at the time and found them of unknown safety/efficacy, including boric acid, mild silver protein, and yellow mercuric oxide. In a later (1983) report the FDA proposed Category II placement for these ingredients.[94] In a final rule the FDA concluded that conjunctivitis is not to be treated with nonprescription products since its symptoms duplicate those of serious disorders (e.g., uveitis, foreign body in the eye).[95] Conjunctivitis also frequently has a viral etiology (the ubiquitous "pink eye") and is also not amenable to nonprescription drug products.[96–100]

Blepharitis and styes involve the eyelid rather than the eye.[95] The FDA concluded that the consumer cannot distinguish infectious blepharitis from noninfectious blepharitis. Further, since the stye is a pustule or abscess within the lumen of a sebaceous or sweat gland in the eyelid, local antiinfectives cannot reach the source of the infection and are useless.[94] For these reasons, the pharma-cist must refer all suspected infections of the eye or eyelid for professional care.

Some patients purchase boric acid solution or powder in a misguided attempt to use it for ophthalmic purposes. (Manu-

FOCUS ON...

MISCELLANEOUS OPHTHALMIC ISSUES

OPHTHALMIC PROSTHESES
Patients with an ophthalmic prosthesis may discover that it requires cleaning beyond that of mere soap and water. The product Enuclene contains tyloxapol, a surfactant that facilitates removal of mucus and other secretions.

EYE PATCHES
Patients who require temporary eye patching may request eye patches. There are two general types:

- A nonsterile, semirigid, black patch with an elastic band that fits around the head
- A sterile, cushioned, nonadhesive or adhesive oval eye pad (The patient should be shown hypoallergenic tapes to secure the patch if the nonadhesive type is chosen.)

OPHTHALMIC VITAMINS
Storz/Lederle is marketing Ocuvite—a vitamin/mineral mix containing vitamins A, C, and E; zinc; copper; and selenium—to people concerned about their vision. The FDA asked the company to halt such claims as preventing and treating senile macular degeneration, night blindness, cataracts, corneal injuries, hemorrhages in the lids, and severe near-sightedness.[103,104]

UNIT-OF-USE PACKAGING
Nonprescription ophthalmic products are available in either bulk packages or unit-of-use packages. Bulk, multiuse containers carry the risk of contamination of contents unless patients are extremely careful not to touch the tips of the droppers to eyes or fingers. The products include a preservative; some patients are allergic to thimerosal, at one time one of the most common preservatives.

Unit-of-use packages are small plastic vials containing a single dose. Any excess is discarded. Unit-of-use packages effectively eliminate the risk of contamination of contents, although they do cost more because of increased packaging.

facturers have included ophthalmic instructions on these packages for many years.) Pharmacists must advise against such home remedies. Boron is an element with well-known toxicities and is only weakly effective as an antiinfective.

The manufacturer of Stye Ointment claimed for many years that it healed styes. Yielding to FDA pressure, the company reformulated it to remove yellow mercuric oxide and substitute white petrolatum and mineral oil. It is presently labeled for relief of the burning, stinging, and itching of styes. Assuming these ingredients are effective for these symptoms, the product could mask them, allowing the consumer to believe that the stye is receding. Rather than recommending this product, pharmacists should refer patients with styes for professional care, which may include an oral antibacterial.

FLASH BURNS FROM WELDING

Arc welding can produce a radiation burn (from ultraviolet radiation) of the eye.[2] OSHA requires protective eyewear, but welders sometimes work without it. The degree of burn damage depends on the type of process, length of the arc, level of current, exposure time, flux used, type of filler material, atmosphere and shielding about the arc, composition of the electrodes, and base metal being welded.[101,102] The symptoms of flash burns include extreme discomfort 3 to 6 hours after exposure such as burning and a sensation of sand in the eye.[2] The face and eyelids may also be burned. The condition is self-limiting and is optimally treated with patching, systemic analgesics, cycloplegics, and antibiotics. See "A Pharmacist's Journal: Where's the Stuff for Eye Burns?"

INSTRUCTIONS FOR USE OF OPHTHALMIC DROPS

In 1989 two faculty members at Northeast Louisiana University examined the adequacy of manufacturers' instructions for the use of nonprescription eye drops (excluding contact lens drops).[105] The instructions were found to be grossly inadequate. Thus, for instance, an individual needing a tear substitute to prevent the medical consequences of dry eye might not obtain those benefits because of improperly using the product. Full instructions for use of an eye solution include the following:

1. Wash the hands thoroughly with an antibacterial soap.
2. Tilt head back and gently pull lower lid forward to create a pouch.
3. As shown in the figure, instill one drop into the pocket without touching the eyelid or lashes with the eyedropper or bottle tip. (Place only one drop at a time because the normal eye can only retain a fraction of the volume of the average eye drop.)
4. Wait a few seconds, then bring the lid forward, look down, and gently lift the lower lid up until it touches the upper lid.
5. Release the lid and keep the eyes closed without blinking or squeezing for 1 to 2 minutes.
6. Apply gentle pressure over the puncta (opening of tear duct at the inner corner of the eye) for 2 minutes to minimize systemic absorption and to prevent drainage of solution from the intended area.
7. Blot area with a clean tissue.

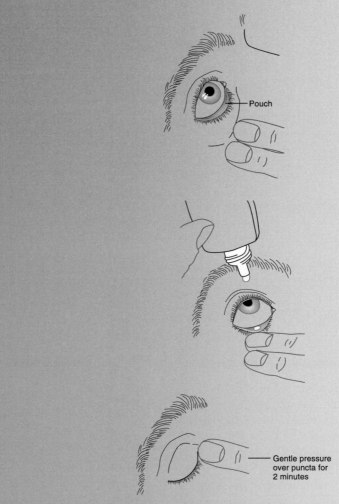

Proper method for applying ophthalmic drops.

SUMMARY

Ophthalmic problems present a challenge to the pharmacist. Any patient presenting with eye pain, changes in vision, continued redness or irritation of the eye, or a condition that worsens or persists more than 72 hours should be referred to an eye-care practitioner. The following conditions are considered to be self-treatable, within FDA-mandated limits:

- Dry eye
- Loose foreign material in the eye
- Redness of the eye caused by minor irritation
- Discomfort caused by minor eye irritation
- Allergic conjunctivitis
- Corneal edema

Left untreated, serious ophthalmic conditions may threaten the patient's sight. For this reason, immediate referral is mandatory for the following conditions:

- Foreign body in the eye
- Ocular trauma
- Chemical exposure
- Infections of the eye and proximal areas
- Flash burns from welding

FOCUS ON...

INSTRUCTIONS FOR USE OF OPHTHALMIC OINTMENTS AND GELS[106]

The patient using an ophthalmic ointment or gel may not be able to understand the methods of use on the manufacturer's package. The pharmacist can help by presenting the following steps:

1. Wash the hands thoroughly with an antibacterial soap.
2. Without touching the tip of the tube, remove the cap from the ointment or gel container.
3. Tilt the head slightly backward.
4. With one finger, pull the eyelid down to form a pouch, as shown in the figure.
5. Squeezing the tube carefully to avoid touching it to the eye, apply the recommended amount of ointment or gel to the pouch inside of the eyelid.
6. Release the eyelid and close the eye, keeping it closed for 1 to 2 minutes.
7. While the eye is closed, distribute the medication by moving the eye, but do not rub the eye with a finger.
8. Replace the cap.

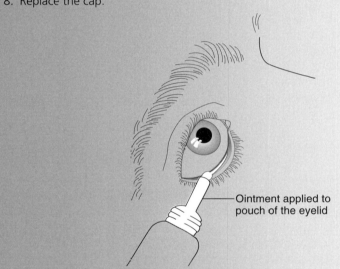

Ointment applied to pouch of the eyelid

Proper method for applying ophthalmic ointments.

A Pharmacist's Journal

"Where's the Stuff for Eye Burns?"

A man in his 30s approached the counter and asked, "Where's the stuff for eye burns?" I noticed that both eyes were red and appeared quite irritated. I asked if he knew what the problem was. He replied, "I looked at an arc welder." I asked if he had used his eye protection. "No, I wasn't actually doing the welding. I was just holding the metal for the other guy. I didn't know when he would strike, so I couldn't close my eyes fast enough. Don't you have that stuff that we used to carry around for eye burns years ago?" He couldn't recall the name of the product, and I certainly could not recall a nonprescription product for ophthalmic burns, so I urged him to see his physician without delay.

AT THE COUNTER

 A patient wants to know if there is anything stronger than the popular ophthalmic vasoconstrictor he has been using.

Interview/Patient Assessment

The patient states that he is on wheat harvest and has an allergy to the wheat pollen. His eyes are red and itching. He has used the vasoconstrictor for 2 weeks, and it helped at first, but is not working as well now. His eyes are watering so badly that he has constant tearing.

Pharmacist's Analysis

1. Can he use a vasoconstrictor that is stronger than the leading brand?

2. What is the likely source of this patient's ophthalmic tearing?
3. What product might be more appropriate for this patient?

This patient describes ophthalmic symptoms that appear to be caused by allergic rhinitis. He has used Visine far beyond the 72-hour use limit for an ophthalmic vasoconstrictor. It may be causing rebound redness.

Patient Counseling

The patient should be advised to discontinue the Visine and consider using one of the specific products approved for allergic conjunctivitis (e.g., antihistamine-vasoconstrictor combinations).

References

1. Fed Reg 43:7076, 1988.
2. Fed Reg 45:30002, 1980.
3. Kaden I, Mayers M. Systemic associations of the dry-eye syndrome. Int Ophthalmol Clin 31:69, 1991.
4. Khurana AK, et al. Tear film profile in dry eye. Acta Ophthalmol 69:79, 1991.
5. Caffery BE, Josephson JE. Is there a better comfort drop? J Am Optom Assoc 61:178, 1990.
6. Golding TR, et al. Soft lens lubricants and prelens tear film stability. Optom Vis Sci 67:461, 1990.
7. Schein OD, et al. Relation between signs and symptoms of dry eye in the elderly. A population-based perspective. Ophthalmology 104:1395, 1997.
8. Mathers WD, et al. Model for ocular tear film function. Cornea 15:110, 1996.
9. Herreras JM, et al. Influence of topical anesthesia on tests diagnostic of blepharitis-associated dry eye syndrome. Ocul Immunol Inflamm 5:33, 1997.
10. Toda I, Shimazaki J, Tsubota K. Dry eye with only decreased tear break-up time is sometimes associated with allergic conjunctivitis. Ophthalmology 102:302, 1995.
11. Gilbard JP. Dry eye: Pharmacological approaches, effects and progress. CLAO J 22:141, 1996.
12. Kjaergaard S. Assessment of eye irritation in humans. Ann NY Acad Sci 641:187, 1992.
13. Anon. Dry eyes and visual acuity (Editorial). Lancet 339:1389, 1992.
14. Patel S, et al. A possible reason for the lack of symptoms in aged eyes with low tear stability. Optom Vis Sci 67:733, 1990.
15. Fassihi AR, Naidoo NT. Irritation associated with tear-replacement drops. S Afr Med J 75:233, 1989.
16. Hecht A. Eyes too dry to cry. FDA Consumer 23(1):26, 1989.
17. Xu KP, Yagi Y, Tsubota K. Decrease in corneal sensitivity and change in tear function in dry eye. Cornea 15:235, 1996.
18. DeCarlo DK, et al. Dry eye among males infected with the human immunodeficiency virus. J Am Optom Assoc 66:533, 1995.

19. Caffery BE. Influence of diet on tear function. Optom Vis Sci 68:58, 1991.
20. Parsons JT, et al. Response of the normal eye to high dose radiotherapy. Oncology 10:837, 1996.
21. Farris RL. Contact lenses and dry eye. Int Ophthalmol Clin 31:83, 1991.
22. Silbert JA. A review of therapeutic agents and contact lens wear. J Am Optom Assoc 67:165, 1996.
23. Pflugfelder SC. Differential diagnosis of dry eye conditions. Adv Dent Res 10:9, 1996.
24. Versura P, et al. Mucus alteration and eye dryness. Acta Ophthalmol 67:455, 1989.
25. Rieger G. Lipid-containing eye drops: A step closer to natural tears. Ophthalmologica 201:206, 1990.
26. Tsubota K, Yamada M. Tear evaporation from the ocular surface. Invest Ophthalmol Vis Sci 33:2942, 1992.
27. Mathers JD, Daley TE. Tear flow and evaporation in patients with and without dry eye. Ophthalmology 103:664, 1996.
28. Charlton JF, Schwab IR, Stuchell R. Tear hyperosmolarity in renal dialysis patients asymptomatic for dry eye. Cornea 15:335, 1996.
29. Yokoi N, Takehisha Y, Kinoshita S. Correlation of tear lipid layer interference patterns with the diagnosis and severity of dry eye. Am J Ophthalmol 122:818, 1996.
30. Mainstone JC, Bruce AS, Golding TR. Tear meniscus measurement in the diagnosis of dry eye. Curr Eye Res 15:653, 1996.
31. Xu KP, et al. Tear function index: A new measure of dry eye. Arch Ophthalmol 113:84, 1995.
32. Trees GR, Tomlinson A. Effect of artificial tear solutions and saline on tear film evaporation. Optom Vis Sci 67:886, 1990.
33. Tsubota K, et al. Quantitative videographic analysis of blinking in normal subjects and patients with dry eye. Arch Ophthalmol 114:715, 1996.
34. Yap M. Tear break-up time is related to blink frequency. Acta Ophthalmol 69:92, 1991.
35. Nakamori K. Blinking is controlled primarily by ocular surface conditions. Am J Ophthalmol 124:24, 1997.

36. Tsubota K. The effect of wearing spectacles on the humidity of the eye. Am J Ophthalmol 108:92, 1989.

37. Korb DR, et al. Effect of periocular humidity on the tear film lipid layer. Cornea 15:129, 1996.

38. Murube J, Murube E. Treatment of dry eye by blocking the lacrimal canaliculi. Surv Ophthalmol 40:463, 1996.

39. MacLeod AM, Robbins SP. Submandibular gland transfer in the correction of dry eye. Aust N Z J Ophthalmol 20:99, 1992.

40. Hara JH. The red eye: Diagnosis and treatment. Am Fam Physician 54:2423, 1996.

41. Fed Reg 63:8888, 1998.

42. Spector SL, Raizman MB. Conjunctivitis medicamentosa. J Allergy Clin Immunol 94:134, 1994.

43. Higgins GL, et al. Pediatric poisoning from over-the-counter imidazoline-containing products. Ann Emerg Med 20:655, 1991.

44. Friedlander MH. Conjunctivitis of allergic origin: Clinical presentation and differential diagnosis. Surv Ophthalmol 38(Suppl):105, 1993.

45. Fujishima H, et al. Allergic conjunctivitis and dry eye. Br J Ophthalmol 80:994, 1996.

46. Trade package. Naphcon A, 1995.

47. Trade package. Opcon-A, 1995.

48. Trade package. Vasocon-A, 1995.

49. Knoop K, Trott A. Ophthalmologic procedures in the emergency department. II. Routine evaluation procedures. Acad Emerg Med 2:144, 1995.

50. de la Hunty D, Sprivulis P. Safety goggles should be worn by Australian workers. Aust N Z J Ophthalmol 22:49, 1994.

51. Thompson CG, et al. Penetrating eye injuries in rural New South Wales. Aust N Z J Ophthalmol 25:37, 1997.

52. Janicke S, Wagner W. Retained pieces of wood in the retromaxillary space: A case report. J Craniomaxillofac Surg 23:312, 1995.

53. Fong LP, Taouk Y. The role of eye protection in work-related eye injuries. Aust N Z J Ophthalmol 23:101, 1995.

54. Waggoner TL, Nishimoto JH, Eng J. Eye injury from tarantula. J Am Optom Assoc 68:188, 1997.

55. Lee LR, Briner AM. Intralenticular metallic foreign body. Aust N Z J Ophthalmol 24:361, 1996.

56. Silverman H, Nunez L, Feller DB. Treatment of common eye emergencies. Am Fam Physician 45:2279, 1992.

57. Janda AM. Ocular trauma. Postgrad Med 90:51, 1991.

58. Catalano RA. Eye injuries and prevention. Pediatr Clin North Am 40:827, 1993.

59. Migneco MK, Simpson DE. Penetrating injury from hammering with subtle ocular damage. J Am Optom Assoc 63:634, 1992.

60. Nichols CJ, et al. Ocular injuries caused by elastic cords. Arch Ophthalmol 109:371, 1991.

61. Levin AV. Eye emergencies: Acute management in the pediatric ambulatory care setting. Pediatr Emerg Care 7:367, 1991.

62. Joseph E. Predictors of blinding or serious eye injury in blunt trauma. J Trauma 33:19, 1992.

63. Cooney MJ, Pieramici DJ. Eye injuries caused by bungee cords. Ophthalmology 104:1644, 1997.

64. Fong LP. Sports-related eye injuries. Med J Aust 160:743, 1994.

65. Napier SM, et al. Eye injuries in athletics and recreation. Surv Ophthalmol 41:229, 1996.

66. Livingston LA, Forbes SL. Eye injuries in women's lacrosse: Strict rule enforcement and mandatory eyewear required. J Trauma 40:144, 1996.

67. Pardhan S, Shacklock P, Weatherill J. Sport-related eye trauma: A survey of the presentation of eye injuries to a casualty clinic and the use of protective eye-wear. Eye 9(Pt 6)(Suppl):50, 1995.

68. Orlando RG, Doty JH. Ocular sports trauma: A private practice study. J Am Optom Assoc 67:77, 1996.

69. Filipe JA, Barros H, Castro Correia J. Sports-related ocular injuries. A three-year follow-up study. Ophthalmology 104:313, 1997.

70. Lynch P, Rowan B. Eye injury and sport: Sport-related eye injuries presenting to an eye casualty department throughout 1995. Ir Med J 90:112, 1997.

71. Zwaan J, Bybee L, Casey P. Eye injuries during training exercises with paint balls. Mil Med 161:720, 1996.

72. Alonso JE, Sanchez FL. Lawn mower injuries in children: A preventable impairment. J Pediatr Orthop 15:83, 1995.

73. Anon. Serious eye injuries associated with fireworks—United States, 1990–1994. MMWR 44:449, 1995.

74. Smith GA, et al. The rockets' red glare, the bombs bursting in air: Fireworks-related injuries to children. Pediatrics 98:1, 1996.

75. Baker RS, et al. Demographic factors in a population-based survey of hospitalized, work-related, ocular injury. Am J Ophthalmol 122:213, 1996.

76. Owen CG, Margrain TH, Woodward EG. Aetiology and prevalence of eye injuries within the United Kingdom fire service. Eye 9(Pt 6)(Suppl):54, 1995.

77. Lee BL, Sternberg P Jr. Ocular nail gun injuries. Ophthalmology 103:1453, 1996.

78. Goel N, et al. Grease gun injuries to the orbit and adnexa. Ophthal Plast Reconstr Surg 10:211, 1994.

79. McDonald TE, Walsh LJ, Savage NW. Analysis of workplace injuries in a dental school environment. Aust Dent J 42:109, 1997.

80. Kutschke PJ. Ocular trauma in children. J Ophthalmic Nurs Technol 13:117, 1994.

81. Chan T, et al. Childhood penetrating eye injuries. Ir Med J 88:168, 1995.

82. Finkelstein M, Legmann A, Rubin PA. Projectile metallic foreign bodies n the orbit: A retrospective study of epidemiologic factors, management, and outcomes. Ophthalmology 104:96, 1997.

83. Marshall DH, et al. Air guns: The main cause of enucleation secondary to trauma in children and young adults in the greater Ottawa area in 1974–93. Can J Ophthalmol 30:187, 1995.

84. Fannin LA, et al. Eye injuries from merchandise display hooks. Am J Ophthalmol 120:397, 1995.

85. Duma SM, et al. Airbag-induced eye injuries: A report of 25 cases. J Trauma 41:114, 1996.

86. Manche EE, Goldberg RA, Mondino BJ. Air bag-related ocular injuries. Ophthalmic Surg Lasers 28:246, 1997.

87. Kuhn F, et al. Epidemiology of motor vehicle crash-related serious eye injuries. Accid Anal Prev 26:385, 1994.

88. Byhr E. Perforating eye injuries in a western part of Sweden. Acta Ophthalmol 72:91, 1994.

89. Pugh EJ, Dang MS, Mackie P. Eye injuries in children caused by aerosols and sprays (Letter). Br J Ophthalmol 76:703, 1992.

90. Watson WA, Stremel KR, Westdorp EJ. Oleoresin capsicum (Cap-Stun) toxicity from aerosol exposure. Ann Pharmacother 30:733, 1996.

91. Nasser RE. The ocular danger of Hibiclens (chlorhexidine) (Letter). Plast Reconstruct Surg 89:164, 1992.
92. Classe JG. Five liability claims involving the cornea and how they could have been prevented. Optom Clin 4:75, 1995.
93. Fed Reg 54:50240, 1989.
94. Fed Reg 48:29788, 1983.
95. Fed Reg 57:60416, 1992.
96. Weiss A. Acute conjunctivitis in childhood. Curr Probl Pediatr 24:4, 1994.
97. Benson WH, Lanier JD. The red eye: Avoiding pitfalls from topical ocular therapy. WV Med J 88:6, 1992.
98. Gigliotti F. Acute conjunctivitis of childhood. Pediatr Ann 22:353, 1993.
99. Weiss A, Brinser JH, Nazar-Stewart V. Acute conjunctivitis in childhood. J Pediatr 122:10, 1993.
100. King RA. Common ocular signs and symptoms in childhood. Pediatr Clin North Am 40:753, 1993.
101. Chou BR, Cullen AP. Evaluation of ocular hazards due to electric arc flash at an inline switch. Health Phys 61:473, 1991.
102. Chou BR, Cullen AP. Ocular hazards of industrial spot welding. Optom Vis Sci 73:424, 1996.
103. What can you do for the aging eye (Advertisement). Am Drugg 201:49, 1990(3).
104. Anon. Zinc supplement action. Hippocrates 4:29, 1990(4).
105. Lisi DM, Fazio A. Instructions provided by manufacturers for proper use of nonprescription ophthalmic drops. Am J Hosp Pharm 48:987, 1991.
106. Ziska DS, Noble SL. Common ophthalmic diseases and their treatment. Drug Topics 139(13):85, 1995.

Otic Conditions

AT THE COUNTER

A young couple with a child in a shopping cart ask if the child's ear can be treated.

Interview/Patient Assessment

The child, who appears to be 4 or 5, is pulling at his ear lobe. The parents relate that for two nights the child has been crying and complaining that his right ear hurts when he lies down to sleep. They add that he used to have frequent ear infections until they had tubes put in when he was 3. They want to buy an ear-cleaning product.

Pharmacist's Analysis

1. Is this child's age appropriate for self-therapy with carbamide peroxide?

2. What is the significance of the tympanostomy (ear) tubes?

3. Should the parents be allowed to treat the child?

There are several problems with this child that contraindicate self-therapy. Carbamide peroxide products are contraindicated under the age of 12. They are also not to be used in patients with perforated eardrums or with tubes in the ears. Finally, they are contraindicated in ear pain.

Patient Counseling

Because of his age, ear tubes, and pain, self-therapy is unsafe for this child, and the child should be referred to a physician, preferably the physician who placed the tubes.

Otic conditions are difficult for the pharmacist to differentiate. Unless he or she is trained to examine the ear, the pharmacist is wholly dependent on the patient's recitation of symptoms. Unfortunately, the same symptoms can be produced by many medical conditions, some dangerous and some minor. There are only two otic conditions for which pharmacists can recommend nonprescription products with certainty. One is cerumen impaction, and pharmacists can only recommend one nonprescription ingredient for cerumen removal—carbamide peroxide. Unless impacted cerumen can be clearly blamed for the symptom(s), however, patients should be referred for physician evaluation.

The other minor condition that is self-treatable is water-clogged ears. The pharmacist may recommend products containing isopropyl alcohol and glycerin for this use.

See Figure 28.1 to review ear anatomy.

PART 1: OTIC CONDITIONS THAT CAN BE SELF-TREATED

CERUMEN IMPACTION

Cerumen, also known as earwax, which has never been the subject of intensive research, plays an important role in ear health.[1] Unfortunately, however, in recent years it has become evident to health professionals that most people mistakenly believe that earwax denotes lack of cleanliness. As a consequence many people attempt to remove earwax, often using dangerous techniques that can compromise hearing and overall health.[2] It is important that pharmacists be aware of the benefits of earwax and understand the safe methods for its removal—when there is a reason to do so (Fig. 28.2).

Cerumen is a mixture of secretions from the **ceruminous gland** (modified apocrine sweat glands in the ear) and sebaceous glands, combined with **desquamated** (the outer layer of skin cells that sheds in the normal process of epidermal-cell migration) sheets of stratum corneum and hair.[3–7] Chemicals composing the glandular secretions include saturated and unsaturated long-chain fatty acids, alcohols, squalene, cholesterol, lysozymes, copper, and immunoglobulins G and A.[6,8–13] Although the desquamated keratinocytes and hair do not provide any health benefits, the glandular secretions help protect against infection.[8]

Cerumen color varies. When first produced, cerumen is colorless and somewhat fluid, but contact with air causes it to darken and become hard.[3,7,14–16] In black and white patients, cerumen is initially pale yellow, then progresses to dark brown as it approaches the outer ear.[1,3,5] However, the cerumen of Asian patients appears dry, gray, and brittle.[1,5] These color differences are a result of racial variations in the ceruminous glands and composition of the cerumen itself.[1]

Cerumen consistency also varies with age.[1] The elderly have drier wax, possibly because of the decline in the number of ceruminous glands and decrease in their secretory powers that occurs with aging.[1,17]

Cerumen provides several benefits to the ear. Conditions in the ear—a warm, moist, dark enclosed tube—naturally favor the growth of microorganisms.[9] Foremost among the functions of cerumen is the antibacterial and antifungal activity of its chemical components.[6] The pH of earwax averages 6.5 in normal patients, which is bactericidal.[18] Suspensions of cerumen demonstrate excellent antimicrobial activity against *Streptococcus pyogenes, Streptococcus viridans, Staphylococcus aureus, Staphylococcus epidermidis, Corynebacterium, Escherichia coli, Propionibacterium acnes,* and *Serratia marcescens.*[18] Because of its water-repellent nature, cerumen provides an oily, mechanical barrier that helps ensure that organisms that enter the ear in water

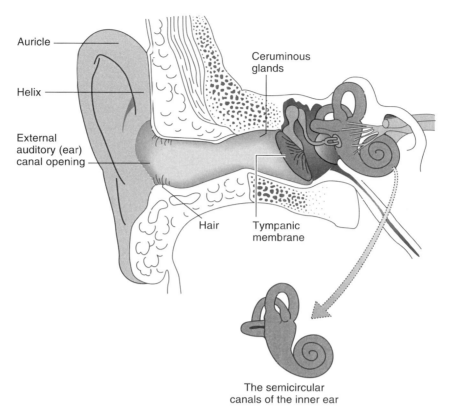

Figure 28.1. Anatomic features of the ear. Note the position of the semicircular canals, important in the etiology of motion sickness (Chapter 6), and the ceruminous glands, which produce cerumen (earwax).

(i.e., when swimming or bathing) do not cause infection.[11,19] (The triglyceride level of cerumen is lower in the summer, which may be a causal factor for the increase in external ear infections during the summer.[5])

Because it is sticky, cerumen also protects the tympanic membrane from penetration by several agents, including insects, dust, and other airborne materials.[11,17] Other factors protecting the ear include the S shape of the canal and the hair located in the canals.[11]

Cerumen lubricates the skin, which helps prevent pruritus in the external ear canal.[3,7,17] This function is critical as people tend to relieve external ear pruritus by scratching with rigid objects (e.g., keys, pencils, and paper clips). If these objects abrade the lining of the ear canal, the individual is more prone to an infection such as external otitis. The patient may also perforate the tympanic membrane with these objects, which may cause severe consequences.

The healthy ear self-cleans through the continual outward migration of cerumen, a process known as ceruminokinesis.[11,20] Movements of the jaw such as eating and talking facilitate ceruminokinesis.[7,17,21] Physicians have asked somewhat rhetorically what happens to cerumen as it approaches the superficial ear canals.[22] What usually happens is that hardened earwax is removed by patients with the use of wash cloth and water, cotton-tipped swabs, soap, and ear drops.[6]

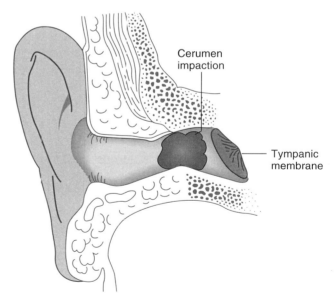

Figure 28.2. When normal ceruminokinesis is disrupted, the patient may develop a cerumen impaction that occludes the ear canal.

PREVALENCE OF CERUMEN IMPACTION

The prevalence of cerumen impaction is open to speculation since many patients do not seek professional help. Overall, the condition is said to be the most common condition of the external auditory canal.[23] Cerumen impaction was the most common otic disorder in first-grade children, experienced by 7.4% of students.[24] More than 4% of students in one school-based study failed an audiologic screening solely because of excess cerumen.[3]

EPIDEMIOLOGY OF CERUMEN IMPACTION

Some patients have ear canals that are abnormally **stenotic** (narrowed) or have more hair than normal in the ear canal—genetic factors that predispose to impaction.[7,25] In one study nonwhites had more ear canal occlusion than whites.[6] The elderly also have increased problems with ceruminokinesis because of the decline with age in the number of cerumen glands, which makes cerumen drier. The hair cells in the external auditory canal also become coarser with age.[26]

Patients with psoriasis have increased amounts of waxy material in the ears and may be more prone to impaction.[1] Mentally retarded adolescents and adults have been found to have higher incidences of impaction than a group of normal adolescents.[25,27] Also, persons with Down syndrome have been found to be more prone to impaction, possibly because of a genetic predisposition to stenotic ear canals.[25]

The likelihood of impaction is increased whenever the process of ceruminokinesis is blocked. For example, people who use hearing aids are more prone to impaction since hearing aids mechanically block ceruminokinesis.[7,28] Likewise, "ear plugs" and other hearing protective devices that are inserted into the ear canals can cause impaction through the same mechanism.[26] Anesthesiologists, who must wear molded stethoscope ear pieces for prolonged periods, often experience impacted cerumen, an occupational hazard.[29] Also, people with any bony growth in the ear canal may experience obstruction to ceruminokinesis.[7,30]

ETIOLOGY OF CERUMEN IMPACTION

Healthy, normal ceruminokinesis can become disrupted for several reasons, perhaps causing an impaction of earwax in the external ear canal. The impaction is often discovered when patients require certain otologic procedures (e.g., hearing assessment and speech testing, ear-mold impression.)[31–33]

Inadequate overall bodily hygiene contributes to impaction.[25] Skin particles and scales that accumulate from inadequate bathing of the head and shampooing of the hair can enter the ear and become trapped in earwax, hampering its normal outward migration. (People with scaling caused by dandruff should use an antidandruff shampoo.) People with seborrheic dermatitis in the ear canals can try nonprescription products to help reduce scaling (e.g., a small amount of hydrocortisone ointment or zinc pyrithione shampoo placed in the ear canal). (However, attempts to attain excellent otic hygiene with the use of cotton-tipped applicators or any

other device placed into the ear to remove cerumen usually worsen the problem of ear impaction. See "Home Hygiene Methods to Remove Cerumen Impaction.")

MANIFESTATIONS OF IMPACTION

Cerumen impaction may cause a feeling of pressure or fullness in the ear, vertigo, partial hearing of certain tones, tinnitus (manifested by occasional noises such as whistles, squeaks, and crackling sounds), and a general feeling of ear discomfort.[1,3,17] Cerumen impaction may cause a chronic cough because of pressure against the tympanic membrane or because of stimulation of the auricular branch of the vagal nerve.[1,7,26,34] Pain is not a normal symptom of impaction.

Patients with ear pain should be referred for initiation of appropriate antibiotic/antibacterial therapy if an ear infection is present.[17]

Cerumen may also cause hearing loss, although considerable controversy exists in the medical literature.[35,36] Some authors state that impaction is the most common cause of conductive hearing loss, while others categorically deny that impaction is a frequent cause of deafness.[27,37] One research study demonstrated a 30- to 40-decibel hearing improvement after wax removal, while another study failed to demonstrate more than a 5- to 10-decibel improvement in hearing after wax removal.[1,2]

Logically, an impaction large enough to occlude the ear canal should produce a conductive hearing loss.[3,4,7,17,25] Research revealed that 55% of a study population over the age of 55 had hearing impairment; 19% of those patients had bilateral cerumen impaction, leading the authors to the conclusion that cerumen removal would be a simple method to improve hearing.[38] Exposure to water sometimes allows a hard, desiccated cerumen plug that is only partially occluding the ear canal to expand, totally occluding the canal.[1,3] Thus reduced hearing may be more noticeable following a shower or swimming.

The patient with a cerumen impaction–induced loss of hearing usually relates a barely perceptible loss of hearing that slowly worsened, as opposed to a sudden hearing loss induced by trauma or other more serious causes of hearing loss.

Cerumen impactions may affect tympanic membrane temperature measurements. (See Chapter 26, Fever, for details on thermometers and taking temperatures.) Cerumen may lower the measured temperature by as much as 0.9°F.[39,40]

Impactions are said to be unilateral in about 75% of patients.[4] However, research in one series of patients indicated that 85% of patients had identical levels of occlusion in both ears.[6] Thus *pharmacists should advise patients to use cerumen-removal products in both ears.*

TREATMENT OF CERUMEN IMPACTION

When suggesting treatment for suspected cerumen impaction, the pharmacist must be careful to differentiate this minor condition from other more serious conditions and should refer the patient when self-treatment is not appropriate. Patient Assessment Algorithm 28.1 illustrates the steps used in this decision process.

Treatment Guidelines

Extreme caution must be taken when placing any foreign ⚠ substance or object in the ear. ***When the pharmacist recommends any method to remove cerumen, it is prudent to reinforce warnings about proper use of the products to ensure that the tympanic membrane is not damaged.***

Nonprescription Medications

🔔 *Carbamide peroxide 6.5% formulated in an anhydrous glycerin vehicle is the only nonprescription ingredient approved by the FDA for cerumen removal* (Table 28.1).[41,42] When placed into contact with tissues that contain **catalase** (a protein that breaks hydrogen peroxide down to water and

oxygen), it releases oxygen. The mechanical effect of this effervescence loosens debris and helps remove earwax. Carbamide peroxide products should not be used with the following conditions or situations[43]:

- Ear drainage or discharge
- Ear pain
- Irritation or a rash in the ear
- Dizziness
- Ear injury
- Perforation in the eardrum
- Recent ear surgery
- Tubes in the ears

The time limit for self-use is 4 days. If earwax remains after this time, a physician must be consulted. A physician must be consulted for children under the age of 12.

Patients should place 5 to 10 drops into each ear twice daily for up to 4 days. If the problem seems to be better (e.g., the feeling of pressure or discomfort eases), the patient may stop using the product before the 4 days is up. (See "In-

Patient Assessment Algorithm 28.1. Cerumen Impaction

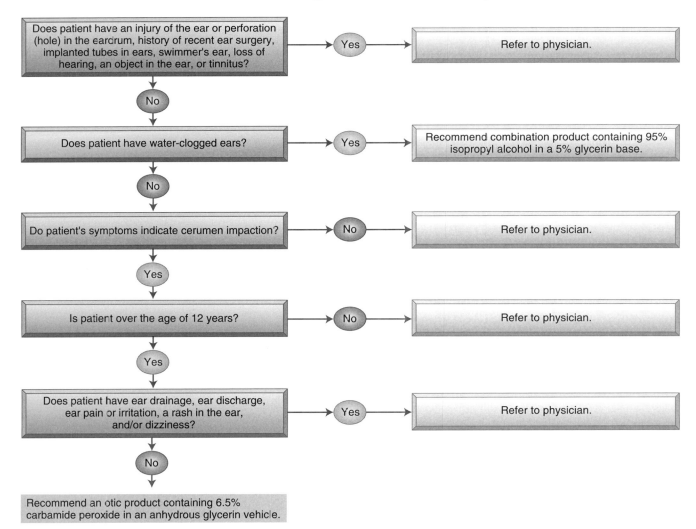

Table 28.1. Representative Products for Cerumen Impaction

PRODUCT	SELECTED INGREDIENTS/COMMENTS
Bausch & Lomb Earwax Removal System	Carbamide peroxide 6.5% in anhydrous glycerin
Debrox	Carbamide peroxide 6.5%, glycerin
E.R.O.	Carbamide peroxide 6.5% in anhydrous glycerin
Murine Ear Wax Removal System	Carbamide peroxide 6.5%, alcohol 6.3%, anhydrous glycerin (available with or without an otic syringe)

structions for Use of Otic Drops.") An ear syringe may help remove the wax softened by otic drops. (See "Instructions for Use of an Otic Syringe.")

Nonpharmacologic Therapies

IRRIGATION TO REMOVE CERUMEN
Pharmacists are familiar with traditional otic irrigation as a gentle cerumen removal method using an otic syringe (See "Instructions for Use of an Otic Syringe"), but the procedure can be dangerous.[44,45] However, patients should see a physician before conducting aural irrigation if the following conditions exist:

- Ear pain
- Congenital external ear abnormalities
- Tympanic membrane perforation—either through accidental means or for medical reasons such as the insertion of myringotomy tubes (irrigation can introduce contamination into the middle ear if the tympanic membrane is perforated[3,7,17])
- External otitis (irrigation often aggravates the condition[7,46])

A physician examination can confirm that the tympanic membrane is not perforated.[31] *A perforation should be suspected when the ear has been subjected to trauma or if the patient has a history of chronic otitis media.*[47] Otitis media can weaken the tympanic membrane, increasing the risk of rupture due to the barotrauma of syringing.[48]

Complications to syringing include perforation, otitis externa, vertigo, and cardiac arrest.[2,49] *Failure to use tepid water can result in dizziness and nystagmus.*[50]

Some patients use oral jet irrigators to cleanse the ears by introducing water into the ear under pressure. Oral jet irrigators have been used in several studies, using low pressure settings and lukewarm water (since water at extreme temperatures can cause nausea and vomiting).[4,25] ***Oral jet irrigators can cause traumatic tympanic membrane rupture with complete neurosensory hearing loss.***[48,51] Because of the proven dangers associated with them, pharmacists should advise against the use of oral jet irrigators for otic cleansing.

HOME HYGIENE METHODS TO REMOVE CERUMEN IMPACTION
Earwax should be removed with a wet, soapy washcloth placed over the finger during normal bathing. Many people clean their own ears or their child's ears with such objects as bobby pins, twisted napkin corners, fingernail files, matches, toothpicks, pencils, and keys in misguided attempts to remove the wax.[52] Others use cotton-tipped applicators.[37] (The label on a package of cotton-tipped applicators states that manufacturers only recommend them for cleansing the outer ear. Most labels warn against inserting the cotton-tipped applicator into the opening of the ear. Their careless use may abrade the ear, resulting in external otitis, or may cause tympanic membrane erythema or perforation.[53,54]) Misusing cotton-tipped applicators (and other objects) can push harder earwax further into the ear canal, where it can harden next to the eardrum. See "Ear Candling Warning."

WATER-CLOGGED EARS

Several companies attempted to gain approval for combination products containing 95% isopropyl alcohol in a 5% glycerin base for prevention of swimmer's ear in 1986.[59] The combination has not been proven effective for swimmer's ear, but instead has been proven safe and effective for drying water-clogged ears.[60] Several products for drying water-clogged ears appear in Table 28.2.

PART 2: OTIC CONDITIONS THAT MUST BE REFERRED TO A PHYSICIAN

SWIMMER'S EAR

Swimmer's ear (also known as diffuse external otitis) is the common name for a type of external otitis that follows prolonged exposure of the ear to water.[59,61] It is most common in the summer, when the ambient air is humid.[41] Swimming and diving are obvious risk factors, but other risk factors include high temperature and local trauma of the ear.[41] Individuals with allergies are also more prone to develop swimmer's ear than those without allergies.[59]

Since the ear canal is a cul-de-sac, it does not easily allow fluids that have been introduced into it to drain. Thus, if swimmers attempt to remove water from the ear after swimming (by using cotton-tipped applicators, keys, or any rigid object), the lining of the external auditory canal can be damaged. If this occurs, organisms can enter the wound, where they will proliferate in the ideal temperature and moist conditions. Further, the pH of the ear may change from the protective acidic value to an alkaline one because of the retained water. The most common organism to take advantage of the more favorable pH is *Pseudomonas aeruginosa*.[59]

Symptoms of swimmer's ear include acute pain, itching, inflammation, and drainage of a foul-smelling watery discharge.[37] Should the accumulated debris occlude the external auditory canal sufficiently, hearing may also be compromised.[59]

The FDA expressed concern in 1986 that patients may not be able to rule out more serious conditions, the symptoms of which might overlap with those of swimmer's ear.[59] Realizing that patients with a previous history of swimmer's ear might be able to reliably recognize recurrences, however, the FDA concluded that any ingredient eventually approved for the condition must include a warning that it is only to be used by individuals with a history of swimmer's ear.[59]

The FDA feels that nonprescription products would be appropriate for treatment of swimmer's ear, yet no ingredient has yet been proven safe and effective in this regard.[59] Specifically, research conducted on glycerin in isopropyl alcohol and a combination product containing isopropyl alcohol and acetic acid was inadequate to prove safety and/or efficacy in swimmer's ear.[60,62]

Mechanical barriers to prevent water from entering the ears while swimming, diving, or bathing are listed in Table 28.3.

FOCUS ON...

INSTRUCTIONS FOR USE OF OTIC DROPS

1. The patient should read the instructions regarding the proper amount of product to be placed into the ear.
2. The patient may hold the bottle in the hand for a few minutes prior to insertion to warm the solution, making application more comfortable.
3. The head should be tilted to the side so that the first ear canal to be treated is pointing toward the ceiling.
4. With one hand, the patient should pull the earlobe upward and back to straighten the ear canal. (A child's earlobe is pulled downward and back.)
5. The other hand should squeeze the bottle of otic drops carefully to expel just the number of recommended drops into the ear canal. The tip of the bottle should not enter the ear canal itself.[43]
6. The patient should move the head until the otic drops reach the tympanic membrane.
7. The drops should remain in the ear for several minutes by keeping the head tilted or placing cotton in the ear.
8. When the head regains the normal position, the patient should hold a tissue next to the outer ear canal to catch any solution that exits.
9. If necessary, the procedure is repeated on the other ear.
10. Gentle and careful use of an ear syringe as directed by the manufacturer may help remove the wax softened by the product. (See "Instructions for Use of an Otic Syringe.")

1. Straighten the ear canal.

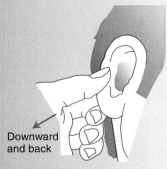

a. Adult method   **b.** Pediatric method

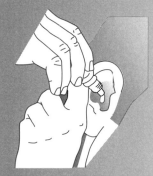 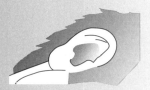

2. Place drops.   **3.** Keep head tilted.

The procedure for instilling ear drops: **1.** Straighten the ear canal of an adult (*1a*) and pediatric patient (*1b*). **2.** Instill drops in the ear. **3.** Keep the head tilted upward following instillation. (See discussion in chapter for full explanation.)

LOSS OF HEARING

Hearing loss has multiple potential causes—some are easily remediable and reversible, while others can result in permanent hearing loss if not promptly diagnosed and treated. Hearing loss indicates serious underlying pathology and is irreversible. Pharmacists must refer all patients with hearing loss to a physician or audiologist for proper diagnosis and treatment.

Hearing loss etiologies fall into two broad categories: sensorineural or conductive[63,64]:

- Sensorineural hearing loss results from exposure to noise, ototoxic medications, idiopathic or degenerative changes (e.g., **presbycusis** [a bilateral hearing loss linked to aging, often occurring with tinnitus]), genetics, and miscellaneous medical conditions (e.g., multiple sclerosis, acoustic neuroma, and Meniere's syndrome)[64–66]
- Conductive hearing loss results from otosclerosis, cerumen impaction, or otitis media[64]

A variety of medications can cause ototoxicity, including erythromycin, aminoglycosides, loop diuretics such as ethacrynic acid; furosemide and bumetanide; quinine; vancomycin; salicylates; and nonsteroidal anti-inflammatory medications.[67–73]

Cerumen impaction is a reversible cause of conductive hearing loss that is common in the elderly, as previously discussed.[74,75] In one study 35% of older patients admitted to a hospital had impacted cerumen in one or both ears.[65] Following its removal, 75% had improved hearing.

Two types of otic injury are attributable to noise, acoustic trauma, and prolonged exposure to noise.[76,77]

- Acoustic trauma occurs when the ear is exposed to sounds exceeding 140 decibels. This in-

FOCUS ON...

INSTRUCTIONS FOR USE OF AN OTIC SYRINGE

Otic syringes (ear syringes) are small rubber appliances used to cleanse the ear canal. The patient should be informed about their proper use at the point of sale. Steps for use include the following:

1. Fill the otic syringe approximately halfway with warm water.
2. If the head is to be upright during the procedure, place a towel underneath the ear to catch solution. Otherwise, the head may be placed over a sink.
3. Straighten the ear canal.
4. Insert the tip of the otic syringe carefully into the first ear to be treated.
5. Check to ensure that the ear opening is not occluded by the syringe.
6. Squeeze the bulb section of the otic syringe gently, allowing solution to enter the ear. Check to ensure that solution runs out of the ear as it enters to prevent **barotrauma** (damage to the tympanic membrane caused by pressure).
7. Tilt the head downward toward the skin to allow the water to drain out of the treated ear.
8. Repeat on the other ear, if necessary.

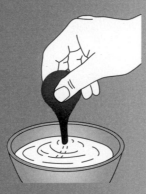

1. Fill the syringe.

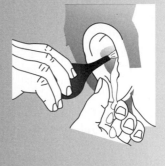

2. Straighten ear canal and instill the water.

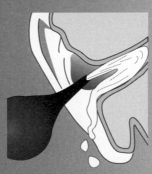

3. Confirm that water leaves the ear as solution enters.

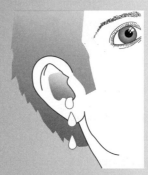

4. Allow the water to drain from the ear.

The procedure for irrigating the ear with an otic syringe: **1.** Fill the syringe. **2.** Instill the water. **3.** Confirm that water exits as it enters. **4.** Allow residual water to drain from the ear. (See discussion in chapter for full explanation.)

jury occurs instantly and is irreversible because it tears delicate tissues of the inner ear, which cannot stretch beyond their elastic limits.[78] Acoustic trauma often is associated with exposure to fireworks, firearms, and explosions.

- Prolonged and repeated exposure to noise from recreational, occupational, or environmental sources, the more common type of noise damage, develops gradually. After exposure to prolonged noise, an individual may notice that he cannot hear well for a short period (e.g., persistent ringing in the ears). Continued exposure causing symptoms such as this can produce a loss of sensory cells in the organ of Corti.[76,77,79,80] Eventually, a permanent hearing loss can result as these cells do not regenerate.[65,81,82]

Occupational noise exposure is a major concern, but sound from hobbies and recreational exposure is also a severe threat. Riding motorcycles, for example, produces low-frequency wind noise caused by turbulent airflow around the helmet. Only 15% of riders surveyed in one study used hearing protection, but 46% had sensorineural hearing loss, compared with age-matched, non–noise exposed controls.[83]

Other potentially dangerous recreational exposure, from highest to lower decibel ratings, include use of automobile "boom boxes," hunting/shooting (including cap pistols), model airplanes, snowmobiles, go carts/ATVs, private planes, and video arcades.[76] Hobbies and workshop exposures that should be of concern include chain saws and power saws, lawn mowers, routers, shop vacuums, and snow blowers.[76,83,84]

Information is emerging that personal stereos and cassettes can be highly dangerous to hearing. While many variables influence hearing loss (e.g., volume chosen, susceptibility of the person's ear to noise damage, and duration of exposure), personal stereos have registered sound levels as high as 128 decibels.[76] Investigators have concluded from several surveys that 5 to 10% of listeners regularly listen at levels high enough for sufficient durations to cause damage and that up to 20% experience indications of a temporary noise-induced hearing loss (ringing in the ears, fullness in the ears).[76] In another survey authors gave free hearing tests to students listening to personal stereos from which sound could be heard as far away as 5 to 10 feet and determined that 87% had hearing loss.[85] Alarmingly, when asked if they would continue to listen as loud if this practice were proven to cause deafness, 25% answered affirmatively.

Several kinds of hearing protectors are available for phar-

FOCUS ON . . .

EAR CANDLING WARNING

Patients occasionally ask about the procedure known as "ear candling" for earwax removal, since devices known as "ear candles" are sold in some pharmacies and health food stores. Reputable medical references do not usually include this topic, which may prompt patients to visit the Internet.[55–57] If one enters "ear and candles," a host of information becomes available.

The ear candle is a hollow cone or tube made of a combustible material. According to literature from several companies, the patient's helper places one end of the candle into the patient's ear, lighting the other end. Supposedly, the heat loosens earwax, which enters the candle because of a suction effect. "Air is drawn up from the eustachian tube into the inner ear then through the porous membrane out into the outer ear," according to a Washington-based company. The absurdity of this becomes quickly evident when one considers that ear tubes are necessary to allow equalization of pressure in legitimate medicine. Indeed, tympanometric measurements confirm that ear candles are unable to produce any negative pressure in the ears.[58] The safety of this quack technique is a further issue.

⚠️ ***Placing a burning object in the ear is not only foolish, but may produce tympanic membrane rupture or other damage.*** A survey of otolaryngologists revealed 21 injuries had occurred from the use of ear candles.[58] See "A Pharmacist's Journal: What Brand of Cigarettes Is Best" and "A Pharmacist's Journal: The Burning Torch."

A Pharmacist's Journal

"What Brand of Cigarettes Is Best?"

A patient once asked me which type of cigarettes is best. Of course, I responded that no brand is best, that they are all killers. He said, "I mean which is best for the ear?" I expressed profound confusion, and he clarified: "Whenever my kids get an earache, I learned from my parents to blow cigarette smoke into their ears until they feel better. I wonder if I should use any particular brand or should I use filtered?" I attempted to explain that one must see a physician for ear pain rather than using this primitive and toxic form of home remedy.

A Pharmacist's Journal

The Burning Torch

A Hispanic student shared the following story with me. When children in her family got an earache, they were taken to an elderly woman who functioned as the "healer." This woman directed the mother to place the child down on a table with the affected ear pointing upward toward the ceiling. The student remembers the healer lacing wet towels all over the patient's head, leaving only the ear opening uncovered. The healer next took a plain sheet of paper and formed a tapering cone, with the small end of the cone being placed directly into the child's ear. The other end of the cone was lit with a match.

As the cone burned downward, the student said observers would see a rush of air out of the cone. If you were the subject, this rush of air was followed by relief from the ear pain. This therapy, known as "the burning torch" is evidently widely practiced in Mexico. The student said the practice is thought to draw out the evil spirits causing the aching ear, and the rush of air from the ear is evidence of the spirits being chased away. I observed that the only thing that would cause a rush of air such as she observed is an actual rupture of the tympanic membrane, which may be in fact the result of this extremely dangerous home remedy. (See "Ear Candling Warning.")

Table 28.2. Representative Products for Drying Water-Clogged Ears

PRODUCT	SELECTED INGREDIENTS/COMMENTS
Auro-Dri	Isopropyl alcohol 95% in anhydrous glycerin (concentration unlabeled)
Swim-Ear	Isopropyl alcohol 95% in anhydrous glycerin 5%

macy sale, including foam inserts and wax ear stoppers (Table 28.4).[78,86] Pharmacists should stock these products and explain their potential benefits for patients at risk of noise-induced hearing loss.

EAR PAIN

Pharmacists often see children (and occasionally adults) suffering from ear pain (otalgia). The usual cause of ear pain is acute otitis media, which is most common in children.[75] At least one-fourth of children will experience earache caused by acute otitis media by the age of 10, with the peak incidence between ages 3 and 6.[87] Earache is more common during the winter months, when otitis media occurs as a sequela of the common cold.[88] The pain is severe, deep, and throbbing and seems to originate from the ear, the temporomandibular joint, or the throat. Symptoms that often accompany the condition are fever, hearing loss, otorrhea, pressure in the ear, dizziness, and irritability. The response to antibiotic therapy is usually dramatic, with rapid improvement within 24 hours.[75] If the condition is left untreated, the tympanic membrane may rupture.[88] The middle ear may not completely recover, and infection can spread, producing sinusitis, labyrinthitis, mastoiditis, sepsis, or meningitis.[88] See

Table 28.3. Representative Products to Keep Water from the Ears While Swimming

PRODUCT	COMMENTS
Flent's Ear Plugs	Rubber ear inserts for water protection
Silaflex 2	Soft silicone ear plugs

"A Pharmacist's Journal: What Brand of Cigarettes is Best?" and "A Pharmacist's Journal: The Burning Torch."

Other causes of otalgia include eustachian-tube dysfunction, edema associated with upper respiratory infection, otitis externa, virally induced myringitis, TMJ disorders, and referred pain from a sore throat or abscessed teeth.[37,75,89–91] Otalgia may also indicate extracranial neoplasms such as nasopharyngeal carcinoma.[92]

During the 1970s nonprescription products containing antipyrine or benzocaine in an oily vehicle were available.[41] Patients often purchased them to treat ear pain. However, they were assigned prescription status by the end of that decade. Some people remember the products and assume that they can still be purchased.

Some customers will purchase olive oil (sweet oil) for ear pain. They may heat the oil prior to insertion. While the oil

Table 28.4. Representative Products for Protecting Hearing

PRODUCT	COMMENTS
Flent's Ear Stoples	Wax inserts
Flent's Quiet! please	Cylindrical foam inserts
Mack's Earplugs	Wax inserts
Silaflex 2	Soft silicone ear plugs

may provide some symptomatic relief by warming the area and coating the external ear canal, it cannot penetrate an intact ear drum and thus it does not affect the cause of most ear pain, even if it had any analgesic effect. Relief of otalgia (however brief) can falsely reassure patients or parents/caregivers that the infection is abating, possibly leading to hearing loss as the bacteria continue to damage the middle ear.

Although nonprescription systemic analgesics may be useful adjuncts in the care of ear pain, the danger in recommending them is that the parent may use them alone and neglect a physician visit. Thus symptoms are masked while the underlying pathologic process proceeds. Prudent pharmacists should not recommend analgesics at the initial contact, but should strongly advise patients or parent/caregivers to see a physician. Pharmacists must attempt to convince patients or parents/caregivers that antibiotic therapy will help alleviate pain and that the physician may prefer a certain analgesic.

The following chain of logic will help support referrals:

1. Nonprescription otic products containing antipyrine and benzocaine are no longer available.
2. The only otic nonprescription products are for cerumen impaction, but the likelihood of ear pain being caused by cerumen impaction is so small as to be virtually nonexistent.
3. Ear pain usually indicates a middle ear infection, for which systemic antibacterial prescription products are necessary, or external otitis, for which a prescription medication is required.
4. Since untreated ear infections can cause long-lasting problems, a physician visit is mandatory.

OBJECTS IN THE EAR

Virtually any object in the ear, whether inserted intentionally or accidentally, is potentially dangerous. Young children, particularly aged 2 to 4, are especially prone to insert objects into their ears.[37] Insects—flying species such as gnats and crawling species such as roaches—occasionally enter the ear.[93] An occupation might present unusual hazards, as in the

case of a construction worker whose ear was filled with concrete being applied with a pneumatic spray device.[94] With patients using hearing aids, the device itself is the foreign object.[37] (Note that leakage of a hearing aid battery can cause chemical trauma to the tissues.) Hair imbedded in cerumen can cause persistent nonproductive cough and should be removed by the physician.[95]

In each of these cases, attempting to remove foreign objects without professional intervention can result in additional trauma and inflammation.[37] Thus pharmacists must refer patients with suspected foreign objects in their ears to physicians, who may choose to remove the object via irrigation, suction, or with the use of a curette.[37]

DRAINAGE

Drainage from the ear may be relatively trivial (e.g., an infected scratch) or more serious (e.g., a perforated eardrum, middle ear infection, cerebrospinal fluid leakage through a fistula, or following head trauma).[37,96–101] Patients with tympanostomy tubes may experience drainage as a result of otitis media or simply from swimming without taking precautions.[102,103] Swimmer's ear also may produce drainage. Pharmacists should refer all patients with otic drainage so the source of the fluid can be determined.

TINNITUS

Tinnitus is an aberrant sensation of sound or a perception of unwanted noise in the ear or head area that originates within the individual in most cases.[104,105] This form of tinnitus may arise as a result of disorders in several locations within the auditory system, including the organ of Corti or the peripheral fibers of the spiral lumina. Otologic causes responsible for tinnitus in more than 90% of patients include presbycusis, noise-induced hearing loss, chronic otitis media, impacted cerumen, and Meniere's disease.[106]

Whereas most people think of tinnitus as ringing in the ears, the actual range of possible sounds is much more varied, including chirping sounds (such as that made by crickets), single or multiple tones, a whooshing or blowing sound, and high-pitched or low-pitched ringing, hissing, buzzing, roaring, whistling, popping, or clicking.[107,108]

Sonic (acoustic) trauma may be responsible for tinnitus, as discussed above.[109] Thus tinnitus may be regarded as one step along the spectrum to permanent hearing loss resulting from continual exposure to noise. Tinnitus sufferers should be given information about the use of ear protection to prevent an increase in symptom severity, even when using home devices such as lawn mowers, chain saws, power tools, and recreational devices such as snowmobiles.[110]

Patients reporting tinnitus should be asked about their medications. Pharmacologic causes of tinnitus are common. Alcohol is the most common cause of temporary, drug-

AT THE COUNTER

A college-aged student at the counter says that his ears feel like they need to be cleaned out.

Interview/Patient Assessment

In answer to the pharmacist's questions, the patient states that he assumes that his ears have too much wax because his ears feel full. He tried to clean them out several weeks ago with a cotton-tipped applicator, and the feeling of fullness began several days after that. He has no other otic symptoms or problems and does not take any medications.

Pharmacist's Analysis

1. What is the probable cause of this patient's ear discomfort?

2. What is the significance of his use of a cotton-tipped applicator?

3. Is a nonprescription product appropriate for this patient?

The patient's unwise use of a cotton-tipped applicator could have disrupted the normal process of ceruminokinesis, leading to the discomfort of a cerumen impaction. His cerumen cannot exit normally and is building up in the proximal ear canal.

Patient Counseling

The patient may be advised to use a carbamide peroxide product twice daily for 4 days, perhaps along with an otic syringe. If the problem persists more than 4 days, he should see a physician.

---

induced tinnitus.[105] Salicylates are the second most common.[104] Additional offenders include aminoglycosides, loop diuretics, quinine, nonsteroidal antiinflammatories, and antidepressants.[105,111,112] Recreational drugs associated with tinnitus include cocaine and marijuana; caffeine, which is often abused, also is associated with tinnitus.

Tinnitus in most cases reflects an underlying abnormality and is not a disease itself.[107] As such, further work is necessary to determine a potential etiology.[113] Thus patients with tinnitus should be referred.

PERFORATED EARDRUM

A perforated eardrum is a tympanic membrane that has an opening in it. Should the patient relate any incident that could have caused perforated eardrum, immediate referral is indicated. For instance, a woman was cleaning her ear with a cotton-tipped applicator when her young child accidentally hit her arm.[114] She experienced sudden onset of pain and mild deafness in that ear. On examination, she was found to have a perforated eardrum with resultant conductive deafness.

SUMMARY

Treatment of the ear with nonprescription products is subject to many limitations, not the least of which is the small number of conditions that can be self-treated. Because of the inability of the pharmacist to assess the ear, recommendations must be based on patients' oral recitation of symptoms. Unless pharmacists can be relatively sure that the problem is cerumen occluding the eardrum or water-clogged ears, pa-

tients should be referred for a complete evaluation and otic examination.

Patients should not self-treat cerumen impaction if under the age of 12 or if experiencing the following:

- Ear drainage
- Ear discharge
- Ear pain
- Irritation within the ear
- Rash in the ear
- Dizziness
- An injury of the ear or perforation of the tympanic membrane
- Recent ear surgery
- Tubes in the ears

Patients who ask for assistance with such problems as swimmer's ear, loss of hearing, ear pain, objects in the ear, ear drainage, tinnitus, and perforated eardrum must all be referred.

References

1. Hanger HC, Mulley GP. Cerumen: Its fascination and clinical importance: A review. J R Soc Med 85:346, 1992.

2. Sharp JF, et al. Ear wax removal: A survey of current practice. BMJ 301:1251, 1990.

3. Ballachanda BB, Peers CJ. Cerumen management. ASHA 34:43, 1992.

4. Roeser RJ, et al. Cerumen management in hearing conservation: The Dallas (Texas) independent school district program. J Sch Health 61:47, 1991.

5. Cipriani C, et al. Production rate and composition of cerumen: Influence of sex and season. Laryngoscope 100:275, 1990.

6. Macknin ML, et al. Effect of cotton-tipped swab use on earwax occlusion. Clin Pediatr 33:14, 1994.

7. Zivic RC, King S. Cerumen-impaction management for clients of all ages. Nurse Pract 18:29, 1993.
8. Okuda I, et al. The organic composition of earwax. J Otolaryngol 20:212, 1991.
9. Megarry S, et al. The activity against yeasts of human cerumen. J Laryngol Otol 102:671, 1988.
10. Lindsey D. It's time to stop washing out ears! (Letter) Am J Emerg Med 9:297, 1991.
11. Overend A, et al. Does earwax lose its pathogens on your auriscope overnight? BMJ 305:1571, 1992.
12. O'Connor PMP. Copper-bottomed earwax (Letter). Nature 344:300, 1990.
13. Sirigu P, et al. Local immune response in the skin of the external auditory meatus: An immunohistochemical study. Microsc Res Tech 38:329, 1997.
14. Robinson AC, et al. The mechanism of ceruminolysis. J Otolaryngol 18:268, 1989.
15. Dummer DS, et al. A single-blind, randomized study to compare the efficacy of two ear drop preparations ('Audax' and 'Cerumol') in the softening of ear wax. Curr Med Res Opin 13:26, 1992.
16. Robinson AC, et al. Impacted cerumen: A disorder of keratinocyte separation in the superficial external ear canal? J Otolaryngol 19:86, 1990.
17. Webber-Jones J. Doomed to Deafness? Am J Nurs 92:37, 1992.
18. Driscoll PV, et al. Characteristics of cerumen in diabetic patients: A key to understanding malignant external otitis? Otolaryngol Head Neck Surg 109:676, 1993.
19. Osborne JE, Baty JD. Do patients with otitis externa produce biochemically different cerumen? Clin Otolaryngol 15:59, 1990.
20. Rodgers RW. Less problems for ears! (Letter) Am J Emerg Med 10:97, 1992.
21. Lyndon S, et al. A comparison of the efficacy of two ear drop preparations ('Audax' and 'Earex') in the softening and removal of impacted ear wax. Curr Med Res Opin 13:21, 1992.
22. Kwok P, Hawke M. Oh where oh where does the ear wax go? And how does it get there? (Letter) J Otolaryngol 22:138, 1993.
23. Kelly KE, Mohs DC. The external auditory canal. Anatomy and physiology. Otolaryngol Clin North Am 29:725, 1996.
24. Swart SM, et al. A survey of ear and hearing disorders amongst a representative sample of grade 1 school children in Swaziland. Int J Pediatr Otorhinolaryngol 32:23, 1995.
25. Crandell CC, Roeser RJ. Incidence of excessive/impacted cerumen in individuals with mental retardation: A longitudinal investigation. Am J Mental Retard 97:568, 1993.
26. Roeser RJ, Crandell C. The audiologist's responsibility in cerumen management. ASHA 33:51, 1991.
27. Brister F, et al. Incidence of occlusion due to impacted cerumen among mentally retarded adults. Am J Ment Defic 91:302, 1986.
28. Lewis-Cullinan C, Janken JK. Effect of cerumen removal on the hearing ability of geriatric patients. J Adv Nurs 15:594, 1990.
29. Liston SL. Ear wax and the otolaryngologist (Letter). Anesthesiology 63:566, 1985.
30. Meador JA. Cerumen impaction in the elderly. J Gerontol Nurs 21:43, 1995.
31. Schuring AG. Cerumen management (Editorial). Am J Otol 13:495, 1992.
32. Anon. External auditory canal examination and cerumen management. ASHA 33:65, 1991.
33. Andaz C, Whittet HB. A in vitro study to determine efficacy of different wax-dispersing agents. ORL J Otorhinolaryngol Relat Spec 55:97, 1993.
34. Raman R. Impacted ear wax—A cause for unexplained cough? (Letter) Arch Otolaryngol Head Neck Surg 112:679, 1986.
35. Evenhius HM. Medical aspects of ageing in a population with intellectual disability: II. Hearing impairment. J Intellect Disabil Res 39(Pt 1):27, 1995.
36. Hatcher J, et al. A prevalence study of ear problems in school children in Kiambu district, Kenya, May 1992. Int J Pediatr Otorhinolaryngol 33:197, 1995.
37. Amundson LH. Disorders of the external ear. Prim Care 17:213, 1990.
38. Flugrath J, et al. Hearing impairment and cerumen impaction in older patients. J Tenn Med Assoc 86:301, 1993.
39. Hasel KL, Erickson RS. Effect of cerumen on infrared ear temperature measurement. J Gerontol Nurs 21:6, 1995.
40. Doezema D, Lunt M, Tandberg D. Cerumen occlusion lowers infrared tympanic membrane temperature measurement. Acad Emerg Med 2:17, 1995.
41. Fed Reg 42:63555, 1977.
42. Fed Reg 47:30011, 1982.
43. Fed Reg 51:28655, 1986.
44. Sorensen VZ, Bonding P. Can ear irrigation cause rupture of the normal tympanic membrane? An experimental study in man. J Laryngol Otol 109:1036, 1995.
45. Thurgood K, Thurgood G. Ear syringing: A clinical skill. Br J Nurs 4:682, 1995.
46. Hall D. Otalgia in general practice. J R Coll Gen Pract 37:562, 1987.
47. Drysdale AJ. Ear wax removal (Letter). BMJ 302:182, 1991.
48. Dinsdale RC, et al. Catastrophic otologic injury from oral jet irrigation of the external auditory canal. Laryngoscope 101(1 Pt 1):75, 1991.
49. Ford GR, et al. Another hazard of ear syringing: Malignant external otitis. J Laryngol Otol 104:709, 1990.
50. Mahoney DF. One simple solution to hearing impairment. Geriatric Nurs 8:242, 1987.
51. Brunk K. (Untitled Letter). Am J Nurs 93:14, 1993.
52. Gregg JB. Ruminations upon cerumen: Dry vs. wet; Indian vs whites. S D J Med 38:23, 1985(5).
53. Sim DW. Wax plugs and cotton buds. J Laryngol Otol 102:575, 1988.
54. Weiss JC, Yates GR, Quinn LD. Acute otitis media: Making an accurate diagnosis. Am Fam Physician 53:1200, 1996.
55. Seely DR, Langman AW. Ear candles (Letter). Arch Otolaryngol Head Neck Surg 121:1068, 1995.
56. Seely DR, Langman AW. Coning candles—An alert for otolaryngologists. Ear Nose Throat J 76:47, 1997.
57. Blakely BW. Coning candles—An alert for otolaryngologists? Ear Nose Throat J 75:585, 1996.
58. Seely DR, Quigley SM, Langman AW. Ear candles—Efficacy and safety. Laryngoscope 106:1226, 1996.
59. Fed Reg 51:27365, 1986.
60. Fed Reg 60:42435, 1995.
61. Bojrab DI, Bruderly T, Abdulrazzak Y. Otitis externa. Otolaryngol Clin North Am 29:761, 1996.
62. Fed Reg 60:8915, 1995.
63. Nadol JB Jr. Hearing Loss. N Engl J Med 329:1092, 1993.

64. Todd NW. At-risk populations for hearing impairment in infants and young children. Int J Pediatr Otorhinolaryngol 29:11, 1994.

65. Smeltzer CD. Primary care screening and evaluation of hearing loss. Nurse Pract 18:50, 1993.

66. Drulovic B, et al. Sudden hearing loss as the initial monosymptom of multiple sclerosis. Neurology 43:2703, 1993.

67. Wallach PM, et al. Erythromycin associated hearing loss in a patient with prior cis-platinum induced ototoxicity. J Fla Med Assoc 79:821, 1992.

68. Scott PMJ, Griffiths MV. A clinical review of ototoxicity. Clin Otolaryngol 19:3, 1994.

69. Rybak LP. Ototoxicity of loop diuretics. Otolaryngol Clin North Am 26:829, 1993.

70. Paintaud G, et al. The concentration-effect relationship of quinine-induced hearing impairment. Clin Pharmacol Ther 55:317, 1994.

71. Jung TTK, et al. Ototoxicity of salicylate, nonsteroidal anti-inflammatory drugs, and quinine. Otolaryngol Clin North Am 26:791, 1993.

72. Karlsson KK, et al. The effect of quinine on psychoacoustic tuning curves, stapedius reflexes and evoked otoacoustic emissions in healthy volunteers. Scand Audiol 20:83, 1991.

73. Brummett RE. Ototoxicity of vancomycin and analogues. Otolaryngol Clin North Am 26:821, 1993.

74. Andrews JC. Hearing loss in the elderly: Causes, impact and treatment. Compr Ther 17:3, 1991.

75. Browning GG. Childhood otalgia: Acute otitis media. BMJ 300:1005, 1990.

76. Clark WW. Hearing: The effects of noise. Otolaryngol Head Neck Surg 106:669, 1992.

77. Chen T-J, Chen S-S. Effects of aircraft noise on hearing and auditory pathway function of school-age children. Int Arch Occup Environ Hlth 65:107, 1993.

78. Bahadori RS, Bohne BA. Adverse effects of noise on hearing. Am Fam Physician 47:1219, 1993.

79. Attias J, et al. Oral magnesium intake reduces permanent hearing loss induced by noise exposure. Am J Otolaryngol 15:26, 1994.

80. Flottorp G. Treatment of noise induced hearing loss. Scand Audiol Suppl 34:123, 1991.

81. Ries PW. Prevalence and characteristics of persons with hearing trouble. Vital Health Stat 188:1, 1994.

82. Smoorenburg GF. Risk of noise-induced hearing loss following exposure to Chinese firecrackers. Audiology 32:333, 1993.

83. Turunen-Rise I, et al. A study of the possibility of acquiring (sic) noise-induced hearing loss by the use of personal cassette players (Walkman). Scand Audiol Suppl 34:133, 1991.

84. Turunen-Rise I, et al. Personal cassette players ('Walkman'). Do they cause noise-induced hearing loss? Scand Audiol 20:239, 1991.

85. Tsumura TK, Dicus G. Degree of hearing loss due to personal stereo use (Letter). J Sch Health 62:119, 1992.

86. McBride D, et al. Noise and the classical musician. BMJ 305:1561, 1992.

87. Bain J. Justification for antibiotic use in general practice. BMJ 300:1006, 1990.

88. Kemp ED. Otitis media. Prim Care 17:267, 1990.

89. Kreisberg MK, Turner J. Dental causes of referred otalgia. Ear Nose Throat J 66:398, 1987.

90. Wazen JJ. Referred otalgia. Otolaryngol Clin North Am 22:1205, 1989.

91. Rareshide EH, Amedee RG. Referred Otalgia. J La St Med Soc 142:7, 1990(6).

92. Thaller SR, De Silva A. Otalgia with a normal ear. Am Fam Physician 36:129, 1987.

93. Schiavone WA, Levine HL. Hair clippings in the external auditory canal: Ah, there's the rub. N Engl J Med 318:54, 1988.

94. Cuomo MD, Sobel RM. Concrete impaction of the external auditory canal. Am J Emerg Med 7:32, 1989.

95. Papay FA, et al. Facial fuzz and funny findings. Cleve Clin J Med 56:273, 1989.

96. Valtonen H, et al. Early post-tympanostomy otorrhea in children under 17 months of age. Acta Otolaryngol 117:569, 1997.

97. Mra Z, MacCormick JA, Poje CP. Persistent cerebrospinal fluid otorrhea: A case of Munchausen's syndrome by proxy. Int J Pediatr Otorhinolaryngol 41:59, 1997.

98. Shetty PG, et al. Cerebrospinal fluid otorhinorrhea in patients with defects through the lamina cribosa of the internal auditory canal. AJNR Am J Neuroradiol 18:478, 1997.

99. Choi D, Spann R. Traumatic cerebrospinal fluid leakage: Risk factors and the use of prophylactic antibiotics. Br J Neurosurg 10:571, 1996.

100. Arienta C, Caroli M, Balbi S. Management of head-injured patients in the emergency department: A practical protocol. Surg Neurol 48:213, 1997.

101. Ostrowski VB, Wiet RJ. Pathologic conditions of the external ear and auditory canal. Postgrad Med 100:223, 1996.

102. Salata JA, Derkay CS. Water precautions in children with tympanostomy tubes. Arch Otolaryngol Head Neck Surg 122:276, 1996.

103. Goldstein NA, Roland JT Jr, Sculerati N. Complications of tympanostomy tubes in an inner city clinic population. Int J Pediatr Otorhinolaryngol 34:87, 1996.

104. Williamson A, Amedee RG. Tinnitus. J La State Med Soc 142:9, 1990(4).

105. Alleva M, et al. Tinnitus. Prim Care 17:289, 1990.

106. Schleuning AJ. Management of the patient with tinnitus. Med Clin North Am 75:1225, 1991.

107. Marion MS, Cevette MJ. Tinnitus. Mayo Clin Proc 66:614, 1991.

108. Berliner KI, et al. Acoustic tumors: Effect of surgical removal on tinnitus. Am J Otol 13:13,1992.

109. Bruins WR, Cawood RH. Blast injuries of the ear as a result of the Peterborough lorry explosion: 22 March 1989. J Laryngol Otol 105:890, 1991.

110. Stouffer JL, et al. Tinnitus as a function of duration and etiology: Counselling implications. Am J Otol 12:188, 1991.

111. Laird LK, Lydiard RB. Imipramine-related tinnitus. J Clin Psychiatry 50:146, 1989.

112. Jastreboff PJ, et al. Quinine-induced tinnitus in rats. Arch Otolaryngol Head Neck Surg 117:1172, 1991.

113. Vernon J, et al. Attributes of tinnitus associated with the temporomandibular joint syndrome. Eur Arch Otorhinolaryngol 249:93, 1992.

114. Warwick-Brown NP. Wax impaction in the ear. Practitioner 230:301, 1986.

Dermatologic Conditions

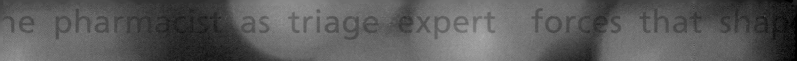

Hyperproliferative Skin Disorders

AT THE COUNTER

A male patient in his 30s asks the pharmacist for help with a coal-tar shampoo. He also wonders if there is anything that is effective that smells better than the shampoo he is interested in.

Interview/Patient Assessment

The pharmacist notices skin scaling on the patient's face, especially in the eyebrows and around the nose. His physician told him he has "a condition like dandruff but not psoriasis." He takes Prevacid for "stomach problems" and a nonprescription herbal product for weight loss. He has no other medical conditions and takes no other medications.

Pharmacist's Analysis

1. What might his skin condition be?

2. Is coal-tar shampoo appropriate for his skin condition or would another product be preferable?
3. Should he see a physician for his problem?

This patient's condition appears to be seborrheic dermatitis.

Patient Counseling

Patients should not use nonprescription products for seborrheic dermatitis that covers large areas of the body, but this patient has a relatively small area of affected skin, so any approved product could be recommended. Coal-tar shampoo would be helpful, but because of several problems with its use (e.g., dermatitis, folliculitis, unpleasant odor, bleaching of skin), other ingredients might be more appropriate, including zinc pyrithione, selenium sulfide, and salicylic acid.

This chapter addresses several related disorders: dandruff, seborrheic dermatitis, psoriasis, and cradle cap. Although they can affect different parts of the body, all of these conditions may result from an abnormality in skin proliferation known as hyperproliferation. These conditions are self-treatable with a diverse group of nonprescription ingredients, with varying degrees of success. Figure 29.1 indicates the common locations and symptoms of the four hyperproliferative disorders addressed in this chapter.

The human skin—which shields lower tissues from contaminants in the outside environment and protects the body from loss of fluids and electrolytes—comprises approximately 10% of the body weight of the average adult.[1] The outermost layer of skin is the epidermis (Fig. 29.2). Beneath the epidermis lies the dermis and then the subcutaneous layer, which includes fat deposits of differing depths (depending on the area of the body). The disorders discussed in this chapter affect the epidermis.

To understand these hyperproliferative conditions, it is necessary to be familiar with the normal process of epidermal cell formation. The epidermis is made up of several layers. The inner layer, next to the dermis, is known as the stratum germinativum or basal layer of the epidermis. This layer is made up of columnar basal cells that reproduce by mitotic division to form daughter cells. The daughter cells continuously migrate upward and outward, passing through subsequent layers of the epidermis until they eventually reach the skin surface.

As cells formed in the stratum germinativum move upward, they enter the next layer of epidermis, known as the stratum spinosum or prickle-cell layer. As the upward cellular migration continues, the cells gradually flatten and develop inner granules of keratohyalin. They then become the next skin layer, known as the stratum granulosum or granular

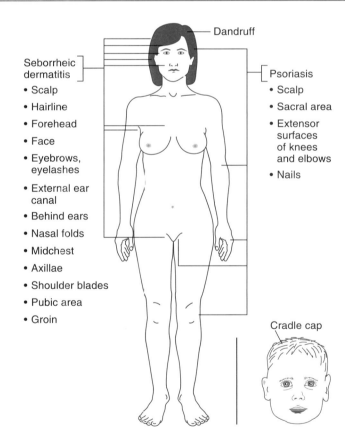

Figure 29.1. Typical sites affected by dandruff, seborrheic dermatitis, psoriasis, and cradle cap.

layer. The cells also begin to die; as they die the keratohyalin granules convert to a chemical known as keratin. The cells then lose their nuclei and enter the outermost layer of epidermis, known as the stratum corneum or horny layer. The

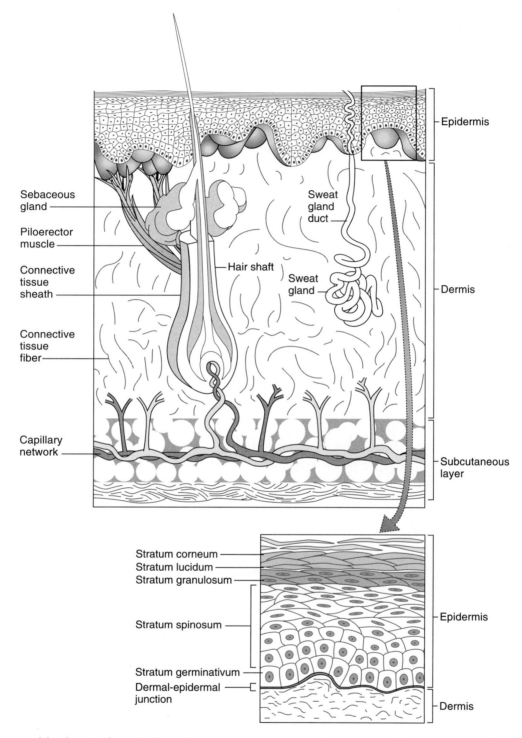

Figure 29.2. Structures of the skin. Epidermal cells undergo a continuous process of renewal, as cells migrate upward from the stratum germinativum to the stratum corneum.

dead cells of the stratum corneum are shed into the environment continually, to be replaced by cells migrating upward.

Normally, 25 to 30 days elapse during cell migration from the stratum germinativum, the inner layer of the epidermis, to the stratum corneum, the outermost horny layer. As cells are shed, they normally are not noticeable. With such conditions as dandruff, seborrheic dermatitis, and psoriasis, however, cellular turnover has accelerated abnormally, producing noticeable shedding. If the hyperproliferative condition is severe (e.g., psoriasis), the accumulated cells typically form plaques that are potentially disfiguring. Cradle cap may also be a result of accelerated cell turnover, although this is debated.

DANDRUFF

Dandruff is a hyperproliferative skin condition resulting from a skin cell turnover rate of approximately double the normal rate.[1] Rather than taking 25 to 30 days to migrate from the stratum germinativum to the outermost horny layer, with dandruff skin cells reach the outermost layer in about 13 to 15 days. Where the scalp of an individual with a normal cell turnover rate has a closely packed keratinized stratum corneum with orderly arrayed cells, the scalp of an individual with dandruff has a disorderly arrangement of cells that build up on the scalp and then flake off (Fig. 29.3). Because of the high turnover rate, dandruff results in fewer cells than normal, some that retain their nuclei.[1] Dandruff is not serious, but it can itch and be unsightly.

See Patient Assessment Algorithm 29.1 for general assessment guidelines for hyperproliferative skin disorders.

Prevalence data for dandruff are sparse, but as many as 50% of Caucasians may experience it at some time in their lives.[2,3] Dandruff is not common until the onset of puberty.[1] In affected individuals, cell turnover increases to peak in the early 20s.[2] Cell turnover decreases thereafter, so that dandruff is rare in the middle-aged and elderly patients. Dandruff does not exhibit any preference for gender. As many as 50% of whites may suffer from dandruff at some time, and a significant portion of other racial groups also experience the condition.[2–4]

ETIOLOGY OF DANDRUFF

The exact reason for the accelerated cell turnover that causes dandruff (and other hyperproliferative skin disorders) is unknown; etiologies such as diet, hormones, and vitamin deficiencies have been explored with little result.[1] There does not appear to be an association between oiliness of the scalp and dandruff.[2]

Increasingly, research on the etiology of dandruff has focused on the role of a fungus normally found on the human scalp and skin (*Pityrosporum ovale*, variously referred to as *Malessezia ovalis, Malessezia furfur, Pityrosporum orbiculare*).[5–12] This organism exerts a lipase activity, which allows it to reduce sebum triglycerides into free fatty acids, which in turn induces scaling.[13] A study revealed that while this organism made up 74% of the scalp flora of patients with dandruff, it constituted only 46% of the flora in healthy individuals.[14] This theoretical etiology may also explain the otherwise puzzling worsening of dandruff in the winter, since fungal organisms may thrive in the warmth and moisture produced on the scalp by sweating while wearing caps and hats.

Several trigger factors have been proposed to explain why *Pityrosporum ovale* transforms from a "ubiquitous **commensal** (an organism that lives in a symbiotic relationship with another without harming it) into a noninvasive pathogenic organism," including a genetic predisposition, emotional stress, changes in the quantity or quality of sebum (an increase in wax esters and short-chain fatty acids), increased alkalinity of the skin, and occlusion of the skin in the scalp.[13,15]

MANIFESTATIONS OF DANDRUFF

The major manifestations of dandruff are scaling and occasional pruritus. The rapidity of cell turnover in dandruff prevents complete keratinization of **desquamated** (shed) cells, which causes dry, white or gray flakes to accumulate on the scalp in small, round patches.[1] Dandruff flakes brush away painlessly as patients scratch them or as they are disturbed by hair brushing, putting on clothes, etc.[2] Some flakes may also cling to hair until it is washed. The crown of the head is the most common location for dandruff, although the entire scalp may be affected. Bare scalp areas, such as those caused by male pattern baldness, are not affected by dandruff.[3]

The borders of dandruff scaling are indistinct, as it is a diffuse condition. Also, although the patients may complain of pruritus in more severe cases, inflammation is not associated with dandruff.[2] Dandruff is more severe from October through December and milder in the summer—a seasonal occurrence that aids in recognition.[1]

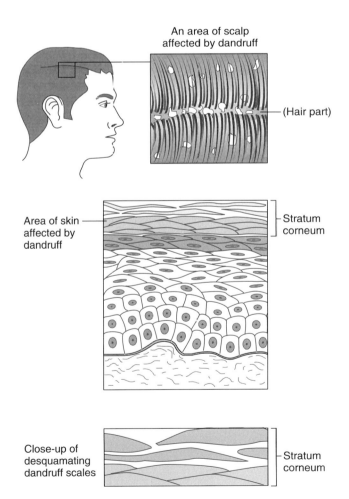

Figure 29.3. Areas of the scalp affected by dandruff exhibit visible flakes of desquamated stratum corneum.

Patient Assessment Algorithm 29.1. Hyperproliferative Disorders

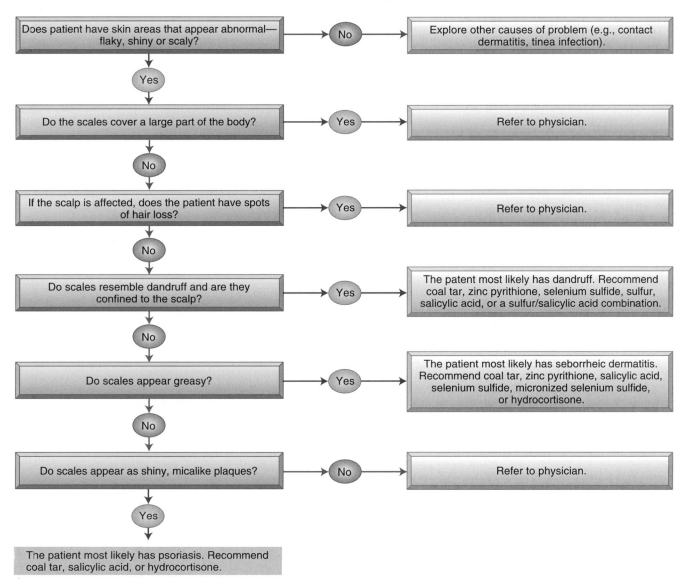

Tinea of the scalp (a superficial fungal infection requiring prescription medications) can mimic dandruff.[2] Persistent dandruff unresponsive to nonprescription products should be referred to a dermatologist for evaluation.

PROGNOSIS OF DANDRUFF

Dandruff is not a serious condition, but left untreated it can be unsightly and embarrassing. The symptoms of mild dandruff can usually be controlled by shampooing daily with a mild, hypoallergenic shampoo and scrubbing the scalp thoroughly. For more severe cases of dandruff, patients can self-treat the condition with several medications that suppress cell turnover. Depending on a patient's age, cell turnover tends to return to an abnormal rate once treatment is stopped, and dandruff scaling will begin again.

TREATMENT OF DANDRUFF

Treatment Guidelines

Patients may choose several dosage forms containing ingredients effective for dandruff. Lotions, creams, or ointments are more difficult to apply and to remove following application. They may need to remain on the head for a certain period, which is uncomfortable. For this reason most patients prefer a shampoo, which can be applied during normal bathing and is removed during the bath/shower. Dandruff responds well to shampooing with certain nonprescription products, but patients must be reminded not to rinse the shampoo for several minutes to maximize epidermal absorption.[2]

The FDA in its final rule in 1991 approved a number of safe and effective ingredients that can help control the itching, flaking, irritation, redness, and scaling associated with *(tip)* dandruff.[16] *Dandruff shampoos are for external use only, and contact with the eyes must be avoided. Should the condition worsen or fail to improve after regular use of the product, the patient should consult a physician.* Dandruff shampoos direct patients to use them at least twice a week or as directed by a physician.[16]

(tip) *Dandruff products not formulated as shampoos (e.g., creams, ointments, lotions, hair grooming aids) are applied to the affected area(s) one to four times daily (or as directed) and left on the skin.*

See "Unapproved Products Marketed for Hyperproliferative Conditions."

Nonprescription Medications

COAL TAR

Crude coal tar (a product of the destructive distillation of bituminous coal) contains at least 10,000 different compounds.[1] Coal tar is refined to produce coal-tar extract, solution, and distillate, all of which retain its various therapeutic properties (e.g., effectiveness against dandruff, seborrheic dermatitis, and psoriasis), although the magnitude of therapeutic effects differ. For hyperproliferative conditions, refined coal tar can reduce the number and size of epidermal cells produced by the body.[1] The FDA allows concentrations of 0.5 to 5% or the equivalent in products containing coal tar (Table 29.1).

(tip) *The labels on shampoos containing coal tar must caution patients not to use coal-tar preparations for long periods without consulting a physician.[16] Unfortunately, the FDA did not further define the phrase "long periods."* Coal-tar preparations can cause **folliculitis** (infectious inflammation of the hair follicles) and allergic or contact dermatitis. They also have an odor often considered to be unpleasant and can stain skin and hair (especially if the hair is blonde, bleached, or gray). Because coal tar can cause photosensitivity reactions, patients should be cautioned against sun expo-

(tip) sure.[1] *The labels on shampoos containing coal tars will state, "Use caution in exposing skin to sunlight after applying this product. It may increase your tendency to sunburn for up to 24 hours after application." In addition, the labels on coal-tar products that are applied and left on the skin (e.g., creams, ointments, and lotions) must carry this warning, "Do not use this product in or around the rectum or in the genital area or groin except on the advice of a doctor."* (This caution is required because of a possible link between coal tar and anogenital cancer.[1])

Table 29.1. Representative Products Containing Coal Tar

PRODUCT	SELECTED INGREDIENTS/COMMENTS
Balnetar Bath	Coal tar 2.5%
Denorex Medicated Shampoo and Conditioner	Coal tar solution 9% (equivalent to 1.8% coal tar)
Denorex Extra Strength Medicated Shampoo and Conditioner	Coal tar solution 12.5% (equivalent to 2.5% coal tar)
DHS Tar Shampoo	Solubilized coal tar extract 2.9% (equivalent to 0.5% coal tar)
Ionil•T Shampoo	Coal tar topical solution 5% (equivalent to 1% coal tar)
Ionil•T Plus	Coal tar distillate 1% (equivalent to 1% coal tar)
MG 217 Intensive Strength Ointment	Coal tar solution 10% (equivalent to 2% coal tar)
Oxipor VHC Lotion	Coal tar solution 25% (equivalent to 5% coal tar)
Pentrax Anti-Dandruff Tar Shampoo	Coal tar extract 7.71% (equivalent to 4.3% coal tar)
Polytar Soap	Solubilized crude coal tar and coal tar solution 2.5% (equivalent to 0.5% coal tar)
Tegrin Dandruff Shampoo	Coal tar solution 7% (equivalent to 1.1% coal tar)
Tegrin Cream	Coal tar solution 5% (equivalent to 0.8% coal tar)
T/Gel Therapeutic Conditioner	Solubilized coal tar extract 2% (equivalent to 0.5% coal tar)
T/Gel Therapeutic Shampoo	Solubilized coal tar extract 2% (equivalent to 0.5% coal tar)
X Seb T Plus Shampoo	Coal tar solution 10% (equivalent to 2% coal tar)
Zetar Shampoo	Whole coal tar 1%

ZINC PYRITHIONE

Zinc pyrithione can be effective in treating dandruff because of its antifungal effect and/or by reducing cell turnover.[1,2] Concentrations of 0.3 to 2% are allowed for shampoos that are washed away after a brief exposure; concentrations of 0.1 to 0.25% may be applied and left on the skin or scalp (Table 29.2). Because most people are more familiar with shampooing, these products are preferable.

SELENIUM SULFIDE

Selenium sulfide 1% is thought to exert a **cytostatic effect** (reducing the rate of turnover of cells) (Table 29.3).[1] Selenium sulfide may also inhibit the growth of *Pityrosporum ovale*.[13] A formulation of micronized selenium sulfide 0.6% is also effective, in which the particle size is reduced through a process of fine grinding to an average size of 5 micrometers.[17,18]

SALICYLIC ACID

Salicylic acid is effective in hyperproliferative disorders because of its ability to lower the pH of tissues (Table 29.4). The lower pH results in an increase in water concentration in epidermal cells, which in turn softens and destroys the stratum corneum.[1] The net effect is to cause the upper skin layer to become inflamed and soft, followed by desquamation. This keratolytic action removes the scales of dandruff when the product concentration is 1.8 to 3%.

SULFUR

Sulfur can be effective in controlling dandruff, possibly by exerting a fungicidal effect. Sulfur is Category I in concentrations of 2 to 5%. Rather than market it as a single-entity product, most manufacturers have opted to combine it with salicylic acid (discussed below). One product containing sulfur alone is Suave Dandruff Control Shampoo, although the concentration is unlabeled.

SULFUR AND SALICYLIC ACID IN COMBINATION

The only combination of ingredients permitted for these products is sulfur and salicylic acid. When a sulfur/salicylic acid combination is used, both ingredients must be limited to concentrations approved by the FDA for their use alone (e.g., salicylic acid, 1.8 to 3%, and sulfur, 2 to 5%). The combination is effective only for dandruff, not for other hyperproliferative conditions.[1] One product containing this combination is Meted Anti-Dandruff Shampoo, with sulfur 5% and salicylic acid 3%.

KETOCONAZOLE

Ketoconazole 1% shampoo is a prescription antifungal product that has been approved for an Rx-to-OTC switch, to be known as Nizoral AD.[19] The product controls the flaking, itching, and scaling of dandruff.[20] The committee that recommended the change suggested label warnings against use in patients younger than 12 and against continued use if the condition fails to improve or worsens in 2 to 4 weeks. In clinical studies twice-weekly application yielded good to excellent results in 80% of dandruff patients after 4 weeks.[21]

Table 29.2. Representative Products Containing Zinc Pyrithione

PRODUCT	SELECTED INGREDIENTS/COMMENTS
Head & Shoulders Dandruff Shampoo	Zinc pyrithione (concentration unlabeled)
Head & Shoulders Dry Scalp Dandruff Shampoo and Conditioner	Zinc pyrithione (concentration unlabeled)
Head & Shoulders 2 in 1 Dandruff Shampoo Plus Conditioner	Zinc pyrithione (concentration unlabeled)
Pert Plus Dandruff Control	Zinc pyrithione (concentration unlabeled)
ZNP Bar	Zinc pyrithione 2%

Table 29.3. Representative Products Containing Selenium Sulfide

PRODUCT	SELECTED INGREDIENTS/COMMENTS
Head & Shoulders Intensive Treatment	Selenium sulfide (concentration unlabeled)
Selsun Blue Shampoo Moisturizing Treatment	Selenium sulfide 1%
Selsun Blue 2-in-1 Treatment Shampoo	Selenium sulfide 1%

Table 29.4. Representative Products Containing Salicylic Acid	
PRODUCT	SELECTED INGREDIENTS/COMMENTS
Ionil Plus Shampoo	Salicylic acid 2%
Neutrogena Healthy Scalp Anti-Dandruff Shampoo	Salicylic acid 1.8%
Scalpicin Liquid	Salicylic acid 3%
Scalpicin Maximum Strength Foam	Salicylic acid 3%
T/Sal Maximum Strength Therapeutic Shampoo	Salicylic acid 3%

SEBORRHEIC DERMATITIS

Seborrheic dermatitis is a hyperproliferative skin condition resulting from a cell turnover rate of approximately three times the normal rate—higher than dandruff but less rapid than with psoriasis.[1] Rather than taking 25 to 30 days to migrate from the stratum germinativum to the outermost horny layer, with seborrheic dermatitis, skin cells reach the outermost layer in as few as 9 to 10 days. Like dandruff, the cells may retain their nuclei.[22]

While the prevalence of seborrheic dermatitis is unknown, one medical article refers to it as one of the most common disorders.[23]

Seborrheic dermatitis, which becomes more common after puberty, affects men six times more commonly than women.[1,3,23] It is worsened by stress and poor health and is more common in atopic individuals.[1,13] As many as 80% of AIDS patients experience seborrheic dermatitis, further substantiating the possible fungal etiology and perhaps facilitating an early diagnosis of HIV infection.[13,23–39]

ETIOLOGY OF SEBORRHEIC DERMATITIS

Seborrheic dermatitis has several potential etiologies. One theory of seborrheic dermatitis causation is related to the propensity of the condition to localize where sebaceous glands are found. In this theory the condition is caused by excessive sebum production, which allows yeasts and bacteria to produce free fatty acids from the sebum.[1,23] The free fatty acids, in turn, irritate the skin. Research, however, has yet to confirm that patients with seborrheic dermatitis do produce excess sebum.[2]

As in dandruff, *Pityrosporum ovale* has been implicated in the etiology of seborrheic dermatitis.[23,31–35] The severity of the seborrheic dermatitis appears to decrease when the count of organisms on the scalp decreases.[14,36] Further, in one study *Pityrosporum ovale* made up 46% of the scalp flora in unaffected persons, and 82% of the scalp flora in those with seborrheic dermatitis.[14]

MANIFESTATIONS OF SEBORRHEIC DERMATITIS

Seborrheic dermatitis produces pruritus, flaking, and redness of the affected skin.[37] Seborrheic dermatitis scales are yellowish and greasy in appearance, unlike the dry scale of dandruff.[1,2] Borders are indistinct, characterized by underlying skin inflammation, as implied by the name.

While dandruff is confined to the scalp, seborrheic dermatitis affects other areas of the body in addition to the scalp. The highest-risk locations either have high concentrations of sebaceous glands or high likelihood of colonization by yeasts and bacteria such as areas covered by hair or in skin folds (intertriginous skin).[1] Common sites for seborrheic dermatitis include the hairline, forehead, face, eyebrows, eyelashes, eyelids, the external ear canal, behind the ears, in the nasal folds, and occasionally nonfacial areas such as the scalp, midchest, axillae, between the shoulder blades, and in the pubic area and groin (Fig. 29.4).[1,3,31,38,39]

PROGNOSIS OF SEBORRHEIC DERMATITIS

Seborrheic dermatitis does not yield to any treatment. It persists for the life of the individual, although—unlike dandruff—its course is characterized by frequent exacerbations and remissions.[1]

TREATMENT OF SEBORRHEIC DERMATITIS

Treatment Guidelines

Seborrheic dermatitis is a more difficult condition to treat than dandruff and not all dandruff medications will help the

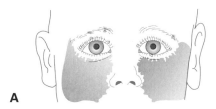

A

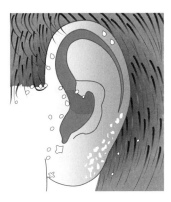

B

Figure 29.4. Seborrheic dermatitis appears as an inflamed area of skin with greasy scaling.

condition. Approved ingredients include coal tar 0.5 to 5% or its equivalent; zinc pyrithione 0.95 to 2% (when washed off after a brief exposure) or 0.1 to 0.25% (when applied and left on the scalp); selenium sulfide 1%; micronized selenium sulfide 0.6%; and salicylic acid 1.8 to 3%. [16] Ingredient labeling for seborrheic dermatitis duplicates the labeling for dandruff with two exceptions: *Products for seborrheic dermatitis must include the warning, "If condition covers a large area of the body, consult your physician before using this product." Also, soaps formulated for seborrheic dermatitis must direct the patient to "Use on affected areas in place of your regular soap."*

See "Unapproved Products Marketed for Hyperproliferative Conditions."

Nonprescription Medications

Several ingredients used for dandruff are also appropriate for seborrheic dermatitis (e.g., coal tar, zinc pyrithione, selenium sulfide, micronized selenium sulfide). See "Treatment Guidelines" under "Dandruff" above and Tables 29.1 through 29.4. In addition, hydrocortisone and antifungals have also been approved for seborrheic dermatitis.

HYDROCORTISONE

Hydrocortisone in concentrations of 0.25 to 1% is also approved for seborrheic dermatitis. The original FDA-appointed panel assigned hydrocortisone Category III status for dandruff, seborrheic dermatitis, and psoriasis. However, in Phase II the FDA evaluated studies that supported the safety and efficacy of hydrocortisone 0.25 to 1% in controlling the inflammation and itching of seborrheic dermatitis and psoriasis and amended the tentative final monograph for external analgesics to add seborrheic dermatitis and psoriasis to the list of conditions for which hydrocortisone is safe and effective.[16,40,41] At the present time no leading product marketed for hyperproliferative conditions contains hydrocortisone.

The use of hydrocortisone for seborrheic dermatitis is potentially dangerous. The original panel report that discussed it in 1979 considered such adverse effects as aggravation of cutaneous bacterial, fungal, or viral infection, striae formation, atrophy of the skin, and telangiectasia.[42] However, it concluded that these adverse effects would be rare. A further point in safety of hydrocortisone is a label warning that prohibits patient self-use for more than 7 days. If the patient is still bothered by seborrheic dermatitis after that time, the patient might switch to an alternative nonprescription product or make a physician appointment.

ANTIFUNGALS

Most authorities assert that it is generally accepted that dandruff and seborrheic dermatitis are fungal in origin.[31] See "Etiology of Dandruff" and "Etiology of Seborrheic Dermatitis." For this reason topical antifungals have been used in both conditions.[43–46] Ketoconazole shampoo, for example, effective for both conditions, is available as a prescription product that has been approved for an Rx-to-OTC switch.[31,19] Many of the products traditionally used for dandruff and seborrheic dermatitis may also be beneficial because of their antifungal effects, including coal tar, zinc pyrithione, selenium sulfide, and sulfur.[5]

PSORIASIS

Psoriasis affects from 1 to 3% of the population of the world.[47,48] About 2% of United States residents have psoriasis.[1,49]

Psoriasis is a hyperproliferative skin condition resulting from a skin cell turnover rate of approximately 10 to 20 times the normal rate—higher than both dandruff and seborrheic dermatitis.[1,50] Rather than taking 25 to 30 days to migrate from the stratum germinativum to the outermost horny layer, with psoriasis skin cells reach the outermost layer in as few as 3 to 4 days.

Within the affected area the thickness of the epidermis increases, nuclei are retained in epidermal cells, and the stratum granulosum is absent. Capillaries beneath the plaque are larger than normal.

There are several subtypes of psoriasis: plaque, pustular, erythrodermic, and guttate.[51–53] This section addresses plaque psoriasis, the most common subtype and the only type of psoriasis that is amenable to self-treatment with nonprescription medications. Plaque psoriasis is also known as psoriasis vulgaris.

Psoriasis is more common in whites than blacks.[1] Studies suggest that individuals aged 16 to 22 and 57 to 60 are most likely to experience the onset of psoriasis.[47,54,55] A genetic predisposition exists for psoriasis both for identical twins (both twins are affected more often than both members of a set of fraternal twins, who do not have an identical genetic makeup) and for those individuals with first-degree relatives (who experience psoriasis in 20 to 30% of cases).[1,55,56]

ETIOLOGY OF PSORIASIS

The development of psoriasis is probably a result of exposure of the skin or the patient to trauma or other triggering factors.[57,58] However, the genetic predisposition to psoriasis must be present before the condition will develop.[59]

The Koebner Phenomenon

The spread of a skin condition into a new area following exposure to an external trigger is known as the Koebner phenomenon.[47,60] Psoriasis plaques often exhibit this phenomenon, appearing at sites of skin trauma such as burns, cuts, sunburn, or contact dermatitis. Lesions usually appear after a latent period of 3 to 18 days (generally 10 to 14 days) after exposure to trauma, with capillary changes either preceding or following appearance of the plaque.

Triggers for Development of Psoriasis

Other than skin trauma, provoking factors for psoriasis include streptococcal infections, medications (e.g., lithium, antimalarials, propranolol and other beta-blockers, NSAIDs, terbinafine, and steroid withdrawal), and emotional stress.[61–63] Stressful incidents reported to cause or exacerbate psoriasis include situations producing anxiety and depression (e.g., marital and financial difficulties, "near-death" experiences).[64,65] Psoriasis may clear completely or improve markedly during pregnancy and then relapse in the postpartum period. Psoriasis improves in hot weather in the majority of patients, and cold weather increases its severity.

MANIFESTATIONS OF PSORIASIS

Plaque psoriasis produces scales (known as plaques) that are silvery on top and pink to dull red beneath.[1] The plaques may be found at any location on the body, although they are more common on the scalp, sacral area, and the extensor surfaces of the knees and elbows (and less common on the face—the opposite of seborrheic dermatitis) (Fig. 29.5).[51] The borders of the plaque are sharp with inflammation surrounding the plaque.[66,67] The plaque tends to flake off in layers, similar to the mineral mica. Each plaque is a dermal immune response to some antigenic stimulus mediated by T-lymphocytes.[47,66,68]

Because the appearances of seborrheic dermatitis and psoriasis are often similar, the fingernails may provide a help-

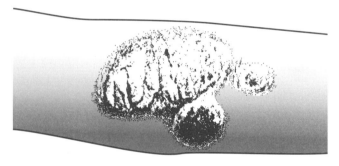

Psoriasis plaque on the elbow and surrounding skin

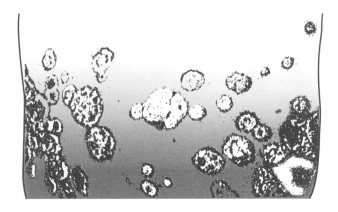

Trunk affected with psoriasis

Figure 29.5. The psoriatic lesion is a shiny, sharply demarcated plaque.

ful clue to the condition.[69] Psoriatic fingernails and toenails undergo hyperproliferation, producing a disordered nail plate. Nails appear distorted and thick with a crumbling surface, embedded with pits and ridges. In some cases the nail will completely separate from the nail bed. The appearance of the affected nail mimics the fungal infection of the nails known as onychomycosis.

PROGNOSIS OF PSORIASIS

Psoriasis is a chronic condition that does not yield to any treatment.[1] Any particular lesion may be intermittent or persist indefinitely, or the entire condition may appear to disappear at times without scarring, only to recur later.[47] Psoriasis severity is determined by the size of the area involved, redness of skin, thickness of the lesion, and extent of scaling.

COMPLICATIONS OF PSORIASIS

Most patients affected with psoriasis have only a mild form of the disease, and it is seldom noticed by friends or coworkers; some patients, however, have psoriasis so severe that it inhibits their social or work life.[70,71] Fortunately, most psoriasis patients have no complications from the condition (e.g., psoriatic arthritis), regardless of the severity. A major cause of morbidity is psoriatic arthritis, which about 7% of patients develop.[49]

TREATMENT OF PSORIASIS

Treatment Guidelines

Skin affected by psoriasis is more permeable to topical medications than normal skin, which facilitates treatment. For this reason markedly abnormal skin often exhibits a rapid improvement, although improvement slows as the skin returns to its normal permeability.

Psoriasis is often greatly improved by simply soaking the affected area in water.[49] *A warm-water bath for about 20 minutes hydrates the upper stratum corneum, especially when a hypoallergenic emollient is also used directly following the bath.*

As psoriasis is the most severe, self-treatable, hyperproliferative condition, only a few ingredients adequately provide relief. These include coal tar 0.5 to 5% (or its equivalent) and salicylic acid 1.8 to 3%; either may be included in shampoos, preshampoo rinses, postshampoo rinses, creams, ointments, lotions, or hairgrooms.[16,72] However, ingredient labeling is the same for psoriasis as it is for dandruff, including the special warnings for seborrheic dermatitis mentioned in that section. Also, hydrocortisone 0.25 to 1% was given FDA approval for psoriasis through the rather convoluted route described under "Hydrocortisone" in the section on seborrheic dermatitis. Should nonprescription products fail to provide relief, pharmacists should refer patients to a dermatologist or physician. Prescription modalities include oral and topical medications, as well as the use of ultraviolet light.[73–78] See

"Unapproved Products Marketed for Hyperproliferative Conditions."

Nonprescription Medications

A number of nonprescription products used for dandruff and seborrheic dermatitis are also appropriate for psoriasis. (See Tables 29.1 and 29.4.)

CRADLE CAP

Cradle cap (infantile seborrheic dermatitis) is included in this chapter because its etiology is thought by some to be partially related to epidermal hyperproliferation.[82] Although cradle cap can occur at any time during infancy, it is most common during the first several weeks of life.[83]

ETIOLOGY OF CRADLE CAP

The child with cradle cap may be well bathed in all areas but the top of the head. Cradle cap is thought to be due to the new parents' fear of thoroughly washing the area over the foramen ovale (popularly known as the "soft spot") where the fontanelles have not yet grown together and fused.[84] If not washed, the skin accumulates skin scales in addition to unremoved vernix caseosa (a fatty material that covered the fetus at birth). Cradle cap may also be found on other poorly washed pediatric locations such as behind the ears, the na-

solabial fold, neck, axillae, umbilicus, and diaper area.[7] While siblings are commonly affected, this tendency is thought to reflect the parents' or caregiver's washing habits rather than any genetic predisposition.[82,85]

Cradle cap may be a pediatric form of seborrheic dermatitis, but simple lack of cleanliness is probably the major cause, since accelerated cell turnover has not yet been demonstrated via research. Further, the condition does not seem to be fungal in etiology.[86]

FOCUS ON...

UNAPPROVED PRODUCTS MARKETED FOR HYPERPROLIFERATIVE CONDITIONS

Several products marketed for hyperproliferative conditions lack FDA approval for safety and efficacy. In some cases the individual ingredients of a combination are approved, but the safety of the combination is unknown. Pharmacists should not recommend these products.

Home remedies and herbal medicines may also be dangerous. One patient used fenugreek paste on the scalp for dandruff, experiencing allergic reactions such as numbness of the head, facial angioedema, and wheezing.[79] In another case a patient given a Chinese medication known as Kamisyoyo-san for seborrheic dermatitis developed adult respiratory distress syndrome, highlighting the dangers of imported ethnic medications that have not been subjected to FDA scrutiny.[80] Other Chinese herbal medicines have induced liver damage when used for skin conditions.[81]

When one enters "psoriasis treatment" as a search term on the Internet, a number of bizarre, unproven, and possibly dangerous psoriasis treatments are promoted:

- An expensive travel package to Turkey that takes the patient to spa pools inhabited by three species of carp: The strikers eat the psoriasis scales, the jabbers puncture the skin, and the lickers seal the holes. (This incredible tale is known as "The Little Fish of Kangal.")
- A homeopathic mixture of nickel and bromide promoted by a dermatologist
- A health center that promises to treat psoriasis by enlivening the inner intelligence of the body
- A company selling Dead Sea salts and mud, banana peels, and flax seed

---

A Pharmacist's Journal

"Where's the Heads & Shoulders?"

A man approached to ask me the location of Head and Shoulders. I asked if it was for simple dandruff. He said it was for his son's cradle cap. I asked how serious the baby's cradle cap was. He said, "He's not a baby. He's in the second grade." I explained that cradle cap is an infant condition and asked what made him think it was cradle cap. He replied, "I haven't looked at his head for several weeks. Today I noticed him scratching. I looked at his head and noticed a hard crust that

is caught in his hair and covers most of the crown of his head." I explained that it sounded like cradle cap, but the child was older than the age range for the condition. The father then volunteered this information: "Well, we had been washing his hair for him up until about a month ago. Then we wanted him to start washing his own hair. I guess he hasn't been doing too good a job, so he's got all of this dirt there. I broke some off, but it was kind or raw underneath." I suggested that the child see a physician since an antibiotic might be necessary.

See "A Pharmacist's Journal: Where's the Head & Shoulders?"

MANIFESTATIONS OF CRADLE CAP

Cradle cap is most commonly located on the scalp, as implied by the name (Fig. 29.6). Scales appear greasy and yellowish brown with indistinct borders. There is an associated inflammation, and the skin is red.[82]

In severe cases the skin scales can be so thickened that a caplike crust forms. This "cap" requires medical intervention for removal.[23]

PROGNOSIS OF CRADLE CAP

Cradle cap usually resolves within a month of birth and does not recur.[82] However, if the accumulated scale develops sufficient thickness, the area beneath is marked by atopic dermatitis with pruritus, papulovesicles, and exudation.[38] The condition may then spread to the cheeks, forehead, and extensor surfaces of the extremities.

TREATMENT OF CRADLE CAP

At this time the FDA does not recognize any ingredient as safe and effective for either the prevention or treatment of cradle cap. However, two pediatric dermatologists suggest the use of a mild, nonmedicated shampoo, followed by the use of coaltar or ketoconazole shampoos for nonresponsive cases.[23] Cra-

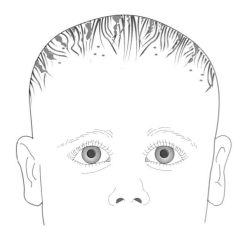

Figure 29.6. Cradle cap may appear as a crusted accumulation on a child's scalp; the scalp may also be affected with open, weeping vesicles.

dle cap that has proceeded to the point of dermatitis, vesicles, papules, or exudate is beyond the realm of nonprescription therapy, requiring a prompt visit to a physician for care.[1]

SUMMARY

Because hyperproliferative skin conditions cannot be cured, the goal of self-treatment with nonprescription products is to suppress symptoms with regular product usage. The self-

---

AT THE COUNTER

 A female patient in her late 20s asks the pharmacist to look at a skin condition on her elbow.

Interview/Patient Assessment

The pharmacist notes a shiny, thickened scale on the tip of her elbow, approximately 1 cm in diameter. She says she has picked it off several times since it first appeared last year, but it always grows back. She confirms that when she removes the "scab," a small pinpoint of bleeding appears almost at the center. She has had this lesion for several months and wonders if she should use Neosporin or a hand lotion on it. She denies any other plaques, states that she has no medical conditions, and is taking oral contraceptives.

Pharmacist's Analysis

1. What condition might this patient have?
2. Would Neosporin or a hand lotion be appropriate for her?

3. Should she see a physician?

This patient appears to have a psoriatic plaque, as noted by the description, pinpoint of bleeding after plaque removal, and location at the site of frequent abrasions. If she indeed has psoriasis, Neosporin or a hand lotion would be of little benefit, if any.

Patient Counseling

The pharmacist should explain the nature of the condition and possible triggering factors. The pharmacist must stress that the condition cannot be cured but that it may be slowed with the help of nonprescription or prescription products containing salicylic acid or coal tar (e.g., shampoos, creams, ointments, or other topical dosage forms) since the condition is relatively minor at this time. The pharmacist should point out that she must see a physician if the condition worsens dramatically or if the products fail to help.

treatable hyperproliferative conditions discussed in this chapter vary in severity from dandruff (the least severe) to severe seborrheic dermatitis to psoriasis. The major defect in all three is thought to be accelerated turnover of epidermal cells, although dandruff and seborrheic dermatitis may have a fungal component.

Self-treatment of dandruff utilizes coal-tar products, zinc pyrithione, selenium sulfide, and salicylic acid and/or sulfur. Seborrheic dermatitis may be successfully treated with coal tar, zinc pyrithione, selenium sulfide or micronized selenium sulfide, salicylic acid, and hydrocortisone. Psoriasis requires hydrocortisone, coal tar, or salicylic acid. Some ingredients produce more severe adverse reactions than others; for instance, coal tar products may cause folliculitis and contact dermatitis. For this reason, the pharmacist should recommend the nonprescription product with the least severe reactions.

References

1. Fed Reg 47:54646, 1982.
2. Lane P. Dandruff. Aust Fam Physician 17:973, 1988.
3. Tooley P. Dandruff: An irritating problem. Practitioner 234:593, 1990.
4. Kelly AP. Aesthetic considerations in patients of color. Dermatol Clin 15:687, 1997.
5. Nenoff P, Haustein UF, Fiedler A. The antifungal activity of a coal tar gel on *Malassezia furfur* in vitro. Dermatology 191:311, 1995.
6. El-Gothamy Z, Ghozzi M. Tinea versicolor of the scalp. Int J Dermatol 34:533, 1995.
7. Broberg A. *Pityrosporum ovale* in healthy children, infantile seborrheic dermatitis and atopic dermatitis. Acta Derm Venereol Suppl 191:1, 1995.
8. Cutsem JV, et al. The in vitro antifungal activity of ketoconazole, zinc pyrithione, and selenium sulfide against *Pityrosporum* and their efficacy as a shampoo in the treatment of experimental pityrosporosis in guinea pigs. J Am Acad Dermatol 22:993, 1990.
9. Danby FW, et al. A randomized, double-blind, placebo-controlled trial of ketoconazole 2% shampoo versus selenium sulfide 2.5% shampoo in the treatment of moderate to severe dandruff. J Am Acad Dermatol 29:1008, 1993.
10. Stenfors LE, Raisanen S. Is *Pityrosporum ovale* a pathogen of the external auditory meatus? Acta Otolaryngol 111:943, 1991.
11. Schmidt A. *Malassezia furfur:* A fungus belonging to the physiological skin flora and its relevance in skin disorders. Cutis 59:21, 1997.
12. Nenoff P, Haustein UF, Munzberger C. In vitro activity of lithium succinate against *Malassezia furfur.* Dermatology 190:48, 1995.
13. McGrath J, Murphy GM. The control of seborrheic dermatitis and dandruff by antipityrosporal drugs. Drugs 41:178, 1991.
14. Peter RU, Richarz-Barthauer U. Successful treatment and prophylaxis of scalp seborrheic dermatitis and dandruff with 2% ketoconazole shampoo: Results of a multicentre, double-blind, placebo-controlled trial. Br J Dermatol 132:441, 1995.
15. Anon. Scales in the balance: Dandruff reconsidered (Editorial). Lancet 2:703, 1985.
16. Fed Reg 56:63554, 1991.
17. Fed Reg 58:17554, 1993.
18. Fed Reg 59:4000, 1994.
19. Anon. J&J OTC Nizoral AD shampoo approved for control of dandruff. Weekly Pharmacy Reports 46(42):2, 1997.
20. Arrese JE, et al. Effect of ketoconazole-medicated shampoo on squamometry and *Malassezia ovalis* load in pityriasis capitis. Cutis 58:235–237, 1996.
21. Go IH, Wientjens DP, Koster M. A double-blind trial of 1% ketoconazole shampoo versus placebo in the treatment of dandruff. Mycoses 35:103, 1992.
22. Amer M, et al. Corneocytes in scaly parakeratotic diseases. Int J Dermatol 35:417, 1996.
23. Janniger CK, Schwartz RA. Seborrheic dermatitis. Am Fam Physician 52;149, 1995.
24. Mahe A, et al. Seborrheic dermatitis as a revealing feature of HIV infection in Bamako, Mali (Letter). Int J Dermatol 33:601, 1994.
25. Odom RB. Common superficial fungal infections in immunosuppressed patients. J Am Acad Dermatol 31(3 Pt 2):S56, 1994.
26. Elmets CA. Management of common superficial fungal infections in patients with AIDS. J Am Acad Dermatol 31(3 Pt 2):S60, 1994.
27. Osterle LS, et al. Skin surface lipids in HIV-positive patients with and without seborrheic dermatitis. Int J Dermatol 35:276, 1996.
28. Myskowski PL, Ahkami R. Dermatologic complications of HIV infection. Med Clin North Am 80:1415, 1996.
29. Hood S, Denning DW. Treatment of fungal infection in AIDS. J Antimicrob Chemother 37(Suppl B):71, 1996.
30. Aly R, Berger T. Common superficial fungal infections in patients with AIDS. Clin Infect Dis 22(Suppl 2):S128, 1996.
31. Ive FA. An overview of experience with ketoconazole shampoo. Br J Clin Pract 45:279, 1991.
32. Faergemann J. Pityrosporum infections. J Am Acad Dermatol 31(3 Pt 2):S18, 1994.
33. Nanda VS. Common dermatoses. Am J Obstet Gynecol 173:488, 1995.
34. Bergbrant IM. Seborrheic dermatitis and *Pityrosporum* yeasts. Curr Top Med Mycol 6:95, 1995.
35. Ross S, Richardson MD, Graybill JR. Association between *Malassezia furfur* colonization and seborrheic dermatitis in AIDS patients. Mycoses 37:9, 1994.
36. Faergemann J. *Pityrosporum* yeasts—What's new? Mycoses 40(Suppl 1):29, 1997.
37. Kasteler JS, Callen JP. Scalp involvement in dermatomyositis. Often overlooked or misdiagnosed. JAMA 272:1939, 1994.
38. English J. Managing scalp conditions. Practitioner 239:48, 1995.
39. Zug KA, Palay DA, Rock B. Dermatologic diagnosis and treatment of itchy red eyelids. Surv Ophthalmol 40:293, 1996.
40. Fed Reg 51:27346, 1986.
41. Fed Reg 51:27360, 1986.
42. Fed Reg 44:69768, 1979.
43. Zeharia A, Mimouni M, Fogel D. Treatment with bifonazole shampoo for scalp seborrhea in infants and young children. Pediatr Dermatol 13:151, 1996.
44. Dobrev H, Zissova L. Effect of ketoconazole 2% shampoo on scalp sebum level in patients with seborrheic dermatitis. Acta Derm Venereol 77:132, 1997.

45. Sei Y, et al. Seborrheic dermatitis: Treatment with anti-mycotic agents. J Dermatol 21:334, 1994.

46. Faergemann J, et al. *Pityrosporum ovale* (*Malassezia furfur*) as the causative agent of seborrheic dermatitis: New treatment options. Br J Dermatol 134(Suppl 46):12, 1996.

47. Greaves MW, Weinstein GD. Treatment of psoriasis. N Engl J Med 332:581, 1995.

48. Zhu JF, et al. Psoriasis: Pathophysiology and oral manifestations. Oral Dis 2:135, 1996.

49. Lebwohl M, et al. Topical therapy for psoriasis. Int J Dermatol 34:673, 1995.

50. Arbiser JL. Angiogenesis and the skin: A primer. J Am Acad Dermatol 34:486, 1996.

51. Lewis HM. Therapeutic progress II: Treatment of psoriasis. J Clin Pharm Ther 19:223, 1994.

52. Prystowsky JH, Cohen PR. Pustular and erythrodermic psoriasis. Dermatol Clin 13:757, 1995.

53. Christophers E, Kiene P. Guttate and plaque psoriasis. Dermatol Clin 13:751, 1995.

54. Swanbeck G, et al. Age at onset and different types of psoriasis. Br J Dermatol 133:768, 1995.

55. Naldi L. Psoriasis. Dermatol Clin 13:635, 1995.

56. Henseler T. The genetics of psoriasis. J Am Acad Dermatol 37(2 Pt 3):S1, 1997.

57. Kandunce DP, Krueger GG. Pathogenesis of psoriasis. Dermatol Clin 13:723, 1995.

58. Ortonne JP. Aetiology and pathogenesis of psoriasis. Br J Dermatol 135 Suppl 49:1, 1996.

59. Guzzo C. Recent advances in the treatment of psoriasis. Dermatol Clin 15:59, 1997.

60. Rosenberg EW, Noah PW, Skinner RB Jr. Psoriasis is a visible manifestation of the skin's defense against micro-organisms. J Dermatol 21:375, 1994.

61. Raychaudhuri SP, Rein G, Farber EM. Neuropathogenesis and neuropharmacology of psoriasis. Int J Dermatol 34:685, 1995.

62. Rotstein H. Psoriasis: Changing clinical patterns. Australas J Dermatol (37 Suppl 1):S27, 1996.

63. Gupta AK, et al. Terbinafine therapy may be associated with the development of psoriasis *de novo* or its exacerbation: Four case reports and a review of drug-induced psoriasis. J Am Acad Dermatol 36(5 Pt 2):858, 1997.

64. Farber EM, Therapeutic perspectives in psoriasis. Int J Dermatol 34:456, 1995.

65. Perez RG, et al. Positive patch tests to zinc pyrithione. Contact Dermatitis 32:118, 1995.

66. Christophers E. The immunopathology of psoriasis. Int Arch Allergy Immunol 110:199, 1996.

67. Van de Kerkhof PC, Gerritsen MJ, de Jong EM. Transition from symptomless to lesional psoriatic skin. Clin Exp Dermatol 21:325, 1996.

68. Griffiths TW, Griffiths CE, Voorhees JJ. Immunopathogenesis and immunotherapy of psoriasis. Dermatol Clin 13:739, 1995.

69. Larko O. Problem sites: Scalp, palm and sole, and nail. Dermatol Clin 13:771, 1995.

70. Penzer R. Psoriasis. Nurs Stand 10:49, 1996.

71. Ginsburg IH. Psychological and psychophysiological aspects of psoriasis. Dermatol Clin 13:793, 1995.

72. Schmid MH, Korting HC. Coal tar, pine tar and sulfonated shale oil preparations: Comparative activity, efficacy and safety. Dermatology 193:1, 1996.

73. Abel EA. Phototherapy. Dermatol Clin 13:841, 1995.

74. Cowen P. New horizons in the treatment of psoriasis and cutaneous fungal infections. Aust Fam Physician 25:317, 1996.

75. Christophers E. Psoriasis: Mechanisms and entry points for possible therapeutic interventions. Australas J Dermatol 37(Suppl 1):S4, 1996.

76. Gonzalez E. PUVA for psoriasis. Dermatol Clin 13:851, 1995.

77. Phillips TJ. Current treatment options in psoriasis. Hosp Pract 31:155, 1996.

78. Katz HI. Topical corticosteroids. Dermatol Clin 13:805, 1995.

79. Patil SP, Niphadkar PV, Bapat MM. Allergy to fenugreek (*Trigonella foenum graecum*). Ann Allergy Asthma Immunol 78:297, 1997.

80. Shiota Y, et al. Adult respiratory distress syndrome induced by a Chinese medicine, Kamisyoyo-san. Intern Med 35:494, 1996.

81. Perharic L, et al. Possible association of liver damage with the use of Chinese herbal medicine for skin disease. Vet Hum Toxicol 37:562, 1995.

82. Mimouni K, et al. Prognosis of infantile seborrheic dermatitis. J Pediatr 127:744, 1995.

83. Singleton JK. Pediatric dermatoses: Three common skin disruptions in infancy. Nurse Pract 22:32, 1997.

84. Feldman MA, et al. Teaching child-care skills to mothers with developmental disabilities. J Appl Behav Anal 25:205, 1992.

85. Philipp R, Hughes A, Golding J. Getting to the bottom of nappy rash. ALSPAC Survey Team. Avon Longitudinal Study of Pregnancy and Childhood. Br J Gen Pract 47:493, 1997.

86. Tollesson A, Frithz A, Stenlund K. *Malassezia furfur* in infantile seborrheic dermatitis. Pediatr Dermatol 14:423, 1997.

CHAPTER 30

Arthropod Stings and Bites, Pediculosis, and Scabies

A young mother asks the pharmacist to help determine how to treat her 4-year-old son.

Interview/Patient Assessment

The family spent the previous day at a lake, and the mother thinks the child has insect bites. The child has several small but inflamed and erythematous papules on the arms, legs, and face. The mother says that the boy had been scratching them so badly that she had to trim his nails.

Pharmacist's Analysis

1. What insect is likely to have caused these bites?
2. Would nonprescription products help this type of bite?
3. Should the child's mother be advised to use nonprescription products?

The bites could be caused by several insects, including chiggers, but the child's proximity to the water when the bites occurred and the resultant pruritus implicate the mosquito. Nonprescription products can help this type of bite, and there are several options from which the pharmacist may choose.

Patient Counseling

The mother should be shown products containing external analgesics, astringents, or skin protectants. For example, the pharmacist might recommend a spray containing benzocaine to provide rapid relief from pruritus. The mother might also be counseled to use a hydrocortisone ointment to reduce the inflammation and shorten the duration of skin irritation. However, if the papules and pruritus persist for more than 7 days from the date of onset, the child should be seen by a physician to rule out a more serious condition. Further, should the child scratch enough to produce a secondary bacterial infection, a prescription antibiotic would be necessary.

Stinging and biting arthropods (including lice and scabies—common parasites that live on the host or on clothing and continually feed on the host's blood [lice] or skin [scabies]) can cause a variety of toxic reactions in humans. Although most individuals only suffer mild, nonthreatening reactions to insect stings and bites, for some, insect venom can be life-threatening. For example, *a single sting from an insect can cause death from* anaphylaxis (*an acute allergic reaction whose features may include bronchospasm and circulatory collapse*) *in a severely allergic individual.*

This chapter discusses stinging and biting arthropods and two parasitic insects, lice and scabies. (Note that the term "arthropod" encompasses insects and noninsect creatures such as spiders and scorpions. Since the term "insect" is used by the lay public for any creature grouped in the phylum *Arthropoda*, however, that term is used in this chapter.)

ARTHROPOD STINGS

Unlike biting insects, stinging insects usually only sting as a defensive reaction. Thus they are not parasitic like many biting insects (e.g., lice, ticks, scabies). The sting usually causes immediate pain, versus the relatively painless feeding of a parasitic biting insect. Most anaphylactic reactions are caused by stinging insects (see "Complications of Arthropod Stings: Anaphylactic Reactions").

PREVALENCE OF ARTHROPOD STINGS

Although the prevalence of insect stings is difficult to ascertain, they do tend to be seasonal in incidence, being worse in late summer and early autumn.[1,2] The incidence of anaphylaxis resulting from insect stings—a serious complication—has been estimated at 0.3 to 3%.[3]

EPIDEMIOLOGY OF ARTHROPOD STINGS

Most stinging arthropods go about their business paying no attention to humans.[3] Individuals who are stung usually have done something to upset an insect such as intruding on the hive/nest or annoying the insect by venturing too close to it.[1,4] Occasionally, individuals disturb an entire colony and suffer multiple stings.[5]

Several researchers have noted that individuals wearing perfume or scented hair sprays are more prone to insect stings.[1]

Data on the incidence of anaphylaxis indicate that stings are more common in those under the age of 20 and may be twice as common in females as in males.[3] Perhaps these data result from age/gender differences in play and leisure pursuits.

ETIOLOGY OF ARTHROPOD STINGS

The order of insects known as *Hymenoptera* of the class Insecta contains 100,000 species. Many of these insects have poison glands, which perhaps evolved as offensive or defensive weapons.[5,6] The order includes the winged vespids (yellow jackets, hornets, wasps), a nonwinged group (ants), and the apids (honeybees, bumblebees).[3,7] Stinging insects envenomate their victims by introducing a foreign substance into the body.

MANIFESTATIONS OF ARTHROPOD STINGS

The consequences of insect stings are so similar that they may be discussed as a group. Insect stings usually produce immediate acute burning pain.[5] Local erythema and edema appear within a few minutes. Localized reactions usually disappear over the following 4 to 6 hours, although patients may develop more severe edema that can last for 7 days.[3,5] Stings may evolve into papules, vesicles, or bullae, and become intensely pruritic or painful.[5] Some patients exhibit late reactions such as flulike symptoms (e.g., fatigue and nausea) occurring 8 to 24 hours after a honeybee sting.[3,5,8] Occasionally, unexpected sequelae occur. For instance, a bee sting in the brow area produced bilateral optic neuritis in a healthy 11-year-old boy; he did not recover full ophthalmic function.[9] A set of three wasp stings precipitated a myocardial infarction in a 50-year-old woman with normal coronary arteries.[10] Two children developed acute renal failure after receiving stings from many wasps, but recovered after several months of peritoneal dialysis and supportive care; two patients developed atrial flutter after bee stings.[11,12] Patients stung by massive numbers of Africanized bees may experience such complications as anaphylaxis, acute renal failure, hypotension, and skin necrosis.[13]

Most ant stings produce itching, pain, and burning that resolves in a short period.[7] However, in some study groups as many as 16% of those stung by fire ants show a systemic reaction, and at least 2% develop anaphylaxis.[14] In rare instances, imported fire ant bites have caused grand mal seizures.

The immediate reaction to a scorpion sting is local pain and burning, followed by cramping, **hyperesthesia** (acute sensitivity to touch), numbness, and tenderness at the bite site. Scorpion venom produces excessive neuronal firing, manifested as central nervous system and neuromuscular dysfunction.[15] The reaction may proceed to lacrimation, salivation, nausea, urinary frequency, speech difficulties, chills, cold sweats, **bradypnea** (slowed respirations), aspiration, and convulsions.[16]

See the individual arthropod sections under "Specific Considerations of Arthropod Stings" for more detail.

SPECIFIC CONSIDERATIONS OF ARTHROPOD STINGS

Wasps, Yellow Jackets, and Hornets

These related species cause painful stings.[5] Yellow jackets are often found nesting on the ground or feeding on food and garbage.[3] Wasps are commonly found under the eaves of houses.[7] Hornets produce paper nests, often in bushes or trees.

Ants

Virtually all ants both bite and sting, but the bite is usually only a means to anchor the ant while it sprays or injects the venom through stinging. Ant stings usually cause only transient discomfort.

The imported fire ant (*Solenopis invicta* and *richteri*) is a notable exception because its bite is more severe.[17,18] Reportedly, fire ants sting 30 to 60% of the population in infested areas each year.[14,19] Fire ants are common in the southern United States, but have been spotted as far north as southern Oklahoma.[5,20] (Sensitivity to colder climates has limited its geographic distribution.[14]) The fire ant first attaches itself to the victim's skin by the mouth. The fire ant then arches its body and pivots around the bite location, stinging many times on the circumference of the resulting circle.[3,21,22] The fire ant bite causes an immediate wheal, accompanied by pain and pruritus.[19] The sterile pustule that develops within 24 hours confirms the diagnosis as a fire ant sting. While most fire ant bites are a response to invasion of their territory, in two documented cases fire ants apparently engaged in organized attacks on humans—one a sleeping diabetic patient and the other an elderly nursing home patient with Alzheimer's-type dementia.[19] The former patient expired as a result of the "attack"; the latter patient suffered over 1000 stings but was successfully treated with intravenous methylprednisolone and cephalothin.

Honeybees

The honeybee's stinger is equipped with several barbs.[1] As the honeybee inserts the stinger into a person, the barbs secure the stinger in the skin. Once it is inserted, the honeybee cannot remove the stinger. This has several implications. Honeybees can only sting once, unlike the other stinging bees and arthropods whose stingers include few or no barbs. Further, the honeybee disembowels itself as it flies away, causing its death.

Bumblebees

The bumblebee is often found close to the ground where their hives are located. Because the bumblebee stinger is not barbed, bumblebees can sting repeatedly.[5]

Africanized Bees

These so-called "killer bees" entered the United States in southern Texas and subsequently migrated to Arizona and California.[3,6,23] While their venom is no more toxic or allergenic than the venom of other bees, Africanized bees are especially noted for their aggressive responses to disruption.[3,24] Even a slight disturbance in the area of the nest can cause swarms of many thousands of "warriors", each capable of stinging many times.[13] The bees have been known to pursue people for over a kilometer.[23] ⚠ **Massive numbers of stings from Africanized bees have caused death from venom toxicity.**[3,25]

Scorpions

The American scorpion (*Centruroides sculpturatus*), a species with a potent venom, is found primarily in warmer states such as Oklahoma, Texas, California, Arizona, Nevada, and New

Mexico.[15,26] These nocturnal arthropods generally are encountered in remote places such as under stones, roots, or other debris on the ground.[16] Most bites occur from April to November, since the arthropod hibernates during the winter.[26]

The venom of the scorpion is neurotoxic and cardiotoxic. (The venom of scorpions in New Mexico, Arizona, and California is more toxic than the venom of scorpions in the south-central portion of the United States.[16]) Reactions to the American scorpion range from painful tingling and burning to cranial nerve abnormalities (e.g., rotary eye movements, blurred vision, loss of pharyngeal muscle control), bleeding disorders, myocardial injury, pulmonary edema, cardiovascular collapse, and pancreatitis.[27,28]

COMPLICATIONS OF ARTHROPOD STINGS: ANAPHYLACTIC REACTIONS

The generalized systemic reaction known as anaphylaxis may begin within 10 to 20 minutes of the sting in an individual previously sensitized to that insect's sting.[3,5] See "A Pharmacist's Journal: I've Just Been Stung by a Bee." The *Hymenoptera* are the most likely insects to cause anaphylaxis because their venom is more highly antigenic.[5,29–31] (See "Etiology of Arthropod Stings.") In the southeastern United States, the imported fire ant has overtaken winged arthropods in frequency of anaphylaxis-producing stings.[17,32]

The most common anaphylactic symptoms are cutaneous: urticaria, angioedema, and flushing.[3] However, anaphylactic shock also includes potentially fatal symptoms such as bronchospasm (manifested as respiratory difficulty or tightness in the chest), circulatory collapse with shock, epileptic attacks, hypotension, and upper-airway edema.[33–35] Patients may also exhibit anxiety, **diaphoresis** (extreme sweating), nausea, vomiting, pallor, and edema.[1,5] While anaphylaxis is

more common in individuals younger than 20, deaths are more common in older patients.[3] Unless an individual has suffered a prior anaphylactic reaction, it is not possible to predict whether they might suffer from anaphylaxis.[3,36–38]

The standard treatment for anaphylaxis is parenteral epinephrine (e.g., subcutaneous in a 1:1000 dilution, 0.2 to 0.5 mL, repeated every 30 minutes as needed). Although once mentioned as a possible Rx-to-OTC switch, parenteral epinephrine remains a prescription medication as of this writing.[39,40] Thus suspected anaphylaxis is a medical emergency necessitating emergency medical transport.[41] When the patient has a prescription filled for future use in anaphylaxis, the pharmacist should advise the patient about use of the product, and provide other emergency precautions. (See "Advice for the Patient with Possible Anaphylaxis to Insect Stings.")

TREATMENT OF ARTHROPOD STINGS

Treatment Guidelines

The first step in treatment depends on the particular arthropod that has stung the patient. (See Patient Assessment Algorithm 30.1.) If the insect (or insects) is likely to cause a serious outcome (e.g., a scorpion, a fire ant, a large number of Africanized bees), medical attention is advisable.[42] More minor stings may be self-treated.

If the insect is a honeybee, the stinger may still be imbedded in the skin and should be removed since it continues to pump venom after it has separated from the bee.[1] For years, conventional wisdom held that the stinger should not be squeezed during removal, since that might increase the volume of venom injected. According to this older theory, the person was to locate a stiff object (such as a credit card) and remove the barbed stinger by scraping. However, experts now suggest that patients remove the stinger by any means

A Pharmacist's Journal

"I've Just Been Stung by a Bee!"

A former student once called to tell me how her work was proceeding. The day before, a woman had entered her small independent Texas store and asked to talk to the pharmacist about a nonprescription product for an insect sting. As the former student approached her, the patient said, "I've just been stung by a bee and I'm not feeling too. . . . ." The patient then collapsed on the pharmacy floor. My former student directed the technician to close and lock

the pharmacy, leaving a note that the pharmacist would be back later. They placed the patient in a car and drove her to the emergency room, where her blood pressure was 0/0. With emergency care, she had a complete recovery. The pharmacist was cited as a heroine by state and regional newspapers and media. At that time, there was no 911 service, but the use of a 911 emergency phone number would be an excellent way to handle this type of situation.

at hand, rather than wasting time hunting for a stiff object to scrape it away.[3,43]

A drug manufacturer requested that diphenhydramine be approved for relief of itching associated with hives resulting from insect bites.[44] However, the FDA responded that hives and pruritic rashes secondary to insect stings and bites are only one component of a systemic anaphylactic reaction, stressing that the use of a nonprescription antihistamine could delay proper care for the reaction.[44] The agency further mentioned that the average person cannot distinguish between a mild allergic reaction and a life-threatening reaction that begins with itching. Since histamine is merely one of the mediators released during mast cell degranulation, blocking its effects may not be sufficient. For these reasons, pharmacists should not recommend nonprescription oral antihistamines for the treatment of insect sting (or bite) symptoms.

Nonprescription Medications

Technically, there is no product approved by the FDA for insect *stings*. Labeling on all insect products refers only to insect bites. For this reason, nonprescription products for treating stings are discussed fully under the section on insect bites in this chapter (see "Treatment of Arthropod Bites"). (It is possible that the FDA meant to use the term "insect bite" as an inclusive term. In one publication regarding insect bite neutralizers, the agency used the wording, "For temporary relief of stings caused by wasps, hornets, bees, mosquitoes, spiders, fleas, chiggers, ticks, and ants."[45] This mingling of stinging and biting insects under one heading suggests that the agency also means to include insect stings in the insect bite monograph. Further, in a phone conversation about this issue, FDA personnel confirmed that the agency included stinging insects in this group.)

If the reaction to the sting is minor, patients can use several topical nonprescription products successfully. Sodium bicarbonate (baking soda) paste may help neutralize the formic acid injected by ants.[7] Also, nonprescription systemic analgesics and systemic antihistamines may reduce the pain of insect stings or bites, but this is not a part of the FDA-approved labeling.

FOCUS ON...

ADVICE FOR PATIENTS WITH POSSIBLE ANAPHYLAXIS TO INSECT STINGS

Pharmacists can provide helpful advice to patients who present a prescription for an anaphylaxis kit or for ampules of epinephrine and syringes to be kept in case of an anaphylactic reaction:.

- Carry a card in the wallet or purse explaining the possibility of an anaphylactic reaction to a sting.
- Wear a medical alert bracelet, necklace, or other visible jewelry on the body that has an inscription warning about the possibility of anaphylaxis.
- If the prescription is for an anaphylaxis kit or epinephrine pen, demonstrate the product at the point of sale; encourage questions and urge the patient to become thoroughly familiar with the kit or pen in advance.
- If the prescription is for separate epinephrine ampules, help the patient select appropriate syringes; demonstrate the technique of opening an ampule and withdrawing its contents. Dispense the ampules to minimize the possibility of breakage (e.g., in a cotton-lined vial)
- Suggest that the patient teach other members of the family and friends how to use the epinephrine products.
- Point out the expiration date on the prescription products and suggest that the patient obtain a refill prior to that date.
- Suggest that the patient carry a current prescription filled out for an epinephrine product in case one is needed in an emergency (e.g., the current product cannot be located or is broken).
- Remind the patient to carry the product in a pocket or purse at all times a sting might be possible.
- Caution against keeping the epinephrine product in a hot car or other location where the temperature would degrade the epinephrine; caution against use if the solution has darkened.
- Urge the patient to inject the product immediately after a sting, rather than waiting for symptoms to begin.

Nonpharmacologic Therapies

Minor local reactions from most stinging insects can be treated with nonprescription products. While some recommend topical application of meat tenderizers, this method has not been assessed for efficacy.[3] For patients with a history of severe local reactions to stings, it might be helpful to remove the venom through suction.[1] Several vacuum devices are marketed to pharmacies and various sports-related retailers, although they are not usually approved for this use as medical devices by the FDA.

Local application of ice may also provide some relief.[1] Various devices used to deliver cryotherapy (described in Chapter 20) are especially useful for larger local reactions.[5]

Electric shock, a folklore remedy for insect stings and bites, is not recommended. See "A Pharmacist's Journal: A Lawnmower Works Best."

PREVENTION OF ARTHROPOD STINGS

The fear of insect stings and anaphylaxis resulting from hymenoptera venom allergy can affect a patient's recreational

Patient Assessment Algorithm 30.1. Arthropod Stings

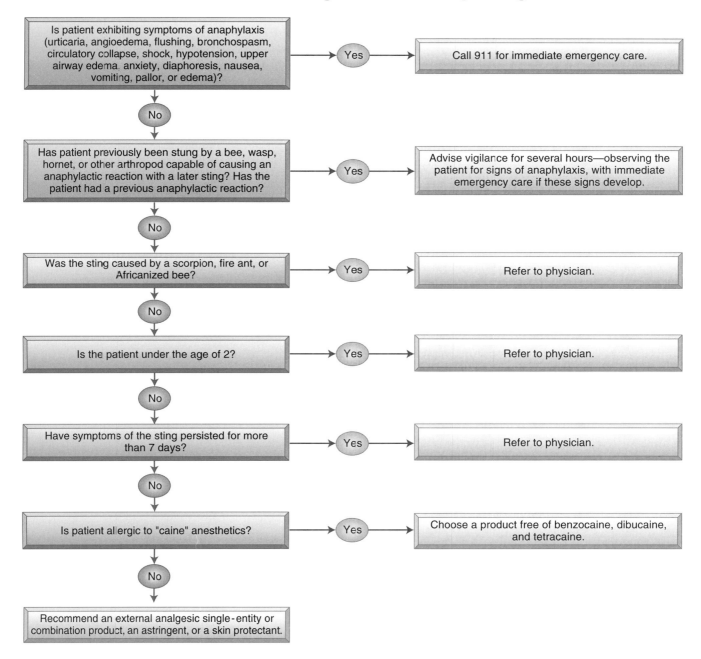

and occupational activities.[46] Several measures can be taken to avoid arthropod stings:

- Do not wear cosmetics or personal grooming aids that emit an odor such as cologne, perfume, or hair sprays.[1]
- When a stinging insect is in the area, stay still or move slowly. In most cases, the insect will buzz around, but will not sting unless it feels threatened.
- Do not run from a stinging insect.
- Do not slap or brush at a stinging insect.
- Be observant for insects when in their territories such as blooming orchards, flower gardens, and fields of clover.

- Wear protective clothing when entering insect territories (e.g., shoes, socks, slacks, long-sleeved shirts, and gloves [when gardening]).[3]
- Wear dark or drab-colored clothing rather than bright colors, pastels, and white materials.[3]
- Use caution during high-risk activities: gardening, mowing lawns, picking flowers, and trimming hedges.
- Periodically inspect your residence for insect infestations, looking under eaves and in out-of-the-way locations. Nests and hives are best located during daylight but treated at night, when all insects have returned and their activity level drops. (A professional exterminator may be needed.)

A Pharmacist's Journal

"A Lawnmower Works Best."

Following a continuing education lecture on insect stings and bites, a pharmacist approached me to share this advice: "The best thing of all for bee and wasp stings is to get electricity to them. A lawnmower works best. I take the wire to the spark plug off and touch it to the sting.

Then I have my wife crank the lawnmower starter. It'll hurt and sometimes it knocks you off your feet, but it sure stops that bee sting!" Of course, this method must never be recommended since it could cause tissue damage and perhaps create systemic dangers.

ARTHROPOD BITES

Whereas insect stings virtually always cause immediate pain, many insect bites (e.g., ticks, spiders) are initially painless, perhaps becoming pruritic over time. Furthermore, repeated bites (such as several mosquito bites over the summer) often sensitize individuals so that the reaction becomes progressively more serious as other bites occur.[47]

PREVALENCE OF ARTHROPOD BITES

Arthropod bites are common, but their prevalence is unknown because most people consider them to be minor and do not report them to a physician or pharmacist. Also, there is no central data collection point for insect bites.

EPIDEMIOLOGY OF ARTHROPOD BITES

The likelihood of arthropod bites ebbs and flows with the season. Most bites occur in summer, the peak activity season for insects, but bites are also common in fall and spring. A harsh winter can kill many ticks, spiders, mosquitoes, and other pests, while a mild winter will allow many insects to survive (which may make the following summer particularly bothersome.)

Generally, children receive more insect bites (e.g., mosquitoes) than adults because of their propensity to play outdoors for sustained periods during the summer, when the insect population is at a peak and their clothing is minimal.[47] Flea bites are most common in those who live with cats and dogs, especially when the animal is allowed to roam freely outside, where it can contact infested animals. Tick bites are most common in outdoor workers.[48]

ETIOLOGY OF ARTHROPOD BITES

Biting insects place a mixture of foreign substances into the human body. Mosquitoes, for instance, inject toxins and allergens.[47] These chemicals usually cause little reaction when

a person is first bitten, although repeated bites over time will cause sensitization with worsening of symptoms.[47]

MANIFESTATIONS OF ARTHROPOD BITES

Because of the large number of biting arthropods, it is difficult to generalize about their manifestations. (Unlike arthropod stings, arthropod bites can produce quite dissimilar reactions.) Some bites are painless initially (e.g., ticks and head lice), while other bites cause almost immediate reactions (e.g., mosquitoes). Arthropod bites also range widely in severity, from trivial (e.g., mosquitoes) to disfiguring or deadly (e.g., certain spiders).

See the individual insect sections under "Specific Conditions of Arthropod Bites" for more detail.

SPECIFIC CONSIDERATIONS OF ARTHROPOD BITES

Mosquitoes

Mosquitoes, a problem in many regions of the world, infest both tropical and temperate zones.[49] Mosquitoes obtain blood from warm-blooded species to incubate their eggs.

The initial symptom of a mosquito bite is usually a wheal-and-flare reaction, which begins about 10 to 15 minutes after the bite and persists for 1 to 2 hours, with severe pruritus being common. Some patients exhibit severe swellings of the skin, which can last for several days.[49] Researchers believe that extreme reactions are immunologic, a classic type I allergic reaction.[47,49]

Fleas

Fleas are most common in areas with warm temperatures and high humidity.[47] Because of the sensitivity of fleas to the environment, flea bites are less common in the winter; pets can be infested with the insects throughout the winter, however, resulting in flea bites during cold seasons.[47,50] See "A Pharmacist's Journal: Do You Have Something for Phlebitis?"

Fleas can live for months without feeding, but require a blood meal to lay eggs. Thus pharmacists in towns with a large transient population (e.g, college towns) often counsel patients with flea bites who do not have a pet. Fleas will remain in houses and apartments when occupants change—even after the infested pet has left—and will then ravenously bite new residents.[47,51]

The first flea bites an individual receives may not cause any reaction.[47] However, repeated bites result in sensitization, causing urticarial papules.[47] Pharmacists may recognize flea bites by their appearance and location (Fig. 30.1). Since fleas can easily jump onto their victim's ankles from the carpet, women—whose legs are exposed more than men's—tend to receive more flea bites than men.[52] Occasionally, flea bites are found on areas where the clothing fits snugly such as under elastic bands and on the shoulders and hips.[47,52]

Pharmacists should advise patients who discover fleas infesting their residences to contact a veterinarian (or pest-control business) for help eradicating fleas from the pet's bedding, the carpets, and household furnishings.[52]

Ticks

Tick bites have little impact, except for the diseases they can spread, including Rocky Mountain spotted fever (RMSF), Lyme disease, and the less common ehrlichiosis and babesiosis.[1] Ticks bite by cutting the skin and inserting their proboscis.[47] The saliva introduced into the wound contains an anesthetic that makes the bite painless, along with digestive juices and chemicals that prevent coagulation of blood.[47] (See "Prevention Guidelines" under "Prevention of Arthropod Bites.")

TICK INSPECTIONS
It is difficult to eliminate tick bites, but with care patients can nearly eliminate disease transmission from ticks. Ticks do not transmit disease until they have been attached to human hosts for several hours.[1] Accordingly, patients should be warned to check for embedded ticks every hour or so when in tick territory. Light-colored clothing facilitates recognition of the ticks.[53] The ticks may be in any body area, even the

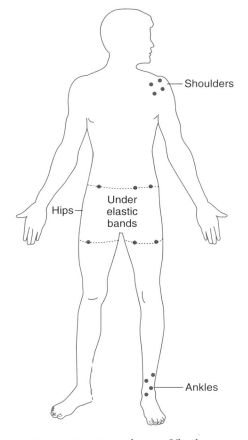

Figure 30.1. Typical sites of flea bites.

eyelid margin.[54] The tick stays attached an average of 29 hours, but may feed for more than 48 hours.[55]

TICK REMOVAL
While some experts still advise traditional tick-removal methods such as covering the tick with kerosene or camp-stove fuel or touching the tick with a hot object (such as a match head), these techniques are unreliable and may actually increase the risk of disease since the tick may expel its infected oral fluids into the patient as it is injured or killed. In-

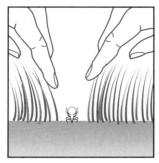

1. Expose attached tick.

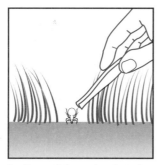

2. Grasp tick as closely to its head as possible with tweezers.

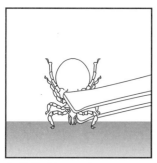

3. Pull with steady pressure, without twisting or undue squeezing. (Tick should release its grip so tick, complete with head, can be removed.)

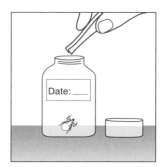

4. Save tick in a labeled jar.

Figure 30.2. Steps in tick removal.

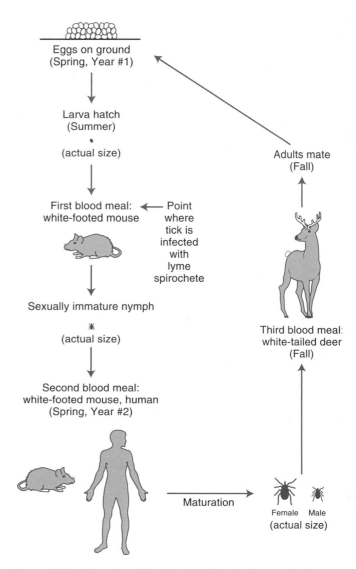

Figure 30.3. Life cycle of the deer tick (*Ixodes dammini*), the vector of Lyme disease.

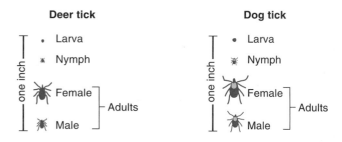

Figure 30.4. Deer tick (Lyme disease vector) compared with dog tick (probable vector of Rocky Mountain spotted fever).

stead, the tick should be removed as illustrated in Figure 30.2. With insistent, steady pulling, the tick should release its grip, and the entire tick (complete with head) can be removed. If the tick's head (or part of the head) remains in the skin, it can cause skin infection and may need to be excised.[47] Ticks should be placed in a jar with a secure screw top, and the date should be written on the jar; later, the ticks can be examined if necessary to confirm a diagnosis of tick-borne disease.

DISEASES TRANSMITTED BY TICKS

Lyme Disease

The pharmacist should be alert to the possibility of Lyme disease in a patient with a recent history of tick bite. As shown in Figure 30.3, Lyme disease is caused by a spirochete that is transmitted by the bite of the extremely small deer tick.[56] (See Figure 30.4 to compare the deer tick with the common dog tick.)

While the first cases were clustered around Lyme, Connecticut, the condition has been diagnosed in more than 48 states.[53] Symptoms of Lyme disease include nonspecific flu-like illnesses, a characteristic rash (a nonpruritic, erythematous, painless maculopapular ring with a defined border and perhaps a clear center, sometimes described as a "bulls-eye"—see Fig. 30.5), malaise, fatigue, lethargy, headache,

fever and chills, multiple circular lesions, stiff neck, **arthralgias** (joint pains), **myalgias** (muscle pains), anorexia, sore throat, nausea, and a malar rash.[56] Suspected patients must be referred to a physician for immediate care; delay can increase the risk of debilitating conditions.[55]

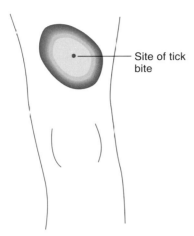

Figure 30.5. The earliest stage of Lyme disease is an expanding round/oval–shaped rash surrounding the tick bite location.

Rocky Mountain Spotted Fever

RMSF is caused by a bacterium belonging to the family Rickettsiaceae. The wood tick, dog tick, and Lone Star tick are thought to be vectors (see Fig. 30.4).[56] RMSF has been reported in nearly every state. The classical symptoms consist of fever (of abrupt onset) and rash in a person with known history of tick bite.[56] The rash begins on the palms, soles, wrists, and forearms, spreading to the trunk, neck, and face. Patients also suffer headache, malaise, myalgias, nausea, and emesis. Pharmacists who suspect RMSF should refer the patients immediately so that care can be instituted.

Chiggers

The chigger mite (also known as the red bug or harvest bug) is a tiny red insect that feeds on human blood, producing a small papule at the site.[57] They are most often found in warmer climates and in woody and grassy areas. Pruritus may last for as long as 7 to 10 days. Bites are common at points where clothing fits snugly such as elastic waist and leg bands, the tops of socks, and brassieres (Fig. 30.6). As in tick-bite prevention, chigger bites can be avoided by wearing clothing that prevents chiggers from contacting skin.

Spiders

Spiders will occasionally bite humans, but generally with only a mild local reaction of little consequence.[1] There are two notable exceptions: the black widow spider and the brown recluse (fiddleback) spider. With both species, only the female is capable of envenomating man.

Other species of spiders have been reported to cause reactions in man after biting, notably *Tegenaria agrestis* (the funnel-web spider) and *Chiracanthium mildei* (the garden spider), both of which may produce a necrotic reaction that is often confused with a brown recluse bite.[58,59] The funnel-web spider is found in the northwestern United States, in states such as Washington, Oregon, and Idaho. The garden

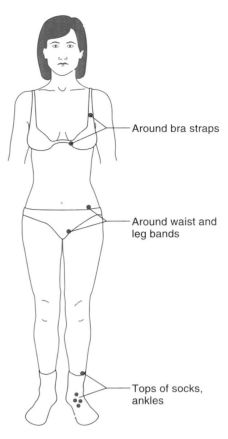

Figure 30.6. Typical sites of chigger bites.

spider is found in Massachusetts, Connecticut, New York, New Jersey, Alabama, Indiana, and Utah.

BLACK WIDOW

The bite of a black widow (*Latrodectus mactans*) produces a condition known as latrodectism. Other species of *Latrodectus* cause similar reactions, including the brown widow (*L. geometricus*), the red-legged widow (*L. bishopi*), *L. variolus*, and *L. hesperus*.[60] The other species differ from *L. mactans* in their markings and color. *L. mactans* is the most significant of these spiders because it is the leading cause of arthropod deaths in the United States.[61] *L. mactans* is identified by its shiny, glossy black color and the red hourglass on its ventral surface (underneath the globular abdomen).[1,62] The fully mature female is about the size of a quarter if the legs are fully extended.[61]

L. mactans, whose range extends throughout the United States, frequents out-of-the-way places—such as woodpiles, garages, barns, basements, the inside of closets or drawers, and the underside of rocks, where it can ambush small insects.[61] Unlike the regular, geometric web of some spiders, the black widow's web is poorly organized.

Black widow bites are seldom noticed by the patient, although some victims perceive a slight pinprick or pinching feeling.[1,61] Also, at least 20% of black widow envenomations show no visible bite mark. Within 20 to 30 minutes, however, a burning, cramping pain develops at the bite site, accompanied by slight erythema, **piloerection** (the hair standing up—"goose bumps"), sweating, and **lymphangitis** (inflammation of the lymph channels).[62] These symptoms gradually spread to involve a larger part of the bitten extremity.[62] About 30 to 60 minutes following the bite, the patient usually experiences severe pain, cramping, and muscle contractions radiating from the bite location.[1,62] During the ensuing 4 to 6 hours, the patient may experience any combination of the following: headache, nausea, **priapism** (a continual erection in which the penis is unable to disengorge), anxiety, fatigue, insomnia, salivation, lacrimation, tremors, tachycardia, bradycardia, vomiting, extreme restlessness, diaphoresis, severe abdominal and back pain, a rigid boardlike abdomen, hypertension, shock, and coma.[62,63] Most of the more minor symptoms generally resolve over 12 to 48 hours.[60] *At least 3 to 5% of patients will die from black widow bites, usually younger and older patients.*[62]

No nonprescription product can provide relief of black widow bites. An ice cube or cryotherapy device may reduce the progression or effects of the venom and perhaps even inactivate it, but patients must be referred to an emergency room since treatment may also involve intravenous calcium gluconate, muscle relaxants (e.g., diazepam), narcotic analgesics (e.g., morphine), and antivenin.[1,60,63,64]

BROWN RECLUSE

The bite of a brown recluse (*Loxosceles reclusa*) produces a condition known as loxoscelism. The brown recluse spider is harder to identify than the black widow since it resembles many brown spiders.[58] However, a trained eye can spot the fiddle-shaped coloration on the dorsal (upper) surface of the cephalothorax, the section to which its legs are attached. The fully mature female is about the size of a quarter with the legs fully extended. The range of *Loxosceles* is limited to the southern states, since it cannot survive harsh winters.[61] A shy, nocturnal spider, it frequents dry, warm, out-of-the-way places such as garages, shoes, gloves, drawers, and woodpiles. (Brown recluse spiders carried inside on logs in the winter will halt their dormancy, exit their protective webbed sheath, and infest the house.)

Brown recluse spider bites often occur when patients put on clothing that had been left on the floor and in which a brown recluse has hidden.[65] If a brown recluse bite is felt at all, the patient usually will only perceive a pinprick sensation. Bites are more common during the months of April through October.[66]

The venom of the brown recluse spider contains nine proteins, all with cytotoxic actions.[66] While symptoms of the black widow bite are mostly systemic, symptoms of the brown recluse bite are mostly local.[1] The location of the bite is a factor in the outcome. If it is in a fatty area, the prognosis is worse than if the bite is in a lean area. The hallmark local reaction is necrosis of the tissue, which is more pronounced with bites in the abdomen, thighs, and buttocks than lean areas such as the fingers or hands. Bites on the face

and neck can produce local edema. The patient may first notice a small **bleb** (fluid-filled lesion—a blister) atop the puncture site. The initial ischemic area evolves into a necrotic lesion within a few hours to several weeks time. The black necrotic lesion is surrounded by a pale halo of ischemic tissue and an area of edema.[67] Gangrenous tissue sloughs to reveal a large crater that can be as deep as 0.75 cm. In its worst manifestation, the ulceration requires debridement and reconstructive surgery.[1]

If sufficient venom is injected the bite of the brown recluse also produces systemic reactions, although these reactions are rare.[66,68] In these instances, within 72 to 96 hours, patients experience any combination of fever, chills, headaches, malaise, joint and muscle tenderness, gastrointestinal distress, rash, hepatic and pancreatic inflammation, hemolytic anemia, thrombocytopenia, and disseminated intravascular coagulation.[66] *Patients may proceed to hemoglobinuria, shock, renal failure, and death.*

Brown recluse bites are not self-treatable, and patients must be referred to an emergency room. See "A Pharmacist's Journal: Where's the Campho-Phenique?" Therapy for the bite of the brown recluse may involve corticosteroids, nitroglycerin patches, dapsone, hyperbaric oxygen, electric shock, packed red blood cells, platelets, and reconstructive surgery.[65–67,69]

While advising patients about a brown recluse bite, *pharmacists should caution against use of heat in any form. Heat worsens the prognosis by stimulating activity of an enzyme that lyses erythrocytes.*[66]

Centipedes

The centipede (*Scolopendra* species) inflicts a painful bite, possibly producing burning, bleeding, edema, and infection at the site.[70–74] There is little information available in United States publications, but in at least one case injection of a local anesthetic was required.[75] Because of the possibility of severe pain, the pharmacist should refer the patient with a centipede bite.

COMPLICATIONS OF ARTHROPOD BITES: SECONDARY INFECTION

Should an insect bite produce pruritus, the patient may be tempted to scratch the area. Unfortunately, excessive scratching can excoriate the skin. Dirt and other debris found on the fingers and beneath the nails can then cause a secondary infection of the skin.

TREATMENT OF ARTHROPOD BITES

Treatment Guidelines

As mentioned under "Treatment of Arthropod Stings" above, nonprescription products are usually labeled only for insect bites but often provide relief of insect stings. The representative nonprescription products discussed should only

A Pharmacist's Journal

"Where's the Campho-Phenique?"

A young mother accompanied by three young children asked me, "Where's the Campho-Phenique?" I asked what the mother needed the product for. (I teach students never to point out a product's location without gathering further information.) She said her child had an insect bite. I asked if it was in a location where I might look at it. The mother asked the child to sit on the counter and pulled back her pants to show me a silver-dollar sized lesion on the upper leg. The lesion was blackened and deeply necrotic. I expressed dismay at the appearance, to which the mother responded, "It really doesn't hurt her." However, as the mother said this, her daughter cringed with pain. I asked when they noticed the bite. "We went to the lake on Saturday, and I think it must have bitten her then, because I only noticed it yesterday," the woman replied. It was Tuesday, so the bite had occurred 2 to 3 days before. A necrosis that develops quickly caused me to suspect the brown recluse spider.

I urged the mother to visit the emergency room immediately, mentioning the possibility that the child might require reconstructive surgery and stressing that time was of the essence in treating a brown recluse bite. The following day, I phoned the emergency room, but discovered no record of her visit. I then phoned the family at home and determined that she had an appointment later in the day. In a follow-up phone call to the mother, I learned that the physician had diagnosed dermonecrosis due to a brown recluse bite. The physician had prescribed an oral antibiotic and pain medication and had mentioned that the child might require surgical correction for disfigurement. Then the mother said, "You know, I've got three kids. This is the first time that a pharmacist cared enough to call me at home. I really appreciate your concern."

The end of the story came several months later when the family returned to the store, and I asked the mother how the daughter was. The mother appeared confused at first but when I reminded her about the spider bite, she asked her daughter to jump up on the counter again. The bite had healed so well that there was no residual evidence of a lesion. I often shudder to think what the outcome might have been if the mother had actually poured a nonprescription product containing camphor and phenol on a necrotic lesion—perhaps deep chemical burns and irreversible scarring.

---

be used for minor stings and bites and when there is no evidence of anaphylaxis. Pharmacists should refer patients for immediate care for any bites that appear serious (e.g., spider bites). (See Patient Assessment Algorithm 30.2.)

Nonprescription Medications

EXTERNAL ANALGESICS
External analgesics are a diverse group of ingredients. Products containing these ingredients should carry this label: "For the temporary relief of pain and itching caused by insect bites." Product labels also warn that the product is for external use only, that contact with the eyes should be avoided, and that the product should not be used on children younger than 2. Further, *if the condition worsens, or if symptoms persist for more than 7 days or clear up and recur within a few days, the patient should discontinue use of the product and consult a physician.*[76–78] All products are approved for use up to 3 to 4 times daily.

Counterirritants
Counterirritant external analgesics, safe and effective when used as directed for insect bites, were discussed in Chapter 20. These products may include allyl isothiocyanate, ammonia water, methyl salicylate, turpentine oil, camphor, menthol, histamine hydrochloride, methyl nicotinate, capsaicin, and capsicum products. Table 30.1 lists several products containing counterirritants.

Topical Anesthetics
Topical anesthetics are also safe and effective when used as directed for insect bites (as well as other uses). These medications penetrate damaged skin to anesthetize pain receptors and other receptors in the skin and also to anesthetize receptors in structures immediately beneath the epithelial layers.[76] Table 30.2 lists products containing topical anesthetics.

Benzocaine 5 to 20%.   Benzocaine is one of the most widely used and safest local anesthetics.[76] Its low degree of water

Patient Assessment Algorithm 30.2. Arthropod Bites

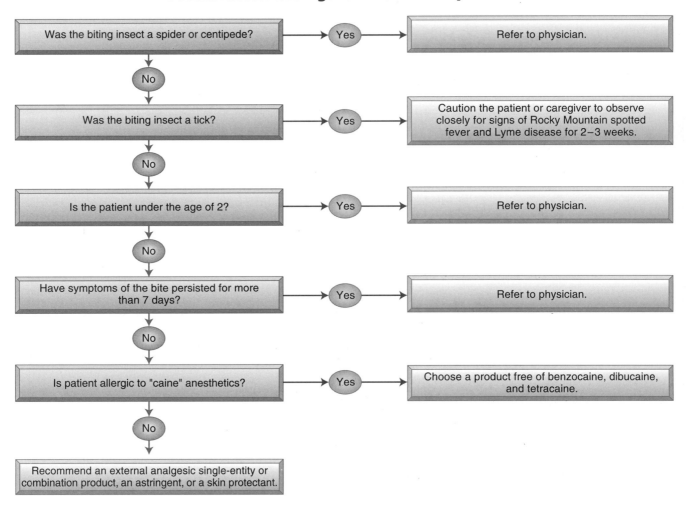

Table 30.1. Representative Products for Insect Bites/Stings That Contain Counterirritants

PRODUCT	SELECTED INGREDIENTS/COMMENTS
Aveeno Anti-Itch Cream	Calamine 3%, pramoxine HCl 1%, camphor 0.3%
Campho-Phenique Pain Relieving Antiseptic Liquid	Phenol 4.7%, camphor 10.8%, eucalyptus oil, light mineral oil
Chigarid Liquid	Camphor 2.8%, phenol 1.5%, menthol 0.1%, in collodion vehicle
Chiggerex Ointment	Benzocaine, camphor, menthol, clove oil, olive oil, peppermint oil (no concentrations labeled for any ingredient)
Dermoplast Hospital Strength Aerosol	Benzocaine 20%, menthol 0.5%
Gold Bond Medicated Anti-Itch Cream	Lidocaine, menthol (no concentration labeled for any ingredient)
Medi-Quik Aerosol	Benzalkonium chloride 0.13%, lidocaine 2%, camphor 0.2%
Rhuli Anti-Itch Gel	Benzyl alcohol 2%, menthol 0.3%, camphor 0.3%
Rhuli Calamine Spray	Benzocaine 5%, calamine 13.8%, camphor 0.7%
StingEze	Benzocaine, camphor, liquefied phenol, diphenhydramine HCl, eucalyptol (all concentrations unlabeled)
Sting-Kill Applicator	Benzocaine 20%, menthol 1%

Table 30.2. Representative Products for Insect Bites/Stings That Contain Topical Anesthetics

PRODUCT	SELECTED INGREDIENTS/COMMENTS
Americaine Aerosol	Benzocaine 20%
Aveeno Anti-Itch Cream	Calamine 3%, pramoxine HCl 1%, camphor 0.3%
Bactine First Aid	Lidocaine 2.5%, benzalkonium chloride 0.13%
Bicozene Cream	Benzocaine 6%, resorcinol 1.67%
Caladryl Lotion	Calamine 8%, pramoxine HCl 1%
Caladryl Clear Lotion	Pramoxine HCl 1%, zinc acetate 0.1%
Chiggerex Ointment	Benzocaine, camphor, menthol, clove oil, olive oil, peppermint oil (no concentrations labeled for any ingredient)
Chigger-Tox Liquid	Benzocaine, benzyl benzoate, soft soap (no concentrations labeled for any ingredient)
Dermoplast Hospital Strength Aerosol	Benzocaine 20%, menthol 0.5%
Foille Spray	Benzocaine 5%, chloroxylenol 0.6% (unapproved ingredient)
Gold Bond Medicated Anti-Itch Cream	Lidocaine, menthol (no concentration labeled for any ingredient)
Itch-X Gel	Benzyl alcohol 10%, pramoxine HCl 1%
Lanacane Cream	Benzocaine 6%, benzethonium chloride 0.2%
Lanacane Maximum Strength Cream	Benzocaine 20%, benzethonium chloride 0.2%
Medi-Quik Aerosol	Benzalkonium chloride 0.13%, lidocaine 2%, camphor 0.2%
Nupercainal Cream	Dibucaine 0.5%
Rhuli Anti-Itch Gel	Benzyl alcohol 2%, menthol 0.3%, camphor 0.3%
Rhuli Calamine Spray	Benzocaine 5%, calamine 13.8%, camphor 0.7%
Solarcaine Aerosol	Benzocaine 20%, triclosan 0.13%
StingEze	Benzocaine, camphor, liquefied phenol, diphenhydramine HCl, eucalyptol (all concentrations unlabeled)
Sting-Kill Applicator	Benzocaine 20%, menthol 1%
Unguentine Plus Cream	Lidocaine 2%, phenol 0.5%

solubility ensures that little of the product is absorbed, so the toxic reactions associated with other "caine" anesthetics (e.g., convulsions and cardiac depression) are absent. Benzocaine does cause allergic reactions in about 5% of patients, mostly minor rashes. Methemoglobinemia resulting from benzocaine ingestion is rare and seldom has significant medical consequences.[76]

Benzyl Alcohol 10 to 23%. Benzyl alcohol does not cause the "caine" toxicities and has less potential for sensitization than benzocaine.[76]

Dibucaine, Dibucaine Hydrochloride (both 0.25 to 1%). Dibucaine is a potent and long-lasting local anesthetic.[76] Dibucaine can produce the "caine" toxicities of central nervous system depression and myocardial depression if too

much is absorbed. For this reason, *products containing dibucaine must carry this precaution: "Do not use in large quantities, particularly over raw surfaces or blistered areas."*[76] Sensitization is extremely rare.

Dyclonine Hydrochloride 0.5 to 1%. Dyclonine does not share the toxicities of the "caine" anesthetics and is very low in sensitization potential.

Lidocaine 0.5 to 4%. Lidocaine does produce toxicities typical of the "caine" anesthetics, including depression leading to drowsiness, nervousness, dizziness, blurred vision, nausea, tremors, convulsions, and respiratory arrest.[76] Myocardial depression, cardiac arrest, hypotension, and intercostal paralysis are also possible. For this reason, *products containing lidocaine must carry this precaution: "Do not use in large quantities, particularly over raw surfaces or blistered areas.*[76] The sensitization potential of lidocaine is lower than benzocaine.

Pramoxine 0.5 to 1%.   Pramoxine does not share the toxicities of the "caine" anesthetics; sensitization is possible, but rare.[76]

Tetracaine, Tetracaine Hydrochloride (both 1 to 2%). Tetracaine and its hydrochloride salt cause greater myocardial depression than other "caine" anesthetics because its detoxification is slower than other local anesthetics. For this (tip) reason, *products containing tetracaine must carry this precaution: "Do not use in large quantities, particularly over raw surfaces or blistered areas.*[76]

Topical Antihistamines

Topical antihistamines also depress cutaneous receptors for pain and itch. Table 30.3 lists products containing topical antihistamines.

Diphenhydramine Hydrochloride 1 to 2%.   Diphenhydramine has topical anesthetic properties that are useful in insect bites.[76]

Hydrocortisone, Hydrocortisone Acetate 0.25 to 1%

Hydrocortisone has antipruritic and antiinflammatory effects that benefit many skin conditions.[76,77,79] The potential for sensitivity or irritation with hydrocortisone is virtually nonexistent. (When hydrocortisone was originally evaluated for nonprescription status, the various agencies that examined its potential for toxic effect concluded that the probability of adverse reactions such as aggravation of infections and striae formation was much lower than with stronger prescription (tip) corticosteroids.[76]) *Products containing hydrocortisone should include a special warning that differs slightly from the external analgesic warning: "If condition worsens or if symptoms persist for more than 7 days or clear up and occur again within a few days, stop use of this product and do not begin use of any other hydrocortisone product unless you have consulted a physician."*[80] Products containing hydrocortisone are listed in Table 30.4.

Phenol, Sodium Phenolate (Both 0.5 and 2%)

Phenol depresses cutaneous receptors, but it can cause (tip) sloughing of tissue in certain conditions. *Products containing phenol must carry this warning: "Do not apply this product to large areas of the body or bandage.*[76,77] This warning is not required for phenolate sodium, however, since it does not have the irritation potential of phenol. Products containing phenol are listed in Table 30.1.

Resorcinol 0.5 to 3%

Resorcinol, also known as resorcin, depresses cutaneous sensory receptors. It can be toxic when ingested or if too much (tip) is applied to the skin. For this reason, *products containing resorcinol must carry this warning: "Do not apply this product to large areas of the body."* Products containing resorcinol are listed in Table 30.2.

Other External Analgesics

Other approved external analgesics that are not currently in widely sold products include camphorated metacresol; the local anesthetics butamben picrate, dimethisoquin hydrochloride, and the antihistamine tripelennamine; and the natural product juniper tar.

COMBINATIONS

The FDA allows combinations of certain external analgesics, as follows:

- "Caine" anesthetics may be combined with alcohol-ketone ingredients (e.g., benzyl alcohol, camphor, camphorated metacresol, juniper tar, menthol, phenol, phenolate sodium, and resorcinol).
- Alcohol-ketone ingredients may be combined with the antihistamines.
- Any two, three, or four counterirritants may be combined, as long as the product does not contain more than one ingredient from any category (e.g., those that produce redness [allyl isothiocyanate, strong ammonia solution, methyl salicylate, turpentine oil]; those that cool [camphor, menthol]; those that vasodilate [histamine HCl, methyl nicotinate]; and those that do not produce redness

Table 30.3. Representative Products for Insect Bites/Stings That Contain Topical Antihistamines	
PRODUCT	SELECTED INGREDIENTS/COMMENTS
Benadryl Itch Stopping Cream	Diphenhydramine HCl 1%, zinc acetate 0.1%
Benadryl Extra Strength Itch Stopping Cream	Diphenhdyramine HCl 2%, zinc acetate 0.1%
Benadryl Itch Stopping Gel	Diphenhydramine HCl 2%, zinc acetate 1%
Benadryl Original Strength Itch Stopping Spray	Diphenhdyramine HCl 1%, zinc acetate 0.1%
Benadryl Extra Strength Itch Stopping Spray	Diphenhdyramine HCl 2%, zinc acetate 0.1%
Benadryl Extra Strength Itch Stopping Stick	Diphenhdyramine HCl 2%, zinc acetate 0.1%
StingEze	Benzocaine, camphor, liquefied phenol, diphenhydramine HCl, eucalyptol (all concentrations unlabeled)

[capsaicin, capsicum, capsicum oleoresin]); however, certain exceptions are allowed (see below).

- Camphor and menthol may be combined with benzyl alcohol, juniper tar, phenol, phenolate sodium, or resorcinol.
- Camphor and phenol may be combined in a light mineral oil vehicle.
- Camphor may be combined with menthol.
- Camphor and menthol may be combined with any one, two, or three ingredients as long as there is no more than one ingredient from each group present.

Table 30.4. Representative Products for Insect Bites/Stings That Contain Hydrocortisone

PRODUCT	SELECTED INGREDIENTS
Caldecort Anti-Itch Cream	Hydrocortisone 1%
Cortaid Cream	Hydrocortisone 0.5%
Cortaid Intensive Therapy Cream	Hydrocortisone 1%
Cortaid Maximum Strength Cream	Hydrocortisone 1%
Cortaid Maximum Strength FastStick	Hydrocortisone 1%
Cortaid Ointment	Hydrocortisone 0.5%
Cortaid Spray	Hydrocortisone 0.5%
Cortizone•5 Cream, Ointment	Hydrocortisone 0.5%
Cortizone•10 Cream, Ointment	Hydrocortisone 1%
Cortizone for Kids Cream	Hydrocortisone 0.5%
KeriCort•10 Cream	Hydrocortisone 1%
Lanacort 10	Hydrocortisone 1%

Combination products are listed in Tables 30.1 and 30.2.

ASTRINGENTS

(tip) Astringents can provide relief from insect bites. *Astringents should not be used longer than 7 days.*[81,82] Pharmacists should advise patients to see a physician if the condition worsens or persists for longer than 7 days. Table 30.5 lists products containing astringents.

Aluminum Acetate

Aluminum acetate is used as a wet dressing, compress, or soak to relieve minor skin irritation caused by insect bites.[45,81,83] Patients should soak the area for 15 to 30 minutes, three times daily, discarding the solution after each use. Patients may also produce a compress or wet dressing by saturating a clean, soft, white cloth (e.g., a diaper or torn sheet) with the solution, gently squeeze, and apply it loosely to the affected area. The cloth should be resaturated every 15 to 30 minutes and applied as often as needed. The wet dressing or compress should not be covered with plastic to prevent evaporation.

Pharmacists should caution patients to keep aluminum acetate out of their eyes.

Witch Hazel

Witch hazel relieves the pain and swelling caused by insect bites. Patients may apply it as often as necessary.[45]

SKIN PROTECTANTS

Treatment of insect bites was not part of the original labeling recommended for skin protectants. However, the FDA proposed such labeling, amending a tentative final monograph to do so.[84] Skin protectants can relieve minor irritation and itching caused by insect bites by providing a mechanical barrier against harmful or annoying stimuli. The only skin protectants allowed to carry this labeling are sodium bicarbonate and colloidal oatmeal. Products containing skin protectants are listed in Table 30.6.

Sodium bicarbonate (baking soda) may be used by patients older than 2 using various methods:

Table 30.5. Representative Products for Insect Bites/Stings That Contain Astringents

PRODUCT	SELECTED INGREDIENTS/COMMENTS
Bluboro Powder	Aluminum sulfate 53.9%, calcium acetate 43% to form aluminum acetate in solution
Domeboro Tablets	Aluminum sulfate 878 mg, calcium acetate 604 mg per tablet to form aluminum acetate when placed in water
T.N. Dickinson's Witch Hazel	Witch hazel distilled 100%

Table 30.6. Representative Products for Insect Bites/Stings Containing Skin Protectants

PRODUCT	SELECTED INGREDIENTS
Aveeno Bath Treatment (Regular)	Colloidal oatmeal 100%
Aveeno Bath Treatment (Moisturizing)	Colloidal oatmeal 43%, mineral oil

- Paste: Add sufficient water to the powder to make a paste.
- Tub soak: Dissolve 1 to 2 cupfuls in warm water and soak for 10 to 30 minutes, then pat dry so that the layer of sodium bicarbonate remains on the skin.
- Wet dressing: Soak a cloth in a saturated solution and apply to the skin as needed, resaturating the cloth every 15 to 30 minutes.

Colloidal oatmeal may be used by patients older than 2 using the following technique:

- Turn on the warm tap in the bathtub full force.
- Sprinkle 1 cup of colloidal oatmeal slowly into the water directly under the faucet.
- Stir any oatmeal not suspended.

tip *Pharmacists should caution patients to be careful when entering and exiting the tub since the oatmeal will make the bottom of the tub slippery.* Patients should soak for 15 to 20 minutes once or twice daily as needed, patting the skin rather than rubbing it dry to allow a thin layer of the active ingredient to remain on the skin.

SKIN ANTISEPTICS

Some products labeled for insect bites contain antiseptics (e.g., benzalkonium chloride or benzethonium chloride) or chemicals with reputed antiseptic effect (e.g., chloroxylenol). However, the labeling of topical antiseptics does not include prevention of infection in insect bites.[85]

ARTHROPOD BITE NEUTRALIZERS

FDA investigators have determined that insect bite neutralizers are ineffective.[45] One such product that was advertised for this purpose contains ammonium hydroxide, which is ineffective as a venom neutralizer.

PREVENTION OF ARTHROPOD BITES

Tips for prevention of arthropod bites are specific, depending on the particular arthropod, its habitat, and living habits. For instance, pharmacists should inform patients to take the following commonsense steps to avoid tick bites when in woods and grasslands[53]:

- Wear long pants and tuck them into socks to prevent ticks from contacting skin.
- Wear long-sleeved shirts with tight wrist closures.
- Wear shoes that cover the entire foot.

n,n-Diethyl-*m*-toluamide (DEET)

The insect repellent *n,n*-Diethyl-*m*-toluamide (DEET) will repel mosquitoes, ticks, and chiggers, as well as several biting flies and gnats.[47,57,86] Products containing it (listed in Table 30.7) are regulated by the Environmental Protection Agency, under the auspices of the 1972 Federal Environmental Pesticide Control Act.[57]

While DEET is safe for the majority of users, pharmacists should advise patients to follow the following guidelines to minimize toxicity[57,87]:

- Use DEET sparingly.
- Do not apply DEET more often than every 4 to 8 hours (or as directed on the package).
- Avoid frequent total-body applications.
- Avoid swimming, sweating, and toweling the skin, which remove DEET.
- Do not inhale DEET.
- Do not apply DEET around the eyes.
- Do not apply DEET to parts of the hands likely to enter the mouth (e.g., the hands or thumbs of a toddler).
- Do not apply DEET to cuts or abrasions.
- Wash off DEET soon after coming indoors.
- Do not apply DEET under a diaper, since the moisture could enhance absorption.

⚠ Adverse reactions to DEET, which are rare, usually involve skin and eye irritation.[57,88,89] *Excessive application to children has produced central-nervous-system reactions such as toxic encephalopathy, seizures, confusion, irritability, and insomnia, and oral ingestion has caused death.*[57,90–93]

Table 30.7. Representative Insect Repellents

PRODUCT	SELECTED INGREDIENTS/COMMENTS
Cutter Stick	30% DEET
Cutter Outdoorsman Aerosol, Stick, Lotion	28.5% DEET
Deep Woods Off! for Sportsmen Pump Spray	100% DEET
Deep Woods Off! for Sportsmen Aerosol	28.5% DEET
Permanone Repel Tick & Mosquito	Permethrin 0.5% (to be applied to clothing only)
Repel Family Formula Aerosol	33.25% DEET
Repel Sportsmen Formula Insect Block 20	19% DEET
Repel Sportsmen Formula Insect Block 29	27.5% DEET

ORAL THIAMIN

Oral thiamin has been evaluated by the FDA for effectiveness as an oral insect repellent, but the efficacy has not been verified. Oral thiamin was placed in Category II for this use.[94–96]

PEDICULOSIS

The louse is an obligate parasite that depends on frequent blood meals for survival.[97,98] Each species of mammal is said to have its own distinct type of louse. Three species of louse prey on the human: the head louse (*Pediculus humanus* var. *capitis*), the body louse (*Pediculus humanus,* var. *corporis*), and the pubic (crab) louse (*Phthirus pubis*)[99,100] (Fig. 30.7).

PREVALENCE OF PEDICULOSIS

During recent decades, pediculosis rates have increased steadily in the United States. In particular, head lice are second only to the common cold in incidence in children; in children, head lice are more prevalent than all other childhood communicable diseases combined.[101] An estimated 6 to 12 million Americans are infested with head lice at any one time.[102,103]

Pubic lice is not a reportable disease, but is one of the most common sexually transmitted diseases.[104]

EPIDEMIOLOGY OF PEDICULOSIS

Epidemiology of Head Lice

As late as the mid 1980s, head lice was considered to be a malady of people who were unclean or poor. Neither income nor cleanliness are considered to be factors in the United

States now, however.[47,99] There is an age stratification. Children are more likely to be affected with head lice than adults, with preschoolers at the highest risk. Females are also at greater risk than males—possibly because boys engage in less "dress-up" play than girls (which often includes sharing of hats and brushes).[99]

Blacks in the United States apparently have infestation rates that are extremely low.[47] In one study, only one black child was found to have head lice out of 4271 children studied.[101] This may be because the predominant United States head louse varieties evolved to grasp the cylindrical European hair.[97] Thus they are unable to grasp tightly curled hair or hair that has the oval cross-sectional shape of African-American hair.[99] By contrast, head lice found in Africa have adapted to the characteristics of the hair of the indigenous populations; accordingly, whites have low infestation rates in Africa. Hispanics or American Indians living in the United States appear to be as prone to contract head lice as whites.[101]

Epidemiology of Pubic Lice

The pubic or crab louse is found on those who are sexually active, unless it is spread to casual contacts through sharing a toilet seat, bed or clothing. Pubic lice infestations most commonly affect women aged 15 to 19 and males aged 20 and over and is commonly spread in jails and brothels.[99,105]

Epidemiology of Body Lice

Unlike head lice and pubic lice, body lice do not live on the skin or in the hair, but instead live in clothing.[47] Body lice are only found on the skin when they require a blood meal from the host; thus, their hosts generally are people who cannot shower and change clothing frequently (e.g., street people and homeless people). The eradication of body lice is simple: change clothing daily and treat infested clothing by boiling or ironing.[47]

Because pharmacists seldom encounter patients with body lice, the discussion in this section focuses on head and pubic lice.

ETIOLOGY OF PEDICULOSIS

As noted in the introduction to pediculosis, the etiologic agents of this condition are insects of three species. Figure 30.8 shows the life cycle of lice that prey on humans. The female louse can lay 8 to 12 eggs daily throughout her life span of 17 to 22 days, cementing them to the host's hair (or clothing in the case of the body louse) with an extremely strong glue (Fig. 30.9).[47]

In the case of the head louse, the 1 mm egg is generally laid next to the scalp, at the scalp/hair-shaft junction, where warmed by body heat it will hatch within 6 to 9 days.[99] Since hair grows an average of 0.35 mm per day, the distance of the egg case from the scalp gives a rough estimate of when the egg was laid. If the ambient air is warm enough, however,

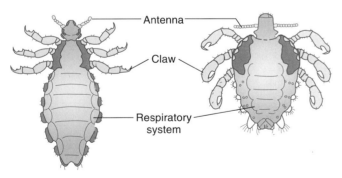

Pediculus humanus
• *Capitis* (head louse)
• *Humanus* (body louse)

Phthirus pubis
(crab or pubic louse)

Figure 30.7. The two anatomically distinct varieties of human lice: **1.** *Pediculus humanus* variety: *capitis* (head louse) and *Pediculus humanus* variety: *corporis* (body louse) are the same species. **2.** *Phthirus pubis* (crab or pubic louse) is a different species from the head and body louse.

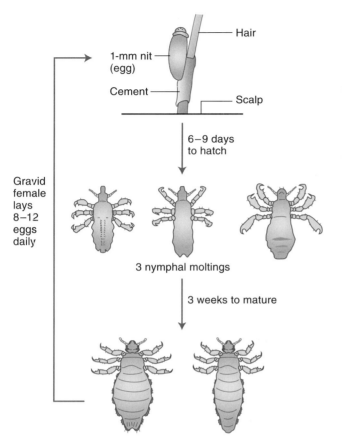

Figure 30.8. Life cycle of the head louse.

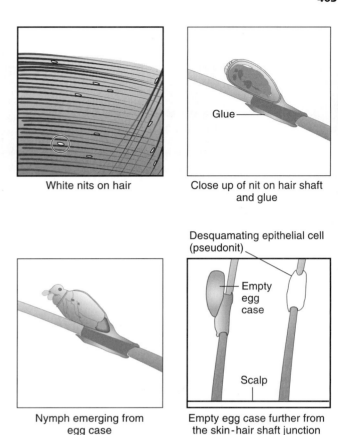

Figure 30.9. **1.** Nits on hair. **2.** Close-up of nit on hair shaft. **3.** Nymph emerging from egg case. **4.** Empty egg case located further from the skin-hair shaft junction, next to hair cast (pseudonit).

the **gravid** (pregnant) female may lay several eggs along the hair shaft.[99] After emerging from the egg, the nymph feeds on the host five to six times daily, undergoing three molts to arrive at the final adult stage—approximately 2 to 4 mm.[100,106] The female louse is able to mate shortly after undergoing her final molting (see Fig. 30.8).[99]

TRANSMISSION OF LICE

Transmission of Head Lice

Head lice are transmitted either by direct contact with the head of an infested individual or through **fomites** (inanimate objects capable of transmitting diseases).[47] Sharing combs, brushes, and head wear, for example, are common transmission routes.[107] Head lice do not have wings and thus cannot fly, nor can they jump from host to host.[102]

Transmission of Pubic Lice

The pubic louse is often transmitted during sexual activity, being therefore classified as a venereal disease.[108] This species of louse has large claws on the middle and hind legs, which permit it to grasp two or more of the more widely spaced pubic hairs.[99,109] However, the insect is also transmitted by fomites (e.g., by sharing the bed or the toilet seat with an infected person).[109] (See "A Pharmacist's Journal: But I Haven't Been with a Girl in Two Years!")

Pubic lice are also found in the hair on the trunk, arms, and legs and in the beard, eyebrows, and eyelashes, in addition to pubic hair.[99]

MANIFESTATIONS OF PEDICULOSIS

Manifestations of Head Louse Infestation

Head lice epidemics are more common at certain times of the year such as late August to early September (after school starts), after prolonged school holidays (e.g., Christmas and Easter), and summer (because of summer camps).[110] Pharmacists may be asked to inspect the heads of individual patients or may be called on to participate in a public-health screening.

Since head louse infestations are often asymptomatic, the gold standard for confirmation of head louse infestation is to see live lice. It is often difficult to locate the flat, gray-brown adult lice, however, since there may only be a few on the individual's head.[99,106] (The ratio of nymphs to adult females is 6:1.) In a survey, 50% of pediatric nurses and physicians had never seen a louse.[97] To check for head lice, a simple set of steps can be followed:

A Pharmacist's Journal

"But I Haven't Been with a Girl in Two Years!"

A young man asked me about products for lice. As we talked, it became apparent that he was describing a case of pubic lice. I mentioned that his sexual contact should also be treated. He said in an anguished voice, "I just can't understand that. I haven't been with a girl for two years. How could I have gotten them?" I in-

formed him about the remote possibility of transfer by fomites. He thought for a second and replied, "You know, I work at a gas station, and I have to use the customer rest rooms. People are always in and out. Could that be how I got them?" I assured him that it was a possibility, and stressed that in any case, prompt treatment would eradicate the infestation.

- The hair must be parted carefully with a wooden paddle or the fingers (while wearing gloves). At the slightest sign of disruption of the hair (perceived by proprioceptors on the insects' legs), the adult louse rapidly moves to deeper hair at a rate of 12 inches/minute, making it difficult to verify the species.[97,99]
- Use of a detection comb with teeth spaced no farther than 0.33 mm apart can aid identification, as it combs out even the smallest newly hatched nymphs.[97]
- When inspecting for lice, the pharmacist must concentrate on the hottest areas of the scalp: the crown, over the ears, and on the lower neck.

Because of the difficulty of finding live lice, it may be more realistic to examine the hair for the presence of attached nits or inspect the scalp for signs of lice.[111] As noted above, lice bite the host to feed five to six times daily, injecting an anticoagulant and an anesthetic and leaving small, red maculopapular or bullous lesions.[47,48,110,112] When bites are located, they appear as papules with a central puncture mark, since the saliva and chemicals injected with each bite stimulate an allergic response. Scratching with unclean fingernails in an attempt to relieve the pruritus can cause secondary infection, with possible impetigo.[97,113] In addition, the powdered feces of head lice may appear as black dust on collars or pillows.[99] (Perspiration inside the collar may reduce the powder to blackish smears.) Pharmacists should ask about the most prominent symptom, scalp pruritus, if inspection is impossible or unfeasible.[97]

With continued, untreated louse infestations, increasing amounts of salivary protein are injected as the lice feed. Patients may suffer a generalized allergic reaction to this protein, manifested by such problems as regional lymphadenopathy of the posterior cervical or occipital nodes, a rise in body temperature, generalized and diffuse allergic rash in noninfested areas, headache, limb heaviness, muscle stiffness, and general lassitude.[99,112]

VIABILITY OF OVA

As mentioned, eggs on the hair are an obvious clue to the presence of head lice (see Fig. 30.9). Whether the eggs are viable or not is crucial. When a nymph hatches from its egg, the empty egg case remains attached to the hair. Although it remains on the head, it is only an indication of a past infection. The egg that is viable is fully capable of causing a new infestation or prolonging the current one. The empty egg case is a white oval speck that stands out from the background hair color, while a viable egg case blends in with the color of hair, making it more difficult to see.[99] Unfortunately, it is difficult for even a trained medical professional to tell the difference between viable and nonviable nits using the naked eye. A microscope provides the magnification necessary to easily differentiate the empty nit from the viable one.

PSEUDONITS

When inspecting patients' hair, pharmacists must be alert to the presence of pseudonits. Many objects in the hair can resemble a nit such as hair spray residue, dandruff, windblown sand, or plant debris. Most of these objects can be easily flicked away with the finger, while the louse egg will remain firmly attached. However, some patients have cylindrical material attached to the hair known as desquamated epithelial cells that is not easily removed (see Fig. 30.9). Unlike nits, this material will slide along the hair shaft if pulled.[99] Pharmacists must learn how to differentiate these pseudonits from nits to prevent unnecessary application of pediculicide.[99]

Manifestations of Pubic Louse Infestation

The pubic louse, which is shorter and wider than the head louse, infests hair in the groin, lower abdomen, thighs, eyelashes, and axilla.[47,110,114] See "A Pharmacist's Journal: Can I Put Someone Who Has Crabs in Jail?" Pruritus of the affected areas is the most common symptom.[109] When an infestation is long-standing or severe, patients may experience

A Pharmacist's Journal

"Can I Put Someone Who Has Crabs in Jail?"

I answered the phone one night to hear a female ask in an angry tone of voice, "How can I tell if someone has crabs?" I described the look of the insect and its residue, but she wasn't satisfied with that answer. "I mean, if I meet someone, how can I tell if they have crabs?" I replied that there is no way to tell just by looking at someone that they have crabs. She continued, "Well, what can I do to someone who has crabs?" I began to describe the treatment options, but she interrupted again, "I mean, can I put someone who has crabs in jail?" I was rather perplexed by the question, but informed her that it is not a criminal act to have pubic lice or to spread them to someone else, but it would be an act of kindness to inform

him of her problem so that he might treat himself. Apparently, she was extremely upset that a casual contact with whom she had sexual activity had given her pubic lice. Once she discovered that he could not be punished, she asked how to treat the problem. It took more than five minutes to describe the roles of combs and nonprescription products. She then asked, "How long will you be there?" I told her I would be at the store until closing. She said, "I'll have on a yellow jumpsuit. Please just sell me all of the things you would recommend, get them in a plain paper bag, and get me out of the store quickly." When she came in later, I was able to quietly point out the products and answer a few of her remaining questions before I rang up her products.

painless subcutaneous blue-colored macules (maculae cerulae) on the abdomen, thighs, or thorax, apparently caused by a reaction of blood cells to salivary protein.[47,99,115] Also, crab louse feces produce rust, red, or black stains on the underwear.[99] Finally, the patient with pubic lice has usually contracted the infestation through sexual activity, so the risk of other sexually transmitted disease is high.[116,117] The patient may also have a heightened risk of cervical cancer.[118]

SPECIFIC CONSIDERATIONS OF PEDICULOSIS: SOCIAL IMPLICATIONS

Louse infestation is a social stigma for patients and other family members. Some patients attempt to enter the pharmacy surreptitiously, hoping to purchase lice-treatment products without detection. Unfortunately, patients who do not ask for assistance miss the counseling that is necessary to ensure that the products are used safely and effectively. Although pediculosis is common in all socioeconomic groups, there remains a feeling that head lice happens to other people, especially those who are unclean. For many people, a family member with lice indicates a failure on the part of the family to adequately control their hygiene. Pharmacists must acknowledge the patient's (or family members') embarrassment, then advise them of these important facts:

- Head lice are found in people from all social and economic groups.

- It should not be embarrassing to catch head lice.
- Responsible patients (or caregivers) must treat the problem so they (or the patient) will not be a source of reinfestation for friends, relatives, fellow students, and/or coworkers.
- It is vital to inform the child's school or play group and parents of the child's friends of the infestation.[119]
- Nonprescription products can eradicate the problem if used correctly.

A cautionary note about pubic lice is in order. When a child is found to be infested with pubic lice, the possibility of sexual abuse by a parent or caregiver must be considered. In one case, a 6-week-old child was found to have pubic lice on the scalp, which may have been caused by this type of situation.[120]

COMPLICATIONS OF PEDICULOSIS: SECONDARY INFECTION

The patient affected with head lice may scratch the scalp to the point of excoriating the skin. Organisms on the hands and under the fingernails can cause secondary infections.

TREATMENT OF PEDICULOSIS

Treatment Guidelines

Pediculosis is a condition that usually is completely curable with nonprescription products. The exceptions include patients with allergies to the nonprescription ingredients and those with lice resistant to the nonprescription ingredients. In these cases, the patient should be referred to the physician for a prescription product such as lindane or malathion:

- Lindane was available as a well-known, trade-named, prescription product (Kwell) for decades for head and crab lice, but those products have been discontinued by the manufacturer. (Generic versions are still available, however.) This prescription ingredient has caused a great deal of concern about possible central nervous system toxicity, blood disorders, and hepatic and renal toxicities.[121] One woman who misused a small amount experienced uncontrolled motor activity.[122] Also, lice have developed resistance to it.
- Malathion is a prescription ingredient for head and crab lice that is somewhat safer than lindane, although its alcoholic vehicle can be irritating to the scalp and is flammable. Available as Ovide, it was also discontinued by the manufacturer, although it may be reintroduced at a future time.

When patients require treatment with either nonprescription or prescription products, pharmacists should also point out the dangers of pesticide sprays and discuss safe alternatives for ridding the environment of lice such as vacuuming and isolating objects in plastic bags. Nit-removal aids—such as nit combs and enzymatic products—should also be discussed with the patient (Fig. 30.10). (See "Patient Assessment Algorithm 30.3 and "Nonpharmacologic Therapies.")

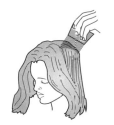

Insert nit comb as
close to scalp as possible.

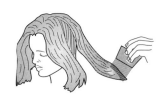

Pull comb firmly away from
scalp to ends of hair.

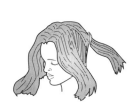

Pin back hair strands after
treatment; continue on all strands.

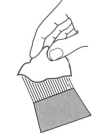

Wipe nit comb with a tissue
after combing each strand.

Figure 30.10. Steps in using nit comb to remove nits.

Nonprescription Medications

Lice products are not prophylactic agents, do not act as louse repellents, and must not be used to prevent a louse infestation.[106,110] Indeed, some lack residual activity so that they would be ineffective as preventive agents. Nonprescription lice products should only be recommended when pharmacists are assured that a patient has an active infestation (Table 30.8). Accordingly, *pharmacists must carefully counsel families and living groups in which one member has a confirmed louse infestation. For example, although fully 50% of head lice patients have at least one other family member with the condition, other family (or living group) members must be carefully inspected to confirm an infestation before treating to prevent unnecessary exposure to chemicals.*[101] Pharmacists should advise other family (or living group) members to be alert for signs of pediculosis, but to withhold treatment until an infestation is confirmed.

SYNERGIZED PYRETHRINS

Pyrethrins are natural chemicals derived from plants such as the *Chrysanthemum*.[99,123] To be effective, the pyrethrins are synergized by the addition of piperonyl butoxide, a petroleum derivative.[99] The synergist inhibits the oxidative breakdown of the pyrethrin by the detoxification systems of lice, in turn killing the lice.[123] *Patients allergic to* Chrysanthemum *plants or to ragweed may have allergies to pyrethrin.*[99] The combination of pyrethrins and piperonyl butoxide is effective for either head or pubic lice.

Pharmacists should counsel patients and caregivers to follow the directions for the use of nonprescription synergized pyrethrins exactly to ensure efficacy:

- If the product label advises shampooing the hair before application of the product, the patient should wash the hair with a mild shampoo and dry the hair.
- If the lice-treatment product is a shampoo, patients should apply to dry hair until the hair is thoroughly wet, then wait 10 minutes.[124]
- Sufficient warm water should be added to make a lather, and the hair should be thoroughly rinsed.
- If the lice-treatment product is not a shampoo, the patient should apply it to the head as a shampoo, but then use a mild shampoo or soap to clear the product from the hair.

After either treatment, a lice/nit comb should be used to remove dead lice and nits. *Since no product is 100% ovicidal, another treatment in 7 to 10 days is mandatory to kill newly hatched nits before they can perpetuate the infestation.* There is no specific age cutoff for use of synergized pyrethrins, but the general age cutoff of 2 years applies.

The FDA requires several labeling precautions for nonprescription lice-treatment products[124]:

- Patients must keep the product away from mucous membranes (e.g., inside the nose, mouth, and vagina).
- Patients must avoid the eyes when applying lice treatment to the hair by closing the eyes and not opening them un-

Patient Assessment Algorithm 30.3. **Head Lice**

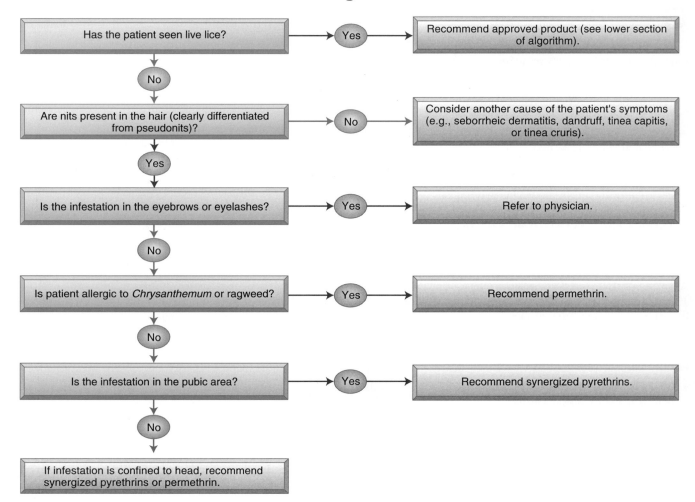

til the product is thoroughly rinsed out and by protecting children's eyes with a washcloth or towel. If the product enters the eyes, patients should flush them immediately with water.

- Should skin irritation or infection exist or develop, patients should not use the product, but see a physician.
- If the infestation is in the eyebrows or eyelashes, a physician should be consulted. Lice in the eyelashes are especially difficult to treat, since pediculicides must be kept away from the eyes. For this reason, some authorities recommend application of petrolatum (e.g., Vaseline) hourly to the eyebrows or eyelashes for 8 days, after which time the nits can be plucked off.[125]

PERMETHRIN

Permethrin is a synthetic chemical derived from pyrethrins. Following application and removal, a residual is left on the hair that enhances its activity.[99] Permethrin is only approved for treating head lice, since its efficacy against crab lice is as low as 57%.[99] Lice resistance to this product has been reported.[126] Although its approval by the FDA was through

Table 30.8. Representative Pediculicides

PRODUCT	SELECTED INGREDIENTS/COMMENTS
A•200 Shampoo	Synergized pyrethrins
Barc Liquid	Synergized pyrethrins
End-Lice Liquid	Synergized pyrethrins
Lice-Enz Foam then Comb	Synergized pyrethrins; a foam
Nix Creme Rinse	Permethrin; not effective for pubic lice
Pronto Concentrate	Synergized pyrethrins
R&C Shampoo	Synergized pyrethrins
Rid Shampoo	Synergized pyrethrins
Triple X Shampoo	Synergized pyrethrins

switching from prescription status, its labeling is quite close to that of the permethrins. *Permethrin should not be used on children younger than 2 months.*

Nonpharmacologic Therapies

Some parents and caregivers react to head lice by shaving their child's head.[127] While this will certainly eliminate head lice, it is unnecessary. The pharmacist can suggest treatments that allow the child to retain his dignity, without appearing abnormal or marked.

Likewise, some patients react to pubic lice by shaving the entire groin. Most patients miss the hair in hard-to-reach areas of the groin, however, making this intervention ineffective.

Patients must avoid home remedies that present dangers to the patient—and whose effectiveness is unknown. (See "Dangerous/Ineffective Treatments of Pediculosis.")

AREA TREATMENT

There are few live lice in the environment. While some authorities recommend use of environmental sprays (such as those listed in Table 30.9) on floors, carpets, furniture, and bedding, pharmacists should discourage the use of these products for two reasons[110]:

- Their safety for humans with this use is questionable. (One can imagine an overzealous parent saturating a mattress and pillow, and a child later sleeping on pesticide-saturated bedding.)
- The environment is not heavily contaminated with either live lice or nits.

As an alternative, thorough vacuuming should be effective in removing the few lice actually present.[97]

FOMITE TREATMENT

When treating a head lice infestation, all clothes, towels, and bed linens should be washed on the hot cycle then dried on the heated-air cycle for at least 20 minutes.[97,124] (Lice and nits cannot live through heat of this magnitude.) *Any clothing that should not be washed (e.g., hats) and items that cannot be washed (e.g., some stuffed animals) should be sealed in a plastic bag for 2 weeks.* (During this time, the adult lice will die, and all viable nits will hatch and expire without access to a blood meal.) Combs and brushes should be cleaned in hot water of at least 130°F for 5 to 10 minutes.[102]

When treating a pubic lice infestation, underwear should be washed as described above.[124] Simple fomite treatment for body lice consists of washing the patient's clothes.[128]

NIT REMOVAL

Total nit removal refers to efforts by the parent, caregiver, or helper to remove each hair to which a nit is attached. In the United States, "nit" refers to an egg that is either viable (unhatched) or nonviable (hatched).[129] (In the United Kingdom, the term "nit" refers only to an empty egg case, but this text will use the term to refer to either viable or nonviable egg cases.) Total nit removal has three objectives:

- Total nit removal is an important method to augment the efficacy of louse treatments, since no nonprescription product is 100% ovicidal (penetrates 100% of the ova to render them nonviable). An effective treatment kills all adult lice, but viable eggs invariably remain. Although the products suggest a second treatment, if it is delayed or neglected, the cycle of louse reinfestation can begin again, with possible spread to other hosts. Therefore judicious use of lice treatments, coupled with total nit removal, is necessary to assure that the infestation is stopped.
- Total nit removal will make it unlikely that nonviable nits will be discovered days, weeks, or months after treatment, raising the suspicion of reinfestation. The result might be another round of exposure to pediculicides. Complete removal of all nits would have prevented this confusion.
- Total nit removal also enhances patients' appearance and self-esteem.

To remove all nits, the patients' hair must be examined closely under a bright light. Each hair to which a nit is attached should be cut with scissors below the location to which the nit is cemented or plucked (if the nit is too close to the scalp). Unfortunately, complete hair examination can take many hours.[99]

To reduce the spread of lice, many schools have adopted a "No Nit" policy, under which schoolchildren with louse infestations are not permitted to return to class until their hair is free of nits.[101] Pharmacists can assist patients and caregivers by describing the various nit-removal aids.

FOCUS ON...

DANGEROUS/INEFFECTIVE TREATMENTS OF PEDICULOSIS

Gasoline and kerosene are sometimes used by uninformed laymen to treat pediculosis, often with deadly results.[99,127] Serious burns and even death have resulted when gasoline has been applied to patients—often young children.

Patients, parents, or caregivers might resort to this dangerous practice for a number of reasons—they do not recognize the danger, they do not know any alternatives, or they are embarrassed to seek medical advice from a pharmacist. Since pharmacists are unable to intervene directly prior to the use of these dangerous substances, it is wise for pharmacists to place a brief note in the local paper at the beginning of the primary head lice season (late August) to warn people against the use of gasoline and kerosene.

Some parents may resort to use of garden pesticides, veterinary pediculicides, or industrial-strength chemicals such as diazinon. All carry a serious potential for toxicity and death.

Table 30.9. Representative Environmental Pediculicides and Kits	
PRODUCT	SELECTED INGREDIENTS/COMMENTS
A•200 Lice Control Spray	Permethrin 0.5%
Pronto Complete Lice Killing System	Box includes shampoo, nit comb, gloves, creme rinse, magnifying glass, environmental spray
Rid Lice Control Spray	Permethrin 0.5%
Rid Lice Elimination Kit	Box includes shampoo, nit comb, environmental spray

Nit Combs

A traditional hair grooming comb is not effective in removing nits because the teeth are spaced too far apart.[129] Most packages of lice products include a small plastic or metal comb known as a nit comb. The closely spaced teeth of the comb are supposedly adequate for the removal of dead adult lice. However, their ability to remove nits attached to the head is questionable at best since their teeth must be spaced so closely that they allow hair to pass but deny passage to a nit attached to the hair (see Fig. 30.10). An excellent comb available from the National Pediculosis Association (the LiceMeister) achieves better nit removal than standard combs.

Formic-Acid Nit-Removal Aid

Vinegar (dilute acetic acid) was a popular nit-removal aid for many years, but its use can cause chemical burns of the face and eyes.[130] Step 2, a commercially available product containing formic acid, is safer than vinegar but works on the same principle. Like vinegar, Step 2 helps dissolve the chitin forming the glue that attaches the nit to the hair. The pharmacist may recommend its careful use followed by use of a nit-removal comb such as the LiceMeister. See "The National Pediculosis Association."

Enzymatic Nit-Removal Aid

Clear, a product containing oxidoreductases, transferases, hydrolases, lyases, isomerases, and ligases, attacks the specific components of the chemical glue binding the nit to the hair.

PREVENTION OF PEDICULOSIS

Prevention of head louse infestation is facilitated by following several commonsense guidelines:

- Never share hats, combs, baseball helmets, scarves, brushes, radio or computer earphones, pillows, or other objects that have touched the hair of another person.
- Be cautious in allowing the head to contact any object where another's head has been (e.g., seat backs in planes or busses).
- Keep coats, hats, and other personal objects separated from those of others.
- If possible, keep one's possessions (e.g., coats, hats, combs) in a separate locker at work or school.
- Arrange for children to sleep separately, if possible.
- Check children often. If live lice are found on a child's head, treat immediately to prevent transfer to other family members.
- Avoid games that involve head-to-head or head-to-body contact such as wrestling.

Prevention of pubic lice may be facilitated by following these guidelines:

- Avoid sexual activity with those who have other partners.
- Avoid sharing towels, washcloths, or any other object that may have contacted another's pubic area.
- Avoid public restrooms whenever possible. If this cannot be avoided, carry disposable alcohol swabs to disinfect the toilet seat or use a disposable paper liner.

If louse infestation occurs, use nonprescription products as indicated, with a second treatment when recommended to avoid reinfestation. Practice total nit removal to prevent reinfestation.

For additional information, see "The National Pediculosis Association."

SCABIES

The mite *Sarcoptes scabiei* burrows beneath the skin by producing a chemical that dissolves stratum corneum. Except

FOCUS ON...

THE NATIONAL PEDICULOSIS ASSOCIATION

An excellent resource for health care professionals is the National Pediculosis Association (P.O. Box 610189, Newton MA, 02161; 617–449-NITS), which maintains a storehouse of unbiased information. A minimal membership fee brings the pharmacist into contact with a network of concerned professionals able to provide such services as examination aids for head lice and a video lending library. They may also be contacted at www.head-lice.org.

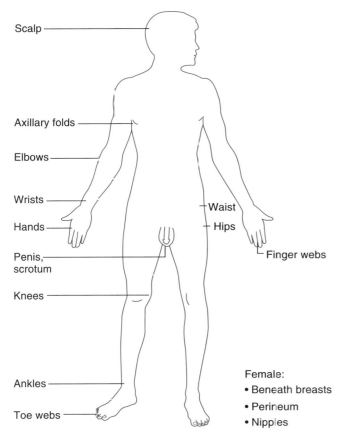

Scalp

Axillary folds

Elbows

Wrists

Hands

Penis,
scrotum

Knees

Waist

Hips

Finger webs

Ankles

Toe webs

Female:
• Beneath breasts
• Perineum
• Nipples

Figure 30.11. Typical sites of scabies infestation.

for fertilization, which occurs on the skin surface, the entire life cycle occurs beneath the skin. Eggs, which are laid under the skin, hatch in 3 to 4 days and mature into adults in 10 days to 2 weeks.[47,51,115]

Scabies are usually transmitted by contacting a person or object on which the scabies mite was located, perhaps through sexual activity or sharing a bed.[109] Even frequent hugging or fondling allows the mite to be transferred.

Pharmacists may recognize scabies by several markers: pruritus (especially nocturnal) is the hallmark symptom, but it is nonspecific.[109,115] For this reason, some pharmacists look for signs of the burrow—about 1 cm long and colored bluish—caused by the feces left by the mite as it burrows. Since the burrow is only visible in 10% of patients, however, pharmacists may have better luck noting the appearance of papules, pustules, vesicles, or nodules on the skin. Scabies mites favor the hands and feet, axillary folds, groin, scalp, and finger webs (Fig. 30.11). Pharmacists must refer suspected cases to a physician since there is no nonprescription product for scabies. A physician will confirm a diagnosis by examining magnified skin scrapings for the mites and their ova.

SUMMARY

Arthropod stings are usually a defensive reaction on the part of the creature. Nonetheless, the sting of the wasp, yellow jacket, hornet, or bumblebee usually only produces pain and

---

AT THE COUNTER

A good friend from the community approaches the pharmacist somewhat hesitantly. He mentions that his youngest son, a 6-year-old, was sent home with a note from his teacher stating that he had head lice.

Interview/Patient Assessment

The pharmacist attempts to discover if other family members are affected. However, the parent denies the possibility and does not understand how his son could have gotten them. "You know us," he said, "We have always made the boys take daily baths. How could we have this problem? How do we treat it? Do we have to go to the doctor?"

If the boy had been present, the pharmacist could don gloves and inspect his scalp to confirm the infestation.

Pharmacist's Analysis

1. Can those with clean habits be infested with head lice, or could this be another insect?
2. What can be done to ease this father's embarrassment?

3. What treatment(s) should the pharmacist suggest?

Clean habits do not prevent head lice. Having a note from the teacher (or school nurse) strongly indicates that a head louse infestation is present.

Patient Counseling

The father's embarrassment can be made less acute by the pharmacist providing reassurance such as, "You know, this is going around right now. Lots of children have head lice. It's not just your child. It's not embarrassing to have lice, but it would be embarrassing not to treat them properly, allowing your child to be the focus of reinfestation of surrounding children." Once the parent understands that head lice are routine for the pharmacist, information provided by the pharmacist can be communicated more effectively. The pharmacist should next point out effective products such as pediculicides, nit combs, and acidic/enzymatic nit-removal aids and should discuss their use. The pharmacist should also provide information regarding the delousing of clothing, bedding, linens, and combs as described in this chapter.

discomfort. For these minor stings, nonprescription products can provide some relief. Treatment options include external analgesics (e.g., counterirritants, topical anesthetics, topical antihistamines, hydrocortisone), astringents, and skin protectants. Scorpion stings may rarely result in severe cardiovascular problems. Some stinging insects such as fire ants and Africanized bees attack in mass, producing more severe reactions. For these reasons, fire ant, Africanized bee, and scorpion stings should be referred. ***Anaphylactic reactions to stings are life-threatening, requiring immediate physician referral.***

Arthropod bites may be defensive, but also occur because certain insects feed on human blood. Many bites are minor, only causing pruritus or other minor discomfort (e.g., chiggers, ticks, fleas). However, tick bites require observation for transmissible disease such as Rocky Mountain Spotted Fever or Lyme Disease. Further, bites of spiders (e.g., the black widow, brown recluse) and centipedes necessitate a visit to an emergency room for physician evaluation. DEET may be used to help prevent attacks by biting insects. Used according to label directions, it helps repel such arthropods as mosquitoes and ticks.

Pediculosis presents a separate set of problems, but can be easily eradicated with judicious pharmacist counseling. Pharmacists may be asked to help patients recognize a present infestation, counsel on prevention of future infections, and recommend effective nonprescription and ancillary products. Nonprescription products containing synergized pyrethrins are effective in the eradication of head, pubic, and body lice, while permethrin is only effective for head lice. Ancillary products such as nit combs and enzymatic nit-removal aids can assist in eradication of an infestation.

References

1. Gluckman SJ. Medicine for the outdoors. Hosp Pract 29:51, 1994.
2. Bischof RO. Seasonal incidence of insect stings: Autumn 'yellow jacket delirium.' J Fam Pract 43:271, 1996.
3. Reisman RE. Insect stings. N Engl J Med 331:523, 1994.
4. Morsy TA, Lashen AH. An unusually severe bee-sting allergic reaction in a bee keeper boy. J Egypt Soc Parasitol 26:539, 1996.
5. Janniger CK, Schutzer SE, Schwartz RA. Childhood insect bite reactions to ants, wasps, and bees. Cutis 54:14, 1994.
6. Cohen SG, Biachine PJ. Hymenoptera, hypersensitivity, and history: A prologue to current day concepts and practices in the diagnosis, treatment, and prevention of insect sting allergy. Ann Allergy Asthma Immunol 74:198, 1995.
7. Green VA, Siegel CJ. Bites and stings of hymenoptera, caterpillar and beetle. J Toxicol Clin Toxicol 21:491, 1983.
8. Annila IT, et al. Bee and wasp sting reactions in current bee-keepers. Ann Allergy Asthma Immunol 77:423, 1996.
9. Berrios RR, Serano LA. Bilateral optic neuritis after a bee sting. Am J Ophthalmol 117:677, 1994.
10. Wagdi P, et al. Acute myocardial infarction after wasp stings in a patient with normal coronary arteries. Am Heart J 128:820, 1994.
11. Vachvanichsanong P, Dissaneewate P, Mitarnum W. Non-fatal acute renal failure due to wasp stings in children. Pediatr Nephrol 11:734, 1997.
12. Law DA, et al. Atrial flutter and fibrillation following bee stings. Am J Cardiol 80:1255, 1997.
13. Ariue BK. Multiple Africanized bee stings in a child. Pediatrics 94:115, 1994.
14. Candiotti KA, Lamas AM. Adverse neurologic reactions to the sting of the imported fire ant. Int Arch Allergy Immunol 102:417, 1993.
15. Sofer S, Shahak E, Gueron M. Scorpion envenomation and antivenom therapy. J Pediatr 124:973, 1994.
16. Burnett JW, Calton GJ, Morgan RJ. Scorpions. Cutis 36:393, 1985.
17. Stafford CT. Hypersensitivity to fire ant venom. Ann Allergy Asthma Immunol 77:87, 1996.
18. Hoffman DR. Reactions to less common species of fire ants. J Allergy Clin Immunol 100:679, 1997.
19. DeShazo RD, Banks WA. Medical consequences of multiple fire ant stings occurring indoors. J Allergy Clin Immunol 93:847, 1994.
20. Moffitt JE, Barker JR, Stafford CT. Management of imported fire ant allergy: Results of a survey. Ann Allergy Asthma Immunol 79:125, 1997.
21. Eagle K. Sting of the fire ant. N Engl J Med 329:1317, 1993.
22. Bloom FL, DelMastro PR. Imported fire ant death. J Fla Med Assoc 71:87, 1984.
23. Winston ML. The Africanized 'killer' bee: Biology and public health. Q J Med 87:263, 1994.
24. Jerrard DA. ED management of insect stings. Am J Emerg Med 14:429, 1996.
25. Graft DF. Stinging insect hypersensitivity in children. Curr Opin Pediatr 8:597, 1996.
26. Rachesky IJ, et al. Treatments for *Centruroides exilicauda* envenomation. Am J Dis Child 138:1136, 1984.
27. Barthwal SP, et al. Myocarditis and hemiplegia from scorpion bite—A case report. Indian J Med Sci 51:115, 1997.
28. Holve S. Treatment of snake, insect, scorpion, and spider bites in the pediatric emergency department. Curr Opin Pediatr 8:256, 1996.
29. Essayan DM, Kagey-Sobotka A, Lichtenstein LM. Nearly fatal anaphylaxis following an insect sting. Ann Allergy 73:297, 1994.
30. van Halteren HK, et al. Discontinuation of yellow jacket venom immunotherapy: Follow-up of 75 patients by means of deliberate sting challenge. J Allergy Clin Immunol 100(6 Pt 1):767, 1997.
31. Tamir R, et al. Risk factors associated with the severity of systemic insect sting reactions. Isr J Med Sci 43:1192, 1996.
32. Freeman TM. Ann Allergy Asthma Immunol 78:369, 1997.
33. Glaspole I, et al. Stinging insect allergies. Assessing and managing. Aust Fam Physician 26:1395, 1997.
34. Stewart AG, Ewan PW. The incidence, aetiology, and management of anaphylaxis presenting to an accident and emergency department. QJM 89:859, 1996.
35. Gonzalo Garijo MA, Bobadilla Gonzalez P, Puyana Ruiz J. Epileptic attacks associated with wasp sting-induced anaphylaxis. J Investig Allergol Clin Immunol 6:277, 1996.
36. van Halteren HK, et al. *Hymenoptera* sting challenge of 348 patients: Relation to subsequent field stings. J Allergy Clin Immunol 97:1058, 1996.

37. Golden DB, et al. Natural history of *Hymenoptera* venom sensitivity in adults. J Allergy Clin Immunol 100(6 Pt 1):760, 1997.
38. Annila IT, Annila PA, Msrsky P. Risk assessment in determining systemic reactivity to honeybee stings in beekeepers. Ann Allergy Asthma Immunol 78:473, 1997.
39. Fortenberry JE, Laine J, Shalit M. Use of epinephrine for anaphylaxis by emergency medical technicians in a wilderness setting. Ann Emerg Med 25:785, 1995.
40. Frazier CA. Epinephrine for anaphylaxis (Editorial). Alaska Med 36:206, 1994.
41. Gelder C, Harris J, Williams D. Allergy to bee and wasp venom. Br J Hosp Med 55:349, 1996.
42. Burnett JW, Calton GJ, Morgan RJ. Centipedes. Cutis 37:241, 1986.
43. Visscher PK, Vetter RS, Camazine S. Removing bee stings. Lancet 348(9023):301, 1996.
44. Fed Reg 57:58356, 1992.
45. Fed Reg 47:39412, 1982.
46. Yee CJ, et al. Acquired immunity to Africanized honeybee (*Apis mellifera*) venom in Brazilian beekeepers. J Investig Allergol Clin Immunol 7:583, 1997.
47. Honig PJ. Bites and parasites. Pediatr Clin North Am 30:563, 1983.
48. Schwartz BS, Goldstein MD. Lyme disease in outdoor workers: Risk factors, preventive measures, and tick removal methods. Am J Epidemiol 131:877, 1990.
49. Reunala T, Brummer-Korvenkontion H, Palosuo T. Are we really allergic to mosquito bites? Ann Med 26:301, 1994.
50. Howard R, Frieden IJ. Papular urticaria in children. Pediatr Dermatol 13:246, 1996.
51. Angarano DW, Parish LC. Comparative dermatology: Parasitic disorders. Clin Dermatol 12:543, 1994.
52. Burns DA. The investigation and management of arthropod bite reactions acquired in the home. Clin Exp Dermatol 12:114, 1987.
53. Lewis R. Getting Lyme disease to take a hike. FDA Consumer 28(5):5, 1994.
54. Samaha A, et al. Tick infestation of the eyelid. Am J Ophthalmol 125:263, 1998.
55. Falco RC, Fish D, Piesman J. Duration of tick bites in a Lyme disease–endemic area. Am J Epidemiol 143:187, 1996.
56. Wright SW, Trott AT. North American tick-borne diseases. Ann Emerg Med 17:964, 1988.
57. Brown M, Herbert AA. Insect repellents: An overview. J Am Acad Dermatol 36(2 Pt 1):243, 1997.
58. Fisher RG, et al. Necrotic arachnidism. West J Med 160:570, 1994.
59. Reifsnyder DN. Spider Bites (Letter). Hosp Pract 29:15, 1994.
60. Handel CC, Izquierdo LA, Curet LB. Black widow spider (*Latrodectus mactans*) bite during pregnancy. West J Med 160:261, 1994.
61. Mack RB. Will the defendant please rise? MC Med J 55:86, 1994.
62. Zukowski CW. Black widow spider bite. J Am Board Fam Pract 6:279, 1993.
63. Suntorntham S, et al. Dramatic clinical response to the delayed administration of black widow spider antivenin (Letter). Ann Emerg Med 24:1198, 1994.
64. Miller TA. Treatment of black widow spider bite (Letter). J Am Board Fam Pract 7:183, 1994.
65. Barrett SM, Romine-Jenkins M, Fisher DE. Dapsone or electric shock therapy of brown recluse spider envenomation? Ann Emerg Med 24:21, 1994.
66. Knapp JF, et al. Case 06–1994: A 10-year-old female with fever, jaundice, and orthostatic hypotension. Pediatr Emerg Care 10:364, 1994.
67. Burton KG. Nitroglycerin patches for brown recluse spider bites (Letter). Am Fam Physician 51:1401, 1995.
68. Phillips S, et al. Therapy of brown spider envenomation: A controlled trial of hyperbaric oxygen, dapsone, and cyproheptadine. Ann Emerg Med 25:363, 1995.
69. Skinner MW, Butler CS. Necrotising arachnidism treated with hyperbaric oxygen. Med J Aust 162:372, 1995.
70. Mumcuoglu KY, Leibovici V. Centipede (*Scolopendra*) bite: A case report. Isr J Med Sci 25:47, 1989.
71. Lin TJ, et al. Features of centipede bites in Taiwan. Trop Geogr Med 47:300, 1995.
72. Uppal SS, et al. Clinical aspects of centipede bite in the Andamans. J Assoc Physicians India 38:163, 1990.
73. Barnett PL. Centipede ingestion by a six-month-old infant: Toxic effects. Pediatr Emerg Care 7:229, 1991.
74. Mohri S, et al. Centipede bites in Japan. Cutis 47:189, 1991.
75. Kunkel DB, Wasserman GS. Editorial comment: Envenomations by miscellaneous animals. J Toxicol Clin Toxicol 21:557, 1983.
76. Fed Reg 44:69768, 1979.
77. Fed Reg 48:5852, 1983.
78. Fed Reg 54:40818, 1989.
79. Fed Reg 55:6932, 1990.
80. Fed Reg 56:43025, 1991.
81. Fed Reg 54:13490, 1989.
82. Fed Reg 47:39436, 1982.
83. Fed Reg 58:54458, 1993.
84. Fed Reg 48:6820, 1983.
85. Fed Reg 56:33644, 1991.
86. Frances SP, et al. Effectiveness of repellent formulations containing DEET against mosquitoes in northeastern Thailand. J Am Mosq Control Assoc 12(2 Pt 1):331, 1996.
87. Mafong EA, Kaplan LA. Insect repellents. What really works? Postgrad Med 102:63, 1997.
88. Osimitz TG, Murphy JV. Neurological effects associated with use of the insect repellent N,N-diethyl-m-toluamide (DEET). J Toxicol Clin Toxicol 35:435, 1997.
89. Fai FY, Lee L. Perception and use of insect repellent among soldiers in the Singapore Armed Forces. Mil Med 161:113, 1996.
90. Stinecipher J, Shah J. Percutaneous permeation of N,N-diethyl-m-toluamide (DEET) from commercial mosquito repellents and the effect of solvent. J Toxicol Environ Health 52:119, 1997.
91. Veltri JC, et al. Retrospective analysis of calls to poison control centers resulting from exposure to the insect repellent N,N-diethyl-m-toluamide (DEET) from 1985–1989. J Toxicol Clin Toxicol 32:1, 1994.
92. Osimitz TG, Grothaus RH. The present safety assessment of deet. J Am Mosq Control Assoc 11(2 Pt 2):274, 1995.
93. Fraser AD, et al. Analysis of diethyltoluamide (DEET) following intentional oral ingestion of Muscol. J Anal Toxicol 19:197, 1995.
94. Fed Reg 47:424, 1982.
95. Fed Reg 48:26986, 1983.

96. Fed Reg 50:25170, 1985.
97. Janniger CK, Kuflik AS. Pediculosis capitis. Cutis 51:407, 1993.
98. Barker SC. Phylogeny and classification, origins, and evolution of host associations of lice. Int J Parasitol 24:1285, 1994.
99. Burgess IF. Human lice and their management. Adv Parasitol 36:271, 1995.
100. Forsman KE. Pediculosis and scabies. Postgrad Med 98:89, 1995.
101. Clore ER, Longyear LA. A comparative study of seven pediculicides and their packaged nit removal combs. J Pediatr Health Care 7:55, 1993.
102. Sokoloff F. Identification and management of pediculosis. Nurse Pract 19:62, 1994.
103. Vander Stichele RH, Dezeure EM, Bogaert MG. Systematic review of clinical efficacy of topical treatments for head lice. Br Med J 311:604, 1995.
104. Billstein SA, Mattalino VJ Jr. The "nuisance" sexually transmitted diseases: Molluscum contagiosum, scabies, and crab lice. Med Clin North Am 74:1487, 1990.
105. Ragheb DA, et al. *In vitro* control of *Phthirus pubis* with four pediculicides: Eurax, Elimite, Licid and Benzanil. J Egypt Soc Parasitol 25:677, 1995.
106. Maunder JW. An update on headlice. Health Visit 66:317, 1993.
107. Olsen CG, et al. The role of the family physician in the day care setting. Am Fam Physician 54:1257, 1996.
108. Turow VD. Phthiriasis palpebrarum: An unusual course of blepharitis. Arch Pediatr Adolesc Med 149:704, 1995.
109. Robinson AJ, Ridgway GL. Sexually transmitted disease in children: Non viral including bacterial vaginosis, *Gardnerella vaginalis*, mycoplasmas, *Trichomonas vaginalis*, *Candida albicans*, scabies, and pubic lice. Genitourin Med 70:208, 1994.
110. Halpern JS. Recognition and treatment of pediculosis (head lice) in the emergency department. J Emerg Nurs 20:130, 1994.
111. Gillis D, et al. Sociodemographic factors associated with *Pediculosis capitis* and *pubis* among young adults in the Israel Defense Forces. Public Health Rev 18:345, 1990–91.
112. Oliver P. Making sense of . . . head lice. Nurs Times 90:34, 1994.
113. Levine GI. Sexually transmitted parasitic diseases. Prim Care 18:101, 1991.
114. Rundle PA, Hughes DS. *Phthirus pubis* infestation of the eyelids. Br J Ophthalmol 77:815, 1993.
115. Martin DH, Mroczkowski TF. Dermatologic manifestations of sexually transmitted diseases other than HIV. Infect Dis Clin North Am 8:533, 1994.
116. Routh HB, et al. Ectoparasites as sexually transmitted diseases. Semin Dermatol 13:243, 1994.
117. Deschenes J, Seamone C, Baines M. The ocular manifestations of sexually transmitted diseases. Can J Ophthalmol 25:177, 1990.
118. Herrero R, et al. Sexual behavior, venereal diseases, hygiene practices, and invasive cervical cancer in a high-risk population. Cancer 65:380, 1990.
119. Scowen P. Head lice: A problem for 1 in 10 primary school children. Prof Care Mother Child 6:139, 1996.
120. Silburt BS, Parsons WL. Scalp infestation by *Phthirus pubis* in a 6-week-old infant. Pediatr Dermatol 7:205, 1990.
121. Brown S, Becher J, Brady W. Treatment of ectoparasitic infections: Review of the English-language literature, 1982–1992. Clin Infect Dis 20(Suppl 1):S104, 1995.
122. Fischer TF. Lindane toxicity in a 24-year-old woman. Ann Emerg Med 24:972, 1994.
123. Fed Reg 47:28312, 1982.
124. Fed Reg 58:65452, 1993.
125. Murtagh J. Treatment of infestations. Aust Fam Physician 24:201, 1995.
126. Burgess IF, et al. Head lice resistant to pyrethroid insecticides in Britain (Letter). Br Med J 311:752, 1995.
127. Magee J. Unsafe practices in the treatment of pediculosis capitis. J Sch Nurs 12:17, 1996.
128. Elgart ML. Pediculosis. Dermatol Clin 8:219, 1990.
129. Burgess I. *Pediculus humanus capitis* in schoolchildren (Letter). Lancet 345:730, 1995.
130. Benmeir P, et al. Facial chemical burn (Letter). Burns 20:282, 1994.

Minor Wounds

The average person suffers many accidents that result in a minor wound each year.[1–3] They include conditions in which the skin is broken (e.g., blisters, scrapes, splinters, insect bites, and small cuts caused by paper or other sharp objects) and some in which the skin is unbroken (such as the minor burn). For purposes of this chapter, a minor wound has the following characteristics:

- It is not an extensive abrasion.
- It would not have caused injury to tendons, nerves, or muscles.
- It is not infected.
- It is not chronic (e.g., it has not lasted more than 1 week).
- It is not in a patient taking corticosteroids or immunosuppressants.

Major wounds, injuries that require physician intervention or emergency care, are not self-treatable. They may be too deep, infected, dirty, or chronic (having lasted more than 1 week).

Insect bites and minor burns are covered in other chapters (See Chapter 30, Arthropod Stings and Bites, Pediculosis, and Scabies, and Chapter 32, Burns).

PREVALENCE OF MINOR WOUNDS

The prevalence of minor wounds such as scratches and scrapes is unknown.[4,5] Many do not need care of any sort and heal without incident. Most minor wounds that require treatment are self-treated successfully.

It is well known that young children are most likely to be injured at home or day care through such accidents as cuts, blows, and burns, although a significant number of injuries also occur in other high-risk sites such as playgrounds.[6–9]

A study of pregnant patients attempted to chart each physical trauma.[10] For every two severe injuries, there were two minor injuries and another 153 classified as "insignificant."

EPIDEMIOLOGY OF MINOR WOUNDS

Information on epidemiology of minor wounds is difficult to locate; however, several studies describe the epidemiology of injuries in general, many of which would be minor wounds.

Injuries demonstrate a bimodal age pattern. One peak occurs at ages 2 to 3 and another during the teenage years (13 to 19).[6] Children younger than 6 months have a low risk of injury. However, the risk increases steadily from that point on. A significant number of elderly patients also suffer minor injury from such accidents as falls.[11]

Research suggests that children of adolescent mothers are injured more often than children of older mothers.[6] A recent study found that children with adolescent mothers had an overall injury rate of 14.9 per 100 person-years.[6]

Males are generally more prone to injury.[12,13] In one child-and-adolescent study group, 19% of males and 18% of females were injured in a 15-month time span.[6] However, falls were more common in boys, and burns were over twice as common in girls.[6] (The higher rate of burns was attributed to the use of hair-grooming devices such as heated rollers and a curling iron.) The rate of injuries in pregnancy is higher than that of other women for such common problems as contusions.[14]

Type of work is a strong predictor of injury. Many agricultural workers, for example, have high risk factors for injury because they often work with equipment in disrepair, sometimes work at night with inadequate sleep, and must labor under all types of adverse environmental conditions.[15] By the nature of their work, emergency rescue workers experience a higher rate of strains, sprains, and laceration/puncture wounds than those in other occupations.[16] Those whose work involves working with sharp objects (e.g., axes) are also more prone to injury.[17] Those who must work with fork-lift trucks also experience minor injuries such as contusions.[18]

Recreational activities, hobbies, and toys also cause injury. Air rifles are highly dangerous, causing many cases of skin penetration since they are sold without regard to age or training and are widely considered to be toys.[19] Air-gun pellets also cause many injuries each year.[20] Off-road bicycling causes numerous minor injuries.[21] Minor trauma is also a common reason for presentation to first-aid stations at rock concerts.[22]

Patients who are frequently intoxicated are more likely to undergo minor injury than other patients, with most having minor trauma above the neck.[23–25]

ETIOLOGY OF MINOR WOUNDS

Minor wounds have a number of causes, accidental and intentional, including falls, brushing against plant thorns, misusing knives and tools, scraping against an object (causing splinters or scrapes), being hit by a dropped or thrown object, etc.[26]

Many accidents cause minor wounds. For example, falls often result in bruises and/or broken skin.[6] Falls are common in children. However, at least 30% of those aged 65 or over living in community dwellings fall yearly.[27] From 8 to 17% of this group fall more than once during the average year. Usually, the falls cause only minor injury such as scrapes and other minor skin breaks. Being struck by a falling object or a thrown object is another common accidental source of minor wounds.[28]

SPECIFIC CONSIDERATIONS OF MINOR WOUNDS: ACUTE VERSUS CHRONIC WOUNDS

Wounds commonly are classified as acute or chronic.[29–31] Acute wounds are caused by trauma, either accidental or intentional, while chronic wounds are injuries that have not healed:

- Acute wounds
  —Accidental: Falls, cuts, bumping, scratches, splinters; animal bites, etc.
  —Intentional: Self-mutilation, body piercing, attempted suicide via cutting, etc.[32]
- Chronic wounds: Pressure ulcers, diabetic ulcers, lower-leg ulcerations, etc.[33,34]

Minor, acute wounds may be self-treated, but chronic wounds should always be referred.

(Generally, wounds that have not healed in 1 week are considered chronic. Chronic wounds often indicate that something is retarding the normal healing processes of the body such as venous disease, arterial disease, diabetes mellitus, or certain medications (e.g., corticosteroids; nonsteroidal anti-inflammatory agents).[15,35]

PROGNOSIS OF MINOR WOUNDS

Factors That Affect Wound Healing

Before recommending a product or products, pharmacists should assess wounds to determine if they are amenable to self-treatment.[36,37] Certain factors signal a wound that will heal more or less slowly, including the type of wound, its anatomic site, the presence of infections, and certain medications taken by the patient.[38]

TYPE OF WOUND

A wound's propensity to heal in the appropriate amount of time is a function of the causative injury. With a minor cut caused by a sharp object (e.g., knife, paper, or razor), the edges can be placed directly together (apposed), which facilitates healing (Fig. 31.1).[39,40] However, an abrasion injury such as from a fall onto gravel or pavement results in irregular edges that cannot be apposed (Fig. 31.2). While puncture wounds (e.g., stepping on a nail) may seem to heal rapidly on the outside, the possibility of anaerobic infection (e.g., gangrene, tetanus) should be remembered.

Pharmacists should only suggest self-therapy for minor wounds caused by sharp objects and minor abrasions. Because of the possibility of damage to tendons, nerves, and

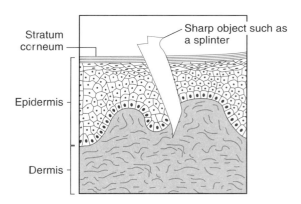

Figure 31.1. Cross-section of skin illustrating minor wound caused by sharp object lacerating the epidermis and superficial dermis. (Note that the edges can be brought into apposition with a bandage.)

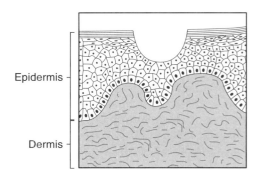

Figure 31.2. Cross-section of skin illustrating minor wound caused by abrasion into the epidermis. (Note that the edges cannot be brought into apposition.)

muscles, deep wounds (e.g., those below the dermis) should be referred. Similarly, extensive abrasions should be referred for cleansing of such material as gravel and dirt.[41]

ANATOMIC SITE

Some areas heal better than others. For example, highly vascular areas such as the head and neck heal more quickly than other areas such as the abdomen or back. Wound areas that are difficult to keep disinfected (e.g., the perineal skin or skin adjacent to the anal opening) should be referred for appropriate care.[42] Minor wounds of the inner ear, **nasolabial fold** (area between the nose and upper lip), temple, concave ear, and **nasal alar crease** (flaring creases at the side of the nostrils) often heal rapidly with no treatment.[39] Nevertheless, minor wounds in other areas can also be self-treated and

should still heal within a normal time unless the wound becomes infected.

PRESENCE OF INFECTION

An infection in the tissues delays wound healing because bacteria secrete **proteases** (enzymes that degrade proteins), which injure tissue.[39,43,44] (See "A Pharmacist's Journal: Will This Help a Splinter?") The classical signs of wound infection, which are known by their Latin names, are tumor (swelling), calor (heat), rubor (redness), and dolor (pain).[45] (See "A Pharmacist's Journal: Will Neosporin Help My Ear?") Other signs include systemic fever, foul odor, and exudate.

Sometimes the cause of the wound can help predict infection. (See "A Pharmacist's Journal: Where's the Alcohol?") For instance, an injury suffered in a barnyard would

A Pharmacist's Journal

"Will This Help a Splinter?"

A woman in her early 20s asked me if Neosporin would help a splinter. I mentioned that it would help prevent infection in small wounds such as a splinter. She told me this story, "My husband got a splinter in his hand, but he couldn't get it out. We wrapped it up and the next morning it came out but it left a hole in his hand." I asked how the hand felt, and she said it was swollen and painful. I asked how it looked and she said it was better and the hole had healed over. She then said, "It doesn't look too bad, except he has red streaks going up his arm." I expressed astonishment at this and urged her to take him

to a physician immediately. She responded, "He won't go. I tried to make him, but he doesn't want to." I asked her to explain the possibility of tetanus to him, and how the tetanus organism can incubate in a wound that appears well. I also explained the need for systemic antibiotics and an examination of the wound site for necrosis or gangrene. I stressed that a surface ointment would be worthless and asked her to have her husband call me if necessary so I might tell him these problems directly. I neglected to ask her name, or I might have called her to check on the progress of the wound. However, I never heard from them again.

A Pharmacist's Journal

"Will Neosporin Help My Ear?"

A young woman about 20 pulled back her hair while I was filling a prescription and asked, "Will Neosporin help my ear?" Her ear lobe was swollen to the size of a golf ball. I asked how long it had been like that. "Since I got my ears pierced about a week ago. It hurts really bad and there's greenish stuff coming out of the hole." I urged her to see her physician, telling her that any surface antibiotic would allow the

infection to spread. She then asked, "What about my earring." I told her not to wear it until the infection subsided. She answered, "I mean, what about the one I was wearing when my ear got infected. It got sucked inside of my ear and I can't get it out. What do I do?" I urged her to tell the physician immediately so the earring could be removed, since it was probably acting as an infective agent in her tissues.

A Pharmacist's Journal

"Where's the Alcohol?"

A woman in her 20s came into the pharmacy asking, "Where's the alcohol?" I noticed that she had a white cloth covering much of her lower arm. I asked what kind of injury she had. She unwrapped the towel, revealing a gash some 6 inches in length along her lower arm. The gash was oozing blood and appeared deeply bruised at the edges. I asked about the cause. She replied, "I cut it on a fence I was building for the pig pen." I asked what she had done so far. "I just washed it out and got the bleeding stopped. Now I want alcohol to kill the germs." I asked about the status of her tetanus immunizations." She appeared puzzled, finally saying, "I don't know. Why is that important?" I told her the greater danger of the injury is tetanus, since she was around farm animals. I also shared with her the story of an uncle who died of tetanus in the 1920s prior to the time of immunizations. She was sufficiently motivated to promise that she would obtain an immunization, stating, "You know, I just never thought of that." I also stressed that emergency room personnel could take a look at the wound to gauge depth and the need for sutures.

be more likely infected than a paper cut suffered in an office in an inner city high-rise.[46] The infected wound must be seen by a physician.

MEDICATION USAGE

Some medications will retard healing. For example, patients taking corticosteroids and immunosuppressants experience slow wound healing because these medications retard proliferation of cells and decrease the healing functions of macrophages, leukocytes, and lymphocytes.[39] Patients taking these medications should be referred.

NUTRITIONAL STATUS

The patient should take in adequate nutrition following a wound. New protein (e.g., collagen fibers) cannot form adequately if the patient does not ingest adequate protein, for instance.[47,48]

Natural Healing of Minor Wounds

The body institutes wound healing in a predictable, stepwise fashion from inflammation to proliferation and ending with the remodeling phase (Fig. 31.3). However, the time needed for certain steps may be shortened by certain treatments. Conversely, the time to healing may be impeded by mistreatment of the wound, poor health, or infection.

INFLAMMATION

The inflammatory phase of wound healing primarily involves platelet coagulation and leukocytes.[27] When the wound occurs, blood vessels are disrupted, and platelets are stimulated to release mediators, resulting in aggregation and the formation of the platelet plug.[39] Platelets also secrete the growth factors that are integral to the healing process.

Coagulation occurs by numerous substeps, which form thrombin, fibrin, and factor X. The steps terminate in the formation of a blood clot. Neutrophil infiltration is triggered by chemotactic factors. Monocytes then enter the wound area and are transformed into macrophages, which in turn help decontaminate the wound.

PROLIFERATION

In the proliferative phase the integrity of the skin is reestablished. Within 12 to 24 hours of injury, keratinocytes migrate from the wound's edges.[33,39] (Moisture is critical in ensuring effective migration. (See "Moist Versus Dry Healing.") Eventually, keratinocytes from both edges meet, allowing the skin to resume its barrier function. **Angiogenesis** (development of blood vessels) also occurs as proliferation progresses. Capillaries adjacent to the wound send fresh buds into the wound, a process also known as **neovascularization.**

Healthy granulation tissue also develops, a process known as fibroplasia. Development of granulation tissue depends on new vessel formation, fibroblast accumulation, and production of elastin/collagen.

The wound may also contract, which minimizes the wound's surface area.[39] Contractions present problems in some anatomic areas that require excellent mobility such as the hands and feet.

REMODELING

Remodeling refers to the continued deposition of collagen in the area of the healing wound and the changes of the wound over time.[57]

TREATMENT OF MINOR WOUNDS

Treatment Guidelines

Patients whose wounds may have damaged tendons, nerves, or muscles should be referred. Wounds that are possibly in-

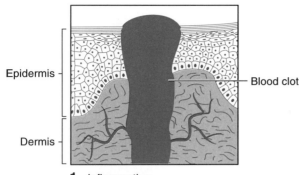

1. Inflammation

Epidermis

Dermis

Blood clot

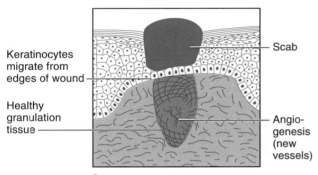

2. Proliferation

Keratinocytes migrate from edges of wound

Healthy granulation tissue

Scab

Angio-genesis (new vessels)

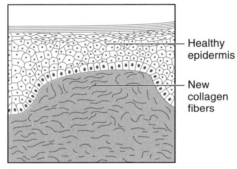

3. Remodeling

Healthy epidermis

New collagen fibers

Figure 31.3. Three stages of wound healing: (1) inflammation, (2) proliferation, and (3) remodeling.

fected (e.g., with presence of swelling, heat, redness, or pain) or were suffered in a contaminated environment (e.g., around farm animals) should also be referred. Patients taking corticosteroids or immunosuppressants should be referred. Generally, patients should only self-treat acute, minor wounds that are clean (minor wounds should not require debridement) and not infected. (See Patient Assessment Algorithm 31.1.) Initial treatment of minor wounds consists of first attempting to cleanse it thoroughly (Fig 31.4).[58,59] Irrigation with tap water is the best alternative in the absence of sterile normal saline in a typical household.[45] (See "Surgical Wounds" for a discussion of the pharmacist's role in helping the patient care for wounds intentionally created during a surgical procedure.)

HEALING PROCESSES

One way of categorizing wound care is by "intention." Different approaches or "intentions" are used, depending on the type of wound.

Primary Intention

With primary intention an attempt is made to bring the edges of the wound back together (i.e., in apposition), as they were prior to the wound.[33] Direct apposition may be accomplished by the physician through the use of sutures or clamps or with bandages that secure the wound edges to each other (in self-treatment only bandages are used). Primary intention promotes healing because migrating epithelial cells need only travel a short distance during reepithelialization.

Pharmacists may help patients achieve primary-intention healing by demonstrating such products as butterfly bandages, which hold wound edges together during healing.

Secondary Intention

If wound edges are not placed in apposition, wounds are said to heal through secondary intention.[61] With secondary intention, the time to reepithelialization is lengthened by such factors as wound depth, location, and shape. For instance, more superficial wounds will heal faster because less tissue has been affected.[33]

Generally, pharmacists advise healing by secondary intention for abrasions and scrapes in which some tissue has been removed and apposition is not possible because of the irregular nature of the edges of the wound.

MINOR-WOUND DRESSINGS

Wound dressings serve several purposes[62–65]:

- Absorb exudates and contaminated wound fluids so they will not contact healthy surrounding tissues (a wicking effect)
- Protect wounds from environmental filth and from bacteria and other organisms found in the ambient air
- Ensure that proper moisture remains in the area
- Prevent patient embarrassment from having an open wound

All wound dressings come in individual packages that are guaranteed sterile until opened. *The patient and/or caregivers should wash hands before applying wound dressings and should not touch the side of the bandage that will face the wound.* (See "When to Bandage a Minor Wound.")

Nonadherent Dressings

Some wound dressings are impregnated with petrolatum emulsion or are constructed from rayon/polyethylene laminate so that they will not adhere to skin (Table 31.1). These nonadhering dressings, which are placed directly on the wound, help prevent any material from becoming encrusted or enmeshed in the wound (Fig. 31.5).[62,63] With a nonadherent dressing, discomfort is minimized during dressing changes and healing tissue is not subjected to the stresses caused by removal of dressings that are "stuck" to the wound or to adjacent healthy skin.

Some nonadherent dressings (e.g., Release, Telfa Pads) absorb light drainage; others (e.g., Adaptic, Vaseline Gauze) cannot absorb drainage; however, because they are porous, drainage can flow through both types to the primary dressing, which is absorbent. Nonadherent dressings are also appropriate for relatively dry wounds such as skin tears, lacerations, abrasions, and superficial burns.

Primary Dressings

Absorbent primary dressings are placed directly over nonadherent dressings if nonadherent dressings are used (Table 31.2). Otherwise, primary dressings are placed directly on the wound and surrounding skin.[62,67] The absorbency of primary dressings wicks exudate up away from wounds. They also serve as protective cushioning for wounds.

Secondary Dressings

Secondary dressings, which are placed over primary dressings, are appropriate when a wound is producing moderate to heavy drainage (Table 31.3).[68] In addition to increasing absorbency, secondary dressings also provide compression (since they are taped to the wound) and extra cushioning protection.

Some secondary dressings are absorbent sponges. If these dressings are the type also known as abdominal pads, they must not be used as a primary dressing because they could introduce cotton fibers into the wound.

Some secondary dressings are called bandages because they help secure the underlying dressings to the wound site. One layer of a secondary dressing will also adhere to a second layer when wrapped around a wound, which facilitates compression while the wound is being taped.

Transparent Films

Transparent films are adhesive dressings useful for some superficial wounds, abrasions, and burns (Table 31.4).[45,69] They may be used as the only dressing; because they are transparent, patients can see the area beneath them and assess the degree of healing of the wound. They do not absorb much moisture, so they may be used in conjunction with a secondary dressing for a heavily draining wound. Their semipermeable nature allows air and moisture to pass through, which maintains the occlusive environment conducive to healing. (See "Moist Versus Dry Healing.") Other miscellaneous types of specialty dressings are listed in Table 31.5.

FOCUS ON...

MOIST VERSUS DRY HEALING

Over the years medical practitioners have observed that blisters heal faster if the overlying skin (the roof) remains intact than if the skin is removed, which allows the underlying skin to dry out.[33] Based on this knowledge, investigators have determined that occlusive dressings reduce healing times greatly when compared to air-exposed wounds.[49–51] Where wounds exposed to air epithelialize in about 2 to 3 days, wounds with occlusive dressings require but 18 to 24 hours.[39,52]

There are several theories for the apparent benefits of occlusive dressings:

- Enhancement of keratinocyte migration and/or maintenance of the natural wound fluids and their associated growth factors
- Prevention of infection by keeping bacteria from the wound[32,39]
- Pain reduction
- Augmentation of the final cosmetic outcome of the wound

In addition, occlusive dressings—as any dressings—help protect wounds from environmental trauma.

If wounds are not kept moist and allowed to dry, a scab will form.[39,53] The scab is formed from necrotic cells, fibrin, blood products, and exposed cells and tissues (e.g., collagen, elastin), which are sacrificed to create a temporary barrier for the wound. The scab also acts as a barrier to wound healing, since migrating epidermal cells are forced to detour under the scab.[54] Healing is further slowed because epidermal cell–derived proteases are forced to loosen the scab.

Despite their many advantages, occlusive dressings are not accepted by some traditional medical practitioners, who hold to the older view that allowing a scab to form provides protection for underlying skin.[54,55] Nevertheless, the advantages of moist dressings should cause pharmacists to recommend it for all wounds.[56]

Occlusive dressings should not be applied to infected wounds and should be used cautiously in immunocompromised patients.[54] (See "When to Bandage a Minor Wound.")

Tapes

Tapes are necessary for both wound closure and for securing nonadhesive dressings over a wound (Table 31.6).[70,71] (See Patient Assessment Algorithm 31.2.) Wounds closed with tape have a lower rate of infection than non–self-treatable wounds closed by sutures or staples.

Hypoallergenic tapes are preferred for all uses in which they contact skin because they lessen the possibility of allergy in broken skin, which complicates healing. Cloth tape should be used over bone, on other difficult-to-tape areas, and with bulky secondary dressings because of its high tensile strength. Plastic tape stretches with movement, making it preferable in areas that require mobility. (They are also transparent, which enhances their cosmetic appearance.) Paper tapes, which are porous and have light adhesive backings, are ideal for tender or painful areas and for wounds that should breathe, although they have low tensile strength and tend to break with movement. To seal out the environment with any type of tape, all four sides of a dressing must be secured to the skin.

Nonprescription Medications

To help determine the appropriate treatment, see Patient Assessment Algorithm 31.3.

Patient Assessment Algorithm 31.1. Minor-Wound Assessment and Dressing

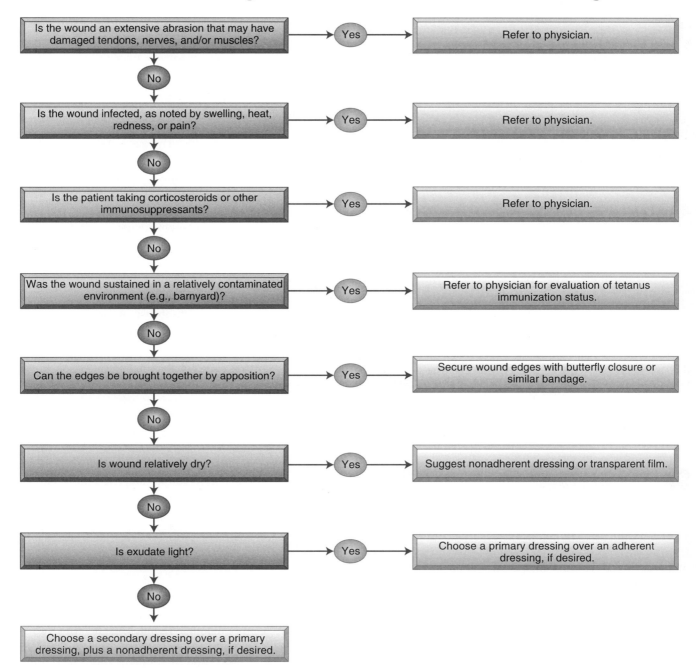

Is the wound an extensive abrasion that may have damaged tendons, nerves, and/or muscles? → Yes → Refer to physician.

No ↓

Is the wound infected, as noted by swelling, heat, redness, or pain? → Yes → Refer to physician.

No ↓

Is the patient taking corticosteroids or other immunosuppressants? → Yes → Refer to physician.

No ↓

Was the wound sustained in a relatively contaminated environment (e.g., barnyard)? → Yes → Refer to physician for evaluation of tetanus immunization status.

No ↓

Can the edges be brought together by apposition? → Yes → Secure wound edges with butterfly closure or similar bandage.

No ↓

Is wound relatively dry? → Yes → Suggest nonadherent dressing or transparent film.

No ↓

Is exudate light? → Yes → Choose a primary dressing over an adherent dressing, if desired.

No ↓

Choose a secondary dressing over a primary dressing, plus a nonadherent dressing, if desired.

FIRST-AID ANTISEPTICS

First-aid antiseptics are applied to the skin to help prevent infection in minor cuts and scrapes.[72] *The label will caution against use in the eyes or over large areas of the body.*[73] (See "A Pharmacist's Journal: We Used to Soak It in Kerosene.") *The label will also caution against use if the patient has a deep wound, puncture wound, or animal bite.* As noted under "Treatment Guidelines" above, all wounds should be cleaned before self-treatment. For most ointments, creams, and liquids, a small amount of the antiseptic can be applied to the wound one to three times daily. (The bandage should be kept wet with the product for compresses.) Sprays generally can be applied one to three times daily.[73] Wounds treated with a first-aid antiseptic may be covered with a sterile bandage, unless the antiseptic contains camphorated metacresol, camphorated phenol, or phenol.[73] *Topical antibiotics and first-aid antiseptics are contraindicated with infected wounds. To discourage patients from treating infected wounds, the FDA mandates this labeling, "Stop use and consult a doctor if the condition persists or gets worse. Do not use longer than 1 week unless directed by a doctor."*[73]

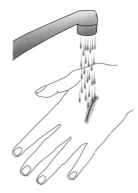

1. Irrigate with tap water.

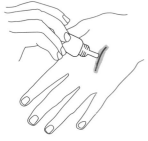

2. Apply first-aid antiseptic.

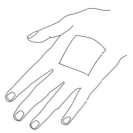

3. Cover wound with suitable dressing.

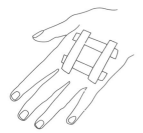

4. Apply tape for nonadhesive dressings.

Figure 31.4. Steps in care of a minor wound.

tip *Topical antibiotics and first-aid antiseptics are also contraindicated if patients have any type of bacterial skin infection, since self-treatment of bacterial skin infections is inappropriate.*[73–76] (See "A Pharmacist's Journal: I Cut Off All of My Cuticles.") Impetigo, for instance, can proceed to acute poststreptococcal glomerulonephritis, and prompt oral antibiotic therapy is mandatory to prevent possible loss of renal function.[74]

Alcohols

Alcohols considered safe and effective as first-aid antiseptics include denatured ethyl alcohol 48 to 95% and isopropyl alcohol 50 to 91.3% (Table 31.7).[73,77] All alcohols, which have Gram-positive, Gram-negative, and antitubercular activity, destroy many viruses and fungi, but lack sporicidal activity.[78,79] Alcohols in the concentrations listed can rapidly reduce cutaneous bacteria, but skin must be cleaned with soap prior to application because their activity is compromised in the presence of organic materials such as mucus, blood, and exudates. (See "Nonantiseptic Uses of Alcohols.")

Camphorated Metacresol

This **complex** (chemical combination) consists of 3 to 10.8% camphor and 1 to 3.6% metacresol in a ratio of 1:3. Products containing this ingredient must carry the warning, "Do not bandage," because irritation of the skin might occur. No major product contains camphorated metacresol at this time.

Camphorated Phenol

This complex consists of 10.8% camphor and 4.7% phenol in a light, mineral oil vehicle. Products containing this ingredient must caution the patient, "Do not bandage." If phenol is bandaged, the incidence of adverse reactions (e.g., skin irritation) increases.[81] A product containing this complex is listed in Table 31.8.

Eucalyptol Combination

This combination is composed of eucalyptol 0.091%, menthol 0.042%, methyl salicylate 0.055%, and thymol 0.063% in 26.9% alcohol. It is essentially the same as the proprietary product Listerine, which is primarily marketed as an oral antiseptic.[73] Although Listerine would function as a first-aid antiseptic, the labeling of the oral product does not include all of the required warnings to allow the patient to safely use it as a first-aid antiseptic, and it should not be recommended for this use.

Hexylresorcinol 0.1%

Hexylresorcinol is fully approved and has no special warnings or precautions associated with its use. A product containing hexylresorcinol is included in Table 31.8.

Hydrogen Peroxide Solution 3%

Hydrogen peroxide cleanses a wound through an effervescent action (Table 31.9). The enzyme catalase found in human tissues releases nascent oxygen when hydrogen peroxide is placed on a wound.[82] However, *hydrogen peroxide should only be used in the initial care of a wound, since it damages viable tissue and inhibits the formation of granulation tissue.*[83] *It must never be used for a deep wound or one with a cul-de-sac.* The bubbles created can produce severe tissue trauma, raising air-filled bullae, which separate epithelium from underlying tissues.[83–85] Bubbles may also produce retroperitoneal gas if the solution is used to irrigate wounds.[82]

Iodine and Iodophors

Iodides have bactericidal, sporicidal, tuberculocidal, fungicidal, and virucidal properties (Table 31.10).[86,87] Tincture of iodine exerts a rapid bactericidal effect through direct toxicity on cells. Tincture of iodine requires alcohol for solubility, however, and thus stings on application and dries skin. Products containing iodine also stain the skin a brownish color.

In complexes known as iodophors, iodine is chemically bound to a large molecule such as povidone in a solution.[78,88,89] The advantages of an iodophor over tincture of iodine are water solubility, reduced skin irritation, and lack of staining. However, at least 2 minutes of contact time with iodophors is needed for the release of free iodine.[78,90] Iodophors do have other drawbacks: in one study povidone-iodine inhibited the formation of granulation tissue, prompting some health-care practitioners to caution against its use in wounds.[83,85]

Iodine and/or iodophors may cause allergic reactions, so pharmacists should inquire about allergies to iodine or povidone-iodine before recommending either one.[91] Despite these problems, the FDA granted iodine and povidone-iodine Category I status in its tentative final monograph for first-aid products.[73]

Solutions known as "colorless iodine" or "decolorized iodine" may be purchased to prevent the well-known staining of tincture of iodine. However, these products are not iodophors. Instead, they contain iodides such as potassium iodide, sodium iodide, and/or ammonium iodide, all of which are useless as antiseptics.[92]

Phenol 0.5 to 1%

Products containing a phenol ingredient must carry the warning, "Do not bandage." If phenol is bandaged, the incidence of adverse reactions such as severe skin irritation under the bandage increases.[81] No leading product contains phenol as a sole antiseptic at this time.

Quaternary Ammonium Compounds

Safe and effective quaternary ammonium surfactants include benzalkonium chloride 0.1 to 0.13%, benzethonium chloride 0.1 to 0.2%, and methylbenzethonium chloride 0.13 to 5%. These compounds are only effective against Gram-positive organisms.[83] A product containing a quaternary ammonium compound is listed in Table 31.8.

Chlorhexidine Gluconate

Chlorhexidine gluconate, found in a 4% concentration in a product known as Hibiclens, is an effective topical antiseptic for disinfecting unbroken skin. Specifically, it is effective against bacteria and fungi, but is relatively ineffective against tubercle bacillus or viruses.[83]

Although chlorhexidine gluconate remains active in wounds containing blood and organic material and has a residual effect that persists for 5 to 6 hours, it has been found to be toxic when applied to wounds.[32] Hard tap water and natural soaps inactivate it.

Chlorhexidine gluconate has not been marketed for first-aid use, so the FDA has classified it as a new drug.[73] It should not be recommended as a first-aid antiseptic until it is proven safe and effective for this use.

Unapproved First-Aid Antiseptics

Some ingredients have been found by the FDA to lack sufficient evidence of safety and/or effectiveness as first-aid antiseptics[73] (Table 31.8):

- Mercurials (e.g., thimerosal and merbromin)
- Benzyl alcohol
- Chloroxylenol

FOCUS ON...

SURGICAL WOUNDS

Self-treatment of wounds has been complicated by the trend to minimize the number of days a patient remains in the hospital following surgery.[60] Patients today are frequently sent home with surgical wounds that are still healing and producing exudate. Quite often, patients are given an insufficient supply of dressing materials and must seek help from a pharmacist. In these instances, where patients are treating wounds under medical supervision, pharmacists should attempt to match the dressing products as closely as possible. When there is a discrepancy between the product used initially and the products routinely stocked by the pharmacy (or available through special order), the pharmacist may request a product recommendation from the physician's office.

FOCUS ON...

WHEN TO BANDAGE A MINOR WOUND

Patients have differing opinions about what type of wound needs bandaging. Generally speaking, virtually all wounds involving a skin break will benefit from bandaging for the reasons discussed in "Moist Versus Dry Healing." However, there are a few exceptions. Minor bruises in which the skin is not broken would not benefit from dressing. Even with a large bruise without an accompanying skin break, the only benefit from a dressing would be to prevent further trauma. A sunburn that does not result in blistered skin benefits little from a dressing.

As described below, when certain medications are placed on the skin, bandaging is not advisable since it can increase the potential for skin irritation.[66] These medications include camphorated metacresol, camphorated phenol, and phenol.

Table 31.1. Representative Nonadherent Minor-Wound Dressings

PRODUCT	COMMENTS
Adaptic Nonadhering Dressing	Nonadhering petrolatum-impregnated dressing
Vaseline Gauze	Nonadhering petrolatum-impregnated dressing
Release Non-Adhering Dressing	Nonadhering nonimpregnated dressing
Telfa Pads	Nonadhering nonimpregnated dressing

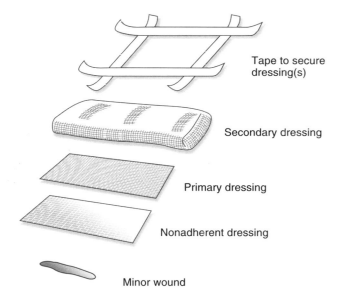

Figure 31.5. Coverage of wound using nonadherent dressing, primary dressing, secondary dressing, and tape to secure the dressings.

- Triclosan
- Poloxamer-iodine complex
- Triple dye

Pharmacists should advise against the use of first-aid antiseptics containing unapproved ingredients and other products not labeled for first-aid antiseptic use; instead they should recommend a safe and effective product.

TOPICAL ANTIBIOTICS

Topical antibiotics may be labeled for the reduction of risk of infection in minor wounds (Table 31.11). The label should advise external use only, should caution against ophthalmic contact, and should tell the consumer not to apply the antibiotic over large parts of the body.[76,93] Labels should also advise, *"Do not use longer than 1 week unless directed by a doctor."* Further, the patient should stop use and consult a physician if a rash or other allergic reaction develops.[76] The label of any product containing bacitracin, neomycin, and polymyxin should contain this slightly modified warning: "Stop use and consult a doctor if the condition persists or gets worse, or if a rash or other allergic reaction

Table 31.2. Representative Primary Minor-Wound Dressings

PRODUCT	COMMENTS
BAND-AID Brand Adhesive Bandage	Primary dressing; nonadherent facing with a tape backing
BAND-AID Brand Antibiotic Adhesive Bandage	Primary dressing; nonadherent facing with a tape backing; pad is impregnated with ointment containing polymyxin B 10,000 units and bacitracin zinc 500 units per gram
BAND-AID Brand Antiseptic Adhesive Bandage	Primary dressing; nonadherent facing with a tape backing, pad is impregnated with benzalkonium chloride
Kerlix Sponge	Primary dressing; appropriate for heavy drainage
SOF-WIK Drain Sponge	Primary dressing; precut (fenestrated) to fit around tubing
SOF-WIK Dressing Sponge	Primary dressing; appropriate for heavy drainage
Steri-Pad	Primary dressing; appropriate for heavy drainage
Topper Dressing Sponge	Primary dressing; appropriate for moderate to heavy drainage

Table 31.3. Representative Secondary Minor-Wound Dressings

PRODUCT	COMMENTS
Kerlix	Secondary dressing
KLING Conforming Gauze Bandage	Secondary dressing; conforming gauze which aids in covering areas such as the head or extremities
KLING-FLUFF Bulky Bandage	Secondary dressing
SURGIPAD Combine Dressing	Secondary dressing; also known as an abdominal pad; provides additional absorbency, compression, and protection

Table 31.4. Representative Transparent Films for Minor-Wound Dressings

PRODUCT	COMMENTS
Bioclusive Transparent Dressing	Hypoallergenic adhesive film which creates an occlusive environment beneath it
OpSite	Water-resistant, semipermeable dressing

Table 31.5. Representative Specialty Minor-Wound Dressings

PRODUCT	COMMENTS
BAND-AID Butterfly Closures	Waterproof closures designed to close and secure small wounds and incisions without adhering to the wound site
Elastikon	Elastic tape with adhesive back; good for hard-to-tape areas
Proxi-Strips	Hypoallergenic closures used to secure small wounds and incisions and secure suture sites

develops. Pharmacists should advise patients to stop using these products if they are allergic to any of the ingredients."[94]

As noted under "Treatment Guidelines," all wounds should be cleaned before self-treatment. These products can be applied one to three times daily, followed by application of a sterile bandage, if desired. (See "When to Bandage a Minor Wound.") Ointments and creams are applied by placing a small amount of product (an amount no larger than the surface area of the tip of a finger) on the wound. Powders are lightly dusted on the area. Aerosols are sprayed in small amounts.

Bacitracin

Bacitracin, a polypeptide antibiotic, is active mostly against Gram-positive organisms.[95] Bacitracin has a low propensity to cause contact dermatitis.

Bacitracin may be marketed as a single-entity product or in combination with neomycin and/or polymyxin (see Table 31.11). The combination of bacitracin, neomycin, and polymyxin is popularly known as "triple antibiotics." In one study triple-antibiotic ointment was found to be more effective than tincture of iodine in disinfecting wounds.[32]

Neomycin

Neomycin, an aminoglycoside, is active against Gram-negative organisms (except *P. aeruginosa*), anaerobes, and some Gram-positive organisms (e.g., staphylococci), but lacks activity against other Gram-positive organisms such as streptococci. Neomycin has a high incidence of allergic contact dermatitis (as high as 3.5 to 19%), which limits its utility.[74,95] Patients with certain conditions (e.g., chronic leg ulcers and stasis dermatitis) experience neomycin allergy prevalences of 20 to 30%. The incidence is higher when a patient has used a product containing neomycin for at least 1 week at any time in the past.[74] Allergy to neomycin produces cross-sensitivity to other aminoglycosides such as gentamicin in some pa-

Table 31.6. Representative Tapes for Minor-Wound Dressings

PRODUCT	COMMENTS
Blenderm	Plastic tape
Dermicare Hypo-Allergenic Tape	Paper tape
Dermicel Hypo-Allergenic Tape	Cloth tape
Dermiclear	Plastic tape
Durapore	Cloth tape
Micropore	Paper tape
Transpore	Plastic tape

tients.[74] If neomycin is applied to large areas of the body, systemic absorption may result in ototoxicity, especially in patients with reduced renal function.[95]

Neomycin may be marketed as a single-entity product or in combination with bacitracin and/or polymyxin (see Table 31.11). (See "Bacitracin" above.)

Polymyxin

Polymyxins are decapeptides that have a Gram-negative activity.[95] Contact dermatitis is rare.

The ingredient may only be marketed in combination with bacitracin or bacitracin and neomycin (see Table 31.11). (See "Bacitracin" above.)

Tetracyclines

Tetracycline, chlortetracycline, and oxytetracycline are safe and effective for nonprescription use as topical antibiotics; however, they are seldom requested by patients (see Table 31.11). They are not highly advertised, and some pharmacists

Patient Assessment Algorithm 31.2. Minor-Wound Dressing Tape

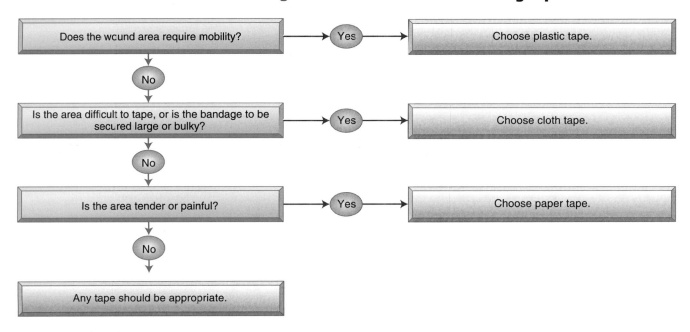

Does the wound area require mobility?	Yes →	Choose plastic tape.
↓ No		
Is the area difficult to tape, or is the bandage to be secured large or bulky?	Yes →	Choose cloth tape.
↓ No		
Is the area tender or painful?	Yes →	Choose paper tape.
↓ No		
Any tape should be appropriate.		

Patient Assessment Algorithm 31.3. Minor-Wound Treatment

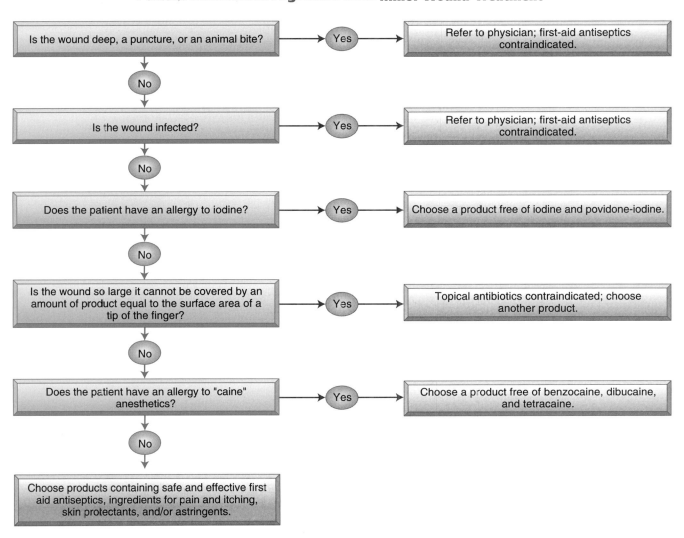

Is the wound deep, a puncture, or an animal bite?	Yes →	Refer to physician; first-aid antiseptics contraindicated.
↓ No		
Is the wound infected?	Yes →	Refer to physician; first-aid antiseptics contraindicated.
↓ No		
Does the patient have an allergy to iodine?	Yes →	Choose a product free of iodine and povidone-iodine.
↓ No		
Is the wound so large it cannot be covered by an amount of product equal to the surface area of a tip of the finger?	Yes →	Topical antibiotics contraindicated; choose another product.
↓ No		
Does the patient have an allergy to "caine" anesthetics?	Yes →	Choose a product free of benzocaine, dibucaine, and tetracaine.
↓ No		
Choose products containing safe and effective first aid antiseptics, ingredients for pain and itching, skin protectants, and/or astringents.		

A Pharmacist's Journal

"We Used to Soak It in Kerosene."

I was giving a lecture on home remedies to a local civic organization. After I had finished, an older gentleman said, "You know what we used to use when we got a nail in our foot? We used to soak it in kerosene. You'd see the blood globules coming out of the hole in your foot, and that meant that the kerosene was sterilizing the wound. By the way, we also ate a tablespoonful of sugar soaked in kerosene when we had the cough. Kerosene's the best medicine of all for things like this." I tried to explain to him that modern medicine would advise strongly against this old home remedy. Kerosene and other petroleum distillates are common causes of poisoning and should never be ingested. In contact with wounds, they might increase healing time and lead to dermatitis; they could be systemically absorbed, causing serious injury.

A Pharmacist's Journal

"I Cut Off All of My Cuticles."

A woman who appeared to be in her late teens came in swinging her hands around in an odd manner. As I approached her in the vicinity of the skin care products, she asked where the topical antibiotics were, swinging her hands all the while. I asked what had happened to her. She replied, "I cut off all of my cuticles. I decided to make my hands look pretty, so I got some cuticle scissors and cut them all off. That's what they're for. Anyway, it hurts when I wash dishes and some of my fingers have stuff leaking from the cuticles." She stopped her frantic hand waving to demonstrate; each nail had an inflamed, erythematous pit where the cuticle should have been. I told her that she appeared to have an infection in the living nail beds, and that she would need to see a physician, who would probably prescribe an oral antibiotic/antibacterial. I also explained that the cuticles function to provide protection for the nail bed and prevent infection, and urged her not to engage in cuticle removal again.

Table 31.7. Representative Alcohol-Containing First-Aid Antiseptics

PRODUCT	SELECTED INGREDIENTS/COMMENTS
Lavacol	Ethyl alcohol 70% with denaturants
Isopropyl Rubbing Alcohol	Isopropyl alcohol 70%
Isopropyl Rubbing Alcohol Gel	Isopropyl alcohol 70% in gel; unapproved dosage form

believe mistakenly that they are prescription products. Allergy is uncommon.

Antibiotic/Anesthetic Combinations

Topical antibiotics may be marketed in combination with local anesthetics, providing the dual benefits of local anesthesia and antisepsis. For instance, bacitracin (combined with neomycin and polymyxin, if desired) may be marketed with "caine" anesthetics or pramoxine (see Table 31.11).[93]

LOCAL ANALGESICS, ANESTHETICS, AND ANTIPRURITICS

Ingredients found in the products listed in Table 31.12 are safe and effective in providing temporary relief for the pain and/or itching of minor wounds[66,96]:

- Camphor and menthol (See Chapter 20, Injuries to Muscles, Ligaments, and Tendons.)
- Topical amines and "caine"-type local anesthetics, including benzocaine, butamben picrate, dibucaine, dimethiso-quin, dyclonine, lidocaine, pramoxine, and tetracaine (See "Treatment of Arthropod Bites" in Chapter 30, Arthropod Stings and Bites, Pediculosis, and Scabies.)
- Alcohol/ketone ingredients,including benzyl alcohol, camphor/phenol, camphor/metacresol, juniper tar, phenol, phenolate sodium, and resorci-

FOCUS ON...

NONANTISEPTIC USES OF ALCOHOLS

tip Alcohols are considered safe when applied to disinfect minor wounds. However, *when applied over large areas, both isopropyl and denatured ethyl alcohols can be toxic.* For example, in some instances children have had toxic reactions when well-meaning parents gave them an "alcohol bath" to bring down fever.[78-80] In other cases, infants wrapped in towels saturated with alcohol or given alcohol baths have been found unconscious or in a stupor after 4 to 8 hours of exposure to ethyl alcohol.[73]

Occasionally, a patient asks to purchase pure ethyl alcohol, not denatured ethyl alcohol. (A denaturant is a chemical that will cause stomach upset and other unpleasant symptoms if the product is ingested. Because the denaturant distills at the same temperature as the ethyl alcohol, pure ethyl alcohol cannot be produced from denatured ethyl alcohol. Accordingly, denatured ethyl alcohol does not carry a federal tax and sells for a fraction of drinkable ethyl alcohol.) Pharmacists cannot sell pure ethyl alcohol without a liquor license (not allowed in many states), so patients requesting that product generally will have to be referred to a liquor store.

Table 31.8. Representative Miscellaneous First-Aid Antiseptics

PRODUCT	SELECTED INGREDIENTS/COMMENTS
Bactine Aerosol	Benzalkonium chloride 0.13%, lidocaine HCl 2.5%
Campho-Phenique Pain Relieving Antiseptic Liquid	Phenol 4.7%, camphor 10.8%, eucalyptus oil, light mineral oil
Corona Ointment	Lanolin 50%, oxyquinoline 0.11% (unapproved antiseptic), beeswax, petrolatum, sodium borate (a veterinary product sometimes used in humans)
Gentian Violet	Gentian violet 1% (unapproved antiseptic)
Medicated Vaseline	White petrolatum, chloroxylenol (unapproved antiseptic; unlabeled concentration)
Mercurochrome	Aqueous merbromin 2% (unapproved antiseptic)
S.T. 37 Antiseptic Solution	Hexylresorcinol 0.1%, glycerin 27.1%
Tincture of Merthiolate	Thimerosal 0.1% (unapproved antiseptic)

Table 31.9. Representative Hydrogen Peroxide–Containing First-Aid Antiseptics

PRODUCT	SELECTED INGREDIENTS/COMMENTS
Hydrogen Peroxide Gel	Hydrogen peroxide 3% in gel; unapproved dosage form
Hydrogen Peroxide Solution	Hydrogen peroxide 3% solution

Table 31.10. Representative Iodine/Iodophor–Containing First-Aid Antiseptics

PRODUCT	SELECTED INGREDIENTS/COMMENTS
Betadine Skin Cleanser	Povidone-iodine 7.5%
Betadine Solution, Ointment	Povidone-iodine 10%
BFI Powder	Bismuth-formic-iodide 16% (unapproved antiseptic), bismuth subgallate, boric acid, potassium alum, thymol, zinc phenolsulfonate
Iodine Tincture	Iodine 2%, alcohol 44–50%
Iodides Tincture (Decolorized Iodine)	Ammonium and potassium iodides in 45% alcohol; unapproved antiseptic iodides

Table 31.11 Representative Topical Antibiotics

PRODUCT	SELECTED INGREDIENTS
Achromycin Ointment	Tetracycline HCl 3%
Baciguent Ointment	Per gram: bacitracin 50 units
Betadine First Aid Antibiotics + Moisturizer Ointment	Per gram: polymyxin B sulfate 10,000 units, bacitracin zinc 500 units
Mycitracin Ointment	Per gram: polymyxin B sulfate 5000 units, bacitracin 500 units, neomycin sulfate equivalent to 3.5 mg neomycin
Mycitracin Plus Pain Reliever Ointment	Per gram: polymyxin B sulfate 10,000 units, bacitracin 500 units, neomycin sulfate equivalent to 3.5 mg neomycin, and pramoxine HCl 10 mg
Lanabiotic Ointment	Per gram: polymyxin B sulfate 10,000 units, bacitracin 500 units, neomycin sulfate 5 mg, lidocaine 40 mg
Myciguent Ointment	Per gram: neomycin sulfate equivalent to 3.5 mg neomycin
Neosporin Ointment	Per gram: polymyxin B sulfate 5000 units, bacitracin zinc 500 units, neomycin 3.5 mg
Neosporin Plus Pain Relief Cream	Per gram: polymyxin B sulfate 10,000 units, neomycin 3.5 mg, lidocaine 40 mg
Neosporin Plus Pain Relief Ointment	Per gram: polymyxin B sulfate 10,000 units, bacitracin zinc 500 units, neomycin 3.5 mg, pramoxine 10 mg
Polysporin Ointment, Powder	Per gram: polymyxin B 10,000 units, bacitracin zinc 500 units

Table 31.12. Representative Analgesics, Anesthetics, and Antipruritics

PRODUCT	SELECTED INGREDIENTS/COMMENTS
Americaine Aerosol	Benzocaine 20%
Bicozene Cream	Benzocaine 6%, resorcinol 1.67%
Dermoplast Hospital Strength Aerosol	Benzocaine 20%, menthol 0.5%
Foille Spray	Benzocaine 5%, chloroxylenol 0.6% (unapproved ingredient)
Gold Bond Medicated Anti-Itch Cream	Lidocaine, menthol (no concentration labeled for any ingredient)
Itch-X Gel	Benzyl alcohol 10%, pramoxine 1%
Lanacane Cream	Benzocaine 6%, benzethonium chloride 0.2%
Medi-Quik Aerosol	Benzalkonium chloride 0.13%, lidocaine 2%, camphor 0.2%
Nupercainal Cream	Dibucaine 0.5%
Rhuli Anti-itch Gel	Benzyl alcohol 2%, menthol 0.3%, camphor 0.3%
Solarcaine Aerosol	Benzocaine 20%, triclosan 0.13%
Unguentine Original Formula Ointment	Phenol 1%
Unguentine Plus Cream	Lidocaine 2%, phenol 0.5%

nol (See Chapter 30, Arthropod Stings and Bites, Pediculosis, and Scabies.)

TOPICAL ANTIHISTAMINES
Topical antihistamines such as diphenhydramine and tripelennamine depress cutaneous receptors for pain and itch.

(See Chapter 30, Arthropod Stings and Bites, Pediculosis, and Scabies.)

SKIN PROTECTANTS
Skin protectants protect minor wounds from harmful or annoying stimuli (Table 31.13). Protectants found to be safe

Table 31.13. Representative Products for Minor Wounds That Contain Topical Protectants

PRODUCT	SELECTED INGREDIENTS/COMMENTS
Aveeno Anti-Itch Cream	Calamine 3%, pramoxine HCl 1%, camphor 0.3%
Benadryl Itch Stopping Cream	Diphenhydramine HCl 1%, zinc acetate 0.1%
Benadryl Extra Strength Itch Stopping Cream	Diphenhdyramine HCl 2%, zinc acetate 0.1%
Benadryl Itch Stopping Gel	Diphenhydramine HCl 2%, zinc acetate 1%
Benadryl Original Strength Itch Stopping Spray	Diphenhdyramine HCl 1%, zinc acetate 0.1%
Benadryl Extra Strength Itch Stopping Spray	Diphenhdyramine HCl 2%, zinc acetate 0.1%
Benadryl Extra Strength Itch Stopping Stick	Diphenhydramine HCl 2%, zinc acetate 0.1%
Caladryl Lotion	Calamine 8%, pramoxine HCl 1%
Caladryl Clear Lotion	Pramoxine HCl 1%, zinc acetate 0.1%
Calamine Lotion	Calamine, zinc oxide, glycerin, bentonite magma, calcium hydroxide, purified water (concentrations unlabeled)
Glycerin, U.S.P.	Glycerin anhydrous U.S.P., 99.5%
Rhuli Calamine Spray	Benzocaine 5%, calamine 13.8%, camphor 0.7%
Vaseline	White petrolatum 100%
Zinc Oxide Ointment	Zinc oxide 20%, mineral oil, white wax, white petrolatum (concentrations unlabeled)

Table 31.14 Representative Products for Minor Wounds That Contain Astringents

PRODUCT	SELECTED INGREDIENTS/COMMENTS
Bluboro Powder	Aluminum sulfate 53.9%, calcium acetate 43% to form aluminum acetate in solution
Domeboro Tablets	Aluminum sulfate 878 mg, calcium acetate 604 mg per tablet to form aluminum acetate when placed in water
T.N. Dickinson's Witch Hazel	Witch hazel distilled 100%

and effective for this use include allantoin, aluminum hydroxide gel, cocoa butter, calamine, dimethicone, glycerin, kaolin, petrolatum, shark liver oil, sodium bicarbonate, zinc acetate, zinc carbonate, and zinc oxide, which may be combined as manufacturers desire.[97] Products containing any of these ingredients must be labeled for external use only, and the label must caution patients to avoid contact with the eyes. If the minor wound worsens or does not improve within 7 days, the patient should consult a physician.[98] Protectants may be purchased as single ingredients (e.g., cocoa butter, petrolatum, and calamine lotion) or combined with other ingredients.

Aloe vera is often used for minor cuts and scrapes, but lacks evidence of effectiveness. Nonmedicated petrolatum slows epithelialization; a thick layer is a barrier to cell migration, perhaps interfering with cell adherence.[39]

ASTRINGENTS

Astringents coagulate protein to minimize oozing, discharge, or bleeding when applied to skin (Table 31.14).[81] Aluminum acetate may be used as a wet dressing, soak, or compress to relieve inflammation associated with minor bruises and minor ulcerations of the skin. Witch hazel helps treat bruises and contusions and protects minor cuts and scrapes. Aluminum sulfate, in the form of a styptic pencil, stops bleeding from minor surface cuts and abrasions such as those that occur during shaving.[99]

SUMMARY

Patients who wish to self-treat a wound present a challenge to the pharmacist. The wound must be assessed to ascertain

AT THE COUNTER

 A woman in her 40s asks for a butterfly bandage.

Interview/Patient Assessment

The pharmacist directs the patient to the bandage products and asks what kind of wound she has. She replies, "It's my son, the 14-year-old. They were playing baseball, and it was too dark to see the ball very well. His brother threw the ball toward him, but he didn't see it and it hit him on the top of the head. It didn't knock him out." The pharmacist asks how the wound looks. "Well, it was bleeding at first, but not a great deal. It's almost stopped now, and I wanted the butterfly bandages to bring the ends of the wound together. Should I use some antibiotic ointment, too?"

Pharmacist's Analysis

1. Is a butterfly bandage appropriate for this type of wound?
2. Is an antibiotic ointment appropriate for this wound?
3. Should this boy see a physician?

This boy seems to have a typical play-associated wound. Although he did not lose consciousness and has no further problems (e.g., sudden onset of severe headache), he should still be watched for signs of a concussion (e.g., nausea, vomiting, pallor, lethargy). In the meantime, the wound can be self-treated. The butterfly bandage allows the edges of the wound to be brought together to speed healing.

Patient Counseling

In addition to recommending the butterfly bandage, the pharmacist should advise the mother to apply an antibiotic ointment to help prevent infection in the wound and help protect the skin from dehydration (which retards the healing process). The pharmacist should suggest covering the wound lengthwise with a primary dressing, which will keep the skin beneath the wound moist. A superficial wound may only need a primary dressing, but if it has more drainage, a secondary dressing would also help control the exudate.

whether it is amenable to self-therapy. Patients should be referred for extensive abrasions that may have damaged tendons, nerves, or muscles; deep cuts; those with heavy bleeding; and for infected wounds. Patients with compromised ability to heal (e.g., taking corticosteroids or immunosuppressants) should also be referred. Wounds likely to require extensive decontamination (e.g., wounds sustained in a heavily contaminated environment) or surgical repair should also be referred.

For minor wounds, pharmacists may recommend several products over several stages in the healing process, including the application of first-aid antiseptics to prevent infection in the wound, anesthetic/analgesics to lessen the pain of the wound, and protectants to protect the skin while it is healing. Appropriate wound dressings may also be recommended, including the use of primary dressings for wounds with light exudate, secondary dressings for moderate exudate, and tape to secure the dressings.

References

1. Howell JM, Chisholm CD. Wound care. Emerg Med Clin North Am 15:417, 1997.
2. McClure RJ. The importance of minor injury. Aust N Z J Public Health 20:97, 1996.
3. Brebner JA, et al. The nurse practitioner: Management of minor trauma. Accid Emerg Nurs 4:43, 1996.
4. Gruen RL, Chang S, MacLellan DG. The point prevalence of wounds in a teaching hospital. Aust N Z J Surg 67: 686,1997.
5. McClure RJ, Douglas RM. The public health impact of minor injury. Accid Anal Prev 28:443, 1996.
6. Jordan EA, Duggan AK, Hardy JB. Injuries in children of adolescent mothers: Home safety education associated with decreased injury risk. Pediatrics 91:481, 1993.
7. Lillis KA, Jaffe DM. Playground injuries in children. Pediatr Emerg Care 13:149, 1997.
8. Laffoy M. Childhood accidents at home. Ir Med J 90:26, 1997.
9. Cummings P, et al. Injuries and their relation to potential hazards in child day care. Inj Prev 2:105, 1996.
10. Holland JG, Hume AS, Martin JN Jr. Drug use and physical trauma: Risk factors for preterm delivery. J Miss State Med Assoc 38:301, 1997.
11. Capezuti E, et al. The relationship between physical restraint removal and falls and injuries among nursing home residents. J Gerontol A Biol Sci Med Sci 53:M47, 1998.
12. Riley AW, et al. Behavior and injury in urban and rural adolescents. Inj Prev 2:266, 1996.
13. Wazana A. Are there injury-prone children? A critical review of the literature. Can J Psychiatry 42:602, 1997.
14. Greenblatt JF, Dannenberg AL, Johnson CJ. Incidence of hospitalized injuries among pregnant women in Maryland, 1979–1990. Am J Prev Med 13:374, 1997.
15. Wright KA. Management of agricultural injuries and illness. Nurs Clin North Am 28:253, 1993.
16. Dellinger AM, Waxweiler RJ, Malonee S. Injuries to rescue workers following the Oklahoma City bombing. Am J Ind Med 31:727, 1997.
17. Muir L, Foucher G, Marian Braun F. Ax injuries of the hand. J Trauma 42:927, 1997.

18. Born CT, et al. Patterns of injury and disability caused by fork-lift trucks. J Trauma 40:636, 1996.

19. Radhakrishnan J, Fernandez L, Geissler G. Air rifles—Lethal weapons. J Pediatr Surg 31:1407, 1996.

20. Amirjamshidi A, Abbassioun K, Roosbeh H. Air-gun pellet injuries to the head and neck. Surg Neurol 47:331, 1997.

21. Rivara FP, et al. Injuries involving off-road cycling. J Fam Pract 44:481, 1997.

22. Erickson TB, et al. Drug use patterns at major rock concert events. Ann Emerg Med 28:22, 1996.

23. Biros MH. The frequency of unsuspected minor illness or injury in intoxicated patients. Acad Emerg Med 3:853, 1996.

24. Ryan CW. Alcohol and minor trauma. Mil Med 162:292, 1997.

25. Bostrom L. Injury panorama and medical consequences for 1158 persons assaulted in the central part of Stockholm, Sweden. Arch Orthop Trauma Surg 116:315, 1997.

26. Singh AJ, Kaur A. Minor injuries in ninth class school children of Chandigarh and rural Haryana. Indian Pediatr 33:25, 1996.

27. O'Loughlin JL, et al. Incidence of and risk factors for falls and injurious falls among the community-dwelling elderly. Am J Epidemiol 137:342, 1993.

28. Gofin R, Liscn M, Morag C. Injuries in primary care practices. Arch Dis Child 68:223, 1993.

29. Flanagan M. A practical framework for wound assessment. I. Physiology. Br J Nurs 5:1391, 1996.

30. van Rijswijk L. Issues in chronic wound care: Where do we go from here? Ostomy Wound Manage 42(10A Suppl):70S, 1996.

31. Gogia PP. Physical therapy modalities for wound management. Ostomy Wound Manage 42:46, 1996.

32. Mertz PM, Ovington LG. Wound healing microbiology. Dermatol Clin 11:739, 1993.

33. Kirsner RS, Eaglstein WH. The wound healing process. Dermatol Clin 11:629, 1993.

34. Laverty D, Mallett J, Mulholland J. Protocols and guidelines for managing wounds. Prof Nurs 13:79, 1997.

35. Wysocki AB. Wound fluids and the pathogenesis of chronic wounds. J Wound Ostomy Continence Nurs 23:283, 1996.

36. Flanagan M. A practical framework for wound assessment. 2: Methods. Br J Nurs 6:6, 1997.

37. van Rijswijk L. The fundamentals of wound assessment. Ostomy Wound Manage 42:40, 1996.

38. Flanagan M, Fletcher J. Wound care: The healing process. Nurs Stand 11(40 Suppl):5, 1997.

39. Moy LS. Management of acute wounds. Dermatol Clin 11:759, 1993.

40. Ger R. Wound management by constant tension approximation. Ostomy Wound Manage 42:40, 1996.

41. Oliver L. Wound cleansing. Nurs Stand 11:47, 1997.

42. Del Pino A, Abcarian H. The difficult perineal wound. Surg Clin North Am 77:155, 1997.

43. Rijswijk LV, Cuzzell JZ. Managing full-thickness wounds. Am J Nurs 91:18, 1991.

44. Thornton FJ, Schaffer MR, Barbul A. Wound healing in sepsis and trauma. Shock 8:391, 1997.

45. Krasner D. Selecting wound dressings by category. NARD J (Spec Educ Suppl): 1992 (10).

46. Polk HC Jr. Factors influencing the risk of infection after trauma. Am J Surg 165(2A Suppl):2S, 1993.

47. Kiy AM. Nutrition wound healing. A bio-psychosocial perspective. Nurs Clin North Am 32:849, 1997.

48. Stotts NA, Wipke Tevis D. Co-factors in impaired wound healing. Ostomy Wound Manage 42:44, 1996.

49. Chang H, Wind S, Kerstein MD. Moist wound healing. Dermatol Nurs 8:174, 1996.

50. Cho CY, Lo JS. Dressing the part. Dermatol Clin 16:25, 1998.

51. Tallon RW. Wound care dressings. Nurs Manage 27:68, 1996.

52. Willey T. Use a decision tree to choose wound dressings. Am J Nurs 92:43, 1992.

53. Larkin T. The story behind the scab. FDA Consumer 19(2):27, 1985 .

54. Cuzzell JZ, Stotts NA. Trial & error leads to knowledge. Am J Nurs 90:53, 1990.

55. Witkowski JA. Rational approach to wound care. Int J Dermatol 31:27, 1992.

56. Kerstein MD. The scientific basis of healing. Adv Wound Care 10:30, 1997.

57. Barr JE, Cuzzell J. Wound care clinical pathway: A conceptual model. Ostomy Wound Manage 42:18, 1996.

58. Jeter KF, Tintle TE. Wound dressings of the nineties. Clin Podiatr Med Surg 8:799, 1991.

59. Young T. Wound care in the accident and emergency department. Br J Nurs 6:395, 1997.

60. Hansis M. Pathophysiology of infection—A theoretical approach. Injury 27(Suppl 3):SC5, 1996.

61. Hon J, Jones C. The documentation of wounds in an acute hospital setting. Br J Nurs 5:1040, 1996.

62. Anon. A Practical Guide to Wound Care. Fort Washington, PA: Johnson & Johnson, 1987.

63. Ryan TJ. Wound Dressing. Dermatol Clin 11:207, 1993.

64. Knight CL. The chronic wound management decision tree: A tool for long-term care. J Wound Ostomy Continence Nurs 23:92, 1996.

65. Maklebust J. Using wound care products to promote a healing environment. Crit Care Nurs Clin North Am 8:141, 1996.

66. Fed Reg 44:69768, 1979.

67. Hanna JR, Giacopelli JA. A review of wound healing and wound dressing products. J Foot Ankle Surg 36:2, 1997.

68. Watret L. Know how...management of wound exudate. Nurs Times 93:38, 1997.

69. Anon. Local applications to wounds. II. Dressings for wounds and ulcers. Drug Ther Bull 29:97, 1991.

70. Rubio PA. Use of adhesive tape for primary closure of surgical skin wounds. Int Surg 75:189, 1990.

71. Chao T-C, Tsaez F-Y. Paper tape in the closure of abdominal wounds. Surg Gynecol Obstet 171:65, 1990.

72. Langford JH, Artemi P, Benrimoj SI. Topical antimicrobial prophylaxis in minor wounds. Ann Pharmacother 31:559, 1997.

73. Fed Reg 56:33644, 1991.

74. Hirschmann JV. Topical antibiotics in dermatology. Arch Dermatol 124:1691, 1988.

75. Carruthers R. Prescribing antibiotics for impetigo. Drugs 36:364, 1988.

76. Fed Reg 47:29986, 1982.

77. Fed Reg 47:22324, 1982.

78. Laufman H. Current use of skin and wound cleansers and antiseptics. Am J Surg 157:359, 1989.

79. Larson E. Guideline for use of topical antimicrobial agents. Am J Infect Control 16:253, 1988.

80. Mangione RA. Potential hazards of rubbing alcohol. Am Pharm NS25:133, 1985.

81. Fed Reg 47:39436, 1982.

82. Swayne LC, Ginsberg HN, Ginsburg A. Pneumoretroperitoneum secondary to hydrogen peroxide wound irrigations. Am J Roent 148:149, 1987.

83. Thomason SS. Front-line antiseptics. Geriatr Nurs 10:235, 1989.

84. Schneider DL, Hebert LJ. Subcutaneous gas from hydrogen peroxide administration under pressure (Letter). Am J Dis Child 141:10, 1987.

85. Oberg MS. Do not put hydrogen peroxide or povidone iodine into wounds! (Editorial). Am J Dis Child 141:27, 1987.

86. Fed Reg 39:33102, 1974.

87. Fleischer W, Reimer K. Povidone-iodine in antisepsis—State of the art. Dermatology 195(Suppl 2):3, 1997.

88. Kunisada T, et al. Investigation on the efficacy of povidone-iodine against antiseptic-resistant species. Dermatology 195 (Suppl 2):14, 1997.

89. Arata T, et al. Antiseptic effects at injection sites. Dermatology 195(Suppl 2):107, 1997.

90. Shindo K. Antiseptic effect of povidone-iodine solution on abdominal skin during surgery and on thyroid-gland–related substances. Dermatology 195(Suppl 2):78, 1997.

91. Niedner R. Cytotoxicity and sensitization of povidone-iodine and other frequently used anti-infective agents. Dermatology 195(Suppl 2):89, 1997.

92. Pesko LJ. Iodine solution. Am Drugg 200(1):60, 1989.

93. Fed Reg 52:47313, 1987.

94. Fed Reg 61:5918, 1996.

95. Kaye ET, Kaye KM. Topical antibacterial agents. Infect Dis Clin North Am 9:547, 1995.

96. Fed Reg 48:5852, 1983.

97. Fed Reg 43:34628, 1978.

98. Fed Reg 48:6820, 1983.

99. Fed Reg 58:54458, 1993.

Burns

A woman in her early 20s asks the pharmacist what product will help a burn.

Interview/Patient Assessment

The pharmacist asks how, when, and where she was burned. The patient replies, "It's not me, it's my husband. He was burned at work." The pharmacist asks if the husband can come in, but she says he doesn't want to. "The burn doesn't really hurt him. It's not blistered, but I'm still kind of worried about it." As she picks up a popular local anesthetic aerosol spray, she asks, "Can't he just spray some of this on it?" In response to further questions, the woman volunteers that the burn was caused by the exhaust of a power unit, and it is on his upper arm.

Pharmacist's Analysis

1. Is it necessary for the pharmacist to see the burn?
2. What does the absence of pain signify?

3. Should the patient be allowed to use a nonprescription product?

Had this burn been caused by electrical or chemical exposure, the patient would require referral. However, a minor thermal burn can be self-treated. Absence of pain is a dangerous sign, since it may indicate loss of nerves in damaged skin layers.

Patient Counseling

The pharmacist should strongly advise the patient not to use a nonprescription product until the severity of the burn can be assessed. The pharmacist should explain that the absence of pain and lack of blistering are cautionary signs, and that great care is required for self-treatment. The pharmacist can also mention that if the burn is minor, suitable nonprescription products include pain control medications, topical antibacterials (first-aid antiseptics), skin protectants, lubricants, and dressings.

Virtually no other trauma wreaks havoc on the body to the degree that a major burn injury can.[1,2] Some of the potential sequelae include loss of livelihood, infection, toxic shock syndrome, disfigurement, contractures, and death.[3,4] Since only minor (e.g., first-degree and minor second-degree) burns caused by thermal agents or sunburn can be self-treated, pharmacists must be able to gauge the extent and severity of the burn injury.[5]

PREVALENCE OF BURNS

About 2 million burns occur yearly in the United States.[6] Fully 500,000 are seen in emergency rooms, 100,000 result in hospitalization, and 20,000 are of sufficient severity to necessitate care in a burn center.[7] Burns are the fourth most frequent cause of death from unintentional injury in the United States—6000 to 20,000 patients annually—and the second most important cause of home deaths for those aged 65 and over.[7-9]

EPIDEMIOLOGY OF BURNS

About one-third of burn patients are individuals with a physical, psychiatric, or alcohol-related problem that contributed to the injury.[10] At least 35% of burn patients are children.[1] (Unfortunately, 10 to 25% of burns to children are intentionally caused by adults, a particularly pernicious form of child abuse.[1,11] Intentional burn victims have a death rate of 30%, as compared with only 2% in accidentally burned children.[1]) Young people aged 17 to 25 are another high-risk

group, perhaps because of more risky behaviors (e.g., high-speed driving).[12] Elderly patients experience more serious burns and suffer greater morbidity than other age groups.[9]

Many burns are the result of hazardous practices such as storing gasoline at home or other misuse of flammable materials.[13,14] Many adults suffer electrical burns in the workplace, but most electrical-burn patients are children, generally younger than 15, who are burned at home.[15,16]

ETIOLOGY OF BURNS

Burns have a number of causes, including thermal agents, ultraviolet (UV) light radiation, chemicals, and electricity (Table 32.1).

Thermal Burns

Thermal burns can be caused by flames, flaming liquids (e.g., alcoholic drinks made with high-proof alcohol and set afire), hot liquids (e.g., water and oil), hot objects (e.g., burners, irons, and pavement), and hot gases (e.g., steam or gases released during airbag deployment).[1,17-20] Flames cause about 50% of all burns seen in emergency rooms.[16] It is difficult to visually assess these burns, as they may be full thickness in the center, but partial thickness around the periphery. (See Figure 32.1 and "Depth" under "Factors in Burn Evaluation" for details on burn thickness.)

Scalds, especially common in children, comprise 30% of all burn injuries.[16] (Pharmacists should suspect child abuse if a child is scalded.[21] See "Scalding and Child Abuse.") Scalds can result from contact with hot liquid in a number of forms,

Table 32.1. Various Burn Classifications and the Proper Method of Treatment

DESIGNATION	DESCRIPTION	MOST APPROPRIATE TREATMENT
Etiology		
Thermal	Due to a heat source	May be self-treatable, depending on degree
Sunburn	Caused by UV radiation	May be self-treatable, depending on degree
Chemical	Considered a major injury by American Burn Assoc.	Recommend emergency first aid, and immediate referral
Electrical	Considered a major injury by American Burn Assoc.	Recommend emergency first aid, and immediate referral
Depth		
First-degree	Limited to epidermis	Self-treatable
Second-degree	Burn extends to dermis	Only self-treatable if a minor second-degree burn
Third-degree	Burn extends to subcutaneous tissue	Referral required
Fourth-degree	Burn involves muscle and bone	Referral required
Thickness		
Partial thickness	First or second-degree burn	Self-treatable unless more than a minor second-degree burn
Full thickness	Third or fourth-degree burn	Referral required

including water boiling on a stove, beverages and foods (e.g., coffee and soup), and hot water from the faucet.[22–24] *Pharmacists should advise patients that all hot-water heaters should be adjusted no hotter than 120 to 130°F.*[25] (See "Prevention of Burns.")

Hot objects cause 5% of all burns, often on the hands and fingers.[16] Sources include stoves, grills, heaters, irons, hair-curling devices, and hot motors.[26] The pharmacist may notice an outline of the object contacted, much like a brand. Some patients suffer foot burns when they walk on hot pavement.[27] Because of extreme temperatures and hazardous processes, workplace thermal burns are generally more severe than other burns.

Sunburn

Unprotected exposure to UV light can cause the well-known sunburn.[28] Sunburn differs from a thermal burn because it is not caused by an abrupt increase in tissue temperature, but rather is produced by the ionizing effects of ultraviolet light radiation. *Sunburn is also one of the few burns that is almost always preventable because generally it results from willful exposure to sunlight.* (See "Skin Damage Caused by Sunburn" and Chapter 33, Sun-Induced Skin Damage.)

Chemical Burns

About 3% of all burns result from exposure to caustic chemicals, such as various acids (e.g., sulfuric, hydrochloric, battery) and alkalis (e.g., cement, drain cleaner, caustic lime, oven cleaners), as well as metallic sodium or potassium.[16,28,30–33] Chemical burns also can result from garlic applied to the skin as a natural remedy.[34]

While immediate first aid for chemical burns is vital, referral to an emergency room is mandatory. (See "First Aid for Chemical Burns.")

Electrical Burns

Ten percent of all burns are electrical in nature.[16] They are caused by such activities as biting through an electrical cord (infants), placing an object into an electrical socket, or touching a wire or appliance.[35] Most electrical burns result from touching the source and thus generally affect the hands. In evaluating electrical burns, both the entrance and exit sites must be located, since high voltage may produce full-thickness injuries, affecting exposed muscle and bone, in both locations.[15,36]

Complications of electrical burns include bone and soft-tissue destruction, renal tubular damage from myoglobinuria, cardiac dysrhythmias, and cardiovascular collapse. Immediate referral to an emergency room is mandatory.

Lightning burns, an extreme type of electrical burn, produce widespread injury that can result in death.[37]

MANIFESTATIONS OF BURNS

Burn symptoms vary, depending on the burn severity. In appearance, burns range from the typical red of a sunburn to the complete skin charring of the fourth-degree burn. Superficial burns of the upper skin are painful because of the tissue damage, while, paradoxically, deep burns may not be painful because of nerve destruction. Also, while the most superficial burns produce reddened skin and more severe burns cause blisters, very severe burns eliminate the layers of skin that produce the blister. As a minor burn wound heals, the patient may develop pruritus that is fairly intense. Signs of an infected burn include erythema, edema in the tissues around the wound, increasing pain, odor, drainage, necrosis, or discoloration from red to violet, dark brown, or black.[38,39] The patient must be urged to visit a physician if these signs appear.

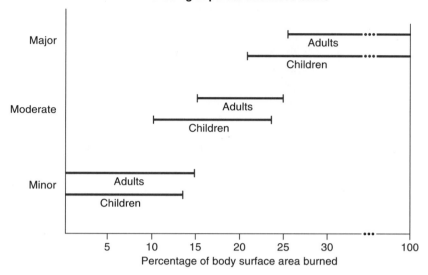

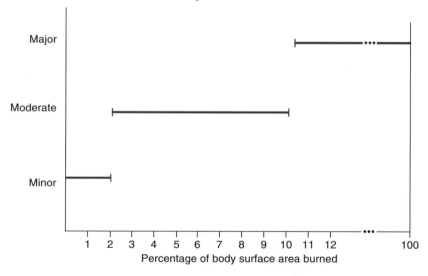

Figure 32.1. Grading of burns by percentage of body surface area burned.

See "Classification of Burn Severity" below for a more detailed method of classifying burns based on the symptoms they produce, their appearance, and other factors.

SPECIFIC CONSIDERATIONS OF BURNS

Classification of Burn Severity

Major burns disrupt the barrier effect of the skin, which can result in severe consequences (e.g., infection and fluid loss).[16] Expert medical opinion from the Advisory Review Panel on Over-the-Counter (OTC) Topical Analgesic, Antirheumatic, Otic, Burn, and Sunburn Prevention and Treatment Drug Products yielded the following statement, ". . . OTC products should be applied only to first-degree and less severe second-degree burns."[40] (See "Depth" under "Factors in Burn Evaluation" below for a discussion of burn degrees.) Consequently, it is critically important for pharmacists to be capable of differentiating burn severity. Note that if any portion of mixed-degree burns exceeds the criteria for self-treatment, patients should be referred, using the FDA's criteria. For example, if the patient has a second-degree burn, but any portion is third-degree, the patient should receive a referral.

Burn assessment is difficult even for trained professionals.[41] The American Burn Association has identified criteria that are useful in judging the severity of burns, as outlined in Table 32.2.[1] As shown, patients with minor thermal burns may be treated as outpatients (except for very young patients).[7] However, the classification used by the American Burn Association (e.g., minor, moderate, or major) is not that used by the pharmacist for a quick judgment to refer a patient (e.g., first-degree or less severe second-degree burn versus more severe second-degree, third-degree, or fourth-degree burns).

Factors in Burn Evaluation

DEPTH

Burn depth can be assessed by several methods, but the pharmacist usually must rely on only visual assessment and a recitation from the patient. The time-honored categorization of burn depth is first-, second-, third-, or fourth-degree (Fig. 32.2) (Table 32.2).[1,42] All types of burns—whether caused by thermal, UV, chemical, or electrical sources—can be first-, second-, third-, or fourth-degree in depth. It is difficult to generalize about the depth to be expected with any one etiology (e.g., chemical) since, with all types of burns, depth depends on the exact agent and the duration of exposure (e.g., 1 minute's exposure to dilute acetic acid, which might produce a first-degree burn, versus several minutes of exposure to lye, which could produce a third-degree burn).

First-Degree Burns

First-degree burns—known as partial-thickness burns (see Table 32.2)—affect the epidermis and associated structures such as hair. First-degree burns—which produce swelling, redness, and pain—blanch when pressure is applied, quickly refilling after pressure is removed.[17] Skin function is not compromised, so the skin continues to serve as a barrier to infection.[2]

First-degree burns heal on their own in 3 to 5 days with no scarring. If patients notice any tissue loss, it is usually a minor flaking of the skin later in the healing phase caused by epithelial shedding such as the "peeling" that occurs after a sunburn.[40,43]

Many of the nonblistering, painful sunburns seen by the pharmacist are first-degree burns.

Second-Degree Burns

Second-degree burns—also called partial-thickness burns—affect the epidermis and the underlying dermis (see Fig. 32.2). Residual epithelium and the associated structures

---

(e.g., hair follicles, sebaceous glands, and sweat glands) eventually regrow to resurface the wound. A minor (self-treatable) second-degree burn will have visible blistering, with loss of **proteinaceous** (possessing proteinlike properties) exudate, redness, and pain. Second-degree burns blanch with pressure, but refill only slowly.[28] (See "A Pharmacist's Journal: How Bad Is My Sunburn?")

Minor, second-degree burns heal in 7 to 10 days and do not require skin grafting, although the skin may not return to normal coloration for 1 to 2 months.[16] More-severe, second-degree burns, which require referral, appear waxy or mottled-white, heal slowly over 8 to 12 weeks, and scar.[44]

Many of the thermal burns seen by pharmacists, including more severe sunburns, are minor, second-degree in depth with pain and blistering.

Table 32.2. American Burn Association Injury Severity Grading System[a]

Minor Burns: May be treated on an outpatient basis. Very young patients may need hospitalization.
1. Less than 15% of the body surface area (BSA) (adults) or 10% of the BSA (children and elderly) if a partial-thickness burn
2. Less than 2% of the BSA if a full-thickness burn
3. Must not present functional or cosmetic risk to areas of specialized function (e.g., face, eyes, ears, hands, feet, and perineum)

Moderate Burns: may be treated in a hospital; does not require a burn facility.
1. 15–25% of the BSA (adults) or 10–20% of the BSA (children and elderly) if a partial-thickness burn
2. 2–10% of the BSA if a full-thickness burn
3. Must not present functional or cosmetic risk to areas of specialized function (e.g., face, eyes, ears, hands, feet, and perineum)

Major Burns: Emergency treatment at a local hospital followed by transport to a regional burn facility for specialized definitive care.
1. More than 25% of the BSA (adults) or more than 20% of the BSA (children and elderly) if a partial-thickness burn
2. More than 10% of the BSA if a full-thickness burn
3. All burns involving the face, eyes, ears, hands, feet, or perineum that may result in functional or cosmetic impairment
4. Burns due to caustic chemical agents
5. High-voltage electrical injury
6. Burns complicated by inhalation injury, major trauma, or poor-risk patients

Adapted from Rieg LS, Jenkins M. Burn injuries in children. Crit Care Nurs Clin North Am 3:457, 1991; and Griglak MJ. Thermal injury. Emerg Med Clin North Am 10:369, 1992.

[a]For detail on BSA (body surface area), see "Body Surface Area." The term "partial-thickness burn" refers to a burn that is either first-degree or second-degree. The term "full-thickness burn" refers to a burn that is either third-degree or fourth-degree.

Third-Degree Burns

Third-degree burns—also called full-thickness burns (see Table 32.2)—destroy layers of the skin (e.g., epidermis, dermis, and subcutaneous tissue), along with all hair follicles, sweat glands, and sebaceous glands. The wounds appear leathery, dry, inelastic, or charred.[7] Patients usually feel little or no pain since nerve endings have also been obliterated. Third-degree burns do not refill following pressure-induced blanching, if the area can be blanched.[28,38] (See "A Pharmacist's Journal: What Do You Have for a Burn?")

Healing can be protracted since **eschar** (dead tissue caused by a burn) slows recovery and the wound is **avascular** (lacking in circulation); skin grafting is usually mandatory.[44] Permanent scarring is the rule (unless the body surface area is less than 1%; see "Body Surface Area"). The skin color of the scarred area seldom matches surrounding skin.[16]

Although the appearance of the third-degree burn causes many patients to prefer a physician, the pharmacist occasionally counsels these patients, who self-assess them as minor because of the lack of pain.

Fourth-Degree Burns

Fourth-degree burns—also known as full-thickness burns— can affect underlying fat, fascia, muscle, and perhaps bone. The appearance of the fourth-degree burn causes virtually all patients to seek emergency care from a source other than a pharmacist.

BODY SURFACE AREA

The body surface area (BSA) of burns helps determine their severity, although the pharmacist does not need it to meet the FDA standard of self-treatable burns. BSA may be

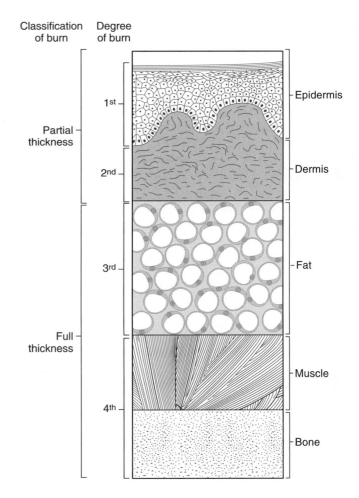

Figure 32.2. Classification of burns by depth of tissue burned.

A Pharmacist's Journal

"How Bad Is My Sunburn?"

A young woman in her late teens or early 20s approached me one summer to ask me to look at her sunburn. I didn't notice any problem with her face and asked her how bad it hurt. She said, "Let me show you." She turned her back to me and pulled her blouse up until her upper back was fully exposed, asking, "How bad is my sunburn?" I've seldom had an ambulatory patient present with a burn as bad. Her entire back looked as though someone had taken a hot iron and repeatedly ironed across it. The only exception was an X-shaped white mark where her sun dress had covered her skin. The skin was covered with large blisters and was ex-

tremely reddened and edematous. She replied that the pain was severe and wondered if a nonprescription product would help. I expressed doubt and asked her how she got the burn. She said she had weeded her yard the previous day and was bent over from sunup until past sunset. She added that the warmth of the sun had deceived her and that her face had been shielded, so it had been spared. I referred her to a local emergency room because of the surface area and extent of the burn. She returned later with prescriptions for silver sulfadiazine and a narcotic analgesic combination product, stating that the physician had diagnosed a deep, second-degree burn.

A Pharmacist's Journal

"What Do You Have for a Burn?"

A young woman appearing to be in her early 20s approached me in the pharmacy and asked what we had for a burn. I asked how she was burned, and she relied that the patient was her husband. I stressed the necessity to see the burn prior to rendering an opinion. She demurred, stating that it really didn't hurt him. I replied that the degree of pain might be less in a more-severe burn, whereupon she promised to bring him in. When she returned with her husband, he showed me a rectangular burn, approximately 5" × 3" in size, on the upper back. He explained that he had been welding a pipe in the

oil fields. When he was climbing from the trench, the handlers dropped the pipe, which trapped him against the side of the trench. The hot weld remained in contact with his back until the pipe could be secured and moved. The burn was grayish in color and appeared to be deep. Blistering had not occurred because of the depth. This burn was beyond nonprescription therapy, and I urged an emergency-room visit. The couple returned later with prescriptions for silver sulfadiazine and systemic analgesics. The physician diagnosed a deep, second- to third-degree burn.

approximated in several ways, but the traditional method is the "Rule of Nines." The "Rule of Nines" is based on a curious finding that BSA can be roughly divided into multiples of the number 9, as described in Table 32.3 and shown in Figure 32.3. BSA percentage figures for children and infants differ from the "Rule of Nines" figures because their head is larger in proportion to the rest of their body. For this reason a different set of percentages is used to estimate BSA for children and infants (Fig.32.4).

Another useful BSA estimation is the "Rule of Palms."

Table 32.3. Body Surface Area Using the "Rule of Nines"

BODY AREA	PERCENTAGE OF BODY SURFACE AREA
Head	9% (4.5% front and 4.5% back)
Trunk	36% (18% front and 18% back)
Arm	9% (4.5% front and 4.5% back)
Leg	18% (9% front and 9% back)
Genitalia	1%

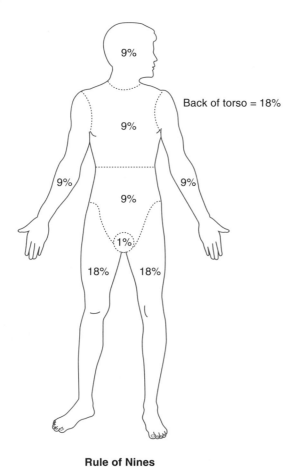

Rule of Nines

Figure 32.3. The "Rule of Nines" for determination of body surface area.

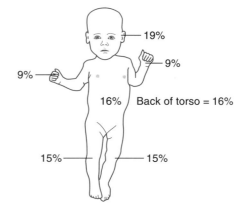

1. Body surface area for children aged 1–4 years

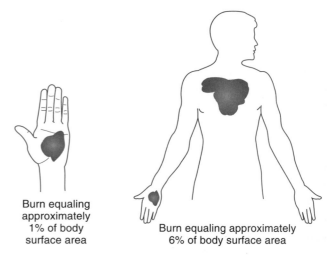

2. Rule of Palms

Figure 32.4. Alternate methods for body surface area determination: (1) Body surface area for children aged 1 to 4 years. (2) The "Rule of Palms."

The patient's own palm (without fingers) is approximately 1% of the total BSA. (However, an entire burned hand is 2.5% of the BSA, apportioned as 1% for the front palm, 1% for the back [exclusive of fingers], and 0.5% for the fingers).[16,45] Using the Rule of Palms, the patient places his palm over the burn area, counting the number of times the palm can cover it (see Fig. 32.4). More recent research indicates that this method underestimates the area and that the entire palm (including fingers) is more accurately placed at 0.8 to 0.85% of the BSA.[45,46]

LOCATION

Burns in certain body areas are more likely to cause complications during treatment and/or healing and should be referred if they are more severe than first-degree or minor, second-degree burns, even if the BSA is relatively small.[1] Problematic body areas include the face, especially the tip of the nose and eyelids; ears; joints; the dorsal surface of the hands; feet; and the perineum (see "Complications of Burns").

PATIENT AGE

The skin of very young and very old patients is thinner than the skin of most other individuals, so a given burn can produce more serious injury in these groups.[7] Therefore, burns to very young and elderly patients should be referred unless the burns are minor.

CAUSATIVE AGENT

The pharmacist should ascertain the offending agent. Brief contact burns are generally superficial such as touching a hot appliance and jerking the hand away rapidly.[7] However, burns with extended contact such as liquid burns can be much more dangerous. (A liquid [e.g., water, oil] at 300°F can cause a deep partial-thickness burn or a full-thickness burn in just 1 second.[38])

PREBURN MEDICAL STATUS

Certain medical conditions worsen the prognosis of burns, including diabetes mellitus, hypertension, and renal disease.[47,48] Conditions such as these impair healing because of a compromised ability to resist infection.[38] These patients should probably be referred for medical care, even if the burn appears to be nothing more than first-degree.

ASSOCIATED TRAUMA

Pharmacists should be alert for associated injury such as pulmonary complications. Patients with an inhalation burn, in addition to a topical burn, for example, have a substantially higher risk of mortality than those with just the topical burns.[7,49–51]

COMPLICATIONS OF BURNS

The risk of complications of burns increases as the severity of the burns increases. While minor burns resolve relatively rapidly with no scarring or residual skin problems, more serious burns can cause residual problems such as nerve injury.[52] The protective function of blistered and deeply damaged skin is compromised, which can lead to skin infections, systemic infections, fluid and electrolyte loss, and shock, which could cause death. For these reasons more-severe, second-degree and all third- or fourth-degree burns must be referred.

The risk of complications also increases with burns on problematic body areas, including the following:

- Tip of the nose—possible necrosis
- Eyelids—skin contraction prevent the lids from closing (resultant exposure keratitis can result in loss of vision)[43]
- Ears—loss of cartilage and the pinna[43,53]
- Joints— skin contractions decrease mobility[1,47]
- Dorsal surface of the hands—damage to thin skin decreases flexible finger motion. (For this reason, all hand injuries should also be medically supervised.[16])
- Feet—loss of function if contractures occur
- Perineum—difficulty in maintaining hygiene and risk of irritation from urine and feces

TREATMENT OF MINOR BURNS

Treatment Guidelines

This section describes self-treatment of first-degree and minor, second-degree burns caused by thermal agents or sunburn. *Patients with more-severe, second-degree, third-degree, and fourth-degree burns—which may necessitate airway assessment, cleansing, debriding, and therapy designed to stabilize fluid shifts, repair major wounds, prevent tetanus, and combat infection—must be referred.[16,54–57] Further, all chemical and electrical burns must be referred, following the application of emergency first-aid measures. (See Patient Assessment Algorithm 32.1.)*

FIRST AID FOR THERMAL BURNS
First aid for a thermal burn begins with removing the patient from the heat source or removing the heat source from the patient since the duration of contact affects the degree of tissue damage.[40]

Next, the burn area should be cooled.[58] Heat destroys tissues through denaturation of native protein and disruption of cell membranes.[43] However, protein that has undergone heat-induced denaturation can refold into its original configuration if cooled rapidly enough.[43] If no effort is made to cool the tissues, the elevated temperature may continue to produce injury for several minutes. Optimally, the burn area either should be immersed in cool water or covered with cool compresses as

quickly as possible (but for no longer than 30 minutes).[47] The burn area should be free of pain both while being cooled and when cooling is discontinued. Still water is preferable because running water can be painful. Also, ice is not advisable since it can cause pain and/or frostbite. Should cold water immersion prevent pain, the wound may not need topical treatment.

Pharmacists should advise patients not to place petroleum jelly, butter, margarine, or other home remedies on burns. Although these substances may decrease pain, they also will compromise sterility and retard healing.

If necessary, first-degree thermal burns can be dressed with a sterile bandage or nonadherent dressing to prevent infection pending assessment by a pharmacist or other qualified medical personnel. (See Chapter 31, Minor Wounds.) Blisters should be left intact to minimize areas of denuded skin that might subsequently become infected.[47]

FIRST AID FOR SUNBURN
The sunburn is not an accidental exposure, but an intentional exposure to ultraviolet radiation without taking proper precautions (e.g., use of sunscreen, protective clothing). Since it is not an accidental burn, first-aid measures are not applicable. The patient may move immediately to active treatment using nonprescription medications.

FIRST AID FOR CHEMICAL BURNS
First aid for chemical burns begins with cleaning the caustic powder or removing/diluting the caustic liquid.[16] Both acids and alkalis absorb progressively into tissue, extending the area of damage. Clothing saturated with the chemical should be removed immediately if possible, and the burn area should be irrigated with copious amounts of water. Patients should be assessed by emergency-room physicians or paramedics as quickly as possible.[7,28]

FIRST AID FOR ELECTRICAL BURNS
First aid for electrical burns begins with a call to 911 (or other emergency service) for help. Patients may require airway support to maintain breathing until they reach an emergency facility or until paramedics arrive. Beyond that, there is little else that can be done at home. ***Immediate care is mandatory.***

Nonprescription Medications

As previously mentioned, FDA panels and the agency itself limit self-treatable burns to first-degree and less-severe, second-degree burns.[40] The discussions refer mainly to thermal burns and sunburn. Electrical burns are not considered to be self-treatable; treatment of burns caused by chemical agents is not specifically recommended.[40,59] For these reasons the pharmacist should recommend referral for electrical and chemical burns after first-aid measures are instituted.

PAIN AND ITCH CONTROL
Self-treatable burns present with more pain than more severe burns since in more severe burns the nerves may have been destroyed.[16,60] Several ingredient categories (e.g., local anesthetics, counterirritants, and antipruritics) affect sensory

Patient Assessment Algorithm 32.1. Burn Therapy

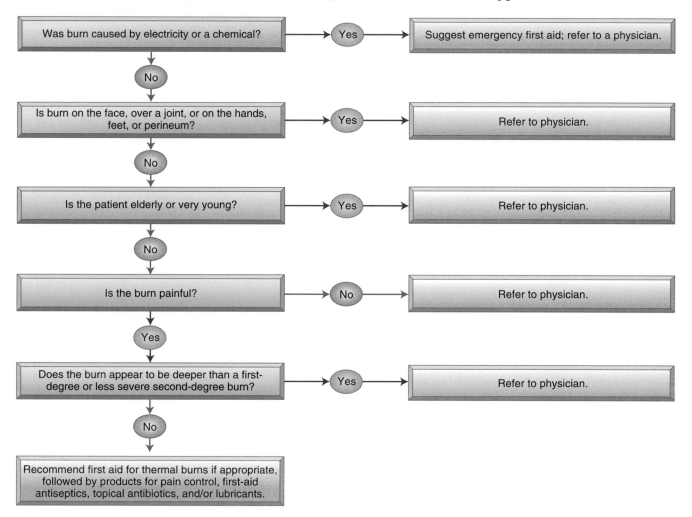

receptors in the skin and are safe and effective for treating minor burns and sunburn (Table 32.4).[59] (Note that the topical anesthetic listing is similar to Tables 30.1 and 30.2 in Chapter 30, Arthropod Stings and Bites, Pediculosis, and Scabies and to Table 31.12 in Chapter 31, Minor Wounds. Products containing ingredients that are not safe/effective for burns—such as hydrocortisone—do not appear in Table 32.4.)

All ingredients in this section are labeled for external use only, and patients are cautioned to avoid contact with their eyes. *If burns worsen or fail to improve after more than 7 days have passed, patients should discontinue self-treatment and consult a physician.[59] These products should not be applied more than three to four times daily and should not be used on patients younger than 2.*

Local Analgesics, Anesthetics, and Antipruritics

These ingredients effectively provide temporary relief for the pain and/or itching of minor burns or sunburn.[59,61] Camphor and menthol are safe and effective for all burns that can be self-treated (see Chapter 20, Injuries to Muscles, Ligaments, and Tendons, for a discussion of these ingredients).

Topical amines and "caine"-type local anesthetics are also safe and effective for burns that can be self-treated, including benzocaine, butamben picrate, dibucaine, dimethisoquin, dyclonine, lidocaine, pramoxine, and tetracaine (see Chapter 30, Arthropod Stings and Bites, Pediculosis, and Scabies, for a discussion of these ingredients). Safe and effective alcohol/ketone ingredients include benzyl alcohol, camphor/phenol, camphor/metacresol, juniper tar, phenol, phenolate sodium, and resorcinol (see Chapter 30, Arthropod Stings and Bites, Pediculosis, and Scabies). Topical antihistamines (e.g., diphenhydramine, tripellenamine) also act to depress cutaneous receptors for pain and itch (see Chapter 30, Arthropod Stings and Bites, Pediculosis, and Scabies).

Hydrocortisone, Hydrocortisone Acetate 0.25 to 0.1%

Many local anesthetics, analgesics, and antipruritics are safe and effective for such conditions as insect bites, poison ivy and oak, and minor burns. However, hydrocortisone has more restricted labeling than the others. Alone among the topical anesthetics, analgesics, and antipruritics, hydrocortisone is approved only for use as a topical antipruritic.[59,61]

Table 32.4. Representative Products for the Pain and Itch Caused by Minor Burns

PRODUCT	SELECTED INGREDIENTS/COMMENTS
Americaine Aerosol	Benzocaine 20%
Aveeno Anti-Itch Cream	Calamine 3%, pramoxine HCl 1%, camphor 0.3%
Bactine First Aid	Lidocaine 2.5%, benzalkonium chloride 0.13%
Benadryl Itch Stopping Cream	Diphenhydramine HCl 1%, zinc acetate 0.1%
Benadryl Extra Strength Itch Stopping Cream	Diphenhdyramine HCl 2%, zinc acetate 0.1%
Benadryl Itch Stopping Gel	Diphenhydramine HCl 2%, zinc acetate 1%
Benadryl Original Strength Itch Stopping Spray	Diphenhdyramine HCl 1%, zinc acetate 0.1%
Benadryl Extra Strength Itch Stopping Spray	Diphenhdyramine HCl 2%, zinc acetate 0.1%
Benadryl Extra Strength Itch Stopping Stick	Diphenhydramine HCl 2%, zinc acetate 0.1%
Bicozene Cream	Benzocaine 6%, resorcinol 1.67%
Caladryl Lotion	Calamine 8%, pramoxine HCl 1%
Caladryl Clear Lotion	Pramoxine HCl 1%, zinc acetate 1%
Campho-Phenique Pain Relieving Antiseptic Liquid	Phenol 4.7%, camphor 10.8%, eucalyptus oil, light mineral oil
Dermoplast Hospital Strength Aerosol	Benzocaine 20%, menthol 0.5%
Foille Spray	Benzocaine 5%, chloroxylenol 0.6% (unapproved ingredient)
Gold Bond Medicated Anti-Itch Cream	Lidocaine, menthol (no concentration labeled for any ingredient)
Itch-X Gel	Benzyl alcohol 10%, pramoxine HCl 1%
Lanacane Cream	Benzocaine 6%, benzethonium chloride 0.2%
Lanacane Maximum Strength Cream	Benzocaine 20%, benzethonium chloride 0.2%
Medi-Quik Aerosol	Benzalkonium chloride 0.13%, lidocaine 2%, camphor 0.2%
Nupercainal Cream	Dibucaine 0.5%
Rhuli Anti-Itch Gel	Benzyl alcohol 2%, menthol 0.3%, camphor 0.3%
Rhuli Calamine Spray	Benzocaine 5%, calamine 13.8%, camphor 0.7%
Solarcaine Aerosol	Benzocaine 20%, triclosan 0.13%
Unguentine Original Formula Ointment	Phenol 1%
Unguentine Plus Cream	Lidocaine 2%, phenol 0.5%

Since minor burns or sunburn are more likely to cause pain than itching, the FDA has ruled that hydrocortisone cannot be labeled for relief of the discomfort from burns or sunburn.

TOPICAL ANTIBACTERIAL AGENTS
Topical antibacterial agents are not considered necessary for minor burns by some physicians who specialize in burns since the skin is unbroken.[7,43] However, they are approved by the FDA for this purpose and are widely used by the lay public.

tip According to the FDA, however, *topical antibacterial agents should only be recommended for the prevention of infection and must never be applied to an infected injury.*[62]

(See "Manifestations of Burns" for a description of infected burns.)

First-Aid Antiseptics
A number of first-aid antiseptics are effective for preventing infection in minor wounds such as burns. These products are discussed in greater detail in Chapter 31 since they are also useful for prevention of infection in minor wounds.

Alcohols. Safe and effective alcohols include ethyl alcohol 48 to 95% and isopropyl alcohol 50 to 91.3%. Products containing alcohols are listed in Table 32.5.

Camphorated Metacresol. This complex consists of 3 to 10.8% camphor and 1 to 3.6% metacresol in a ratio of 1:3. When camphorated metacresol is used, the area should not be bandaged to prevent possible irritation to the skin. No leading product contains camphorated metacresol at this time.

Camphorated Phenol. This complex consists of 10.8% camphor and 4.7% phenol in a light, mineral oil vehicle. When camphorated phenol is used, the area should not be bandaged to prevent possible skin irritation. A product containing camphorated phenol is listed in Table 32.6.

Eucalyptol Combination. This combination is composed of eucalyptol 0.091%, menthol 0.042%, methyl salicylate 0.055%, and thymol 0.063% in 26.9% alcohol. It is essentially the same as the proprietary product Listerine, although that product is not labeled for burns and should not be recommended for burns.

Hexylresorcinol 0.1%. Hexylresorcinol is safe and effective for treatment of minor burns, with no specific warnings necessary for its use. A product containing hexylresorcinol is listed in Table 32.6.

Hydrogen peroxide solution 3%. Hydrogen peroxide is safe and effective for treatment of minor burns. (See Chapter 31,

Minor Wounds.) Products containing hydrogen peroxide are listed in Table 32.7.

Iodine Derivatives. Safe and effective iodine derivatives include iodine topical solution, povidone-iodine complex 0.5 to 10%, and iodine tincture. Tincture of iodine contains 1.8 to 2.2 g of iodine and 2.1 to 2.6 g of sodium iodide in 100 mL of 44 to 50% ethyl alcohol or denatured alcohol.[63,64] Products containing iodine and/or iodophors are listed in Table 32.8.

Phenol 0.5 to 1%. When phenol is used, the area should not be bandaged to prevent skin irritation. No leading product contains phenol as a sole ingredient at this time.

Quaternary Ammonium Compounds. Safe and effective quaternary ammonium surfactants include benzalkonium chloride 0.1 to 0.13%, benzethonium chloride 0.1 to 0.2%, and methylbenzethonium chloride 0.13 to 5%. A product containing a quaternary ammonium compound is listed in Table 32.6.

First-Aid Antiseptics That Lack Proof of Safety and/or Efficacy for Burns. Some ingredients have been found to lack sufficient evidence of safety and/or effectiveness as first-aid antiseptics.[65] Some are listed in Table 32.6; others include the following:

Table 32.5. Representative Alcohol-Containing First-Aid Antiseptics for Minor Burns

PRODUCT	SELECTED INGREDIENTS/COMMENTS
Lavacol	Ethyl alcohol 70% with denaturants
Isopropyl Rubbing Alcohol	Isopropyl alcohol 70%
Isopropyl Rubbing Alcohol Gel	Isopropyl alcohol 70% in gel; unapproved dosage form

Table 32.6. Representative Miscellaneous First-Aid Antiseptics for Minor Burns

PRODUCT	SELECTED INGREDIENTS/COMMENTS
Bactine Aerosol	Benzalkonium chloride 0.13%, lidocaine HCl 2.5%
Campho-Phenique Pain Relieving Antiseptic Liquid	Phenol 4.7%, camphor 10.8%, eucalyptus oil, light mineral oil
Corona Ointment	Lanolin 50%, oxyquinoline 0.11% (unapproved antiseptic), beeswax, petrolatum, sodium borate (a veterinary product sometimes used in humans)
Gentian Violet	Gentian violet 1% (unapproved antiseptic)
Medicated Vaseline	White petrolatum, chloroxylenol (unapproved antiseptic; unlabeled concentration)
Mercurochrome	Aqueous merbromin 2%
S.T. 37 Antiseptic Solution	Hexylresorcinol 0.1%, glycerin 27.1%
Tincture of Merthiolate	Thimerosal 0.1% (unapproved antiseptic)

Table 32.7. Representative Hydrogen Peroxide–Containing First-Aid Antiseptics for Minor Burns

PRODUCT	SELECTED INGREDIENTS/COMMENTS
Hydrogen Peroxide Gel	Hydrogen peroxide 3% in gel; unapproved dosage form
Hydrogen Peroxide Solution	Hydrogen peroxide 3% solution

Table 32.8. Representative Iodine/Iodophor–Containing First-Aid Antiseptics for Minor Burns

PRODUCT	SELECTED INGREDIENTS/COMMENTS
Betadine Skin Cleanser	Povidone-iodine 7.5%
Betadine Solution, Ointment	Povidone-iodine 10%
BFI Powder	Bismuth-formic-iodide 16% (unapproved antiseptic), bismuth subgallate, boric acid, potassium alum, thymol, zinc phenolsulfonate
Iodine Tincture	Iodine 2%, alcohol 44–50%
Iodides Tincture (Decolorized Iodine)	Ammonium and potassium iodides in 45% alcohol; unapproved antiseptic iodides

- Chlorhexidine gluconate (not included in the approved ingredient list because the manufacturer has not marketed it for use in first-aid applications)
- Mercurials (e.g., thimerosal, merbromin)
- Benzyl alcohol
- Chloroxylenol
- Triclosan
- Poloxamer-iodine complex
- Triple dye

Topical Antibiotics

Topical antibiotics are labeled for the reduction of risk of infection in burns (Table 32.9). Labels should advise external use only, caution against ophthalmic contact, and tell patients not to apply the product to sizable areas.[65,66] *Labels should also direct patients, "In case of serious burns, consult a physician."* Patients should discontinue using topical antibiotics and consult a physician if the burn does not improve in more than 1 week, if it worsens, or if a rash or other allergic reaction develops.[66]

Topical antibiotics can be applied one to three times daily. Ointments and creams are applied by placing a small amount of product (an amount no larger than the surface area of the tip of a finger) on the wound; powders should be lightly dusted on the area; and aerosols should be sprayed in small amounts. A sterile bandage may be applied if desired.

Bacitracin. Bacitracin is a polypeptide antibiotic that is active mostly against Gram-positive organisms.[67] Its propensity to cause contact dermatitis is low. It may be marketed as a single-entity product, or in combination with neomycin and/or polymyxin.

Products containing bacitracin must caution the patient: "Stop use and consult a doctor if the condition persists or gets worse, or if a rash or other allergic reaction develops. Do not use this product if you are allergic to any of the ingredients."

Neomycin. Neomycin, an aminoglycoside, is active against Gram-negative organisms (except *P. aeruginosa*), anaerobes, and staphylococci, but lacks activity against other Gram-positive organisms such as streptococci.[67] Although effective, its utility is limited by a high incidence of allergic contact dermatitis, which has been found to be as high as 3.5 to 19% in the general population and as high as 20 to 30% in patients with certain conditions (e.g., chronic leg ulcers, stasis dermatitis).[67,68] If neomycin is applied to large areas of the body, systemic absorption may result in ototoxicity, especially in patients with reduced renal function.[67]

Neomycin may be marketed as a single-entity product or in combination with bacitracin and/or polymyxin. Products containing neomycin must caution the patient: "Stop use and consult a doctor if the condition persists or gets worse, or if a rash or other allergic reaction develops. Do not use this product if you are allergic to any of the ingredients."

Polymyxin. Polymyxins are decapeptides that have a Gram-negative activity.[67] Contact dermatitis is rare. Products containing polymyxin may only be marketed in combination with bacitracin or bacitracin and neomycin. Products containing polymyxin must caution the patient: "Stop use and consult a doctor if the condition persists or gets worse, or if a rash or other allergic reaction develops. Do not use this product if you are allergic to any of the ingredients."

Tetracyclines. Tetracycline, chlortetracycline, and oxytetracycline are safe and effective for nonprescription use as topical antibiotics, but they are seldom requested by pa-

Table 32.9. Representative Topical Antibiotics for Minor Burns

PRODUCT	SELECTED INGREDIENTS
Achromycin Ointment	Tetracycline HCl 3%
Baciguent Ointment	Per gram: bacitracin 50 units
Betadine First Aid Antibiotics + Moisturizer Ointment	Per gram: polymyxin B sulfate 10,000 units, bacitracin zinc 500 units
Mycitracin Ointment	Per gram: polymyxin B sulfate 5000 units, bacitracin 500 units, neomycin sulfate equivalent to 3.5 mg neomycin
Mycitracin Plus Pain Reliever Ointment	Per gram: polymyxin B sulfate 5000 units, bacitracin 500 units, neomycin sulfate equivalent to 3.5 mg neomycin, lidocaine 40 mg
Lanabiotic Ointment	Per gram: polymyxin B sulfate 10,000 units, bacitracin 500 units, neomycin sulfate 5 mg, lidocaine 40 mg
Myciguent Ointment	Per gram: neomycin sulfate equivalent to 3.5 mg neomycin
Neosporin Ointment	Per gram: polymyxin B sulfate 5000 units, bacitracin zinc 500 units, neomycin 3.5 mg
Neosporin Plus Pain Relief Cream	Per gram: polymyxin B sulfate 10,000 units, neomycin 3.5 mg, lidocaine 40 mg
Neosporin Plus Pain Relief Ointment	Per gram: polymyxin B sulfate 10,000 units, bacitracin zinc 500 units, neomycin 3.5 mg, pramoxine 10 mg
Polysporin Ointment, Powder	Per gram: polymyxin B 10,000 units, bacitracin zinc 500 units

tients, perhaps because they are seldom if ever advertised to patients or pharmacists.

Antibiotic/Anesthetic Combinations

Topical antibiotics may be marketed in combination with local anesthetics, thus providing the dual benefits of local anesthesia and antisepsis (see Table 32.9). For instance, in Mycitracin Plus Pain Reliever Ointment, bacitracin, neomycin, and polymyxin B are combined with lidocaine.[65]

SKIN PROTECTANTS FOR BURNS

Skin protectants that are safe and effective for first-degree and minor, second-degree, thermal burns and sunburn include allantoin, aluminum hydroxide gel, cocoa butter, calamine, dimethicone, glycerin, kaolin, petrolatum, shark liver oil, sodium bicarbonate, zinc acetate, zinc carbonate, and zinc oxide (Table 32.10).[40] These ingredients may be combined with each other (e.g., petrolatum plus cocoa butter) as manufacturers desire. *Products containing skin protectants for burns must be labeled "for external use only" and must caution patients to avoid contact with the eyes. Also, if the burn worsens or does not improve within 7 days, patients should consult a physician.*[69]

Aloe vera, often used as a skin protectant for burns, lacks evidence of effectiveness.

ASTRINGENTS

Although early FDA publications regarding astringents included labeling for treatment of sunburn, current reviews do not allow astringents to be labeled for treatment of sunburn or other burns.[70–73]

SKIN LUBRICATION

Lotions and other skin moisteners can help the skin feel less dry, and the pharmacist may recommend them for that purpose. Some skin protectants (e.g., cocoa butter, glycerin, petrolatum) also lubricate the skin, providing dual benefit (see Table 32.10). However, the value of vitamin E oil, as opposed to other lubricants, has not been demonstrated, although some people claim that it can help eliminate scarring from burns. Other substances are used to lubricate or treat burns, but are ineffective and may be dangerous (see "Myths in Burn Care").

PREVENTION OF BURNS

Pharmacists may choose to assume an important role in preventing burns by educating patients, parents, caregivers, and the community at large. When electrical devices are sold in the pharmacy (e.g., steam vaporizers), pharmacists should discuss their safe operation. Pharmacists might also print and disseminate a list of burn prevention guidelines for customers to read such as the following:

- When cooking, make sure all children are supervised or restrained, so they cannot accidentally touch hot surfaces.
- Turn off stoves, deep fat fryers, and hot plates immediately after use.

Table 32.10. Representative Products for Minor Burns That Contain Topical Protectants

PRODUCT	SELECTED INGREDIENTS/COMMENTS
Aveeno Anti-Itch Cream	Calamine 3%, pramoxine HCl 1%, camphor 0.3%
Benadryl Itch Stopping Cream	Diphenhydramine HCl 1%, zinc acetate 0.1%
Benadryl Extra Strength Itch Stopping Cream	Diphenhdyramine HCl 2%, zinc acetate 0.1%
Benadryl Itch Stopping Gel	Diphenhdyramine HCl 2%, zinc acetate 1%
Benadryl Original Strength Itch Stopping Spray	Diphenhdyramine HCl 1%, zinc acetate 0.1%
Benadryl Extra Strength Itch Stopping Spray	Diphenhdyramine HCl 2%, zinc acetate 0.1%
Benadryl Extra Strength Itch Stopping Stick	Diphenhydramine HCl 2%, zinc acetate 0.1%
Caladryl Lotion	Calamine 8%, pramoxine HCl 1%
Caladryl Clear Lotion	Pramoxine HCl 1%, zinc acetate 1%
Calamine Lotion	Calamine, zinc oxide, glycerin, bentonite magma, calcium hydroxide, purified water (concentrations unlabeled)
Glycerin, U.S.P.	Glycerin anhydrous U.S.P., 99.5%
Rhuli Calamine Spray	Benzocaine 5%, calamine 13.8%, camphor 0.7%
Vaseline	White petrolatum 100%
Zinc Oxide Ointment	Zinc oxide 20%, mineral oil, white wax, white petrolatum (concentrations unlabeled)

- Protect hands when removing items from the oven and/or microwave.
- Test the temperature or food carefully before taking a full bite or a full swallow.
- Keep vaporizers out of traffic flow patterns and instruct household members and visitors to stay 4 feet away from the steam outlet. (See Chapter 16, Humidity Deficit.)
- Never use gasoline or kerosene to treat head lice.
- Keep electrical cords of all appliances (e.g., lamps, coffee makers, hot plates, slow cookers, and irons) from dangling where a toddler can reach them.
- Take up the slack of electrical cords and secure them so toddlers cannot reach them (and possibly chew or pull on the cords).
- Never leave children unattended with any source of heat or fire.
- Use heating pads and other thermotherapy devices with care (see Chapter 20, Injuries to Muscles, Ligaments, and Tendons).
- Take appropriate precautions to prevent sunburn (see Chapter 33, Sun-Induced Skin Damage).
- Secure all chemicals that can damage skin (or cause poisoning) and ensure that the contents of containers are clearly identified.

FOCUS ON...

MYTHS IN BURN CARE

Many common home remedies are used to treat burns. Unfortunately, these "therapies" range from the innocent to the disfiguring. Placing butter, honey, or lard on burns lubricates the skin but provides no active treatment.[74] Using kerosene on burns is irrational since it may further irritate the burn; it is also dangerous since it could start a fire if a source of flame is in close proximity. Rubbing ashes into burns can produce permanent, blackish-colored scars.

- Reduce the temperature of the hot-water heater to 120 to 130°F.
- Always test bath water carefully before bathing children or immersing the whole body.
- Never walk on hot pavement or other surfaces without foot protection.
- Never add additional starter fluid to charcoal or to a fire that has already been lit.

SUMMARY

Burn injuries range from minor to devastating. Correct first aid can be vitally important in limiting the extent of injury. Pharmacists must be familiar with first aid for burns to properly advise patients. In particular, pharmacists must be sufficiently familiar with burn categorization to know when to re-

AT THE COUNTER

 A young woman in her late teens and her mother ask the pharmacist about a burn on the girl's leg.

Interview/Patient Assessment

The girl says the burn was caused by a curling iron about 45 minutes earlier. She explained that she was using the curling iron while sitting in a chair. The curling iron started to fall, and she tried to grab it. She missed, and the curling iron fell onto her leg. The burn is approximately one palm size. It appears red, and the girl says it is quite painful. There are no blisters. The girl wants to stop the pain so she can get her homework done. She denies use of medications and has no health conditions.

Pharmacist's Analysis

1. How is the burn classified?
2. Would first aid still be effective?
3. Are nonprescription products appropriate?

The burn was caused by a brief contact with a hot object, so it is more likely to be first-degree than a burn caused by a hot liquid. The absence of blisters and presence of pain are characteristics of a first-degree burn. The burn area is only 1% of the BSA (or less). When all of these factors are taken into consideration, the burn appears to qualify for self-treatment.

Patient Counseling

The pharmacist should mention the utility of cool water in limiting the extent of the burn, although this burn is probably beyond the time that cooling would be helpful. The pharmacist should discuss appropriate nonprescription products. Since the skin is unbroken, the value of an antibacterial/antibiotic is debatable. However, a local anesthetic would help with her pain. A skin protectant would also help keep the skin soft and lessen her discomfort. The pharmacist should explain the method of use and precautions associated with both products.

fer patients and to allow appropriate patient triage. Patients who are elderly, very young, or who have sustained burns on the face, hands, feet, perineum, or over a joint should always be referred. Likewise, patients with burns caused by chemical exposure or electricity should always be referred.

Patients with first-degree and less-severe, second-degree burns caused by the sun or exposure to a thermal source may use several nonprescription products such as local anesthetics for pain and skin protectants for prevention of discomfort. Further, the application of first-aid antiseptics or topical antibiotics can help prevent infection in the burn.

References

1. Rieg LS, Jenkins M. Burn injuries in children. Crit Care Nurs Clin North Am 3:457, 1991.
2. Greenhalgh DG. The healing of burn wounds. Dermatol Nurs 8:12, 1996.
3. Mast BA, Newton ED. Aggressive use of free flaps in children for burn scar contractures and other soft-tissue defects. Ann Plast Surg 36:569, 1996.
4. Blomqvist L. Toxic shock syndrome after burn injuries in children. Scand J Plast Reconstr Surg Hand Surg 31:77, 1997.
5. Mertens DM, Jenkins ME, Warden GD. Outpatient burn management. Nurs Clin North Am 32:343, 1997.
6. Parsons L. Office management of minor burns. Lippincotts Prim Care Pract 1:40, 1997.
7. Griglak MJ. Thermal injury. Emerg Med Clin North Am 10:369, 1992.
8. Mallonee S, et al. Surveillance and prevention of residential-fire injuries. N Engl J Med 335:27, 1996.
9. Lilley JM, Arie T, Chilvers CED. Special review—Accidents involving older people. A review of the literature. Age Aging 24:346, 1995.
10. Partridge J, Robinson E. Psychological and social aspects of burns. Burns 21:453, 1995.
11. Jessee SA. Orofacial manifestations of child abuse and neglect. Am Fam Physician 52:1829, 1995.
12. Wrigley M, et al. Factors relating to return to work after burn injury. J Burn Care Rehabil 16:445, 1995.
13. Wilson DI, Bailie FB. Petrol—Something nasty in the woodshed? A review of gasoline-related burns in a British burns unit. Burns 21:539, 1995.
14. Cox MJ, et al. Severe burn injury from recreational gasoline use. Am J Emerg Med 14:39, 1996.
15. Garcia CT, et al. Electrical injuries in a pediatric emergency department. Ann Emerg Med 26:604, 1995.
16. Drueck C III. Emergency department treatment of hand burns. Emerg Med Clin North Am 11:797, 1993.
17. Tiernan E, Harris A. Butter in the initial treatment of hot tar burns. Burns 19:437, 1993.
18. Still J, et al. An unusual mechanism of burn injury due to flaming drinks. Am Surg 63:252, 1997.
19. Hallock GG. Mechanisms of burn injury secondary to airbag deployment. Ann Plast Surg 39:111, 1997.
20. Brown RL, Greenhalgh DG, Warden GD. Iron burns to the hand in the young pediatric patient: A problem in prevention. J Burn Care Rehabil 18:279, 1997.
21. Dedovic Z, et al. Epidemiology of childhood burns at the Burn Centre in Brno, Czech Republic. Burns 22:125, 1996.
22. Ray JG. Burns in young children: A study of the mechanism of burns in children aged 5 years and under in the Hamilton, Ontario burn unit. Burns 21:463, 1995.
23. Burvin R, et al. Female breast burns: Conservative treatment with a reconstructive aim. Isr J Med Sci 32:1297, 1996.
24. Watts AM, McCallum MI. Acute airway obstruction following

facial scalding: Differential diagnosis between a thermal and infective cause. Burns 22:570, 1996.

25. Rosenfeld RM, Sandhu S. Injury prevention counseling opportunities in pediatric otolaryngology. Arch Otolaryngol Head Neck Surg 122:609, 1996.

26. Schieber RA. Injuries from propane gas grills. JAMA 275:886, 1996.

27. Harrington WZ, et al. Pavement temperature and burns: Streets of fire. Ann Emerg Med 26:563, 1995.

28. Edwards K. Burns. Nurs Stand 10:36, 1995.

29. Guercio-Hauer C, McFarlane DF, Deleo VA. Photodamage, photoaging and photoprotection of the skin. Am Fam Physician 50:327, 1994.

30. Luong KVQ, Nguyen LTH. Cement burn. J Fam Pract 41:601, 1995.

31. Kuckelkorn R, et al. Poor prognosis of severe chemical and thermal eye burns: The need for adequate emergency care and primary prevention. Int Arch Occup Environ Health 67:281, 1995.

32. Erdmann D, Hussmann J, Kucan JO. Treatment of a severe alkali burn. Burns 22:141, 1996.

33. Rider MA, Tarar MN. Burns caused by domestic alkalis. J Accid Emerg Med 12:130, 1995.

34. Farrell AM, Staughton RCD. Garlic burns mimicking herpes zoster (Letter). Lancet 347:1195, 1996.

35. Zubair M, Besner GE. Pediatric electrical burns: Management strategies. Burns 23:413, 1997.

36. Haberal M, et al. Visceral injuries, wound infection and sepsis following electrical injuries. Burns 22:158, 1996.

37. Graber J, Ummenhofer W, Herion HJ. Lightning accident with eight victims: Case report and brief review of the literature. J Trauma 40:288, 1996.

38. Klein DG, Fritsch DE, Amin SG. Wound infection following trauma and burn injuries. Crit Care Nurs Clin North Am 7:627, 1995.

39. Judson R. Minor burns: Modern management techniques. Aust Fam Physician 26:1023, 1997.

40. Fed Reg 43:34628, 1978.

41. Smith S, et al. Emergency room management of minor burn injuries: A quality management evaluation. J Burn Care Rehabil 18(1 Pt 1):76, 1997.

42. Heimbach D, et al. Burn depth: A review. World J Surg 16:10, 1992.

43. Ahrenholz DH, Clayton MC, Solem LD. Burns and wound management. Otolaryngol Clin North Am 28:1039, 1995.

44. Duncan DJ, Driscoll DM. Burn wound management. Crit Care Nurs Clin North Am 3:199, 1991.

45. Sheridan RL, et al. Planimetry study of the percent of body surface represented by the hand and palm: Sizing irregular burns is more accurately done with the palm. J Burn Care Rehabil 16:605, 1995.

46. Perry RJ, et al. Determining the approximate area of a burn: An inconsistency investigated and re-evaluated. BMJ 312:1338, 1996.

47. Griffin P, Leitch I. Initial burn management in the primary care situation. Aust Fam Physician 24:129, 1995.

48. Raff T, Germann G, Barthold U. Factors influencing the early prediction of outcome from burns. Acta Chir Plast 38:122, 1996.

49. Flint L. What's new in trauma and burns. J Am Coll Surg 182:177, 1996.

50. Darling GE, et al. Pulmonary complications in inhalation injuries with associated cutaneous burn. J Trauma 40:83, 1996.

51. Kornberger E, et al. Inhalation injury treated with extracorporeal CO_2 elimination. Burns 23:354, 1997.

52. van der Lan L, Goris RJ. Reflex sympathetic dystrophy after a burn injury. Burns 22:303, 1996.

53. Lee D, Sperling N. Initial management of auricular trauma. Am Fam Physician 53:2339, 1996.

54. Jordan MH. Management of head and neck burns. Ear Nose Throat J 71:219, 1992.

55. Camilleri IG, Milner RH. Human papilloma virus proliferation in a healing burn. Burns 22:162, 1996.

56. Sheridan RL, et al. Candidemia in the pediatric patient with burns. J Burn Care Rehabil 16:440, 1995.

57. Hollinworth H. Management of burns. Nurs Times 91:74, 1995.

58. Hill MG, Bowen CC. The treatment of minor burns in rural Alabama emergency departments. J Emerg Nurs 22:570, 1996.

59. Fed Reg 44:69768, 1979.

60. Pal SK, Coritella J, Herndon D. Adjunctive methods of pain control in burns. Burns 23:404, 1997.

61. Fed Reg 48:5852, 1983.

62. Fed Reg 56:33644, 1991.

63. Fed Reg 39:33102, 1974.

64. Fed Reg 47:29986, 1982.

65. Fed Reg 52:47312, 1987.

66. Fed Reg 61:5918, 1996.

67. Kaye ET, Kaye KM. Topical antibacterial agents. Infect Dis Clin North Am 9:547, 1995.

68. Hirschmann JV. Topical antibiotics in dermatology. Arch Dermatol 124:1691, 1988.

69. Fed Reg 48:6820, 1983.

70. Fed Reg 47:39412, 1982.

71. Fed Reg 47:39436, 1982.

72. Fed Reg 54:13490, 1989.

73. Fed Reg 58:54458, 1993.

74. Hall M. Minor burns and hand burns: Comparing treatment methods. Prof Nurse 12:489, 1997.

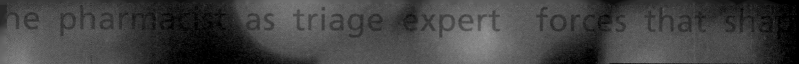

Sun-Induced Skin Damage

A man and woman with a baby just a few weeks old, who are planning a vacation to Florida, ask the pharmacist about sunscreens.

Interview/Patient Assessment

In response to questioning, the pharmacist determines that both parents have Type III skin, which is quite sensitive to the sun. The infant's skin is quite pale, and he has blond hair and blue eyes. The parents want to know if they can take him to the beach if they use a sunscreen with a high SPF (sun protection factor) value or a sunblocking agent.

Pharmacist's Analysis

1. What is the significance of the parent's skin type?
2. What is the significance of the infant's complexion and hair and eye color?
3. Should the infant be given a sunscreen with a high SPF value?
4. Would a sunblocking agent be appropriate for the baby?

The parents should be adequately protected by using a maximal value SPF sunscreen or sunblock, along with adequate clothing, as long as they follow all other instructions on the package to avoid sun damage.

Patient Counseling

The pharmacist should caution the parents that sunscreens are contraindicated for children younger than 6 months and should explain that children under the age of 6 months must not be exposed to the sun since their melanin content is minimal and they are at a high risk of burning. (The pharmacist should also mention that children that young cannot sweat, cannot move to the shade voluntarily, and cannot verbalize their discomfort, which makes sun exposure even more risky.) The sun may also damage the child's eyes. Recommending sunscreen use may give the parents a false sense of security about exposing this young child to the sun. The pharmacist should also discuss the risks of reflected sun (e.g., sunlight reflected from the sand, even under a beach umbrella) and the dangers of cloudy days, in which one can still burn badly. Further, the pharmacist should remind the parents that this information is important any time the baby is taken into the sun (e.g., a trip to Disney World or a state park).

Skin damage resulting from exposure to the ultraviolet (UV) radiation in sunlight ranges from sunburn to a number of long-term conditions such as photoaging, pigmentary changes, solar keratosis, various carcinomas, and premature aging. (See Chapter 39, Skin Hyperpigmentation). This chapter is concerned with the damage induced by long-term sun exposure, mainly to the skin (but to a lesser degree also to the eyes). The focus is not sunburn, which is covered in Chapter 32 (See "Sunburn" and "Skin Damage Caused by Sunburn" in Chapter 32, Burns).

A number of techniques can be used to prevent or reduce sun-induced skin damage, including avoiding the sun and using sunscreens. Sunscreens differ from most other nonprescription products because they are marketed to prevent a condition, not treat it. The judicious use of sunscreen can prevent relatively minor problems such as sunburn (see "Sunburn" in Chapter 32, Burns) and premature aging of the skin (see Chapter 39, Skin Hyperpigmentation), as well as conditions that can cause permanent disfigurement and even death such as basal-cell and squamous-cell carcinomas. Ingredients known as sun blockers are also covered in this chapter. These ingredients screen virtually all of the sun's UV radiation.

Despite the risks of sun exposure, and the severity of sun-induced skin damage, many physicians fail to discuss sun exposure with their patients. For example, a survey of pediatricians revealed that few warned patients about UV exposure and none could name five risk factors for melanoma.[1] This finding underscores the importance of pharmacists' advice in avoiding sun exposure. It is important when advising patients about sun exposure to understand that patients should not become fearful of the sun. (See "Sunlight: How Much Is Enough?")

ETIOLOGY OF SUN-INDUCED SKIN DAMAGE: THE WAVELENGTHS OF SOLAR RADIATION

The etiology of sun-induced skin damage has focused on the role of UV radiation, the shortest wavelengths of the solar spectrum.[4,6] Damage due to UV radiation increases yearly around the world because of the continuing loss of stratospheric ozone.[7,8] The ozone loss over Antarctica, which has perhaps been created by the widespread usage of chlorofluorocarbons, may eventually extend to nonpolar areas, increasing the amount of UV radiation reaching the earth.[9]

Researchers have arbitrarily divided UV radiation into UVA (320 to 400 nanometers), UVB (290 to 320 nm), and UVC (200 to 290 nm) (Fig. 33.1).[2,10] The different wavelengths of UV radiation damage skin differently:

- Longer wavelengths generally penetrate skin more deeply than shorter wavelengths (Fig. 33.2).[2] UVA radiation alters pigmentation, tanning the skin and penetrating the dermis, but does not produce the erythema of sunburn as severely as UVB.

- UVB radiation produces sunburn, a condition that peaks in intensity from 6 to 20 hours after exposure.[11] Sunburn also results in tanning, so UVB radiation is also responsible for this visible type of skin damage.
- UVC radiation, the most carcinogenic of the three UV radiations, does not reach the earth, but artificial sources (e.g., certain types of bulbs) can produce it.[4,11] UVC radiation reddens the skin but does not induce tanning.

UVB radiation is one thousand times more powerful than UVA radiation in burning skin, but 10 to 100 times more UVA radiation reaches the surface of the earth.[2] Thus both of these wavelength ranges should be protected against. Skin damage caused by UV radiation occurs because of radiation absorption by molecules in the skin known as chromophores.[2] These molecules absorb the energy of certain UV radiation wavelengths; permanent changes may occur as a result. DNA is a chromophore that absorbs UVB radiation (causing the eventual development of skin cancers); proteins and lipids absorb UVA radiation.[12] Melanin and hemoglobin are affected by both UVA and UVB radiation.

MANIFESTATIONS OF SUN-INDUCED SKIN DAMAGE

Exposure to UV radiation causes numerous skin problems; one of the most immediate is sunburn.[13] (See "Sunburn" and "Skin Damage Caused By Sunburn" in Chapter 32, Burns.) UV radiation also results in numerous long-term problems. *UV radiation is a cumulative poison that begins with one's first exposure to the sun and continues throughout life.*[14] The most common manifestations of sun-induced skin damage include photoaging, pigmentary changes, basal cell carcinoma, squamous cell carcinoma, and melanoma.

Sunlight can also induce recurrence of herpes simplex labialis. (See "Herpes Simplex Labialis," Chapter 4, Oral Problems.)

Photoaging

Photoaging, also known as premature aging or dermatoheliosis, is a long-term response to chronic, continued UV exposure.[2,5] The skin is chronically inflamed, a state known as heliodermatitis.[2] The changes, caused by the action of UVB on DNA and detectable on histologic examination, differ from chronologic (also known as intrinsic) aging.[15] Although each cell has the capacity to repair its damaged DNA, with intense and continued UVB exposure, this capability is over-

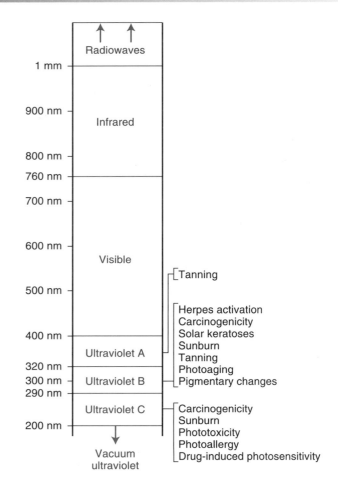

Figure 33.1. Divisions of solar radiation. Various ultraviolet wavelengths cause different types of damage, as illustrated.

whelmed (Fig. 33.3).[16] Photoaging does not manifest until decades have passed, leading to the myth of "safe tanning."

Photoaged skin shows epidermal changes such as wrinkles, coarsening, scaling, laxity, dryness, mottled hyperpigmentation, bruising, and **telangiectasias** (visible veins under the skin) (Fig. 33.4).[2,16,17] The degree of photoaging one

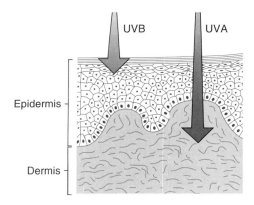

Figure 33.2. Penetration of skin by UVA and UVB radiation.

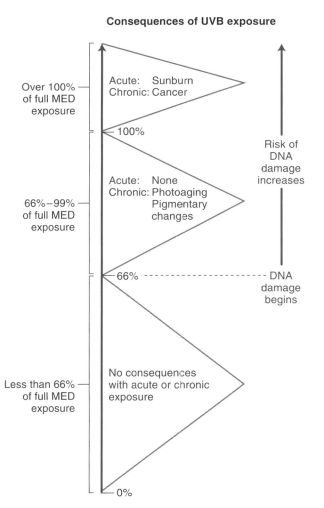

Figure 33.3. Consequences of receiving fractional amounts of a patient's minimal erythema dose (MED).

has can be roughly estimated by comparing two areas: the skin of the buttocks and the skin of the face or arms.[18] Although their chronologic age is identical, these areas usually appear markedly different.

Solar elastosis is a type of photodamage that occurs more deeply in the skin than the epidermis, affecting the der-

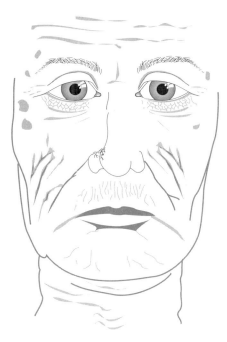

Figure 33.4. Manifestations of photoaging include wrinkles, scaling, laxity (sagging skin on the neck and cheeks), mottled hyperpigmentation (scattered blotches), bruising, and telangiectasias (fine blood vessels visible under the skin).

mis.[2,19] Elastic fibers normally present in the dermis give skin its elasticity.[20,21] With continued sun damage, however, these fibers mutate into a mass of tangled, thick fibers that have lost their full elasticity.[2,22] As these fibers accumulate, skin becomes thicker. Other effects of photoaging include degeneration of collagen, the development of deep furrows and wrinkles on the face, and the appearance of a yellowish discoloration on the forehead and back of the neck.[17,23,24] Participants in one study routinely overestimated the ages of photoaged women when showed their photographs.[9]

Patients suffer from photoaging in different degrees. Light-skinned whites are most prone to experience this skin damage, while the most dark-skinned people are least likely to suffer from it. (Even in low-risk, dark-skinned patients, photodamage may be clinically apparent if UV protection is disregarded completely.[9]) Photoaging also is a greater risk for patients involved in certain activities and occupations such as driving for long periods (the left side of the face is more damaged than the right side, which is shaded by the vehicle); working in the construction, fishing, and farming industries; and recreational tanning.[25] (Zealous recreational tanners now approach the risk level of patients with occupational exposure.[9])

Interventions such as dermabrasion and tretinoin may provide some relief from certain symptoms of photodamage (e.g., improvement of wrinkles).[26,27] (Tretinoin currently is not labeled for this indication, however.) Pharmacists should advise patients that the best "treatment" is still prevention.

Pigmentary Changes

Chronic exposure to UV radiation can result in increased or decreased pigmentation.

HYPERPIGMENTARY CHANGES

Hypermelanosis (increased pigmentation) is seen as solar lentigo, irregular spots of mottled hyperpigmentation on sun-exposed areas, popularly known as liver spots or age spots (Fig. 33.5).[9] These spots can be found on over 90% of whites aged 70 or more.[2] Hydroquinone, an FDA-approved hypopigmenting agent that can help reduce their visibility, is discussed in Chapter 39, Skin Hyperpigmentation. Ephelides or freckles, small benign macules that darken after sun exposure, can also be treated with hydroquinone.

HYPOPIGMENTARY CHANGES

Sun exposure causes small white scar-like lesions—known as spontaneous stellate pseudoscars—on the backs of the head and forearms of many individuals older than 60.[2] Idiopathic guttate hypomelanosis is a sun-induced condition that produces multiple white macules on the lower extremities, abdomen, and arms.

Solar Keratoses

Solar **keratoses** (epidermal lesions in which the upper layer of skin has hypertrophied) usually appear as dry, scaly lesions, pink-to-red in color and usually less than 1 cm in diameter.[10,23] Rare symptoms include irritation or tenderness.[10]

More than 80% of these lesions are found on chronically sun-exposed areas such as the face, head and neck, forearms, and back of the hands, underscoring the role of UV radiation in solar keratoses. (Not surprisingly, solar keratoses are also known as "actinic" keratoses, or keratoses related to rays in the UV spectrum.)[10]

Prevalence rates (patients with at least one solar keratosis) in the United States are 5.5% of females and 13.9% of males.[10] Because solar keratoses are more common with increasing age (denoting accumulated sun exposure) and with fair skin, lesions are seen in 50% of middle-aged, fair-complexioned individuals.[2,10] Individuals with darker skin have more natural protection than individuals with lighter skin since melanin absorbs some hazardous UV radiation.[28]

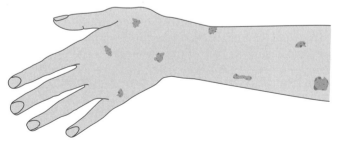

Figure 33.5. Typical distribution of hypermelanosis on the arm and hand.

Solar keratoses are more common at lower latitudes, again implicating UV radiation in sunlight, which is strongest at the equator.[10] Individuals whose occupations require outdoor work are two to three times more prone to develop solar keratoses than individuals who work indoors.[10]

Solar keratoses should be a concern because of their propensity to turn from benign lesions to nonmelanoma skin tumors (especially squamous cell carcinomas) without warning.[29] Estimates of the risk of this range from 0.1 to 20%.[10] Researchers estimate that as many as 60% of squamous cell carcinomas began as solar keratoses.[29] *Solar keratoses should always be watched closely for any changes (e.g., size, shape, or color).*

Basal Cell Carcinoma (BCC)

The major environmental factor responsible for inducing BCC is UV radiation, especially intermittent bursts of high exposure.[7,30,31] BCC ranks highest in incidence of all cancers diagnosed in white patients in North America, Europe, and Australia.[7,28]

A survey revealed that individuals most at risk for BCC have mothers of Celtic, English, or Scandinavian origin, blue/hazel eyes, freckles, medium or light skin, and red hair.[7] Individuals over 40 are also at higher risk than younger persons.[28] Childhood sun exposure also has been found to be an extremely important risk factor: individuals who suffered two or more episodes of childhood sunburn severe enough to cause pain for 2 or more days experienced a risk of basal cell carcinoma nearly five times that of those who do not have this history.[7]

BCC is most often found on the face, upper body, scalp, and neck.[28] Most BCC does not metastasize and is easily treated if diagnosed within the first few months of appearance.[32]

Squamous Cell Carcinoma (SCC)

The link between SCC and UV radiation has been well established in that total sun exposure increases the risk.[33] Individuals at high risk for SCC have light skin and red or blonde hair, burn rather than tan, and cannot develop a tan, even after a week of sun exposure.[34] The risk is doubled for individuals whose mother is Celtic, English, or Scandinavian. Freckles in childhood also increase risk.

The most frequent locations of SCC are the backs of the hands, the forearms, the head, and the neck.[28] Like BCC, SCC rarely metastasizes and is easily treated if caught early.[32]

Melanoma

Melanoma is less common than both SCC and BCC, but the incidence of this deadly cancer has doubled every decade for the past several decades.[32,35] Tragically, melanoma is the most rapidly increasing cancer in young people, shortening many lives. Melanoma ranks second only to lung cancer in rate of increase of mortality.

Unlike BCC and SCC, the exact contribution of UV radiation to melanoma is unclear. However, a history of three or more blistering sunburns before the age of 19 increases the risk of melanoma, so that acute exposure to UV radiation rather than chronic exposure may be the triggering factor.[36,37] The value of sunscreen in melanoma prevention is also less clear.[32,38]

Melanoma can be diagnosed by a physician prior to biopsy using several visible indicators[32]:

- Asymmetry of the lesion
- Irregular border
- Color variation from normal skin to black, brown, or bluish-red
- Diameter greater than 6 mm

Accordingly, change in the appearance of a lesion is a key indicator for melanoma. Pharmacists should urge patients to see a physician or dermatologist if the patients report that a lesion has enlarged, darkened, become elevated, begun scaling, or started itching.[14,35]

Melanoma risk factors are the qualities of the "Irish Lass" complexion: light-colored eyes (blue or green), blonde or red hair, fair complexion, tendency to freckle after sun exposure, sunburn rather than tanning on sun exposure, and moles on the body.[32] Moles known as atypical or dysplastic moles are also associated with a higher risk of developing melanoma.[35,36] Individuals who lived in sunny areas during childhood and young adulthood are at higher risk, as are individuals who worked outdoors 3 or more years during summer jobs as a teenager.[39,40]

Common sites for melanoma are the head, neck, and upper back.[35] For unknown reasons, the lesions are often found on sun-protected areas. Melanoma undergoes a noninvasive phase that may last for several years.[32] Detection during this phase can allow biopsy and removal while the lesion is in Stage I (confined to the skin). Prognoses at Stage II (positive lymph nodes) or Stage III (distant metastases) are quite poor.

SPECIFIC CONSIDERATIONS OF SUN-INDUCED SKIN DAMAGE: THE TANNING PHENOMENON

In the 1800s porcelain skin was seen as the ideal, as it showed that an individual was able to enjoy leisure time indoors, rather than being forced to work outside as a common laborer. However, in the early 1900s Europeans began to use the sun as therapy, and within a few years sunbathing spread to the United States.[5] Over the next several decades, untanned skin became associated with factory work, while tanned skin showed that one had the leisure time to "lay out" in the sun.[5,9] During the 1930s babies as young as 1 month were thought to require daily sun exposure. In the 1940s and 1950s this **heliotherapy** (exposure to the sun as a medical therapy) was scientifically exposed as dangerous, but the public has seemingly neither understood nor heeded this message.[5]

Tanning occurs in two phases[41]:

- First, skin exhibits an immediate darkening, which fades to be replaced by a delayed, longer-lasting tan.[2,5] UVA is thought to produce the immediate tan through oxidation of melanin that is present in the epidermis, while the delayed response is caused by UVB and its ability to increase the number and/or size of melanocytes. UVB also promotes melanogenesis, the production of new melanin.[42]
- Second, the long-term tan begins 48 to 72 hours after UVA or UVB exposure, peaking in discoloration within 7 to 10 days, and may not fade for several weeks or months.[41]

Tanning is a widespread pastime. One survey revealed that 43% of women sunbathed at least once weekly, as compared with 15% of men.[43] When asked, 61% of patients who tan stated that they do so because it prepares them for vacations (to look better during the vacation), while another 35% tan to obtain a darker skin tone.

Tanning Myths

Health professionals who attempt to spread the message of sun dangers must confront a number of myths and beliefs.[5] Foremost is the myth that tanned skin connotes good health.[44,45] The exact opposite is true. There is absolutely no health benefit to tanning.[43] *To the contrary, tanned skin is damaged skin that actually indicates individuals who will be at high risk of skin damage—possibly cancer—in later years.* For many people, sunburn is the limiting factor in tanning.[46] Their rationale for using sunscreens is simply to allow them to remain in the sun to tan for longer periods, while preventing burning. The myth in this behavior is that *irreversible DNA damage begins when sunbathers have received 60 to 70% of the UV dose necessary to cause sunburn.*[16]

Next is the belief that tans make the individuals more attractive and desirable.[5,37] Many ads featuring bronzed bodies perpetuate this pernicious stereotype, although a slow backlash of publicity has disseminated the message that one's own natural untanned skin color should be seen as the goal for all individuals. Nevertheless, many young people are unmotivated to protect themselves from damaging UV radiation. In fact one survey revealed that 27% of a group of 13- to 18-year-olds considered the use of sunscreen and hats to be "uncool."[1]

A final myth also relates to the healthy tan. Many people who are aware of the risk of skin cancer perceive their own risk to be small and acceptable.[5] Even providing concrete evidence of tanning dangers may not be sufficiently convincing. In one survey, 10% of the respondents stated that they would continue to tan even if the practice were proven to cause skin cancer.[43]

Tanning Parlors (Salons)

Tanning parlors are poorly regulated in most areas of the United States, although federal law states that maximal exposure time must not exceed four times the minimal erythema dose (also known as MED, the smallest dose of UV radiation that will cause minimal erythema—skin reddening) for Type II skin (see "Matching Skin Type to SPF" for a definition of Type II skin).[43] Further, the FDA requires sunlamps to carry the warning "Danger—Ultraviolet Radiation."[47] The FDA does not allow tanning parlor operators to state that their establishments produce "no harmful rays."[48] Despite these regulations, tanning parlors still cause direct harm to customers.[35] Most tanning parlors use UVA radiation sources rather than UVB sources, but the UVA sources still emit some UVB.[2,40,49] (At one time, some equipment in tanning parlors was found to emit five times more UVA than the sun's rays at the equator.[41])

Aside from the risk of long-term skin damage, tanning bed users have reported such acute adverse effects as burning, itching, rash, nausea, and warts.[43] Also, neglecting the FDA-mandated protective goggles can produce corneal burns.[43,49] Like natural UV radiation, the radiation in tanning booths also suppresses the immune system, which can result in an increased number of common colds and outbreaks of cold sores.[40,50,51]

In the words of the FDA, ". . . many experts would cheerfully ban tanning salons . . ."[47]

Tanning Pills, Artificial Tan Products, and Tan Accelerators

A number of products are marketed as tanning aids (Table 33.1). These products range from safe, in the case of artificial tan products, to unsafe and deceptive, in the case of canthaxanthin. Regardless of their safety, however, none of them have SPF values and thus they do not provide UV radiation protection. For this reason, the FDA requires a warning on any approved tanning aid that does not also contain a sunscreen: "Warning—this product does not contain a sunscreen and does not protect against sunburn."[42]

TANNING PILLS

For many years, health food stores, tanning parlors, and mail-order ads in magazines advertised oral tablets that purport to provide the user a tan without the sun. These unapproved products usually contain canthaxanthin, a chemical approved by the FDA in extremely low doses as a food and medication colorant.[52] When ingested, the chemical produces a pink-to-tan-to-orange color in epidermal fat cells.[53,54]

One company submitted canthaxanthin for FDA approval, but withdrew the application when adverse reactions such as crystal deposition in the eye surfaced.[53] Thus the FDA has not approved canthaxanthin as safe in the doses used in tanning pills, and has also not approved the use of oral products for tanning.[40] The agency has routinely seized products containing canthaxanthin, but this has not stopped their widespread sale and use since enforcement efforts are limited.[55] Because canthaxanthin is related to beta-carotene, some companies list the main ingredient of their products as beta-carotene, which is misleading.[56] *The Skin Cancer Foundation urges people to report these illegal products to the FDA and/or the U.S. Postal Service (if a catalog was received through the mail).*

Canthaxanthin products cause nausea, stomach cramps, diarrhea, severe itching, skin eruptions, night blindness, and drug-induced hepatitis.[42,55] In a widely reported case, a 20-year-old woman purchased an unknown number of

Table 33.1. Representative Artificial Tan Products and Tan Extenders

PRODUCT	SELECTED INGREDIENTS/COMMENTS
Bain De Soleil Sunless Tanning Creme	Dihydroxyacetone (unlabeled concentration)
Banana Boat Sunless Tanning Lotion	Dihydroxyacetone (unlabeled concentration)
Banana Boat Sunless Tanning Spray	Dihydroxyacetone (unlabeled concentration)
Clear Bronze Sunless Self-Tanning Lotion	Dihydroxyacetone (unlabeled concentration)
Coppertone Moisturizing Self Tanner Spray	Dihydroxyacetone (unlabeled concentration)
Coppertone Oil Free Sunless Tanner Lotion	Dihydroxyacetone (unlabeled concentration)
Eurotan Liquid Tan Liquid	Dihydroxyacetone (unlabeled concentration)
Eurotan Optimizer Lotion	Acetyl tyrosine
Eurotan Tanning Bed Accelerator Spray	Tyrosine
L.A. Express X Solarator Lotion	Tyrosine, aminophylline, ginseng extract, grapefruit extract
Neutrogena Glow Sunless Tanning Spray	Dihydroxyacetone (unlabeled concentration)
Vaseline Intensive Care Moisturizing Sunless Tanning Lotion	Dihydroxyacetone, titanium dioxide (unlabeled concentrations)

canthaxanthin pills from a tanning parlor.[57] After ingesting some of the pills her skin turned deep orange. Several weeks later she noticed increased fatigue and bruising. Four months after ingesting the unapproved, illegally distributed pills, she was diagnosed with aplastic anemia; she died 17 days after diagnosis.

ARTIFICIAL TAN PRODUCTS

These products stain the skin with an ingredient such as synthetic color or walnut juice. Known as "bronzers," these products are fully washable with soap and water and are not harmful.[40]

Artificial tan "extenders" chemically affect the protein of the skin to darken it, producing a golden color. Unless applied evenly, extenders may result in streaking.[53] The FDA has approved dihydroxyacetone for this purpose.[40]

Extenders have no SPF value although some dihydroxyacetone products are marketed in combination with sunscreens.[58] The sunscreen lasts only as long as the time period indicated by its rated SPF, but the skin discoloration may last for several days. For this reason, patients must be carefully counseled to ensure that they understand the need for reapplication of sunscreen before the next sun exposure, even though the skin is still discolored.

TAN ACCELERATORS

These products, also known as tan promoters, claim to speed up the process of obtaining a natural tan.[59] Their major ingredient is the amino acid tyrosine, an essential precursor for the formation of melanin. A tan results when tyrosine is converted to melanin through oxidation and other intermediary steps. Tan accelerators are unapproved new drugs, however, with unproven efficacy and safety.[40,42,47,53] Research designed to demonstrate efficacy showed no difference from controls.[40]

Although some people have taken the prescription psoralens to accelerate tanning, topical use of psoralens combined with UVA radiation is cytotoxic, carcinogenic, and mutagenic.[5,16] This practice induces the formation of **thymidine-psoralen adducts** (complexes of psoralen with thymidine), which greatly enhance DNA damage, exceeding the ability of repair systems to compensate.[16]

COMPLICATIONS OF SUN-INDUCED SKIN DAMAGE

Some patients react abnormally to sun exposure. Some are ingesting medications or have medical conditions that worsen sun exposure, and some have medical conditions that are exacerbated by the sun (e.g., photosensitive epilepsy).

Photosensitivity

Some patients have photosensitivity, an exaggerated risk of damage when exposed to the sun. Some are taking medications that induce photosensitivity by absorbing UV radiation, and others have certain medical conditions that worsen the effects of sun exposure.

MEDICATION-INDUCED PHOTOSENSITIVITY

In one study of adverse effects of medications, 8% were photosensitivity reactions, in which the medication enhances the effect of the sun to increase the susceptibility to burn and may produce such serious reactions as toxic epidermal necrolysis (these reactions may also be known as photoallergy or phototoxicity).[60–63] Certain medications place patients at a higher risk of photosensitivity. These include the following:

- Antipsychotics (chlorpromazine)[64,65]
- Antidepressants[64]
- Quinolones (e.g., norfloxacin) [66,67]
- St. John's Wort[68]
- Flutamide (a nonsteroid androgen used for prostate cancer)[69]
- Pyridoxine[70]
- Oral hypoglycemics (e.g., chlorpropamide, glipizide)[71]
- Diuretics (e.g., furosemide, chlorothiazide, hydrochlorothiazide)[71]
- Nonsteroidal, antiinflammatory medications (e.g., ketoprofen, naproxen, ibuprofen)[72,73]
- Antilipemics (e.g., gemfibrozil)[74]

The pharmacist should explore the possibility of photosensitivity when counseling the patient with a sunburn.[64] Cosmetics and plants also cause photodermatitis.[63,75]

PHOTOSENSITIVITY INDUCED BY CERTAIN MEDICAL CONDITIONS

Medical conditions that cause photosensitivity include serious systemic diseases such as systemic lupus erythematosus or dermatomyositis.[76,77] A small number of genetic conditions also cause photosensitivity, including the porphyrias, xeroderma pigmentosum, Cockayne syndrome, Bloom syndrome, and Rothmund-Thomson syndrome.[76,78]

Solar Urticaria

Solar urticaria, more common in atopic patients, is a reddened, pruritic, and urticarial rash that occurs immediately after sun exposure or up to 30 minutes later.[79–82] The V of the neck and arms are the most common sites. Physicians may prescribe antihistamines or cyclosporin.[83]

Photosensitive Epilepsy

A certain group of epileptics experience a heightened risk of seizures in the sunlight.[84,85] Many outgrow this reaction by the late 20s.[86]

TREATMENT OF SUN-INDUCED SKIN DAMAGE

Sunburn is a type of sun-induced skin damage that is self-treatable, unless the skin is broken or blistered. (See "Treatment of Minor Burns" in Chapter 32, Burns.) Also, hyperpigmentary changes caused by sun exposure are self-treatable. (See Chapter 39, Skin Hyperpigmentation.) However, more severe skin changes such as basal cell carcinoma and photoaging are not self-treatable. (See Patient Assessment Algorithm 33.1.)

Patient Assessment Algorithm 33.1. Sunscreen

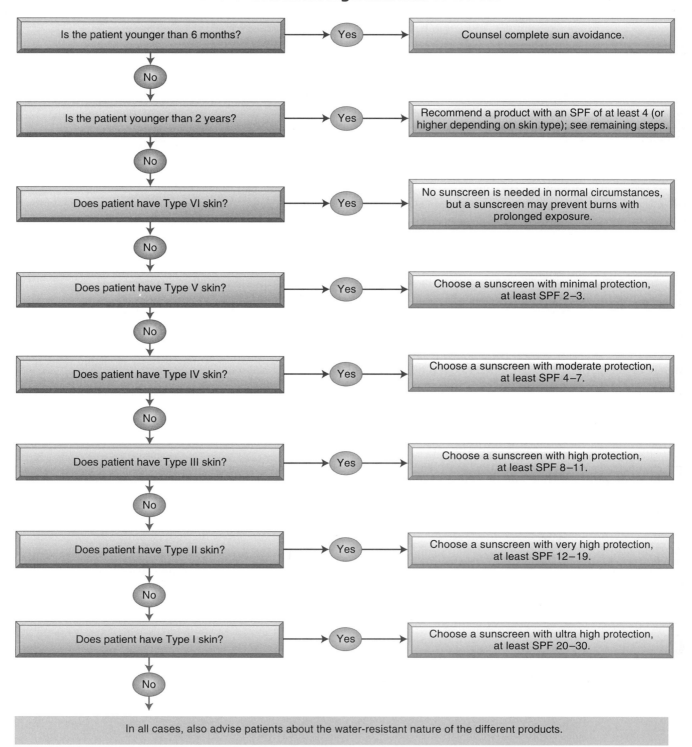

Is the patient younger than 6 months? → Yes → Counsel complete sun avoidance.

No ↓

Is the patient younger than 2 years? → Yes → Recommend a product with an SPF of at least 4 (or higher depending on skin type); see remaining steps.

No ↓

Does patient have Type VI skin? → Yes → No sunscreen is needed in normal circumstances, but a sunscreen may prevent burns with prolonged exposure.

No ↓

Does patient have Type V skin? → Yes → Choose a sunscreen with minimal protection, at least SPF 2–3.

No ↓

Does patient have Type IV skin? → Yes → Choose a sunscreen with moderate protection, at least SPF 4–7.

No ↓

Does patient have Type III skin? → Yes → Choose a sunscreen with high protection, at least SPF 8–11.

No ↓

Does patient have Type II skin? → Yes → Choose a sunscreen with very high protection, at least SPF 12–19.

No ↓

Does patient have Type I skin? → Yes → Choose a sunscreen with ultra high protection, at least SPF 20–30.

No ↓

In all cases, also advise patients about the water-resistant nature of the different products.

PREVENTION OF SUN-INDUCED SKIN DAMAGE

Prevention of sun-induced skin damage may be achieved through use of nonprescription medications (e.g., sunscreens, sun blockers) and various nonpharmacologic interventions.

FDA-mandated labeling for products to prevent sun-induced skin damage (e.g., sunscreens, sun blockers) cautions consumers not to ingest the product and to avoid contact with the eyes and suggests discontinuation if a rash occurs. Pharmacists should advise patients to consult a physician if the rash persists or worsens. The FDA requires all sunscreens to carry this warning: "SUN ALERT: The sun causes skin damage. Regular use of sunscreens over the years may reduce the chance of skin damage, some types of skin cancer, and other harmful effects caused by the sun."

Nonprescription Medications

Prevention of sun-induced skin damage is facilitated with nonprescription products known as sunscreens or sun blockers.

MECHANISM OF ACTION

Sunscreens reduce the amount of UV radiation reaching the skin by either chemical or physical means.[11] Sunscreens acting by chemical means absorb portions of the UV spectrum, while those acting through physical means reflect or scatter certain UV rays (those that completely block UV radiation are therefore known as sun blockers).[2,11] *The ideal sunscreens protect against exposure to both UVA and UVB radiation, thereby reducing the risk of photoaging, melanoma, and other skin cancers.[2,87] Use of these "broad-spectrum" sunscreens is recommended by the American Academy of Dermatology.[40,42]*

SUN-PROTECTION FACTOR (SPF): MEASURING THE EFFECTIVENESS OF SUNSCREENS

Sunscreen efficacy is indicated by the Sun Protection Factor (SPF), a ratio calculated by comparing the amount of time needed to produce minimal skin reddening with sunscreen to the time required to produce the same degree of reddening without sunscreen.[2,4] For example, consider a person who burns after 20 minutes in the sun without protection. A product with an SPF of 2 will protect this person for two times that exposure, or 40 minutes, while a product with an SPF of 12 will protect this person for twelve times that exposure, or 240 minutes (4 hours). Importantly, these exposure times assume that the product is not washed or sweated off, and that an adequate layer was applied. Also, the person should go inside when the exposure time is reached. Reapplication of sunscreen in an attempt to further extend the allowable time outdoors is futile and self-deceiving. Reapplication does not extend the total allowable time in the sun.[88] To stay outside longer, a product with a higher SPF should be applied. Note, *two back-to-back applications of SPF 12 do not equal one application of SPF 24.* Even reapplying at noon does not extend the time in the sun in any way. Reapplication is only helpful if the product has been washed, sweated, or toweled off.

When an individual reaches the MED, any further sun will produce the erythema of sunburn. Thus patients should stay out of the sun until the effects of any earlier exposure have abated. While the recovery time is highly individual, the pharmacist might advise the patient to stay out of the sun for several days to ensure that the MED is not exceeded on another day. The goal is to prevent the occurrence of UV-induced erythema (which is a marker for increased skin cancer risk).[89]

The FDA allows designations for sunscreen products, based on their SPF, as shown in Table 33.2. The minimal SPF recommended by the American Academy of Dermatol-

ogy is 15.[40] With use of this product, tanning can still be achieved by diehard sun bathers, but it will be attained slowly and without burning.[90] As noted in Table 33.1, SPF 20 to 30 products may also be called sunblocks.

MATCHING SKIN TYPE TO SPF

Although it is desirable for everyone to use ultra-high-protection products at all times, the FDA recognizes the need to balance optimal health with the reality of the tanning behaviors of consumers. Accordingly, the FDA has issued SPF recommendations for various skin types[42]:

- Type I skin. Highly sensitive, always burns (in as little as 10 minutes of exposure), will not tan. Individuals with Type I skin are of Celtic background, usually with blue eyes and freckles. Their unexposed skin is white.[42,91,92] Pharmacists should recommend an ultra high protection sunscreen for these patients (SPF 20 to 30).[42]
- Type II skin. Quite sensitive, and burns easily, tans to a small degree. Individuals with Type II skin are usually fair-skinned, with red or blonde hair, and often blue or hazel eyes. Their unexposed skin is also white. They should choose a very high protection sunscreen (SPF 12 to 19), at the least.
- Type III. Burns moderately, tans gradually. This is average white-blend skin that is white on unexposed areas. Individuals with Type III skin tan to light brown skin. Pharmacists should recommend at least a high protection sunscreen for them (SPF 8 to 11).
- Type IV skin. Burns little, always tans well to a moderate brown color. Individuals with Type IV skin are of Mediterranean, Asian, or Hispanic background. Their unexposed skin is white to light brown. Pharmacists should recommend a moderate protection sunscreen for them (SPF 4 to 7).
- Type V skin. Rarely burns, tans profusely. Individuals with Type V skin are of American Indian, East Indian, and Hispanic background. Their unexposed skin is brown, and dark brown when tanned. Pharmacists should recommend a minimal protection product for them (SPF 2 to 3).
- Type VI skin. Does not burn, except in the most extreme cases of exposure. Individuals with Type VI skin are of

Table 33.2. Sun Protection Factors and Their Utility

SPF VALUE	DESCRIPTION OF THE PROTECTION PROVIDED
2–3	Minimal protection; permits tanning
4–7	Moderate protection; permits some tanning
8–11	High protection; permits limited tanning only
12–19	Very high protection; permits little or no tanning
20–30	Ultra high protection; does not permit tanning; may be referred to as sunblocks

Adapted from Fed Reg 58:28194, 1993.

African, African-American, Australian aboriginal, and South Indian background. Their deeply pigmented skin is black on unexposed areas. Pharmacists should normally not recommend a sunscreen for them, although long exposure times may produce a sunburn. If long exposures are anticipated, a product with an SPF of 2 to 3 should be sufficient.

PROTECTION AFFORDED BY SUNSCREENS

Regular sunscreen use reduces photoaging and the incidence of precancerous skin lesions (solar keratoses).[29,93,94] In animal studies, UV-induced skin tumors (e.g., basal cell carcinomas, squamous cell carcinomas) are also reduced by sunscreens.[2,28] Experts estimate that a 78% reduction in basal cell and squamous cell skin cancers would occur if all individuals used sunscreen regularly from childhood through adolescence.[2] Despite this, a large percentage of the United States population neglects the use of sunscreens.[95,96]

AGE AND SUNSCREEN USE

 Sunscreens are contraindicated for infants younger than 6 months for several reasons:

- Infants younger than 6 months cannot move themselves to a place of shade if they are uncomfortable.[97]
- The dermal melanin content of very young children is low, so their protection from UV radiation is far less than that of adults and older siblings.
- Most babies cannot sweat to reduce body heat, increasing their risk of heat prostration.
- The metabolic and excretory systems of infants are not fully developed.[42]

Recommending sunscreens for infants may give parents or caregivers a false sense of safety. Therefore, babies must be kept out of the sun and sunscreens should not be used on them. Pharmacists can assure parents and caregivers who are concerned about lack of sunlight causing vitamin D deficiency that typical infant vitamin supplements contain adequate vitamin D.[97] Even if a baby is not taking a supplement, the typical baby will obtain sufficient sun from routine short exposures (e.g., being carried to and from the automobile, etc.).

Children between 6 months and 2 years should use a sunscreen with an SPF of at least 4, regardless of skin type.[42] If a sunscreen of only 2 to 3 is used, it may not provide adequate protection, increasing the risk of skin cancers in later life.

Elderly patients are also at higher risk than younger patients for sun-induced skin damage. After the age of 30, melanocyte counts in skin plummet, rendering elderly individuals much less able to endure ultraviolet radiation than younger adults.[98] Consequently, many older persons cannot tan as easily or as evenly as in youth.[99] (Ironically, many elderly elect to retire to states with warm climates and correspondingly high UV exposures such as Florida and California.[98])

Elderly individuals must also consider the risk of light sensitivity with medications. Many elderly patients take medications that cause photosensitivity and can suffer severe reactions if they obtain too much sun exposure.[53] (See "Medication-Induced Photosensitivity.")

SUNSCREEN INGREDIENTS

Some sunscreen products approved in original FDA monographs were withdrawn because of lack of interest in establishing United States Pharmacopeia monographs.[100] The currently approved sunscreen ingredients are discussed below. Representative products containing these ingredients appear in Table 33.3.

Chemical Sunscreens

Benzophenones. Oxybenzone, dioxybenzone, and sulisobenzone, the sunscreens in this class, absorb UVB and as much as 60% of UVA, with spectra of 270 to 350 nm (oxybenzone), 260 to 380 nm (dioxybenzone), and 270 to 360 nm (sulisobenzone).[41,42,101] Trade packages may use the name benzophenone-3 as a synonym for oxybenzone.[11]

Aminobenzoic Acids. Aminobenzoic acid (also known as para-aminobenzoic acid or PABA) and its esters (glyceryl aminobenzoate and padimate O) absorb UVB and some UVA radiation.[41,102] PABA was once used quite widely, but its use has diminished because of skin irritation and the propensity to stain clothing.[50] (The esters do not stain or sting as much as aminobenzoic acid.) Aminobenzoic acid penetrates the stratified corneum approximately 1/2 to 2 hours after application.[102] Once this has occurred, it stays on the skin well despite washing or swimming. Padimate O may also be labeled under its alternate name, octyl dimethyl PABA.

Cinnamates. Chemicals in this class include cinoxate, diethanolamine methoxycinnamate, and octyl methoxycinnamate (the latter with a spectrum of 290 to 380 nm). They absorb mainly in the UVB range, but may possess some UVA activity.[41,42] These chemicals do not bind to the stratum corneum and are easily washed off so they must be formulated in adhesive vehicles.[102] Trade packages often list one of the ingredients as ethylhexyl *p*-methoxycinnamate, the older synonym for octyl methoxycinnamate.[42]

Salicylates. Octyl salicylate, homosalate, and trolamine salicylate are also UVB absorbing agents.[41] Trade packages often list one of the ingredients as 2-ethylhexyl salicylate, an older synonym for octyl salicylate.[42]

Other Chemical Sunscreens

Additional ingredients include menthyl anthranilate (a weak absorber of UVB and good absorber of UVA, with a spectrum of 290 to 360 nm), octocrylene (a spectrum of 290 to 360 nm), and phenylbenzimidazole sulfonic acid (a selective UVB filter).[102,103] At least one trade package lists an alternative name for octocrylene, 2-ethylhexyl 2-cyano-3, 3 diphenylacrylate.[11]

Physical Sunscreens

Physical sunscreens reflect or scatter UV radiation because of their opaque nature. However, they are often considered

Table 33.3. Representative Sunscreens[a]

PRODUCT (SPF)	SELECTED INGREDIENTS
Banana Boat Baby Sunblock Lotion (50)	Octocrylene, octyl methoxycinnamate, oxybenzone, octyl salicylate
Banana Boat Express Atomic Gel (4)	Phenylbenzimidazole sulfonic acid
BioSun Oil Free Gel (30)	Avobenzone, octyl methoxycinnamate, octyl salicylate, oxybenzone, homosalate
Club Bronze Dark Tanning Lotion (4)	Octyl methoxycinnamate, oxybenzone
Coppertone Waterproof Moisturizing Sunblock Lotion UVA/UVB (15)	Octyl methoxycinnamate, oxybenzone
Coppertone 30 All Day UVA/UVB Waterproof Moisturizing Sunblock Lotion (30)	Octyl methoxycinnamate, octyl salicylate, homosalate, oxybenzone
Coppertone Bug & Sun (30)	DEET 9.5%, octocrylene, octyl methoxycinnamate, oxybenzone
Coppertone Gold Exotic Lotion (2)	Homosalate
Coppertone Kids Colorblock 6 Hour Waterproof Lotion (30)	Octyl methoxycinnamate, oxybenzone, octyl salicylate, homosalate
Coppertone SHADE Sunblock Lotion UVA/UVB (45)	Octyl methoxycinnamate, octyl salicylate, oxybenzone, homosalate
Coppertone Water Babies UVA/UVB Lotion (30)	Octyl methoxycinnamate, oxybenzone, octyl salicylate, homosalate
Hawaiian Tropic 15 Plus UVA/UVB/IR Sunblock All Day Waterproof (15)	Octyl methoxycinnamate, octyl salicylate, titanium dioxide
Hawaiian Tropic 45 Plus UVA/UVB/IR Sunblock All Day Waterproof (45)	Octyl methoxycinnamate, octyl salicylate, titanium dioxide
Hawaiian Tropic Baby Faces 50 Sunblock All Day Waterproof (50)	Octyl methoxycinnamate, octyl salicylate, titanium dioxide
Panama Jack Dark Tanning Lotion (4)	Octyl methoxycinnamate
PreSun Block UVA/UVB Cream (28)	Titanium dioxide 16%
PreSun for Kids Spray Mist (23)	Padimate O, octyl methoxycinnamate, oxybenzone, octyl salicylate
PreSun Moisturizing Sunscreen (46)	Padimate O, oxybenzone

[a]Sunscreen manufacturers do not often list concentrations of the active ingredients on the containers.

to be cosmetically unacceptable, so that patients tend to use them less often.[104]

Titanium Dioxide. Titanium dioxide is an opaque chemical that physically reflects or scatters UV radiation.[90,92,105] The UV radiation protection range of titanium dioxide is 290 to 700 nm.[42] The particulate nature of titanium dioxide causes a high coloration, which limits acceptability to many patients, although those exposed to constant sun (e.g., lifeguards) often apply titanium dioxide to high-risk areas such as the nose, shoulders, helix of the ears, neck, and lips.[106]

Zinc Oxide. Zinc oxide is currently being considered as an FDA-approved sunblocking agent, although no official notice of approval has appeared in the *Federal Register* as of this writing.[107]

Avobenzone

Avobenzone (Parsol 1789) was not approved by the FDA OTC Review panels, but on individual application from a manufacturer via the New Drug Application process.[53] Avobenzone (both in a concentration of 3% as a single-entity ingredient or 2 to 3% in combination products) has an absorption band that protects against UVA.[108–110]

ADVERSE REACTIONS TO SUNSCREENS

Sunscreen-Induced Contact Dermatitis

Some patients exhibit allergic reactions to sunscreens (or to specific inactive ingredients).[111–113] This sunscreen-induced contact dermatitis may be worsened by the sun, giving the allergic reaction the more precise name of photocontact allergic dermatitis.[114] Generally, sunscreen allergy is more common in patients with atopic dermatitis.[92]

Oxybenzone sensitivity has been reported, with one patient exhibiting an itching, burning sensation that evolved into an erythematous, papulovesicular eruption where the sunscreen had been applied.[114]

Allergy to aminobenzoic acid and its esters manifests as redness and itching about 24 hours after application.[50,115] This aminobenzoate allergy is more likely in patients who have preexisting allergies to benzocaine, thiazides, or other sulfonamides.[92] The likelihood of allergy to aminobenzoic acid and its esters prompted the FDA to suggest use of alternative agents such as benzophenones or anthralinates.

Allergies to cinnamates have also been reported, as has allergy to avobenzone.[88,116–118]

CORRECT APPLICATION OF SUNSCREEN

Sunscreens are formulated as solutions, lotions, or creams. The dosage form is not as critical as the SPF value, however. When applying sunscreen a thickness of 2 mg/cm^2 is suggested by physicians to obtain the rated SPF value. Sufficient product must be used because thin applications may not protect completely, particularly if washed or sweated away. An adult should use the following amounts[41]:

- Face and neck: 1/2 teaspoonful
- Arms and shoulders: 1 teaspoonful
- Torso: 1 teaspoonful
- Legs and tops of feet: 2 teaspoonfuls

Health professionals have long suspected that the average person does not apply sufficient sunscreen to ensure that the rated product's SPF is valid—in fact, may apply as little as 0.5 to 1 mg/cm^2, reducing the SPF by 50%.[4,119–121] Researchers confirmed this perception by directing patients to apply lotion containing a fluorescent chemical to the face as though it were sunscreen. Exposure to Wood's light revealed that most of the patients underapplied sunscreen to the periorbital area, ears, perioral area, and nasolabial region, with the hairline and nose the next areas most commonly missed.[120] By contrast, most patients adequately covered the forehead and cheeks. As a result of this study, researchers concluded the following:

- Patients should be taught to use the fingertips to apply sunscreen to ensure even and total application.
- Patients should apply sunscreen to one area at a time, completely and correctly covering that area before progressing.
- Patients with thinning hair must not neglect the top of the head.[5]
- Patients should use a lip balm containing sunscreen to prevent actinic cheilitis, which may become infected with Candida in elderly patients.[9]

Many patients only apply sunscreen after reaching the place of sun exposure (e.g., a beach) or after an initial swim.[121] *Sunscreens should be applied 30 minutes before sun exposure,* which allows time for the chemical to bind to the skin.[2] The product should be applied to every sun-exposed area and, to replace sunscreen that might be washed, sweated, or wiped away, should be reapplied frequently during the time outdoors.[2] However, reapplication is only necessary to ensure that the product meets its original SPF time; it does not allow the patient to stay in the sun longer than the SPF value allows. (See "Sun Protection Factor SPF: Measuring the Effectiveness of Sunscreens.")

WATER-RESISTANT NATURE OF SUNSCREENS

Since the typical sunscreen user is at a beach or pool, a product that washes off easily with water is impractical. The importance of water-resistant sunscreens is even more pronounced for children, who sweat more heavily than adults and tend to enter the water more frequently than adults.[50] The FDA defines a "very water resistant" product as one that allows 80 minutes of sweating or water activity before its activity is compromised through becoming too thin to fully protect the patient.[42] A "water resistant" product only allows 40 minutes of activity before becoming partially inefficient.

LIP PROTECTION

The lips are more sensitive to UV radiation than outer skin. Lips have at best an extremely thin layer of stratum corneum, and may have none in some spots. Further, they lack melanin; thus they cannot tan but can burn easily. Finally, although patients may cover the arms and legs, the lips are virtually always exposed to the sun. Despite this, patients seldom apply lotion or cream sunscreens to the lips. A better alternative is the use of lip balms with a high SPF value, as listed in Table 33.4. Lip balms are formulated to be acceptable when applied to the lips and may prevent sun-induced skin damage to this vulnerable area.

PRODUCTS RESEMBLING SUNSCREENS

Major sunscreen manufacturers have marketed several products under the traditional name of their sunscreen line that do not contain sunscreens (Table 33.5). Unless the patient reads the label carefully, they could be mistakenly used during sun exposure, leading to severe burning. They include several products that claim to help hold the tan for "weeks longer" or to "prevent peeling to prolong your tan." They also include several "tanning oils," which are to be used by those with a good or dark tan, one of which promises "more glistening power." The role of these oils is unknown; the misleading nature of their trade names coupled with the absence of a sunscreen argues against their use by those who wish to obtain sun exposure.

Nonpharmacologic Therapies

The American Academy of Dermatology developed a marker of potential risk of UV exposure known as the Ultraviolet Index (UVI), which is a measure of the strength of the sun's rays.[122] Reported by television weather forecasters and newspapers, it can help guide the American public in choosing appropriate nonpharmacologic therapies in addition to judicious use of sunscreens and sunblocker. Nonpharmacologic therapies include avoiding or limiting sun exposure, and covering the skin when outdoors.

Table 33.4. Representative Lip Balms Containing Sunscreens

PRODUCT	SELECTED INGREDIENTS/COMMENTS
Blistex Lip Balm (10)	Padimate O 6.6%, oxybenzone 2.5%, dimethicone 2%
Blistex Lip Tone (15)	Octyl methoxycinnamate 7.3%, menthyl anthralinate 4%, dimethicone 2%
Blistex Ultra Protection (30)	Octyl methoxycinnamate, oxybenzone, octyl salicylate, menthyl anthralinate, homosalate, dimethicone (unlabeled concentrations)
ChapStick Lip Moisturizer (15)	White petrolatum 33%, octyl methoxycinnamate 7.5%, oxybenzone 3.5%
ChapStick Ultra 30 (30)	White petrolatum 30%, oxybenzone 10%, octyl methoxycinnamate 7.5%, octyl salicylate 5%, oxybenzone 5%
Face Sense (30)	Octyl methoxycinnamate, oxybenzone, titanium dioxide (unlabeled concentrations)
Mentholatum Natural Ice (14)	Padimate O 8%; dimethicone 1%
Natural Ice Extreme (30)	Octyl methoxycinnamate 7.5%, octyl salicylate 5%, avobenzone 3%, dimethicone 1%

Table 33.5. Representative Products Resembling Sunscreens

PRODUCT	SELECTED INGREDIENTS/COMMENTS
Coppertone Aloe Aftersun Lotion	Water, propylene glycol, mineral oil, glyceryl stearate SE, cocoa butter (company advertises that product prevents peeling to prolong the tan)
Hawaiian Tropic Aloe After Sun Moisturizer Forever Tan	Aloe vera extract, mineral oil, propylene glycol, stearic acid (company promises that product helps hold a tan for weeks longer)
Hawaiian Tropic Dark Tanning Oil	Mineral oil, coconut oil, cocoa butter, aloe, lanolin (company suggests use by those with a good tan) (contains no sunscreen)
Hawaiian Tropic Tan Amplifier Oil	Mineral oil, isocetyl alcohol (company suggests use by those with a dark tan; "more glistening power") (contains no sunscreen)

AVOIDING OR LIMITING EXPOSURE

The best way to prevent sun-induced skin damage is to avoid sun exposure altogether.[28,123,124] Obviously, avoiding exposure to the sun would be impractical if not impossible for most people. Health professionals, however, do suggest limiting exposure to the sun during times when UV irradiation is at a maximum. In the early morning (e.g., before 11:00 am) and late afternoon (e.g., after 3:00 pm), for instance, the intensity of UV radiation is 25% of the intensity at noon because of the lower angle of the sun (Fig. 33.6).[11,125] The most common rule of thumb is to avoid sun exposure from 10 am to 3 pm, when the angle is highest—although it is possible to burn at other times.[2,126] Another technique for limiting exposure to UV radiation is to follow the "shadow rule": If your shadow is shorter than your height, the sun is too high and you should take measures to limit exposure.[127,123] (The rule, as illustrated in Figure 33.6, is also phrased, "Short shadow? Seek shade.")

Any reflective surface can direct ultraviolet rays to skin surfaces. Snow reflects 85% of UV radiation and water re-flects up to 100%.[41] Cement and sand also reflect as much as 25% of UV radiation.[5,35] At best, a beach umbrella may only reduce ultraviolet radiation by 50%.[5] Reflected UV radiation can actually heighten the effects of exposure, so that patients would require a sunscreen with a higher SPF value.[2]

The season also affects the intensity of UV radiation. Because of the angle of the sun, summer UV radiation is many hundreds of times more intense than winter sun.[35] This does not mean that participants in winter sports can neglect proper protection, however, because snow and ice can reflect a great deal of UV radiation onto exposed skin.

Latitude also is a critical determinant of the intensity of UV radiation. For example, on a June day, the average white-skinned person (skin Type I or II) with no sunscreen and no tan will experience redness in 21 minutes and painful sunburn in 80 minutes in New Jersey, but will experience redness in 10 minutes and painful sunburn in only 50 minutes in the Florida keys.[11] Cloud coverage is little help in reducing exposure to UV radiation. Thin clouds reduce UV radiation by only 20 to 40%. Considering that people often remain out-

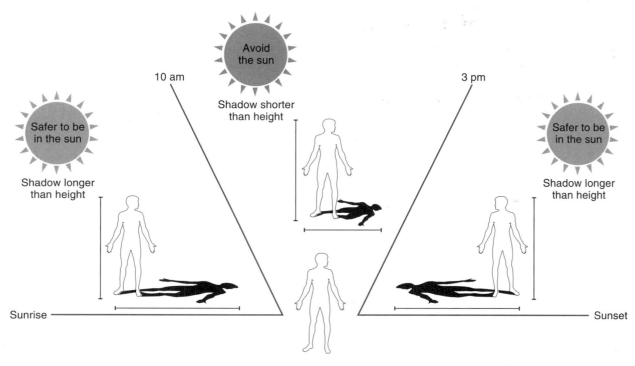

Figure 33.6. The dangerous angles of the sun and the results of using the "shadow rule" to guide sunlight exposure.

side longer on a cool, cloudy day than when the sun is hot, cloud cover can actually increase the risk of overexposure.[5] Smog can help screen out UV radiation somewhat, but it is a poor alternative, since it has adverse effects on respiration and is inconsistent from day to day.

SKIN COVERING STRATEGIES

Clothing that is wisely chosen can reduce the amount of ultraviolet radiation reaching the skin. Pharmacists should remind patients that effective skin covering strategies include long sleeves, long pants, and hats.[10] The typical beachwear (such as T-shirts, with an SPF of 5 to 9) will not protect the skin adequately.[9] Also, when this lightweight, loose-weave clothing is wet, the SPF is reduced further, allowing as much as 20 to 30% of UV rays to penetrate to skin.[2,5,35] Tightness of weave is a major factor determining UV transmission.[129] (Sun Precautions of Everett ,WA, offers a line of clothing that is manufactured to minimize ultraviolet penetration.[130,131] These fabrics were reviewed by the FDA as medical devices, and found to possess SPF values in excess of 30.) Covering strategies can also include sunglasses to prevent ophthalmic problems. See "Ultraviolet-Radiation–Related Ophthalmic Diseases."

FOCUS ON...

ULTRAVIOLET-RADIATION–RELATED OPHTHALMIC DISEASES

Ocular diseases include conditions for which sun is one of the causal factors—such as age-related macular degeneration, pterygium, photokeratitis, cancer of the periocular skin, and age-related cataracts, the leading cause of blindness worldwide.[18,132] The primary method of preventing these conditions is to avoid UV radiation, but sunglasses and hats can help reduce the amount of UV radiation reaching the ocular tissues.[132] Sunglasses have also been shown to block UV radiation.[133]

Under a voluntary labeling program developed by the Sunglass Association of America in cooperation with the FDA, nonprescription glasses are now labeled as cosmetic (blocking 70% of UVB, 20% of UVA and less than 60% of visible light), general purpose (blocking 95% of UVB, 60% of UVA, and 60 to 92% of visible light), and special purpose (blocking 99% of UVB, 60% of UVA, and 20 to 97% of visible light).[134] Pharmacists should discuss the need to take care of the eyes with patients at the same time that sunscreens are purchased.

SUMMARY

Although exposure to the sun is unavoidable at some level for most people, and can be beneficial (e.g., helping ensure adequate vitamin D stores), sun-induced skin damage is responsible for a variety of adverse health consequences, including photoaging, pigmentary changes, solar keratosis, and basal cell and squamous cell carcinomas. Sun exposure also may play a role in melanoma, although the role of the sun is not as clearly defined.

AT THE COUNTER

Two teenaged girls ask the pharmacist where the tincture of iodine is located.

Interview/Patient Assessment

When the pharmacist inquires about its potential use, the girls say they mix it with baby oil and use it as a tanning oil. They ask whether it is as good as their friends say it is in helping them tan while preventing damage to the skin.

Pharmacist's Analysis

1. What is the rationale for tincture of iodine mixed with baby oil?
2. What is the SPF value of this mixture?
3. What advice should the pharmacist give these patients?

Tincture of iodine mixed with baby oil has been a popular teen tanning mixture for many years. The tincture of iodine discolors the skin to produce a somewhat browner appearance, while the baby oil moisturizes the skin, preventing the tight, dry feel of sunburned skin. Unfortunately, the mixture has no SPF value, so those using it are essentially "deep-fat-frying" their skin as they tan excessively. The false sense of security given by the product promotes burning and sun-induced skin damage.

Patient Counseling

The patients should be urged to modify their tanning behaviors. They should be made aware that tanning can produce short-term damage such as sunburn and long-term damage such as skin cancer and prematurely aged skin. If this information does not dissuade them from tanning, they must be cautioned to use a high SPF value sunscreen at all times.

The tanning phenomenon is a pernicious trend that greatly increases the risk of skin damage—and even cancer—in individuals who seek the "perfect tan." Rather than tanning, patients must be encouraged to begin a program of sun protection. Sunscreens are vitally important components of this program. Used properly, sunscreens can screen different parts of the sun's UV spectrum, preventing both long-term and short-term damage to the skin. Whenever the patient will accept them, sunscreens—or sun blockers—with maximal SPF values are always preferable to those with lower SPF values.

Pharmacists can help combat the lack of general knowledge about the hazards from sun exposure and should help patients choose appropriate sunscreen products. Pharmacists should suggest other interventions such as avoiding the sun during times of peak danger, wearing appropriate clothing, and understanding the hazards of reflected light and the presence of risk during cloudy days.

References

1. Nguyen GT, Topilow AA, Frank E. Protection from the sun: a survey of area beachgoers. N J Med 91:321, 1994.
2. Guercio-Hauer C, McFarlane DF, Deleo VA. Photodamage, photoaging and photoprotection of the skin. Am Fam Physician 50:327, 1994.
3. Sollitto RB, Kraemer KH, DiGiovanna JJ. Normal vitamin D levels can be maintained despite rigorous photoprotection: Six years' experience with xeroderma pigmentosum. J Am Acad Dermatol 37:942, 1997.
4. Goldhar JNH, Yong PY. Photodamaged skin. Can Fam Physician 39:352, 1993.
5. Taylor CR, et al. Photoaging, photodamage and photoprotection. J Am Acad Dermatol 22:1, 1990.
6. Kawada A, et al. A new approach to the evaluation of broad-spectrum sunscreens against ultraviolet and visible light-induced delayed tanning. J Dermatol 21:571, 1994.
7. Gallagher RP, et al. Sunlight exposure, pigmentary factors, and risk of nonmelanocytic skin cancer. I. Basal cell carcinoma. Arch Dermatol 131:157, 1995.
8. Kaminester LH. Current concepts. Photoprotection. Arch Fam Med 5:289, 1996.
9. Browder JF, Beers B. Photoaging. Postgrad Med 93(8):74, 1993.
10. Frost CA, Green AC. Epidemiology of solar keratoses. Br J Dermatol 131:455, 1994.
11. Fed Reg 43:38206, 1978.
12. Ley RD, Reeve VE. Chemoprevention of ultraviolet radiation-induced skin cancer. Environ Health Perspect 105(Suppl 4):981, 1997.
13. Noda T, et al. The relationship among minimal erythema dose, minimal delayed tanning dose, and skin color. J Dermatol 20:540, 1993.
14. McCarthy JT. Prevent cancer. Cutis 54:11, 1994.
15. Farmer KC, Naylor MF. Sun exposure, sunscreens, and skin cancer prevention: A year-round concern. Ann Pharmacother 30:662, 1996.
16. Raab WP. Photodamaged skin: a medical or a cosmetic concern? J Int Med Res 18(Suppl 3):2C, 1990.
17. Warren R, et al. Age, sunlight, and facial skin: a histologic and quantitative study. J Am Acad Dermatol 25(5 Pt 1):751, 1991.
18. Young RW. The family of sunlight-related eye diseases. Optom Vis Sci 71:125, 1994.
19. Bernstein EF, et al. Evaluation of sunscreens with various sun protection factors in a new transgenic mouse model of cutaneous photoaging that measures elastin promoter activation. J Am Acad Dermatol 37(5 Pt 1):725, 1997.
20. McCallion R, Wan Po AL. Dry and photo-aged skin: manifestations and management. J Clin Pharm Ther 18:15, 1993.

21. Green LJ, McCormick A, Weinstein GD. Photoaging and the skin. Dermatol Clin 11:97, 1993.
22. Farnes SW, Setness PA. Retinoid therapy for aging skin and acne. Postgrad Med 92:191, 1992.
23. Bolognia JL. Dermatologic and cosmetic concerns of the older woman. Clin Geriatr Med 9:209, 1993.
24. West MD. The cellular and molecular biology of skin aging. Arch Dermatol 130:87, 1994.
25. Singer RS, et al. Association of asymmetrical facial photodamage with automobile driving. Arch Dermatol 130:121, 1994.
26. Sendagorta E, et al. Topical isotretinoin for photodamaged skin. J Am Acad Dermatol 27(6 Pt 2):S15, 1992.
27. Benedetto AV, et al. Dermabrasion: therapy and prophylaxis of the photoaged face. J Am Acad Dermatol 27:439, 1992.
28. Kaplan RP. The aging skin. Compr Ther 17:59, 1991.
29. Naylor MF, et al. High sun protection factor sunscreens in the suppression of actinic neoplasia. Arch Dermatol 131:170, 1995.
30. Kricker A, et al. A dose-response curve for sun exposure and basal cell carcinoma. Int J Cancer 60:482, 1995.
31. Kricker A, et al. Does intermittent sun exposure cause basal cell carcinoma? A case-control study in western Australia. Int J Cancer 60:489, 1995.
32. Wong JG, Feussner JR. Screening for melanoma. N C Med J 55:142, 1994.
33. English DR, et al. Sunlight and cancer. Cancer Causes Control 8:271, 1997.
34. Gallagher RP, et al. Sunlight exposure, pigmentation factors, and risk of nonmelanocytic skin cancer. II. Squamous cell carcinoma. Arch Dermatol 131:164, 1995.
35. Sagebiel RW. Cutaneous malignant melanoma—the party line and more—with a word on "safe sun." Compr Ther 19:225, 1993.
36. White E, Kirkpatrick CS, Lee JAH. Case-control study of malignant melanoma in Washington state. I. Constitutional factors and sun exposure. Am J Epidemiol 139:857, 1994.
37. Anon. Program educates teens about killer tans. Tex Med 89:52, 1993.
38. Farmer KL, Goller M, Lippman SM. Prevention of non-melanoma skin cancer. Standard and investigative approaches. Clin Plast Surg 24:663, 1997.
39. Stern RS. Sunscreens for cancer prevention. Arch Dermatol 131:220, 1995.
40. Greeley A. Dodging the rays. FDA Consumer 27(6):30, 1993.
41. Prawer SE. Sun-related skin diseases. Postgrad Med 89:51, 1991.
42. Fed Reg 58:28194, 1993.
43. Mawn VB, Fleischer AB. A survey of attitudes, beliefs, and behavior regarding tanning bed use, sunbathing, and sunscreen use. J Am Acad Dermatol 29:959, 1993.
44. Jones JL, Leary MR. Effects of appearance-based admonitions against sun exposure on tanning intentions in young adults. Health Psychol 13:86, 1994.
45. Novick M. To burn or not to burn: Use of computer-enhanced stimuli to encourage application of sunscreens. Cutis 60:105, 1997.
46. Boldeman C, et al. Sunbed use in relation to phenotype, erythema, sunscreen use and skin diseases. A questionnaire survey among Swedish adolescents. Br J Dermatol 135:712, 1996.
47. Greeley A. No safe tan. FDA Consumer 25(4):16, 1991.
48. Thompson RC. Out of the bronzed age. FDA Consumer 21(5):21, 1987 .
49. Anon. Burns, eye injuries from tanning devices. FDA Consumer 23(8):3, 1989.
50. Sweet CA. "Healthy tan"—A fast fading myth. FDA Consumer 23(5):11, 1989.
51. Hurks HM, et al. Differential effects of sunscreens on UVB-induced immunomodulation in humans. J Invest Dermatol 109:699, 1997.
52. Anon. Warning about tanning pills. Pharm Times 57(1):95, 1991.
53. Pine D. Cool tips for a hot season. FDA Consumer 26(5):20, 1992.
54. Stewart DS. Indoor tanning. Cancer Nursing 10:93, 1987.
55. Anon. Tanning pills may cause severe side effects. US Pharm 17(4):12, 1992.
56. Anon. Beware of tanning pills. Pharm Times 58(5):16, 1992.
57. Bluhm R, et al. Aplastic anemia associated with canthaxanthin ingested for "tanning" purposes. JAMA 264:1141, 1990.
58. Anon. No longer ugly orange, self-tanning agents offer choice. Drug Topics 137(6):71, 1993 (March 22).
59. Generali JA. What are tan accelerators and are they effective? US Pharm 14(7):67, 1989.
60. Selvaag E. Clinical drug photosensitivity. A retrospective analysis of reports to the Norwegian Adverse Drug Reactions Committee from the years 1970–1994. Photodermatol Photoimmunol Photomed 13:1, 1997.
61. Gonzalez E, Gonzalez S. Drug photosensitivity, idiopathic photodermatoses, and sunscreens. J Am Acad Dermatol 35:871, 1996.
62. Redondo P, et al. Photo-induced toxic epidermal necrolysis caused by clobazam. Br J Dermatol 135:999, 1996.
63. Augustin C, Collombel C, Damour O. Use of dermal equivalent and skin equivalent models for identifying phototoxic compounds in vitro. Photodermatol Photoimmunol Photomed 13:1, 1997.
64. Harth Y, Rappaport M. Photosensitivity associated with antipsychotics, antidepressants, and anxiolytics. Drug Saf 14:252, 1996.
65. Garnis Jones S. Dermatologic side effects of psychopharmacologic agents. Dermatol Clin 14:503, 1996.
66. Kimura M, et al. Photosensitivity induced by fleroxacin. Clin Exp Dermatol 21:46, 1996.
67. Bilski P, et al. Photosensitization by norfloxacin is a function of pH. Photochem Photobiol 64:496, 1996.
68. Brockmoller J, et al. Hypericin and pseudohypericin: Pharmacokinetics and effects on photosensitivity in humans. Pharmacopsychiatry 30(Suppl 2):94, 1997.
69. Leroy D, Dompmartin A, Szczurko C. Flutamide photosensitivity. Photodermatol Photoimmunol Photomed 12:216, 1996.
70. Morimoto K, et al. Photosensitivity from pyridoxine hydrochloride (vitamin B6). J Am Acad Dermatol 35(2 Pt 2):304, 1996.
71. Selvaag E. Evaluation of phototoxic properties of oral antidiabetics and diuretics. Photohemolysis model as a screening method for recognizing potential photosensitizing drugs. Arzneimittelforschung 47:1031, 1997.
72. Leroy D, et al. Photodermatitis from ketoprofen with cross-reactivity to fenofibrate and benzophenones. Photodermatol Photoimmunol Photomed 13:93, 1997.
73. Becker L, Eberlein Konig B, Przybilla B. Phototoxicity of non-steroidal anti-inflammatory drugs: in vitro studies with visible light. Acta Dermatol Venereol 76:337, 1996.

74. Diemer S, Eberlein Konig B, Przybilla B. Evaluation of the phototoxic properties of some hyperlipemics in vitro: Fenofibrate exhibits a prominent phototoxic potential in the UVA and UVB region. J Dermatol Sci 13:172, 1996.

75. Juckett G. Plant dermatitis. Possible culprits go far beyond poison ivy. Postgrad Med 100:159, 1996.

76. Garzon MC, DeLeo VA. Photosensitivity in the pediatric patient. Curr Opin Pediatr 9:377, 1997.

77. Callen JP. Management of skin disease in lupus. Bull Rheum Dis 46:4, 1997.

78. Sinclair PR, et al. Ascorbic acid deficiency in porphyria cutanea tarda. J Lab Clin Med 130:197, 1997.

79. Ryckaert S, Roelandts R. Solar urticaria. A report of 25 cases and difficulties in phototesting. Arch Dermatol 134:71, 1998.

80. Harris A, Burge SM, George SA. Solar urticaria in an infant. Br J Dermatol 136:105, 1997.

81. Tsien A, Schanker H. Solar urticaria: A case report. Cutis 57:87, 1996.

82. Alora MB, Taylor CR. Solar urticaria: Case report and phototesting with lasers. J Am Acad Dermatol 38(2 Pt 2):341, 1998.

83. Edstrom DW, Ros AM. Cyclosporin A therapy for severe solar urticaria. Photodermatol Photoimmunol Photomed 13:1, 1997.

84. Nezu A, et al. Two cases of essential myoclonus, epilepsy, mental retardation and anxiety disorders. Brain Dev 19:433, 1997.

85. Besag FM. Modern management of epilepsy: Adolescents. Baillieres Clin Neurol 5:803, 1996.

86. Harding GF, Esdon A, Jeavons PM. Persistence of photosensitivity. Epilepsia 38:663, 1997.

87. Naylor MF, Farmer KC. The case for sunscreens. A review of their use in preventing actinic damage and neoplasia. Arch Dermatol 133:1146, 1997.

88. Anon. Sunscreens. Med Lett Drugs Ther 30(768):61, 1988.

89. Naylor MF. Erythema, skin cancer risk, and sunscreens (Editorial). Arch Dermatol 133:373, 1997.

90. Warshauer DM, Steinbaugh JR. Sunlight and protection of the skin. Am Fam Physician 27(6):109, 1983.

91. Schreiber MM. Exposure to sunlight: effects on the skin. Compr Ther 12(5): 38, 1986.

92. Pathak MA. Sunscreens and their use in the preventive treatment of sunlight-induced skin damage. J Dermatol Surg Oncol 13:739, 1987.

93. Schiraldi FG. Common dermatologic manifestations in the older patient. Clin Podiatr Med Surg 10:79, 1993.

94. Augustin C, Collombel C, Damour O. Measurements of the protective effect of topically applied sunscreens using in vitro three-dimensional dermal and skin equivalents. Photochem Photobiol 66:853, 1997.

95. Hall HI, et al. Sun protection behaviors of the U.S. white population. Prev Med 26:401, 1997.

96. Robinson JK, et al. Summer sun exposure: Knowledge, attitudes, and behaviors of Midwestern adolescents. Prev Med 26:364, 1997.

97. Morelli JG, Weston WL. What sunscreen should I use for my 3-month-old baby? Pediatrics 92:882, 1993.

98. O'Donoghue MN. Cosmetics for the elderly. Dermatol Clin 9:29, 1991.

99. Kurban RS. Bhawan J. Histologic changes in skin associated with aging. J Dermatol Surg Oncol 16:908, 1990.

100. Fed Reg 59:29706, 1994.

101. Schallreuter KU, et al. Oxybenzone oxidation following solar irradiation of skin: Photoprotection versus antioxidant inactivation. J Invest Dermatol 106:583, 1996.

102. Roelandts R, et al. A survey of ultraviolet absorbers in commercially available sunscreens. Int J Dermatol 22:247, 1983.

103. Murphy GM, Hawk JML. Sunscreens. J R Soc Med 79:254, 1986.

104. Diffey BL, Grice J. The influence of sunscreen type on photoprotection. Br J Dermatol 137:103, 1997.

105. Tan MH, et al. A pilot study on the percutaneous absorption of microfine titanium dioxide from sunscreens. Australas J Dermatol 37:185, 1996.

106. Pathak MA, et al. Principles of photoprotection in sunburn and suntanning, and topical and systemic photoprotection in health and diseases. J Dermatol Surg Oncol 11:575, 1985.

107. Fed Reg 61:42398, 1996.

108. Johnson JA, Fusaro RM. Protection against long ultraviolet radiation: topical browning agents and a new outlook. Dermatologica 175:53, 1987.

109. Fed Reg 62:23350, 1997.

110. Fed Reg 61:48645, 1996.

111. Urbach F. Risk of contact dermatitis from UV-A sunscreens. Contact Dermatitis 29:220, 1993.

112. Trevisi P, et al. Sunscreen sensitization: a three-year study. Dermatology 189:55, 1994.

113. Schauder S, Ippen H. Contact and photocontact sensitivity to sunscreens. Review of a 15-year experience and of the literature. Contact Dermatitis 37:221, 1997.

114. Collins P, Ferguson J. Photoallergic contact dermatitis to oxybenzone. Br J Dermatol 131:124, 1994.

115. Ricci V, et al. Contact sensitization to sunscreens. Am J Contact Dermat 8:165, 1997.

116. English JSC, White IR, Cronin E. Sensitivity to sunscreens. Contact Dermatitis 17:159, 1987.

117. Stitt WZ, et al. Multiple chemical sensitivities, including iatrogenic allergic contact dermatitis, in a patient with chronic actinic dermatitis: Implications for management. Am J Contact Dermat 7:166, 1996.

118. Ang P, Ng SK, Goh CL. Sunscreen allergy in Singapore. Am J Contact Dermat 9:42, 1998.

119. Warrick PP. Current views on sunscreen protection. Cutis 39:540, 1987.

120. Loesch H, Kaplan DL. Pitfalls in sunscreen application. Arch Dermatol 130:665, 1994.

121. Wulf HC, Stender IM, Lock Anderson J. Sunscreens used at the beach do not protect against erythema: A new definition of SPF is proposed. Photodermatol Photoimmunol Photomed 13:129, 1997.

122. Geler AC, et al. Evaluation of the Ultraviolet Index: Media reactions and public response. J Am Acad Dermatol 37:935, 1997.

123. Morison WL. Sunlight: An environmental toxin for humans. A primer to advise patients. Md Med J 46:227, 1997.

124. Donawho C, Wolf P. Sunburn, sunscreen, and melanoma. Curr Opin Oncol 8:159, 1996.

125. Everett SA, Colditz GA. Skin cancer prevention: A time for action. J Community Health 22:175, 1997.

126. Schultz BC, Sweltzer JS. Sun between 3 PM and 4 PM can burn! J Am Acad Dermatol 29:658, 1993.

127. Holloway L. Shadow rule for sun protection. J Am Acad Dermatol 31(3 Pt 1):517, 1994.

128. Schultz BC. Reply. J Am Acad Dermatol 31(3 Pt 1):517, 1994.

129. Gies HP, et al. Ultraviolet radiation protection factor for clothing. Health Phys 67:131, 1994.

130. Menter JM, et al. Protection against UV photocarcinogenesis by fabric materials. J Am Acad Dermatol 31(5 Pt 1):711, 1994.

131. Strange CJ. Thwarting skin cancer with sun sense. FDA Consumer 29:10, 1995.

132. West SK. Daylight, diet, and age-related cataract. Optom Vis Sci 70:869, 1993.

133. Diddie KR. Do sunglasses protect the retina from light damage? West J Med 161:594, 1994.

134. Hale E. Shielding your eyes from the sun. FDA Consumer 23(10):27, 1989–1990.

Acne

A young man in his late teens or early 20s asks for help with the acne products.

Interview/Patient Assessment

The pharmacist notes pustular acne on the face in excess of one dozen lesions, and his cheeks appear to be scarred. He says the acne is also on his back and upper arms. He has been using a nonprescription benzoyl peroxide product, but it doesn't seem to be helping anymore. The pharmacist notes that the product in question contains only 5% benzoyl peroxide. The patient denies use of any medications and denies the presence of any diagnosed medical condition.

Pharmacist's Analysis

1. What is the significance of the appearance and number of lesions?

2. Should the patient be switched to a 10% benzoyl peroxide product?

3. Should the patient receive an alternate acne product?

4. Should the patient be referred?

From the appearance of the acne and the information given, this patient's acne would be rated as Type 3. Acne that is greater than Type 1 in severity requires prescription treatment. (Therefore, there is little likelihood that any nonprescription product will be helpful.)

Patient Counseling

The patient should be referred to a physician for evaluation.

Acne vulgaris, more commonly known as acne, is a condition that occurs in virtually all adolescents, appearing at the time of puberty or shortly thereafter.[1–3] The word "acne" is thought to derive from the Greek word "akme," which refers to the highest point, which is appropriate because acne manifests during the prime years of growth.[4–6]

In most cases acne does not produce severe problems—either psychologic or physical. However, in its more severe forms it can produce devastating psychologic consequences and permanent scarring.[7] Nonprescription products may provide benefit for those with the more minor forms of acne, but patients with more severe involvement should be referred for prescription products.

PREVALENCE OF ACNE

The exact incidence of acne is unknown, although one 1997 paper reported a prevalence of 35 to 90% of adolescents.[2] All teens surveyed in one research study had acne by age 14 in girls and age 16 in boys; another reference suggested that almost 100% of adolescents have comedones.[2,8] Other figures are only slightly more optimistic, with only 95% of 16-year-old boys and 83% of 16-year-old girls being affected in another study.[9] The incidence may be as low as 80 to 85%.[4,10–12] As many as 30% of teens' acne is so severe that medical treatment is needed.[13]

EPIDEMIOLOGY OF ACNE

Age and gender are primary epidemiologic factors in acne, as discussed below. Genetic factors may also play a role in acne, although this hypothesis is poorly documented.[9,11] Studies indicate that white patients are more likely to experience moderate-to-severe acne than black patients.[6]

Patients who rate their health as good or excellent are less likely to have acne than those who only rate their health as fair or poor. Patients who rate themselves as nervous tend to suffer more from acne.[6]

Age Variation

Because of the etiology of acne, the strongest epidemiologic variable in occurrence of acne is age. Although neonatal acne does occur (maternal androgenic hormones can stimulate a newborn's sebaceous glands, producing the characteristic acne lesions), it is rare.[11] Acne lesions normally begin in late childhood or in the early teen years, although some patients experience onset in adulthood.[10,12] Patients seeking advice from pharmacists are most likely to be between the ages of 15 and 18.[5,12]

Interestingly, teenagers living in the South and West are more likely to have acne than teens in the Northeast or Midwest.[6] Also, the likelihood of a child having acne is inversely proportional to the parents' years of education.[6]

Gender Variation

Acne occurs earlier in females than males, but is less severe and less common in females.[2,10,12] In one study 27% of women and 34% of men had active acne.[14] Only 1.9% of the affected women had severe acne, as opposed to 4.3% of the males.

A low-grade, late-onset, persistent acne exists in as many as 40 to 50% of adult females.[8,10] In some of these patients it is thought to be caused by excess androgens secreted by either the ovaries or adrenal cortex.[15–17] Females with acne, hirsutism (abnormal amounts of hair growth), and **androgenic alopecia** (genetic baldness) should be evaluated to determine the cause of **hyperandrogenism** (symptoms of excessive androgenic stimulation).[18–20]

ETIOLOGY OF ACNE

Acne develops in the **pilosebaceous unit** (the area relating to the hair follicle and its associated sebaceous glands) (Fig. 34.1).[1,21] The pilosebaceous unit consists of a cell-lined hair follicle containing a rudimentary **vellus hair** (the fine, non-pigmented hairs that cover most of the body) and a sebaceous gland.[10,11] The sebaceous gland's secretions pass upward through the duct that carries the hair to the surface.[6]

The pilosebaceous unit is fairly quiescent prior to the onset of puberty.[22] Stratified squamous epithelial cells that are shed from the lining of the follicle pass smoothly out of the ductal opening, carried by the sebum flow.[10,11,13] At puberty, this process is disrupted, because the desquamated epithelial cells develop an abnormal cohesion (Fig. 34.2).[10] As these keratinized cells accumulate and narrow the ductal lumen—a process known as hypercornification—sebum outflow is retarded.[5,13] Concurrently, androgens provoke the sebaceous glands to become **multilobular** (having several lobules), which results in an increased sebum output.[4,23–25] Thus sebum production increases just as its drainage channel narrows. Eventually, the desquamated cornified cells can combine with bacteria, sebum, and hair fragments to block the opening of the follicle (Fig. 34.3).[26] As sebum accumulates behind the keratotic plug, dilation distorts the normal follicular architecture, forming a **microcomedo** (small whitehead) (Fig. 34.4A).[11,20] As it grows, the microcomedo evolves

into the closed comedo, also known as a whitehead (a small, pale nodule that lies just beneath the skin surface) (Fig. 34.4B).[6,23] This microcomedo is the primary lesion of acne vulgaris, the precursor lesion from which all others eventually develop.[12,13]

Should sufficient material accumulate behind the keratotic plug, the closed pilosebaceous unit pore opens. This is the genesis of the noninflamed, open comedo, an eruption 1 to 3 millimeters in diameter that is commonly known as a blackhead (Fig. 34.4C).[13] The typically dark color of the blackhead is not caused by dirt, as most individuals believe, but a combination of oxidized lipids, melanin, and keratinocytes.[10]

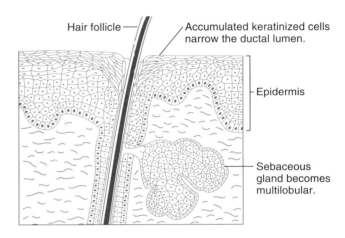

Figure 34.2. Changes in the pilosebaceous unit in puberty. Accumulated keratin cells narrow the ductal lumen. The sebaceous gland becomes multilobular, producing more sebum.

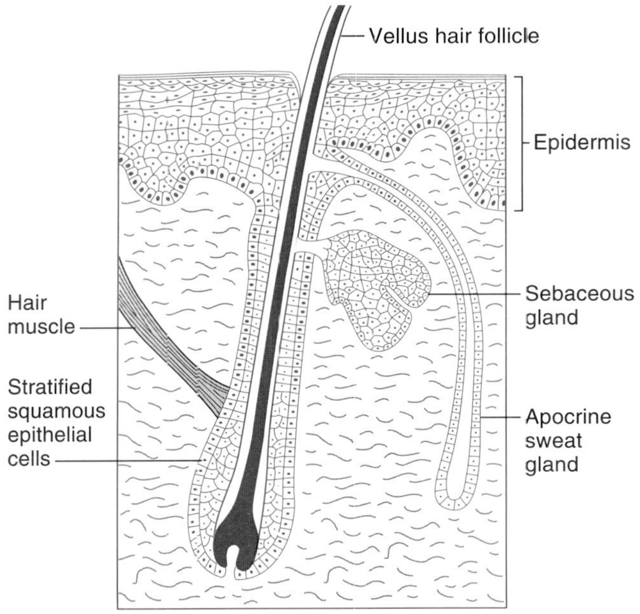

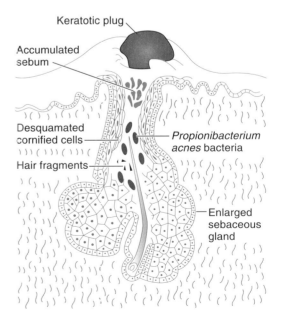

Figure 34.1. Normal structure of the pilosebaceous unit.

Figure 34.3. As a keratotic plug occludes the ductal lumen, a microcomedo begins to form.

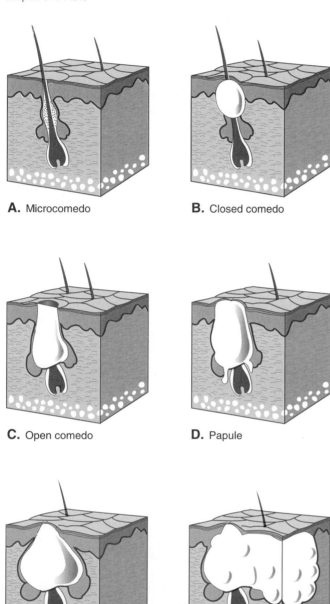

A. Microcomedo

B. Closed comedo

C. Open comedo

D. Papule

E. Pustule

F. Nodule

Figure 34.4. Progression of acne from (A) the microcomedo to (B) the closed comedo, (C) the open comedo, (D) the papule, (E) the pustule, and (F) the nodule.

Bacteria play a fundamental role in the evolution of the comedo and especially the more serious inflammatory lesions of acne. All pilosebaceous units contain small numbers of the anaerobic diphtheroid bacillus *Propionibacterium acnes,* an organism that requires glycerol for subsistence.[10–12] Prior to puberty, the pilosebaceous unit does not produce sufficient sebum to support widespread proliferation of any bacteria.[20] However, heightened sebum production at puberty enhances the organism's inherent toxicity.[27] Patients with acne have higher levels of the organism in the pilose-

baceous units.[20] To obtain glycerol, *P. acnes* produces lipases, which act on the triglyceride component of sebum.[10] Free fatty acids produced as by-products irritate tissue.[11,12] The tissue irritation in combination with the organism's elaboration of chemotactic products culminate in leukocyte migration.[11,23] The neutrophils produce hydrolytic enzymes (proteases, hyaluronidase), which damage the cellular wall, allowing free fatty acids and enzymes to pour through.[4,11,13] The free fatty acids and enzymes irritate dermal tissues, producing the well-known inflammatory lesions of acne.

Follicular rupture, which occurs to an inflamed pilosebaceous unit, results in formation of a papule, pustule, or cyst (nodule) (Fig. 34.4, *D–F*). Rupture of the follicle in the superficial dermis forms a papule, an erythematous, raised lesion of less than 5 millimeters in size (Fig. 34.4D).[10] Pustules occur when follicular rupture occurs in more superficial layers of the skin, allowing purulent material to be visible in the center of the lesion (Fig. 34.4E). If the inflammation is sufficiently severe and rupture occurs deeper in the dermis, a painful acne cyst can develop, which usually results in pigmentary changes in the skin (Fig. 34.4F).[10,13] (Acne cysts are not true cysts, but rather are sterile abscesses.[11]) These cysts may grow to incorporate more than one pilosebaceous unit.[20] All lesions that become inflamed can produce scarring.[20]

MANIFESTATIONS OF ACNE

Location of Lesions

Pilosebaceous units are not located uniformly across the skin surface.[24] Acne, which occurs only in pilosebaceous units, appears to shift locations slightly with age.[5,27] For instance, early acne involves the mid-forehead, nose, medial cheeks, and chin.[20] Over time, the lesions spread out laterally from these initial foci. In the late teens to early 20s the disease seems to favor the lower third of the face—such as the chin, jawline, and neck areas—as well as the midline chest and back.[11,13]

Severity Ratings for Acne

Acne treatment must be guided by severity of the condition at the time the patient is seen. Dermatologists and other researchers have created several taxonomies for grading acne, but none has gained acceptance by all concerned parties. According to one such popular grading system, pharmacists may assess such factors as lesion type, location of lesions, and number and status of irreversible sequelae (scarring).[10]

- Type 1: Comedones only, fewer than 10 lesions on the face, no lesions on the trunk, and no scarring
- Type 2: Papules, 10 to 25 lesions on the face and trunk, mild scarring
- Type 3: Pustules, more than 25 lesions, moderate scarring
- Type 4: Nodules or cysts, extensive scarring

SPECIFIC CONSIDERATIONS OF ACNE

Factors That Exacerbate Acne

Acne is worsened by a variety of exogenous and endogenous factors (Table 34.1). Endogenous factors include emotional stress and menses.[8,10] Some females experience flares of acne during the premenstrual period because of increased obstruction of the sebaceous duct orifices at this time.[10]

Exogenous factors include mechanical trauma, a friction-induced rupture of the pilosebaceous unit, which is worsened by occlusive clothing that does not allow evaporation from the skin.[10] This acne variant, termed acne mechanica, can be induced by athletic equipment such as football helmets (the chin and nape of the neck are the most common sites) and the heavy protective padding and headgear worn by hockey players.[28,29] Wearing a clean, absorbent, cotton garment under a uniform or athletic equipment can help reduce friction, pressure, occlusion, and buildup of heat. Leotards worn during aerobic dance or exercise classes also can produce acne mechanica, as can plastic-covered weight benches that constantly contact the backs of weight lifters. The lower lateral areas of the back are sometimes affected in golfers who carry their bags. The foreheads of wrestlers, too, are common sites.[29]

Environmental factors that can trigger acne include humid environments, which produce heavy sweating.[10] (Paradoxically, some patients report improvement during the summer.[6]) Air pollution may also aggravate the condition.

Harsh scrubbing and zealous washing both can be harmful through damaging the pilosebaceous unit.[4] Patients often engage in these deleterious behaviors because they believe that acne is caused by blocked pores that can be opened and cleansed by excessively abrading the skin.[11] Such actions may have a detrimental effect through friction-induced rupture of the pilosebaceous unit.[4,8] *Thus abrasive acne lotions and facial scrubbing sponges are counterproductive.[10] Further, plain unmedicated soap is of little use in acne since*

sebum and bacteria on the skin surface have no role in the pathogenesis of acne.[4]

Any oil-based product placed on the skin can occlude the pilosebaceous unit. Oil-based cosmetics and hair sprays exacerbate existing acne or induce acnelike lesions, a condition known as acne cosmetica (or pomade acne when oil-based pomades are the cause).[10] To prevent acne cosmetica, water-based products should be used.[8] Several tanning products contain oils, perhaps with or without a sunscreen. They should be avoided.

Working with oils can induce occupational acne, known as acne venenata. Occupational contact with oil results in problems for machine-tool operators; auto, truck, and aircraft mechanics; roofers; ship's engineers; oil well drillers; and road pavers.[30,31] Exposure to grease when fat frying hamburgers can cause acne that has been nicknamed, "McDonald's acne."[30]

Certain medications can produce **acneiform** (similar to acne) lesions such as oral contraceptives (particularly contraceptives with high progestin levels), lithium, azathioprine, dantrolene sodium, hydantoins, and rifampin.[5,13,30,32,33] Topical and inhaled corticosteroids (e.g., beclomethasone,) are also responsible.[34,35] In an unusual case a woman who sought dietary advice from a health-food store in regard to stress related to marital separation was advised to take 50 times the recommended daily allowance of pyridoxine, over 16 times the RDA for cyanocobalamin, and twice the RDA for vitamin A, plus zinc picolinate.[36] As a result, she developed facial acne within a few weeks. The condition resolved promptly with discontinuation and recurred with rechallenge.

Although diet is widely assumed to have an effect on acne vulgaris, experts believe that diet has little effect on either the course of acne or its severity.[4] For example, acne is not found to be worsened by chocolate, fried foods, nuts, or carbohydrates.[8] Pharmacists should advise patients to eat a healthy, well-balanced diet and not worry excessively about food.[10] (Overemphasis on diet as a causative factor in acne exacerbated a patient's eating disorders in at least one case.[27])

Another myth concerning acne is its relationship to sexual activity.[8] The temporal link is the most probable reason for this misconception. Acne worsens at the precise time that many teenagers initiate sexual activity. However, both are induced by the underlying hormonal changes.

Social Impact of Acne

For teens affected with acne, the condition can be devastating since the body image is critical during adolescence.[37] Ridicule from schoolmates and coworkers leads to social isolation for some patients.[8] The majority of patients of all ages report shame, embarrassment, and anxiety. Many report depression.[8,38,39]

Acne also can affect employment, and unemployment levels are significantly higher among acne patients than nonaffected controls.[8,9] For example, employers sometimes deny

Table 34.1. Factors That Increase Acne Severity

RISK FACTOR	HOW IT INCREASES ACNE SEVERITY
Endogenous factors	
Emotional stress	Unknown
Premenstrual phase	Unknown
Exogenous factors	
Mechanical trauma	Traumatizes the skin
Occlusive clothing	Prevents evaporation from skin
Humidity	Causes heavy sweating
Air pollution	Unknown
Harsh scrubbing of skin	Traumatizes the skin
Oils on the skin	Occludes the pilosebaceous unit
Medications	Various etiologies

fashion-store positions to applicants with acne; skin irritation with chemicals makes laboratory positions unwise.[8]

Acne patients are often denied the "sick role" and are unable to obtain time off to see a physician for a problem that is misperceived as trivial.[8]

Because of the significant social impact of acne, pharmacists must exercise a high level of tact and patience when helping patients afflicted with acne.

PROGNOSIS OF ACNE

In most cases acne resolves by the mid 20s. Few teenagers affected by Types 2 to 4 acne escape scarring, but it can be minimized if they seek appropriate treatment in the early stages of the condition.[40,41]

TREATMENT OF ACNE

Acne cannot be cured with nonprescription products.[42] However, judicious use of nonprescription products for Type 1 acne can reduce the extent and severity of the condition. For many teens with minor acne, that would be sufficient. When the patient has Types 2, 3, or 4 acne, referral can allow the physician to prescribe more powerful medications that can also allow a marked improvement in these more severe variants of acne.[43]

Treatment Guidelines

Acne treatments can produce a variety of adverse reactions such as dryness, irritation, or peeling. For this reason therapy is graded, with Type 1 acne being treated with nonpre-scription products (which have a level of safety greater than prescription products), and more severe acne being treated with prescription products. (See Patient Assessment Algorithm 34.1) Pharmacists should tell patients that no product (except isotretinoin) shortens the duration of acne or provides a cure.[13] Thus acne medications must be continued until the patient's underlying susceptibility decreases naturally with time.

The following treatment taxonomy is useful, but physicians may choose a different approach to therapy[44,45]:

- Type 1 Acne. Type 1 acne can usually be treated successfully with nonprescription products such as benzoyl peroxide, salicylic acid, or sulfur/resorcinol combinations.[9,10] Physicians also may prescribe azelaic acid or tretinoin.
- Type 2 Acne. Type 2 acne requires referral. Topical antibiotics are often chosen for moderate papular acne such as topical clindamycin, tetracycline, meclocycline, or erythromycin.[46]
- Type 3 Acne. Type 3 acne requires referral. Moderate pustular acne usually requires oral antibiotics in addition to topical therapy. Tetracycline, erythromycin, minocycline, doxycycline, or co-trimoxazole may be prescribed, depending on the particular physician's experience with the agents.
- Type 4 Acne. Type 4 acne requires referral. Severe acne presenting with nodules and cysts requires isotretinoin or systemic hormones.[38,47–49]

Nonprescription Medications

Patients with acne that is more severe than Type 1 should be referred to a physician (a dermatologist would be the optimal

Patient Assessment Algorithm 34.1. Acne

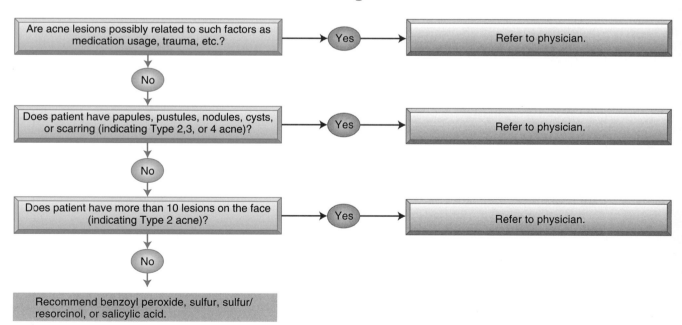

choice) for evaluation.[50] Lesions that clearly are not acne vulgaris (e.g., lesions possibly related to medication usage, trauma, or other causes) should also be referred. Pharmacists should always caution patients that since nonprescription medications will only lessen the severity of the condition, not shorten the duration of the condition, therapy must continue until the condition has resolved.[13] Also, pharmacists should advise patients that the response to therapy is slow, and a noticeable change may not occur for a few months.

The FDA requires several general labels on all acne products, including those stating that the products are indicated to clear up or dry up acne blemishes (e.g., blackheads, whiteheads), allowing the skin to heal, and that they help keep the skin clear of new blemishes by helping to prevent the eruption of new lesions. The labels on acne medications should caution patients that use of other topical acne medications concurrently with the product purchased can increase dryness and thus irritate the skin; if this occurs, one of the medications should be discontinued.

The labels on acne medications should direct patients to clean the skin before applying the medication. The entire affected area should be covered with a thin layer of product once daily when a product is first used to reduce the possibility of excessive skin dryness. Patients can gradually increase to two or three times daily, as needed. *If dryness or peeling occurs, patients should reduce applications.* The manufacturer may choose to inform the consumer that a sensitivity test may be conducted by applying the product sparingly to one to two small areas for 3 days; if there is no discomfort, it may be applied to the entire affected area.

Patients often wish help in choosing a specific dosage form. There are many: gels, creams, soaps, washes, and pads. All that contain effective ingredients can work equally well when used as directed, but the teen may feel more comfortable with one versus the other. For instance, the teen who is already familiar with the use of soap may prefer this method of application. Pads are also simple to use. Unless the teen has an allergy or contraindication to a specific ingredient, there is little difference between them in regard to potential effectiveness.

BENZOYL PEROXIDE 2.5 TO 10%

Benzoyl peroxide, the most frequently used acne drug, acts by releasing oxygen to destroy the anaerobic *P. acnes*.[11,51] Organisms do not become resistant to benzoyl peroxide.[9] Benzoyl peroxide also acts as an exfoliant, peeling the outer layers of the skin. It may be used concurrently with the prescription medication erythromycin to prevent the development of resistance to the latter agent.[9] The 2.5% concentration appears to be therapeutically equivalent to the 5% and 10% concentrations, while producing less irritation (Table 34.2).[5,10]

FDA labeling provides the following precautions[52]:

- Patients with very sensitive skin or those with a demonstrated sensitivity to benzoyl peroxide should not use the product.

Table 34.2. Representative Benzoyl Peroxide Products for Acne

PRODUCT	SELECTED INGREDIENTS
Clearasil Maximum Strength Vanishing Cream	Benzoyl peroxide 10%
Exact Vanishing Cream	Benzoyl peroxide 5%
Neutrogena Oil-Absorbing Acne Mask	Benzoyl peroxide 5%
Neutrogena On-the-Spot Acne Treatment	Benzoyl peroxide 2.5%
Noxzema Anti-Acne Lotion	Benzoyl peroxide 10%
Oxy Balance Deep Action Night Formula	Benzoyl peroxide 2.5%
Oxy Balance Emergency Spot Treatment	Benzoyl peroxide 5%
Oxy 10 Balance Emergency Spot Treatment	Benzoyl peroxide 10%
Oxy 10 Balance Maximum Medicated Face Wash	Benzoyl peroxide 10%
Panoxyl Bar	Benzoyl peroxide 5 or 10%
PersaGel	Benzoyl peroxide 5%
PersaGel Maximum Strength	Benzoyl peroxide 10%
Zapzyt Gel	Benzoyl peroxide 10%

- Benzoyl peroxide may cause redness, burning, itching, peeling, or swelling. If any of these reactions occur, patients should use the ingredient less frequently or choose a lower concentration. Should the irritation become severe, patients should discontinue the product. If irritation persists following discontinuation, a physician should be consulted.
- Do not allow benzoyl peroxide to contact the eyes, lips, or mouth.
- Benzoyl peroxide may bleach hair or dyed fabrics.
- Avoid unnecessary sun exposure and use a sunscreen during use of benzoyl peroxide. The sunscreen should be applied after the benzoyl peroxide product dries, following the directions on the sunscreen labeling. If patients develop irritation or sensitivity, both products should be discontinued.[53]

The panel originally assigned to acne products gave benzoyl peroxide Category I status.[6] The FDA concurred in its tentative final monograph.[51] However, in an amendment to the tentative final monograph, the FDA reclassified benzoyl peroxide as Category III, citing concerns regarding its capability to produce skin tumors in mice.[52] The final monograph for acne products, published 9 days later, omitted benzoyl peroxide completely from the list of approved ingredients, pending resolution of the concerns.[54] A subsequent publication stated that marketing of benzoyl peroxide could continue, pending evaluation of additional studies of tumorigenic potential.[53] This publication also related the opinion of the Dermatologic Drugs Advisory Committee, which unanimously voted to allow the ingredient to remain available as a nonprescription product during its evaluation. As of this writing, the issue has not been resolved.

Little benzoyl peroxide is absorbed systemically following topical administration; the dangers of greater absorption are unknown.[5] Approximately 1 to 3% of patients develop contact dermatitis following application, which underscores the importance of advising the patient with demonstrated prior sensitivity to choose another product.[5,12]

SULFUR 3 TO 10%

Sulfur medications often lessen the severity of acne, presumably because of keratolytic and antibacterial action (Table 34.3).[6] Sulfur can cause slight ophthalmic and dermatologic irritation, so acne medications that incorporate sulfur must caution patients to avoid eye contact. Pharmacists should advise patients to discontinue use and consult a

Table 34.3. Representative Acne Products Containing Sulfur or Sulfur and Resorcinol

PRODUCT	SELECTED INGREDIENTS/COMMENTS
Clearasil Adult Care Cream	Sulfur, resorcinol (unlabeled concentrations)
SAStid Soap	Precipitated sulfur 10%

Table 34.4. Representative Single-Entity Salicylic Acid Products for Acne

PRODUCT	SELECTED INGREDIENTS/COMMENTS
Clearasil Clearstick Maximum Strength	Salicylic acid 2%
Clearasil Clearstick Regular Strength	Salicylic acid 1.25%
Clearasil Clearstick Sensitive Skin	Salicylic acid 2%
Clearasil Acne-Fighting Pads Regular Strength	Salicylic acid 2%
Neutrogena Oil-Free Acne Wash	Salicylic acid 2%
Noxzema 2 in 1 Pads Regular Strength	Salicylic acid 0.5%
Noxzema 2 in 1 Pads Maximum Strength	Salicylic acid 2%
Oxy Balance Deep Pore Cleanser	Salicylic acid 0.5%
Oxy Balance Deep Pore Cleansing Pads	Salicylic acid 0.5%
Oxy Balance Facial Cleansing Wash	Salicylic acid 2%
Stri-Dex Dual Textured Pads	Salicylic acid 2%
Stri-Dex Maximum Strength Pads	Salicylic acid 2%
Stri-Dex Regular Strength Pads	Salicylic acid 0.5%

physician if sulfur products cause excessive irritation.[54]

SULFUR 3 TO 8% AND RESORCINOL/RESORCINOL MONOACETATE

The FDA Review Panel found that resorcinol enhances the activity of sulfur, approving this combination.[51] Labels on nonprescription medications containing resorcinol and sulfur in combination must contain the sulfur cautions noted above and must caution that the product should only be applied to affected areas and not on large areas of the skin or on broken skin.[54] (See Table 34.3.)

SALICYLIC ACID 0.5 TO 2%

The FDA Review Panel assigned salicylic acid to Category III because of insufficient evidence of efficacy.[6] (Presumably, its mechanism is keratolytic.) Subsequently, studies submitted to the agency allowed reassignment to Category I status in the tentative final monograph and final monograph (Table 34.4).[51,54] Products containing salicylic acid require nothing more than the standard labeling found on all acne products, as presented under "Nonprescription Medications" above.[54]

Nonpharmacologic Therapy

Patients with acne often ask how the severity can be lessened. Pharmacists can advise patients to attempt the following:

- Wear clothing that allows the skin to breathe.
- Avoid sports equipment that rubs against the skin with friction; if this is not possible, wear a clean, absorbent cotton pad or garment under the equipment.
- Avoid humid environments.
- Wash no more than once in the morning and once in the evening, from the jawline to the hairline (avoid harsh scrubbing and zealous washing of the skin; even a rough washcloth can produce damage).
- Avoid abrasive acne products and facial scrubbing sponges.
- Avoid the use of oil-based facial products, cosmetics, and hair sprays.
- Avoid oil-based tanning aids.
- Avoid occupations that involve contact with oils.
- Keep the hands away from the face; cupping the chin in a hand while reading can produce acne lesions.
- Avoid such habits as rubbing or handling the skin of the

face; it responds with hyperkeratosis that may induce acne.
- Wash the face after a meal to remove excess oils from the food that remain about the mouth.
- Don't manipulate, pick, or squeeze acne lesions; all of these can actually worsen the lesion and prolong its existence on the face.
- Avoid products that have not been proven safe and effective for acne. (See "Acne Products of Unproven Safety and/or Efficacy.")

FOCUS ON...

ACNE PRODUCTS OF UNPROVEN SAFETY AND/OR EFFICACY

Quite often, manufacturers of acne products market facial cleansers that carry the trade name of actual acne products (e.g., Clearasil, Oxy, Stri-Dex), yet they do not contain safe and effective acne ingredients. If the patient uses them instead of actual acne ingredients, the condition may worsen. Several of these products are listed in the table.[54]

Representative Products of Unproven Safety and/or Efficacy for Acne

PRODUCT	SELECTED INGREDIENTS/COMMENTS
Acne-Aid Cleansing Bar	Soap (contains ingredients not approved for acne treatment)
Clearasil Antibacterial Soap	Triclosan (unlabeled concentration; not approved for acne treatment)
Clearasil Daily Face Wash	Triclosan 0.3% (ingredient not approved for acne treatment)
Cuticura Medicated Antibacterial Soap	Triclocarban 1% (ingredient not approved for acne treatment)
Oxy Balance Facial Cleansing Bar	Triclosan 1% (ingredient not approved for acne treatment)
Sea Breeze Facial Cleansing Bar	Soap (contains ingredients not approved for acne treatment)
Stri-Dex Antibacterial Cleansing Bar	Triclosan 1% (ingredient not approved for acne treatment)

SUMMARY

Acne is a common condition, but it need not cause undue hardship for the patient. Early and continued treatment with agents that are proven safe and effective is the key to minimizing severity. Pharmacists can recommend self-treatment for Type 1 acne, which is characterized by fewer than 10 lesions on the face, no lesions on the trunk, comedones only, and no scarring. Nonprescription medications effective for this mild type of acne include benzoyl peroxide, sulfur, sulfur/resorcinol combinations, and salicylic acid. These ingredients are safe and effective for clearing up acne lesions such as blackheads and whiteheads, although the precautions associated with each must be pointed out to patients (e.g., keep

AT THE COUNTER

 A 13-year-old boy and his parents ask for advice on acne products.

Interview/Patient Assessment

The pharmacist notes five to six scattered comedones on the forehead and in the eyebrow area, but does not see any pustules, nodules, or scarring. The patient confirms that his back, arms, and chest are free of lesions. He has not used any acne treatment product to date, is taking no medications, and has no diagnosed medical conditions.

Pharmacist's Analysis

1. How is this patient's acne rated as to severity?
2. Are nonprescription products appropriate for him?
3. When should he see a physician?

This patient's acne is rated as Type 1. Thus he may use nonprescription products.

Patient Counseling

The patient may use such medications as benzoyl peroxide 2.5 to 10%, sulfur 3 to 10%, sulfur 3 to 8% and resorcinol/resorcinol monoacetate in combination, or salicylic acid 0.5 to 2%. Any of these are appropriate, unless the patient has an allergy or a specific contraindication to one of them.

Pharmacists should explain that if the acne worsens, nonprescription medications may no longer be appropriate. Pharmacists should describe Type 2 acne—papules, with 10 to 25 lesions on the face and trunk and mild scarring—and should advise the parents that if their son's acne reaches this severity, he should see a physician.

out of the eyes and away from lips). In all cases patients should begin with one application daily and gradually increase to two to three applications daily. Patients must also take care not to aggravate the pilosebaceous unit by undue trauma or scrubbing.

References

1. Gollnick HPM, et al. Pathogenesis and pathogenesis related treatment of acne. J Dermatol 18:489, 1991.
2. Stathakis V, Kilkenny M, Marks R. Descriptive epidemiology of acne vulgaris in the community. Australas J Dermatol 38:115, 1997.
3. Landow K. Dispelling myths about acne. Postgrad Med 102:94, 1997.
4. Matsuoka LY. Acne and related disorders. Clin Plast Surg 20:35, 1993.
5. Syken NL Jr, Webster GF. Acne. Drugs 48:59, 1994.
6. Fed Reg 47:12430, 1982.
7. Alster TS, West TB. Treatment of scars: A review. Ann Plast Surg 39:418, 1997.
8. Lowe JG. The stigma of acne. Br J Hosp Med 49:809, 1993.
9. Healy E, Simpson N. Acne vulgaris. BMJ 308:831, 1994.
10. Nguyen QH, Kim YA, Schwartz RA. Management of acne vulgaris. Am Fam Physician 50:89, 1994.
11. Eichenfield LF, Leyden JJ. Acne: Current concepts of pathogenesis and approach to rational treatment. Pediatrician 18:218, 1991.
12. Zander E, Weisman S. Treatment of acne vulgaris with salicylic acid pads. Clin Ther 14:247, 1992.
13. Kumasaka BH, Odland PB. Acne vulgaris. Postgrad Med 92:181, 1992.
14. Stern RS. The prevalence of acne on the basis of physical examination. J Am Acad Dermatol 26:931, 1992.
15. Aizawa H, Niimura M. Adrenal androgen abnormalities in women with late onset and persistent acne. Arch Dermatol Res 284:451, 1993.
16. Derman RJ. Androgen excess in women. Int J Fertil Menopausal Stud 41:172, 1996.
17. Derman RJ. Effects of sex steroids on women's health: Implications for practitioners. Am J Med 98:1A:137S, 1995.
18. Rosenfield RL, Lucky AW. Acne, hirsutism, and alopecia in adolescent girls. Endocrinol Metab Clin North Am 22:507, 1993.
19. Jurzyk RS, Spielvogel RL, Rose LI. Antiandrogens in the treatment of acne and hirsutism. Am Fam Physician 45:1803, 1992.
20. Lucky AW. Hormonal correlates of acne and hirsutism. Am J Med 98(1A):89S, 1995.
21. Thiboutot DM. Acne. An overview of clinical research findings. Dermatol Clin 15:97, 1997.
22. Burdon-Jones D. New approaches to acne. Aust Fam Physician 21:1615, 1992.
23. Anon. Topical antibiotics for acne. Drug Ther Bull 30:33, 1992.
24. Millikan LE, Shrum JP. An update on common skin diseases. Postgrad Med 91:96, 1992(6).
25. Aizawa H, Niimura M. Serum hormone levels in men with severe acne. J Dermatol 19:404, 1992.
26. Weiss JS. Current options for the topical treatment of acne vulgaris. Pediatr Dermatol 14:480, 1997.
27. Gupta MA, et al. Bulimia nervosa and acne may be related: A case report. Can J Psychiatry 37:58, 1992.
28. Harris H. Acne keloidalis aggravated by football helmets. Cutis 50:154, 1992.
29. Basler RSW. Acne mechanica in athletes. Cutis 50:125, 1992.
30. Kokelj F. Occupational acne. Clin Dermatol 10:213, 1992.
31. Svendsen K, Hilt B. Skin disorders in ship's engineers exposed to oils and solvents. Contact Dermatitis 36:216, 1997.
32. Kanzaki T. Acneiform eruption induced by lithium carbonate. J Dermatol 18:481, 1991.
33. Darney PD. OC practice guidelines: Minimizing side effects. Int J Fertil Womens Med (Suppl 1):158, 1997.
34. Hughes JR, Higgins EM, Du Vivier AWP. Acne associated with inhaled glucocorticosteroids (Letter). BMJ 305:1000, 1992.

35. Monk B. Acne induced by inhaled corticosteroids. Clin Exp Dermatol 18:148, 1993.

36. Sheretz EF. Acneiform eruption due to "megadose" vitamins B_6 and B_{12}. Cutis 48:119, 1991.

37. Lim C-CL, Tan T-C. Personality, disability and acne in college students. Clin Exp Dermatol 16:371, 1991.

38. Layton AM, Cunliffe WJ. Guidelines for optimal use of isotretinoin in acne. J Am Acad Dermatol 27(6 Pt 2):S2, 1992.

39. Hull SMc, Cunliffe WJ, Hughes BR. Treatment of the depressed and dysmorphophobic acne patient. Clin Exp Dermatol 16:210, 1991.

40. Layton AM, Henderson CA, Cunliffe WJ. A clinical evaluation of acne scarring and its incidence. Clin Exp Dermatol 19:303, 1994.

41. Strasburger VC. Acne. What every pediatrician should know about treatment. Pediatr Clin North Am 44:1505, 1997.

42. Usatine RP, Quan MA, Strick R. Acne vulgaris: A treatment update. Hosp Pract (Off Ed) 33:111, 1998.

43. Jansen T, Plewig G. Advances and perspectives in acne therapy. Eur J Med Res 2:321, 1997.

44. Gibson JR. Rationale for the development of new topical treatments for acne vulgaris. Cutis 57(1 Suppl):13, 1996.

45. Thiboutot DM. An overview of acne and its treatment. 57 (1 Suppl):8, 1996.

46. Eady EA, et al. Effects of benzoyl peroxide and erythromycin alone and in combination against antibiotic-sensitive and -resistant skin bacteria from acne patients. Br J Dermatol 131:331, 1994.

47. Goulden V, Layton AM, Cunliffe WJ. Long-term safety of isotretinoin as a treatment for acne vulgaris. Br J Dermatol 131:360, 1994.

48. Kauffman RE, et al. Retinoid therapy for severe dermatologic disorders. Pediatrics 90(1 Pt 1):119, 1992.

49. Layton AM, et al. Isotretinoin for acne vulgaris—10 years later: A safe and successful treatment. Br J Dermatol 129:292, 1993.

50. Stern RS. Acne therapy. Medication use and sources of care in office-based practice. Arch Dermatol 132:776, 1996.

51. Fed Reg 50:2172, 1985.

52. Fed Reg 56:37622, 1991.

53. Fed Reg 60:9554, 1995.

54. Fed Reg 56:41008, 1991.

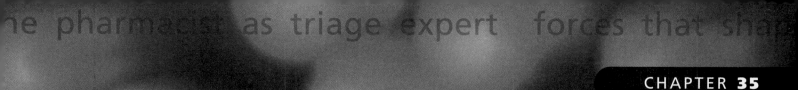

Fungal Skin Infections

A young man about college age asks the pharmacist to look at his athlete's foot. "I get it every year, ever since I first got it in high school. The itching is what bothers me the most. I just can't take my shoe off in class and scratch it, but I would like to. Sometimes I use a hairbrush because it itches so badly. I think I may have worn off some skin."

Interview/Patient Assessment

The pharmacist notes an active, red, inflammatory infection with broken skin on both feet, especially on the soles and around the toes. Both large toenails appear whitened and brittle, with flaking ends.

Pharmacist's Analysis

1. Does this young man appear to have tinea pedis (athlete's foot)?

2. What is the cause of a recurrent tinea pedis?
3. Is this patient's condition self-treatable?

This patient's symptoms suggest tinea pedis, and the description of the condition is also indicative of this minor fungal infection. A recurrent tinea pedis is often caused by a reservoir that persists from year to year such as tinea colonization of shoes that are worn each summer or a toenail infection. In this case a toenail infection appears to be the reinfective locus. Treating the infection on the skin would be counterproductive since the nail will reseed the infection whenever conditions are conducive to its spread.

Patient Counseling

The patient must be referred. Although tinea pedis is self-treatable, no nonprescription product will eradicate a nail infection.

This chapter addresses fungal skin infections—known as tineas—that are caused by the fungi known as dermatophytes. Dermatophytes invade the dead cells of the stratum corneum layer of the skin and also invade the hair and nails, digesting keratin.[1-3] Unlike *Candida,* a common cause of oral and vaginal fungal infections, these dermatophytes cannot exist on unkeratinized mucous membranes.[2,4,5]

The antifungal medications used for these superficial skin conditions accomplish more than most nonprescription products.[6] While most nonprescription medications either prevent certain conditions or treat symptoms of medical problems, nonprescription antifungals actually cure the conditions. The nonprescription antifungal medications must be used properly, however, to effect a complete cure.

PREVALENCE OF FUNGAL SKIN INFECTIONS

Dermatophytic skin infections are some of the most common infections seen in patients since the causative organisms are found in many familiar locations such as homes, offices, and athletic facilities.[7-10] Perhaps as many as 10 to 20% of the population of the United States is affected by a dermatophyte at any one time.[11] The prevalence varies by type of tinea:

- Tinea pedis is the most common dermatophyte, occurring in up to 70% of adults.[2,11-13]
- The two next most common fungal infections are tinea corporis and tinea cruris.[14]
- The incidence of tinea capitis has shown a sharp decline in recent decades, with the exception of large urban areas.[2]
- Data on prevalence of other types of tinea (e.g., unguium,

versicolor, nigra) is lacking, but, of the three, versicolor and unguium appear to be the most common.
- Because of its limited geographic distribution, nigra is not often seen.

Infection with any of the tineas does not provide immunity, so that the individual may be infected simultaneously at several skin sites or by several different fungal genera or species.[2]

EPIDEMIOLOGY OF FUNGAL SKIN INFECTIONS

Common dermatophytic fungi prefer conditions of high temperature (e.g, the high 80s and up) and high humidity. For this reason they have a geographic distribution that tends toward tropical and subtropical areas.[1] Common dermatophytic fungi also are generally more common in patients who are immunocompromised.[15,16] In most cases mild skin trauma or skin maceration through occlusion is necessary for successful fungal implantation.[7]

Tinea Pedis

Tinea pedis—also known as athlete's foot or ringworm of the foot—is rare in blacks but common in white urban dwellers.[1] Tinea pedis is more common in adults from the ages of 15 to 40 years than in prepubertal children and is more prevalent in males than females.[8,11,17-19] Individuals who must use communal bathing facilities (e.g., swimming pools, summer camps, sports clubs, and gyms) face a higher risk of tinea pedis than the general population.[20-22] In addition, sports such as marathon running cause a constant foot trauma that predisposes participants to tinea pedis.[20-22]

Following inoculation, tinea pedis survives best in patients who wear socks and shoes, as opposed to patients who go barefoot or wear sandals, practices that allow the feet to remain dry and cool most of the time.[1,2,23]

Tinea pedis may occur if an individual or a family member has tinea capitis caused by a species that thrives on human-tissue fungi.[11]

Tinea Corporis

Tinea corporis—also known as tinea circinata, or ringworm of the body—is spread through person-to-person contact when it is caused by anthropophilic fungi.[1] Tinea corporis is also caused by fungi that prefer animal tissues, having been contracted when the child played with an infected dog or cat.[8,11,24]

Tinea corporis is more prevalent in patients with tinea capitis caused by anthropophilic pathogens.[11] The patient with tinea corporis may spread the infection to other body areas or to other family members.

The most common prepubertal tinea infection, tinea corporis is often transmitted at day-care centers.[25] The fungi is more common in warmer climates than in cooler climates.[2] It also appears to occur more often in patients who are overweight or under stress.[12]

Tinea corporis is not common after puberty, but there are exceptions such as "tinea corporis gladiatorum." The lesions of this condition, which is spread through wrestling, appear on the arms, shoulders, trunk, head, and neck, a distribution that corresponds to the body-to-body wrestling contacts.[26-28]

Tinea Cruris

Tinea cruris—also known as jock itch—is a common summer infection of the groin area. Tinea cruris can also occur in the winter if the skin is kept sufficiently moist and warm through sweating or by wearing wet clothing for a prolonged time.[2]

A factor contributing to tinea cruris is the **intertriginous skin** (any part of the body where opposing skin surfaces remain in contact with each other much of the time, preventing evaporation of accumulated moisture) in the groin.[8] Opposing skin surfaces constantly rub against each other, trapping moisture and fostering the warm, moist environment that promotes the spread of fungi. Because the scrotal skin folds increase the surface area of the groin, males are more prone to this condition than females. Occlusive undergarments are also contributory.[12] Tinea cruris is rare in prepubertal children.

Males aged 18 to 40 years are the highest risk group.[19] Women may be infected by an infected sleeping partner and vice versa.[2,29]

Tinea Capitis

Tinea capitis—also known as ringworm of the scalp—is more common in children than in adults because of the poorer hygiene habits and the increased chances of contacting infected individuals.[2,30-36] When tinea capitis does occur in adults, however, it is more severe because the androgen-associated increase in sebaceous activity occurring at puberty and thereafter produces conditions favorable for fungal proliferation.[1]

The tinea capitis fungus can be spread by using infected brushes and combs, toys, or telephones; wearing infected clothing; sleeping in infected beds; and using infected furniture.[37,38] It may also be transmitted by contacting areas inhabited by a cat or dog.[39] An infected individual also may directly spread the fungus to others.[40]

Tinea capitis is more common in black female children than black males or white children, possibly because of the use of occlusive hair dressings and tight braiding utilized by some black women.[41-43]

Tinea Unguium

Tinea unguium—sometimes referred to as onychomycosis—is a fungal infection of the toenails or fingernails that affects as many as 30% of individuals older than 60.[16,44] Tinea unguium is commonly seen in the toenails of patients who concomitantly suffer from tinea pedis, although it also appears in patients who have no other fungal skin infection.[2]

Tinea Versicolor

Tinea versicolor is an infection of the skin surfaces.[45,46] Not surprisingly, tinea versicolor is more common in geographic areas with warm, humid weather.[47] Patients with an underlying immune deficiency are more commonly affected by tinea versicolor. Patients whose skin is excessively oily or greasy and those with **hyperhidrosis** (excessive sweating of the feet) are also at greater risk since the organism requires excess oils and moisture for optimal growth.

Tinea Nigra

A rare condition, tinea nigra is occasionally seen in the temperate Americas (e.g., along the Atlantic coastal area).[48] It is more common in young people and more common in females. It occurs in the palms and soles, and is apparently spread by contact with either human or nonhuman sources.[49-54]

ETIOLOGY OF FUNGAL SKIN INFECTIONS

Three fungal pathogen genera are responsible for the various superficial tinea infections: *Trichophyton*, *Microsporum*, and *Epidermophyton*.[55] These dermatophytes are not highly contagious; however, their transmission varies from species to species within each genus[1,2,56]:

- **Anthropophilic fungi** (infecting man rather than other animals) are transmitted from person–to–person.
- **Zoophilic fungi** (preferring animals other than man, but capable of infecting man) are transmitted from animal–to–person. Individuals who work on farms, in zoos, in laboratories with animals, and in veterinary practices are more likely to contract a zoophilic fungus.[11]

- **Geophilic fungi** (preferring soil, although they are capable of infecting man) are transmitted from soil–to–person.[20] Geophilic fungi normally digest keratin shed from animals.[2] Individuals who garden with bare skin in the soil, for example, increase their risk of becoming infected by geophilic fungus.[11]

Of the three methods of spread, person–to–person, animal–to–person, and soil–to–person, person–to–person is most common.

A fourth pathogen, *Exophiala (Hortaea) werneckii*, causes the rare fungal condition known as tinea nigra.[51]

Table 35.1 presents some common fungi in the United States, their origins, and the conditions they cause. The most common dermatophyte in the United States is *T. rubrum*, which produces the majority of nonscalp tinea infections.[11,57] The organism most likely to cause tinea capitis in this country is *T. tonsurans*.[29] The other most prevalent organisms found in the United States are *T. mentagrophytes*, *T. verrucosum*, *M. canis*, *M. gypseum*, and *E. floccosum*.

MANIFESTATIONS OF FUNGAL SKIN INFECTIONS

Pharmacists should be able to recognize several superficial fungal infections and recommend self–treatment. Generally, the origin of the fungi provides clues. *Fungal infections with anthropophilic sources present with little inflammation.*[1] *Conversely, fungal infections with zoophilic and geophilic origins are often acutely inflamed when seen by the pharmacist.*[2] Inflammation is caused by an allergic response to the fungal antigens that reach living epidermis.

Corticosteroids are inappropriate as sole therapy for tineas since they would not affect the tinea and might contribute to its spread by suppressing the inflammatory response. Further, nonprescription corticosteroids are neither recommended or labeled for fungal infections. Inappropriate treatment of a tinea by patients who obtain nonprescription steroids may cause an unusual condition known as tinea incognito.[58] (See "Tinea Incognito.")

Tinea Pedis

Tinea pedis (athlete's foot or ringworm of the foot) presents in three forms (Fig. 35.1)[61,62]:

- Skin between the toes is macerated, boggy, whitened, and thick, with a foul odor and intense pruritus—a condition also known as intertriginous tinea pedis.[1,18,63,64]
- Acute vesicular infection, with inflammation and fissuring that predisposes to secondary bacterial infections, accompanied by a foul odor and intense pruritus.[65] (See "A Pharmacist's Journal: Do You Have Surgical Scissors?") Vesicular tinea pedis can reduce patient mobility to the extent of virtual disability.[12]
- Fine scale over the plantar surface, absent of vesicles. Known as the moccasin type of tinea pedis because it covers the totality of the plantar surface. Caused by an anthropophilic fungus, it may persist in this chronic form for many years unless treated.[11]

Tinea pedis may flare during the summer months, but remain largely asymptomatic during the colder winter months.

Occasionally, patients with tinea pedis also experience a tinea of one or both hands, known as tinea manuum.[11,66] If it is seen on one hand only, the condition is sometimes known as "one hand, two foot" syndrome.[12,67,68] The affected hand(s) may appear dry, red, and scaly. Tinea pedis also may produce a secondary allergic reaction on the hands. These noninfectious eruptions are known as dermatophytid or id

Table 35.1. Fungi of Tropical Americas, Their Origins, and the Conditions They Cause

FUNGAL PATHOGEN	ORIGIN	TINEA CAUSED
Epidermophyton floccosum	Anthropophilic	Corporis, pedis, cruris
Microsporum canis	Zoophilic	Corporis, capitis, cruris
Microsporum gypseum	Geophilic	Capitis, corporis, cruris, pedis
Pityrosporum ovale	Probably anthropophilic	Versicolor
Trichophyton concentricum	Anthropophilic	Imbricata[a]
Trichophyton mentagrophytes	Anthropophilic, zoophilic	Pedis, capitis, corporis, cruris, unguium
Trichophyton rubrum	Anthropophilic	Corporis, pedis, manuum[a], capitis, cruris, unguium
Trichophyton schoenleinii	Anthropophilic	Capitis
Trichophyton tonsurans	Anthropophilic	Capitis, corporis
Trichophyton verrucosum	Zoophilic	Capitis, pedis, corporis
Trichophyton violaceum	Anthropophilic	Capitis, corporis

Adapted from Kemma ME, Elewski BE. A U.S. epidemiologic survey of superficial fungal diseases. J Am Acad Dermatol 35:539, 1996; and Mercantini R, et al. Epidemiology of dermatophytoses observed in Rome, Italy, between 1985 and 1993. Mycoses 38:415, 1995.

[a]See "Manifestations of Fungal Skin Infections" for a description of these tineas.

reactions.[69] As these lesions arise from autosensitization, they are free of organisms.

Tinea Corporis

Tinea corporis (tinea corporis or ringworm of the body) refers to superficial fungal infections that do not involve the scalp, hands, feet, groin, ears, or face. Tinea corporis, which usually occurs on **glabrous** (smooth and bare) skin, typically is an oval, scaly patch with an inflammatory border (Fig. 35.2).[11] The skin in the central lesion often appears somewhat normal, hypopigmented, or light brownish.[2,26,27] (This appearance gave rise to the common name of "ringworm," since it appears that a worm has formed a ring beneath the skin.[2] However, there is no worm involved at any stage of tinea corporis.) The infection begins with the development of flat scales. The patient may have one lesion or as many as 15 to 20 or more lesions scattered over the body. Adjacent lesions may coalesce to produce a single, large lesion that has overlapping inflammatory borders and appears to be **polycyclic** (composed of several, overlapping, roughly circular lesions).

Tinea imbricata is an unusual variant of tinea corporis. In this condition, *T. concentricum* produces concentric rings of scale that begin on the trunk and extend to other areas, producing conjoined, polycyclic lesions.[1,56]

Tinea Cruris

Tinea cruris (jock itch) is a groin condition of sharply defined lesions with inflamed borders and reddish-brown centers.[2] It usually begins in the skinfolds of the groin area, but can spread to form large lesions in the surrounding skin such as the perineum, proximal medial thighs, and buttocks.[11,12] Pruritus is intense, proceeding to pain as sweat accumulates to further macerate skin.[2] Secondary bacterial infections result from continued maceration and excoriation. Hair follicles may also be infected.[11]

Tinea Capitis

While the initial lesion of tinea capitis (ringworm of the scalp) is usually a circular patch of scaling skin with a restricted area of alopecia, the condition eventually produces one of several different appearances (Fig. 35.3).[1,2,37] Most commonly, the patient has a scaly, dry, noninflammatory dermatosis, with either patchy areas or total scalp involvement.[2] Common areas of hair loss include the crown, the occipital, and the parietal regions.[41] Pharmacists may notice "black dots," which are infected hairs that have been broken off at the scalp.[70,71] Tinea capitis may also extend to the eyelashes, eyebrows, and beard.[41]

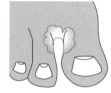
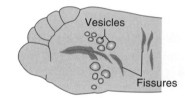

A. Between toes

B. Acute vesicular infection

Vesicles

Fissures

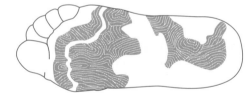

C. Moccasin scale

Figure 35.1. The three types of tinea pedis (athlete's foot): (A) between the toes, (B) acute vesicular infection, and (C) moccasin-type scale over the plantar surface of the foot.

Patients with tinea capitis may also present with an active, inflamed, weeping lesion known as the kerion. The kerion produces a purulent, thick exudate, which builds to crusts.[2] The scalp affected by a kerion usually scars, with hair follicles in the area unable to regenerate. Patients with kerion often also have cervical lymphadenopathy and secondary bacterial infections. This type of tinea capitis also occasionally produces the dermatophytid reaction in which papules or vesicles occur on the trunk or extremities.

Tinea capitis may also produce a **favus** (chronic fungal infection of the scalp, usually when the infecting organism is *T. schoenleinii*).[56] In favus the patient has cup-shaped crusts centered around several hairs, which may coalesce to involve the entire scalp. A mousy odor emanates from the affected scalp. Affected areas inevitably scar if not properly treated.

Tinea Unguium

Nails affected by tinea unguium (or onychomycosis) lose their normal shiny appearance, becoming opaque and yellow.[2] As the infection continues, the nails thicken because of the buildup of waste products and the proliferation of stratum corneum (Fig. 35.4).[12] As it becomes progressively more brittle and crumbled, the nail is lifted from underlying living tissues. Eventually, the nail may be lost altogether. (See "A Pharmacist's Journal: I Tried to See the Half-Moons of My Fingernails.")

Tinea Versicolor

Tinea versicolor is easily recognized by its hallmark description, "versi-" or changing (Fig. 35.5). The causative fungus depigments skin, possibly through the production of dicarboxylic acids such as azaleic acid.[1] Affected skin has many irregular blotches that seem to grow darker in the winter months but lighter as the summer progresses. Lesions are mainly located on the chest, abdomen, upper extremities, and back.[72]

Tinea Nigra

Tinea nigra presents as a black or brownish discoloration, most often on the palm.[48] The lesions begin as small patches, but may coalesce to form larger lesions. They do not scale and are painless and nonpruritic.

TREATMENT OF FUNGAL SKIN INFECTIONS

Treatment Guidelines

Prior to suggesting antifungal therapy, the pharmacist should be relatively sure that the lesions are fungal in origin.[73–75]

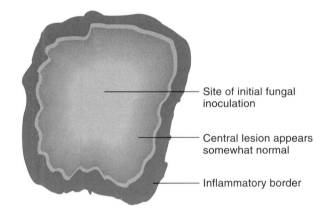

Site of initial fungal inoculation

Central lesion appears somewhat normal

Inflammatory border

Figure 35.2. Appearance of a typical lesion of tinea corporis (ringworm of the body).

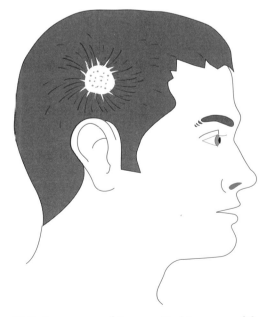

Figure 35.3. Appearance of tinea capitis (ringworm of the scalp).

They should conform to the descriptions of the tineas above. They should also not appear to be caused by other dermatologic conditions covered in this section of the text. Further, the pharmacist should discover whether the patient is taking any medication or has an underlying medical condition, either or both of which might have caused a dermatologic reaction resembling a superficial tinea infection.

Superficial dermatophytes may be treated with topical or systemic therapy, but topical therapy is preferred when it is effective since the patient avoids the adverse reactions common

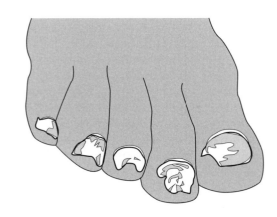

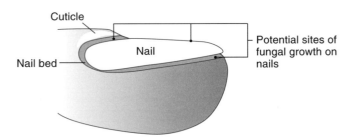

Figure 35.4. Onychomycosis affects one or more nails, producing a cosmetically unacceptable look to the nail. As shown, onychomycosis can affect the nail at three potential sites.

with systemic agents such as griseofulvin and ketoconazole.[76,77] Nonprescription antifungals come in several dosage forms: creams, ointments, liquids, and powders. Creams are preferred to ointments by many patients because of their nongreasy feel. However, the therapeutic effect of ointments is longer than creams; also, ointments help scaly, dry skin return to normal more rapidly.[2] Aerosol liquids and powders are simple to use and provide good skin coverage; they also may be applied into shoes to kill residual fungi responsible for tinea pedis. Solutions in applicator bottles are more difficult to apply to affected skin than other dosage forms (e.g., sprays, creams).

As discussed in the following sections only three of these fungal skin conditions are appropriate for self-treatment: tinea pedis, tinea corporis, and tinea cruris. (See Patient Assessment Algorithm 35.1.) Pharmacists should warn patients not to discontinue treatment prematurely.[12] Although improvement of symptoms may suggest a cure, topical antifungals are fungistatic, so premature discontinuation virtually assures recurrence.

The patient should continue treatment for the full course of therapy suggested, unless the development of new symptoms (e.g., a rash) suggests that the patient is allergic to the product.

TINEA PEDIS

Tinea pedis is self-treatable with nonprescription products.[1] Should topical therapy fail to produce a cure, however, oral antifungals may be necessary. Also, any secondary bacterial infection present requires a physician recommendation, since no bacterial skin infection may be self-treated with nonprescription products. Some physicians recommend the application of antiperspirants such as aluminum chloride to the feet to reduce sweating and hamper the growth of moisture-sensitive dermatophytes. This might be preventive, and would aid in curing an existent infection.

Even with treatment, tinea pedis recurs in 70% of patients.[11] For this reason pharmacists should advise patients to take appropriate preventive steps. (See "Prevention of Fungal Skin Infections.")

A Pharmacist's Journal

"I Tried to See the Half-Moons of My Fingernails."

A female in her 60s asked about the usefulness of nonprescription products for a fingernail infection. I asked why she thought her fingernails were infected. She related this story: "When I was a young girl, we were taught to groom all of our fingernails so that you could see the little half-moon on each nail. About a month ago I realized that I hadn't done that for about 40 years, so I got a fingernail stick and tried to push all of my cuticles down. I found some half-moons but I couldn't find them all so I kept pushing. Over the next several days, I noticed infection in my nails." I noticed that her nails appeared opaque, cracked, and brittle and suggested that she visit a physician for assessment. She returned with a prescription for an oral antifungal.

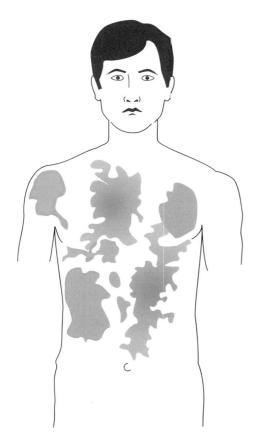

Figure 35.5. Possible distribution of tinea versicolor.

TINEA CORPORIS

Tinea corporis is self-treatable with nonprescription products, although some physicians assert that only noninflammatory tinea corporis should be treated topically.[1,11]

🛈 *Should the condition fail to clear, it may instead be caused by psoriasis, eczema, medication-induced eruptions, or other more severe fungal pathogens.*

TINEA CRURIS

Tinea cruris is self-treatable with nonprescription products. This condition responds more rapidly to therapy than either tinea pedis or tinea corporis.[8]

TINEA CAPITIS

Tinea capitis must be differentiated from other conditions that also cause hair loss such as seborrheic dermatitis, psoriasis of the scalp, genetic alopecia, alopecia areata, and psychiatric conditions (such as trichotillomania, compulsive hair pulling).[1,78] Although some of the other conditions respond to nonprescription therapy, topical nonprescription therapy is ineffective in treating tinea capitis because topical medications cannot penetrate the hair follicles.[7,79] For this reason pharmacists must refer all patients with suspected cases of tinea capitis to a dermatologist or physician for oral therapy.[2] Distant id reactions may require topical corticosteroids.

TINEA UNGUIUM

Tinea unguium does not respond to nonprescription medications, despite ads to the contrary (Fungi-Nail, for in-

Patient Assessment Algorithm 35.1. Fungal Skin Infections

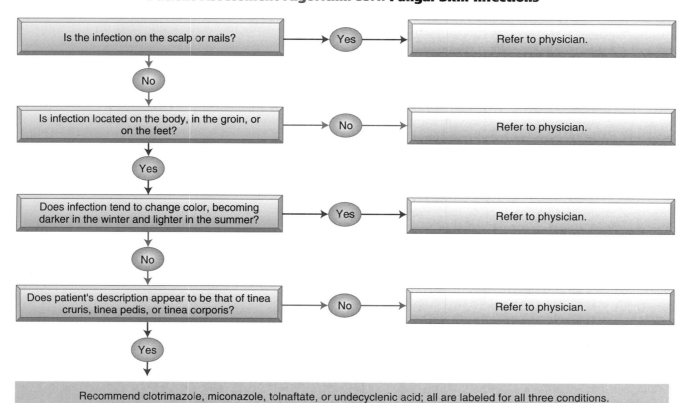

Is the infection on the scalp or nails? → Yes → Refer to physician.

No

Is infection located on the body, in the groin, or on the feet? → No → Refer to physician.

Yes

Does infection tend to change color, becoming darker in the winter and lighter in the summer? → Yes → Refer to physician.

No

Does patient's description appear to be that of tinea cruris, tinea pedis, or tinea corporis? → No → Refer to physician.

Yes

Recommend clotrimazole, miconazole, tolnaftate, or undecylenic acid; all are labeled for all three conditions.

stance, carries a misleading trade name that implies activity against nail fungus).[80] Oral therapy is mandatory since topical products do not penetrate the nail to reach the fungi.[2,7,29,81] If tinea unguium is not treated appropriately, the nail plate may be destroyed permanently.[82]

TINEA VERSICOLOR

Tinea versicolor does not respond to nonprescription medications. Thus, while tinea versicolor is easily recognized, pharmacists must refer patients for prescription medications.[1]

TINEA NIGRA

Tinea nigra, which does not respond to nonprescription medications, must be differentiated from such hyperpigmenting conditions as malignant melanoma by a dermatologist. Pharmacists must refer patients to a physician.

Nonprescription Medications

As noted above, *nonprescription antifungal medications as listed in Table 35.2 are only effective for tinea pedis, tinea corporis, and tinea cruris.*[8,83,84] Adults should supervise children using these products.[84] Labels must caution patients that they are for external use only, and that contact with the eyes must be avoided. *The labels on products used to treat tinea pedis or tinea corporis should advise patients that the products should be used for 4 weeks; labels on products used to treat tinea cruris should advise patients that the product should be used for 2 weeks. If the problem persists longer than these guidelines, patients should discontinue use and consult a physician.* These products must also include a warning that they are not effective on the scalp or nails.[8,83–85]

The skin should be cleaned with a mild soap and dried before products are applied. A thin layer should be applied morning and night. Products labeled for prevention of athlete's foot (tinea pedis) should direct the patient to apply (or spray) a thin layer to clean, dry feet one to two times daily, with special attention to the toenails and interdigital spaces.[83]

CLIOQUINOL 3%

Formerly known as iodochlorhydroxyquin, clioquinol is safe and effective in the treatment of the three superficial tineas. However, it is not widely available, nor is any product containing it highly publicized. Restrictions were imposed on the ingredient when used orally because of an adverse reaction known as subacute myelo-optic neuropathy, which resulted in optic atrophy and permanent visual loss.[86] Products containing it must caution against use in children younger than 2 years of age to reduce the risk of this adverse reaction.[84]

HALOPROGIN 1%

This ingredient has been given FDA approval as a nonprescription ingredient for superficial tinea.[8,83,84] While it was

Table 35.2. Representative Antifungals

PRODUCT	SELECTED INGREDIENTS/COMMENTS
Aftate Spray, Liquid, Powder	Tolnaftate 1%
Blue Star Ointment	Camphor (unlabeled concentration, unapproved ingredient)
Cruex Antifungal Cream	Total undecylenate 20% as undecylenic acid and zinc undecylenate
Cruex Antifungal Spray Powder	Total undecylenate 19% as undecylenic acid and zinc undecylenate
Cruex Prescription Strength Spray Powder	Miconazole nitrate 2%
Desenex AF Prescription Strength Cream	Clotrimazole 1%
Desenex Antifungal Ointment	Total undecylenate 25% as undecylenic acid and zinc undecylenate
Desenex Antifungal Powder	Total undecylenate 25% as undecylenic acid and zinc undecylenate
Dr. Scholl's Fungi Solution	Tolnaftate 1%
Fungi Cure Gel	Tolnaftate 1%
Fungi Cure Liquid	Undecylenic acid 10%
Lotrimin AF Cream, Solution	Clotrimazole 1%
Lotrimin AF Spray Powder, Dusting Powder	Miconazole nitrate 2%
Micatin Antifungal Cream, Powder Liquid Spray	Miconazole nitrate 2%
Odor-Eaters Medicated Antifungal Foot Powder	Tolnaftate 1%
ProClearz Liquid	Tolnaftate 1%
Tinactin Cream, Spray, Solution	Tolnaftate 1%

once available as a prescription product, the company was unable to obtain the ingredient (derived from a Japanese plant), and its manufacture was discontinued in the early 1990s.[87] Thus it was never marketed as a nonprescription product; it is unlikely ever to be reintroduced.

IMIDAZOLES
Imidazoles destroy fungal cells by interfering with synthesis of ergosterol, which is an essential component needed for a fungal cell to create cell membranes.[2,76]

Clotrimazole 1%
Clotrimazole became a nonprescription product in 1989. Most patients can use it without adverse reactions, although it may occasionally cause burning, stinging, peeling, or other minor local reactions.[88]

Miconazole Nitrate 2%
This ingredient was originally assessed by the FDA Panel and found to be safe and efficacious for superficial tinea.[8] However, the FDA warned pharmaceutical companies that marketing would be at the company's risk since the agency wished to gather further information before approving that decision. No company chose to market miconazole as a non-prescription product at that time, but the ingredient was the subject of an Rx-to-OTC switch in the 1980s. It has been available as a nonprescription product since that time. The ingredient occasionally causes irritation and burning, but is otherwise well tolerated.[88]

POVIDONE-IODINE 10%
Povidone-iodine was found to be effective for superficial tinea during the second phase of the FDA OTC review, as described in the Notice of Proposed Rulemaking.[83] However, no major manufacturer has labeled a povidone-iodine product with an antifungal indication. It is available as a first-aid antiseptic, but the patient would not be fully informed of appropriate use if the product with first-aid antiseptic labeling were recommended for athlete's foot.

TOLNAFTATE 1%
Tolnaftate was a prescription medication from its introduction in 1963 until it was switched to OTC status in 1971. This thiocarbamate is extremely safe, but may cause irritation if the skin is excoriated.[2,89] *Tolnaftate is the only ingredient proven to prevent recurrences of tinea pedis indefinitely with regular daily use.*[6] Labels of products that promote tolnaftate as preventive therapy must warn patients to discontinue use and consult a physician if irritation occurs[83]

UNDECYLENIC ACID
Undecylenic acid and its salts (zinc, copper, and/or calcium undecylenate) are common ingredients in nonprescription antifungals. The total undecylenate concentration must equal 10 to 25% to be effective.[8] The ingredient is generally well tolerated with a small risk of irritation. Some patients find the odor slightly unpleasant.

PREVENTION OF FUNGAL SKIN INFECTIONS

Patients who experience a fungal skin infection often ask how a future infection can be prevented. With most of these conditions preventive steps can reduce the chance of reinfection.

Tinea Pedis
Several steps are useful in preventing tinea pedis[90–93]:
- Keep the feet clean and dry.
- Dry the feet thoroughly after bathing or showering (especially between the toes).
- Go barefoot whenever possible (unless walking where another's feet have been); also wear open sandals or shoes with porous soles and uppers, to allow the feet to dry whenever possible.
- Use thongs when walking at public facilities or common bathing facilities where other's feet have been (e.g., dorm or hotel/motel showers, swimming pools, summer-camp shower stalls, sports clubs, workout gyms, etc.).
- Change the shoes and socks daily.
- Use antifungal powders on the foot following a bath or shower.[18]
- Never share footwear.
- If a toenail becomes infected, see a physician for a cure.
- If a condition recurs from season to season, consider preventive tolnaftate.
- If a tinea is present in another area of the body, do not wash or dry the feet with the same cloths used to bathe that area of the body.[18]
- Wear several different pairs of shoes so that each pair may dry out thoroughly between wearings.
- Try to avoid wearing socks so thick that the foot sweats; wear cotton socks that allow sweat to evaporate.
- Apply an antiperspirant to the feet.

Tinea Corporis
Patients can help prevent tinea corporis by observing the following guidelines:
- Always wash and dry the body with different cloths than those used to wash and dry the feet.
- Never play with a strange cat or dog (since it is difficult to tell if a particular animal is infected).
- Avoid contact with affected individuals until their skin is healed.
- Lose weight to minimize areas of intertriginous skin where moisture accumulates.
- Dry thoroughly after bathing, especially in intertriginous areas (e.g., beneath pendulous breasts).
- Never garden in the soil without protecting the skin that comes into close contact with freshly turned earth (e.g., the knees); wash promptly after such activity.

Tinea Cruris

Prevention of tinea cruris is facilitated by the following:

- Lose weight to minimize the presence of intertriginous skinfolds.
- Always wash and dry the groin area with different cloths than used to dry the feet if one has tinea pedis.
- Avoid sexual contact with someone who has tinea cruris until their skin is healed.
- Wear underclothing that does not allow moisture to accumulate in the groin area.

Tinea Capitis

Tinea capitis may be prevented by following several steps.

- Obtain cures for other tineas promptly.
- Avoid touching the head if another tinea infection is present on the body.
- Observe excellent hygiene on the scalp.
- Never share objects that have contacted the head of another person.
- Avoid contact with cats and dogs.
- Avoid contacting the head with any cloth or towel that has contacted areas of the body with an active tinea infection.

Tinea Unguium

Tinea unguium may be avoided if an individual obtains prompt treatment of tinea pedis. Patients should also follow all steps suggested to prevent tinea pedis.

Tinea Versicolor

Tinea versicolor may be avoided by not sharing towels, wash cloths, clothing, or other objects that have come into contact with others. Excellent hygiene with removal of skin oils also helps avoid the problem.

Tinea Nigra

Because of its rarity, preventive steps for tinea nigra are unknown.

SUMMARY

Superficial fungal infections present an excellent opportunity to the pharmacist to recognize and cure an infection. Fungi thrive in the moisture and heat found in several areas of the body, including the groin, feet, and intertriginous body surfaces. Tinea cruris, pedis, and corporis are easily recognizable and usually readily cured by various safe and effective nonprescription ingredients such as clotrimazole, miconazole, tolnaftate, or undecylenic acid. Other, more serious fungal infections, however, such as infection of the nails (tinea unguium), hair (tinea capitis), or tinea versicolor require physician supervision and must be referred.

AT THE COUNTER

 A woman in her early 30s approaches the pharmacist and asks, "Do you have anything for itching 'down there'."

Interview/Patient Assessment

The pharmacist asks if she is referring to the groin region, to which she replies in the affirmative. When asked if this is a vaginal fungal infection, she replies, "No, it's more in the area around my vagina and also in the back around my hips." She describes the infection as being "really itchy around the edges." The pharmacist asks if she has a sexual partner who is also affected with a fungus, and she answers, "My boyfriend has athlete's foot and some itching around the scrotum."

Pharmacist's Analysis

1. Does this patient have vaginal candidiasis or a tinea infection?

2. What is the significance of her boyfriend's conditions?
3. Is this condition amenable to self-treatment?

This patient appears to have a superficial infection known as tinea cruris, which affects the skinfolds around the groin area, but does not migrate intravaginally. The margins of tinea cruris are red and pruritic, while the central lesions often appear relatively healthy. The boyfriend may have transmitted the infection to her through scratching the feet or groin, then touching her.

Patient Counseling

The infection is self-treatable with several nonprescription antifungals. While a solution dosage form would be impractical, either a cream, ointment, spray powder, or spray liquid would be acceptable, depending on patient preference. However, should it fail to clear in 2 weeks, she should see a physician.

References

1. Shrum JP, Millikan LE, Bataineh O. Superficial fungal infections in the tropics. Dermatol Clin 12:687, 1994.

2. Bergus GR, Johnson JS. Superficial tinea infections. Am Fam Physician 48:259, 1993.

3. Mercantini, et al. Epidemiology of dermatophytoses observed in Rome, Italy, between 1985 and 1993. Mycoses 38:415, 1995.

4. Dean DA, Burchard KW. Fungal infections in surgical patients. Am J Surg 171:374, 1996.

5. Assaf RR, Weil ML. The superficial mycoses. Dermatol Clin 14:57, 1996.

6. Kovacs SO, Hruza LL. Superficial fungal infections. Getting rid of lesions that don't want to go away. Postgrad Med 98:61, 1995.

7. Wagron O. 3. Tinea of the skin, hair and nails. Med J Aust 164:552, 1996.

8. Fed Reg 47:12480, 1982.

9. Crissey JT. Common dermatophyte infections: A simple diagnostic test and current management. Postgrad Med 103:11, 1998.

10. Fleischer AB Jr, Feldman SR, McConnell RC. The most common dermatologic problems identified by family physicians, 1990–1994. Fam Med 29:648, 1997.

11. Drake LA, et al. Guidelines for care of superficial mycotic infections of the skin: Tinea corporis, tinea cruris, tinea faciei, tinea manuum, and tinea pedis. J Am Acad Dermatol 34(2 Pt 1):282, 1996.

12. Odom R. Pathophysiology of dermatophyte infections. J Am Acad Dermatol 28(5 Pt 1):S2, 1993.

13. Evans EG. Tinea pedis: Clinical experience and efficacy of short treatment. Dermatology 194(Suppl 1):3, 1997.

14. Lester M. Ketoconazole 2 percent cream in the treatment of tinea pedis, tinea cruris, and tinea corporis. Cutis 55:181, 1995.

15. Elewski BE. Sullivan J. Dermatophytes as opportunistic pathogens. J Am Acad Dermatol 30:1021, 1994.

16. Zaias N, Glick B, Rebell G. Diagnosing and treating onychomycosis. J Fam Pract 42:513, 1996.

17. Kearse HL, Miller FO III. Tinea pedis in prepubertal children: Does it occur? J Am Acad Dermatol 19:619, 1988.

18. Murtagh J. Tinea pedis. Aust Fam Physician 19:245, 1990.

19. Marchisio VF, Preve L, Tullio V. Fungi responsible for skin mycoses in Turin (Italy). Mycoses 39:141, 1996.

20. Aly R. Ecology and epidemiology of dermatophyte infections. J Am Acad Dermatol 31(3 Pt 2):S21, 1994.

21. Auger P, et al. Epidemiology of tinea pedis in marathon runners: Prevalence of occult athlete's foot. Mycoses 36:35, 1993.

22. Griffin LY. Common sports injuries of the foot and ankle seen in children and adolescents. Orthop Clin North Am 25:83, 1994.

23. Masri Fridling GD. Dermatophytosis of the feet. Dermatol Clin 14:33, 1996.

24. Ginter G. Microsporum canis infections in children: Results of a new oral antifungal therapy. Mycoses 39:265, 1996.

25. Wichmann KM. Pediatric management problems. Pediatr Nurs 20:478, 1994.

26. Beller M, Gessner BD. An outbreak of tinea corporis gladiatorum on a high school wrestling team. J Am Acad Dermatol 31(2 Pt 1):197, 1994.

27. Stiller MJ, et al. Tinea corporis gladiatorum: An epidemic of Trichophyton tonsurans in student wrestlers. J Am Acad Dermatol 27:632, 1992.

28. Hradil E. An epidemic of tinea corporis caused by Trichophyton tonsurans among wrestlers in Sweden. Acta Dermatol Venereol 75:305, 1995.

29. Commens CA. Superficial mycoses: A practical approach. Med J Aust 158:470, 1993.

30. Terragni L, Lasagni A, Oriani A. Tinea capitis in adults. Mycoses 32:482, 1989.

31. Barlow D, Saxe N. Tinea capitis in adults. Int J Derm 27:388, 1988.

32. Gianni C, et al. Tinea capitis in adults. Mycoses 38:329, 1995.

33. Elewski B. Tinea capitis. Dermatol Clin 14:23, 1996.

34. Cremer G, et al. Tinea capitis in adults: Misdiagnosis or reappearance? Dermatology 194:8, 1997.

35. Aste N, Pau M, Biggio P. Tinea capitis in adults. Mycoses 39:7, 1996.

36. Pomeranz AJ, Fairley JA. The systematic evaluation of the skin in children. Pediatr Clin North Am 45:49, 1998.

37. Babel DE, Rogers AL, Beneke ES. Dermatophytosis of the scalp: Incidence, immune response, and epidemiology. Mycopathologica 109:69, 1990.

38. Howard R, Frieden IJ. Tinea capitis: New perspectives on an old disease. Semin Dermatol 14:2, 1995.

39. Thomas P, et al. Microsporum canis infection in a 5-year-old boy: Transmission from the interior of a second-hand car. Mycoses 37:141, 1994.

40. Snider R, Landers S, Levy ML. The ringworm riddle: An outbreak of Microsporum canis in the nursery. Pediatr Infect Dis J 12:145, 1993.

41. Schwartz RA, Janniger CK. Tinea capitis. Cutis 55:29, 1995.

42. Lobato MN, Vugia DJ, Frieden IJ. Tinea capitis in California children: A population-based study of a growing epidemic. Pediatrics 99:551, 1997.

43. Laude TA. Skin disorders in black children. Curr Opin Pediatr 8:381, 1996.

44. Summerbell RC. Epidemiology and ecology of onychomycosis. Dermatology 194(Suppl 1):32, 1997.

45. Savin R. Diagnosis and treatment of tinea versicolor. J Fam Pract 43:127, 1996.

46. Hacker SM. Common disorders of pigmentation: When are more than cosmetic cover-ups required? Postgrad Med 99:177, 1996.

47. Drake LA, et al. Guidelines of care for superficial mycotic infections of the skin: Pityriasis (tinea) versicolor. J Am Acad Dermatol 34(2 Pt 1):287, 1996.

48. Severo LC, Bassanesi MC, Londero AT. Tinea nigra: Report of four cases observed in Rio Grande do Sul (Brazil) and a review of the literature. Mycopathologica 126:157, 1994.

49. Sayegh-Carreno R, Abramovits-Ackerman W, Giron GP. Therapy of tinea nigra plantaris. Int J Dermatol 28:46, 1989.

50. Uijthof JM, et al. Polymerase chain reaction–mediated genotyping of Hortaea werneckii, causative agent of tinea nigra. Mycoses 37:307, 1994.

51. Gottlich E, et al. Cell-surface hydrophobicity and lipolysis as essential factors in human tinea nigra. Mycoses 38:489, 1995.

52. Hughes JR, Moore MK, Pembroke AC. Tinea nigra palmaris. Clin Exp Dermatol 18:481, 1993.

53. DeHoog GS, Gerrits van den Ende AH. Nutritional pattern and eco-physiology of Hortaea werneckii, agent of human tinea nigra. Antonie Van Leeuwenhoek 62:321, 1992.

54. Burke WA. Tinea nigra: Treatment with topical ketoconazole. Cutis 52:209, 1993.

55. Babel DE. How to identify fungi. J Am Acad Dermatol 31(3 Pt 2):S108, 1994.

56. Barnetson RStC. Skin diseases in the tropics. Med J Aust 159:321, 1993.

57. Jones HE. Immune response and host resistance of humans to dermatophyte infection. J Am Acad Dermatol 28(5 Pt 1):S12, 1993.

58. Solomon BA, Glass AT, Rabbin PE. Tinea incognito and "over-the-counter" potent topical steroids. Cutis 58:295, 1996.

59. Fisher DA. Adverse effects of topical corticosteroid use. West J Med 162:123, 1995.

60. Burton JA. Tinea incognito. Practitioner 233:271, 1989.

61. Rao A, Forgan-Smith R. Superficial mycoses: A strategic approach. Med J Aust 158:476, 1993.

62. Omura EF, Rye B. Dermatologic disorders of the foot. Clin Sports Med 13:825, 1994.

63. Leyden JL. Tinea pedis pathophysiology and treatment. J Am Acad Dermatol 31(3 Pt 2):S31, 1994.

64. Leyden JJ. Progression of interdigital infections from simplex to complex. J Am Acad Dermatol 28(5 Pt 1):S7, 1993.

65. Brooks KE, Bender JF. Tinea pedis: Diagnosis and treatment. Clin Podiatr Med Surg 13:31, 1996.

66. Skogstad M, Levy F. Occupational irritant contact dermatitis and fungal infection in construction workers. Contact Dermatitis 31:28, 1994.

67. Piletta P, Pasche-Koo F, Saurat JH. Contact dermatitis from tioconazole mimicking "one hand two feet syndrome." Contact Dermatitis 28:308, 1993.

68. Daniel CR 3rd, et al. Two feet–one hand syndrome: A retrospective multicenter survey. Int J Dermatol 36:658, 1997.

69. Veien NK, Hattel T, Laurberg G. Plantar *Trichophyton rubrum* infections may cause dermatophytids on the hands. Acta Derm Venereol 74:403, 1994.

70. Elewski BE, Silverman RA. Clinical pearl: Diagnostic procedures for tinea capitis. J Am Acad Dermatol 34:498, 1996.

71. Drake LA, et al. Guidelines for care of superficial mycotic infections of the skin: Tinea capitis and tinea barbae. J Am Acad Dermatol 34(2 Pt 1):290, 1996.

72. Silva-Lizama E. Tinea versicolor. Int J Dermatol 34:611, 1995.

73. Brodell RT, Elewski B. Superficial fungal infections. Errors to avoid in diagnosis and treatment. Postgrad Med 101:279, 1997.

74. Pierard GE, Arrese JE, Pierard Franchimont C. Treatment and prophylaxis of tinea infections. Drugs 52:209, 1996.

75. Hammarstrsm B, Wessling A, Nilsson JL. Pharmaceutical care for patients with skin diseases: A campaign year at Swedish pharmacies. J Clin Pharm Ther 20:327, 1995.

76. Smith EB. Topical antifungal drugs in the treatment of tinea pedis, tinea cruris, and tinea corporis. J Am Acad Dermatol 28(5 Pt 1):S24, 1993.

77. van Heerden JS, Vismer HF. Tinea corporis/cruris: New treatment options. Dermatology 194(Suppl 1):14, 1997.

78. Elewski BE, Hay RJ. International summit on cutaneous antifungal therapy, focus on tinea capitis, Boston, Massachusetts. Pediatr Dermatol 13:69, 1996.

79. Abdel Rahman SM, Nahata MC. Treatment of tinea capitis. Ann Pharmacother 31:338, 1997.

80. Del Rosso JQ. Advances in the treatment of superficial fungal infections: Focus on onychomycosis and dry tinea pedis. J Am Osteopath Assoc 97:339, 1997.

81. Brautigam M, et al. Randomised double blind comparison of terbinafine and itraconazole for treatment of toenail tinea infection. BMJ 311:919, 1995.

82. Dover JS, Arndt KA. Dermatology. JAMA 273:1668, 1995.

83. Fed Reg 54:51136, 1989.

84. Fed Reg 58:49890, 1993.

85. Fed Reg 58:46744, 1993.

86. Gilman AG, et al., eds. The Pharmacological Basis of Therapeutics. 8th ed. New York: Pergamon Press, 1990; p. 1001.

87. Westwood-Squibb Pharmaceuticals (Telephone call). November 14, 1996.

88. McEvoy GK, ed. AHFS 96 Drug Information. Bethesda, MD: American Society of Health-System Pharmacists, 1996.

89. Degreef HJ, DeDoncker PRG. Current therapy of dermatophytosis. J Am Acad Dermatol 31(3 Pt 2):S25, 1994.

90. Rogers D, Kilkenny M, Marks R. The descriptive epidemiology of tinea pedis in the community. Australas J Dermatol 37:178, 1996.

91. Mast EE, Goodman RA. Prevention of infectious disease transmission in sports. Sports Med 24:1, 1997.

92. King MJ. Dermatologic problems in podiatric sports medicine. Clin Podiatr Med Surg 14:511, 1997.

93. Kamihama T, et al. Tinea pedis outbreak in swimming pools in Japan. Public Health 111:249, 1997.

94. Kemna ME, Elewski BE. A U.S. epidemiologic survey of superficial fungal diseases. J Am Acad Dermatol 35:539, 1996.

95. Mercantini R, et al. Epidemiology of dermatophytoses observed in Rome, Italy, between 1985 and 1993. Mycoses 38:415, 1995.

Warts

AT THE COUNTER

A middle-aged man enters the pharmacy and asks about nonprescription wart products.

Interview/Patient Assessment

When the pharmacist asks him to describe the location and appearance of the warts, he pulls back the hair of the forehead to reveal numerous flat warts on the forehead. He states that they have been present since he was in college, but that they are starting to move downward toward his eyes. He wants to know which product is better, a liquid or a plaster.

Pharmacist's Analysis

1. Are solutions and plasters both effective for warts?
2. Should this patient be allowed to use a nonprescription product?

3. What is the prognosis for spontaneous regression of these warts?

Solutions and plasters containing salicylic acid are both effective for warts. Product choice is dictated by patient preference. However, nonprescription products are not to be used for warts on the face, so this patient must be referred for physician evaluation. The long duration of these warts means that they will probably not resolve without treatment, as spontaneous regression is rare in long-standing warts.

Patient Counseling

The pharmacist should explain that nonprescription medications are not appropriate for use on the face and should advise the patient to see a physician.

Warts (verrucae) result from an infectious disease, the human papilloma virus (HPV). Although considered by many to be trivial, warts can be cosmetically disfiguring, since the epidermis becomes **hyperplastic** (a thickening of the epidermis in response to viral attack). Therapy for warts ranges from nonprescription medications to surgery, with many myths and folk remedies also touted as being effective.

Warts may be **exophytic** (growing outward) or **endophytic** (growing inward). They also exist in several forms (e.g., common, plantar, anogenital), not all of which can be treated with nonprescription products. For this reason pharmacists should try to determine which type of wart the patient has. The most common wart is verruca vulgaris, also known as the common wart. Other frequently occurring warts include flat warts (verruca plana), plantar warts (verruca plantaris), and anal and genital warts.

PREVALENCE OF WARTS

The prevalence of warts is not well described, but they are widely considered to be more common than most people think.[1,2] The prevalence may be as high as 2 to 20% for school children.[3,4] It has also been estimated at 10% for children and young adults, and 16% in the general population.[5–8] Slaughterhouse workers, who are at greater risk, have an incidence in excess of 40%.[9]

EPIDEMIOLOGY OF WARTS

Studies on the epidemiology of warts often seem contradictory. This may partially be because of the finding that the

specific type of human papilloma virus helps determine the epidemiology for a type of wart.[10]

Immunocompromised patients exhibit a propensity for infection with HPV.[11] Immunosuppressants used for prevention of posttransplant rejection, for example, have resulted in a wart incidence as high as 43%.[5] Also, widespread warts are a dermatologic sign of AIDS in the pediatric patient, and HIV-positive patients have significantly more warts on the face, hands, and feet than patients not affected with HIV.[5,12] Cell-mediated immunity may influence the host response to HPV contact since warts are more common in patients with cell-mediated immune deficiency such as lymphoma, chronic lymphatic leukemia, and Hodgkin's disease.

Warts exhibit a correlation with age. The peak incidence of most types of warts is between the ages of 12 and 16, and warts are uncommon in elderly patients.[5,7,13,14]

A gender difference is also seen with warts. Some researchers assert that nongenital warts are more common in females; one series of patients had a male:female ratio of 58:72.[13,15]

When one family member has warts, other family members are placed at higher risk of developing warts.[16] In one case the older sister of a patient with severe, intractable, common warts on the hands and feet had similar warts in the same locations. The presence of warts is also a risk factor for developing additional warts: warts occur three times more often in patients who already have them.[8]

Individuals who work with raw meat suffer a predisposition to hand and finger warts, a type of common wart known as the butcher's wart.[5,17] The combination of trauma (e.g., small cuts to the hands and fingers) and maceration is thought to be causal in the development of butcher's warts.[6,18,19] The fomite may be the protective gloves or the equipment used in processing the meat.[17] Most develop the warts within 2 years of beginning to work with raw meat.

Diabetic patients are at high risk of developing plantar warts.[8] The reason may be impaired circulation to the foot with a lowered ability to resist infection.

Attempts to discover serum antibodies to human papilloma viruses or wart tissue antigens in patients infected with warts have been negative.[5] Because it is located in the outer epidermis, HPV may be shielded from the immune system.[5] HPV may also avoid antibody destruction by forcing cells to produce abnormally low amounts of protein that would form antigen.[20]

ETIOLOGY OF WARTS

HPV, the cause of warts, is an **epithelialtrophic** (preferring upper epithelial tissues) virus, a double-stranded DNA virus.[21–23] Researchers have used several techniques to demonstrate the existence of almost 70 subtypes of HPV, including nucleic acid hybridization, DNA cleavage through the use of restriction endonucleases, and DNA cloning with recombinant molecules in bacteria.[5,11,24–27] All human warts are caused by members of the *Papovaviridae* family of viruses, which stimulate basal cell division to produce the characteristic lesion (Fig. 36.1).[3,5]

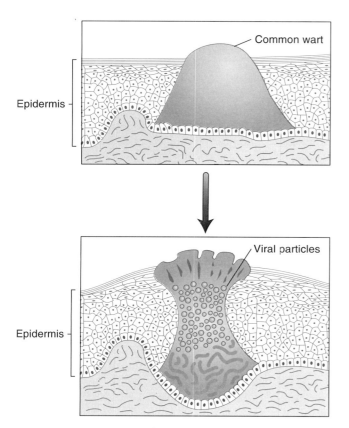

Figure 36.1. Cross-section of a common wart; this view illustrates the viral particles in the epidermal layers.

It is safe to say that the old folk myth that warts are caused by handling frogs or toads is entirely false.

TRANSMISSION OF WARTS

Studies of wart transmission are hampered by the fact that HPV affects only humans. There is no animal host for HPV because of the high species specificity of the papillomaviruses.[22] Furthermore, HPV cannot be grown in laboratories.[20]

Patients generally understand that warts are caused by some type of infection. In one survey 38% of patients attending a hospital wart-therapy clinic sought treatment because of their worry that the warts were infectious.[15] Fully 74% sought treatment from fear that the warts would spread extensively.

HPV is transmitted through skin-to-skin contact with an infected individual.[1] However, contact with an infected person's shed skin cells may also transmit the virus.[5] Evidently, HPV particles aggregate in the nuclei of keratinocytes prior to their release into the environment.[20]

Many viruses have a heat-sensitive lipid coating that does not allow survival in the environment for any period of time, but HPV has a heat-stable protein coating that fosters its survival for long periods, pending transmission to an unsuspecting host. The virus is also resistant to desiccation and prolonged storage, allowing fomites such as towels and clothing to infect additional hosts.[11,22] Tanning beds, finger-puncturing devices for self–blood glucose testing, and electrolysis procedures have been implicated as fomites for the spread of common warts.[28,29] Once any HPV has penetrated skin, the usual incubation period is 1 to 6 months; the incubation period for genital warts is 4 to 6 weeks.[5,11]

The plantar wart is most often spread through use of shower stalls or swimming facilities without protective footwear.[13] These wet environments are ideal for transmitting shed plantar wart virus, especially to patients who have a small skin break on a foot.[30] *Patients with plantar warts should stand on a personal bath mat, dry with a clean towel that will not be used by another person, and constantly keep the feet covered when in public places.*[6] Because it is impossible to be sure of the hygienic habits of others, pharmacists should recommend that patients without warts take these protective steps for their own good.[14]

Researchers believe that intact skin is a barrier to HPV infection.[31] This hypothesis is supported by the **Koebnerization** (Koebnerization refers to the Koebner phenomenon, a process in which warts occur in damaged skin) of flat warts in damaged skin (e.g., knees, hands, and feet).[5] Everyone experiences microabrasions of the skin from time to time.[20] Viral contact with microabraded skin, coupled with maceration, facilitates contact of the virion with the replicating epidermal layer.[20] More intrusive skin breaks increase the risk of warts.[32] For example, in one case a convict who had a tattoo applied with a staple, saliva, and ball-point pen ink developed numerous warts in the areas where the skin had been broken after a latency period of 8 years.[33] In another case a tattoo-induced crop of warts was reported after an incubation of 10 years.[34] The reason for the phenomenally long incubation periods in these warts is unknown.

Patients who already have warts are three times more likely to contract new warts as patients who are not infected with HPV.[35] The process of spreading warts to oneself is known as **autoinoculation.** *This spread of warts is most likely the result of intentional or accidental trauma to the original wart, which allows viral particles to contact uninfected skin, penetrate skin breaks, and begin new lesions.[5] For this reason pharmacists should caution children and their parents or caregivers that they must not bite, scratch, or pick warts.* A primary example of this transmission is the child who bites a wart on the finger and later notices new lesions developing on the mouth and lips. Nail biting can transfer HPV to the nails.[16] Nail warts are known as periungual (or subungual if they occur underneath the nail).[36]

MANIFESTATIONS OF WARTS

Warts are more prone to develop in certain sites, depending on the specific HPV subtype (Fig. 36.2). See Table 36.1 for various types of warts, their locations(s), their appearances, and other comments.

Common Warts (Verruca vulgaris)

As many as 70% of warts are common warts, which appear as rough, keratotic papules or nodules (Fig. 36.3).[5,22] The common wart is usually found on the dorsum of the fingers and hands of adults and children and on the knees in children, either as a single lesion or in groups.[5,37] Common warts appear as flesh-colored exophytic or endophytic papules and then enlarge to 1 cm or larger.[22]

Common warts are produced by infection with HPV subtypes 1, 2, 4, and 26 to 29, among others.[5] Infection may extend to the nailbed; these warts, known as periungual or subungual warts, produce abnormalities in nail growth. Occasionally, the Koebner phenomenon is responsible for their spread.

Flat Warts (Verruca plana)

Flat warts (also known as plane warts) are most often found on the face, hands, and legs of children in groups of lesions. Flat warts appear as small, hard growths, with a surface texture that resembles a cauliflower.[3] Their color may be that of the patient's flesh, or may appear as tan/pink to gray or brown. Flat warts are mostly endophytic, and their slight elevation and small size (usually less than 5 mm) helps in identification.[22]

Flat warts can be produced by HPV subtypes 2, 3, 10, 26 to 29, and 41, among others.[5] Shaving causes the Koebnerization of flat warts, as implied when they occur in a linear pattern.[22]

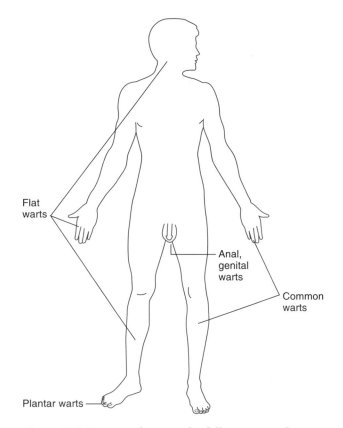

Figure 36.2. Common locations for different types of warts.

Table 36.1. Warts and Their Characteristics

TYPE OF WART	TYPICAL LOCATION(S)	APPEARANCE	COMMENTS
Common	Dorsum of fingers and hands; knees in children	Flesh-colored; rough papules or nodules	Single or grouped
Flat	Face, hands, and legs	Small, hard, with a cauliflower surface; usually do not protrude above skin surface	May grow outward with fingerlike projections
Plantar	Sole of the foot	Rough surface, usually do not protrude above foot surface	Produce pain on walking
Anal, genital	Anal and genital areas	Moist; protrude above the skin surface	A sexually transmitted disease

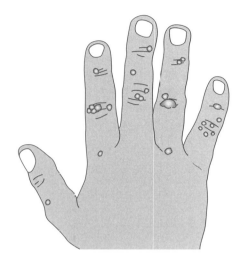

Figure 36.3. Appearance of common warts on the hand.

Some flat warts grow outward into surrounding skin with fingerlike projections rather than remaining round in shape. This flat wart subtype is known as the filiform wart (verruca filiformis).[8]

Plantar Warts (Verruca plantaris)

Plantar warts comprise about 24% of all warts.[5] Plantar warts are found on the sole of the foot, usually directly over weight-bearing areas such as the heel or metatarsal heads (Fig. 36.4).[3,5,38,39] Some plantar warts appear to have black dots scattered across their surface, which is coagulated capillary blood. The rough surface of these warts is surrounded by a rim of thickened skin. Because of their location, plantar warts can cause pain each time the patient places weight on the foot, much like having a small rock in the shoe. Because of the sometimes debilitating pain, plantar warts produce the most discomfort of all warts, except for genital warts.[13,14]

HPV subtypes 1, 2, 4, and 60 are among the viruses responsible for plantar warts.[40] Plantar warts are usually endophytic, except in patients who are not ambulatory.[22] In patients who are not ambulatory, plantar warts protrude from the skin surface. The endophytic nature of most plantar warts makes them difficult to treat.

In some cases several plantar warts on the surface of the foot will grow together to form one large lesion, known as a mosaic wart (Fig. 36.5).[5] (The term mosaic warts has also been used to refer to multiple warts on the knuckles, hands, or periungual areas.[22])

Anal and Genital Warts

Perhaps as many as 1% of sexually active persons suffer from genital warts.[11,41] Common locations include the glans penis, urethral meatus, anal mucosa, labia, and perianal surfaces.[42,43]

Some of the HPV subtypes that can cause anal and genital warts include 6, 11, 16, 18, and 51 to 55.[44,45] These growths are considered to be sexually transmitted diseases

because sexual contact with an infected person is the mode of transmission in 60% of cases.[3,11,46] Genital warts in a gravid female may affect the neonate during birth.[47]

When seen in children, anal and genital warts are possible indications of sexual abuse.[5,48]

Extracutaneous Manifestations of the Human Papilloma Virus (HPV)

HPV infections are not confined to cutaneous sites, but also occur on intraoral surfaces (usually the hard palate), intranasal mucosa, inside the conjunctiva, in the laryngeal area, and on cervical surfaces.[5,49,50] When warts occur in these locations, it is usually the result of such autoinoculation techniques as biting the wart, or allowing an infected finger to contact the eye, inside of the nose, or vagina.

PROGNOSIS OF WARTS

Warts are benign in most cases, causing nothing more than minor discomfort or annoyance and periodic minor embarrassment. For example, 92% percent of patients attending a hospital wart clinic sought therapy because the lesions were unsightly.[15] Warts can, however, produce much more severe problems, as recognized by 11% of attendees, who indicated that they were worried that warts were dangerous to their health. Some warts such as plantar warts can be painful, but other warts such as common warts are usually painless.[3]

Warts can restrict patients' activities. In one case the warts on the hands and feet of a 26-year-old male were so severe that the patient was unable to wear shoes or perform manual labor as an iron worker.[37]

Warts may transform into malignant lesions (e.g., squamous cell carcinoma), especially when they are caused by HPV types 5, 8, 14, 17, and 20.[22,37,51–53] Also, in recent years cancer of the cervix has been increasingly linked to infection with HPV.[5,18]

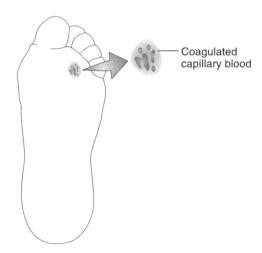

Figure 36.4. Appearance of plantar warts.

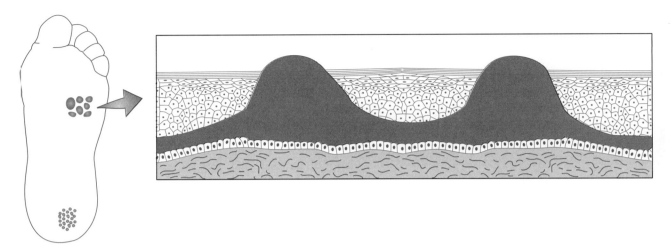

Figure 36.5. Appearance of the mosaic form of plantar warts; cross-section of skin illustrating their coalescence beneath the surface of the skin.

Spontaneous Regression

Many warts will spontaneously disappear if left alone, an occurrence termed spontaneous regression.[3] While exact figures are unknown, research indicates that about 66% of warts in children will disappear within 2 years.[5,22,54]

Flat warts are especially prone to regress. These warts appear red, pruritic, and swollen while shrinking, and a surrounding halo of depigmentation may appear around the flat wart as it disappears. Several additional flat warts often involute at the same time, so all flat warts can disappear within a few weeks.[22]

Plantar and anogenital warts are less likely to regress.[3] When plantar and common warts regress, they do not exhibit inflammation, but appear darker, with the wart becoming either dry or liquid in consistency.[5]

While the reason for spontaneous regression is unknown, patients experiencing it demonstrate IgG antibodies, sometimes combined with IgM antibodies.[5] Spontaneous regression usually takes about 2 months for completion after IgG antibodies develop. It is most likely in those whose warts have been present for only 6 months to 2 years. The immune system in patients whose warts are present for 10 years may be unable to begin the process of regression.

Regardless of their tendency to regress, all warts should be actively treated. Relying on spontaneous regression while neglecting legitimate therapy is misguided.[25] During any time without active treatment, the prevalence of warts can increase greatly as the untreated warts spread to uninfected skin or to other hosts.

Wart-Free Periods

Following regression of one or more warts, some patients may enjoy a wart-free period that lasts for days or years, while others may experience new warts immediately.[11] The reason why some individuals never experience a recurrence and others have new growths before tissues have healed is unknown.

TREATMENT OF WARTS

Treatment Guidelines

Nonprescription products should only be used to treat common and plantar warts.[35] (See Patient Assessment Algorithm 36.1.) Common and plantar warts are easily identified by patients: The common wart has the characteristic "cauliflower-like" surface, while the plantar wart is located only on the bottom of the foot, where it causes tenderness and interrupts the footprint pattern. By contrast, a flat wart mimics other, more serious skin conditions such as malignant melanoma.

(tip) Pharmacists should counsel patients that *if the wart or warts do not improve in 12 weeks, they must discontinue the product and see a physician.* Patients can detect a complete cure by examining the skin ridges. When they have been restored, the area is considered cured.[8]

(tip) Pharmacists should caution patients *not to treat warts on the mucous membranes, face, or genitals.*[55] Skin in these areas is extremely sensitive; in addition, skin on the face should be treated with a method that does not cause scarring.[3,56] With the exception of the wart presoak, patients with warts on the hands should be cautioned to keep the hands as dry as possible as long as warts are present, since softening of the upper layer of keratin contributes to release of viral particles.[16] For the same reason patients with plantar warts should keep the feet dry with the use of cotton socks and shoes that prevent sweating of the feet as long as the wart is present. Nonprescription wart-treatment products must not be applied to moles, birthmarks, or unusual warts with hair growing from them because of the possibility that the patient actually has a premalignant or malignant lesion rather than a wart.[35] These products also should also not be applied to skin that is irritated, infected, or reddened; should be discontinued if they cause irritation; and must be kept away from the eyes.[57] (If collodions contact the eyes, they should be flushed with water for 15 minutes.[55])

Patient Assessment Algorithm 36.1. Warts

```
┌─────────────────────────────────────────────┐        ┌──────────────────────────────────────────────┐
│ Does the patient have diabetes or poor       │──Yes──▶│              Refer to physician.               │
│ circulation?                                  │        └──────────────────────────────────────────────┘
└─────────────────────────────────────────────┘
                     │ No
                     ▼
┌─────────────────────────────────────────────┐        ┌──────────────────────────────────────────────┐
│ Is the skin irritated, inflamed, or reddened?│──Yes──▶│              Refer to physician.               │
└─────────────────────────────────────────────┘        └──────────────────────────────────────────────┘
                     │ No
                     ▼
┌─────────────────────────────────────────────┐        ┌──────────────────────────────────────────────┐
│ Is the wart located on the face, genitals, or│──Yes──▶│              Refer to physician.               │
│ mucous membranes?                             │        └──────────────────────────────────────────────┘
└─────────────────────────────────────────────┘
                     │ No
                     ▼
┌─────────────────────────────────────────────┐        ┌──────────────────────────────────────────────┐
│ Does the area appear to be a mole or          │──Yes──▶│              Refer to physician.               │
│ birthmark, or is it an unusual wart such as a │        └──────────────────────────────────────────────┘
│ wart with hair growing from it?               │
└─────────────────────────────────────────────┘
                     │ No
                     ▼
┌─────────────────────────────────────────────┐        ┌──────────────────────────────────────────────┐
│ Is the wart a common wart or plantar wart?    │──No───▶│              Refer to physician.               │
└─────────────────────────────────────────────┘        └──────────────────────────────────────────────┘
                     │ Yes
                     ▼
┌─────────────────────────────────────────────┐
│ Recommend salicylic acid plaster or collodion.│
└─────────────────────────────────────────────┘
```

tip *Patients with diabetes mellitus or poor circulation should not use wart products without physician direction.*[35] These patients are more prone to infections from the chemical destruction of skin caused by nonprescription, wart-therapy medications.

Collodion formulations contain ether, which evaporates rapidly.[35] For this reason the bottles must be tightly capped **tip** and kept away from fire or flame while in use. *Bottles with visible crystals indicate excessive evaporation of solvent and precipitation of salicylic acid. They must be discarded.* Pharmacists should caution patients not to inhale the vapors of collodion-based products.

Nonprescription Medications

The sole approved ingredient for wart therapy is salicylic acid (Table 36.2).[35] Salicylic acid acts through a keratolytic action to chemically remove epidermal cells that are infected with HPV. The ingredient may also induce inflammation, which induces an immune response. (See "A Pharmacist's Journal: Which Aspirin Do I Use?")

Salicylic acid usually is formulated as plasters in 12 to 40%

concentrations and flexible collodion or collodion-like vehicles in 5 to 17% concentrations, but salicylic acid 15% in a karaya-gum, glycol-plaster vehicle was also given monograph status.[57] The effect of salicylic acid depends on adequate moisture, and these dosage forms promote skin hydration by occluding the **tip** skin. *Pharmacists should advise patients to prepare the wart by washing the area or soaking it in warm water for 5 minutes and then drying the skin thoroughly.*

Liquid products are applied once or twice daily, using an applicator, brush, or dropper, to the wart only (not to the surrounding skin).[58,59] When using a dropper, one drop at a time is applied until each wart is covered, and then they are al-**tip** lowed to dry. *Liquid dosage forms may be kept away from surrounding skin by circling the wart with a ring of petrolatum.*

Plasters are cut to the size of the wart, applied, kept on for 48 hours, and then replaced.

The product formulated as a karaya-glycol plaster is applied at bedtime after the wart has been gently smoothed with an emery file, left on for 8 hours, and removed in the morning. The procedure should be repeated each night for up to the limit of 12 weeks.[21,57]

Table 36.2. Representative Wart Products

PRODUCT	SELECTED INGREDIENTS/COMMENTS
Clear-Away	Salicylic acid 40% discs
Clear-Away Plantar	Salicylic acid 40% discs (larger in diameter than Clear-Away)
Dr. Scholl's Clear-Away Gel	Salicylic acid 17%
Compound W	Salicylic acid 17% in collodion
Compound W Gel	Salicylic acid 17% in collodion; gel dosage form
Compound W Medicated Pads	Salicylic acid 40%
Duofilm	Salicylic acid 17% in collodion
DuoPlant Gel	Salicylic acid 17% in collodion; gel dosage form
Off-Ezy Warts	Salicylic acid 17% in collodion
Tina Med Plantar Patch	Salicylic acid 40%
Wart-Off	Salicylic acid 17% in collodion

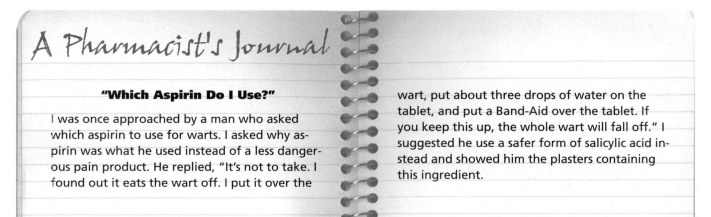

A Pharmacist's Journal

"Which Aspirin Do I Use?"

I was once approached by a man who asked which aspirin to use for warts. I asked why aspirin was what he used instead of a less dangerous pain product. He replied, "It's not to take. I found out it eats the wart off. I put it over the wart, put about three drops of water on the tablet, and put a Band-Aid over the tablet. If you keep this up, the whole wart will fall off." I suggested he use a safer form of salicylic acid instead and showed him the plasters containing this ingredient.

Other Professional Treatment

PHYSICAL METHODS

Cryotherapy

Cryotherapy for warts consists of freezing the lesions with liquid nitrogen (boiling point = −196°C).[15,16,60,61] While this procedure is well tolerated by most patients, it is expensive and painful, and not all lesions respond to treatment.[15,60,62] Further, in one study 11% of patients were unable to go to work, do housework, or take part in other regular activities on the day of treatment and the following day.[15] Cryotherapy is not advisable for patients younger than 10 or 11 because of the discomfort.[30,56]

Electrosurgical Removal

This method requires local anesthesia because of the pain it produces.[56] Because of the scarring associated with this treatment and the risk of infection, it is best limited to small warts.

Surgical Excision

Wart removal through surgery scars the host and commonly causes recurrence.[16] (The resulting scar is often as disfiguring as the wart was.[56,60]) This procedure is reserved for plantar warts that cause acute pain and hamper mobility.

Laser Therapy

Carbon-dioxide laser surgery, which has cure rates ranging from 54 to 100%, causes less pain and scarring than electrosurgery.[56]

CHEMOTHERAPY

Numerous medications have been used to chemically eradicate warts. Some treatments attack the hyperkeratotic tissue itself, rather than the viral cause of the hyperkeratosis, including the irritating or erosive agents salicylic acid, lactic acid, trichloroacetic acid, and podophyllin.[5,11] Recurrence rates following these destructive methods range from 7.5 to 33%, and they often scar or blister the skin.[5,56] Other chemicals that show promise include bleomycin, interferon, 5-fluorouracil, and retinoids.[5,8,63–65]

CIMETIDINE

Cimetidine seems to improve warts when administered orally.[66,67] In one study of high-dose oral cimetidine, 84% of patients with recalcitrant common warts experienced im-

A Pharmacist's Journal

"I Can Heal Warts!"

Whenever I lecture about warts, I can count on several people approaching me after the lecture to share their own personal wart eradication methods such as rubbing the wart with castor oil, mineral oil, onions, potatoes, etc. However, it would be hard to top the sure cure that an older friend confided to me one night at church. "I can heal warts," he shared confidentially. Then he went on to say that several years ago

he had a wart on his wrist that had defied treatment. In frustration, he went outside on a sunny day with a magnifying glass. He trained the rays of the sun on the wart. He said it only hurt for the first few seconds, and then flames began to erupt from the wart. According to my friend, the burned wart went away, never returned, and did not scar the skin. Of course, the hazards of a dangerous method such as this outweigh any potential benefit.

provement or disappearance of the warts.[68] However, the nonprescription product does not carry this indication, so pharmacists should not recommend it for this purpose.

CONTACT IMMUNOTHERAPY

Contact immunotherapy consists of placing a sensitizing chemical on the wart to induce a hypersensitivity response.[69] As the body reacts, the wart is destroyed through the "innocent bystander" theory. Presumably, the sensitizing chemical elicits a cell-mediated process that triggers wart destruction. Dinitrochlorobenzene, a chemical used for this purpose, is first applied in an initial sensitizing application, and then is reapplied to produce a specific area of contact dermatitis.[56,70] Other physicians use *Toxicodendron* plants to achieve the same objective.

OTHER METHODS

Wart removal has been the subject of numerous folk cures over the years. However, most lack any proof of efficacy as measured by placebo-controlled, double-blind studies. (See "Suggestive and Alternative Wart Removal Methods.") (See "A Pharmacist's Journal: I Can Heal Warts!")

PREVENTION OF WARTS

The key to preventing warts is to eliminate possible modes of transmission:

- Avoid skin-to-skin contact with infected individuals.
- Avoid contacting surfaces where others may have been present without protective clothing (e.g., shower floors, locker room floors and benches, tanning beds, community beach chairs, etc.).

FOCUS ON...

SUGGESTIVE AND ALTERNATIVE WART REMOVAL METHODS

Rooted for decades in the realm of "folk healers" or "wart charmers," suggestive wart-treatment techniques include interventions that do not use any active pharmacologic agent, but which attempt to plant in the patient a mental suggestion that warts will disappear.[8,71–73] Hypnosis, which can facilitate the process, has demonstrated positive results in limited research.[49,74,75] In one case a 4-year-old girl taught self-hypnosis experienced regression of 82 warts during four biweekly sessions, a result unexpected for routine spontaneous regression.[75]

In regard to alternative wart removal methods, homeopathy was no better in treating warts than placebo in a controlled study.[76]

- Never enter any area with bare feet where another person may have been in bare feet.
- Treat existing warts immediately to avoid spreading and autoinoculation.
- To avoid autoinoculation, never bite, scratch, or pick a wart.
- If warts are present on the body, use separate towels and wash cloths on affected skin to prevent transfer to new sites.
- Never attempt to remove warts with any kind of device; damaging the wart can contribute to spread.

SUMMARY

Warts are annoying, sometimes painful, and occasionally debilitating common invaders of the skin that are caused by HPV. Frequently occurring warts include the common wart, plantar wart, flat wart, and anal/genital wart.

Nonprescription products using salicylic acid are safe and effective for removing common warts and plantar warts. Other types of warts—such as flat and anogenital warts—should be seen by a physician because they are not as easily recognized as warts by the patient.

AT THE COUNTER

 A grade-school boy is brought in by his father to speak to the pharmacist.

Interview/Patient Assessment

The boy has a wart on the skin of the lower thumb. The wart is raised above the skin surface and appears yellowish in color. The father says the child bites and picks at it during the day. His neighbor says he should take his son to the doctor since surgery will cure the problem. He wonders if the nonprescription products would hurt less.

Pharmacist's Analysis

1. Is this type of wart treatable with nonprescription products?
2. What dangers are inherent in biting or picking at a wart?
3. What are the relative advantages/disadvantages of surgery and nonprescription products?

This child's wart appears to be a common wart, which is treatable with nonprescription, salicylic acid products. If the boy continues to bite or pick the wart, he may autoinoculate to uninfected areas such as the lips, tongue, or adjoining digits. Surgery is rapid, but it is painful and expensive, and HPV may inoculate along the suture lines. Although nonprescription, salicylic-acid products are slow, they cause little pain, are inexpensive, and do not cause spread of HPV.

Patient Counseling

The father should be shown all directions associated with plasters and solutions to allow him to choose a dosage form. The white collodion remaining on the wart after its vehicle has evaporated might not be acceptable to the child because of possible teasing, but an opaque bandage over the wart may prevent this. Also, the difficulty of applying the collodion to the wart without contacting surrounding skin should be mentioned. For this reason a plaster, which is easier to apply and looks more natural, might be preferable.

Generally, the viruses that cause warts can be avoided by following certain commonsense steps. Basically, avoiding contact with the viruses is the best prevention.

References

1. OBrien JM. Common skin problems of infancy, childhood, and adolescence. Prim Care 22:99, 1995.
2. Feldman SR, Fleischer AB Jr, McConnell RC. Most common dermatologic problems identified by internists, 1990–1994. Arch Intern Med 158:726, 1998.
3. Hall A, Murtagh J. Warts. Aust Fam Physician 18:1432, 1989.
4. Kilkenny M, Marks R. The descriptive epidemiology of warts in the community. Australas J Dermatol 37:80, 1996.
5. Cobb MW. Human papillomavirus infection. J Am Acad Derm 22:547, 1990.
6. Benton C. The management of viral warts. Practitioner 232:933, 1988.
7. Parish LC, Monroe E, Rex IH Jr. Treatment of common warts with high-potency (26%) salicylic acid. Clin Ther 10:462, 1988.
8. Bolton RA. Nongenital warts: Classification and treatment options. Am Fam Physician 43:2049, 1991.
9. Aziz MA, Bahamdan K, Moneim MA. Prevalence and risk factors for warts among slaughterhouse workers. East Afr Med J 73:194, 1996.
10. Rubben A, et al. Clinical features and age distribution of patients with HPV 2/27/57–induced common warts. Arch Dermatol Res 289:337, 1997.
11. Beutner KR. Bridging the gap. Arch Derm 126:1432, 1990.
12. Prose NS, et al. Widespread flat warts associated with human papillomavirus type 5: A cutaneous manifestation of human immunodeficiency virus infection. J Am Acad Derm 23:978, 1990.
13. Johnson LW. Communal showers and the risk of plantar warts. J Fam Pract 40:136, 1995.
14. Esterowitz D, et al. Plantar warts in the athlete. Am J Emerg Med 13:441, 1995.
15. Keefe M, Dick DC. Cryotherapy of hand warts—A questionnaire survey of "consumers." Clin Exp Derm 15:260, 1990.
16. Steele K. Management of cutaneous warts. Aust Fam Physician 17:950, 1988.
17. Melchers W, et al. Human papillomavirus and cutaneous warts in meat handlers. J Clin Microbiol 31:2547, 1993.
18. Keefe M, et al. Cutaneous warts in butchers. Br J Dermatol 130:9, 1994.
19. Keefe M, et al. Butchers' warts: No evidence for person to person transmission of HPV7. Br J Dermatol 130:15, 1994.
20. Androphy EJ. Human papillomavirus (Editorial). Arch Dermatol 125:683, 1989.
21. Fed Reg 59:60315, 1994.
22. Melton JL, Rasmussen JE. Clinical manifestations of human papillomavirus infection in nongenital sites. Dermatol Clin 9:219, 1991.
23. Prasad CJ. Pathobiology of human papillomavirus. Clin Lab Med 15:685, 1995.
24. Lewis R. Genital warts. FDA Consumer 29(4):18, 1995.
25. Janniger CK. Childhood warts. Cutis 50:15, 1992.
26. Chen S-L, et al. Characterization and analysis of human papilloma viruses of skin warts. Arch Dermatol Res 285:460, 1993.
27. Ratoosh SL, et al. Mastication of verruca vulgaris associated with esophageal papilloma: HPV-45 sequences detected in oral and cutaneous tissues. J Am Acad Dermatol 36 (5 Pt 2):853, 1997.
28. Perniciaro C, Dicken CH. Tanning bed warts (Letter). J Am Acad Derm 18:586, 1988.

29. Roach MC, Chretien JH. Common hand warts in athletes: Association with trauma to the hand. J Am Coll Health 44:125, 1995.

30. Rhind P, Lindsay D, Catterall M. Verrucae. Practitioner 233:300, 1989.

31. Khan JI, Frame JD. Koebner's phenomenon in burns: Another complication following thermal injury. Burns 19:249, 1993.

32. Long GE, Rickman LS. Infectious complications of tattoos. Clin Infect Dis 18:610, 1994.

33. Ragland HP, et al. Verruca vulgaris inoculated during tattoo placement. Int J Dermatol 33:796, 1994.

34. Miller DM, Brodell RT. Verruca restricted to the area of black dye within a tattoo. Arch Dermatol 130:1453, 1994.

35. Fed Reg 45:65609, 1980.

36. Moghaddas N. Periungual verrucae: Diagnosis and treatment. Clin Podiatr Med Surg 12:189, 1995.

37. Tanigaki T, Kanda R. Severe intractable common warts associated with human papillomavirus 2, 3, and 20. Dermatologica 181:159, 1990.

38. Landsmann MJ, Mancuso JE, Abramow SP. Diagnosis, pathophysiology, and treatment of plantar verruca. Clin Podiatr Med Surg 13:55, 1996.

39. Omura EF, Rye B. Dermatologic disorders of the foot. Clin Sports Med 13:825, 1994.

40. Kashima M, et al. A case of peculiar plantar warts. Human papillomavirus type 60 infection. Arch Dermatol 130:1418, 1994.

41. Galloway DA. Human papillomavirus vaccines: A warty problem. Infect Agents Dis 3:187, 1994.

42. Anon. 1998 guidelines for treatment of sexually transmitted diseases. Centers for Disease Control and Prevention. MMWR 467(RR-1):1, 1998.

43. Hippelainen MI, et al. Clinical course and prognostic factors of human papillomavirus infections in men. Sex Transm Dis 21:272, 1994.

44. Handsfield HH. Clinical presentation and natural course of anogenital warts. Am J Med 102:16, 1997.

45. Beutner KR, Tyring S. Human papillomavirus and human disease. Am J Med 102:9, 1997.

46. Herman-Giddens ME, et al. Association of coexisting vaginal infections and multiple abusers in female children with genital warts. Sex Transm Dis 15:63, 1988.

47. Carson S. Human papillomavirus infection update: Impact on women's health. Nurse Pract 22:24, 1997.

48. Bingham EA. Significance of anogenital warts in children. Br J Hosp Med 52:469, 1994.

49. Spanos NP, Stenstrom RJ, Johnston JC. Hypnosis, placebo, and suggestion in the treatment of warts. Psychosom Med 50:245, 1988.

50. Kundu A, Wade AAH. Warts in the oral cavity. Genitourin Med 71:195, 1995.

51. Guadara J, et al. Transformation of plantar verruca into squamous cell carcinoma. J Foot Surg 31:611, 1992.

52. Baker GE, Tyring SK. Therapeutic approaches to papillomavirus infections. Dermatol Clin 15:331, 1997.

53. Sober AJ, Burstein JM. Precursors to skin cancer. Cancer 75(Suppl):645, 1995.

54. Kimble Haas S. Primary care treatment approach to nongenital verruca. Nurse Pract 21:29, 1996.

55. Fed Reg 47:39102, 1982.

56. Taylor MB. Successful treatment of warts. Postgrad Med 84:126, 1988.

57. Fed Reg 55:33246, 1990.

58. Fed Reg 52:9992, 1987.

59. Fed Reg 57:44494, 1992.

60. Millikan LE, Shrum JP. An update on common skin diseases. Postgrad Med 91:96, 1992.

61. Hewitt WR Jr. Liquid nitrogen treatment of hand and plantar warts. J Am Coll Health 40:288, 1992.

62. Hopkins P. Treatment of warts with liquid nitrogen (Letter). JR Coll Gen Pract 39:173, 1989.

63. Kirby P. Interferon and genital warts: Much potential, modest progress (Editorial). JAMA 259:570, 1988.

64. Berman A, Berman JE. New concepts in viral wart infection. Compr Ther 14:19, 1988.

65. Beutner KR, Ferenczy A. Therapeutic approaches to genital warts. Am J Med 102:28, 1997.

66. Ronna T, Lebwohl M. Cimetidine therapy for plantar warts (Letter). J Am Podiatr Med Assoc 85:717, 1995.

67. Wargon O. Cimetidine for mucosal warts in an HIV positive adult. Australas J Dermatol 37:149, 1996.

68. Glass AT, Solomon BA. Cimetidine therapy for recalcitrant warts in adults. Arch Dermatol 132:680, 1996.

69. Naylor MF, et al. Contact immunotherapy of resistant warts. J Am Acad Derm 19:679, 1988.

70. Shah KC, Patel RM, Umrigar DD. Dinitrochlorobenzene treatment of verrucae plana. J Dermatol 18:639, 1991.

71. Burns A. "Warts and all"—The history and folklore of warts: A review. JR Soc Med 85:37, 1992.

72. Steele K. Wart charming practices among patients attending wart clinics. Br J Gen Pract 40:517, 1990.

73. Dudley W. The psychological impact of warts on patients' lives. Prof Nurs 11:99, 1995.

74. Spanos NP, Williams V, Gwynn MI. Effects of hypnotic, placebo, and salicylic acid treatments on wart regression. Psychosom Med 52:109, 1990.

75. Noll RB. Hypnotherapy of a child with warts. J Dev Behav Med 9:89, 1988.

76. Kainz JT, et al. Homeopathic versus placebo therapy of children with warts on the hands: A randomized, double-blind clinical trial. Dermatology 193:318, 1996.

Contact Dermatitis and Poison Ivy/Oak/Sumac

AT THE COUNTER

A patient asks the pharmacist about an area of broken skin on her lips.

Interview/Patient Assessment

The patient has developed a vesicular reaction on the colored section of the upper and lower lips (known as the vermilion border). The lips are itching and inflamed. There is no pain and the skin is not cracked. She has no history of aphthous stomatitis (canker sores) or herpes simplex (fever blisters). She denies use of any medication and has no other medical condition. The lips began to itch early in the morning of the previous day. As the day progressed, small bumps appeared on the lips, proceeding to vesicles.

Pharmacist's Analysis

1. What are possible causes of this patient's condition?
2. What measures should the patient take to discover the cause of the condition?
3. Are nonprescription products recommended for this condition?

The patient's symptoms are consistent with contact dermatitis.

Patient Counseling

The pharmacist should urge the patient to recall any incident or product that could have caused this reaction. Had she had a minor case of chapped lips, which she began to lick, irritating the skin? Had she been using lipstick, lip balm, or sunscreen and had a reaction to some ingredients, causing an irritant contact dermatitis or allergic contact dermatitis? If she suspects some product(s) caused the reaction, the pharmacist should advise her not to use the product(s) on her lips until the reaction subsides. When the dermatitis is gone, she may reintroduce the suspected product(s) into her cosmetic regimen slowly to help detect the offending product(s). When the reaction recurs, the ingredient list of the newly reintroduced product should be examined closely. She should attempt to purchase products that do not contain those ingredients. Since most skin-care products contain many ingredients, this may not be possible, but she should try to choose one that has as few of the suspect ingredients if possible. Should the reaction recur, she can then more closely narrow the list of ingredients that might be responsible. Over time, she may be able to experiment with different products to discover exactly which ingredient is causing the reaction. All other products containing that ingredient should be avoided in the future.

To help deal with the discomfort caused by the reaction, the pharmacist can recommend hydrocortisone 0.5 to 1%, which will help the skin return to normal sensation and appearance. An ointment would be preferred since a cream would be more quickly removed by the movements of the lips.

"Dermatitis," a general term for several types of skin irritation, may be subdivided into endogenous and exogenous forms[1]:

- Endogenous forms such as nummular eczema, stasis dermatitis, and neurodermatitis are induced by an internal disorder and are typified by **atopic dermatitis** (a skin eruption usually manifesting during childhood, associated with asthma and allergic rhinitis).[2–6]
- Exogenous forms, which are known as "contact dermatitis," are caused by contact with some substance.

The skin is a primary immunologic site, for both endogenous and exogenous dermatitis, with keratinocytes able to participate in inflammatory and nonspecific immune responses.[7]

This chapter addresses exogenous dermatoses (e.g., contact dermatitis) and some of its most common forms, poison ivy/oak/sumac, since the pharmacist is most often asked to advise patients about them.

CONTACT DERMATITIS

Contact dermatitis is an umbrella term that encompasses several adverse skin reactions that result from contact with some substance[8]:

- Irritant contact dermatitis. Irritant contact dermatitis occurs when skin undergoes mechanical or chemical trauma on exposure to an irritating substance(s). The skin reaction is not a result of sensitization, but of direct toxicity to tissues.[9] For example, cacti, rose hips, comfrey, borage, and tulip bulb sheaths all have fine hairs that can induce this damage by mechanical trauma. Likewise, plants with large thorns and slicing blades also can induce irritant contact dermatitis.[10] Hot peppers, tobacco, garlic, and buttercups produce irritant contact dermatitis through a direct action of the chemicals they contain. Sodium lauryl sulfate, found in carpet cleaners, toothpastes, and many other formulations, causes an irritant contact dermatitis that does not resolve for approximately 4 weeks.[11] Irritant contact dermatitis reactions recur with increasing severity on subsequent exposures, and the condition occurs with greater frequency on thin skin (the finger webs and backs of the hands are more common sites than the palms).[12] Diaper dermatitis is a subtype of irritant contact dermatitis. (See Chapter 38, Diaper Dermatitis.)
- Allergic contact dermatitis. The allergic type of contact dermatitis occurs in several steps, involving a process of sensitization with a reaction on elicitation.[5,10] First, an individual contacts some chemical to which he was not previously

allergic. The chemical binds to the skin, producing an allergen. Epidermal Langerhans cells form haptens with T lymphocytes over a 2- to 3-week period, sensitizing the individual to that chemical.[13,14] When the person is reexposed to the chemical at some later time, memory T cells aggregate at the site of skin contact in a cell-mediated immune reaction, which is known as the elicitation phase of the allergic reaction. This produces the symptoms typical of allergic contact dermatitis. Allergic contact dermatitis is virtually synonymous with the condition known as "poison ivy," (see below), although it is produced by other plants such as ragweed.[15]

PREVALENCE OF CONTACT DERMATITIS

Dermatitis is responsible for over 20% of referrals to dermatology departments, and affects 20% of children at one time or another.[1,16,17] One-half of these patients suffer from contact dermatitis, of which one-third to one-half is caused by allergic contact dermatitis.[16] Researchers estimate that contact dermatitis is responsible for at least 7% of occupationally related illnesses, making it the most common occupational skin disease.[7,18] Nickel sensitivity, for example, is seen in 6% of the population and is more common in those who have pierced ears along with gold allergy.[19–21]

EPIDEMIOLOGY OF CONTACT DERMATITIS

Certain characteristics predispose individuals to contact dermatitis: fair skin, especially with red hair; advanced age, when skin is usually drier; atopy; and a preexisting dermatitis at any body site.[22–24]

Gender

Postpartum females are at higher risk of contact dermatitis than other people.[24] Other gender-related aspects of contact dermatitis reflect differing exposures. For instance, nickel sensitivity is 10 times more common in females than in males.[7] This may represent the higher likelihood of exposure to nickel in females as a result of wearing jewelry; sensitization is one of the many complications of ear piercing.[24] Heavy use of ingredient-rich cosmetics is also a contributing factor to the high incidence of contact dermatitis in females.[12]

Occupation

Patients whose occupations require chemical exposure are more likely to manifest contact dermatitis. Common examples include the following[24,26–33]:

- Cosmetologists (exposure to permanent solution and acrylic nails)
- Homemakers, housekeeping personnel (exposure to various cleaning solvents)
- Chemical-manufacturing personnel[34]
- Builders and plasterers (exposure to chromates in cement and plaster)
- Automobile mechanics (exposure to paints, engine fluids, and battery acids)[35]
- Electronics assembly workers (exposure to epoxy resins and hardeners)
- Mechanics and soldiers in the armored or artillery divisions (hand dermatoses from contact with fuel or oil)
- Health-care workers and others who wear natural rubber gloves (exposure to latex or other components of the gloves) (see "Latex Allergy")
- Lawn-care workers (exposure to lawn-care chemicals such as fungicides)[36,37]
- Undertakers (exposure to several allergenic chemicals)
- Those who work with wood[38]

Less common examples include the following[39,40]:

- Bartenders (reactions to malt and yeast in beer)
- Laboratory technicians (one worker caring for cockroaches developed an allergy to them)

ETIOLOGY OF CONTACT DERMATITIS

Items and substances that produce contact dermatitis include topical medications (e.g., benzocaine, zinc pyrithione, neomycin, sodium bisulfite or phenylephrine in ophthalmic drops, and corticosteroids); cosmetic ingredients (e.g., diazolidinyl urea and imidazolidinyl urea); perfume ingredients (e.g., cinnamic aldehyde, balsam of peru, and cinnamic alcohol); buttons, jewelry, earrings, wristwatches, and other adornments (nickel); shoe leather; and rubber.[7,51–58] These allergens share the ability to bind to cutaneous protein.

MANIFESTATIONS OF CONTACT DERMATITIS

The dermis and subcutaneous tissues respond with a variety of symptoms when challenged with allergens. Patients may experience pruritus prior to any visible dermatologic change. Within a short period the skin may begin to redden and a variety of lesions may appear, from raised wheals to fluid-filled vesicles. The same area of skin may have both wheals and vesicles. A rash may also be evident, manifested as crops of small solid lesions.

Body sites most likely to manifest contact dermatitis include the hands, face, legs, ears, eyes, and the anogenital area.[59] These sites are those most often exposed to the various allergens (Figs. 37.1 and 37.2). Recognition of immediate contact dermatitis is facilitated by the fact that the skin reacts instantly following exposure.[10]

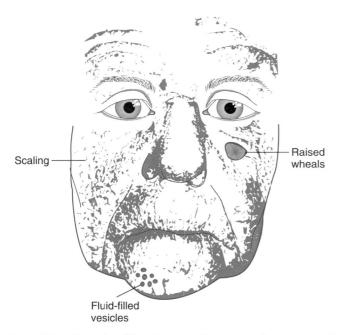

Figure 37.1. Example of facial contact dermatitis, showing raised wheals, fluid-filled vesicles, and scaling.

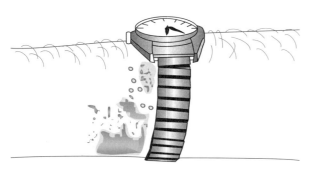

Figure 37.2. Example of contact dermatitis caused by nickel in a watch band.

SPECIFIC CONSIDERATIONS OF CONTACT DERMATITIS: PHYTOMEDICINALS

The growing popularity of herbal medicine can expose patients to plant preparations that may have unknown therapeutic value. This can be troubling because patients may develop contact dermatitis to these unapproved products.[60] Pharmacists should take great care when stocking and recommending unapproved "phytomedicinals." It would be prudent to require that manufacturers provide evidence of FDA approval for the indications placed on the package and clearly state all product ingredients.

TREATMENT OF CONTACT DERMATITIS

See "Treatment of Contact Dermatitis and Poison Ivy/Oak/Sumac."

PREVENTION OF CONTACT DERMATITIS

See "Prevention of Contact Dermatitis and Poison Ivy/Oak/Sumac."

POISON IVY/OAK/SUMAC

The term "poison ivy" is used by the lay public and the medical community to refer to an allergic contact dermatitis caused by poison ivy, poison oak, and poison sumac. Thus this text will discuss poison ivy/oak/sumac as a model of allergic plant dermatoses, but the principles and treatments will be the same for other plants that induce allergic contact dermatitis.

The literature on poison ivy is more complete, so much of the discussion centers around it. However, poison oak and sumac are similar in virtually all respects to poison ivy, except in the differences discussed below.

PREVALENCE OF POISON IVY/OAK/SUMAC

Poison ivy, poison oak, and poison sumac, the most common causes of contact dermatitis, affect millions of Americans each year.[61] At least 50 to 70% of the population is sensitive to **catechols** (the allergenic components of poison ivy, poison oak, and poison sumac).[62]

EPIDEMIOLOGY OF POISON IVY/OAK/SUMAC

Age

Children do not often exhibit poison ivy sensitivity until grade school age.[61] (Since children and infants can be sensitized, this finding is probably because younger children simply are not as likely to contact poison ivy as older children.)

By the ages of 6 to 8 years, however, at least 85% of children can be sensitized.[63] Adults who are not sensitized have only a 50% risk of sensitization, since they are less likely to come into contact with the plant.

Occupation

Individuals who work outdoors are more likely to be exposed to poison ivy than those who work inside.[62] The condition is more common in forestry workers and fire fighters than in farm workers. In the U.S. Forestry Service poison ivy causes more than 10% of all lost time.[62]

Poison ivy accounts for 0.11% of all workers' compensation claims and in California for 1% of the budget for workers' compensation.[63]

Geographic Location

The incidence of sensitivity mirrors the opportunity for individuals to contact plants (Fig. 37.3). While 50 to 75% of the general population is sensitive to poison ivy, those living in areas free of the plants would experience much lower sensitivity. (The plants are not found in such areas as the Rockies [they do not survive above 4000 feet], most of Nevada and Idaho, desert areas [e.g., much of Arizona], and in the Washington state rain forests.)

Atopy

Although they are generally more prone to other types of dermatitis, individuals who suffer from atopic dermatitis are less likely to experience poison ivy.[62] The reason is unknown.

ETIOLOGY OF POISON IVY/OAK/SUMAC

The plants producing poison ivy, poison oak, and poison sumac were assigned at one time to the *Rhus* family, but this is no longer a current term. Nevertheless, the term *Rhus* dermatitis is still used. Currently, these plants are assigned to the *Toxicodendron* genus of the Anacardiaciae family.[61] *All three plants produce greenish-white berries along the stem in the fall.*[10]

Knowing the characteristics and geographic locations of these plants helps differentiate between them:

- Poison ivy is found in two subtypes. (1) A climbing vine (*Toxicodendron radicans*) is located in the eastern-northeastern United States. Robust and hairy-stemmed, the vine also grows in hedges and through grass. (2) A dwarf shrub (*T. rydbergii*) is found in the northern and western United States. The shrub is usually less than 3 feet tall, with three (or as many as five, seven, or nine) shiny or dull leaflets near the tops of the stems (Fig. 37.4A).[10,63] Areas around lakes and along streams are especially favored by the vine and shrub forms of poison ivy.
- Poison oak, a bush or small tree (in sunlight) or vine (in shade), appears as an eastern type (*T. toxicarium*) and a western type (*T. diversilobum*). The leaflets, lobed rather than smooth, resemble white oak leaves (Fig. 37.4B). Leaflets occur in clusters of three up to as many as 11, arising toward the top of the stem.[61]
- Poison sumac (*T. vernix*) is a small shrub or tree mostly confined to swampy and humid climates in the eastern and midwestern United States. Leaves have 7 to 13

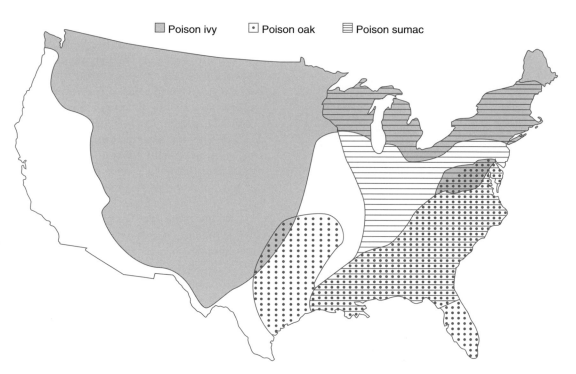

Figure 37.3. Approximate geographic distributions of poison ivy, poison oak, and poison sumac.

A. Poison Ivy

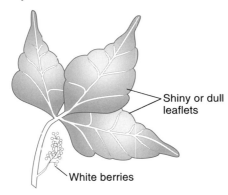

Shiny or dull leaflets

White berries

B. Poison Oak

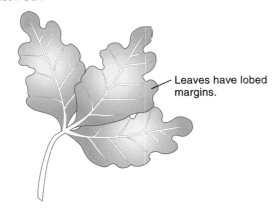

Leaves have lobed margins.

C. Poison Sumac

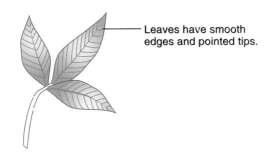

Leaves have smooth edges and pointed tips.

Figure 37.4. Illustrations of common examples of (**A**) poison ivy, (**B**) poison oak, and (**C**) poison sumac.

leaflets with smooth edges and pointed tips (Fig. 37.4C).[61,63] Poison sumac can be differentiated from non-poisonous sumac by the telltale greenish-white berries.

The above generalities concerning plant appearance and location are variable. Pharmacists must become familiar with the appearance of these plants in the particular location and climate in which they work.

All three plants exude a sap when damaged. This sap, a resinous material meant to seal damaged areas of the plant,

contains **urushiol** (an allergenic mixture of antigenic catechols). *The catechols from the three plants are cross-reactive, so patients allergic to one plant will react to others as well.* Individuals must contact a damaged plant to contact urushiol; those who insist that they only have to be close to a plant to catch poison ivy are misinformed. Touching a nondamaged plant would not cause sensitivity, but the plants are fragile and easily damaged, so the risk of contacting urushiol should cause the allergic individual to avoid all poison ivy, oak, and sumac plants whether they appear to be damaged or not.

Poison ivy and oak can be further identified by carefully breaking a leaf or stem (while wearing disposable plastic or rubber gloves) and touching the end to a white paper. Within the next 30 minutes or so, urushiol in the sap will oxidize to produce a color progression: creamy to brownish and then reddish to black. This color change, known as the "black spot sign," can be used to confirm the identity of the plants.[10]

The antigenic catechols are thought to produce dermatologic reactions through reaction with carrier proteins on the surface of the skin (e.g., Langerhans cells).[61] Susceptible patients in the area of burning plants can develop severe dermatitis of exposed skin (e.g., head, neck, and arms) and can suffer acute respiratory failure.[61,64]

Other plants that cause a similar allergic contact dermatitis (although they are not in the *Toxicodendron* genus) include ragweed, chamomile, chicory, sunflower, dandelion, marigold, primrose, and English ivy.

MANIFESTATIONS OF POISON IVY/OAK/SUMAC

The first sensitizing exposure to poison ivy/oak/sumac may not produce symptoms or may produce symptoms 5 to 21 days following the exposure (Fig. 37.5).[65] In these latter cases the exposure sensitizes the person, and lesions result from residual allergen on the skin. After this initial sensitizing incident, future *Toxicodendron* exposure elicits a dermatitis response about 48 to 72 hours following plant contact.[7]

Initially, patients report pruritus and erythema.[10] The skin then becomes eczematous and vesicular.[61] Lesions may overlie an **urticarial plaque** (a relatively large, elevated area of skin that results from dermal edema). Several vesicles may coalesce as the reaction proceeds to form large, fluid-filled lesions (Fig. 37.6). Eventually, lesions weep, crust, and become edematous. Secondary infections can occur if scratching excoriates the skin and the abrasions become infected.

Sites of lesions are the exposed areas of the body such as the hands, arms, face, and legs. However, allergen on the skin can be transferred from one part of the body to another such as when a male touches the penis while urinating.[10] Similarly, the dermatitis can form on the perineum and intragluteal crease when the individual performs personal hygiene with contaminated hands.[65] (See "A Pharmacist's Journal: Can You Help Our Dermatitis?")

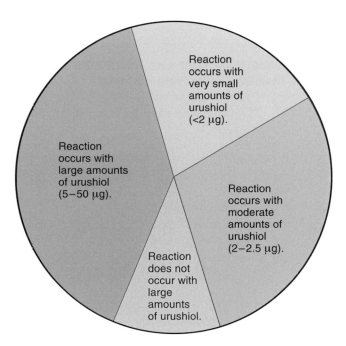

Figure 37.5. Percentages of United States citizens who suffer reactions to poison ivy with exposure to different amounts of urushiol.

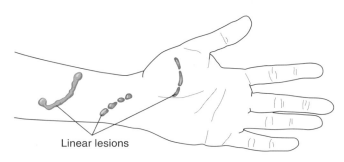

Figure 37.6. Typical presentation of poison ivy lesions when caused by direct contact.

New lesions can appear for up to 3 weeks after exposure. There are two possible reasons for this extended reaction:

- Different areas of skin may have different lag times between exposure to catechol and lesion development because of differing characteristics inherent in the skin such as depletion of Langerhans cells because of chronic sun exposure.[62]
- The patient may have exposed some of the skin areas when initially coming into contact with the plant. However, other skin areas may be exposed later through contact with objects that retain the catechols (e.g., golf clubs, shoes, etc.).

Although it might appear that lesions develop at different times because the vesicles spread from scratching, this is untrue. Intravesicular fluid contains body fluids rather than catechols.

Often, lesions appear in a linear pattern, representing the areas where a bruised plant has brushed across the skin as the individual pushed through undergrowth. Patients exposed through indirect contact (e.g., petting an animal who has rolled in poison ivy or handling contaminated clothing), however, will more often exhibit a diffuse dermatitis.

Poison ivy can last for as long as 3 weeks after lesions appear.[61] During this time pruritus can become so severe that the patients are virtually incapacitated. After healing, the skin is usually completely normal without pigmentary changes.[10] Scarring does not occur unless the skin is secondarily infected while the patient scratches.[65]

About 25 to 40 million Americans (10 to 16% of all who suffer from poison ivy) are extremely sensitive to poison ivy and require medical care whenever it develops.[63] In the worst cases extremely sensitive individuals may undergo sleep deprivation and **impetiginization** (infection of scratches with *Staphylococcus* and *Streptococcus*, producing impetigo).[61,66] Impetiginization can result in renal complications, such as glomerulonephritis or acute tubular necrosis.

A Pharmacist's Journal

"Can You Help Our Dermatitis?"

A young male and female, who appeared to be college students, approached me one summer. They both had dermatitis. I identified it as a contact dermatitis of some type, asking them if they had been out in the woods. They confirmed that they had taken a walk in the outer fringes of a nearby state park. The pattern was of interest. The male had poison ivy on the elbows and lower arms, as well as the penis and front of the legs. The female had poison ivy on the back of her legs, arms, and head, as well as her back and buttocks. Apparently, they had chosen the wrong location to take their "walk." I recommended a benzocaine-menthol spray and hydrocortisone ointment, cautioning them that they might need prescription products if the problem worsened.

SPECIFIC CONSIDERATIONS OF POISON IVY/OAK/SUMAC

Cross-Allergenicity

Several other plants are also in the *Toxicodendron* genus and can cause similar reactions in patients sensitive to poison ivy, including the cashew plant, gingko, mango, Japanese lacquer tree (found in furniture and floor varnish imported from Asia), and Indian marking nut (found in clothing).[61,67-69] Properly cured cashews do not produce allergies, but poorly processed nuts contaminated with oils can produce severe gastrointestinal allergic reactions.[61] Gingko and mango fruits may be safely ingested if the patient avoids exposure to the skin of the fruit while peeling it (e.g., wearing gloves).

Winter Poison Ivy

Poison ivy is more common in the summer when outdoor hobbies and recreation increase the chances of plant contact.[61] However, poison ivy can occur in the winter as a result of the following:

- Pulling plants from the ground
- Handling dried plants
- Handling shoes or other objects that have been contaminated with urushiols
- Bringing logs into the house that are wrapped in poison ivy vines
- Burning logs in the fireplace along with poison ivy vines

Immunity to Poison Ivy

Many people claim to be insensitive to poison ivy. In most instances these individuals have just not yet had a sensitizing exposure and must still take care to avoid the plants. Only about 10 to 15% of United States citizens are actually tolerant to poison ivy and cannot be sensitized.[63]

TREATMENT OF POISON IVY/OAK/SUMAC

See "Treatment of Contact Dermatitis and Poison Ivy/Oak/Sumac."

PREVENTION OF POISON IVY/OAK/SUMAC

See "Prevention of Contact Dermatitis and Poison Ivy/Oak/Sumac."

FOCUS ON...

FOLK REMEDIES AND ALTERNATIVE METHODS FOR POISON IVY TREATMENT AND PREVENTION

Patients may hear and ask about folk advice for poison ivy prevention. One of these is eating the poison ivy plants to prevent reactions. This is based on the theory that oral ingestion of antigens will bypass Langerhans cells, perhaps allowing the patient to develop suppressor T cells. The "evidence" cited is the immunity to mango sensitivity by native Hawaiians, who eat the mango, which contains urushiols.[62] However, this practice would be dangerous at best and could actually produce life-threatening esophageal and tracheal inflammation.

Patients should also avoid medications containing *Toxicodendron* as a purported therapeutic ingredient. *Toxicodendron* has no FDA-approved usage, so the use of this ingredient is highly questionable. At least two patients have suffered reactions to such products.[77] (One of the products was "homeopathic"—a therapeutic teaching that offers uncertain efficacy. Although highly diluted, the homeopathic product contained sufficient urushiol to provoke a reaction.)

Jewelweed is claimed to treat poison ivy/oak dermatitis, but a double-blind, placebo-controlled study did not show any benefit to its use.[78]

See "A Pharmacist's Journal: I Cauterize Them with Cigarettes."

CONTACT DERMATITIS AND POISON IVY/OAK/SUMAC

See above for prevalence, epidemiology, etiology, manifestations, and specific considerations of contact dermatitis. See above for prevalence, epidemiology, etiology, manifestations, and specific considerations of poison ivy/oak/sumac.

TREATMENT OF CONTACT DERMATITIS AND POISON IVY/OAK/SUMAC

Treatment Guidelines

Contact dermatitis may be suspected when the patient's lesions include wheals and vesicles and are accompanied by pruritus. If the patient can recall a specific exposure to an irritating or allergenic substance, the recognition is more sure. To help confirm cases of poison ivy/oak/sumac dermatitis, pharmacists should look for a linear arrangement of lesions, should inquire about past plant exposure, and should consider the areas in which the offending plants grow. For instance, a dermatitis is more likely to be poison ivy when found on patients in the rural Southwest than when found on patients in the inner neighborhoods of large cities.[65] Although poison ivy is found in large cities (e.g., growing as vines on houses), the incidence is rare.

There are no specific guidelines regarding when to refer a patient with contact dermatitis or poison ivy/oak/sumac. However, several logical decision points would seem appropriate. (See "Folk Remedies and Alternative Methods for Poison Ivy Treatment and Prevention.") It would be appropriate to refer the patient with contact dermatitis in the following situations:

A Pharmacist's Journal

"I Cauterize Them with Cigarettes"

A male patient of about 30 asked me to inspect some bumps on his arm. I noticed 8 to 10 small vesicles scattered on each arm. He said, "They itch so bad that I wake up scratching." I began to consider different types of contact dermatitis, and asked him how long they had been present. He replied, "They've been there a long time. I've been to a lot of doctors, and they say I'm allergic to the sun because they are worse when I work out in the sun." He then showed me one particular lesion on the lower arm, which he said he breaks periodically, when a clear fluid comes out, followed by blood.

I told him he really should see a dermatologist, to which he replied, "I've been to the doctors, and all they do is give me hydrocortisones. The blisters started about 4 years ago when I got shingles around my waist. Sometimes they itch terribly, but I can usually stop them by putting a lit cigarette on each blister to cauterize them. That stops the itching for a long, long time." I advised him that he was probably causing severe burns that resulted in relief since he was burning away nerves each time he "cauterized" them. He did not appear to believe me and, before leaving the store, said he might go to a doctor.

- The patient complains of severe pruritus.
- The dermatitis covers a large portion of the body.
- The patient has one or more underlying medical conditions that might be affected by the contact dermatitis or its treatment with topical nonprescription medications (e.g., Type 1 diabetes mellitus).
- The patient has used nonprescription medications, but they do not relieve the problem.
- The problem has persisted for more than 7 days.
- The rash appears to clear and then worsen again.
- The rash is on a body location that presents problems in caring for it (e.g., around the eyes, the conjunctiva, inner nostrils, otic canal, or vagina).

Nonprescription Medications

Various categories of ingredients may be useful in contact dermatitis and poison ivy/oak/sumac. They include external analgesics (e.g., counterirritants, topical anesthetics, topical antihistamines, phenol, and resorcinol), skin protectants, and astringents. (See Patient Assessment Algorithm 37.1.)

EXTERNAL ANALGESICS

External analgesics carry approved labeling for relief of pain and/or itching associated with minor skin irritations or rashes caused by poison ivy, poison oak, or poison sumac. Hydrocortisone carries FDA-approved labeling that is more specific, for the "relief of itching associated with minor skin irritations, inflammation, and rashes caused by eczema; poison ivy, poison oak, or poison sumac; soaps; detergents; cosmetics; and jewelry." Representative products closely identified with poison ivy are listed in Table 37.1, although many other

safe and effective products appear in Tables 30.3 to 30.4. *The FDA has proposed a warning not to use topical diphenhydramine on poison ivy (or on chicken pox, sunburn, or large areas of the body or to broken, blistered, or oozing skin) to prevent toxic psychosis, which has occurred in patients aged 19 months to 9 years.*[70] Symptoms included dilated pupils, flushed face, hallucinations, ataxic gait, and urinary retention.

For a full discussion of external analgesics, see Chapter 30, Arthropod Stings and Bites, Pediculosis, and Scabies.

SKIN PROTECTANTS

Skin protectants carry the FDA-suggested labeling, "Dries the oozing and weeping of poison ivy, poison oak, and poison sumac." Approved skin protectants for this use include aluminum hydroxide gel, calamine, kaolin, zinc acetate, zinc carbonate, and zinc oxide.[71] *These skin protectants will carry a label that cautions patients to see a physician if the condition worsens or does not improve in 7 days.* Products containing aluminum hydroxide gel will caution parents not to use it in children under 6 months of age; products containing zinc acetate will warn against use in children under the age of 2 years.

Colloidal oatmeal and sodium bicarbonate provide temporary skin protection from exposure to the external environment and relieve minor irritation and itching caused by poison ivy, poison oak, and poison sumac.[72] Representative products closely identified with poison ivy and containing skin protectants are listed in Table 37.1, although many other safe and effective products appear in Tables 30.6 and 31.13. For a discussion of sodium bicarbonate and colloidal oatmeal, see Chapter 30, Arthropod Stings and Bites, Pediculosis, and Scabies.

Patient Assessment Algorithm 37.1. Contact Dermatitis

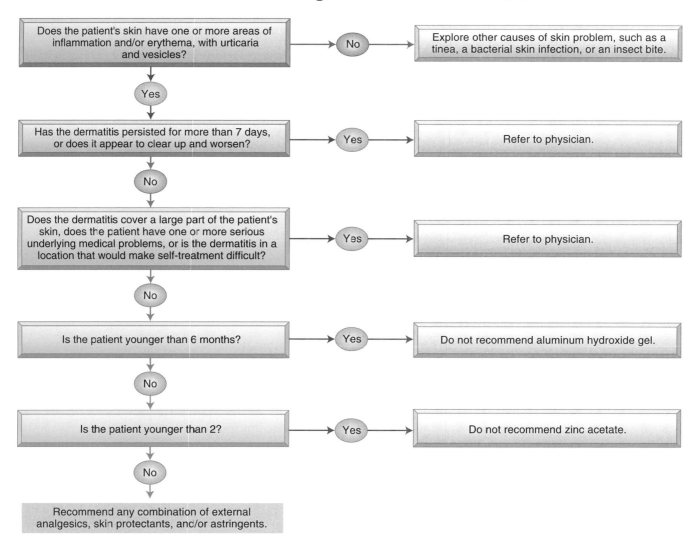

Table 37.1. Representative Products for Relief of Poison Ivy Symptoms	
PRODUCT	SELECTED INGREDIENTS/COMMENTS
Caladryl Lotion	Calamine 8%, pramoxine HCl 1%
Caladryl Clear Lotion	Pramoxine HCl 1%, zinc acetate 0.1%
Ivarest Medicated Cream	Calamine 14%, diphenhydramine HCl 2%
Ivy-Dry Liquid	Zinc acetate, glycerin, acetic acid
Ivy Super Dry Liquid	Zinc acetate, benzyl alcohol
Rhuli Calamine Spray	Benzocaine 5%, calamine 13.8%, camphor 0.7%

Astringents: Aluminum Acetate

As a wet dressing, compress, or soak, aluminum acetate temporarily relieves rashes caused by soaps, detergents, cosmetics, or jewelry and minor skin irritations caused by poison ivy, poison oak, or poison sumac.[73–75] In the form of Burow's solution, it reduces weeping, aids in removal of crusts, and soothes the skin.[61] Pharmacists should counsel patients that if the problem persists for more than 7 days or worsens, they should consult a physician. Table 30.5 lists representative products containing aluminum acetate.

For a full discussion of astringents, see Chapter 30, Arthropod Stings and Bites, Pediculosis, and Scabies.

Other Professional Treatment

Poison ivy is frequently so severe that nonprescription medications are of little benefit. When the patient has used nonprescription products, but is still experiencing severe pruritus, pharmacists should refer the patient to a physician. Quite often, oral corticosteroids in a decremental dosage package (e.g., Medrol Dosepak) cause the lesions to remit.[10] However, the condition may recur as the action of the corticosteroid fades, necessitating a repetition of the dosage pack.[76] For this reason some physicians prefer to prescribe prednisone 20 to 40 mg daily for 10 to 14 days. Adverse reactions to low-dose corticosteroids given for a brief period are not common, but may include sodium retention, nausea, vomiting, headache, vertigo, euphoria, and mood swings.

PREVENTION OF CONTACT DERMATITIS AND POISON IVY/OAK/SUMAC

The best prevention advice for contact dermatitis and poison ivy is to avoid exposure to offending substances completely, minimize exposure when avoidance already has occurred, and use barrier products. Folk remedies and alternative methods for prevention of contact dermatitis and poison ivy should be avoided until they are proven to be safe and effective. (See "Folk Remedies and Alternative Methods for Poison Ivy Treatment and Prevention.")

Avoidance of Exposure

The most important step in preventing contact dermatitis and poison ivy is avoiding exposure to the antigen. When patients' skin resembles possible contact dermatitis, pharmacists should first assist patients in recalling possible antigen exposures. If offending antigens can be identified, patients should try to avoid them. In this sense pharmacists function as detectives, using various clues such as recent activities (e.g., outdoor recreation in the case of suspected poison ivy) or specific body distribution of lesions (e.g., facial dermatitis in the case of female cosmetic allergy).[79,80] Pharmacists can challenge the patient to recall any provoking incidents such as exposure to the following:

- New brands of perfume, eyeliner, mascara, or other facial cosmetic[81–83]
- New laundry detergent, fabric softener, or bleach
- Household detergent, dishwashing detergent, glass cleaner, dusting polish, or toilet cleaners[84,85]
- Exotic woods, varnish, shellac, paint, or stripping chemicals (e.g., "fiddler's neck" caused by prolonged neck contact with a stringed instrument)[86–88]
- Glues or cements[56]
- Dyes or coloring chemicals
- Artificial nails, nail polishes, or nail polish removers[89]
- New personal-hygiene products (e.g., toothpaste, antiperspirant, shampoo, or soap)
- New undergarments with metal components (e.g., brassieres)
- Topical medications such as creams, ointments, gels, lotions, or transdermal patches[90]

- Fertilizers, plants, and pesticides[91]
- Adhesive tapes and wound dressings applied to the skin[92,93]
- Essential oils (used in the unproven therapy known as aromatherapy)[94]
- Neoprene (found in computer keyboard wrist rests)[95]

Pharmacists can point out that some of these products come in fragrance-free or low-allergenicity formulas.[96] If patients are unable to recall a specific allergenic exposure, pharmacists can refer patients to a physician, who can use patch testing to provide definitive identification.[7,97,98]

To prevent poison ivy dermatitis, patients should remove plants from all living areas such as yards and fields.[99] However, defoliants or other herbicides are the preferred method of plant control. Pulling the plants out exposes one to the resin, and burning spreads toxin.[64] (The patient must note that even dead plants can still contain urushiol and cause dermatitis.)

Minimize Exposure

Contact dermatitis and poison ivy/oak/sumac can be prevented if the time of exposure is minimized. For instance, poison ivy can be aborted if the patient washes exposed skin with soap and water within 15 minutes of exposure.[65] After this time urushiol is irreversibly bound with protein, rendering washing and scrubbing useless. Fingernails should also be trimmed and the areas underneath cleaned thoroughly.[99] Clothes should be washed in hot water with adequate soap to prevent further allergen contact.[65]

Barrier Products

Various **organoclay** (organic products formulated using a clay base) products have been investigated for their effectiveness as skin barriers to poison ivy.[100–101] One ingredient, bentoquatam, received FDA approval for this indication.[102,103] A quaternary ammonium salt of sodium bentonite, bentoquatam is more effective than other potential barrier products (e.g., silicone lotion).[103]

Bentoquatam is marketed in a 5% solution as the product IvyBlock lotion. *The bentoquatam product should be applied at least 15 minutes before possible plant contact, and a smooth wet film should be visible on skin following application.* Reapplication every 4 hours helps maintain the barrier. The barrier formulation can be removed with soap and water after exposure ceases. IvyBlock should not be used on children under the age of 6 without physician approval, nor should it be used if patients have an existing poison ivy dermatitis. Patients who have been around poison ivy/oak/sumac and who have the skin covered with IvyBlock may have traces of urushiol over the IvyBlock barrier and should avoid skin contact with other potentially sensitive persons until the skin is thoroughly washed to remove all traces of urushiol.

SUMMARY

Contact dermatitis is a term used for the skin reactions resulting from contact with an irritating or allergenic substance

AT THE COUNTER

A male patient who appears to be in his 40s asks the pharmacist about a rash on his abdomen, arms, and legs.

Interview/Patient Assessment

The pharmacist notes that the abdomen, arms, and legs are covered with multiple vesicular streaks. Some of the vesicles have ruptured. The patient is concerned about the severe pruritus and says that he is scratching so hard he is afraid he will scar his skin. The eruptions began shortly after he went fishing the previous week. The lesions have been present for 5 to 6 days. In response to the pharmacist's suggestion that he has poison ivy, the patient replies, "It can't be that. I've never had poison ivy before. It's all around the fishing pond. In fact, I have to crawl through it to get to my favorite spot." The patient has no medical conditions and is taking no medications.

Pharmacist's Analysis

1. Could poison ivy be the cause of the lesions?
2. Will the skin scar? What is the prognosis?
3. What therapies should be recommended for this patient?

Patient Counseling

While there are other possible causes of this patient's problem (e.g., allergy to laundry soap, bath soap, etc.), the recent fishing trip helps implicate poison ivy. The proximity of the plants to the area also helps the pharmacist recognize *Toxicodendron* allergy.

The pharmacist should explain that poison ivy allergy can begin at any point in one's life. The triggering factor in this patient may have been a previous trip to the fishing spot. Crawling through the plants during this episode produced these lesions. The pharmacist also should counsel that, if the problem is poison ivy, he will not scar unless he scratches enough to excoriate the skin, allowing staphylococcal/streptococcal organisms to impetiginize the lesions. The pharmacist should note that the lesions could be present for as long as two more weeks.

To help him during this episode, the pharmacist can recommend a combination of local anesthetics, astringents, and skin protectants. For instance, he might use a topical aerosol containing benzocaine, as well as a hydrocortisone ointment.

Finally, the pharmacist should caution the patient to avoid exposure to poison ivy/oak/sumac for the rest of his life.

---

that either irritates the skin or produces an immune response. The skin reactions may be categorized as irritant contact dermatitis or allergic contact dermatitis. Affected skin may exhibit wheals, rash, vesicles, inflammation, or erythema. Contact with many substances can produce dermatitis, including medications, cosmetics, perfumes, jewelry, shoe leather, and rubber. Among the most common causes of dermatitis are plants, chief of which are plants in the genus *Toxicodendron,* such as poison ivy, poison oak, and poison sumac. Allergy to this plant group is popularly known as "poison ivy."

Poison ivy dermatitis is characterized by multiple vesicles, often in a linear pattern, on exposed areas of the body. The reaction may continue for 3 weeks after symptoms appear. Generally, poison ivy heals without scarring. Nonprescription therapy can consist of external analgesics, skin protectants, and astringents, but patients should be referred for oral corticosteroids if the skin reaction is severe and nonprescription products do not provide relief. Prevention of exposure through avoidance is the optimal method of dealing with *Toxicodendron* allergy. A newly developed barrier cream may help prevent the allergenic elements of the plants from contacting the skin.

References

1. Perkins P. The management of eczema in adults. Nurs Stand 10: 49, 1996.
2. Rothe MJ, Grant-Kels JM. Atopic dermatitis: An update. J Am Acad Dermatol 35:1, 1996.
3. Boguniewicz M, Leung DYM. New concepts in atopic dermatitis. Compr Ther 22:144, 1996.
4. Herd RM, et al. Prevalence of atopic eczema in the community: The Lothian Atopic Dermatitis Study. Br J Dermatol 135:18, 1996.
5. Zug KA, McCay M. Eczematous dermatitis: A review. Am Fam Physician 54:1243, 1996.
6. Hogan PA. 6. Atopic dermatitis. Med J Aust 164:736, 1996.
7. Fox RW. Allergic skin diseases. J Fla Med Assoc 83:394, 1996.
8. Beltrani VS, Beltrani VP. Contact dermatitis. Ann Allergy Asthma Immunol 78:160, 1997.
9. Zug KA, Palay DA, Rock B. Dermatological diagnosis and treatment of itchy red eyelids. Surv Ophthalmol 40:293, 1996.
10. Juckett G. Plant dermatitis. Postgrad Med 100:159, 1996.
11. Lee JY, Effendy I, Maibach HI. Acute irritant contact dermatitis: Recovery time in man. Contact Dermatitis 36:285, 1997.
12. White IR. Occupational dermatitis. BMJ 313:487, 1996.
13. Kalish RS, Wood JA. Induction of hapten-specific tolerance of human CD8+ urushiol (poison ivy)–reactive T lymphocytes. J Invest Dermatol 108:253, 1997.
14. Belsito DV. The rise and fall of allergic contact dermatitis. Am J Contact Dermat 8:193, 1997.
15. Fisher AA. Esoteric contact dermatitis. Part III: Ragweed dermatitis. Cutis 57:199, 1996.
16. Memon AA, Friedmann PS. Studies on the reproducibility of allergic contact dermatitis. Br J Dermatol 134:208, 1996.

17. Weston WL. Contact dermatitis in children. Curr Opin Pediatr 9:372, 1997.

18. Rietschel RL. Occupational contact dermatitis. Lancet 349:1093, 1997.

19. Haudrechy P, et al. Nickel release from stainless steels. Contact Dermatitis 37:113, 1997.

20. Nakada T, et al. Role of ear piercing in metal allergic contact dermatitis. Contact Dermatitis 36:233, 1997.

21. Armstrong DK, Walsh MY, Dawson JF. Granulomatous contact dermatitis due to gold earrings. Br J Dermatol 136:776, 1997.

22. Stolz R, Hinnen U, Elsner P. An evaluation of the relationship between 'atopic skin' and skin irritability in metalworker trainees. Contact Dermatitis 36:281, 1997.

23. Lugovic L, Lipozencic J. Contact hypersensitivity in atopic dermatitis. Arh Hig Rada Toksikol 48:287, 1997.

24. Shaw S. Managing contact dermatitis. Practitioner 240:16, 1996.

25. Lawton S. Living with eczema: The dermatology patient. Br J Nurs 5:600, 1996.

26. Freeman S, Lee M-S, Gudmundsen K. Adverse contact reactions to sculptured acrylic nails: 4 case reports and a literature review. Contact Dermatitis 33:381, 1995.

27. Kawamura T, et al. Lichen planus-like contact dermatitis due to methacrylic acid esters. Br J Dermatol 134:358, 1996.

28. Van Der Walle HB, Brunsveld VM. Dermatitis in hairdressers. Contact Dermatitis 30:217, 1994.

29. Wolf R, Movshowitz M, Brenner S. Supplemental tests in the evaluation of occupational hand dermatitis in soldiers. Int J Dermatol 35:173, 1996.

30. Packham C. Gloves: The last resort. Occup Health 48:164, 1996.

31. Fein JA, Selbst SM, Pawlowski NA. Latex allergy in pediatric emergency department personnel. Pediatric Emerg Care 12:6, 1996.

32. Rademaker M. Allergic contact dermatitis to Toxicodendron succedaneum (rhus tree): An autumn epidemic. NZ Med J 108:121, 1995.

33. Desciak EB, Marks JG Jr. Dermatoses among housekeeping personnel. Am J Contact Dermat 8:32, 1997.

34. Heron RJ. Worker education in the primary prevention of occupational dermatoses. Occup Med (Oxf):47:407, 1997.

35. Bernstein DI. Allergic reactions to workplace allergens. JAMA 278:1907, 1997.

36. Mathias CG. Allergic contact dermatitis from a lawn care fungicide containing dyrene. Am J Contact Dermat 8:47, 1997.

37. OMalley MA. Skin reactions to pesticides. Occup Med 12:327, 1997.

38. Cook DK, Freeman S. Allergic contact dermatitis to multiple sawdust allergens. Australas J Dermatol 38:77, 1997.

39. Gutgesell C, Fuchs T. Contact urticaria from beer. Contact Dermatitis 33:436, 1995.

40. Kanerva L, et al. Occupational allergic contact urticaria caused by cockroach (*Blaberus giganteus*). Contact Dermatitis 33:445, 1995.

41. Gliniecki CM. Management of latex reactions in the occupational setting. AAOHN J 46:82, 1998.

42. Young MA, Meyers M. Latex allergy: Considerations for the care of pediatric patients and employee safety. Nurs Clin North Am 43:169, 1997.

43. Hamann CP, et al. Natural rubber latex hypersensitivity: Incidence and prevalence of type I allergy in the dental professional. J Am Dent Assoc 129:43, 1998.

44. Sussman GL, et al. Incidence of latex sensitization among latex glove users. J Allergy Clin Immunol 101(2 Pt 1):171, 1998.

45. Woods JA, et al. Natural rubber latex allergy: Spectrum, diagnostic approach, and therapy. J Emerg Med 15:71, 1997.

46. Cowperthwaite B, et al. Latex allergy in the nursing population. Can Oper Room Nurs J 15:23, 1997.

47. Douglas R, et al. Prevalence of IgE-mediated allergy to latex in hospital nursing staff. Aust N Z J Med 27:165, 1997.

48. Tarlo SN, Sussman GL, Holness DL. Latex sensitivity in dental students and staff: A cross-sectional study. J Allergy Clin Immunol 99:396, 1997.

49. Burton AD. Latex allergy in health care workers. Occup Med 12:609, 1997.

50. Kam PC, Lee MS, Thompson JF. Latex allergy: An emerging clinical and occupational health problem. Anaesthesia 52:570, 1997.

51. Liden C, Menne T, Burrows D. Nickel-containing alloys and platings and their ability to cause dermatitis. Br J Dermatol 134:193, 1996.

52. Nilsson EJ, Knuttsson A. Atopic dermatitis, nickel sensitivity and xerosis as risk factors for hand eczema in women. Contact Dermatitis 33:401, 1995.

53. Nagayama H, Hatamochi A, Shinkai H. A case of contact dermatitis due to sodium bisulfite in an ophthalmic solution. J Dermatol 24:675, 1997.

54. Scheinman PL. Is it really fragrance-free? Am J Contact Dermat 8:239, 1997.

55. Moreno Ancillo A, et al. Allergic contact reactions due to phenylephrine hydrochloride in eyedrops. Ann Allergy Asthma Immunol 78:569, 1997.

56. Cohen DE, Brancaccio RR. What is new in clinical research in contact dermatitis. Dermatol Clin 15:137, 1997.

57. Nielsen NH, Menne T. Allergic contact dermatitis caused by zinc pyrithione associated with pustular psoriasis. Am J Contact Dermat 8:170, 1997.

58. Lutz ME, el Azhary RA. Allergic contact dermatitis due to topical application of corticosteroids: Review and clinical implications. Mayo Clin Proc 72:1141, 1997.

59. Landow K. Hand dermatitis: The perennial scourge. Postgrad Med 103:141, 1998.

60. Mateo MP, et al. Erythema-multiforme–like eruption following allergic contact dermatitis from sesquiterpene lactones in herbal medicine. Contact Dermatitis 33:449, 1995.

61. Guay DRP. An update on plant-related contact dermatitis. J Pract Nurs 43:24, 1993.

62. Williford PM, Sherertz EF. Poison ivy dermatitis. Arch Fam Med 3:184, 1994.

63. Epstein WL. Occupational poison ivy and oak dermatitis. Dermatol Clin 12:511, 1994.

64. Kollef MH. Adult respiratory distress syndrome after smoke inhalation from burning poison ivy (Letter). JAMA 274:358, 1995.

65. Baer RL. Poison ivy dermatitis. Cutis 46:34, 1990.

66. D'Mello DA, MacAuley L. Poison ivy dermatitis and secondary mania. J Nerv Ment Dis 182:116, 1994.

67. Rademaker M, Duffill MB. Allergic contact dermatitis in families—Simultaneous occurrence. Contact Dermatitis 32:111, 1995.

68. Hamilton TK, Zug KA. Systemic contact dermatitis to raw cashew nuts in a pesto sauce. Am J Contact Dermat 9:51, 1998.

69. Oelrichs PB, et al. Isolation and characterisation of urushiol components from the Australian native cashew (*Semecarpus australiensis*). Nat Toxins 5:96, 1997.

70. Fed Reg 62:45767, 1997.

71. Fed Reg 48:6820, 1983.

72. Fed Reg 54:40808, 1989.

73. Fed Reg 47:39436, 1982.

74. Fed Reg 54:13490, 1989.

75. Fed Reg 58:54458, 1993.

76. Ives TJ, Tepper RS. Failure of a tapering dose of oral methylprednisolone to treat reactions to poison ivy (Letter). JAMA 266:1362, 1991.

77. Sasseville D, Nguyen KH. Allergic contact dermatitis from *Rhus toxicodendron* in a phytotherapeutic preparation. Contact Dermatitis 32:182, 1995.

78. Long D, Ballentine NH, Marks JG Jr. Treatment of poison ivy/oak allergic contact dermatitis with an extract of jewelweed. Am J Contact Dermat 8:150, 1997.

79. Wooldridge WE. Acute allergic contact dermatitis. Postgrad Med 87:221, 1990.

80. Ophaswongse S, Maibach HI. Allergic contact cheilitis. Contact Dermatitis 33:365, 1995.

81. Parkinson RW. Eyelid dermatitis. Postgrad Med 100:231, 1996.

82. de Groot AC, Frosch PJ. Adverse reactions to fragrances. A clinical review. Contact Dermatitis 36:57, 1997.

83. Rotstein E, Rotstein H. The ear-lobe sign: A helpful sign in facia contact dermatitis. Australas J Dermatol 38:215, 1997.

84. Grammer-West NY, et al. Comparison of the irritancy of hand dishwashing liquids with modified patch testing methods. J Am Acad Dermatol 35(2 Pt 1):258, 1996.

85. Payling KJ. Occupational skin disorders. Prof Nurs 11:393, 1996.

86. Moreno JC, et al. Fiddler's neck. Am J Contact Dermat 8:39, 1997.

87. Rackett SC, Zug KA. Contact dermatitis to multiple exotic woods. Am J Contact Dermat 8:114, 1997.

88. Hausen BM. Allergic contact dermatitis from a wooden necklace. Am J Contact Dermat 8:185, 1997.

89. Hemmer W, et al. Allergic contact dermatitis to artificial fingernails prepared from UV light-cured acrylates. J Am Acad Dermatol 35(3 Pt 1):377, 1996.

90. Quirce S, et al. Allergic contact dermatitis from estradiol in a transdermal therapeutic system. Allergy 51:62, 1996.

91. Spettoli E, et al. Contact dermatitis caused by sesquiterpene lactones. Am J Contact Dermat 9:49, 1998.

92. Dwyer P, Freeman S. Allergic contact dermatitis to adhesive tape and contrived disease. Australas J Dermatol 38:141, 1997.

93. Sasseville D, Tennstedt D, Lachapelle JM. Allergic contact dermatitis from hydrocolloid dressings. Am J Contact Dermat 8:236, 1997.

94. Weiss RR, James WD. Allergic contact dermatitis from aromatherapy. Am J Contact Dermat 8:250, 1997.

95. Johnson RC, Elston DM. Wrist dermatitis: Contact allergy to neoprene in a keyboard wrist rest. Am J Contact Dermat 8:172, 1997.

96. Scheman A. Contact allergy testing alternatives: 1996. Cutis 57:235, 1996.

97. Rajagopalan R, Anderson RT. The profile of a patient with contact dermatitis and a suspicion of contact allergy (history, physical characteristics, and dermatology-specific quality of life). Am J Contact Dermat 8:26, 1997.

98. Guin JD, et al. Patch testing for contact dermatitis. Dermatol Nurs 9:178, 1997.

99. O'Brien JM. Common skin problems of infancy, childhood, and adolescence. Prim Care 22:99, 1995.

100. Smith WB, Baunchalk JM, Grabski WJ. Lack of efficacy of a barrier cream in preventing rhus dermatitis (Letter). Arch Dermatol 129:787, 1993.

101. Grevelink SA, Murrell DF, Olsen EA. Effectiveness of various barrier preparations in preventing and/or ameliorating experimentally produced *Toxicodendron* dermatitis. J Am Acad Dermatol 27(2 Pt 1):182, 1992.

102. Max B. Creeping where no life is seen. A rare old plant is the ivy green. Trends Pharmacol Sci 9:48, 1988.

103. Marks JG Jr. Prevention of poison ivy and poison oak allergic contact dermatitis by quaternium-18 bentonite. J Am Acad Dermatol 33(2 Pt 1):212, 1995.

Diaper Dermatitis

Diaper dermatitis is a general term used to describe a variety of cutaneous inflammatory conditions that share the common anatomic location under the area covered by an infant's diaper. The term "diaper dermatitis" is also referred to as diaper rash; the terms will be used interchangeably in this chapter. A form of diaper dermatitis can also affect adults who must wear an undergarment that is similar to a diaper, usually because of incontinence. See "Incontinence Dermatitis (Adult Diaper Dermatitis, Perineal Dermatitis)."

PREVALENCE OF DIAPER DERMATITIS

Diaper rash is one of the most common dermatitis conditions of infancy.[6–8] Research suggests that probably all children suffer at least one episode of diaper dermatitis in infancy.[9] A survey of parents discovered that 25% of infants had diaper rash.[10] As many as 20% of pediatric dermatologic appointments are caused by diaper dermatitis.[10]

EPIDEMIOLOGY OF DIAPER DERMATITIS

Diaper rash can occur in any infant or young child who wears a diaper.[6] Significant factors that increase the risk of diaper rash include the child's age, presence of atopic dermatitis, diarrhea, the type of diaper worn, and nutritional factors, as discussed below. Other less well researched factors include the following[6]:

- Bowel frequency (the more often feces contact the skin, the greater the incidence of skin breakdown)
- Other infectious diseases

- Antibiotic therapy (may increase the frequency of bowel movements); promotility agents (e.g., cisapride increases the bile acid content of feces, causing irritation)[11]
- Gender (the incidence was slightly higher in females in one study, but the difference was not statistically significant)
- Day-care center attendance (the incidence of diaper dermatitis was higher in diapered infants attending day-care centers as opposed to those at home[12])
- Tooth eruption. Some parents and caregivers seem to notice an episode of diaper dermatitis whenever a tooth erupts. This association is mostly an anecdotal and poorly documented observation.

Age

Age is a determinant of diaper-rash incidence. Infants younger than 2 months often experience diaper rash.[13] Infants between the ages of 3 and 6 months are at higher risk than older children.[6,7] Over the age of 18 months, the risk of diaper rash drops since the child is gaining greater muscular control and does not urinate or defecate as often.[6]

Atopic Dermatitis

In one study 30% of infants with atopic dermatitis had diaper rash, as opposed to only 16% of those who did not have atopic dermatitis.[6] This effect was noted only in infants aged 3 to 6 months rather than older children. Perhaps the presence of atopic dermatitis is indicative of a propensity for that patient's skin to break down more easily.

Diarrhea

Researchers have found diarrhea to be a major predictor of diaper rash, resulting in a diaper rash incidence of 45%, as opposed to an incidence of only 15% in those without diarrhea.[6] Each diarrheal episode exposes the skin to feces, and the feces are more liquid, spreading more readily across the skin surfaces to produce damage.[14]

Type of Diaper

At one time, reusable cloth diapers, which can be used as many as 50 to 100 times and then recycled (as cleaning cloths, for instance), were the norm.[15] Generally a cloth diaper is folded then placed on the changing area. The child's bottom is placed on the diaper, the diaper is pulled up between the child's legs, and the diaper is secured around the child's waist with pins or Velcro fasteners. Waterproof plastic pants are often used to cover the diapers. However, the introduction of disposable diapers in 1961 forever changed diapering.[15] The typical disposable diaper contains an inner surface that is placed next to the infant's skin for cushioning and reduction of friction stress.[16] A cellulose core of pulp absorbs moisture from urine and feces. The outer diaper surface is a thin layer of waterproof plastic such as polyethylene. (The disposable diaper is used much the same as a reusable diaper but without folding and usually with preattached adhesive to secure it.)

The superabsorbent diaper with a hydrogel makeup is a recent diaper innovation.[6,16] High-molecular-weight polymers in the fiber core incorporate fluid from urine and feces within the absorbent matrix, isolating it from the skin.[6] These diapers also isolate urine from feces, so that the pH beneath the diaper does not favor the activation of fecal enzymes.[17]

As many as 80% of babies in the United States are diapered with disposables.[15] Studies generally indicate that infants using disposables are slightly less likely to suffer diaper rash than those using reusables.[15,18,19] Cloth reusable diapers may be more prone to produce diaper dermatitis if home laundering does not remove all traces

FOCUS ON...

INCONTINENCE DERMATITIS (ADULT DIAPER DERMATITIS, PERINEAL DERMATITIS)

Diaper rash is not limited to children. Any individual whose condition mimics the diapered infant (e.g., an incontinent adult) can also experience an identical skin irritation.

Incontinence dermatitis, a more appropriate name for adult patients, affects as many as 33% of adults who are hospitalized.[1-3] The predisposing factors and etiology are the same as diaper rash: exposure of occluded skin in the perianal area to urine and feces. Added factors increase the risk in older patients. Older skin, which like babies' skin is thinner in the dermal and subcutaneous layer, does not regenerate or heal as rapidly as the skin of younger individuals, has reduced barrier capability, and reduced sensory perception.[4] Also, elderly patients' skin is drier, so that crevices that foster bacterial growth proliferate.

Adults who are incontinent of urine and feces are the primary victims of incontinence dermatitis.[5] Urinary incontinence affects at least 10 million Americans, especially patients who are elderly, disoriented, or severely ill.[2]

Incontinence dermatitis leads to skin breakdown if not prevented or treated sufficiently. The costs of managing a single pressure ulcer to complete healing were once estimated to be as high as $27,000. Based on this estimate, it makes sense to prevent skin breakdown at all costs.

PREVENTION OF INCONTINENCE DERMATITIS

For incontinent patients, numerous steps must be taken to prevent incontinence dermatitis, including the following[4]:

- Give incontinent patients a complete skin inspection at least once daily, noting the early signs of skin breakdown (e.g., erythema and swelling).
- Clean skin as soon as soiling occurs.
- Avoid hot water.
- Use a mild cleansing agent that minimizes dryness and skin irritation.
- Minimize force and friction during cleaning.
- Keep skin moist by keeping humidity levels in the residence above 40% if possible (see Chapter 16, Humidity Deficit).
- Avoid exposing skin to cold, which can be drying.
- Apply moisturizers to keep skin properly hydrated.
- Minimize skin exposure to urine and feces by the use of underpads or briefs made of materials that absorb moisture to help keep skin dry.

INCONTINENCE DEVICES

A variety of adult incontinence devices are available, as listed in the table. As pictured, these devices come in a variety of styles and sizes to meet the specific needs of each patient. Patients should first match the device to the type of incontinence (e.g., urine only or urine and feces). Next, the absorbency level should be estimated. The patient who has only slight leakage of urine, with some bladder control remaining should first try a regular absorbency product, since it will be less bulky. If the patient has little urine control, an extra absorbency product might be preferable. Also, if it is difficult for the caregiver to change the product often, extra absorbency will wick the urine up from the skin, helping prevent dermatitis.

Continued

of ammonia and feces; commercial laundering is preferred.[17]

Thus today's parent is presented with an overwhelming display of disposable diapers with differing absorbencies and sizes. Disposables generally cost less than reusables when such factors as the energy and water costs associated with laundering are considered.[20] However, disposables are not environmentally friendly since they introduce raw sewage into landfills.[12,15,20,21]

Nutritional Factors

Research has implicated several nutritional conditions in the genesis of diaper dermatitis such as **kwashiorkor** (malnutrition, usually caused by protein deficiency), **acrodermatitis enteropathica** (defective zinc metabolism, causing numerous dermatologic problems), and zinc deficiency.[9] For example, the incidence of diaper rash decreased significantly when infants were given zinc supplementation in one study.[22]

Bottle-fed infants suffer from the condition more commonly than those that are breast-fed.[16,17] The incidence does not appear to be higher in infants who are introduced to solid food at an early age.[23]

ETIOLOGY OF DIAPER DERMATITIS

The contributing causes that predispose to diaper rash and skin breakdown include occlusion, humidity, and friction; contact irritation; skin pH and fecal enzymes; candidal overgrowth; and certain medical conditions (Fig. 38.1).[6]

Occlusion, Humidity, and Friction

The combination of occlusion, moist skin, and friction between skin and diaper material is the major reason that skin responds with a rash.[7,24,25] When skin is wetted,

Representative Incontinence Devices

PRODUCT	COMMENTS
Compose System	Washable panty with disposable pads; three sizes available
Depend Shields Regular Absorbency	Urine only; adhesive backed to adhere to underwear
Depend Shields Extra Absorbency	Urine only; adhesive backed to adhere to underwear
Depend Fitted Briefs	Urine and feces; undergarment with elastic waist; secured with six refastenable tapes
Depend Guards for Men	Urine only; adhesive backed to adhere to underwear
Depend Undergarments Regular Absorbency	Urine and feces; has a strap to fit hip sizes up to 65 inches
Depend Undergarments Regular Absorbency EasyFit with Velcro Fasteners	Urine and feces
Depend Undergarments Extra Absorbency	Urine and feces; has a strap to fit hip sizes up to 65 inches
Depend Undergarments Extra Absorbency EasyFit with Velcro Fasteners	Urine and feces
Depend Undergarments Extra Absorbency Non-Elastic Leg	Urine and feces
Poise Light Absorbency Thin Pads	Urine only; for light leakage; adhesive backed to adhere to underwear
Poise Pads Regular Absorbency	Urine only; light leakage; adhesive backed to adhere to underwear
Poise Pads Extra Absorbency	Urine only; adhesive backed to adhere to underwear
Poise Pads Extra Plus Absorbency	Urine only; adhesive backed to adhere to underwear
Poise Pads Ultra Absorbency	Urine only; adhesive backed to adhere to underwear
Stayfree Serenity Bladder Protection	Urine only; for light leakage; adhesive backed to adhere to underwear
Stayfree Serenity Bladder Protection Pads	Urine only; light to moderate leakage; adhesive backed to adhere to underwear
Stayfree Serenity Bladder Protection Extra Absorbency Curved Pads	Urine only; light to moderate leakage; adhesive backed to adhere to underwear
Stayfree Serenity Bladder Protection Extra Plus Absorbency Curved Pads	Urine only; for moderate leakage; adhesive backed to adhere to underwear
Stayfree Serenity Bladder Protection Guards Regular Absorbency	Urine only; for moderate leakage; adhesive backed to adhere to underwear
Stayfree Serenity Bladder Protection Guards Regular Absorbency	Urine only; for moderate leakage; adhesive backed to adhere to underwear
Stayfree Serenity Bladder Protection Guards Super Absorbency	Urine only; for moderate to heavy leakage adhesive backed to adhere to underwear
Stayfree Serenity Bladder Protection Guards Super Plus Absorbency	Urine only; for heavy leakage; adhesive backed to adhere to underwear

Continued

the frictional coefficient of the skin increases, making it more prone to damage from minor abrasion.[12,16] Friction becomes a more significant factor as children begin to gain mobility.[26] The type of noninfected diaper rash caused by these factors is sometimes referred to as "irritant" or "chafing" diaper rash.[9]

Contact Irritation

When skin is moist, the normal barrier to contact irritants is reduced since wet skin has an increased permeability.[16,26] Therefore, wet skin allows urine and stool to accelerate the skin breakdown that results in diaper dermatitis.[27] Laundry soap, fabric softeners, or bleaches used to wash reusable diapers also may cause an irritant contact dermatitis on the diaper area.

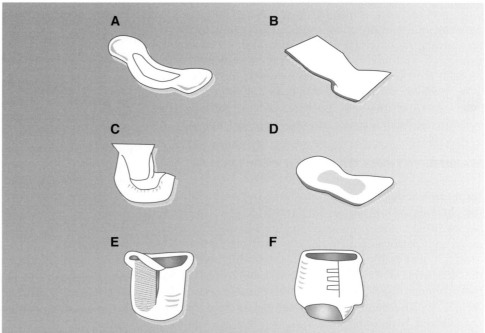

Products for adult incontinence. **A** and **B.** Pads and shields for light drainage of urine. **C** and **D.** Guards for frequent leakage of small amount of urine. **E.** Undergarments for moderate leakage of urine. **F.** Fitted briefs with refastenable tapes for heavy or continuous urine leakage.

Skin pH and Fecal Enzymes

Normal skin pH is 4 to 5.5.[4,16] Skin occlusion elevates surface pH. Bacteria on the skin metabolize urine to form ammonia, which also raises normal skin pH. When the pH of stool is raised through contact with the higher pH of skin or the ammonia from urine, lipases and proteases found in feces are activated, which hastens skin breakdown through a proteolytic action.[7,22,26,28]

The association between fecal enzymes and diaper dermatitis is the probable explanation for the observed rise in incidence of diaper dermatitis in infants with diarrhea. Fecal enzymes also increase the permeability of skin to bile salts, which irritate the skin.[12]

Candidal Overgrowth

Some investigators feel that *Candida albicans* is a primary cause of diaper dermatitis, while others believe that it is an opportunistic invader.[26] Broad-spectrum oral antibiotics predispose patients to diaper rash.[29] The logical conclusion is that *Candida albicans* has extended from its gastrointestinal reservoir to affect the diaper area. The reservoir may be anal organisms, although infected mothers' nipples have also been implicated.[30,31] Researchers recovered *Candida* from 40 to 85% of infants with active diaper rash, whereas it is only infrequently found on the skin of an unaffected infant.[29] Some authorities feel that a diaper dermatitis over 2 to 3 days old will invariably exhibit secondary *Candida* colonization.[7,9,13] Research shows that once an infant has a bout of candidal diaper dermatitis, recurrences are likely.[13]

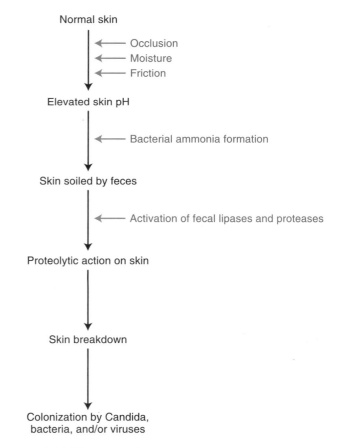

Figure 38.1. The factors that contribute to the development of diaper dermatitis.

Medical Conditions

Some medical conditions may cause a dermatitis in the diaper area such as psoriasis, atopic dermatitis, and seborrheic dermatitis.[27,32] Pharmacists can recognize these conditions as causal if they are observed at other sites on the body.[22] Importantly, *infants affected by other dermatitis will likely experience a worsening of the condition if the lesions are also affected with the contact dermatitis of diaper rash.*[26]

MANIFESTATIONS OF DIAPER DERMATITIS

Most cases of diaper rash are mild and cause no symptoms; the child apparently has no discomfort.[9] When diaper rash begins to be bothersome for the child, he will tend to cry more, especially when he is cleansed at changing time. The most frequent visible symptom of diaper rash is erythema of the skin, seen as shiny, erythematous patches on the buttocks, upper thighs, abdomen, and pubic regions (Fig. 38.2).[6,7,9,33] The skinfolds of the inguinal creases often are not affected, perhaps because urine and feces cannot easily contact them.[34] Skin affected by diaper rash is usually inflamed and may exhibit lesions.[6] Mild scaling is common, but papules, eczema, or open ulcerations are rare.[9] Perineal ulcerations, vesicles, and erosions signal possible bacterial infection (e.g., staphylococcus, streptococcus) or viral complications such as herpes or cytomegalovirus.[27,33,35–37]

A *Candida*-infected diaper dermatitis is recognized by a sharp border with satellite lesions and intense, beefy-red erythema within the border.[7,22] In addition, children with *Candida*-infected diaper rash will often begin violent crying just following urination or defecation.[9] The inguinal creases are invariably affected, given that the fungus prefers warmth and moisture, the condition found in opposing skin surfaces. Occasionally, the fungus causes large, firm, eroded nodules on the diaper area.[38]

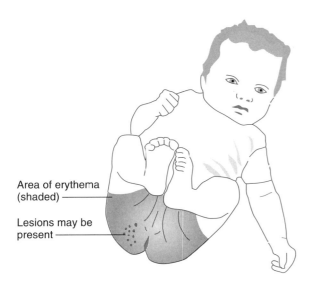

Area of erythema (shaded) —

Lesions may be present —

Figure 38.2. The typical sites of erythematous diaper dermatitis; the appearance of early diaper dermatitis lesions.

COMPLICATIONS OF DIAPER DERMATITIS

If diaper dermatitis is not treated promptly, the skin may excoriate, which is the entry point for viral, bacterial, or fungal infection. (See "Manifestations of Diaper Dermatitis.")

Diaper rash may be complicated by—or coexist with—miliaria, also known as prickly heat. Miliaria occurs whenever eccrine sweat duct outflow is disrupted or when sweat is retained (as in the newborn whose sweat ducts are immature).[17,39,40] When the skin beneath the diaper becomes overheated, it may appear as papules with erythema in varying degrees, depending on the degree of sweat retention. (Miliaria is also seen with fever, working in hot environments, and overdressing.)[41,42] The protectant medications recommended for diaper dermatitis will also provide relief from miliaria.

TREATMENT OF DIAPER DERMATITIS

Treatment Guidelines

Diaper dermatitis often resolves rapidly once it is recognized by the caregiver, who then will change the infant more often and cleanse the diaper area more carefully.[9] After the child is toilet trained, it seldom recurs. One exception is adults who are incontinent and must wear some type of adult diaper or pad that causes skin occlusion. The clinical picture in these patients is virtually identical to the contact irritation of diaper rash.[43] (See "Incontinence Dermatitis [Adult Diaper Dermatitis, Perineal Dermatitis].)

The pharmacist should assess the child to help ensure that diaper dermatitis is the cause of the condition. Diaper rash that is self-treatable is limited to mild skin redness; it should not exhibit broken skin or any type of lesions. Signs of bacterial or fungal infection (e.g., ulcerations, vesicles, erosions, or satellite lesions) require referral. If the child has lesions outside of the diaper area, the chances of another condition are multiplied (e.g., seborrheic dermatitis), necessitating physician referral. If the condition has been present for more than 7 days, it may also be secondarily infected with *Candida*, especially if the skin is broken. If candidal involvement is suspected, the patient should be referred. (See Patient Assessment Algorithm 38.1.)

Many ingredients that are safe and effective when used on older children and adults for other conditions may not be appropriate for diaper rash. Several factors make diaper rash care for infants potentially more serious, including absorption of medications, metabolic inefficiency, and skin area involved[44]:

- The occlusive nature of diapers helps facilitate transcutaneous absorption of medications. When the stratum corneum is damaged, its barrier function is compromised. In addition, since the skin of infants is only one-half the thickness of adult skin, absorption is further facilitated.
- Infants do not metabolize or detoxify medications as well as adults. Many enzyme systems are absent or deficient in the neonate.

Patient Assessment Algorithm 38.1. Diaper Rash

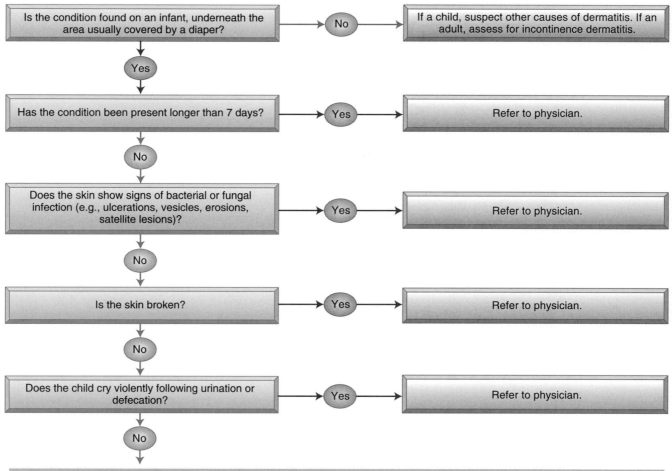

• The diaper area is a relatively large percentage of the infant's body surface area.

Because of all of these factors, pharmacists must take great care to only recommend products containing ingredients proven to be safe and effective. As examples, boric acid, phenol, and mercury preparations are prohibited since to treat diaper rash they would have to be applied over a relatively large part of the body, which could be hazardous since they are all toxic when absorbed.

Labels of nonprescription diaper dermatitis products must caution parents that the product is for external use only and must be kept out of the eyes.[44] *All nonprescription product labels also must advise that, should the condition worsen or fail to improve after 7 days, a physician should be consulted.* Parents and caregivers should be instructed to first change wet and soiled diapers promptly, cleanse the diaper area, allow the diaper area to dry, and then apply the product liberally with each diaper change. Pharmacists should underscore the importance of applying diaper rash medication at bedtime or at any other time when prolonged exposure to wet diapers is anticipated. *If a powder is used, the parent will be cautioned to not use on broken skin and to keep it away from the child's face to avoid the dangers of inhalation pneumonia.* Powder can be used more safely by applying it close to the body or carefully shaking it into the diaper or into the hand before applying to the diaper area.

Nonprescription Medications

The only ingredients considered safe and effective for diaper rash are protectants. The parent should avoid the use of antifungals, antibacterials, external analgesics, hydrocortisone, and dangerous ingredients.

SKIN PROTECTANTS

The FDA considered numerous skin protectants for diaper rash and found several to be safe and effective (Table 38.1).[45] They are effective by covering skin surfaces, protecting them from drying out and exposure to various irritating substances. Some

Table 38.1. Representative Products for Diaper Dermatitis[a]

PRODUCT	SELECTED INGREDIENTS/COMMENTS
A + D Original Ointment	Petrolatum 80.5%, lanolin 15.5%, cod liver oil, light mineral oil
A + D Ointment with Zinc Oxide	Dimethicone 1%, zinc oxide 10%, aloe, cod liver oil, light mineral oil
Desitin Creamy Ointment	Zinc oxide 10%
Desitin Diaper Rash Ointment	Zinc oxide 40%, cod liver oil, lanolin, petrolatum, talc
Diaperene Corn Starch Baby Powder	Topical starch (corn starch), inactive ingredients include possibly allergenic plants, such as extracts of aloe vera, matricaria (chamomile), evening primrose
Flanders Buttocks Ointment	Zinc oxide, peruvian balsam
Gold Bond Cornstarch Plus Medicated Baby Powder	Cornstarch, zinc oxide, kaolin
Gold Bond Medicated Baby Powder	Talc, zinc oxide
Johnson's Baby Oil	Mineral oil, vitamin E
Johnson's Baby Powder	Talc
Johnson's Baby Powder Pure Cornstarch	Topical starch (cornstarch)
Mexsana Medicated Powder	Corn starch, zinc oxide, kaolin, benzethonium chloride (unapproved antibacterial), camphor (unapproved external analgesic), eucalyptol (unapproved ingredient)
Suave Baby Care Oil	Mineral oil
Suave Baby Care Powder	Corn starch
Vaseline Nursery Jelly	White petrolatum

[a]For the most part, only ingredients examined by the FDA are listed, even if the company labels them as inactive ingredients. Products typically contain other formulation ingredients such as fragrance. Companies often do not list concentrations of active ingredients.

products contain two safe and effective skin protectants.[46] Skin protectants may be used at the first sign of erythema. They are also useful in preventing diaper rash through their actions in excluding wetness, preventing dryness, and protecting against intertriginous contact of opposing skin surfaces (see "Skin Hydration"). Only skin protectants that are proven safe and effective should be recommended for the infant. (See "Skin Protectants Lacking Proof of Safety and/or Efficacy.")

Allantoin 0.5 to 2%

Allantoin, a product of purine metabolism, is produced synthetically.[46] It acts to form complexes with many sensitizing agents to render them harmless to the skin.

Calamine 1 to 25%

Calamine, a mixture of ferrous oxide and zinc oxide, has absorbent properties.[46]

Cod Liver Oil 5 to 13.56%

Products containing cod liver oil must yield to the skin within a 24-hour period; 10,000 U.S.P. units of vitamin A and 400 U.S.P. units of cholecalciferol.[45]

Dimethicone 1 to 30%

Dimethicone is a water-repellent silicone oil. Its demulcent properties are useful for diaper rash because it adheres well to skin.[46]

Kaolin 4 to 20%

Kaolin is a native, hydrated aluminum silicate that absorbs excessive moisture and perspiration.[46]

Lanolin 15.5%

Lanolin is allergenic in concentrations normally used (e.g., 15.5%), although the incidence is low.[45] It is slightly irritating to skin of all patients if the concentration is 20% or more. Lanolin may only be used in combination with other products since its efficacy alone remains undemonstrated.

Mineral Oil 50 to 100%

Mineral oil coats the skin with a water barrier, which also provides an emollient action.[45] The FDA discussed the fact that mineral oil is a hydrocarbon that is not metabolized, so that it remains on the skin indefinitely until it is physically removed. Chronic irritation and folliculitis could result. The agency proposed a warning on all diaper-rash products to cleanse the diaper area before application, which it felt would prevent the problem of mineral-oil accumulation on the skin.[45]

Petrolatum 30 to 100%/White Petrolatum

Petrolatum is a purified mixture of semisolid hydrocarbons obtained from petroleum. White petrolatum has been partially or completely decolorized. Both substances are oleaginous ointment bases, providing emollient and lubricant actions on the skin.[46]

Talc 45 to 100%

Talc is a natural hydrous magnesium silicate that has a barrier-like action and emollient effect on skin.[45] As such, it also prevents chafing and irritation by helping lubricate areas where skin is directly apposed (e.g., the buttocks and groin). It also absorbs sweat. However, *talc must not be applied to broken skin since it can cause crusting, infection, and skin granulomas.*

⚠ *Inhalation of powders such as talc can produce severe injury or death as a result of chemical-inhalation pneumonia.*[45] A survey of mothers of children younger than 2 revealed that 42% did not know of the dangers of powder inhalation, explaining the relatively high incidence of baby-powder inhalation. The majority of cases occur in babies younger than 1. Most incidents occur while a baby is having a diaper change. In one incident a 3-year-old sibling poured talcum powder into the nose and mouth of a 1-month-old, who went into cardiopulmonary arrest, but survived after resuscitation. In another case a 22-month-old boy playing with talcum powder expired from intractable cardiopulmonary failure caused by respiratory distress and perioral cyanosis.[45] The FDA proposed the warnings listed above in an attempt to ensure proper use of the ingredient.

Because of the problems associated with talc usage, the FDA has joined with the International Society of Regulatory Toxicology and Pharmacology to hold public hearings on its safe use in the consumer population.[47]

Corn Starch 10 to 98%

Also known as topical starch, corn starch is composed of granules from the mature grain of the corn plant.[46] It protects skin through absorbent actions.[33] ⚠ *Corn starch must be used with caution since it is a powder and could cause breathing problems similar to those seen with talc.*

Zinc Oxide 1 to 25%/Zinc Oxide Ointment 25 to 40%

The FDA evaluated zinc oxide, recommending a 1 to 25% concentration be labeled as safe and effective in any dosage form. However, safety and efficacy information only supported zinc oxide concentrations above 25% for ointments, with a maximum concentration of 40%.

ANTIFUNGALS

An FDA Review Panel considered the use of antifungals on diaper rash as early as 1982.[43] In a later publication the agency stressed that a fungal complication of diaper rash must be diagnosed and treated by a physician.[48] The agency suggested that if fungal infection is suspected, analysis of skin scrapings from the affected area should be done, as it is the only precise method of determining the cause of a secondary infection.[48] For these reasons

 no ingredient is safe or effective for self-treating a diaper dermatitis that is complicated by fungal infection.[49]

ANTIBACTERIALS

The FDA considered numerous antimicrobials for use in diaper rash, including benzalkonium chloride, benzethonium chloride, boric acid, calcium undecylenate, chloroxylenol, hexachlorophene, methylbenzethonium chloride, oxyquinoline, *p*-chloromercuriphenol, phenol, resorcinol, sodium propionate, and triclosan.[44,50] *However, no antimicrobial product is considered safe and effective for nonprescription use in diaper dermatitis. Further, if the skin is broken, it is in danger of secondary bacterial or fungal infection and must not be self-treated. If diaper dermatitis is presently infected, it is also beyond self-treatment.*

For many years boric acid was included in diaper-rash products, supposedly as an antibacterial (or perhaps a protectant). However, it has been deemed unsafe since several fatalities have resulted from its absorption.[1] It is still found in several regional products as of this writing and older boxes of major brands that may still be on the shelves.

An anecdotal report illustrates the dangers of using antibacterial ingredients and formulations that have not been proven safe and effective. Oxyquinoline is an antibacterial that lacks such assurance. A mother applied it to her female infant in the form of Corona Ointment, which is a product intended solely for veterinary use.[51] When seen by her physician at the age of 8.5 months, the child had developed coarse, dark pubic hair, and breasts enlarged to 2 centimeters, a condition known as precocious puberty. The breast tissue was firm and attached to slightly darkened areolae. Her physician suspected an estrogenlike substance found in the beeswax base of Corona Ointment. Patients must be questioned carefully when purchasing this product or other veterinary products (e.g., "bag balms") to ensure that they do not intend to use them on humans. (See "Clioquinol, Dangerous Diaper Rash Ingredient.")

EXTERNAL ANALGESICS

External analgesics intended for pain and itching could be dangerous if used in diaper rash. The occluded moist skin beneath the diaper facilitates absorption of medication. In these conditions, external analgesics could produce erosions on infants' skin.[53] Therefore, *external analgesics are generally contraindicated for children younger than 2 and are not to be used in diaper rash at any time.*

⚠️ *Several fatalities have been caused by camphor absorption through the skin.[1]*

In one case a 6-day-old boy developed methemoglobinemia (cyanosis with blue mucous membranes) as a result of the mother's use of Vagisil Cream for diaper rash.[54] The product contains benzocaine and resorcinol, neither of which is safe for use on diaper rash. His symptoms resolved after injection of 3 mg of methylene blue.

HYDROCORTISONE

Steroids should be avoided in diaper rash.[43] Potent fluorinated steroids are known to thin the skin, cause striae, and facilitate bruising, especially when they are applied under an occlusive dressing such as a diaper. While hydrocortisone is less prone to cause these problems, diaper rash is not one of its labeled indications. Its safety and efficacy for diaper rash have not yet been demonstrated. Further, its label clearly prohibits use under the age of 2 years.[1] It could cause skin atrophy and might be systemically absorbed, given that it is applied over a relatively large area of the baby's skin and that the damaged skin has a compromised barrier function.[55]

PREVENTION OF DIAPER DERMATITIS

Role of the Diaper

Diapers create an environment of occlusion, humidity, and friction. To keep urine and feces out of this environment, and thus prevent diaper rash, diapers must be changed frequently.[26,33] Also, since the outer plastic pants often placed over cloth diapers can exacerbate the humidity of the environment, parents and caregivers can promote evaporation of moisture under diapers by leaving these covers off when possible.[1,26]

As noted above, the issue of which type of diaper is less prone to cause diaper dermatitis is fraught with controversy. In one study, however, highly absorbent disposable diapers were found to cause less dermatitis than disposables with normal absorbency.[7,16]

Since the diaper is thought to be a predisposing factor, some authorities advise lying babies on an open, dry diaper during naps to allow the skin to thoroughly dry.[1] With this technique, diapers can be checked frequently and changed if soiled during sleep.

Cleanliness

When urine and feces mix, the stage is set for diaper rash. Keeping these excreta separated is thus a potent weapon against skin breakdown.[7] Washing and drying the skin in the diaper area helps diaper rash to subside.[43,56] Following urination, the area should simply be rinsed with water to avoid exposure to chemicals such as those found in diaper wipes, which may irritate the skin further.[22]

FOCUS ON . . .

CLIOQUINOL, DANGEROUS DIAPER RASH INGREDIENT

At one time, medical professionals advised use of clioquinol (iodochlorhydroxyquin) on diaper rash as a topical antibacterial/antifungal. This ingredient, marketed as Vioform, can cause serious ophthalmic and nerve damage, especially when used in babies with diaper rash. Its neurotoxicity argues against its use.[52]

Some parents and caregivers use detergents or soaps that can cause allergic dermatitis when cleansing feces.[26] Baby wipes containing alcohol can cause pain when applied to inflamed skin.[7] Following defecation, the skin instead should be washed with warm water and mild soap or other gentle cleansers. Excessive scrubbing further damages fragile skin.

Skin Hydration

While the skin must not be overhydrated, which leads to **maceration** (liquid softening of the skin, which can hasten breakdown of skin), it also should be kept appropriately moist through the use of emollients, creams, or mild oil protectants (e.g., petrolatum).[57,58]

SUMMARY

Diaper dermatitis is a condition caused by a combination of factors:

- Diaper occlusion elevates skin pH above the normal values of 4 to 5.5.
- Urine in contact with the skin causes maceration, compromising the skin's barrier function and increasing the potential for abrasion.
- Normal bacterial skin residents break down urine urea to ammonia, which further raises normal skin pH.
- Feces contain lipases and proteases, which are activated at the higher pH found on diapered skin.
- Activated fecal proteases hasten skin breakdown.
- Skin breakdown facilitates bacterial and candidal overgrowth.

While most cases of diaper rash are mild, the condition ranges from mild erythema to severe conditions with secondary bacterial and/or fungal infections. When the skin is broken, or the pharmacist suspects bacterial or candidal overgrowth, children should be referred to a physician. For mild cases of diaper rash, the pharmacist may recommend safe and effective protectants such as allantoin, calamine, cod liver oil, dimethicone, kaolin, lanolin, mineral oil, petrolatum, talc, corn starch, and zinc oxide. Pharmacists should not recommend antifungals and antibacterials for self-treatment of diaper rash, nor should hydrocortisone and products containing external analgesics be recommended. Skin that is broken or infected mandates physician referral. Also, if the

AT THE COUNTER

 A man with a baby in his arms asks the pharmacist where the Lotrimin is.

Interview/Patient Assessment

The pharmacist asks what the Lotrimin is to be used for, to which the man replies, "It's for my baby's diaper rash." The pharmacist asks why that particular product is being requested. The father mentions that his mother-in-law said to get some. The pharmacist asks if the skin is broken. The father shows the pharmacist several weeping lesions at the upper edge of the diaper area. The lesions are bright red. Finally, the pharmacist asks how long the rash has been present. The father thinks it started about 10 days before. He adds that the child cries almost constantly, especially when his diaper is dirty. The child is taking no medication and has no medical condition.

Pharmacist's Analysis

1. Does the baby's problem sound like diaper rash?
2. What is the significance of the baby's crying?

3. Should the pharmacist recommend nonprescription products for the diaper rash?
4. Is Lotrimin AF indicated for diaper rash?

The location of the lesions resembles that of diaper rash. Several clues indicate that the skin is infected with *Candida* and therefore is not treatable with nonprescription products. For instance, the child usually cries following urination or defecation, and the lesions are bright red as with *Candida*. Further, the skin is broken and the problem has persisted for more than 7 days, reinforcing the presence of a candidal infection.

Patient Counseling

The pharmacist should caution the father that the child may have a fungal infection of the diaper area. Although Lotrimin AF is a topical antifungal, the father should be warned that the product has never been proven to be either safe or effective for diaper rash. The pharmacist should strongly advise the father to see a pediatrician.

---

condition persists beyond 7 days, patients should be seen by a physician.

Prevention of diaper rash is the most effective therapy. However, optimal prevention consists of keeping the skin totally dry by changing the diaper immediately after urine or feces are passed. Since this is not possible for most parents or caregivers, diaper rash will continue to be a common problem of childhood.

References

1. Farrington E. Diaper dermatitis. Pediatr Nurs 18:81, 1992.
2. Brown DS, Small S, Jones D. Standardizing skin care across settings. Ostomy Wound Manage 41:40, 1995.
3. Brown DS. Perineal dermatitis risk factors: Clinical validation of a conceptual framework. Ostomy Wound Manage 41:46, 1995.
4. Fiers SA. Breaking the cycle: The etiology of incontinence dermatitis and evaluating and using skin care products. Ostomy Wound Manage 42:32, 1996.
5. Boiko S, Diapers and diaper rashes. Dermatol Nurs 9:33, 1997.
6. Longhi F, et al. Diaper dermatitis: A study of contributing factors. Contact Dermatitis 26:248, 1992.
7. Sires UI, Mallory SB. Diaper dermatitis. Postgrad Med 98:79, 1995.
8. Singleton JK. Pediatric dermatoses: Three common skin disruptions in infancy. Nurse Pract 22:32, 1997.
9. Rasmussen JE. Classification of diaper dermatitis: An overview. Pediatrician 14 Suppl 1:6, 1987.
10. Philipp R, Hughes A, Golding J. Getting to the bottom of

nappy rash: ALSPAC Survey Team. Avon Longitudinal Study of Pregnancy and Childhood. Br J Gen Pract 47:493, 1997.
11. White CM, Gailey RA, Lippe S. Cholestyramine ointment to treat buttocks rash and anal excoriation in an infant. Ann Pharmacother 30:954, 1996.
12. Wong DL, et al. Diapering choices: A critical review of the issues. Pediatr Nurs 18:41, 1992.
13. Gokalp AS, et al. Relation between the intestinal flora and diaper dermatitis in infancy. Trop Geogr Med 42:238, 1990.
14. Haugen V. Perineal skin care for patients with frequent diarrhea or fecal incontinence. Gastroenterol Nurs 20:87, 1997.
15. Sutton MB, Weitzman M, Howland J. Baby bottoms and environmental conundrums: Disposable diapers and the pediatrician. Pediatrics 88:386, 1991.
16. Lane AT, Rehder PA, Helm K. Evaluations of diapers containing absorbent gelling material with conventional disposable diapers in newborn infants. Am J Dis Child 144:315, 1990.
17. McLaurin CI. Pediatric dermatology in black patients. Derm Clin 6:457, 1988.
18. Seitz ML. Disposable diapers vs the environment (Letter). Pediatrics 89:523, 1992.
19. Scott N. Diaper debate continues (Letter). Pediatrics 90:654, 1992.
20. Moran EJ. Cost of reusable vs. disposable diapers in dispute. Hospitals 64:84, 1990.
21. Primomo J, Greenstreet PK. Influencing policy on diapering: Not for babies only. J Perinatol 13:140, 1993.
22. Collipp PJ. Effect of oral zinc supplements on diaper rash in normal infants. J Med Assoc Ga 78:621, 1989.
23. Forsyth JS, et al. Relation between early introduction of solid food to infants and their weight and illnesses during the first two years of life. Br Med J 306:1572, 1993.

24. Pierard-Franchimont C, Letawe C, Pierard GE. Tribiological and mycological consequences of the use of a miconazole nitrate-containing paste for the prevention of diaper dermatitis: An open pilot study. Eur J Pediatr 155:756, 1996.

25. Konya J, Gow E. Granuloma gluteale infantum. Australas J Dermatol 37:57, 1996.

26. Gallichio V. Nappy rash. Aust Fam Physician 17:971, 1988.

27. Thiboutot DM, et al. Cytomegalovirus diaper dermatitis. Arch Dermatol 127:396, 1991.

28. Preston SL, Bryant BG. Etiology and treatment of diaper dermatitis. Hosp Pharm 29:1086, 1994.

29. Honig PJ, et al. Amoxicillin and diaper dermatitis. J Am Acad Derm 19(2 Pt 1):275, 1988.

30. Darwazeh AMG, Al-Bashir A. Oral candidal flora in healthy infants. J Oral Pathol Med 24:361, 1995.

31. Tanguay KE, McBean MR, Jain E. Nipple candidiasis among breastfeeding mothers. Can Fam Physician 40:1407, 1994.

32. Bosch-Banyeras JM, et al. Diaper dermatitis. Clin Pediatr 27:448, 1988.

33. Janniger CK, Thomas I. Diaper dermatitis: An approach to prevention employing effective diaper care. Cutis 52:153, 1993.

34. Jethwa K. Nappy rash: A pharmaceutical approach. Prof Care Mother Child 4:219, 1994.

35. Jenson HB, Shapiro ED. Primary herpes simplex virus infection of a diaper rash (Letter). Pediatr Infect Dis J 6:1136, 1987.

36. Brook I. Microbiology of secondarily infected diaper dermatitis. Int J Dermatol 31:700, 1992.

37. Simon HK, Steele DW. Varicella: Pediatric genital/rectal vesicular lesions of unclear origin. Ann Emerg Med 25:111, 1995.

38. Enta T. Dermacase. Can Fam Physician 40:232, 1994.

39. Shuster S. Duct disruption, a new explanation of miliaria. Acta Derm Venereol 77:1, 1997.

40. Wenzel FG, Horn TD. Nonneoplastic disorders of the eccrine glands. J Am Acad Dermatol 38:1, 1998.

41. Lillywhite LP. Investigation into the environmental factors associated with the incidence of skin disease following an outbreak of Miliaria rubra at a coal mine. Occup Med 42:183, 1992.

42. Koh D. An outbreak of occupational dermatosis in an electronics store. Contact Dermatitis 32:327, 1995.

43. Fed Reg 47:39464, 1982.

44. Fed Reg 55:25246, 1990.

45. Fed Reg 55:25204, 1990.

46. Fed Reg 43:34628, 1978.

47. Fed Reg 59:2319, 1994.

48. Fed Reg 55:25240, 1990.

49. Fed Reg 57:60430, 1992.

50. Fed Reg 47:39406, 1982.

51. Healy CE. Precocious puberty due to a diaper ointment. Indiana Med 77:610, 1984.

52. Yaffe SJ. Clioquinol (iodochlorhydroxyquin, Vioform) and iodoquinol (diiodohydroxyquin): Blindness and neuropathy. Pediatrics 86:797, 1990.

53. Fed Reg 57:60426, 1992.

54. Tush GM, Kuhn RJ. Methemoglobinemia induced by an over-the-counter medication. Ann Pharmacother 30:1251, 1996.

55. Faucher MA, Jackson G. A review of drugs commonly used during the neonatal period. J Nurse Midwifery 37(2 Suppl):74S, 1992.

56. Fed Reg 47:39415, 1982.

57. Scowen P. Skin care and nappy rash. Prof Care Mother Child 5:138, 1995.

58. Courtenay M. Preparations for skin conditions. Nurs Times 94:54, 1998.

Skin Hyperpigmentation

A Caucasian male patient who appears to be in his 50s asks the pharmacist about products to lighten a dark spot on his cheek.

Interview/Patient Assessment

The patient says that the lesion has been present "for at least 10 years or so." The patient states that there are similar lesions on his arms, but they do not concern him as much as the facial lesion. The lesion is about 1/2 centimeter in diameter, with slightly irregular borders, and is light brown in color. The patient says it does not crust, bleed, peel, or change in any way. It does seem to darken in the summer, however. He is not taking any medications and has no current medical conditions. He has not treated the lesion before.

Pharmacist's Analysis

1. What significance do location, size, shape, and color play in recognition of this lesion?
2. What significance does patient age play in recognition of this lesion?
3. What ancillary instructions should be given with the

nonprescription product that is effective for this condition?

The location, size, shape, and color are consistent with that of a solar lentigo. The condition becomes more common with advancing age and is more likely to be seen on sun-exposed areas such as the face. The fact that the patient has additional lesions on other sun-exposed areas helps in identifying the condition as solar lentigo. However, it is not possible to confirm this recognition visually; therefore, if the lesion does not fade appropriately, he should see a physician.

Patient Counseling

The pharmacist should show the patient products containing hydroquinone, which is safe and effective for lightening solar lentigines when used as directed. The pharmacist also should caution the patient to keep the product away from his eyes and urge the patient to use a sunscreen or sunblock on the area while it is being treated and after treatment to prevent recurrence of the hyperpigmentation. He should also be given general advice regarding regular use of sunscreens. (See Chapter 33, Sun-Induced Skin Damage.)

Human skin has a normal pigmentation that is characteristic of the individual. **Melanocytes** (pigment-producing cells distributed throughout the basal layer of the epidermis) are responsible for maintaining this normal pigmentation. Melanocytes project upward into the upper epidermal layers. They synthesize the colored pigment known as melanin, which they then conduct upward into keratinocytes in the upper epidermal layers to produce skin coloration. Melanin is formed from the oxidation of tyrosine.[1] Many conditions can result in skin **hyperpigmentation** (excess skin pigmentation), also known as melanosis.[2] Causes of hyperpigmentation with serious medical ramifications include endocrine imbalance, hyperthyroidism, cirrhosis, and ingestion of certain medications.[3] In most cases, however, the causes of skin hyperpigmentation are not serious, and the condition has little medical significance.[2] Three minor types of hyperpigmentation may be self-treated:

- Solar lentigines
- Ephelides
- Melasma (when caused by pregnancy or oral contraceptive use)

While these conditions are not dangerous in and of themselves, they do cause cosmetic concern to patients when they appear on the face, hands, and other visible areas of skin.[2]

SOLAR LENTIGINES

Solar lentigo (the plural form is solar lentigines) is also known as actinic lentigo, senile lentigo, and age spot (Fig. 39.1).[3–5] Despite another common name—liver spots—this condition is not associated with hepatic pathology.[6]

PREVALENCE OF SOLAR LENTIGINES

Solar lentigines are found in over 90% of individuals of Caucasian descent who are 70 or older.[7]

EPIDEMIOLOGY OF SOLAR LENTIGINES

Several factors affect the occurrence of solar lentigines, including the age of the patient, the patient's history of ultraviolet light exposure, and the presence of ephelides.

Age

Solar lentigines are strongly associated with age, usually manifesting after the age of menopause or the male **climacteric** (the male equivalent of the female's menopausal period).[3,8] In one study 75% of subjects over 40 had solar lentigo, as compared with only 33.5% of those under 40.[4]

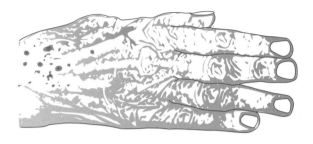

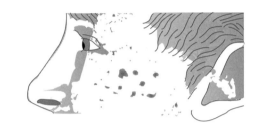

Figure 39.1. Drawing showing typical solar lentigo.

Ultraviolet Light

Solar lentigines are one of the manifestations of photodamaged skin, along with wrinkles, actinic keratoses, and various malignancies. (See Chapter 33, Sun-Induced Skin Damage.)[9] According to one study, the risk of solar lentigines increases by a factor of 1.6 for patients who had two or more sunburns after age 20.[4]

Ephelides

Individuals who have a high number of ephelides, or freckles, as adolescents are 2.5 times more likely to develop actinic solar lentigines as adults.[4]

Other Factors

Solar lentigines do not exhibit a gender preference. Also solar lentigines are seen in equal proportions in those with light or dark skin types.[7]

ETIOLOGY OF SOLAR LENTIGINES

The etiology of solar lentigines is inherent in the name: photodamage as a result of unprotected exposure to the sun, specifically ultraviolet B (UVB) radiation.[10,11] Chronic sun exposure results in melanocyte proliferation, so that there are more than twice as many pigment-producing cells as in nonaffected skin, which thereby doubles the amount of melanin in the area of the lentigines.[12–14] **Keratinocytes** (epidermal cells that produce keratin) also become hyperplastic.[13]

Occasionally, lesions resembling solar lentigo may be seen on patients exposed to ionizing radiation.[15] However, these lesions are not self-treatable.

MANIFESTATIONS OF SOLAR LENTIGINES

Solar lentigines manifest as multiple lesions on sun-exposed skin areas such as the face, dorsae of the hands, and extensor surfaces of the forearms.[7,16,17] Solar lentigines vary in size from a few millimeters to more than 1 cm in diameter, and several close lentigines may coalesce to form a larger lesion. Singularly or combined, solar lentigines can have irregular or regular borders.

Solar lentigines generally are dark brown, but lesions can also exhibit black, yellow, or light brown varieties. Also, within a single lesion there may be several colors or several shades of brown.

SPECIFIC CONSIDERATIONS OF SOLAR LENTIGINES: RISK FACTOR FOR MELANOMA

Although the solar lentigo itself is harmless, the number of solar lentigines is a predictor for malignant melanoma.[4,7] Researchers find that the melanocyte proliferation typical of solar lentigines is present in the epidermal tissues adjacent to 75 to 88% of melanomas.[18,19]

PROGNOSIS OF SOLAR LENTIGINES

Solar lentigo lesions do not scale, desquamate, or become hyperkeratotic. However, following exposure to sunlight, they darken more than healthy skin adjacent to them.[20] Thus for most patients they are only a minor cosmetic annoyance, yielding easily to treatment with nonprescription products in most instances. Lasers may be used to reduce their color if nonprescription agents are ineffective.[21,22]

TREATMENT OF SOLAR LENTIGINES

See "Treatment of Hyperpigmented Skin Conditions."

EPHELIDES

Ephelides (the singular form of the term is ephelis) are also referred to as freckles, "sunburn" freckles, and sun-induced freckles (Fig. 39.2).[16]

PREVALENCE OF EPHELIDES

The prevalence of ephelides is unknown for the population at large, although one survey of white children aged 6 to 18 of European descent revealed that 2.8% of participants had ephelides.[16]

EPIDEMIOLOGY OF EPHELIDES

Ephelides are more commonly seen in individuals of white European descent than in individuals of Asian background.[16]

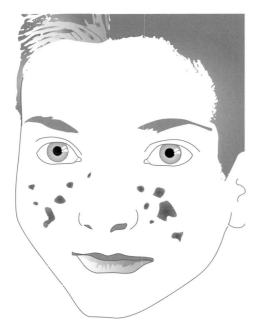

Figure 39.2. Drawing showing typical sun-induced freckles.

The incidence in other racial groups is unknown, although ephelides appear to be generally less common as the skin becomes darker (according to racial makeup).[16] Risk factors include light skin and propensity to burn rather than tan. In one study males aged 6 to 18 had a prevalence of 4.5%, compared with only 1.2% of females.[16]

ETIOLOGY OF EPHELIDES

Ephelides appear as a result of UVB exposure.[16] Unlike solar lentigo, there are actually fewer melanocytes in skin affected with ephelides. However, the melanocytes that are present are larger and more active in production of melanosomes.

MANIFESTATIONS OF EPHELIDES

Ephelides appear as small, medium-brown **macules** (flattened discolorations) scattered across the skin in sun-exposed areas.[23] Larger and darker than typical freckles, ephelides are larger than 4 mm in diameter and darker brown.[16,24] Color within the lesion is evenly distributed, but the borders can be notched or irregular.

Ephelides become darker when exposed to the sun.[7]

PROGNOSIS OF EPHELIDES

Ephelides can fade or disappear entirely when sun exposure is discontinued.[25] However, propensity to freckle as an adult is a risk factor for melanoma and may also be rarely associated with cardiac abnormalities.[26–30]

TREATMENT OF EPHELIDES

See "Treatment of Hyperpigmented Skin Conditions."

MELASMA

Melasma, an acquired, patterned hyperpigmentation of the skin, is also known as chloasma (Fig. 39.3).

PREVALENCE OF MELASMA

Melasma occurs in 50 to 70% of pregnant females and in 5 to 34% of females who take oral contraceptives.[31]

EPIDEMIOLOGY OF MELASMA

The epidemiology of melasma varies according to skin type, pregnancy, ingestion of certain medications, gender, and sunlight exposure.

Skin Type

Melasma has a familial tendency. Melasma affects dark-skinned individuals more frequently than light-skinned individuals, showing a predilection for skin types IV, V, and VI. (See Chapter 33, Sun-Induced Skin Damage, for descriptions of the different skin types.)[5,32] Hispanics, Asians, and African-Americans all have higher rates of melasma than whites.[1,32]

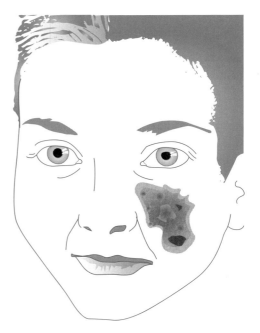

Figure 39.3. Drawing showing typical melasma.

Pregnancy

Melasma is so frequently associated with pregnancy across skin types that it has acquired the specific name melasma gravidarum, chloasma gravidarum, or gravidaric mask (popularly referred to as the "mask of pregnancy"). Melasma gravidarum is more common in the pregnant female with darker skin (up to 80% of pregnant Hispanic women develop melasma).[31,33]

Medication Ingestion

Melasma can be induced by ingestion of oral contraceptives, progestins, or estrogens.[31,33]

Gender

Most patients with melasma are female, largely because of its association with pregnancy and the ingestion of estrogens and/or progestagens.[34] Approximately 10% of sufferers are males.[1,32]

Sunlight

Melasma is especially common in patients who live in areas that receive heavy amounts of UVB radiation and do not take proper skin protection.[32]

ETIOLOGY OF MELASMA

The tendency to suffer from melasma is inherited.[35] Some females begin to experience the condition as a result of puberty-induced hormonal rises. In others, the hormonal changes of pregnancy are the probable cause (e.g., melasma gravidarum).[31] Melanocytes possess estrogen receptors that stimulate hyperactivity.[35] Both estrogen and progesterone stimulate melanogenesis through this mechanism, and both are elevated during pregnancy. Ingestion of oral contraceptives and estrogen supplements produce melasma through the same mechanism.

Melasma is exacerbated by sun exposure, which accounts for its heightened incidence in those who receive greater amounts of UVB radiation.[5,31]

The etiology in males is less well understood, but is not thought to be related to hormonal causes.[32]

MANIFESTATIONS OF MELASMA

Hyperpigmented areas affected with melasma usually appear as blotchy patches.[31] Melasma patches are not elevated above the level of the skin, but appear as flattened discolorations of tan or as any shade of brown from light to dark.[31,32]

Melasma is most frequently noticed on sun-exposed areas of the face, especially the cheeks, forehead, upper lip, nose, and chin.[31,32,36] Other areas such as the hands and arms may also be affected.[1,37] Melasma gravidarum is also likely to oc-

cur on other areas of the body such as the areolae, axillae, and genitalia.[31] Scars and moles located inside of a melasma patch may also undergo progressive darkening.

PROGNOSIS OF MELASMA

Melasma is usually a self-limited condition.[38] In cases of melasma gravidarum, hyperpigmented areas generally lighten within 1 year or so after delivery or discontinuation of estrogen-containing medications.[31] In some cases of melasma gravidarum, however, hyperpigmentation may persist for 5 or more years after delivery or discontinuation of estrogen-containing medications.[1,32]

The prognosis is poorer in some subpopulations; over one-third of Hispanic patients will have lifelong melasma.[33]

TREATMENT OF MELASMA

See "Treatment of Hyperpigmented Skin Conditions."

HYPERPIGMENTED SKIN CONDITIONS

TREATMENT OF HYPERPIGMENTED SKIN CONDITIONS

See above for prevalence, epidemiology, etiology, manifestations, specific considerations, and prognosis of solar lentigines. See above for prevalence, epidemiology, etiology, manifestations, and prognosis of ephelides. See above for prevalence, epidemiology, etiology, manifestations, and prognosis of melasma.

Treatment Guidelines

When patients wish to treat skin hyperpigmentation, pharmacists should examine the skin discoloration(s) carefully to ensure that it is solar lentigines, ephelides, or melasma caused by pregnancy or the use of oral contraceptives. (See Patient Assessment Algorithm 39.1.) Because of the seriousness of some similar conditions (e.g., melanoma), pharmacists should use caution in recommending self-treatment.[39] (See "Melanoma" in Chapter 33, Sun-Induced Skin Damage.)

Nonprescription Medication: Hydroquinone

MECHANISM OF ACTION

Hydroquinone, a hydroxyphenol, is thought to inhibit conversion of dopa to melanin by inhibiting the enzyme tyrosinase (which converts tyrosine to melanin). Thus hydroquinone slowly reduces the degree of pigmentation in hypermelanized areas.[2,32] Laboratory studies on guinea pigs have demonstrated that melanocytes are degraded by hydroquinone. Thus, although these products are known as "bleaching creams" (a name adopted by the FDA), they do not actually bleach the skin, but lighten it by slowly allowing it to fade (Table 39.1).[2]

Patient Assessment Algorithm 39.1. Skin Hyperpigmentation

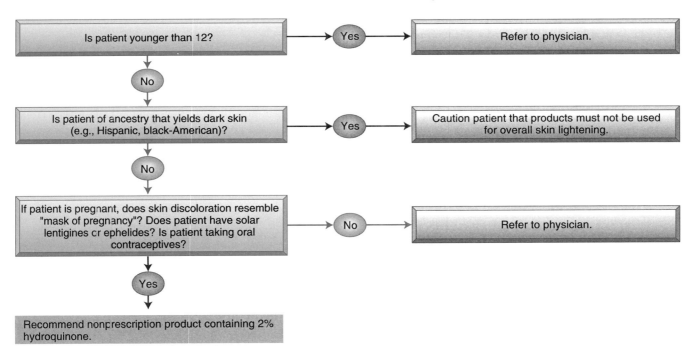

Table 39.1. Representative Nonprescription Products for Hyperpigmentation	
PRODUCT	SELECTED INGREDIENTS/COMMENTS
Esoterica Skin Discoloration Fade Cream Facial with Sunscreen	Hydroquinone 2%, octyl dimethyl PABA 3.3% (padimate O), benzophenone-3 2.5% (oxybenzone)
Esoterica Skin Discoloration Fade Cream Regular	Hydroquinone 2%
Porcelana Medicated Fade Cream Normal Skin with Sunscreen	Octyl methoxycinnamate 2.5%, hydroquinone 2%
Porcelana Original Formula Medicated Fade Cream	Hydroquinone 2%
Nudit Fade Cream	Hydroquinone 2%

For this reason hydroquinone is better termed a hypopigmenting agent.

At least 5 to 6 million people in the United States each year use OTC products containing hydroquinone.[32]

ONSET OF ACTION

Hydroquinone does not affect surface skin, but interacts with melanin production in the lowest layers of the epidermis. These lowest layers of skin require time to rise to upper epidermal layers (the process of cellular turnover). For this reason patients should not expect a rapidly perceptible response. The time of onset of skin changes ranges from 3 weeks to 3 months, averaging about 4 weeks.[3]

Products containing hydroquinone must be labeled, "If no improvement is seen after 3 months of treatment, use of this product should be discontinued."[40] Further, patients with very dark skin may not notice any perceptible lightening during the 3 months allowed.

USE PRECAUTIONS

Products containing hydroquinone direct patients to apply a small amount of the product as a thin layer on affected areas twice daily, avoiding contact with the eyes. Because of unknown safety in children, these products should not be used on patients under 12.[40] Patients are instructed on product labels to limit sun exposure during treatment by using a sunscreen, sunblock, or protective clothing and to cover bleached skin forever following treatment to prevent recurrence.[40] Hyperpigmentation products that contain a sunscreen must be labeled, "This product is not for use in the prevention of sunburn." Patients of black descent should be cautioned that these products are not for overall skin lightening. Furthermore, pharmacists should caution all patients to avoid the sun during treatment with hydroquinone, since exposure to the sun promotes melanin production, working against the hydroquinone.[33]

ADVERSE EFFECTS

The major adverse effect of hydroquinone is irritation.[2] Contact dermatitis also can occur with use.[32] Transient **leukoderma** (complete depigmentation of the treated area and surrounding normal skin) also can result, but the skin color usually returns to normal after the product is discontinued.[2] The labels on products containing hydroquinone should caution patients, "Some users of this product may experience a mild skin irritation. If skin irritation becomes too severe, stop use and consult a doctor."[40] Occasionally, patients may experience nail discoloration from frequent contact during application of the product to the skin.[41]

Ochronosis, an ochre (blue-black) discoloration of the skin, is a more serious adverse reaction to hydroquinone (Fig 39.4). (The condition is best described as a sooty hyperpigmentation of the cheeks, forehead, nose, sides of the neck, and areas surrounding the eyes.) Ochronosis was initially reported in South African females who applied hydroquinone in strong concentrations to achieve a lighter skin tone.[32] Paradoxically, hydroquinone used for overall skin lightening for a prolonged period can actually darken the skin. Researchers in the United States have reported cases in patients of black and Hispanic lineage caused by the commercially available 2% nonprescription products. For these reasons pharmacists should question dark-skinned patients carefully about their proposed use of hydroquinone-containing products.

SUMMARY

Skin hyperpigmentation may result from both serious medical conditions and conditions with little medical consequence. Three minor types of skin discoloration may be safely self-treated: solar lentigines, ephelides, and melasma resulting from pregnancy or ingestion of oral contraceptives:

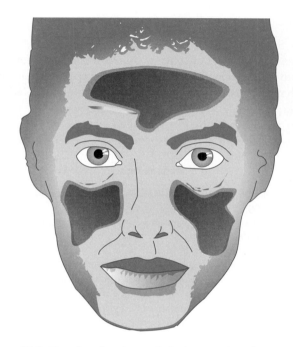

Figure 39.4. Drawing showing typical pigmentation changes with exogenous ochronosis.

AT THE COUNTER

 A pregnant female approaches the pharmacist to ask about a facial discoloration.

Interview/Patient Assessment

The pharmacist notes a uniform, brownish discoloration of the face, extending from below the jawline up to the margins of the scalp. The patient says that she has never had this problem before. She also says that this is her first pregnancy. She is taking a standard prenatal vitamin/mineral combination, and she has no medical conditions other than pregnancy.

Pharmacist's Analysis

1. Is this patient's condition self-treatable?
2. What is the prognosis of this condition?

3. What instructions should this patient be given by the pharmacist?

This patient's condition is consistent with melasma gravidarum, the "mask of pregnancy."

Patient Counseling

The pharmacist should explain that her condition may be a benign discoloration of the skin known as the "mask of pregnancy." The condition usually disappears within a few months after termination of the pregnancy and does not necessarily require treatment. However, should she wish to treat it, she may use any of several nonprescription products containing hydroquinone. The pharmacist should caution the patient to avoid exposure to the sun during treatment.

- Solar lentigines are discolorations of skin on sun-exposed areas. Strongly associated with age and ultraviolet exposure, they do not usually fade in the absence of sun exposure.
- Ephelides, or freckles, are also more likely to be found on sun-exposed areas, but generally fade in the absence of sun exposure.
- Melasma, a discoloration that may be found on the face and other areas, is caused by many factors, including genetic predisposition, ultraviolet exposure, pregnancy, or ingestion of estrogens and/or progestins. When caused by pregnancy or oral contraceptive use, it is self-treatable.

The three conditions may be helped somewhat by hydroquinone, a safe and effective nonprescription ingredient that reduces the production of melanin. Used appropriately, nonprescription products containing hydroquinone slowly fade the hyperpigmented lesions. During use, however, the patient must reduce exposure of the treated area to the sun, either through the use of sunscreens, sunblock, or protective clothing.

References

1. Hacker SM. Common disorders of pigmentation. Postgrad Med 99:177, 1996.
2. Yi K. Use of hydroquinone as a bleaching cream. Ann Pharmacother 27:592, 1993.
3. Fed Reg 43:5156, 1978.
4. Garbe C, et al. Associated factors in the prevalence of more than 50 common melanocyti nevi, atypical melanocytic nevi, and actinic lentigines: Multicenter case-control study of the Central Malignant Melanoma Registry of the German Dermatological Society. J Invest Dermatol 102:700, 1994.
5. Griffiths CEM, et al. Topical tretinoin (retinoic acid) improves melasma. A vehicle-controlled, clinical trial. Br J Dermatol 129:415, 1993.
6. Pray WS. Topical therapy of pigmented skin lesions. U.S. Pharmacist Skin Care Suppl 18(6):42, 1993.
7. Ortonne JP. Pigmentary changes of the ageing skin. Br J Dermatol 122(Suppl 35):21, 1990.
8. Bologna JL. Reticulated black solar lentigo ('ink spot') lentigo. Arch Dermatol 128:934, 1992.
9. Humphrey TR, et al. Treatment of photodamaged skin with trichloroacetic acid and topical retinoid. J Am Acad Dermatol 34:638, 1996.
10. Rafal ES, et al. Topical tretinoin (retinoic acid) treatment for liver spots associated with photodamage. N Engl J Med 326:368, 1992.
11. Gilchrest BA. A review of skin ageing and its medical therapy. Br J Dermatol 135:867, 1996.
12. Stern RS, et al. Laser therapy versus cryotherapy of lentigines: A comparative trial. J Am Acad Dermatol 30:985, 1994.
13. Andersen WK, Labadie RR, Bhawan J. Histopathology of solar lentigines of the face: A quantitative study. J Am Acad Dermatol 36(3 Pt 1):444, 1997.
14. Kopera D, Hohenleutner U, Landthaler M. Quality-switched ruby laser treatment of solar lentigines and Becker's nevus: A histopathological and immunohistochemical study. Dermatology 194:338, 1997.
15. Peter RU, et al. Radiation lentigo. A distinct cutaneous lesion after accidental radiation exposure. Arch Dermatol 133:209, 1997.
16. McLean DI, Gallagher RP. "Sunburn" freckles, cafe-au-lait macules, and other pigmented lesions of schoolchildren: The Vancouver Mole Study. J Am Acad Dermatol 32:565, 1995.
17. Grekin RC, et al. 510-nm pigmented lesion dye laser. Its characteristics and clinical uses. J Dermatol Surg Oncol 19:380, 1993.
18. Skender Kalnenas TM, English DR, Heenan PJ. Benign melanocytic lesions: Risk markers or precursors of cutaneous melanoma. J Am Acad Dermatol 33:1000, 1995.
19. Stern JB, et al. Malignant melanoma in xeroderma pigmentosum: Search for a precursor lesion. J Am Acad Dermatol 28:591, 1993.
20. Adhoute H, et al. Chromametric quantification of pigmentary changes in the solar lentigo after sunlight exposure. Photodermatol Photoimmunol Photomed 10:93, 1994.
21. Shimbashi T, Kamide R, Hashimoto T. Long-term follow-up in treatment of solar lentigo and cafe-au-lait macules with Q-switched ruby laser. Aesthetic Plast Surg 21:445, 1997.
22. Day TW, Pardue CC. Preliminary experience with a flash-lamp-pulsed tunable dye laser for treatment of benign pigmented lesions. Cutis 51:188, 1993.
23. Fritschi L, Green A. Sun damage in teenagers' skin. Aust J Public Health 19:383, 1995.
24. Holze E. Pigmented lesions as a sign of photodamage. Br J Dermatol 127(Suppl 41):48, 1992.
25. Rhodes AR, et al. Sun-induced freckles in children and young adults. Cancer 67:1990, 1991.
26. Bliss JM, et al. Risk of cutaneous melanoma associated with pigmentation characteristics and freckling: Systematic overview of 10 case-control studies. Int J Cancer 62:367, 1995.
27. Rolle F, et al. Cutaneous lentigines, freckles, and atrial myxoma (Letter). Ann Thorac Surg 59:267, 1995.
28. Cummings SR, Tripp MK, Herrmann NB. Approaches to the prevention and control of skin cancer. Cancer Metastasis Rev 16:309, 1997.
29. Maia M, Proenca NG, de Moraes JC. Risk factors for basal cell carcinoma: A case-control study. Rev Saude Publica 29:27, 1995.
30. Martin RH. Relationship between risk factors, knowledge and preventive behavior relevant to skin cancer in general practice patients in south Australia. Br J Gen Pract 45:365, 1995.
31. Errickson CV, Matus NR. Skin disorders of pregnancy. Am Fam Physician 49:605, 1994.
32. Grimes PE. Melasma. Arch Dermatol 131:1453, 1995.
33. Dominguez-Soto L, et al. Pigmentary problems in the tropics. Dermatol Clin 12:777, 1994.
34. Kimbrough-Green CK, et al. Topical retinoic acid (tretinoin) or melasma in black patients. Arch Dermatol 130:727, 1994.
35. Garcia A, Fulton JE. The combination of glycolic acid and hydroquinone or kojic acid for the treatment of melasma and related conditions. Dermatol Surg 22:443, 1996.
36. Kanwar AJ, Dhar S, Kaur S. Treatment of melasma with potent topical corticosteroids. Dermatology 188:170, 1994.
37. OBrien TJ, Dyall Smith D, Hall AP. Melasma of the forearms. Australas J Dermatol 38:35, 1997.
38. Breathnach AS. Melanin hyperpigmentation of skin: Melasma, topical treatment with azelaic acid, and other therapies. Cutis 57(1 Suppl):36, 1996.
39. Torres JE, Torres SM, Sanchez JL. Melanoma in situ on facial skin damaged by sunlight. Am J Dermatopathol 16:171, 1994.
40. Fed Reg 47:39108, 1982.
41. Coulson IH. 'Fade out' photochromonychia. Clin Exp Dermatol 18:87, 1993.

Foot Problems

A middle-aged female asks the pharmacist for help with a corn on her foot.

Interview/Patient Assessment

The pharmacist notes that patient is experiencing difficulty walking. She says that her corn is so painful that she cannot walk without a limp. She shows the pharmacist a shiny, raised protrusion between the fourth and fifth toe of the right foot. She also has a visibly inflamed bunion on that foot. In response to the pharmacist's questions, she says she is taking several medications for asthma, allergies, and hypertension.

Pharmacist's Analysis

1. Does the patient appear to have a corn?
2. What is the significance of her bunion?

3. Are corn-removal products contraindicated for this patient?

The patient appears to have a corn.

Patient Counseling

The corn is caused by pressure and friction. The bunion may have caused the great toe to become misaligned. This increased pressure on the lesser toes may have been the friction that induced the hyperkeratosis known as a corn. Corn products are contraindicated in patients with diabetes or poor circulation, but should be safe for this patient. The pharmacist should recommend use of a collodion, plaster, disk, or pad containing salicylic acid to produce a gradual desquamation of the skin. The pharmacist might also recommend helpful steps in preventing recurrence of the corn such as seeing a podiatrist for bunion surgery and purchasing shoes that allow ample room for the toes.

The foot does an incredible amount of work in an average day, carrying the weight of the body through many impacts with the ground. A 150-pound person walking just one mile forces each foot to endure a total of 60 tons of force.[1,2] A mile of running increases the force to 110 tons per foot because of the increased pressure on the foot. It is no wonder that 10% of Americans have some type of foot problem, reflected in 17 million visits yearly to physicians for foot ailments.[3] Common foot problems will be discussed—corns and calluses, bunions, blisters, hammertoes, and high arches. Occasionally, patients ask about other, less common foot problems (Table 40.1). (See "Tired Feet" and "Foot Odor.")

CORNS AND CALLUSES

The hard corn (heloma durum), soft corn (heloma molle), and callus (callosity) are all **hyperkeratoses** (excessive growths of the upper, keratinized layer) of the skin. These conditions differ from the hyperkeratoses known as warts because they are not infectious in etiology. Since the etiologies and treatments of corns and calluses are similar, they are discussed together.

PREVALENCE OF CORNS AND CALLUSES

The prevalence of corns and calluses is unknown, although they are said to be virtually universal, especially in older women.[9] Callus was present on the feet of 51% of diabetics in one study.[10]

EPIDEMIOLOGY OF CORNS AND CALLUSES

Age

Elderly patients undergo a general atrophy of **adipose** (the fatty layer) tissue; since fat cushions other tissues, its loss on the bottom of the foot increases the risk of corns.[11]

In addition, feet often become distorted with age, displacing metatarsal heads downwards. This places great pressure on the skin between that metatarsal head and the sole of the shoe, further increasing the risk of corns.

Diabetes Mellitus

Patients with diabetes may have increased incidence of calluses on the feet because of loss of sensation, which allows them to endure pressure that other patients would find uncomfortable.[12,13]

ETIOLOGY OF CORNS AND CALLUSES

The primary triggering factors in the development of corns are pressure and friction against one or more of the many bony prominences of the feet (e.g., the **condyles** [rounded surface of a bone] of the heads and bases of the metatarsals and phalanges).[11,14] Typically, corns are caused by the trauma of the shoe or another part of the foot rubbing against an area repeatedly while walking. Contributing factors are improper weight distribution and bunions, which force the great toe inwards.[15]

Pressure and friction are also responsible for calluses (and they occur in other body sites in addition to the feet). Since the upper cornified layer functions as a protective skin layer,

Table 40.1. Representative Miscellaneous Nonprescription Products and Devices for the Feet	
PRODUCT	SELECTED INGREDIENTS/COMMENTS
Fungal Nail Revitalizer	Water, calcium carbonate, PEG-8, urea, stearyl alcohol, mineral oil; cream placed on a toenail affected with fungus; a brush provided is used to scrub the nail for 1 minute; treatment produces cosmetic improvement in the foot (e.g., reduces discoloration and smoothes out the nail)
Ingrown Toenail Relief Strips	Adhesive strips with a ridge to separate the affected toenail from the skin
Toe Cap/Sleeve	Cylindrical foam cap placed over a toe to provide protection (e.g., bruised toe, toe with corn)

it responds to these minor traumas by increasing the rate at which upper cells are shed, which in turn accelerates mitotic activity of the columnar basal cells of the stratum germinativum.[15] The skin thus produces a thicker layer of keratin that is more resistant to future pressure or friction-induced trauma. A callus may result from shear stress of a prominent bone against shoewear that does not fit well when walking or from excessive standing.[16]

MANIFESTATIONS OF CORNS AND CALLUSES

Corns and calluses exhibit increased thickness of the horny layer of the skin.[11] The upper cells do not **desquamate** (shed or peel off as layers of epidermal scale) as they should, so a thicker layer of skin accumulates.

Corns

The corn causes pain when its core is pressed into the dermis by the opposing toes or footwear, much like walking with a small pebble in the shoe (Fig. 40.1).[14,17] Pain can be disabling. They range from millimeters to centimeters in diameter.[15] There are three types of corns: hard corns, soft corns, and plantar corns.

HARD CORNS

Hard corns are a **hyperkeratotic** (thickened area of the outer layer of the skin) lesion with a visible translucent central core shaped like a cone.[11,14] Hard corns are usually found on skin directly overlying a bony prominence such as the toes and bottom of the foot. (See "A Pharmacist's Journal: I've Got a Corn.") Corns can be as small as a pencil eraser or as large as a dime. The size, weight, and texture of shoes are determining factors in development of hard corns. For instance, the side of the small toe bears much of the pressure of shoes and is a common corn site.[1]

SOFT CORNS

Soft corns develop between the toes, especially the fourth and fifth toes.[11] For this reason, soft corns are also known as interdigital corns.[14,18] Soft corns appear as elevated, soft, white growths in the web spaces of the toes. Narrow shoes force the fourth and fifth toes to abut, so metatarsal bones and pha-

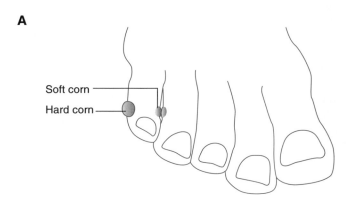

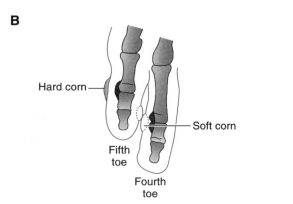

Figure 40.1. A. Common locations of hard and soft corns. **B.** Bony prominences that produce the hard and soft corn.

langes are in constant apposition, producing pressure and friction. Moisture in the area causes this corn to be soft.

PLANTAR CORNS

Corns occasionally occur on the soles of the feet. These corns, which are extremely painful, are especially common in golfers. Because of intermittent use, golfers' shoes wear slowly, but their feet change. Eventually, their shoes fit poorly, causing corns.[19]

Calluses

Calluses are superficial patches of hornified epidermis that are flattened, but thickened somewhat, lacking a central core

(Fig. 40.2).[11,14] Calluses extend slightly above surrounding skin, but taper imperceptibly toward the edges into normal skin.[20] Calluses are yellowish-white or darker. They vary widely in size because they are caused by many kinds of friction, ranging from millimeters to centimeters in diameter.[15] Calluses are usually found on areas where the upper layers of skin are naturally thick such as the soles of the feet (and palms of the hands). Skin lines proceed across the callus without interruption.[14,21]

Calluses are often found on the heel or balls of the feet, as well as other body areas where pressure is repeated (see "Calluses Related to Hobbies and Occupations").[11,22,23] Individuals with Morton's toe (a long second or third toe) may find that these toes buckle when inside shoes, forcing the metatarsal heads down and inducing calluses.[19]

Unlike corns, calluses on the bottom of the feet do not usually cause pain since they are a protective hyperkeratosis.[16] However, if calluses fissure, patients may report burning pain when ambulating. Further, they may affect the gait as the person attempts to compensate for callus pain by walking differently.[14]

PROGNOSIS OF CORNS AND CALLUSES

Corns and calluses will not disappear if left alone. Corns will continue to cause pain until removed, while calluses will continue to protect against pressure and friction as long as it is present and the contributing factors continue (e.g., poorly fitting footwear). However, in some cases, calluses may cause pain if they continue to grow. The central thicker keratin of the growing callus may cause underlying nerves to be painfully stimulated.[14] If hyperkeratosis proceeds unchecked, the plantar callus thickness eventually may

FOCUS ON...

TIRED FEET

Those whose work involves standing or walking may experience foot fatigue at the end of the workday. To prevent foot fatigue, patients may choose several cushioning products to absorb some of the shock of walking such as those in the table. Cushions placed inside the shoe may be made of foam rubber or other materials. Several manufacturers also market shoe liners that are filled with a fluid or gel to cushion the foot during ambulation.

Representative Products to Provide Cushioning for the Foot During Walking and Standing

PRODUCT	COMMENTS
Air-Pillo Insoles	Shoe inserts; men or women's, trimmed to size
BackGuard Insoles	Shoe inserts; men or women's, trimmed to size
Ball-O-Foot Cushions	Latex foam cushions with a loop placed over the second toe so that the cushion is located beneath the ball of the foot; cushions against foot shock
Donut Heel	Foam device placed under the heel to ease pain caused by heel spurs, bruises, or calluses
DynaStep Shoe/Sneaker Inserts	Shoe inserts that cup the heel and support the arch; men or women's
Gel Ball of Foot Cushion	Gel-filled cushion placed beneath the ball of the foot
Half Insoles	Thin cushion placed under the ball of the foot to absorb shock
Massaging Gel Insoles	Shoe inserts; men or women's, trimmed along an outer rim to size
Maximum Comfort Sport Replacement Insoles	Shoe inserts; men or women's, trimmed to size
Maximum Comfort Work/Casual Insoles	Shoe inserts; men or women's, trimmed to size

Tired feet may be eased with simple foot massage, warm soaks (see table), or placing the feet up on a chair at the end of the day. Several products are sold for use as foot soaking solutions, although they have not been proven to provide any benefit beyond that of plain warm water.

Representative Products to Soak the Feet

PRODUCT	SELECTED INGREDIENTS/COMMENTS
Johnson's Foot Soap	Powder packets containing soap, sodium sesquicarbonate, sodium borate, sodium bicarbonate, caramel, potassium iodide, bran, iodoform; patient creates a foot soak by placing 1 packet in 2 quarts of comfortably hot water
Soap'n Soak	Powder packets containing soap, sodium bicarbonate, sodium borate, sodium sesquicarbonate, bran, etc.; patient creates a foot soak by placing 1 packet in 2 quarts of warm water

cause tissues to become entrapped between the shoe and bony prominences. The patient then can be trapped in a vicious cycle in which the callus no longer protects the skin and in which increased shear forces can result in inflammation, hemorrhage, skin breakdown, and ulcer formation.

COMPLICATIONS OF CORNS AND CALLUSES

A greatly thickened and improperly treated callus can fissure, causing inflammation, infection, or cellulitis, especially in elderly patients (whose skin breaks down more readily).[11]

In diabetic patients, calluses allow pressure to affect underlying tissues without the patient's knowledge, as diabetic feet often lack normal sensation because of neuropathy.[16,29,30] Thus diabetic patients do not always know when they are repeatedly injuring the foot. **⚠ *Infection resulting from repeated trauma, which is especially common in diabetics, could lead to amputation.*** Bleeding within a plantar callus is also common in the diabetic.[31]

TREATMENT OF CORNS AND CALLUSES

Treatment Guidelines

Treatment of corns and calluses may be instituted with nonprescription products and devices in

many instances. However, if there is any doubt about self-treatment because of lack of assurance that the problem is actually a corn or callus, pharmacists should refer the patient to a podiatrist. (See Patient Assessment Algorithm 40.1.)

Calluses protect underlying skin from further pressure and friction.[15] Because of this, their removal may cause the underlying skin to be sensitive. For instance, removing calluses on the bottoms of the feet and toes will produce pain when walking. Reduction of the callus should be gradual, through

FOCUS ON...

FOOT ODOR

Pharmacists occasionally receive questions about foot odor. When foot odor occurs, it has been ascribed to excessive sweating, short-chain fatty acids, or certain organisms (e.g., staphylococci, aerobic corynebacterium).[4,5] The eccrine sweat glands of the foot may produce excess sweat, a condition known as hyperhidrosis.[6,7]

Patients are often acutely embarrassed by foot odor; health professionals hesitate to work with odorous feet.[8] The pharmacist can point out several sprays used to deodorize the foot or shoes, and powders to absorb moisture as shown in the table.

Representative Products to Prevent Foot and/or Shoe Odor

PRODUCT	SELECTED INGREDIENTS/COMMENTS
Desenex Foot & Sneaker Spray	Spray to stop foot odor
Medicated Powder	Cornstarch, zinc oxide, kaolin, benzethonium chloride
Odor Destroyers Deodorant Powder	Cornstarch, zinc oxide, sodium bicarbonate, kaolin
Odor Destroyers Deodorant Spray	Spray to stop foot odor
Odor Destroyers Insoles	Shoe inserts; trimmed to size
Odor-Eaters Sneaker Tamer Insoles	Shoe inserts; trimmed to size
Original Foot Powder	Powder containing talc, salicylic acid, methyl salicylate; use may cause peeling of skin

A Pharmacist's Journal

"I've Got a Corn."

A woman approached the pharmacy counter and inquired, "Can you help a corn?" I asked her to describe the corn. She said, "I've got a large swelling on the joint of my first toe." As I questioned her further, it became clear that she had a bunion. I began to explain the problem, "You appear to have a bunion. I have products to protect the bunion from shoe pressure, but you will need to see a podiatrist or physician to receive proper care for the bunion. In any case, it doesn't sound like a corn." She appeared puzzled and replied, "I know about the bunion, but I've got a corn growing on top of the bunion, and I want to get that corn off." Although I had never heard of a corn growing on a bunion, I stressed that it would be possible because of the friction against the bunion and pointed out several products useful for care of corns.

the use of mild nonprescription products, rather than files, pumice stones, or razors. Ideally, the shoes that caused the problem should be changed to prevent recurrence.

Nonprescription Medications

SALICYLIC ACID
Mechanism of Action
Salicylic acid possesses keratolytic action, which means it softens and then destroys the outer layer of skin by increasing its hydration.[15] This action is caused by lowering of the pH of outer skin, which causes it to swell, soften, and be shed.

Dosage Forms
Salicylic acid is effective for corns and calluses when formulated in flexible collodion, plasters, disks, or pads (Table 40.2).

Flexible Collodion. Flexible collodion consists of **pyroxylin** (nitrocellulose) in a mixture of ether and alcohol, along with various plasticizers such as castor oil or camphor.[15] Salicylic acid is present in a 12 to 17.6% concentration. The pyroxylin remains on the skin following evaporation of ether and alcohol, forming a flexible, water-repellent film that adheres tightly to the skin. The film retards evaporation of water from the skin, contributing to the efficacy of the formulation. Other collodion-like vehicles act in a similar manner.[32]

Patients should follow these steps for applying products formulated in flexible collodion:

1. Wash and dry the area. If desired, presoak the area in warm water for 5 minutes to facilitate proper maceration and desquamation.[33,34]
2. Apply one drop at a time or apply with a brush to cover each corn and/or callus. Do not allow the liquid to contact surrounding unaffected skin. If the product contacts healthy skin, it should be removed by wiping off immediately. *To facilitate proper application, patients with poor eyesight or various conditions that cause shaking or tremor should ask for assistance.*[35]
3. Allow product to dry.
4. Repeat the process once or twice daily for up to 14 days.

Flexible collodion is highly flammable. Containers must be kept from heat and flame and must be tightly capped to prevent evaporation. If a bottle has visible crystals, it must be discarded. *Inhaling the volatile ingredients could cause illness.*

Plasters, Disks, and Pads. Plasters, disks, or pads containing 12 to 40% salicylic acid are adhesive-backed, which facilitates proper placement over the corn or callus.[15] They also tend to cause the skin to retain moisture (although perhaps not as effectively as collodion-based products), enhancing the effect of the salicylic acid.

Patients should follow these steps for applying plasters, disks, and pads:

1. Wash and dry the area. If desired, presoak the area in warm water for 5 minutes to facilitate proper maceration and desquamation.[33,34]
2. Cut the plaster disk or pad to size, if necessary.
3. Remove the adhesive backing and apply the product to the skin.
4. Remove the product after 48 hours.
5. Repeat the procedure every 48 hours for up to 14 days.[33]

Precautions With Salicylic Acid
Salicylic acid products are absolutely prohibited for patients with diabetes—or any other patients with

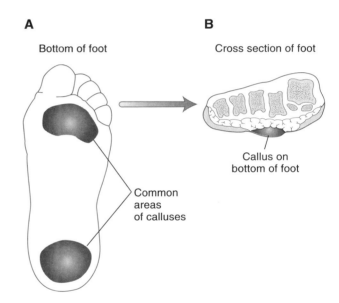

Figure 40.2. A. Typical locations of calluses (over the weight-bearing sections of the foot). **B.** Cross-section illustrating the diffuse nature of the plantar callus.

FOCUS ON...

CALLUSES RELATED TO HOBBIES AND OCCUPATIONS
Certain hobbies and occupations that subject a body part to repetitive friction and trauma will produce calluses on those parts.[24] For instance, weight lifters experience extensive calluses on the thumbs from "hooking," a practice in which thumbs are squeezed tightly between fingers and the bar.[25] Barbell pressure also produces calluses on the palms. Occupations that require sustained use of a screwdriver (e.g., electronics assembly) often cause a particular callosity on the palm.[26] Even a practice such as sustained sitting in a cross-legged position can produce callosities.[27,28] Should the pharmacist be confronted with these calluses, it is best to refer the patient to a physician for evaluation of the problem, since nonprescription callus products are only to be used on feet.

Patient Assessment Algorithm 40.1. Corns and Calluses

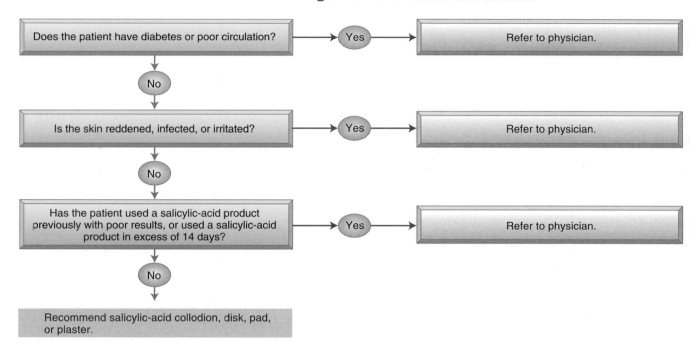

Does the patient have diabetes or poor circulation? → Yes → Refer to physician.

↓ No

Is the skin reddened, infected, or irritated? → Yes → Refer to physician.

↓ No

Has the patient used a salicylic-acid product previously with poor results, or used a salicylic-acid product in excess of 14 days? → Yes → Refer to physician.

↓ No

Recommend salicylic-acid collodion, disk, pad, or plaster.

Table 40.2. Representative Corn and Callus Products Containing Salicylic Acid

PRODUCT	SELECTED INGREDIENTS/COMMENTS
Callus Removers (Extra Thick)	40% salicylic acid disks (adhesive-backed) packaged with adhesive-backed felt covers (approx. 2″ × 1.5″ in size)
Corn Removers	40% salicylic acid disks (adhesive-backed) packaged with adhesive-backed felt covers; regular or small sizes available; regular pad is 1″ × 0.75″ in size (approx.)
Cushlin Gel Corn Removers	40% salicylic acid in a rubber-based vehicle
Freezone Corn and Callus Remover	13.6% salicylic acid liquid to remove corns and calluses
Liquid Corn/Callus Remover	12.6% salicylic acid liquid packaged with small circular adhesive-backed foam cushions to place around a corn
Mediplast	40% salicylic acid plaster; cut to size
One Step Callus Remover	40% salicylic acid in a rubber-based vehicle placed on a round medicated pad
One Step Corn Removers	40% salicylic acid in a rubber-based vehicle placed on an adhesive strip
Soft Corn Removers	40% salicylic acid disks (adhesive-backed) packaged with adhesive-backed felt covers with a central hole which encircles the corn
Ultra-Thin Corn Removers	40% salicylic acid in a rubber-based vehicle placed on a medicated pad; thinner pad for tight shoes
Waterproof Corn Removers	40% salicylic acid in a rubber-based vehicle placed on a waterproof pad that stays dry during a bath

poor circulation because reduced sensation in the foot delays awareness of skin breakdown or sepsis.[15,32,33] In one study, the consequences of seven diabetic patients who incorrectly applied salicylic acid to cure corns were reported.[36] They developed ulcers, cellulitis, necrosis, and/or abscess that required amputation in three cases and skin grafting in one.

Salicylic acid should not be applied to irritated, infected, or reddened skin.[33] If the discomfort persists after using a salicylic acid product for 14 days, the patient should see a physician or podiatrist.

If a collodion-based salicylic acid product contacts the eyes, the patient should flush with water for 15 minutes.

FIRST AID ANTISEPTICS AND/OR LOCAL ANESTHETICS

If a callus fissures, it would produce a minor wound (see Chapter 31, Minor Wounds), self-treatable with products containing first aid antiseptics or antibiotics and/or local anesthetics. (See Tables 31.7 to 31.12.) A product specifically promoted for cracked heels is Dr. Scholl's Cracked Heel Relief Cream, containing 2% lidocaine and 0.13% benzalkonium chloride.

Nonpharmacologic Therapies

In addition to nonprescription products that exert a pharmacologic effect, patients may wish to treat corns and calluses through the use of padding and mechanical removal.

MECHANICAL REMOVAL

Gentle paring, which may help manage such lesions as the soft corn, should only be attempted by a podiatrist or physician.[11] *Patients should never attempt reduction of calluses.* Pharmacists should advise patients that self-use of such drastic devices as razor blades or files to reduce the corn or callus is improper and could cause infection or hemorrhage. Table 40.3 lists several products that pharmacists should advise patients not to use. If calluses are trimmed too completely, underlying tender skin will be painful and more prone to tear.[37]

Pumice Stones

The pumice stone is a rough rock that some people rub against the skin to sand away rough spots and calluses.[14] Presoaking a callus in warm water for 20 minutes or so facilitates removal. Patients must avoid overzealous removal of skin with pumice stones. *Patients with diabetes or other circulatory problems should avoid pumice stones altogether.* Patients should be advised not to use them for corns or calluses.

Corn Files

Corn files are rough filelike tools with a handle that can be used to file away the skin of corns or calluses. Their rough texture can cause pain during this process, however. Also, patients may remove too much skin at a sitting without realiz-

ing that they are doing so. For these reasons, corn files should not be recommended.

Corn Planes

Corn planes contain a razor blade (perhaps in a curved shape). Holding the handle of the plane, the patient draws the razor blade over the corn or callus, removing a slice of epidermis with each stroke. *The patient should be cautioned against use of these products as home use of razor blades to slice skin is unsafe at best and hazardous at worst.*

PADDING

Several products are used to pad the foot and shoe to treat corns and calluses. See Table 40.4 for examples of these products.

Corn Padding

Patients may choose to apply small donut-shaped cushioned pads to corns to relieve pressure from shoes.[38] Each pad has a central hole through which the corn can protrude. These pads are also useful while a corn is being removed with salicylic acid or after a corn has been removed by a physician through paring.[17]

Moleskin adhesive padding can be cut to size to relieve pressure. If desired, patients can cut a hole in the middle of each moleskin for the corn.

To prevent corn-inducing friction, the toes can be separated with lamb's wool placed between the toes.

Callus Padding

If the callus has been reduced by a physician through paring or with salicylic acid, adhesive felt pads or foam pads can be placed around the callus to lessen the risk of recurrence. They may need to be used indefinitely.

PREVENTION OF CORNS AND CALLUSES

Proper Shoes

 A great deal can be done to prevent corns and calluses by simply choosing shoes that do not produce friction

---

Table 40.3. Representative Devices for Corn and Callus Removal Through Mechanical Means

PRODUCT	COMMENTS
Callus Reducer	Stainless steel grater-like device with a handle is rubbed across the hard skin or callus, giving an abrasive removal
Corn File	Plastic-handled file used to file off corns and small calluses
Corn Plane	Plastic-handled device with a head that accepts curved razor blades; used to cut away corns and calluses
Dual Action Swedish File	Plastic device with two abrasive surfaces (coarse or fine) and a handle to allow the patient to remove hard, callused, or rough skin
Pumice Stone: Beauty Stone	Rough stone, which is rubbed over hard or callused skin; also available as a "contoured file," which is a pumice stone with a handle

Table 40.4. Representative Devices to Provide Padding for Corns and Calluses

PRODUCT	COMMENTS
Cushlin Gel Callus Cushion	Polymer gel self-adhering cushion placed over the callus to prevent pain and discomfort
Cushlin Gel Corn Cushion	Polymer gel self-adhering cushions with a central hole placed over the corn to relieve pain
Cushlin Gel Corn Wraps	Polymer gel self-adhering cushions that encircle the toe which has a corn
Callus Cushions	Adhesive-backed foam circles placed over a callus on the foot to cushion shoe pressure
Corn Cushions	Adhesive-backed foam circles that encircle the corn to cushion shoe pressure; available in regular or small sizes; also a tapered cushion for soft corns
Foot and Shoe Padding	Adhesive-backed cloth that can be cut to size and placed on the shoe and/or foot to prevent friction
Heel Liners	Adhesive-backed liner which fits in the heel of the shoe to prevent heel slipping and rubbing
Lamb's Wool	Soft lamb's wool placed where necessary to prevent friction and pressure (e.g., between toes, atop toes)
Molefoam	Adhesive-backed, soft latex foam padding that can be cut to size
Moleskin	Adhesive-backed cotton flannel that can be cut to size and placed on the foot where pressure or friction are problematical
Moleskin Plus	Adhesive-backed cotton flannel that can be cut to size and placed on the foot where pressure or friction are problematical; softer than Moleskin; also available in a roll

or pressure on the feet.[11] Generally, shoes that are least likely to produce corns and calluses have a high toe box that is not pointed or tapered, are made from soft and malleable uppers, and have low heels. Open-toed shoes or sandals also can be effective (although patients with diabetes should not wear open-toed shoes or sandals because of the risk of injury).[1]

Shoe/Foot Padding

Tight areas of shoes may be padded with soft material such as cushioned pads or moleskin to prevent the friction that causes corns and calluses (Table 40.4).[39] Also, soft insoles can reduce the friction caused by a hard inner sole.[29] Shock-absorbing inserts relieve weight from the condyle that could result in a callus.[1]

BUNIONS

Bunions (also known as hallux valgus deformities) result from **hypertrophy** (growth beyond normal parameters) of the bone and soft tissues around the middle of the great toe.[1] As a result the large toe is abducted and rotated.[40]

PREVALENCE OF BUNIONS

The prevalence of bunions is unknown, but they are commonly seen in orthopedic practices.[41] In one study, 8% of diabetic patients had bunions.[10]

EPIDEMIOLOGY OF BUNIONS

Gender

The bunion is ten times more common in females than males, clearly the result of wearing tight shoes with high heels.[1] These shoes may exacerbate a genetic tendency to bunions by placing excessive pressure on the first metatarsal.

Age

The bunion is usually considered a condition of older patients, usually aged in the 40s to 60s and beyond.[42] However, juvenile bunions also occur.[43]

Genetics

There is usually a positive family history in patients with bunions, although some inciting factor is required to produce bunions, in most cases (e.g., tight footwear).[44]

Rheumatoid Arthritis

Patients with rheumatoid arthritis have an increased risk of bunions.[44]

Occupational Dancers

Dancers whose great toes bear much body weight tend to experience bunions more rapidly than nondancers.[45]

ETIOLOGY OF BUNIONS

While various qualities of the foot (e.g., the construction of the great toe) may predispose to bunions, tight shoes are a significant causative factor in bunion development.[40,42,46,47] Shoes that are particularly troublesome are those with a narrow toebox and elevated heel.

MANIFESTATIONS OF BUNIONS

The bunion can be exquisitely painful, limiting function and activities (Fig. 40.3).[1] Pain arises from pressure from shoes on the side of the first metatarsal head.[40,42] Bunions are most often bi-lateral, which would be expected if shoes are the primary causal factor.[46] A bunion can cause the great toe to deviate from its normal direction, so it is displaced in a lateral direction.[3]

PROGNOSIS OF BUNIONS

Left untreated, the bunion continues to cause pain when walking. It rarely proceeds to debilitate the patient completely, but can restrict normal ambulation.

TREATMENT OF BUNIONS

Treatment Guidelines

The patient with bunions should be referred to a podiatrist or physician. Pending their visit, they may find several non-prescription devices helpful in relieving pain and pressure.

Nonpharmacologic Therapies

The most common treatment for bunions is to change to shoes that provide sufficient room between the bunion and the shoe.[1] Sandals fill this requirement, as do athletic shoes that have soft and flexible toe boxes (although the diabetic should not wear sandals because of an increased risk of accidental foot trauma). Some people elect to have the front section of the shoe(s) stretched by a shoe repair shop. (It may be necessary to return several times until the desired stretch is accomplished.)

Pharmacists may recommend several bunion products (Table 40.5). A bunion guard composed of polymer gel may provide relief from bunion pain and discomfort when worn over the bunion. Patients may also place an adhesive-backed soft foam cushion around a bunion to ease the pressure of the shoe. Adhesive-backed felt pads that cover the entire bunion may provide relief.[48]

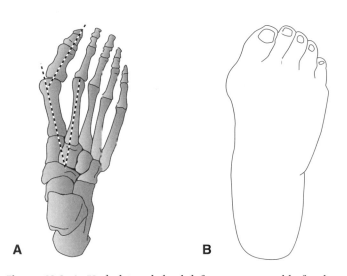

Figure 40.3. A. Underlying skeletal deformity responsible for the bunion. **B.** The appearance of the foot affected with a bunion.

Table 40.5. Representative Devices to Provide Cushioning for Bunions

PRODUCT	COMMENTS
Bunion Guard	Polymer gel self-adhering dome placed over the bunion to relieve pain and discomfort
Bunion Cushion (Felt)	Thick felt pad (adhesive-backed) that covers the bunion to relieve shoe pressure
Bunion Cushion (Foam)	Adhesive-backed foam circle placed around the bunion to relieve shoe pressure
Foot and Shoe Padding	Adhesive-backed cloth that can be cut to size and placed on the shoe and/or foot to prevent friction
Lamb's Wool	Soft lamb's wool placed where necessary to prevent friction and pressure (e.g., between toes, atop toes)
Molefoam	Adhesive-backed, soft latex foam padding that can be cut to size
Moleskin	Adhesive-backed cotton flannel that can be cut to size and placed on the foot where pressure or friction are problematical
Moleskin Plus	Adhesive-backed cotton flannel that can be cut to size and placed on the foot where pressure or friction are problematical; softer than Moleskin; also available in a roll

Table 40.6. Representative Products to Protect Blistered Skin	
PRODUCT	SELECTED INGREDIENTS/COMMENTS
New-Skin	Pyroxylin solution, alcohol 6.7%, oil of cloves, 8-hydroxyquinolone; liquid placed over blister to protect the area with a flexible covering of collodion
No Sting Skin Protectant	Acrylate terpolymer, hexamethyldisiloxane; liquid placed on irritated skin to prevent friction, forming a clear film protective barrier between the skin and the source of friction

Other Professional Treatment

Podiatrists and physicians utilize several treatments for bunions. They include splints, excision **arthroplasty** (reconstruction of a joint), **osteotomy** (removal of bone), and the use of orthotic devices to support the foot and cushion the bunion from pressure.[40,49–52]

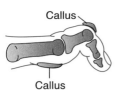

Figure 40.4. Skeletal deformity of the hammertoe and sites where calluses develop because of the increased pressure against the shoes.

BLISTERS

The blister, a fluid-filled sac that lifts the epidermis from the dermis, is a response to damage caused by mechanical friction.[37,53–55] The damage may be caused by horizontal, vertical, backward, or forward shearing frictional forces.[39] Usually, thin skin is spared of blisters because the stratum corneum cannot form a blister roof.[21]

Blisters are most commonly found on the feet, where they can inhibit ambulation.[56,57] (Blisters may also occur on the hands with certain sports such as tennis or racquet ball players.) Common causes are early season exercises, the use of new or borrowed shoes, and carrying of a poorly loaded backpack.[39,58–60] Those who wear acrylic socks may be less prone to blisters than those wearing cotton socks.[61] *If a blister is still closed, pharmacists should caution patients not to break it, since the overlying skin (roof) acts as a barrier to protect the denuded skin beneath.*[62] If a blister is open,

the skin beneath the roof may be protected with a protectant fluid (Table 40.6). Also, if a blister is located on the foot, the corresponding area of the shoe can be padded to prevent trauma. Limited research demonstrates that the use of an antiperspirant on the foot may reduce the incidence of blisters.[63]

HAMMERTOES

Occasionally, such practices as wearing fashionable footwear cause a deformity known as hammertoes, in which the distal joint of one or more toes undergoes contracture to point downwards (Fig. 40.4).[38,64,65] The second toe is at high risk when it is the longest toe. The deformity may be a permanent bilateral problem that causes pain on the tip of the distal toe and on the top of the distal joint as both areas rub

Table 40.7. Representative Products to Cushion Hammertoes	
PRODUCT	COMMENTS
Foam-Ease Hammer Toe Pad	Foam devices that slip over a toe to cushion against shoe friction and pressure
Foot and Shoe Padding	Adhesive-backed cloth that can be cut to size and placed on the shoe and/or foot to prevent friction
Lamb's Wool	Soft lamb's wool placed where necessary to prevent friction and pressure (e.g., between toes, atop toes)
Molefoam	Adhesive-backed, soft latex foam padding that can be cut to size
Moleskin	Adhesive-backed cotton flannel that can be cut to size and placed on the foot where pressure or friction are problematical
Moleskin Plus	Adhesive-backed cotton flannel that can be cut to size and placed on the foot where pressure or friction are problematical; softer than Moleskin; also available in a roll

against shoes during ambulation.[46] Hammertoes were present in 32% of diabetic patients in one study.[10]

Hammertoe pads—soft cushions that encircle the affected toe to provide comfort at the distal joint—protect a hammertoe from pressure against the shoe (Table 40.7). Also, a soft insole may reduce pressure and pain on the tip of the toe(s).[29]

HIGH ARCH

Foot shape can be described in three ways (Fig. 40.5)[40,66]:

- The neutral foot becomes rigid during walking, but is supple when at rest.
- The flatfoot remains supple as the foot attempts to push off during walking.
- The cavus foot, with a high arch, is rigid during walking and at rest.

Arch supports that aid in distributing weight are especially helpful for the cavus foot. An example of a product designed to accomplish this is the Flexo Foam Arch Support, a molded leather shoe insert that provides support for the longitudinal and metatarsal arches.

SUMMARY

Feet are constantly assailed. Walking, for example, causes repetitive pressure and friction. Occasionally, pressure and friction result in the formation of corns, which can produce pain when walking. Skin affected by repeated pressure becomes hyperkeratotic as a protective response, forming a cal-

lus. Calluses protect against pain, unless they thicken to the point of exacerbating the pressure. Various cushions and pads relieve pressure on the corn or callus. Both corns and calluses can be removed by regular application of salicylic

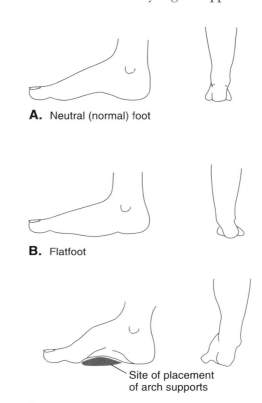

A. Neutral (normal) foot

B. Flatfoot

Site of placement of arch supports

C. Cavus foot

Figure 40.5. A. Neutral (normal) foot is rigid when walking but supple at rest. **B.** Flatfoot is supple at rest, but remains supple when attempting to walk. **C.** Cavus foot is rigid both when walking and at rest.

AT THE COUNTER

An elderly male patient asks the pharmacist whether a corn plane or corn file would help him remove a callus on the bottom of his foot.

Interview/Patient Assessment

The patient says that the callus bothers him when he walks, since it is directly under the part of the foot that he puts his weight on when he takes a step. His skin is too thick, and he wishes to file or cut it off. He is a Type 2 diabetic stabilized on Glucophage and Novolin 70/30.

Pharmacist's Analysis

1. Does the problem appear to be a callus?
2. Why do some people use corn files or corn planes on corns or calluses?

3. Should this patient be allowed to use a nonprescription product or device on his callus?

Patient Counseling

The location of the thickened skin is consistent with a callus, the area of the foot exposed to pressure and friction. Some people attempt to reduce the size of corns or calluses by filing them off with corn files or cutting them away with razor blades encased in handles known as corn planes. These products are dangerous for unsupervised use since the patient may become overzealous, causing bleeding or other skin damage. In any case, because this patient has diabetes, products used for self-treatment of foot problems are contraindicated. He should be referred to a physician or podiatrist for proper care.

acid, which is available as a collodion, or as plasters, disks, or pads. Reducing corns or calluses with planes, pumice stones, or files is potentially dangerous. *To prevent foot injury, patients with diabetes mellitus or poor circulation must not use any product or device for reduction of a corn or callus* and should be referred.

The bunion is an inflamed joint. As such, its treatment must be coordinated by a physician or podiatrist. However, pharmacists may recommend various cushioning devices to reduce pain pending medical resolution of the problem.

Blisters result from short-term pressure or friction. Blisters often occur on the foot as a result of ill-fitting footwear. Various cushioning pads or adhesive-backed cloth devices may prevent the blister. Protectant fluids form a flexible covering over the blister, easing discomfort.

Hammertoes, caused by certain footwear, may be helped with pads or cushions.

A high arch of a cavus foot may be helped by arch supports, which help distribute weight more evenly over the bottom of the foot.

References

1. Silfverskiold JP. Common foot problems. Postgrad Med 89:183, 1991.
2. Nork SE, Coughlin RR. How to examine a foot and what to do with a bunion. Prim Care 23:281, 1996.
3. Manusov EG, et al. Evaluation of pediatric foot problems. I. The forefoot and the midfoot. Am Fam Physician 54:592, 1996.
4. Kanda F, et al. Elucidation of chemical compounds responsible for foot malodour. Br J Dermatol 122:771, 1990.
5. Marshall J, Holland KT, Gribbon EM. A comparative study of the cutaneous microflora of normal feet with low and high levels of odour. J Appl Bacteriol 65:61, 1988.
6. Wenzel FG, Horn TD. Nonneoplastic disorders of the eccrine glands. J Am Acad Dermatol 38:1, 1998.
7. Manusov EG, Nadeau MT. Hyperhidrosis: A management dilemma. J Fam Pract 28:412, 1989.
8. Christensen MH, et al. Effectiveness of a foot care education program on attitudes and behaviors of staff nurses. J Contin Educ Nurs 21:177, 1990.
9. Richards RN. Calluses, corns, and shoes. Semin Dermatol 10:112, 1991.
10. Holewski JJ, et al. Prevalence of foot pathology and lower extremity complications in a diabetic outpatient clinic. J Rehabil Res Dev 26:35, 1989.
11. George DH. Management of hyperkeratotic lesions in the elderly patient. Clin Podiatr Med Surg 10:69, 1993.
12. Cavanagh PR, Ulbrecht JS, Caputo GM. Biomechanical aspects of diabetic foot disease: Aetiology, treatment, and prevention. Diabetic Med 13(Suppl 1):S17, 1996.
13. Smith DG, et al. Prevalence of radiographic foot abnormalities in patients with diabetes. Foot Ankle Int 18:342, 1997.
14. Singh D, Bentley G, Trevino SG. Callosities, corns and calluses. BMJ 312:1403, 1996.
15. Fed Reg 47:522, 1982.
16. Collier JH, Brodbeck CA. Assessing the diabetic foot: Plantar callus and pressure sensation. Diabetes Educ 19:503, 1993.
17. Omura EF, Rye B. Dermatologic disorders of the foot. Clin Sports Med 13:825, 1994.
18. Day RD, Reyzelman AM, Harkless LB. Evaluation and management of the interdigital corn: A literature review. Clin Podiatr Med Surg 13:201, 1996.
19. Sheard C. Simple management of plantar cavi. Cutis 50:138, 1992.
20. Thomas SE, Dykes PPJ, Marks R. Plantar hyperkeratosis: A study of callosities and normal plantar skin. J Invest Dermatol 85:394, 1985.
21. Samitz MH. Repeated mechanical trauma to the skin: Occupational aspects. Am J Ind Med 8:265, 1985.
22. Mann RA. Pain in the foot. Postgrad Med 82:154, 1987.
23. Colagiuri S, et al. The use of orthotic devices to correct plantar callus in people with diabetes. Diabetes Res Clin Pract 28:29, 1995.
24. Villano PA, Ruocco V, Pisani M. The cameo engraver's corn. Int J Dermatol 29:424, 1990.
25. Scott MJ Jr, Scott NI, Scott LM. Dermatologic stigmata in sports: Weightlifting. Cutis 50:141, 1992.
26. Koh D, Jeyaratnam J, Aw TC. An occupational mark of screwdriver operators. Contact Dermatitis 32:46, 1995.
27. Cox NH, Finlay AY. Crossed-leg callosities. Acta Dermatol Venereol 65:559, 1985.
28. Verbov JL, Monk CJE. Talar callosity—A little-recognized common entity. Clin Exp Dermatol 16:118, 1991.
29. Shenaq SM, Klebuc MJA, Vargo D. How to help diabetic patients avoid amputation. Postgrad Med 96:177, 1994.
30. Young MJ, et al. The effect of callus removal on dynamic plantar foot pressures in diabetic patients. Diabetic Med 9:55, 1992.
31. Rosen RC, et al. Hemorrhage into plantar callus and diabetes mellitus. Cutis 35:339, 1985.
32. Fed Reg 52:5412, 1987.
33. Fed Reg 55:33528, 1990.
34. Fed Reg 57:44493, 1992.
35. Berliner H. Aging skin. II. Am J Nurs 86:1259, 1986.
36. Foster A, et al. Corn cures can damage your feet: An important lesson for diabetic patients. Diabetic Med 6:818, 1989.
37. Cabrera JM, McCue FC III. Nonosseus athletic injuries of the elbow, forearm, and hand. Clin Sports Med 5:681, 1986.
38. Coughlin MJ. Lesser toe deformities. Orthopedics 10:63, 1987.
39. Bergfeld WF, Taylor JS. Trauma, sports, and the skin. Am J Ind Med 8:403, 1985.
40. Bordelon RL. Management of disorders of the forefoot and toenails associated with running. Clin Sports Med 4:717, 1985.
41. Scranton PE Jr, McDermott JE. Prognostic factors in bunion surgery. Foot Ankle Int 16:698, 1995.
42. Coughlin MJ. Hallux valgus. J Bone Joint Surg Am 78:932, 1996.
43. Coughlin MJ. Juvenile hallux valgus: Etiology and treatment. Foot Ankle Int 16:682, 1995.
44. Michelson J, et al. Foot and ankle problem in rheumatoid arthritis. Foot Ankle Int 15:608, 1994.
45. Quirk R. Common foot and ankle injuries in dance. Orthop Clin North Am 25:123, 1994.
46. Thompson GH. Bunions and deformities of the toes in children and adolescents. Instr Course Lect 45:355, 1996.
47. Schoenhaus HD, Cohen RS. Etiology of the bunion. J Foot Surg 31:25, 1992.

48. Holmes GB Jr. Surgical management of foot disorders: Bunions and bunionettes. Curr Opin Rheumatol 3:98, 1991.

49. Resch S. Hallux valgus. Acta Orthop Scand 67:84, 1996.

50. Canale PB, et al. The Mitchell procedure for the treatment of adolescent hallux valgus. J Bone Joint Surg Am 75:1610, 1993.

51. Baxter DE. Treatment of bunion deformity in the athlete. Orthop Clin North Am 25:33, 1994.

52. Gordon GM, Cuttic MM. Exercise and the aging foot. South Med J 87:S36, 1994.

53. Knapik JJ, et al. Friction blisters. Pathophysiology, prevention and treatment. Sports Med 20:136, 1995.

54. Reynolds K, et al. Effects of an antiperspirant with emollients on foot-sweat accumulation and blister formation while walking in the heat. J Am Acad Dermatol 33:626, 1995.

55. Buchman JS. Blistering diseases of the skin. Clin Podiatr Med Surg 13:91, 1996.

56. Dicker GD. Traumatic skin conditions in the athlete. Aust Fam Physician 17:1057, 1988.

57. Akers WA. Measurements of friction injuries in man. Am J Ind Med 8:473, 1985.

58. Patterson HS, Woolley TW, Lednar WM. Foot blister risk factors in an ROTC summer camp population. Mil Med 159:130, 1994.

59. Knapik JJ, et al. Soldier performance and strenuous road marching: Influence of load mass and load distribution. Mil Med 162:62, 1997.

60. Linko PE, Blomberg HK, Frilander HM. Orienteering competition injuries: Injuries incurred in the Finnish Jukola and Venla relay competitions. Br J Sports Med 31:205, 1997.

61. Herring KM, Richie DH Jr. Friction blisters and sock fiber composition. A double-blind study. J Am Podiatr Med Assoc 80:63, 1990.

62. Klein AW. Sports related skin problems. Compr Ther 18:2, 1992.

63. Darrigrand A, et al. Efficacy of antiperspirants. Mil Med 157:256, 1992.

64. Cracchiolo A 3rd, Kitaoka HB, Leventen EO. Silicone implant arthroplasty for second metatarsophalangeal joint disorders with and without hallux valgus deformities. Foot Ankle 9:10, 1988.

65. Oliver TP, et al. The combined hammer toe–mallet toe deformity with associated double corns: A retrospective review. Clin Podiatr Med Surg 13:263, 1996.

66. Cowan DN, et al. Consistency of visual assessments of arch height among clinicians. Foot Ankle Int 15:213, 1994.

Hair Loss

AT THE COUNTER

 A male patient in his mid 20s asks the pharmacist if Rogaine will help him.

Interview/Patient Assessment

The pharmacist asks about the patient's hair loss. The patient began to notice a receding hair line when he graduated from high school. It worsened during college and has continued since. The pharmacist notes hair loss receding symmetrically in the frontal location, as well as a thinning on the remaining areas, particularly on the **vertex** (uppermost area of the head). The patient denies use of any medication and claims to have no medical conditions. He recalls a maternal grandfather with the same pattern of hair loss, although his father has retained all of his hair.

Pharmacist's Analysis

1. What significance does symmetrical hair loss have?
2. What are the chances that all areas of hair loss will respond to minoxidil?
3. Is the family history significant?

The patient appears to have typical **androgenetic alopecia** (genetically determined hair loss caused by androgens).

Patient Counseling

The pharmacist should advise the patient that his alopecia appears to be genetic in cause (i.e., androgenetic). The family history (one generation back) and symmetrical nature of the loss are vital clues. Since he has approximately a 7-year history of loss, he is not as likely to respond to Rogaine as a patient whose loss is only recent. Further, while 26% of patients show dense-to-moderate growth, one-third of patients using Rogaine experience only minimal growth. As an alternative, the pharmacist could recommend Rogaine Extra Strength for Men.

If the patient decides to try Rogaine, the pharmacist should suggest that he apply the product in the recommended dose twice daily, using either the dropper or spray applicator. The pharmacist should advise the patient that hair growth may not be noticeable until 4 months have passed (or 2 months if the patient chooses Rogaine Extra Strength for Men). The pharmacist should also tell him that should he decide to discontinue the product, any regrown hair will gradually fall out over a 3- to 4-month period.

People have sought cosmetic relief of hair problems for many centuries. Too often, hair does not grow where it is desired or when it is desired. Head hair, in particular, has strong emotional and psychologic connections, as typified by the story of Samson and Delilah. A full head of hair automatically confers such attributes as youth, vigor, health, and power.[1,2] On the other hand, baldness can communicate sickness, fading youth and vigor, and unattractiveness.

Patients with hair loss undergo various mental stresses such as lack of self-esteem (men) or fear and anxiety about their physical appearance (women). Pharmacists are often asked about **alopecia** (loss of hair) and possible reasons for this condition. While some patients choose surgical methods to treat hair loss, pharmacists may recommend a safe and effective nonprescription ingredient.[3]

See Figure 41.1 to review the anatomy of a hair and its associated structures.

PREVALENCE OF HAIR LOSS

An estimated 23 to 87% of men in the United States experience unwanted hair loss at some time.[4] As many as one-third of females with genetic predisposition also lose hair before the age of 50.[5,6] These figures translate into as many as 40 million men and 20 million women in the United States with some type of hair loss. As a result, many millions of dollars are spent yearly to attempt to prevent hair loss and regrow lost hair.

A less common cause of hair loss, alopecia areata, affects 1% of United States residents by the age of 50.[7]

EPIDEMIOLOGY OF HAIR LOSS

Gender

Because of its etiology, hair loss has an obvious gender preference for males. Although hair loss is less common in women than men, it can nevertheless be problematic, particularly for older women.[1]

Childbirth

Recent childbirth can induce temporary female hair loss.

Weight Loss

Patients who attempt crash diets or otherwise undergo rapid weight loss may also lose hair because of inadequate protein ingestion.

ETIOLOGY OF HAIR LOSS

Hair loss can be subcategorized using several systems. One is scarring versus nonscarring hair loss[1,8]:

- Nonscarring alopecia
  —Androgenetic alopecia, also called common baldness

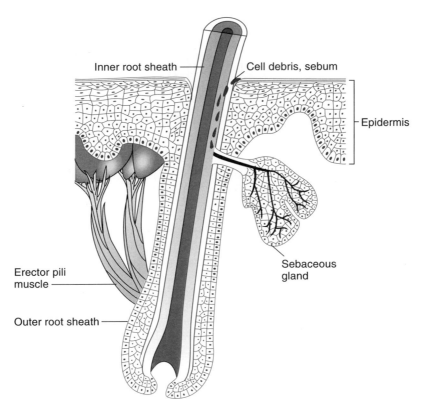

Figure 41.1. Anatomy of hair and its surrounding structures.

—Alopecia areata
- Scarring
  —Traumatic alopecia
  —Alopecia caused by tinea capitis (see Chapter 35)
  —Alopecia caused by syphilis, sarcoidosis, and lupus erythematosus.[9]

Androgenetic Alopecia

The most common type of hair loss in both sexes, androgenetic alopecia occurs in genetically predisposed individuals and is responsible for 95% of hair loss.[10–12] Androgen promotes growth of hair in the beard, axillae, pubis, and on various other parts of the body.[1] Androgens do not promote growth of scalp hair, however, but actually contribute to its premature loss.[13] An enzyme known as 5-alpha-reductase converts androgen to dihydrotestosterone. (Some patients have higher levels of 5-alpha-reductase than others, producing higher levels of dihydrotestosterone.) This chemical binds preferentially to receptors in the hair follicles on the scalp, causing them to produce progressively thinner hair, until the follicles eventually cease activity altogether.[14]

Patients with androgenetic alopecia usually have a positive family history, with the father and/or grandfather(s) and/or great-grandfather(s) with identical patterns of hair loss. Female patients should look to the mother, grandmothers, and great-grandmothers to examine their pattern of hair loss as predictive of their potential hair loss pattern.[10,15]

In approximately 5 to 10% of female patients, androgen excess produces hair patterns similar to the male, resulting in **hirsutism** (excessive hair growth) on some parts of the body (e.g., mustache, arms, nipples) and male-pattern alopecia on the scalp, causing great psychologic distress for many.[1,16–20] Female androgenetic alopecia may be categorized in three grades[11,21]:

- Grade 1: Uniform thinning over the crown with the frontal margin maintained
- Grade 2: More pronounced loss than Grade 1
- Grade 3: Total baldness of the crown, with loss on the sides but retention of the frontal margin

Alopecia Areata

Alopecia areata is a hair loss of unknown etiology, although it is sometimes associated with autoimmune diseases.[1,22–25] It is also occasionally seen in patients with Down syndrome, atopic dermatitis, vitiligo, and endocrine disease; some patients with the condition have abnormal thyroid function tests.[1,7,26,27]

Medical Conditions

Alopecia may be caused by both autoimmune diseases (e.g., systemic lupus erythematosus) and endocrine dysfunction.[1,28] Endocrine imbalances that produce alopecia include hypoparathyroidism, hypothyroidism, hyperthyroidism, and hypopituitarism.

Other physical stresses can also cause alopecia, including iron deficiency anemia; infections, often accompanied by tenderness and pruritus; and fungal infections, which can produce nonreversible hair loss if allowed to proceed to a scarring state. (See Chapter 35, Fungal Skin Infections, for a discussion of tinea capitis.)

Psychological/Psychiatric Disturbances

STRESS

Stress can induce hair loss, although the exact reason is unknown.[1] Stress hair loss can result in a vicious cycle whereby the loss of hair causes stress for the patient, which in turn accelerates the hair loss. Alopecia areata may be exacerbated by stress, especially when the stress is coupled with depressive illness.[29]

TRICHOTILLOMANIA

Trichotillomania (compulsively pulling out one's own hair), somewhat common in children, usually indicates serious psychological problems in adults such as an impulse control disorder.[1,30] Patients with trichotillomania obsessively pull hair from the scalp, eyelashes, and/or eyebrows.[11,31]

Medications/Medical Therapy

The propensity of many chemotherapeutic regimens to cause hair loss (anagen effluvium) is well-known, including medications (e.g., anticoagulants, antihyperlipidemics, zidovudine, lithium, valproate, carbamazepine, cyclophosphamide, doxorubicin), vaccinations, and radiation.[32–40]

Cosmetic Trauma

Hair-care habits can also induce alopecia.[1] Pulling the hair tightly for a sustained period, for example, as in "cornrowing" hair, creating tight ponytails, and using hot combs can contribute to hair loss.[41]

Chemical Toxicity

Occasionally, hair loss is caused by exposure to a toxic workplace chemical such as selenium, which is used in the manufacture of photocopy machine drums.[42] It may also be the result of intentional poisoning with a toxic chemical such as thallium.[43,44]

MANIFESTATIONS OF HAIR LOSS

Androgenetic Alopecia

In both males and females, androgenetic alopecia is characterized by years of gradually accelerating hair loss, with thinning in the **temporal** (over the temples) and **parietal** areas (at the sides of the head).[1] Male patients eventually may have only a horseshoe-shaped fringe of hair around the sides and back of the head.[10] Typically, female patients retain frontal hair, but lose hair over the crown (vertex).

Androgenetic alopecia usually begins in the teens in males and in the teens, 20s, or 30s in females.[5,11] By the 40s it is fully active in most cases for both men and women.

Alopecia Areata

Alopecia areata is typified by acute-onset hair loss from the scalp or other areas.[26,45] Sites may be oval or patchy, with little or no inflammation. Alopecia areata is characterized by **exclamation point hairs** (hairs that taper at the base, are narrower and shorter than normal, and can be pulled out easily because of root disorders) around the borders of the bald spot.[1,11]

SPECIFIC CONSIDERATIONS OF HAIR LOSS

Normal Hair Growth

At 8 months of gestation, **lanugo** hairs (fine fetal hairs) are replaced by **vellus** hairs (fine, nonpigmented hairs that are found on most body surfaces). During puberty, vellus hairs are replaced by terminal hairs on the scalp, pubis, axillae, and beard.

Phases of Hair Growth

Hair growth occurs in a three-phase cycle:

- Anagen phase: An active growth phase, with 85 to 90% of scalp hairs in this phase at any one time[1]
- Catagen phase: A 6-week period during which the lower follicle regresses and thins
- Telogen phase: A 2- to 4-month period during which the hair attachment thins and the hair is lost

Finally, the hair falls out (the average individual loses about 100 hairs daily) and an anagen hair emerges to begin a new cycle.[46–48]

TREATMENT OF HAIR LOSS

Treatment Guidelines

Pharmacists must ensure that patients only treat androgenetic alopecia. *Nonprescription therapy is neither safe nor effective for hair loss resulting from any cause except androgenetic alopecia.* (See Patient Assessment Algorithm 41.1.) Clues to hair loss that is not self-treatable include the following:

- Inflammation
- Erythema and scaling (indicating lupus erythematosus or fungal infection)
- Broken-off hair shafts (indicating trichotillomania or fungal infection)
- Fever/lymphadenopathy (indicating bacterial/viral infection)
- Skin lesions on other parts of the body (indicating lupus erythematosus or syphilis)

Patient Assessment Algorithm 41.1. Part 1 Hair Loss

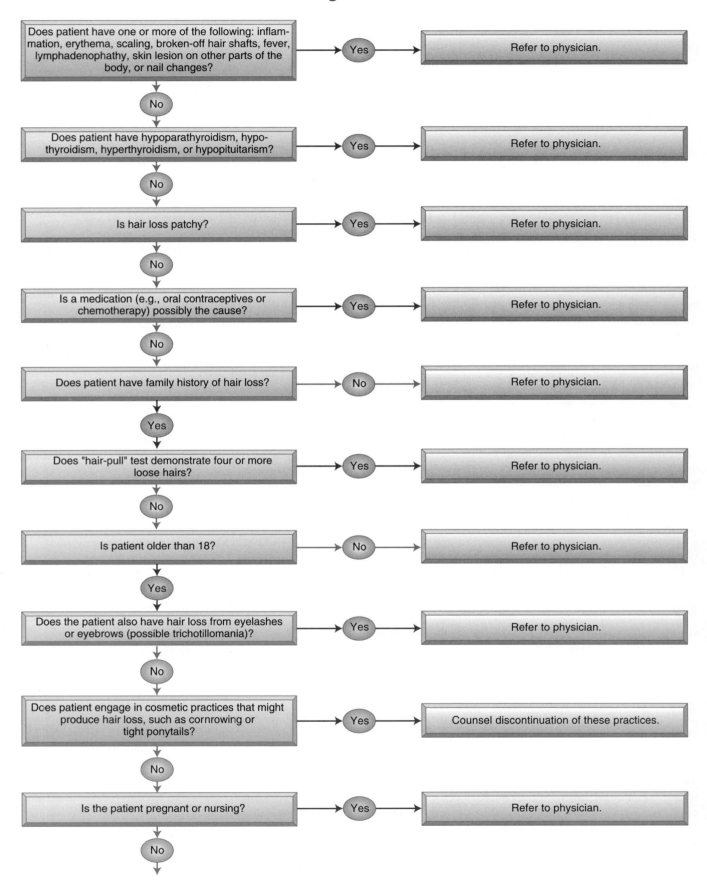

Patient Assessment Algorithm 41.1. Part 2 Hair Loss

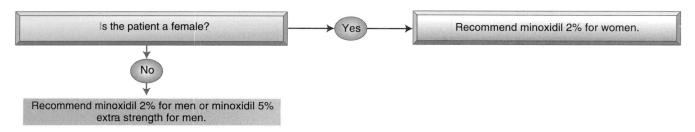

• Nail changes (indicating alopecia areata and lichen planus)

Physicians can evaluate hair loss through scalp biopsy and microscopic examination of hair shafts and bulbs.[8,49] However, pharmacists can ask patients to conduct the "hair-pull" test, in which eight to ten hairs are pulled gently.[1,50] Having one to two hairs loosen is normal, but if four or more hairs are easily removed, an abnormal condition is occurring and further diffuse hair loss will probably occur.

Nonprescription Medications

Although many products have been promoted for hair growth over the years, the FDA banned them in 1989 after extensive study.[10,51–53] In 1996 minoxidil 2% solution became the first OTC product for baldness when it was allowed to switch from Rx status. Minoxidil was also the first FDA-approved cosmetic medication.[54] The product carries the trade name Rogaine, although several generic versions are also available. In 1998 Rogaine Extra Strength for Men (minoxidil 5%) was also approved for nonprescription sales by the FDA (Table 41.1).

INDICATION

Minoxidil is approved only for androgenetic alopecia.[55] Further, it is the only agent approved for this condition.[56] *Patients with no family history of gradual thinning of hair or gradual hair loss—male or female—should be referred to a physician.* The mechanism of minoxidil is not known, but minoxidil causes an increase in cutaneous blood flow to the scalp, which may be responsible.[56]

EFFICACY

Patients will not be able to grow back all of the hair that has been lost.[57,58] Patients who respond more favorably are those who have lost hair for only a short period and those who have little hair loss.

The company sponsoring the RX-to-OTC switch (Upjohn) reported studies in which white males aged 18 to 49 with moderate hair loss used minoxidil.[57,58] Twenty-six percent experienced moderate to dense hair regrowth after 4 months of use. Another 33% experienced minimal regrowth. In females aged 18 to 45 with mild to moderate hair loss, 19% reported moderate regrowth after 8 months, and 40% had minimal regrowth.

Normal hair grows about 0.5 to 1 inch a month, so re-

growth may not become apparent until 4 months have passed with 2% minoxidil or 2 months with 5% minoxidil.[57–59] During the first 2 weeks of use, hair may continue to fall out, but eventually patients should notice soft, downy, colorless hair that eventually becomes the same color and thickness as other scalp hair. The best response may not occur until patients have used the product twice daily for 12 months (males) or 8 months (females). *Patients who do not notice new growth in 12 months (male) or 8 months (female), should discontinue using minoxidil.*[57,58] *Males using Rogaine Extra Strength for Men who do not notice results in 4 months should discontinue the product.*[60]

If patients who do have results with a minoxidil product discontinue use, hair that has been regrown or otherwise retained in the scalp because of minoxidil will fall out over a period of 3 to 4 months. Thus the patient who obtains results with Rogaine or Rogaine Extra Strength must continue using it forever to maintain growth.

USE LIMITATIONS

Minoxidil has only been proven effective for patients with gradually thinning hair or hair loss on the crown (Figs. 41.2 and 41.3). Minoxidil is not approved for frontal hair loss, nor is it appropriate for patchy hair loss, which indicates a serious condition (e.g., alopecia areata, trichotillomania) that should be seen by a physician (Fig. 41.4). Patients with hair loss caused by certain other problems (e.g., medication-induced alopecia, pregnancy, low iron stores, vitamin A excess, chemotherapy, discontinuation of oral contraceptives, hypothyroidism) also should be referred to a physician.

Minoxidil will not improve hair loss caused by hair-care products that scar or deeply burn the scalp or cosmetic practices such as cornrowing or wearing ponytails in which the hair is pulled tightly back from the scalp.

Minoxidil is more effective for younger patients and patients whose hair loss is recent.[10] Minoxidil is contraindicated for patients younger than 18 and must never be applied to babies or children with hair loss or perceived slow hair growth.[57,58] Minoxidil cannot be used to prevent hair loss.

Minoxidil 2% and 5% should be avoided in patients with an allergy to minoxidil and women who are pregnant or nursing since its effects on a fetus or infant are unknown.

Minoxidil 5% topical solution should be avoided in all women since it does not produce better results than the 2% product; women may also grow facial hair with its use.

Table 41.1. Representative Products for Hair Loss

PRODUCT	SELECTED INGREDIENTS/COMMENTS
Rogaine for Men	Minoxidil 2%, alcohol 60%, propylene glycol, purified water
Rogaine for Women	Minoxidil 2%, alcohol 60%, propylene glycol, purified water
Rogaine Extra Strength for Men	Minoxidil 5%, alcohol 30%, propylene glycol 50%, purified water
Minoxidil Topical Solution 2% for Men	Supplied by several manufacturers (e.g., Goldline, HealthGuard)

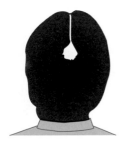

A. Mild vertex hair loss

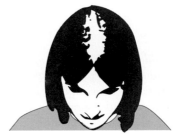

A. Mild vertex hair loss

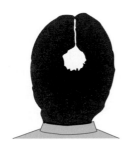

B. Moderate vertex hair loss

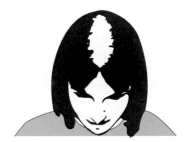

B. Moderate vertex hair loss

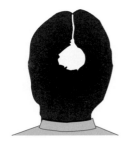

C. More advanced vertex hair loss

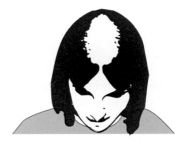

C. More advanced vertex hair loss

Figure 41.2. Typical appearance of various stages of vertex hair loss in male. If hair loss is more advanced than shown, minoxidil may not be effective.

Figure 41.3. Typical appearance of various stages of vertex hair loss in female. If hair loss is more advanced than shown, minoxidil may not be effective.

METHOD OF USE

Minoxidil is applied topically in a dose of 1 mL twice daily each day.[57,58] Typically, patients will use one 60-mL bottle each month. The product may be applied to hair without regard to shampooing, but patients who wish to shampoo before application may use any mild shampoo. *Minoxidil is absorbed over a 4-hour period. Therefore, for 4 hours after application, patients should not swim, shampoo, or walk in the rain, or otherwise wet the scalp.* Minoxidil should be allowed to become visibly dry (which will occur before the full 4-hour absorption period has passed) before styling products are applied. Further, minoxidil should be applied at least 4 hours before bedtime to avoid its being rubbed off on a pillow.

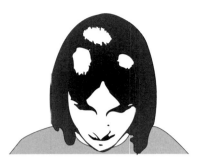

Figure 41.4. Typical appearance of patchy hair loss that should be referred to a physician.

 Patients should wash the hands after application to prevent unwanted absorption. Packages for male patients have two applicators that can be screwed onto the top of the bottle—a dropper and a sprayer. Packages for female patients have two applicators—a sprayer and extended sprayer. The extended spray attachment allows female patients to more easily reach the area beneath long hair.[58] When using the dropper, the patient simply fills it to the indicated 1-mL mark on the dropper. When using the spray attachments, a patient pumps the applicator six times to deliver 1 mL. *Patients should not inhale the mist to prevent pulmonary deposition and possible systemic absorption.*

Minoxidil should not be applied more often than the twice-daily dose, even if patients miss doses. Applying the product more frequently (or in higher quantities) does not appear to speed up hair growth and can increase the incidence of adverse reactions.

ADVERSE REACTIONS

Topical minoxidil is a safe medication for the majority of users.[54] The alcoholic vehicle may cause burning or irritation of sensitive skin or the eyes. *It should not be applied to skin that is infected, irritated, red or inflamed, or painful to touch (e.g., sunburned).* Occasionally, patients experience pruritus, dryness, and flaking or scaling. Local irritation or irritant dermatitis does not usually require discontinuation. Minoxidil rarely produces allergic contact dermatitis, although the propylene glycol in the formulation can produce this reaction.[61] The 5% solution is more likely to produce scalp irritation than the 2% solution.

Pharmacists should caution patients to stop the use of minoxidil and contact a physician if any of the following symptoms occur:

- Chest pain
- Rapid heartbeat
- Faintness and/or dizziness
- Sudden, unexplained weight gain
- Swollen hands or feet
- Redness or irritation on treated scalp areas

Although tachycardia and palpitations are rare adverse reactions, minoxidil should be recommended only with caution for patients with cardiac diseases.[62,63] If applied excessively or to areas other than the scalp, minoxidil may cause localized **hypertrichosis** (excessive hair growth) or generalized hypertrichosis.[64] Should the patient experience generalized hypertrichosis, likely sites are the chest, forearms, ear rim, back, and face.[54] The hair growth is asymmetric.

SUMMARY

Patients may wish to grow hair in locations where it has been lost prematurely. Hair growth can only be attempted for androgenetic alopecia, a hair loss caused by the action of an-

AT THE COUNTER

 A female patient who appears to be in her 30s asks the pharmacist whether Rogaine 5% solution is available for women.

Interview/Patient Assessment

The pharmacist asks the patient about her problem; she has noticed the hair on the top of her head thinning out for the past several years. Her mother also experienced the problem. She is not taking any medications and has no disease conditions.

Pharmacist's Analysis

1. What is the most likely cause of this patient's hair loss?
2. Should the patient be advised to use minoxidil 5% topical solution?

3. What nonprescription product(s) are available for her hair loss?

The patient appears to have typical female androgenetic alopecia.

Patient Counseling

The patient should be advised that her alopecia appears to be from genetic causes. However, she should be advised against use of the topical 5% minoxidil. Its action is no better than the 2% in females. Further, it may grow facial hair. Rather, she should be urged to purchase the 2% topical solution packaged for females. The pharmacist should demonstrate the use of the spray and extended spray attachments. The pharmacist should also urge her to continue use twice daily as directed, despite the fact that she may not see results for 8 months.

drogens. Hair loss from other causes such as alopecia areata, trichotillomania, cosmetic practices, or medications cannot be self-treated.

Androgenetic alopecia is treated with topical minoxidil solution, 2% or 5%, which produces results in up to 40% of patients. Once therapy with minoxidil is begun, however, treatment must continue or the hair will gradually fall out. The product must be used properly or the patient can experience adverse reactions such as chest pain, rapid heartbeat, faintness, dizziness, sudden weight gain, swollen hands or feet, and redness or irritation of treated areas.

References

1. Nielsen TA, Reichel M. Alopecia: Diagnosis and management. Am Fam Physician 51: 1513, 1995.
2. Harris MB. Growing old gracefully: Age concealment and gender. J Gerontol 49:P149, 1994.
3. Stough DB, Miner JE. Male pattern alopecia. Surgical options. Dermatol Clin 15:609, 1997.
4. Bergfeld WF. Androgenetic alopecia: An autosomal dominant disorder. Am J Med 98(1A):95S, 1995.
5. DeVillez RL, et al. Androgenetic alopecia in the female. Arch Dermatol 130:303, 1994.
6. Rushton DH. Management of hair loss in women. Dermatol Clin 11:47, 1993.
7. Sahn EE. Alopecia areata in childhood. Semin Dermatol 14:9, 1995.
8. Templeton SF, Santa Cruz DJ, Solomon AR. Alopecia: Histologic diagnosis by transverse sections. Semin Diagn Pathol 13:2, 1996.
9. Takahashi H, et al. Sarcoidosis presenting as a scarring alopecia: Report of a rare cutaneous manifestation of systemic sarcoidosis. Dermatology 193:144, 1996.
10. Hanover L. Hair replacement. FDA Consumer 31(3):7, 1997.
11. Callan AW, Montalto J. Female androgenetic alopecia: An update. Australas J Dermatol 36:51, 1995.
12. Roberts JL. Androgenetic alopecia in men and women: An overview of cause and treatment. Dermatol Nurs 9:379, 1997.
13. Walsh DS, et al. Improvement in androgenetic alopecia (stage V) using topical minoxidil in a retinoid vehicle and oral finasteride. Arch Dermatol 131:1373, 1995.
14. Sawaya ME, Price VH. Different levels of 5-alpha-reductase type I and II, aromatase, and androgen receptor in hair follicles of women and men with androgenetic alopecia. J Invest Dermatol 109:296, 1997.
15. Rubin MB. Androgenetic alopecia. Battling a losing proposition. Postgrad Med 102:129, 1997.
16. Derman RJ. Androgen excess in women. Int J Fertil Menopausal Stud 41:172, 1996.
17. Redmond GP. Androgenic disorders of women: Diagnosis and therapeutic decision making. Am J Med 98(1A):120S, 1995.
18. Pucci E, Petraglia F. Treatment of androgen excess in females: Yesterday, today and tomorrow. Gynecol Endocrinol 11:411. 1997.
19. Sawaya ME. Clinical updates in hair. Dermatol Clin 15:37, 1997.
20. Whiting DA. Chronic telogen effluvium: Increased scalp hair shedding in middle-aged women. J Am Acad Dermatol 35:899, 1996.
21. Wong WM. Minoxidil use in female alopecia. Ann Pharmacother 28:890, 1994.
22. Dressel D, et al. Alopecia areata but not androgenetic alopecia is characterized by a restricted and oligoclonal T-cell receptor-repertoire among infiltrating lymphocytes. J Cutan Pathol 24:164, 1997.
23. McDonagh AJ, Messenger AG. The aetiology and pathogenesis of alopecia areata. J Dermatol Sci 7(Suppl):S125, 1994.
24. McDonagh AJ, Messenger AG. The pathogenesis of alopecia areata. Dermatol Clin 14:661, 1996.
25. Tobin DJ, et al. Antibodies to hair follicles in alopecia areata. J Invest Dermatol 102:721, 1994.
26. Schwartz RA, Janniger CK. Alopecia areata. Cutis 59:238, 1997.
27. Puavilai S, et al. Prevalence of thyroid diseases in patients with alopecia areata. Int J Dermatol 33:632, 1994.
28. Yell JA, Mbuagbaw J, Burge SM. Cutaneous manifestations of systemic lupus erythematosus. Br J Dermatol 135:355, 1996.
29. Gupta MA, Gupta AK, Watteel GN. Stress and alopecia areata: A psychodermatologic study. Acta Dermatol Venereol 77:296, 1997.
30. Christenson GA, Crow SJ. The characterization and treatment of trichotillomania. J Clin Psychiatry 57(Suppl 8):42, 1996.
31. Trueb RM, Cavegn B. Trichotillomania in connection with alopecia areata. Cutis 58:67, 1996.
32. Hopkins SJ. Investigating drug induced alopecia. Nurs Stand 7:38, 1993.
33. Sitzia J, Hughes J, Sobrido L. A study of patients' experiences of side-effects associated with chemotherapy: Pilot stage report. Int J Nurs Stud 32:580, 1995.
34. Prussick R. Adverse cutaneous reactions to chemotherapeutic agents and cytokine therapy. Semin Cutan Med Surg 15:267, 1996.
35. Geletko SM, Segarra M, Mikolich DJ. Alopecia associated with zidovudine therapy. Pharmacotherapy 16:79, 1996.
36. McKinney PA, Finkenbine RD, DeVane CL. Alopecia and mood stabilizer therapy. Ann Clin Psychiatry 8:183, 1996.
37. Pickard Holley S. The symptom experience of alopecia. Semin Oncol Nurs 11:235, 1995.
38. Wise RP, Kiminyo KP, Salive ME. Hair loss after routine immunizations. JAMA 278:1176, 1997.
39. Martin F, et al. Side-effects of intravenous cyclophosphamide pulse therapy. Lupus 6:254, 1997.
40. Tosi A, et al. Drug-induced hair loss and hair growth. Incidence, management and avoidance. Drug Saf 10:310, 1994.
41. Nicholson AG, et al. Chemically induced cosmetic alopecia. Br J Dermatol 128:537, 1993.
42. Srivastava AK, et al. Generalized hair loss and selenium exposure. Vet Hum Toxicol 37:468, 1995.
43. Herrero F, et al. Thallium poisoning presenting with abdominal colic, paresthesia, and irritability. J Toxicol Clin Toxicol 33:261, 1995.
44. Meggs WJ, et al. Thallium poisoning from maliciously contaminated food. J Toxicol Clin Toxicol 32:723, 1994.
45. Shapiro J. Alopecia areata. Dermatol Clin 11:35, 1993.
46. Courtois M, et al. Hair cycle and alopecia. Skin Pharmacol 7:1, 1994.
47. Rebora A. Telogen effluvium. Dermatology 195:209, 1997.
48. Sawaya ME. Biochemical mechanisms regulating human hair growth. Skin Pharmacol 7:1, 1994.
49. Courtois M, et al. Ageing and hair cycles. Br J Dermatol 132:86, 1995.

50. Rietschel RL. A simplified approach to the diagnosis of alopecia. Dermatol Clin 14:691, 1996.

51. Fed Reg 45:73955, 1980.

52. Fed Reg 50:2190, 1985.

53. Fed Reg 54:28772, 1989.

54. Savin RC, Atton AV. Minoxidil. Dermatol Clin 11:55, 1993.

55. Jacobs JP, Szpunar CA, Warner ML. Use of topical minoxidil therapy for androgenetic alopecia in women. Int J Dermatol 32:758, 1993.

56. Sasson M. Status of medical treatment for androgenetic alopecia. Int J Dermatol 32:701, 1993.

57. Trade Package, Rogaine for Men: 1996.

58. Trade Package, Rogaine for Women: 1996.

59. Shrank AB. Minoxidil lotion over the counter. BMJ 311:526, 1995.

60. Trade Package, Rogaine Extra Strength for Men: 1998.

61. Ebner H, Muller E. Allergic contact dermatitis from minoxidil. Contact Dermatitis 32:316, 1995.

62. Karam P. Topical minoxidil therapy for androgenic alopecia in the middle east. Int J Dermatol 32:763, 1993.

63. Baral J. Concerns about medical treatment for androgenetic alopecia (Letter). Int J Dermatol 33:600, 1994.

64. Gonzalez M, et al. Generalized hypertrichosis after treatment with topical minoxidil. Clin Exp Dermatol 19:157, 1994.

Unwanted Hair

Unwanted hair is not a medical condition per se, but in some societies hair is not considered cosmetically acceptable in certain locations. Pharmacists can advise patients who ask about hair removal on the use of several nonprescription products and therapies, in addition to professional treatments.

EPIDEMIOLOGY OF UNWANTED HAIR

The epidemiology of unwanted hair can be addressed by reviewing the instances in which hair removal is desired in patients with normal hair growth.

Style-Conscious Patients

Unwanted hair may interfere with personal and work activities, but the major reason for removal of hair is cosmetic.[1] Depending on the culture in which one was reared, it is often considered desirable to see certain areas of the body denuded of hair (Fig. 42.1). For example, typical American women wish to remove normal hair growth from their underarms and legs. Should hair appear on the upper lip, chin, or nipples, it too is often removed. The bikini line is also a popular target for removal.

Typical American men remove some or all of the facial and frontal neck hair. In addition, some men remove chest and back hair, particularly if they engage in such events as bodybuilding competitions.

Surgery Patients

Shaving operative areas began in the late eighteenth century.[2] At that time physicians thought that wounds would heal more rapidly if hair was not allowed to enter the wound site and suture areas. Later, however, physicians determined that shaving with a razor increases infection rates by a factor of 10.[3–5] In current preoperative skin preparation, hair is only removed from operative areas if it will interfere with bring-

ing the wound edges together.[6–8] For example, hair would be problematic in an especially hirsute patient whose wound must be stapled or sutured. Removal of hair from the staple or suture area would facilitate placement of the staples/sutures. A common example of an operative procedure requiring grafting is coronary artery bypass grafting in which the chest of the male must be shaved.[9]

ETIOLOGY OF UNWANTED HAIR

The etiology section does not describe situations in which patients simply wish to remove normal hair, as discussed in "Epidemiology of Unwanted Hair" above. Rather, this section focuses on conditions that cause abnormal hair growth.

Medical Conditions

Several medical conditions cause hirsutism for which the patient may seek relief from nonprescription products. The pharmacist should refer patients in whom hair growth is rapid, especially the female who may be experiencing polycystic ovary syndrome or an ovarian tumor.[10]

HYPERANDROGENEMIA
Excess androgens can cause hirsutism, usually resulting in a rapid hair growth.[11,12] In most patients the cause of the hyperandrogenemia is polycystic ovary syndrome, which is the most common overall cause of female hirsutism.[11,13–15] However, hyperandrogenemia is rarely caused by an adrenal tumor, hyperinsulinism, or congenital adrenal hyperplasia. Hyperandrogenemia may also result in anovulation, irregular menses, and Type 2 diabetes mellitus.[12]

TUMORS
Hirsutism may be caused by an ovarian or adrenal tumor in which an unusually rapid hair growth is noticed.[11,16,17]

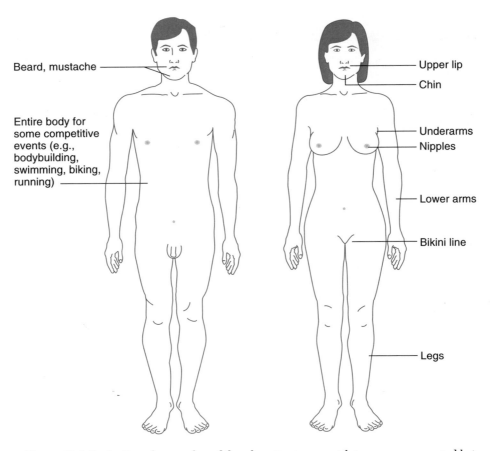

Figure 42.1. Body sites where male and female patients may wish to remove unwanted hair.

CUSHING'S SYNDROME

Hirsutism may be caused by Cushing's syndrome.[11]

Medication-Induced Hair Growth

Excess hair growth may be induced by administration of testosterone, danazol, corticotropin (ACTH), anabolic steroids, glucocorticoids, diazoxide, cyclosporine, and minoxidil (see Chapter 41, Hair Loss).[18]

TREATMENT OF UNWANTED HAIR

Treatment Guidelines

Chemicals and waxes used to remove hair are not handled by the regular FDA OTC agency but rather by the Office of Cosmetics and Colors in the FDA Center for Food Safety and Applied Nutrition (Table 42.1).[19] Thus these depilatories are strictly classified as cosmetics, despite the fact that they alter body hair and can produce adverse reactions. (See Patient Assessment Algorithm 42.1.)

Nonprescription Medications: Depilatories

Depilation is a term for removal of hair at the surface. Chemicals that accomplish depilation are known as depilatories.

MECHANISM OF ACTION

Depilatories contain highly alkaline chemicals such as calcium or sodium thioglycolate (pH of 11.5 to 12.5).[2,19] Applied in the form of gels, lotions, creams, aerosols, or roll-ons, these chemicals dissolve the protein structure of hair. After a short period (usually 4 to 15 minutes) hair becomes a mass of dissolved gel that is easily removed from the skin.

ADVANTAGES OF CHEMICAL DEPILATION

Studies comparing different methods of hair removal demonstrate that depilatories do not cause visible injuries, unlike other methods (e.g., clippers, shaving).[2] Chemical depilation is also the most efficient and rapid hair removal method. The labor and time saved through their use can make up for the greater expense in use of chemical depilatories. Chemical depilation does not increase the microflora of the skin, unlike shaving.[20,21]

ADVERSE REACTIONS

Depilatories cannot discriminate between skin and hair. If the patient fails to follow directions, the product can produce irritant contact dermatitis or chemical burns, manifested as erythema, vesicle formation, and perhaps open, weeping lesions.[19,22,23] This is especially common when they are used to denude genital hair, as the genital region is more sensitive to irritation than many other body sites. *Patients*

Table 42.1. Representative Depilatories[a]

PRODUCT	SELECTED INGREDIENTS/COMMENTS
Nair Roll-On Hair Remover	Calcium thioglycolate, sodium thioglycolate, mineral oil, calcium hydroxide, cetearyl alcohol
Nair Lotion with Baby Oil	Calcium thioglycolate, sodium thioglycolate, mineral oil, calcium hydroxide, cetearyl alcohol
Nair Warm Wax Hair Remover Kit	Rosin, wax, paraffin; product is heated before application
Neet Hair Remover Lotion	Mineral oil, cetearyl alcohol, ceteareth 20, calcium hydroxide, thioglycolic acid, sodium hydroxide
Neet Cream	Potassium thioglycolate, urea, cetearyl alcohol, calcium hydroxide
Hair Off Mitten	Mitten that fits over the hand; claims to remove hair by massaging with the mitten
Sally Hansen Brush-on Facial Hair Remover	Calcium hydroxide, calcium thioglycolate
Sally Hansen Gel Hair Remover	Sodium thioglycolare, potassium thioglycolate
Sally Hansen Hair Remover Wax Strip Kit	Wax strips that are pressed on and then peeled off to remove hair
Sally Hansen Lotion Hair Remover	Calcium hydroxide, calcium thiogycolate, mineral oil
Sally Hansen Natural Cold Wax Hair Remover Kit	Imidazolidinyl urea; soft wax that is pressed over the hair

[a]Manufacturers of depilatories seldom include concentrations of active ingredients.

Patient Assessment Algorithm 42.1. Unwanted Hair

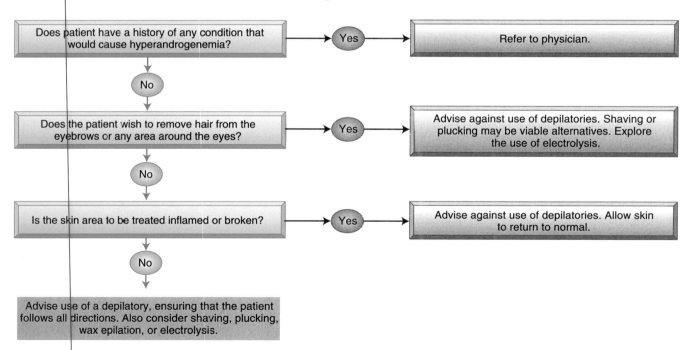

should carry out a preliminary skin test to ensure that they are not unusually sensitive or allergic to a depilatory. Patients also should only use products labeled for the specific site to be treated. Higher concentrations are only safe for the legs, while lower concentrations are used for underarms, the face, and the bikini line. *Depilatories should not be applied to the eyebrows or any other area around the eyes or to inflamed or broken skin.*[19]

Because of the risk of skin irritation, most patients are best advised to continue to shave routine areas where hair removal is desired (e.g., the beard for males and the legs and underarms for females).

Nonpharmacologic Therapies

SHAVING

Millions of Americans shave unwanted hair each day.[19] Common shaving sites include the beard area for males and the underarms and legs in females.

When used for presurgical hair removal, razors can cause gross skin cuts, multiple slices that occur in a perpendicular orientation relative to the line of the blade.[2] Shaving also predisposes the patient to contact dermatitis through creating small wounds that allow penetration by allergenic substances.[24] Shaving also alters the patient's body image.[25] Razor shaving is also associated with a higher postoperative wound-infection rate.[9] Being shaved in a barbershop can transmit hepatitis A and B.[26]

Despite these drawbacks, patients report that shaving is the most helpful and frequent method of hair removal used.[1] Shaving does not speed growth of hair or change its color or texture, despite myths to the contrary.[27]

CLIPPERS

Clippers (both manual and electric) are occasionally used to remove hair prior to surgery, but can nip loose skin, causing minor wounds.[2] Nevertheless, they are efficient for heavy hair growth and cause less postoperative wound infections than shaving.[9]

PLUCKING

Plucking, or epilation, removes hair from below the surface. Plucking yields a longer effect than depilation via chemicals or shaving, with new growth from the root not visible until several weeks.[19] Most females pluck to shape eyebrows or remove facial hair, although removal of individual hairs with tweezers is not well tolerated by many women who use it because of the minor pain it produces.

Plucking may produce such adverse effects as hyperpigmentation, scarring, ingrown hairs, and distorted follicles.[1,27] Also, hair shafts commonly fracture during plucking, which increases the incidence of adverse reactions.

WAX

Waxing has a great variation of hair-removal efficiency, with some sites responding better than others.[27] A painful method of epilation, waxing is usually used by women for the eyebrows, chin, and upper lip, although it may also be used for the bikini line, legs, and underarms.[19] Males may wax to remove chest or back hair for body building competitions.

Patients may purchase hot or cold waxes:

- Hot waxes (e.g., Zip Wax) require the patient to apply a thin layer of heated wax to the skin after fluffing the hair up. The hair is embedded in the wax as it cools.
- With cold waxes the patient applies strips that are precoated with wax, eliminating the heating step.

After the wax hardens with hot wax or immediately after application with cold wax, the patient pulls it from the skin, along with the mass of hair trapped in it. Referred to as "mass plucking," waxing is quite painful. Patients should pretreat a small area of skin to ensure that unusual sensitivity or allergic reactions do not occur.

Waxes should not be used by patients with diabetes mellitus or circulatory problems, as they may irritate the skin and cause infection.[19] Also, waxes should not be applied to skin that has moles or warts or over varicose veins. Patients should not apply waxes to the eyelashes, inside the nose or ears, on nipples or the genital areas, or to irritated, sunburned, chapped, or injured skin as they may cause damage to the more sensitive epidermis or mucous membranes in these areas.

Other Professional Treatment

ELECTROLYSIS

Electrolysis is a professional method of hair removal. (Electrolysis requires from 120 to 1100 hours of training.[19,28] Thirty-one states require licensing to practice.[27]) Electrologists use two methods to remove hair:

- Galvanic electrolysis—Multiple or single needles are inserted into each hair follicle, after which direct electric current is connected to the needle for a minute or more. Electricity reacts with tissue saline to produce caustic sodium hydroxide, which destroys the hair bulb. Despite its slowness, it is the most effective electrolysis method (Fig. 42.2).
- Thermolysis (diathermy, high radio frequency, shortwave)—High-frequency, alternating current is conducted through needles to generate heat that destroys the hair bulb in only a few seconds.[29] Thermolysis is not as consistently effective as galvanic electrolysis and does not work well for thick hairs.

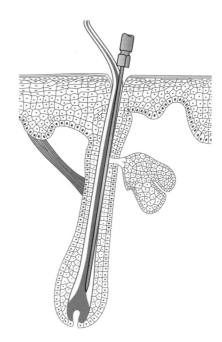

Figure 42.2. Cross-section of hair follicle illustrating insertion of an electrolysis needle.

AT THE COUNTER

A female patient appearing to be in her late teens asks about a hair removal product containing calcium thioglycolate.

Interview/Patient Assessment

The patient has become increasingly self-conscious about hair appearing on her body. She asks whether the product is appropriate for the upper lip, underarms, legs, and bikini lines. She wants to know if the product is safe for use in all of those areas.

Pharmacist's Analysis

1. What precautions are associated with calcium thioglycolate?
2. Is this type of product appropriate for all body areas?
3. What alternative methods of hair removal might she use?

Patient Counseling

Alkaline products containing calcium thioglycolate safely remove hair by dissolving its protein structure within 4 to 15 minutes after application. The pharmacist should advise the patient to carefully follow the directions regarding the time of exposure and other ancillary precautions. The products can produce irritant contact dermatitis in sensitive regions, so the pharmacist should caution her to use care with bikini line growth and to avoid the eyebrows, areas around the eyes, and any inflamed or broken skin. The pharmacist should suggest that she consider shaving or electrolysis as an alternative for her bikini lines. Also, the pharmacist should explain that the upper lip might also be more appropriately treated with a permanent method of removal such as electrolysis.

Many electrologists use a "blend" method, combining both galvanic electrolysis and thermolysis.[30]

Electrolysis is popular among female patients for removal of female facial hair. Unfortunately, the face contains 730 follicles per square centimeter, making hair removal a lengthy process. Further, sensitivity of areas such as the upper lip limits acceptance. Electrolysis can cause postprocedure erythema; occasionally, wheals, bruising, and edema occur.

Electrolysis requires a series of appointments. A forearm may require weekly visits for an entire year to catch hair in different phases of the growth cycle.[19] Male patients use it for hair between the eyebrows and around the outside of the ears and the shoulders. Female patients prefer to treat the lip, chin, eyebrows, neck, bikini line, abdomen, breasts, forearms, and underarms.

LASER

The FDA approved the first laser for hair removal in 1995. As a prescription device, the technique of argon laser ablation is restricted to use under a physician's care.[19,31]

SUMMARY

Patients may wish to remove hair from locations where it is considered to be cosmetically unacceptable. Also, in some cases operative areas are shaved. Some patients have hair growth caused by medical conditions or the ingestion of prescription medications.

Patients who wish to remove unwanted hair may use several interventions. Products containing alkaline chemicals such as calcium, sodium, or potassium salts of thioglycolate will dissolve the protein structure of hair, forming an easily

removed gel. Shaving can cause skin wounds and can increase the risk of infections. Plucking can produce hyperpigmentation, scarring, ingrown hairs, and distorted follicles. Waxing is painful and should be avoided around or on the eyelashes, genitals, nipples, and inside the nose or ears. Electrolysis, a permanent method of hair removal, can be a lengthy process.

References

1. Richards RN, Uly M, Meharg G. Temporary hair removal in patients with hirsutism: A clinical study. Cutis 45:199, 1990.
2. McIntyre FJ, McCloy R. Shaving patients before operation: A dangerous myth? Ann R Coll Surg Engl 76:3, 1994.
3. Rojanapirom S, Danchaivijitr S. Pre-operative shaving and wound infection in appendectomy. J Med Assoc Thai 75(Suppl 2):20, 1992.
4. Kovach T. Nip it in the bud. Controlling wound infection with preoperative shaving. Today's OR Nurse 12:23, 1990.
5. Winston KR. Hair and neurosurgery. Neurosurgery 31:320, 1992.
6. Braun V, Richter HP. Shaving the hair—Is it always necessary for cranial neurosurgical procedures? Acta Neurochir 135:1, 1995.
7. Viney C, Cheater F. Pre-operative shaving in gynaecology. Nurs Stand 7:25, 1992.
8. Ilankovan V, Starr DG. Preoperative shaving: Patient and surgeon preferences and complications for the Gillies incision. J R Coll Surg Edinb 37:399, 1992.
9. De Geest S, et al. Clinical and cost comparison of three postoperative skin preparation protocols in CABG patients. Prog Cardiovasc Nurs 11:4, 1996.
10. Marshburn PB, Carr BR. Hirsutism and virilization: A systematic approach to benign and potentially serious causes. Postgrad Med 97:99, 1995.

11. Sakiyama R. Approach to patients with hirsutism. West J Med 165:386, 1996.

12. Dumesic DA, Herrmann RR, OBrien AM. Estimated prevalence of undiagnosed glucose intolerance from hyperandrogenic anovulation among women requesting electrolysis. Int J Fertil Womens Med 42:255, 1997.

13. Barth JH. Investigations in the assessment and management of patients with hirsutism. Curr Opin Obstet Gynecol 9:187, 1997.

14. Kalve E, Klein JF. Evaluation of women with hirsutism. Am Fam Physician 54:117, 1996.

15. Knochenhauer ES, Azziz R. Advances in the diagnosis and treatment of the hirsute patient. Curr Opin Obstet Gynecol 7:344, 1995.

16. Gilchrist VJ, Hecht BR. A practical approach to hirsutism. Am Fam Physician 52:1837, 1995.

17. Young R, Sinclair R. Hirsutes. I. Diagnosis. Australas J Dermatol 39:24, 1998.

18. Tosi A, et al. Drug-induced hair loss and hair growth. Incidence, management and avoidance. Drug Saf 10:310, 1994.

19. Segal M. Hair today, gone tomorrow. FDA Consumer 30(7):21, 1996.

20. Jaffray B, et al. Bacterial colonization of the skin after chemical depilation. J R Coll Surg Edinb 35:243, 1990.

21. Benmeir P, et al. Stitch removal from hair-bearing areas: A simple method. Ann Plast Surg 26:604, 1991.

22. Gaffoor PMA. Sexually induced dermatoses. Cutis 57:252, 1996.

23. Keira T, et al. Adverse effects of colophony. Ind Health 35:1, 1997.

24. Edman B. The influence of shaving method on perfume allergy. Contact Dermatitis 31:291, 1994.

25. Price B. Dignity that must be respected. Body image and the surgical patient. Prof Nurse 8:670, 1993.

26. Mele A, et al. Beauty treatments and risk of parenterally transmitted hepatitis: Results from the hepatitis surveillance system in Italy. Scand J Infect Dis 27:441, 1995.

27. Richards RN, Meharg GE. Electrolysis: Observations from 13 years and 140,000 hours of experience. J Am Acad Dermatol 33:662, 1995.

28. Wagner RF Jr. Medical and technical issues in office electrolysis and thermolysis. J Dermatol Surg Oncol 19:575, 1993.

29. Wagner RF Jr. Physical methods for the management of hirsutism. Cutis 45:319, 1990.

30. Urushibata O, Kase K. A comparative study of axillar (sic) hair removal in women: Plucking versus the blend method. J Dermatol 22:738, 1995.

31. Elder MJ. Anatomy and physiology of eyelash follicles: Relevance to lash ablation procedures. Ophthal Plast Reconstr Surg 13:21, 1997.

Miscellaneous Medical Conditions and Situations

Problems Related to Sexual Activity

AT THE COUNTER

The pharmacist notices a young man looking at the condoms. He appears embarrassed and anxious and glances frequently at the pharmacist as though he needs help. The pharmacist approaches him and asks if he needs assistance.

Interview/Patient Assessment

The patient confides that he needs to purchase a condom, but doesn't know the difference between all of the brands or if they come in different sizes. He adds that he isn't sure how to use them either.

Pharmacist's Analysis

1. Are the differences among the condom types important?
2. What is the importance of lamb skin versus latex or polyurethane condoms?
3. Are there special condom options that the pharmacist should recommend?
4. What use instructions should be given to the patient?

Patient Counseling

The patient should be approached in a nonthreatening and nonjudgmental way, with the pharmacist appearing open and willing to provide all of the information needed for condom selection and use.

⚠ *The differences among condom types are critical and can make the difference between life and death. Only latex or polyurethane condoms prevent STDs such as acquired immunodeficiency syndrome (or acquired immune deficiency syndrome, also known as AIDS).* Although lamb skin is suitable for condoms when they are used for birth control, it does not prevent STDs, and condoms made of it should not be recommended for anyone at risk of contracting an STD.

The pharmacist should discuss the various condom options: lubrication, spermicide, receptacle end, strength, and size. Lubrication eases insertion and makes the sexual act more pleasurable. The receptacle end helps prevent breakage during ejaculation, reducing the risk of unwanted pregnancy and transmission of STDs. Spermicides (included as a component of the lubricant) help prevent pregnancy. Condoms advertised as "extra strong" also may resist breakage. Should a regular size condom be too tight, a larger condom may be desirable. After explaining about types of condoms, the pharmacist should offer to provide instruction on condom use. (See "Steps in Condom Use.")

This chapter addresses four problems related to sexual activity: unwanted pregnancy, sexually transmitted diseases (STDs), premature ejaculation, and insufficient vaginal lubrication.

Sexual intercourse is a complicated interplay of psychologic, emotional, and physical factors. (Figure 43.1 shows the anatomy of the male and female reproductive systems.) Because the median age at first intercourse is so low (younger than 18 in many countries), many individuals who are quite young, and possibly quite immature, experience problems related to sexual activity, most notably unwanted pregnancy and STDs. Problems related to sexual activity are not confined to youth, however. Unwanted pregnancy occurs as long as the female is fertile, and there is no age limit on the possibility of contracting an STD. Further, even patients in the ninth and tenth decades of life may require counseling in areas related to sexuality.

Nonprescription products and devices related to sexual activity are optimally utilized in the *prevention* of pregnancy and STDs. The *treatment* of pregnancy and STDs is not discussed, since it does not involve nonprescription products or devices

There is a small degree of overlap between problems related to sexual activity and female genital problems (see Chapter 44, Female Genital Conditions). For instance, in-

sufficient vaginal lubrication, which affects females in areas other than sexual, has been categorized under problems related to sexual activity because of its profound impact in this aspect of the patient's life.

UNWANTED PREGNANCY

Unwanted pregnancy is a universal problem that crosses all epidemiologic categories and affects women of all ages between menarche and menopause.[1] The young ages at which sexual activity begins mitigate against well-informed choices regarding the consequences of lack of contraception. By age 15, 33% of males and 26% of females are sexually active.[2] Research suggests that at least 79% of college students are sexually active.[3] One million pregnancies occur in females who are younger than 20 each year in the United States.[4]

PREVALENCE OF UNWANTED PREGNANCY

At least 60% of all pregnancies in the United States are unplanned, an estimated 6 million unplanned pregnancies yearly.[5,6]

Female

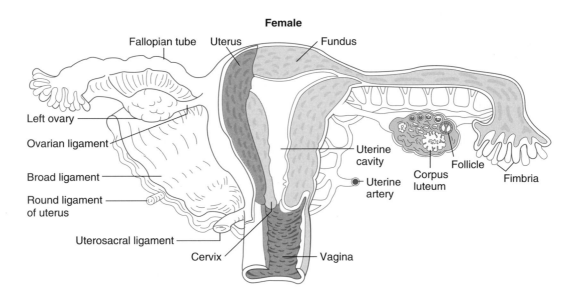

Male

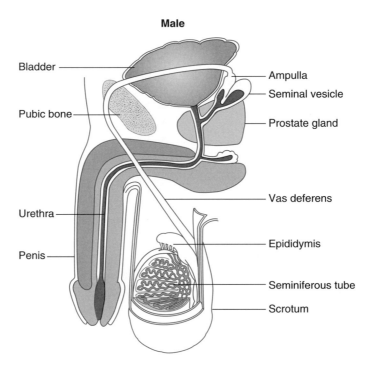

Figure 43.1. Male and female reproductive organs.

EPIDEMIOLOGY OF UNWANTED PREGNANCY

Age

About one-third of unwanted pregnancies occur in females aged 15 to 19.[7–9] At least 42% of pregnancies in women aged 30 to 34 are unintended.[5]

Other Epidemiologic Factors

Black females undergo almost twice as many pregnancies as white women, with the difference being almost solely caused by unintended pregnancies.[10] Unintended pregnancies ex-

hibit a greater increase in the less educated and the poor.[10] Women with schizophrenia tend to experience a higher rate of unintended pregnancies.[11]

ETIOLOGY OF UNINTENDED PREGNANCY

A combination of several factors can cause unintended pregnancy. They include the following:

- Failure to use an appropriate contraceptive device
- Misusing the contraceptive device (e.g., using a condom only when ejaculation is imminent)

- Failure of the contraceptive device
- Willful misrepresentation of one's fertility (e.g., falsely stating that one is sterile)
- Incest or rape[12]

PROGNOSIS OF UNWANTED PREGNANCY

Unwanted pregnancies in general have a less favorable prognosis, since they more commonly occur in females who are younger, less educated, and poor.

Pregnancy in a very young female has a more severe prognosis since it is more likely to be a first birth (hence, more risky) and since the young mother is more likely to be undereducated, poorly nourished, poor, and unable to seek out proper prenatal care.[4] Further, unintended pregnancy can continue a cycle of intergenerational poverty and child abuse.[13]

COMPLICATIONS OF UNWANTED PREGNANCY

Complications of unwanted pregnancy are the same as those in any pregnancy, including hypertension, cephalopelvic disproportion, iron-deficiency anemia, and the dangers of unsafe abortions obtained in an attempt to terminate the pregnancy.[4,14] As noted under "Prognosis," however, many unwanted pregnancies are first pregnancies, and first pregnancies are considered to be higher risk than subsequent pregnancies because many females with hazardous first births elect not to have additional children (that is, those who have more than one child more often had a relatively uneventful first birth). In addition, financial complications can be substantial when such factors as high-risk pregnancy and newborn care are included.[15]

PREVENTION OF UNWANTED PREGNANCY

The optimal method of preventing pregnancy is sexual abstinence.[16] This method is effective and safe, but it is not realistic for a growing majority of youth, as well as for many adults.

Pregnancy prevention is possible through the use of contraceptives, including products that reflect relatively recent advances in contraceptive technology.[15] The many reasons for avoiding conception include the following:

- Some women (e.g., those with chronic diseases such as advanced renal failure) should not become pregnant because of risk to the mother.
- Couples wish to delay starting a family until economic, family, and psychologic factors are all optimal.
- Unmarried but sexually active individuals may not wish to conceive until circumstances are more favorable (e.g., being in a long-term relationship).

Prevention Guidelines

Prevention of unwanted pregnancy involves a wide range of nonprescription products. The prevention method used is a highly personal decision determined by such factors as the individuals' health status, frequency of sexual activity, apprehension about sexually transmitted disease, socioeconomic status (some methods are less expensive than others), number of partners, and desire to have children at some future time.[5,17] Pharmacists must understand that many individuals who purchase contraceptives are young, unmarried adults. These patients generally find it difficult to obtain products and information for several reasons:

- Lack of professional guidance (because they are usually healthy and do not regularly visit health-care providers)
- Unfamiliarity with locations to obtain contraceptive products
- Ignorance about contraceptive product features and what is involved in purchasing these products
- Lack of transportation to the pharmacy or other provider
- Inability to pay for contraceptive products

Although contraceptive devices are sold in a number of outlets, many patients purchase contraceptives in pharmacies. The advantages of pharmacy purchase include the following:

- Convenience
- No appointment needed
- No records kept
- Wide choice of products
- Free choice of pharmacies
- Free information and advice
- Confidentiality and anonymity
- The pharmacist will not notify parents or custodians

Nonprescription Products

The pharmacist may recommend a variety of nonprescription contraceptive agents, varying widely in their use instructions and effectiveness. (See Patient Assessment Algorithm 43.1.) Table 43.1 compares these products in regard to their effectiveness.

MALE CONDOM

The male condom, a flexible sheath placed over the penis, is a barrier to sperm that exit the penis during ejaculation. *The male condom is the optimal contraceptive for sexually active young adults,* a group that faces an especially high risk of both unintended pregnancy and transmission of STDs.[4] The only temporary method of contraception available to males, the condom is simple to use, inexpensive (30 to 40 cents each for latex), easy to purchase in a variety of locations, and provides effective protection against both pregnancy and STDs. Table 43.2 lists examples of different condoms.

Table 43.1 compares the failure rate of condoms to other nonprescription products and devices. (See "A Pharmacist's Journal: They're for My Boyfriend.")

Historical Perspective

The male condom is the oldest contraceptive device still in use.

Patient Assessment Algorithm 43.1. Unwanted Pregnancy Prevention

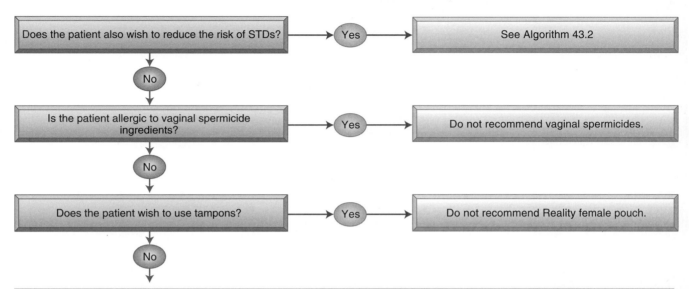

When vulcanized rubber became available in the late 1800s, it was used to make condoms. Although pharmacies stocked condoms, they were not placed out where the consumer could see them, but were kept in such out-of-the-way locations as in drawers, safes, or other locations inaccessible to consumers.[18] This reluctance to place them in visible locations was a concession to once-prevalent moral values that did not allow "polite society" to admit awareness of such objects. Thus they were not considered to be self-service items, and the consumer was required to ask the pharmacist for them. Many customers simply elected not to be embarrassed by asking for condoms, purchasing them from such anonymous locations as vending machines in gas station bathrooms. Their major uses during these early years were mainly to prevent STDs, rather than to prevent pregnancy. During this time male condoms were seldom advertised in any media.

The marketing of condoms changed with the onset of the acquired immunodeficiency syndrome (AIDS) crisis in the 1980s. The Surgeon General of the United States affirmed in 1987 that male condoms should be regarded not as objects of derision but as valuable tools in the fight against STDs.[16,19–21] Subsequently, condom advertisements began to appear in popular magazines and on billboards, television, and radio. Along with this new respectability as STD preventives, male condoms were increasingly seen as valid birth-control options as well.[22] Because of this widespread shift in attitude toward male condoms, the typical pharmacist is confronted with a wide range of condom purchasers. Older male patients often exhibit embarrassment when making condom purchases and may not buy them from female pharmacists, while younger male purchasers tend to have a more cavalier attitude about condom purchase (and

Table 43.1. Nonprescription Contraceptive Products and Their Effectiveness

PRODUCT	FAILURE RATE[a]
Male Condom (Lambskin/Latex)	12–15%
Female Pouch	21–26%
Vaginal Spermicides	20–30%
Periodic Abstinence (Using a device such as the basal body temperature thermometer)	14–47%

[a]Failure rate is provided in terms of the risk of pregnancy in 1 year for a couple using the method as a typical couple would.

use). Also, condoms are purchased by females in an increasing frequency; where only 12% of condom purchasers were female in the mid 1970s, 25 to 30% were female in the mid 1980s.[18,23] (See "A Pharmacist's Journal: I Need Some Propa-plastics.")

The efficacy of the condom as a sperm barrier in the prevention of pregnancy is not the same as its role in the prevention of STDs. See "Male Condoms" under "Prevention of Sexually Transmitted Diseases."

Composition

Condoms are made of several materials:

- Latex rubber has been the traditional material, which gives these devices their popular nickname "rubbers."
- Some condoms are made from lamb intestines, thus the nickname "lambskins." (Trade names include Fourex and Kling-Tite Naturalamb.)

Table 43.2. Representative Condoms and Their Features[a]

PRODUCT	SELECTED FEATURE(S)
Class Act Ultra-Thin and Sensitive	Reservoir end; lubricated with or without spermicide
Lifestyles Assorted Colors	Colors; lubricated
Lifestyles Studded	Lubricated; condom has "hundreds of raised rubber studs"
Lifestyles Ultra Sensitive	Thin; lubricated with or without spermicide
Lifestyles Ultra Thin	Thin; lubricated with or without spermicide
Lifestyles Xtra Pleasure	Lubricated; oversized tip
Naturalamb	Lubricated; lamb membrane composition
Sheik Fiesta	Colored
Sheik Super Thin	Lubricated with or without spermicide
Sheik Super Thin Ribbed	Lubricated with or without spermicide
Trojan-Enz Large Spermicidal Lubricant	Large condom; lubricant contains nonoxynol; reservoir end
Trojan-Enz Lubricated	Lubricant; reservoir end
Trojan-Enz Spermicidal Lubricant	Lubricant contains nonoxynol-9; reservoir end
Trojan Non-Lubricated	Rounded end; no lubrication
Trojan Ribbed	Ribbed to increase pleasure; reservoir end; reservoir end lubricated with or without spermicide
Trojan Shared Sensation	Bumps and ridges to increase pleasure; reservoir end; lubricated with or without spermicide
Trojan Ultra Pleasure	"Unique shape"; reservoir end; lubricated with or without spermicide
Trojan Ultra Texture	Lubricated; reservoir end; "delicately raised spiral and microdot textures"
Trojan Ultra Thin	Reservoir end; lubricated with or without spermicide

[a]Unless otherwise mentioned, the condoms listed are made of latex rubber.

A Pharmacist's Journal

"They're for My Boyfriend."

I once watched a young woman pull a shopping cart up to the condom display shelf and begin to load the condoms in. As I rang up her purchase, I noticed she had bought one box each of 15 to 18 popular brands, with 12 condoms in each box. She asked me, "I suppose you want to know why I need all of these?" She then told me, "Tomorrow's my boyfriend's birthday. I figured I might as well get him something I know he'll use."

- Polyurethane condoms have been available since 1994 (under the trade name Avanti), with an efficacy comparable to that of latex rubber.[5,24,25]

Size
The typical male condom sold in the United States is approximately 7.5 inches in length and 1 inch in width. However, extra large condoms are available. See "Extra Large."

Condom Options
Some condoms offer special features such as lubrication, the addition of a spermicide, a receptacle end, extra strength, enhanced protection, extra size, thinness, colors, textured sur-

A Pharmacist's Journal

"I Need Some Propa-plastic."

A young woman once came to the pharmacy window of the chain store where I worked and asked, "Where is the propa-plastic?" I didn't quite understand and asked her to repeat her request, which was not any more clear. I then remembered that a recent product called "Propa pH" had just debuted. I asked her, "Is this something you put on your face?" At that question, she colored several shades of red, her shoulders slumped, and she looked helplessly behind her. A man who had been standing some distance away walked up with a disgusted look on his face and said, "She wants rubbers." Evidently, he had been too hesitant to purchase them himself and sent his partner instead.

faces, and/or extra sensitivity. Generally, patients prefer one or more of the popular options that reduce the risk of pregnancy, ease the sexual act, or simply provide novelty—especially lubrication and receptacle ends. Several companies market lines of condoms with several options (such as Trojan, Sheik, and Ramses brands).

Lubrication. Some condoms are lubricated by the manufacturer. The addition of a lubricant primarily eases vaginal insertion and provides extra comfort during sex. A lubricant also may lessen the possibility of condom rupture. Lubrication is one of the popular condom options; marketing terms for lubricated condoms include "Ramses Sensitol" and "Naturalube."

Spermicidal Lubricant. Some condoms have a spermicide included in the jelly that lubricates the condom.[26] The spermicide, 5% nonoxynol-9, acts to reduce or destroy the mobility of sperm. The FDA stresses that the addition of spermicide has not yet been proven to augment the effectiveness of the condom used alone.[5] Some women have complained that spermicidal condoms have an unpleasant taste.[27]

Receptacle End. The standard condom tip is shaped to fit tightly against the head of the penis. However, the pressure of ejaculate may induce rupture. *For this reason, many condoms have a small receptacle built into the tip to catch the ejaculate.* Marketing terms for this popular condom option include "receptacle-end," "reservoir end," and "Trojan-Enz."

Extra Strength. The standard condom is labeled for vaginal intercourse. Because anal intercourse causes greater resistance to penetration by the penis, increasing the risk of condom rupture, some condoms are purported to be extra strong to prevent rupture during that sex act, although the validity of this claim is questionable.[16,28]

Enhanced Protection. A two-piece male condom is available that is marketed as being superior in preventing STDs. Called the Mentor, the condom consists of two nested pieces of latex that are unrolled onto the penis. Then—before the sex act is begun—the outer piece is gripped firmly, rotated back and forth gently, and then removed, leaving the inner condom in place over the penis. The gentle rotation spreads an adhesive on the inside of the inner condom, approximately half-way up the penile shaft. The adhesive forms a safety seal around the penile shaft, helping ensure that ejaculate and infected fluids do not leak out of the open end of the condom where they might reach vaginal tissues, possibly resulting in pregnancy and/or STDs.

Extra Large. Some males cannot fit comfortably inside the standard male condom, which may make them reluctant to use it. Large-size condoms are available under such trade names as Trojan Magnum and Trojan-Enz Large.

Thin. Some condoms are marketed as being thinner than regular condoms for greater sensitivity. Both Sheik Super Thin and Trojan Very Thin are claimed to be 64% of the thickness of regular latex condoms.

Colors. As a novelty some condoms are marketed in colors. Colored varieties include Trojan Ribbed (gold), Sheik Fiesta, and Rubber Ducky (blue, green, yellow, and red).

Textured Surface. The outer surface of the male condom may be covered with small concentric circles of raised latex. These "textured" or "ribbed" condoms are said to offer greater satisfaction for the female. Textured condoms include Trojan Ultra Texture, Class Act, and Excita Extra Ultra-Ribbed.

Special Shape. The manufacturer of Trojan Very Sensitive promises that its special shape increases sensitivity. The condom also has lubrication and a receptacle end.

Steps in Condom Use

Condoms should be stored in a cool, dry place.[16,29] (The FDA requires this label: "Heat and light accelerate the degradation of latex films. Store unopened containers away from heat and light.")[30] Do not use condoms if they are sticky, discolored, brittle, or damaged. (See "A Pharmacist's Journal: How Do I Use a Condom?")

The pharmacist should advise patients to follow the steps below for safe and effective condom use:

1. Check the condom package before use. Inspect the box in which the condoms were purchased to ensure that the expiration date has not passed. Ensure that it is not torn or otherwise damaged.

2. Open the condom wrapper carefully to avoid damaging the condom with the fingernails. If the condom does not contain a spermicidal lubricant, add a small amount of spermicidal contraceptive (e.g., 2 to 3 mL) inside the condom tip if desired.

3. Place the condom on the penis prior to any vaginal penetration.[31] Identify which side of the condom unrolls over the penis—the inside of the condom—prior to touching the penis. (If a condom is unrolled incorrectly and then reversed, preejaculate may be inadvertently introduced into the vagina.) Next place the condom over the penis. Pull back the foreskin of an uncircumcised penis prior to applying the condom. Finally, unroll the condom completely to reach the base of the penis. If the condom does not have a receptacle end, leave 1/2 inch of empty space at the end to contain the ejaculate, but air should be squeezed out of this space during condom application.

4. Apply lubricant and/or spermicide, if desired. If a lubricant is desired, a water-soluble lubricant must be used (e.g., KY Jelly or other feminine lubricants marketed **(tip)** specifically for condom use). *Use of oil-based products may weaken condoms, perhaps causing them to rupture during sexual activity (e.g., baby oil, petroleum jelly, lotions, massage oils, butter, margarine, cold cream, ointment, mineral oil, cooking oils).*

5. Be alert for condom failure. Should a condom rupture during use, the male should withdraw immediately and vaginal spermicide should be applied to the vagina.

6. Withdraw penis and condom. Immediately after ejaculation and before withdrawing the penis from the vagina, hold the condom at its base to prevent spillage of ejaculate, and then withdraw the penis and the condom from **(tip)** the vagina at the same time. *Withdrawing the penis without holding the condom may result in the condom remaining in the vagina, possibly spilling its contents over the outer or inner labia.* Should the male remain in the vagina until the penis begins to undergo **detumescence** (loss of penile rigidity), the chances of the condom remaining in the vagina are greatly increased.

7. **(tip)** Dispose of condom. *A condom must not be used more than once.* Wrap the used condom in tissue and dispose of it in a secure trash container where others cannot handle it. If flushed, a condom may plug plumbing. Wash the hands with soap and water following disposal.

Condom-using couples must use condoms during every act that involves penis-vaginal contact. If they do not do so, they incorporate guesswork, which reduces the effectiveness of the condom.

Condom Failures

Condoms rarely rupture during use when used properly. Perhaps one condom ruptures per 50 to 200 acts of intercourse.[32-34] **(tip)** *Factors associated with condom rupture include a low level of vaginal lubrication (possibly resulting from insufficient foreplay) and use of petroleum jelly as a lubricant (since oil-based products destroy rubber).*[16] Polyurethane condoms may also break more readily than latex.[35]

Condom Misuse

A more common reason for condom ineffectiveness is improper use—or no use at all.[16] Male dislike of the products leads to poor compliance.[36,37] (Fewer than 60% of adoles-

A Pharmacist's Journal

"How Do I Use a Condom?"

I was working when a phone call came in from a young male. He sounded distressed and said he had just bought some condoms from us, but didn't know how to use them. I had started at this store only a few days before and was anxious to help our patients. I took several minutes advising him on the proper application of condoms. He asked several serious questions and sounded confident. As I hung up, I felt I had performed a significant public health service. However, I turned around and several clerks and another pharmacist were all smiling at me. I asked what was so funny, since I was just helping a young patient. One of my coworkers replied, "You got the 'rubber boy.' He calls here about every week or so trying to get one of us to talk to him about condoms. You were the lucky fish this week!"

cents use a condom at their first act of intercourse.[38]) Many males complain that condoms reduce penile sensitivity, which decreases sexual pleasure.[36,39] Because of this some males attempt to initiate coitus without a condom, intending to apply a condom prior to ejaculation.[40] Unfortunately, prior to full ejaculation the penis can emit a semen-rich fluid known as preejaculate. Thus waiting to put on a condom until after initial vaginal penetration increases the risk of pregnancy (in the presence of a viable ovum) and disease.

Males also complain about the interruption of sexual activity needed to apply the condom because it reduces the spontaneity of the sex act. Also, some males do not wish to send a message that they might be "unclean" or that they perceive their partner to be infected with an STD.[16]

Condom Allergies

Lambskin condoms are a poor choice for individuals—men and women—who are allergic to lanolin, wool, or other sheep-derived products.[41] For these people the pharmacist should recommend latex rubber or polyurethane condoms. On the other hand, allergies to latex rubber can cause fatal anaphylaxis. (The FDA is monitoring the increasing incidence of latex sensitivity, perhaps as a result of past exposure to latex gloves, footwear, or condoms.[16]) Those allergic to latex rubber might choose polyurethane condoms, since lambskin condoms do not protect against AIDS.[25] For some individuals—men and women—spermicidal lubricants may cause a reaction; they should choose condoms without spermicidal lubricants.[41]

FEMALE POUCH

The female pouch (also known as the female condom or intravaginal pouch) was approved by the FDA in 1993 (Fig. 43.2A).[42] The only product currently available is trade-named the Reality pouch. A 6-inch-long, prelubricated, polyurethane sheath with an inner lumen somewhat larger than the male condom, the Reality pouch covers the vagina and a portion of the perineum when properly inserted.[43,44] Its primary appeal is the ability of the female to reduce the risk of pregnancy and sexually transmitted disease with one product.[36,45,46]

If a couple is using the female pouch as their birth control method, it should be used at every act of intercourse to maximize its effectiveness. *A pouch can be used when pregnant, menstruating, or following a recent childbirth, but cannot be used when a tampon is in place. The female pouch should not be used with a condom because the friction could cause one or both devices to become dislodged.*

The pharmacist should recommend the steps below for proper use of the female pouch:

1. Check the pouch before use. Inspect the box to ensure that the product has not passed its expiration date. Inspect the individually wrapped female pouch to ensure that the outer wrapper is not torn or damaged in any way. Remove the pouch from its package carefully.
2. Unfold the pouch to its full length, which allows the user

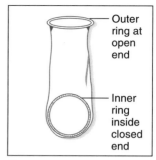

A. Female pouch

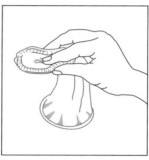

B. Preparing pouch for insertion

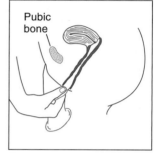

C. Inserting pouch

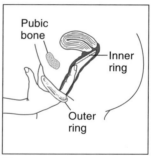

D. Checking pouch placement

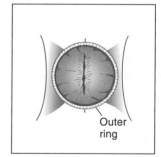

E. Pouch properly inserted (external view)

Figure 43.2. Use of female pouch: **A.** Parts of the pouch. **B.** Preparing pouch for insertion. **C.** Insertion of the pouch. **D.** Checking for proper pouch placement. **E.** An external view of a properly positioned pouch following insertion.

to locate a flexible plastic ring inside the pouch's closed end and a flexible plastic ring around the open end.
3. Insert the pouch (up to 8 hours before intercourse to ensure full protection). Squeeze the sides of the inner ring together and insert it well into the vagina (Figs. 43.2B and C). *Practice insertion during a nonstressful time, before the product is actually used.*
4. Check the pouch after insertion to ensure that the inner ring is past the pubic bone (Fig. 43.2D) and that the open end protrudes from the vagina so that plastic partially covers the labia (Fig. 43.2E). Also check that the pouch has not become twisted during insertion.

5. Apply lubricant, if needed. Begin with only two drops of liquid or two pea-sized amounts of gel; add additional lubricant if the penis does not move freely inside the pouch, if the outer ring is moved into the vagina, if there is noise associated with friction inside the product, or if it is ejected from the vagina during use.

6. Be alert for pouch failure. Remove the pouch if it rips or tears, if the outer ring enters the vagina, or if the product bunches up inside the vagina. Keep in mind that even when the female pouch has been applied as directed, the thrusting penis may slip outside, which can negate its effectiveness.[36]

7. **tip** Dispose of pouch. *A pouch should only be used once.* Remove the pouch from the vagina before standing by squeezing and twisting the outer ring. Wrap the used pouch in tissue and dispose of it in a secure trash container where others cannot handle it. Do not dispose of a used pouch in a toilet because it could plug plumbing.

VAGINAL SPERMICIDES

Vaginal spermicides are placed in the vagina prior to intercourse to prevent pregnancy.[47] (Vaginal spermicides are included in condoms, as discussed under "male condom" above.) Vaginal spermicides are added to a delivery vehicle such as a foam, jelly, film, suppository, or cream (Table 43.3). Males may not be compliant with condoms for many reasons (e.g., cost, loss of sensitivity during coitus, and general dislike); vaginal spermicides give women the ability to control reproductive behavior with an uncooperative male.[48]

Spermicides function by two methods: first, they present a physical barrier to entry of the spermatozoa into the cervical os and further to the ova.[49] Secondly, they destroy sperm through their actions as **nonionic surfactants** (surface-active agents).[47,50] (A detergent action attacks the lipid components of the midpiece and tail of spermatozoa, rendering them nonmotile and incapable of impregnation. The chemicals also compromise the ability of the sperm to metabolize fructose—a lethal change in itself.[47]) The most commonly used spermicide is nonoxynol-9, although octoxynol is occa-

sionally utilized in these products.[44] In early 1995 the FDA issued a ruling that all manufacturers of nonprescription vaginal spermicides must prove efficacy of their specific formulation.[51] The products have been allowed to remain on the market pending receipt of that information.

Spermicides may cause vaginal irritation and inflammation through their detergent action on vaginal mucosa.[52] **tip** *Patients who experience a burning sensation or irritation with their use should discontinue them.* Spermicides can cause oral irritation when used in oral sexual activity.[53]

Females must not douche too soon after ejaculation to avoid flushing out the relatively lighter spermicide while allowing the more viscous ejaculate to remain in the vagina. **tip** *The FDA requires the following precaution: "If douching is desired, always wait at least 6 hours after intercourse before douching."*[47]

Foams

Cans of spermicide foam should be shaken vigorously up and down 20 times or more to thoroughly mix the spermicide with its vehicle and ensure full production of foam. Some foams begin to lose their foamy consistency if they are allowed to sit unused in the applicator after removal from the aerosol can. Thus the applicators of such products as Delfen and Emko Foams should not be loaded until just prior to application (Fig. 43.3). Should the foam product come in a preloaded applicator, its wrapper should only be removed just prior to vaginal insertion.[7] Intercourse may proceed with no waiting period after insertion of a foam product (Fig. 43.4). If intercourse is not initiated within 1 hour, another dose of foam should be inserted. Another dose is also inserted before any subsequent sexual acts.

Jellies (Gels)

Jellies are popular vehicles for vaginal spermicides as they are easily washed from the external vaginal area at the end of the sexual act. Jellies should not be applied more than 1 hour prior to intercourse, and sexual activity may commence directly after application. One gel, Advantage 24, is composed of nonoxynol-9 in a polycarbophil-based vehicle that has

PRODUCT	SELECTED INGREDIENTS
Table 43.3. Representative Vaginal Spermicides	
Encare Insert	Nonoxynol-9 100 mg
K-Y Plus Jelly	Nonoxynol-9 2.2%
Ortho Options Conceptrol Gel	Nonoxynol-9 4%
Ortho Options Delfen Foam	Nonoxynol-9 12.5%
Ortho Options Gynol II Jelly	Nonoxynol-9 2%
Ortho Options Ortho-Gynol Jelly	Octoxynol-9 1%
VCF Vaginal Contraceptive Film	Nonoxynol-9 28%

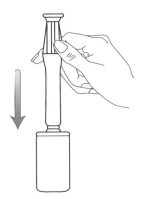

Figure 43.3. Method of filling an applicator with vaginal spermicide foam: After applicator is placed over the top of the foam can, applicator is filled by either pressing down or laterally on the can's nozzle.

been found to be effective for up to 24 hours following application.[54,55] (See "A Pharmacist's Journal: Why Do You Have Purple Vaginal Secretions?")

Films

Vaginal films are inserted by the female so that the film covers the cervical os. The hands should be thoroughly dry to prevent the film from adhering to the fingers during insertion. One vaginal film product, VCF, consists of nonoxynol-9 impregnated on a 2.25-inch-square film.

The film is folded in half, placed over the fingertips, then inserted directly over the cervix, not less than 15 minutes before and not more than 1 hour before intercourse (Fig. 43.5). If more than 1 hour elapses, another film should be inserted. One film only protects for one act, but several films can be inserted in a 24-hour period. The film does not require removal following intercourse, as it dissolves.

Suppositories

Suppositories must be removed from the wrapper and inserted as closely as possible to the cervix. Couples must wait 10 to 15 minutes for the suppository to dissolve and spread

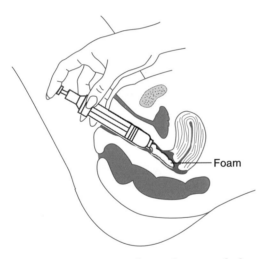

Figure 43.4. Insertion of vaginal spermicide foam.

to cover vaginal mucosa, which can interrupt spontaneity. (Semicid requires 15 minutes; Encare and Conceptrol Inserts require 10 minutes.) Suppositories only protect patients for 1 hour and for a single act of intercourse.[7] Some females complain that vaginal spermicide suppositories cause discomfort, pain, or itching during use or shortly thereafter.[48]

Creams

Creams are uncommon vehicles for vaginal spermicides.

BASAL BODY TEMPERATURE MEASUREMENT

Basal body temperature measurement (BBTM) is a fertility-awareness technique for identifying "safe" days for unprotected intercourse. The method employs a special thermometer sold in pharmacies or other outlets. (The basal temperature is a reading taken under basal conditions such as 12 hours after eating, after a restful sleep, without exercise, without emotional excitement, and with fairly constant air temperature).

The BBTM is based on the ovulation cycle. Because most females experience a drop in body temperature prior to ovulation and a rise of 0.4 to 0.8°F after ovulation, body temperature theoretically indicates when it is safe to engage in sex. The female should take her temperature each day of the month to note these rather modest temperature changes. The female uses contraception approximately for the first half of her cycle. Then, 3 days after the rise is noted, she may assume that her fertile period has ended and not use contraception. A simple chart is included with the basal thermometer that allows the female to better visualize the low and high temperatures.

Fertility-awareness techniques such as BBTM have a low success rate for many reasons, including the following:

- Sperm ejaculated into the female retain the ability to impregnate an egg for up to 7 days.
- Each egg is fertile for 24 hours.[5]
- The day of ovulation is typically day 14 of the menstrual cycle (day 1 being the first day of flow), but ranges from day 8 to day 19.
- Body temperature is affected by loss of sleep or illness.[32]

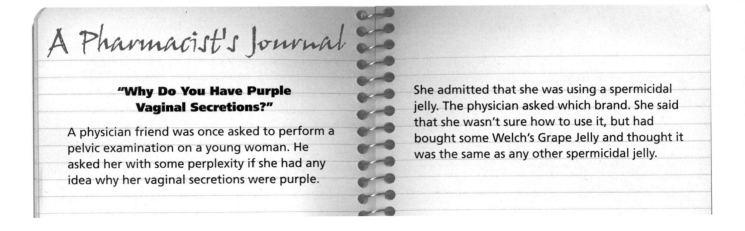

A Pharmacist's Journal

"Why Do You Have Purple Vaginal Secretions?"

A physician friend was once asked to perform a pelvic examination on a young woman. He asked her with some perplexity if she had any idea why her vaginal secretions were purple.

She admitted that she was using a spermicidal jelly. The physician asked which brand. She said that she wasn't sure how to use it, but had bought some Welch's Grape Jelly and thought it was the same as any other spermicidal jelly.

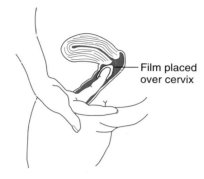

Figure 43.5. Insertion of vaginal spermicide film.

These variables make it difficult to avoid pregnancy using fertility-awareness techniques such as the BBTM, but a highly motivated couple may be successful.

To increase the effectiveness of this method, patients should rigidly adhere to the following guidelines:

- Take the temperature before eating, drinking, smoking, urinating, or arising from bed every day of the month, at the same time each day.
- Take the temperature for a full 5 minutes.
- If an electric blanket is used, it should be at the same setting every night while basal temperatures are being taken.
- Take the temperature in the same location each time (e.g., oral or rectal).
- Do not use a fever thermometer. (The fever thermometer range is 92 to 106°, and its accuracy is only 0.2° per calibration.) Use a glass basal thermometer (e.g., Becton-Dickinson or other manufacturers) with a range of 95 to 100° and calibrations of 0.1° each. Optionally, a digital basal may be used (e.g., manufactured by Becton-Dickinson).

CONTRACEPTIVE SPONGE

A vaginal contraceptive sponge impregnated with spermicide was marketed until 1995, when the manufacturer (Whitehall-Robins Healthcare) voluntarily halted its sale. The cost to correct problems identified by the FDA was deemed too costly to continue manufacture.[56] It is still approved by the FDA and could be marketed in the future.

SEXUALLY TRANSMITTED DISEASES

There are a host of sexually transmitted diseases. They include gonorrhea, viral hepatitis (B and perhaps also C), syphilis, chlamydia, genital herpes, and genital warts.[57,58] Over the last 20 years, chlamydia and viral agents have assumed primary importance as STDs, including AIDs.[59-61] A core of individuals are either frequently infected or transmit the infection to others.[62]

The most alarming STD today is AIDS, eclipsing the once-feared genital herpes. Several factors have combined to cause this nearly universal fear. Carriers of HIV may not know they can transmit the virus; their potential partners have no visible clue to use in detecting the presence of HIV.[63] If the carrier develops AIDS, it is an incurable condition that will cause an early death in virtually all cases. Finally, AIDS has spread rapidly since it became known in the 1980s. (See "Facts About Aids.")

PREVALENCE OF SEXUALLY TRANSMITTED DISEASES

Each year at least 250 million people around the world contract STDs, with 66% of those being under the age of 25.[4,65,66] In the United States 2.5 million teenagers contract an STD yearly.[67] As of 1997 there have been over 600,000 cases of AIDS reported to the Centers for Disease Control.[68] Genital herpes antibody is carried by over 16% of the United States population.[69] Pelvic inflammatory disease is often related to an STD such as gonorrhea or chlamydia. Although it is not a reportable disease, approximately 1% of women aged 15 to 25 develop pelvic inflammatory disease each year.[70,71] As many as 6% of males are positive for chlamydia, which is said to be the most common STD in the United States.[72,73]

EPIDEMIOLOGY OF SEXUALLY TRANSMITTED DISEASES

Age

Young people (e.g., 10 to 19 years) are more prone to contract STDs because, when compared with adults, they lack knowledge, tend to use preventive measures more inconsistently, and are more likely to have multiple partners.[4,74] In the United States, females aged 15 to 19 contract gonorrhea more than other age groups with males aged 15 to 19 being the second-highest group.[4] Patients younger than 25 account for over 5% of AIDS cases with many contracting AIDS before age 20.[68]

College students, in particular, are prone to high-risk sexual activity such as refusal to use condoms while engaging in sex with multiple partners and experimenting with drugs.[65] These problems, coupled with a refusal to practice safe sex practices, places them at higher risk of STDs. In a survey one-fifth of college students had already contracted an STD.[75]

Gender

Females face the highest risk of contracting AIDS by heterosexual transmission because the prevalence of AIDS in males is 1 in 100 as opposed to only 1 in 800 for females (511,934 cases in males by 1997, as opposed to only 92,242 in women).[68,76,77] Almost 20% of females have antibody to genital herpes, as compared with 13% of men.[69]

Racial Group

AIDS has a characteristic racial distribution. A majority of women in the United States with AIDS are black or Hispanic, despite the fact that these groups only represent 20% of females in the United States.[78]

ETIOLOGY OF SEXUALLY TRANSMITTED DISEASES

Sexually transmitted diseases are caused by infective agents. Some are bacterial in nature (e.g., syphilis, gonorrhea), some are viral (e.g., AIDS, genital warts, genital herpes), and some are fungal (e.g., candidal infection).

TRANSMISSION OF SEXUALLY TRANSMITTED DISEASES

The mode of transmission of medical conditions referred to as sexually transmitted diseases occurs through sexual activity in most cases, although a small percentage of patients contract them through other means—such as patients who contract AIDS through maternal-infant transfer, injection of illicit drugs, or the administration of medications for hemophilia.

Patients who contract an STD through sexual activity may do so through heterosexual penis-vaginal intercourse, anal intercourse, and oral-genital contact among either heterosexual or homosexual partners.

MANIFESTATIONS OF SEXUALLY TRANSMITTED DISEASES

Some STDs produce early and visible signs of infection such as vaginitis and cervicitis.[79] Syphilis results in the well-known chancre, and gonorrhea causes a painful burning on urination. Genital warts manifest as moist protrusions from the genital and perianal skin. Genital herpes produces a periodic set of painful lesions. HIV infection may cause

FOCUS ON...

FACTS ABOUT AIDS

Acquired immune deficiency syndrome (or acquired immunodeficiency syndrome), also known as AIDS, has captured headlines since the mid 1980s. Pharmacists may counsel AIDS patients and wonder what actions are safe or unsafe. (If you need information on universal precautions for patients with AIDS or other bloodborne diseases, see Universal Precautions When Counseling Patients in Chapter 1.)

The following short discussion on AIDS presents basic concepts regarding the patient with AIDS.[64] For further information, the pharmacist may contact such Internet sites as the United Methodist Church General Board of Global Ministries at http://gbgm-umc.org/cam/aidsinfo.html; the AIDS Education Global Information System at http://www.aegis.com/search/index.html; or the National AIDS Information and Education Project at http://www.qcfurball.com/cat/aids/kidsaids.html.

Human immunodeficiency virus (HIV), the causative organism for AIDS, may be contracted through several routes. They include sharing of needles, sexual activities (intercourse—both vaginal and anal, and oral-genital sexual contact). Some contract it through maternal-fetal transfer or breast-feeding or when transfusion of blood derivatives is necessary (e.g., hemophiliacs), although the risk of this latter occurrence has been virtually eliminated since 1985 when screening of blood began.

HIV virus selectively infects T-helper cells, but also resides in B cells, macrophages, and nerve cells. Eventually, T cells are destroyed in such high numbers that an immune deficiency becomes evident, and the person is said to have AIDS. When AIDS develops, the person first notices minor symptoms such as recurrent vaginal fungal infections (see Chapter 44, Female Genital Conditions). However, at some point the condition becomes more evident, including such problems as pneumonia, tuberculosis, oral candidiasis, and ophthalmic infections.

The AIDS patient requires more pharmacy counseling than the average patient, because of the greater number of infections that occur. Patients at risk of HIV infection also see the pharmacist to purchase various contraceptive devices and to purchase home test kits to monitor for the presence of HIV. (See Chapter 48, Home Test Kits.)

There is little cause to fear the AIDS patient who requires counseling. The following are some of the critical truths about HIV-positive patients and patients with AIDS:

- AIDS is not spread through the air, food, water, insects, animals, dishes, or toilet seats.
- You cannot get AIDS by touching a patient. Casual contact with the AIDS patient does not transmit HIV. Counsel them just as you would any other patient.
- Be cautious if you are carrying out any type of screening program (e.g., blood glucose testing) that requires removing blood, since the blood of an HIV-positive patient is infective. Take universal precautions with all patients.
- Be careful (e.g., wear gloves) when handling any patient's body fluid containing blood (such as bloody stool), vaginal secretions, or ejaculate; wash the hands with soap and water after removing the gloves.
- Do not allow any patient's blood or body fluid to splash onto skin, into the eyes, or onto mucous membranes.
- Any personnel with chickenpox should avoid being in the same room with an AIDS patient to prevent transmission of chickenpox to the AIDS patient, which could be deadly.
- Avoid contact with herpes simplex labialis lesions in the AIDS patient, as this can transmit AIDS.
- For more information, call the Centers for Disease Control National AIDS Hotline at 1-800-342-AIDS (English), 1-800-344-7432 (Spanish), or 1-800-243-7889 (TDD-Deaf access).

frequent vaginal infections, increasing frequency of genital herpes outbreaks, and pelvic inflammatory disease.[78] However, *Chlamydia trachomatis* is often asymptomatic.[80]

PROGNOSIS OF SEXUALLY TRANSMITTED DISEASES

STDs can result in infertility through damage to fallopian tubes or to the male reproductive tract, pelvic inflammatory disease, and death.[4,79,81] Chlamydia infections, perhaps the most common cause of pelvic inflammatory disease, causes infertility in many cases.

STDs in the pregnant female can also cause adverse effects on the fetus (e.g., congenital syphilis, ophthalmia neonatorium, or chronic hepatitis B carrier status) and may increase the risk of preterm birth.[82,83]

Syphilis and gonorrhea, the classic STDs, can result in damage to major organs (e.g., brain, kidney) if untreated.[81] Herpes infection may infect an infant during a delivery, inducing herpetic encephalitis.[50] Gonorrhea and chlamydia can both produce ophthalmia neonatorium in a newborn, following delivery through a diseased birth canal.[50] The human papillomavirus strains responsible for genital warts can also induce cervical cancer.[78]

In the year 2000 an estimated 40 million people will carry HIV infection, and 1.8 million will die of AIDS.[36] AIDS is the fourth leading cause of death among women aged 25 to 44 in the United States and is the leading cause of death in that age group in such highly developed urban areas as New York City and northern New Jersey.[78]

PREVENTION OF SEXUALLY TRANSMITTED DISEASES

The best prevention for STDs is sexual abstinence prior to a mutually monogamous relationship with an uninfected partner.[16,84] However, these goals are not realistic for many people. Prevention of sexually transmitted diseases in those who are sexually active is possible with certain nonprescription devices. (See Patient Assessment Algorithm 43.2.)

Male Condom

The male condom is the most effective method available for reducing the risk of infection from sexually transmitted disease in those who are sexually active (see Table 43.2).[5,16,41,85–88] (See "Male Condom" in "Prevention of Unwanted Pregnancy" above.) However, *to prevent STDs the condom must be placed on the erect penis before vaginal, oral, or anal contact.*

The composition of the condom assumes paramount importance when STD transmission is considered. Because lambskin condoms are porous and allow the passage of viral particles, manufacturers must include the following warning or a similar warning on the label, "Not to be used for prevention of sexually transmitted diseases (STDs). To help reduce the risk of catching or spreading many STDs, use only latex condoms."[82,89]

Latex condoms have no pores and are impervious to the passage of organisms responsible for STDs; thus latex condoms function effectively to prevent STDs when used as directed (including HIV and hepatitis B virus).[49,50,90] The virus responsible for AIDS measures approximately 100 nanometers, as opposed to the relatively large 3000 nanometer head of a sperm (Fig. 43.6).[89] With approximately 1% of patients, latex allergies can result in anaphylaxis and death; thus latex must be avoided by these patients.[91] Polyurethane condoms are a viable alternative to latex condoms since they are also free of pores.[5]

Polyurethane or latex condoms can be used to help prevent STDs when a couple is using a contraceptive that does not provide such protection (e.g., oral contraceptives, diaphragms, IUDs).[92] However, condoms should not be used with a female pouch (see below).

Patient Assessment Algorithm 43.2. STD Prevention

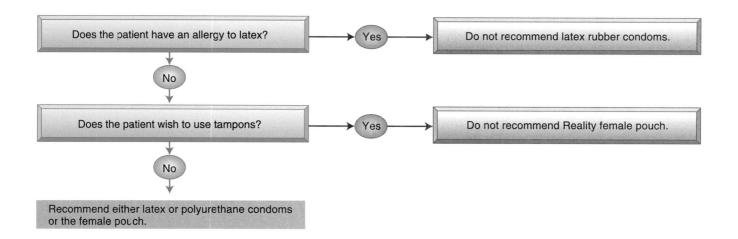

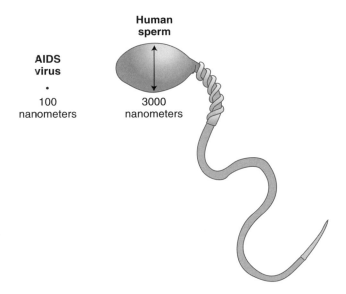

Figure 43.6. Relative sizes of a human sperm head and the AIDS virus.

Female Pouch

The barrier effect of the female pouch (discussed in detail in "Prevention of Unwanted Pregnancy"), allows it to prevent STDs in the same manner as the male condom.[5] However, the pouch is not as effective as the male condom, perhaps because ejaculate is not as tightly encapsulated as in the condom.[49]

Vaginal Spermicides

Vaginal spermicides may have action against the organisms that cause STDs through the same detergent action that destroys sperm.[82,93] However, this ability is not yet sufficiently well proven for the FDA to permit labeling to that effect.[94,95]

PREMATURE EJACULATION

Premature ejaculation is a form of sexual dysfunction in which the male ejaculates when the penis contacts the vulva, during the process of inserting the penis into the vagina, or immediately after penile introduction. This premature ending of the sexual act for the male does not allow the sustained thrusting required by most females to reach orgasm. This leads to dissatisfaction for both the female and male.[96] Premature ejaculation may be quantified as an inability to control the ejaculatory process for a sufficient length of time to satisfy the partner for at least 50% of their coital connections.

PREVALENCE OF PREMATURE EJACULATION

Premature ejaculation is the most common sexual dysfunction of males.[97–99] In one survey it was noted by 31% of males.[100] As many as 75% of males ejaculate within 2 min-

utes of vaginal penetration.[96,101] In a large number of men, the time to ejaculation is only 10 to 20 seconds.

EPIDEMIOLOGY OF PREMATURE EJACULATION

Premature ejaculation may be more common in those who experience a long period of sexual inactivity.[101] (For these men, sexual activity leads to a heightened excitement, which in turn causes ejaculation at low levels of sexual stimulation. Premature ejaculation is the second most common complaint of elderly men (just behind erectile problems).[1]

ETIOLOGY OF PREMATURE EJACULATION

Premature ejaculation—which is seldom caused by a serious underlying organic pathology such as prostatitis or a urinary tract infection—has several common causes[96,102]:

- Hypersensitivity of the glans penis, which excessively stimulates the sexual center[101,103]
- Inflammation of the trigger mechanism that regulates ejaculation (a problem that may be addressed by urologists)
- A psychoneurosis that produces performance anxiety
- Venous leakage, arterial insufficiency[104]
- Hormonal abnormalities[105]

With some couples, the male's ejaculation is not premature, and the male does not suffer from any abnormality.[106] Rather, there is a perceived prematurity that results from the well-established, slower sexual response of the female.[101,107] Couples striving toward simultaneous climax must understand that only an estimated 75% of couples ever reach this goal at some time during coitus.

TREATMENT OF PREMATURE EJACULATION

The impulse to ejaculate originates in the glans penis.[101] Thus, if an anesthetic is applied to this area, resistance to ejaculation is raised, prolonging the sexual act. Nonprescription penis anesthetizing products are known as male genital desensitizers. Should they fail to be effective, physicians may perform surgery or prescribe prescription products such as topical anesthetics (e.g., prilocaine/lidocaine), clomiphene, sertraline, fluoxetine, or other antidepressants.[107–113]

Treatment Guidelines

Patients should be cautioned that premature ejaculation may be caused by a serious condition requiring physician consultation. If the product does not work when used as directed, a physician should be seen. *If either partner develops rash, irritation, burning, or itching, the patient should discontinue the product.*[114,115] To prevent the development of an allergic reaction, the male should wash male genital desensitizers away following sexual activity.

Nonprescription Medications

BENZOCAINE

Benzocaine 3 to 7.5% in a water-soluble base safely and effectively prolongs time to ejaculation without anesthetizing the female partner's clitoris or vaginal tissues.[101] Patients are directed to apply a small amount of this male genital desensitizer to the head and shaft of the penis prior to intercourse. Table 43.4 lists products for premature ejaculation that contain benzocaine.

LIDOCAINE

Lidocaine, in a metered spray designed to deliver 10 mg per spray, is also considered to be safe and effective as a male genital desensitizer. The patient applies three or more sprays to the head and shaft of the penis prior to intercourse. The patient should not use more than 10 sprays per sexual act.

INSUFFICIENT VAGINAL LUBRICATION

PREVALENCE OF INSUFFICIENT VAGINAL LUBRICATION

Insufficient vaginal lubrication affects as many as 40 million United States females; in one study 30 of 73 sexually active females (average age of 56) experienced it.[116,117]

EPIDEMIOLOGY OF INSUFFICIENT VAGINAL LUBRICATION

Vaginal dryness, which exhibits a strong age link, is experienced by as many as 60% of women older than 40, compared with approximately 40% of women younger than 40.[118–122]

ETIOLOGY OF INSUFFICIENT VAGINAL LUBRICATION

Most females experience insufficient vaginal lubrication as a result of either low estrogen concentrations secondary to menopause or **oophorectomy** (surgical removal of the ovaries). However, estrogen levels drop in the postpartum period because of loss of estrogen in the placenta, also causing vaginal dryness. In addition, breast-feeding releases prolactin, which suppresses release of estrogen from the ovaries, resulting in insufficient vaginal lubrication.[123] Sjögren's syndrome, diabetes mellitus, and systemic lupus erythematosus can all produce vaginal dryness.[124–127]

Vaginal dryness may occur during menses or when women are stressed or fatigued. Strenuous exercise, endometriosis, and diabetes mellitus may also reduce vaginal moisture.

The anticholinergic effects of prescription and nonprescription medications (e.g., antihistamines, tricyclic antidepressants, antipsychotics) induce vaginal dryness.[128] Adverse local effects of products applied vaginally (e.g., soaps, douches, perfumed sanitary products) may also result in vaginal dryness. Finally, tamoxifen, danazol, certain antibiotics, chemotherapy, and radiation may cause vaginal dryness.

MANIFESTATIONS OF INSUFFICIENT VAGINAL LUBRICATION

Dry vaginal tissues can result in impaired sexual arousal, pain during intercourse, vaginal pruritus, burning or irritation, and/or a malodorous discharge.[116,129] Women also may suffer genital inflammation or abrasion.[130]

TREATMENT OF INSUFFICIENT VAGINAL LUBRICATION

Treatment Guidelines

Insufficient vaginal lubrication is mainly of concern during sexual intercourse. Vaginal lubricants provide temporary relief, but must be reapplied when sexual activity is to be carried out again. Should nonprescription lubricants prove ineffective or inadequate, the patient should be referred to her physician. Oral estrogen prescribed by a physician is often helpful.

Nonprescription Medications

Vaginal lubricants, which contain such ingredients as water, glycerin, cellulose derivatives, parabens, and glycols, are considered to be cosmetics by the FDA (Table 43.5). For this reason adequate scientific data are often lacking, but some studies show effectiveness.[131–133] Comparative information is generally unavailable, and company claims are difficult to evaluate objectively.

Vaginal lubricants can be warmed to body temperature prior to application. The majority of products are water soluble; if they are not effective, oil-based products are available (e.g., petroleum jelly), although rubber products (e.g., the male condom, female pouch, and diaphragm) are incompatible with them.

Table 43.4. Representative Products for Premature Ejaculation

PRODUCT	SELECTED INGREDIENTS
Detane Gel	Benzocaine 7.5%, carbomer 940, polythylene glycol 400
Maintain	Benzocaine 7.5%, carbomer, polyethylene glycol

Vaginal lubricants may inhibit sperm motility and should perhaps be avoided by the couple attempting to attain a pregnancy.[134]

PREVENTION OF INSUFFICIENT VAGINAL LUBRICATION

Regular sexual activity maintains the female's vaginal lining in a state that is more capable of producing appropriate lubrication during sexual arousal.[119]

SUMMARY

Problems related to sexual activity that can be addressed by nonprescription products and devices include unwanted pregnancy, STDs, premature ejaculation, and insufficient vaginal lubrication.

At least 6 million unwanted pregnancies occur yearly in the United States, many in females too young to adequately care for a child. Pharmacists can help prevent unwanted pregnancies through proper patient counseling on the nonprescription

Table 43.5. Representative Vaginal Lubricants

PRODUCT	SELECTED INGREDIENTS/COMMENTS
Astroglide	Purified water, glycerin, propylene glycol; can also be used to lubricate condoms, tampons, rectal thermometers, and enema and douche nozzles
K-Y Jelly	Chlorhexidine gluconate, glycerin, purified water; can also be used to lubricate condoms, tampons, rectal thermometers, and enema and douche nozzles
K-Y Liquid	Glycerin, propylene glycol, sorbitol; a liquid that is compatible with condoms
K-Y Long Lasting	Purified water, glycerin, mineral oil; pre-filled applicators; lasts for 2–3 days; company claims compatibility with condoms
Lubrin Suppository	PEG-6-32, PEG-20, caprylic/capric triglyceride, glycerin, PEG-40 stearate, polysorbate-80, silica; must be inserted at least 5 minutes prior to intercourse; concurrent use with condom not mentioned in product literature
Replens	Purified water, glycerin, mineral oil, polycarbophil; only requires 2–3 applications weekly
Vagisil Intimate Moisturizer	Purified water, glycerin, propylene glycol

AT THE COUNTER

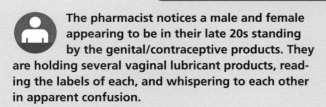 **The pharmacist notices a male and female appearing to be in their late 20s standing by the genital/contraceptive products. They are holding several vaginal lubricant products, reading the labels of each, and whispering to each other in apparent confusion.**

Interview/Patient Assessment

The pharmacist asks if he can help the couple. The male is silent at first, but the female volunteers that she is unable to take birth control tablets and has been recently fitted for a diaphragm. However, she has insufficient vaginal lubrication and wonders if plain petroleum jelly would be less expensive than the vaginal lubricant products.

Pharmacist's Analysis

1. Why is the choice of a vaginal lubricant important for the patient using a diaphragm?

2. Would petroleum jelly be acceptable for use with a diaphragm?
3. Which vaginal lubricants would be appropriate for this couple?

Patient Counseling

The choice of a vaginal lubricant is critical when the couple is using latex rubber products such as a diaphragm or condom. Oil-based products such as petroleum jelly or mineral oil degrade rubber and could cause rupture of the diaphragm or condom during use. For this reason the couple should be advised to use a product specifically labeled for use as a vaginal lubricant.

products and devices that prevent conception such as male condoms, the female pouch, vaginal spermicides, and basal thermometers. Condoms, which are available with several options such as lubrication and a receptacle end, are simple to use and offer the highest efficacy of all nonprescription contraceptive products. The female pouch, a similar product, gives women greater control over conception. Vaginal spermicides, which provide the dual actions of a barrier to sperm and a detergent effect that destroys sperm, can be purchased as foams, gels, films, suppositories, and creams. The basal thermometer may also be used to help the female discover the time of ovulation so she can decide when to use a contraceptive product.

The prevention of sexually transmitted diseases is more difficult than the prevention of conception, since any partner-to-partner contact with genitals (e.g., anal, oral, genital) may transmit the human immunodeficiency virus and other diseases and since viral agents can pass through some barrier-type contraception devices such as lambskin condoms. For these reasons only latex condoms, polyurethane condoms, or the female pouch can be considered to protect against STDs at this time.

Premature ejaculation, a problem usually associated with hypersensitivity of the head of the penis, may improve with application of benzocaine-containing, nonprescription products.

Vaginal dryness resulting from insufficient vaginal lubrication, a condition related to aging, may be improved with the application of vaginal moisturizers.

References

1. Petersen R, Moos MK. Defining and measuring unintended pregnancy: Issues and concerns. Women Health Issues 7:234, 1997.
2. Anon. Condom availability for adolescents. J Adolesc Health 18:380, 1996.
3. Gabbay M, Gibbs A. Does additional lubrication reduce condom failure? Contraception 53:155, 1996.
4. Anon. Meeting the needs of young adults. Popul Rep J (41):1, 1995.
5. Nordenberg T. Protecting against unintended pregnancy. FDA Consumer 31(3):20, 1997.
6. Morgan KW, Deneris A. Emergency contraception: Preventing unintended pregnancy. Nurse Pract 22:34, 1997.
7. Pray WS. Vaginal spermicides. US Pharmacist 17(5):17, 1992.
8. Gold MA. Emergency contraception: A second chance at preventing adolescent unintended pregnancy. Curr Opin Pediatr 9:300, 1997.
9. Goldfarb AF. Adolescent sexuality. Ann N Y Acad Sci 816:395, 1997.
10. Mosher WD, Bachrach CA. Understanding U.S. fertility: Continuity and change in the National Survey of Family Growth, 1988–1995. Fam Plann Perspect 28:4, 1996.
11. Miller LJ. Sexuality, reproduction and family planning in women with schizophrenia. Schizophren Bull 23:623, 1997.
12. Lathrop A. Pregnancy resulting from rape. J Obstet Gynecol Neonatal Nurs 27:25, 1998.
13. Moskowitz E, Jennings B. Directive counseling on long-acting contraception. Am J Public Health 86:787, 1996.
14. Henshaw SK, Kost K. Abortion patients in 1994–1995: Characteristics and contraceptive use. Fam Plann Perspect 28:140, 1996.
15. Trussell J, et al. The economic value of contraception: A comparison of 15 methods. Am J Public Health 85:494, 1995.
16. Pray WS. Condoms and prevention of HIV transmission. US Pharmacist 17(11):37, 1992.
17. Benagiano G, Cottingham J. Contraceptive methods: Pitfalls for abuse. Int J Gynaecol Obstet 56:39, 1997.
18. Anon. Pharmacists and family planning. Popul Rep J (37):1, 1989.
19. Anon. Condom availability for adolescents. J Adolesc Health 18:380, 1996.
20. Schuster MA, et al. Students' acquisition and use of school condoms in a high school condom availability program. Pediatrics 100:689, 1997.
21. Brown NL, Pennylegion MT, Hillard P. A process evaluation of condom availability in the Seattle, Washington public schools. J Sch Health 67:336, 1997.
22. Ellen JM, et al. Types of adolescent sexual relationships and associated perceptions about condom use. J Adolesc Health 18:471, 1996.
23. Santelli JS, et al. Stage of behavior change for condom use: The influence of partner type, relationship and pregnancy factors. Fam Plann Perspect 28:101, 1996.
24. Anon. Avanti polyurethane condom. Wkly Pharm Rep 46 (34):1, 1997.
25. Farr G, et al. Safety, functionality and acceptability of a prototype polyurethane condom. Adv Contracept 13:439, 1997.
26. Fihn SD, et al. Association between use of spermicide-coated condoms and *Escherichia coli* urinary tract infection in young women. Am J Epidemiol 144:512, 1996.
27. Donovan B. Condoms and the prevention of sexually transmissible disease. Br J Hosp Med 54:575, 1995/96.
28. Silverman BG, Gross TP. Use and effectiveness of condoms during anal intercourse. A review. Sex Transm Dis 24:11, 1997.
29. Free MJ, et al. Latex rubber condoms: Predicting and extending shelf life. Contraception 53:221, 1996.
30. Anon. Latex condoms; user labeling; expiration dating. Fed Reg 61:26140, 1996.
31. Silverstone T. Condoms: Still the most popular contraceptive. Prof Care Mother Child 7:108, 1997.
32. Heath CB. Helping patients choose appropriate contraception. Am Fam Physician 48:1115, 1993.
33. Rosenberg MJ, Waugh MS. Latex condom breakage and slippage in a controlled clinical trial. Contraception 56:17, 1997.
34. Rugpao S, et al. Multiple condom use and decreased condom breakage and slippage in Thailand. J Acquir Immune Defic Syndr Hum Retrovirol 14:169, 1997.
35. Anon. New data on plastic condoms. Consum Rep 60(8):506, 1995.
36. Short RV. Contraceptives of the future in light of HIV infection. Aust NZ J Obstet Gynaecol 34:330, 1994.
37. Hiltabiddle SJ. Adolescent condom use, the health belief model, and the prevention of sexually transmitted disease. J Obstet Gynecol Neonatal Nurs 25:61, 1996.
38. Nguyen MN, Saucier J-F, Pica LA. Factors influencing the intention to use condoms in Quebec sexually inactive male adolescents. J Adolesc Health 18:48, 1996.

39. Rosenberg MJ, et al. The male polyurethane condom: A review of current knowledge. Contraception 53:141, 1996.

40. Quirk A, Rhodes T, Stimson GV. 'Unsafe protected sex': Qualitative insights on measures of sexual risk. AIDS Care 100:105, 1998.

41. VanUlsen J, et al. Allergy to spermicidal lubricant in a contraceptive. Contact Dermatitis 17:115, 1987.

42. McCabe E, Golub S, Lee AC. Making the female condom a "reality" for adolescents. J Pediatr Adolesc Gynecol 10:15, 1997.

43. Gollub EL, Stein Z, El-Sadr W. Short-term acceptability of the female condom among staff and patients at a New York City hospital. Fam Plann Perspect 27:155, 1995.

44. Shoupe D. Contraception in the 1990s. Curr Opin Obstet Gynecol 8:211, 1996.

45. Gollub EL, Stein Z, El-Sadr W. Power and the female condom (Reply to Letter). Fam Plann Perspect 28:78, 1996.

46. Elias CJ, Coggins C. Female-controlled methods to prevent sexual transmission of HIV. AIDS 10(Suppl 3):S43, 1996.

47. Fed Reg 45:82014, 1980.

48. Hira SK, et al. Spermicide acceptability among patients at a sexually transmitted disease clinic in Zambia. Am J Public Health 85(8 Pt 1):1098, 1995.

49. Goldberg MS. Choosing a contraceptive. FDA Consumer 27(7):18, 1993.

50. Kirkman R, Chantler E. Contraception and the prevention of sexually transmitted diseases. Br Med Bull 49:171, 1993.

51. Fed Reg 60:6892, 1995.

52. Cohen D, et al. Influencing spermicide use among low-income minority women. J Am Med Wom Assoc 50:11, 1995.

53. McGroarty JA, Reid G, Bruce AW. The influence of nonoxynol-9 containing spermicides on urogenital infection. J Urol 152:831, 1994.

54. Poindexter AN III, et al. Comparison of spermicides on vulvar, vaginal, and cervical mucosa. Contraception 53:147, 1996.

55. Sangi Haghpeykar H, Poindexter AN 3rd, Levine H. Sperm transport and survival of a new spermicide contraceptive. Advantage 24 Study Group. Contraception 53:353, 1996.

56. Anon. Today sponge discontinued. FDA Consumer 29(3):4, 1995.

57. Buzby M. Viral hepatitis: A sexually transmitted disease? Nurse Pract Forum 7:10, 1996.

58. Wang Q. Sexually transmitted diseases: Incidence and distribution. Chin Med Sci J 11:56, 1996.

59. Catchpole MA. The role of epidemiology and surveillance systems in the control of sexually transmitted diseases. Genitourin Med 72:321, 1996.

60. Brugha R, et al. Genital herpes infection: A review. Int J Epidemiol 26:698, 1997.

61. Wold C, et al. Unsafe sex in men who have sex with both men and women. J Acquir Defic Syndr Hum Retrovirol 17:361, 1998.

62. Thomas JC, Tucker MJ. The development and use of the concept of a sexually transmitted disease core. J Infect Dis 174(Suppl 2):S134, 1996.

63. Pyett PM, Warr DJ. Vulnerability on the streets: Female sex workers and HIV risk. AIDS Care 9:539, 1997.

64. Anon. The immune system and HIV. U.S. Department of Health and Human Services. http://www.qcfurball.com/cat/aids/kidsaids.html. 1998.

65. Wendt SJ, Solomon LJ. Barriers to condom use among heterosexual male and female college students. J Am Coll Health 44:105, 1995.

66. Anon. Popul Rep L (9):1, 1993.

67. Krowchuk DP. Sexually transmitted diseases in adolescents: What's new? South Med J 91:124, 1998.

68. Anon. Centers for Disease Control and Prevention. http://cdc.gov/nchstp/hiv-aids/stats/cumulati.htm. 1998.

69. Swanson JM, Dibble SL, Trocki K. A description of the gender differences in risk behaviors in young adults with genital herpes. Public Health Nurs 12:99, 1995.

70. Jossens MOR, Schachter J, Sweet RL. Risk factors associated with pelvic inflammatory disease of differing microbial etiologies. Obstet Gynecol 83:989, 1994.

71. Quan M. Pelvic inflammatory disease: Diagnosis and management. J Am Board Fam Pract 7:110, 1994.

72. Ku L, et al. The promise of integrated representative surveys about sexually transmitted diseases and behavior. Sex Transm Dis 24:299, 1997.

73. Ferreira N. Sexually transmitted Chlamydia trachomatis. Nurse Pract Forum 8:70, 1997.

74. Brabin L. Providing accessible health care for adolescents with sexually transmitted disease. Acta Trop 62:209, 1996.

75. Beckman LJ, Harvey SM, Tiersky LA. Attitudes about condoms and condom use among college students. J Am Coll Health 44:243, 1996.

76. Daly CC, et al. Contraceptive methods and the transmission of HIV: Implications for family planning. Genitourin Med 70:110, 1994.

77. Frank ML, et al. A cross-sectional survey of condom use in conjunction with other contraceptive methods. Women Health 23:31, 1995.

78. Cu-UIvin S, et al. Human immunodeficiency virus infection and acquired immunodeficiency syndrome among North American women. Am J Med 101:316, 1996.

79. Creatsas G. Sexually transmitted diseases and oral contraceptive use during adolescence. Ann N Y Acad Sci 816:404, 1997.

80. Tait IA, et al. Silent upper genital tract chlamydial infection and disease in women. Int J STD AIDS 8:329, 1997.

81. Willis JL. Preventing STDs. FDA Consumer 27(5):33, 1993.

82. U.S. Preventive Services Task Force. Counseling to prevent HIV infection and other sexually transmitted diseases. Am Fam Physician 41:1179, 1990.

83. Goldenberg RL, et al. Sexually transmitted diseases and adverse outcomes of pregnancy. Clin Perinatol 24:23, 1997.

84. O'Connell ML. The effect of birth control methods on sexually transmitted disease/HIV risk. J Obstet Gynecol Neonatal Nurs 25:476, 1996.

85. Anderson JE, Brackbill R, Mosher WD. Condom use for disease prevention among unmarried U.S. women. Fam Plann Perspect 28:25, 1996.

86. King G, et al. Substance use, coping, and safer sex practices among adolescents with hemophilia and human immunodeficiency virus. The Hemophilia Behavioral Intervention Evaluative Project Committee. J Adolesc Health 18:435, 1996.

87. Pinkerton SD, Abramson PR. Effectiveness of condoms in preventing HIV transmission. Soc Sci Med 44:1303, 1997.

88. Sanchez J, et al. Sexually transmitted infections in female sex workers: Reduced by condom use but not by a limited periodic examination program. Sex Transm Dis 25:82, 1998.

89. Anon. Condoms relabeled for accuracy. FDA Consumer 26(1):42, 1992.

90. d'Oro LC, et al. Barrier methods of contraception, spermicides, and sexually transmitted diseases: A review. Genitourin Med 70:410, 1994.

91. Tan BB, et al. Perioperative collapse: Prevalence of latex allergy in patients sensitive to anaesthetic agents. Contact Dermatitis 36:47, 1997.

92. Evans BA, Bond RA, MacRae KD. Sexual relationships, risk behaviour, and condom use in the spread of sexually transmitted infections to heterosexual men. Genitourin Med 73:368, 1997.

93. Cook RL, Rosenberg MJ. Do spermicides containing nonoxynol-9 prevent sexually transmitted infections? A meta-analysis. Sex Transm Dis 25:144, 1998.

94. Hiar SK, et al. Condom and nonoxynol-9 use and the incidence of HIV infection in serodiscordant couples in Zambia. Int J STD AIDS 8:243, 1997.

95. Anon. Recommendations for the development of vaginal microbicides. AIDS 10:1, 1996.

96. Fein RL. Intracavernous medication for the treatment of premature ejaculation. Urology 35:301, 1990.

97. St Lawrence JS, Madakasira S. Evaluation and treatment of premature ejaculation: A critical review. Int J Psychiatry Med 22:77, 1992.

98. Kindler S, et al. The treatment of comorbid premature ejaculation and panic disorder with fluoxetine. Clin Neuropharmacol 20:466, 1997.

99. Metz ME, et al. Premature ejaculation: A psychophysiological review. J Sex Marital Ther 23:3, 1997.

100. Read S, King M, Watson J. Sexual dysfunction in primary medical care: Prevalence, characteristics and detection by the general practitioner. J Public Health Med 19:387, 1997.

101. Fed Reg 47:39420, 1982.

102. Xin ZC, et al. Somatosensory evoked potentials in patients with primary premature ejaculation. J Urol 158:451, 1997.

103. Xin ZC, et al. Penile sensitivity in patients with primary premature ejaculation. J Urol 156:979, 1996.

104. Ozturk B, et al. Erectile dysfunction in premature ejaculation. Arch Ital Urol Androl 69:133, 1997.

105. Cohen PG. The association of premature ejaculation and hypogonadotropic hypogonadism. J Sex Marital Ther 23:208, 1997.

106. Rowland DL, Cooper SE, Slob AK. Genital and psychoaffective response to erotic stimulation in sexually functional and dysfunctional men. J Abnorm Psychol 105:194, 1996.

107. Haensel SM, Rowland DL, Kallan KT. Clomipramine and sexual function in men with premature ejaculation and controls. J Urol 156:1310, 1996.

108. Ludovico GM, et al. Paroxetine in the treatment of premature ejaculation. Br J Urol 77:881, 1996.

109. Segraves RT, et al. Clomipramine versus placebo in the treatment of premature ejaculation: A pilot study. J Sex Marital Ther 19:198, 1993.

110. Mendels J, Camera A, Sikes C. Sertraline treatment for premature ejaculation. J Clin Psychopharmacol 15:341, 1995.

111. Berkovitch M, Keresteci AG, Koren G. Efficacy of prilocaine-lidocaine cream in the treatment of premature ejaculation. J Urol 154:1360, 1995.

112. Kara H, et al. The efficacy of fluoxetine in the treatment of premature ejaculation: A double-blind placebo controlled study. J Urol 156:1631, 1996.

113. La Pera G, Nicastro A. A new treatment for premature ejaculation: The rehabilitation of the pelvic floor. J Sex Marital Ther 22:22, 1996.

114. Fed Reg 50:40260, 1985.

115. Fed Reg 57:27654, 1992.

116. O'Connell MB. Vaginal dryness. US Pharmacist 19(9):80, 1994.

117. Weber AM, et al. Vaginal anatomy and sexual function. Obstet Gynecol 86:946, 1995.

118. Debrovner D. The New VD. Am Drugg 207(4):39, 1993.

119. Deamer RL, Thompson JF. The role of medications in geriatric sexual function. Clin Geriatr Med 7:95, 1991.

120. Natchigall LE. Comparative study: Replens versus local estrogen in menopausal women. Fertil Steril 61:178, 1994.

121. Barlow DH, et al. Urogenital ageing and its effect on sexual health in older British women. Br J Obstet Gynaecol 104:87, 1997.

122. Leiblum SR, Baume RM, Croog SH. The sexual functioning of elderly hypertensive women. J Sex Marital Ther 20:259, 1994.

123. Bachmann G. Urogenital ageing: An old problem newly recognized. Maturitas 22(Suppl):S1, 1995.

124. Marchesoni D, et al. Gynaecological aspects of primary Sjögren's syndrome. Eur J Obstet Gynecol Reprod Biol 63:49, 1995.

125. Mulherin DM, et al. Sjögren's syndrome in women presenting with chronic dyspareunia. Br J Obstet Gynaecol 104:1019, 1997.

126. Sreebny LM, et al. Xerostomia in diabetes mellitus. Diabetes Care 15:900, 1992.

127. Curry SL, et al. The impact of systemic lupus erythematosus on women's sexual functioning. J Rheumatol 21:2254, 1994.

128. Baird DD, et al. Vaginal douching and reduced fertility. Am J Public Health 86:844, 1996.

129. Levin RJ. VIP, vagina, clitoral and periurethral glans—An update on human female genital arousal. Exp Clin Endocrinol 98:61, 1991.

130. Civic D, Wilson D. Dry sex in Zimbabwe and implications for condom use. Soc Sci Med 42:91, 1996.

131. Bygdeman M, Swahn ML. Replens versus dienoestrol cream in the symptomatic treatment of vaginal atrophy in postmenopausal women. Maturitas 23:259, 1996.

132. Loprinzi CL, et al. Phase III randomized double-blind study to evaluate the efficacy of a polycarbophil-based vaginal moisturizer in women with breast cancer. J Clin Oncol 15:969, 1997.

133. Heimer G, Samsioe G. Effects of vaginally delivered estrogens. Acta Obstet Gynecol Scand Suppl 163:1, 1996.

134. Kutteh WH, et al. Vaginal lubricants for the infertile couple: Effect on sperm activity. Int J Fertil Menopausal Stud 41:400, 1996.

Female Genital Conditions

AT THE COUNTER

A woman asks the pharmacist whether a popular douche product is better than hydrocortisone cream for vaginal pruritus.

Interview/Patient Assessment

The pharmacist asks the patient about her symptoms. She has experienced vaginal itching for 2 to 3 days.

Pharmacist's Analysis

1. Has the vaginal itch persisted too long to recommend self-treatment?
2. What symptoms would contraindicate self-therapy for vaginal itch?
3. Should the pharmacist recommend a douche product or hydrocortisone cream for this patient?

The patient appears to have vaginal itch that is self-treatable.

Patient Counseling

The patient may use self-medication for vaginal itch that does not exceed 7 days in duration. Thus this patient may use an appropriate nonprescription product for another 4 to 5 days before she should see a physician. However, if redness, swelling, or pain develops, she should stop use of the nonprescription product and see a physician.

Douche products have not been found to be safe and effective in relieving vaginal itch. However, hydrocortisone 0.25 to 1% relieves pruritus of the genital areas safely and effectively, unless the patient has a vaginal discharge. The pharmacist may recommend hydrocortisone vaginal cream, cautioning the patient about the maximum recommended duration of use and about ceasing use if the new symptoms listed above develop. Further, should the problem clear up and recur within a few days, she should also see a physician.

This chapter describes several conditions particular to the female: inadequate vaginal hygiene, vaginal fungal infections, and vaginal irritation and pruritus. Perhaps the most troublesome is the vaginal fungal infection, which also can be embarrassing. Further, recurrent vaginal fungal infections signal the possible presence of diabetes mellitus or AIDS. Inadequate vaginal hygiene, which may result in irritation and pruritus, may be treated with such nonpharmacologic agents as nonmedicated douches. Vaginal irritation and pruritus may also be caused by allergy and can be safely self-treated with several ingredients.

INADEQUATE VAGINAL HYGIENE

Inadequate vaginal hygiene is not a medical condition per se, but is caused by a lack of cleanliness. Vaginal hygiene is in large part based on personal perception. For example, female patients may perceive vaginal uncleanliness following sexual activity, as a result of a vaginal infection, or even for unspecified reasons. One author suggested that to avoid the perception of inadequate vaginal hygiene, women must maintain scrupulous cleanliness of the external vaginal genitalia at all times, especially when experiencing vaginal discharge.[1] If vaginal hygiene becomes extremely poor, it may cause irritation and pruritus. (See "Vaginal Irritation and Pruritus.")

PREVALENCE OF INADEQUATE VAGINAL HYGIENE

As a poorly defined problem, the prevalence of inadequate vaginal hygiene is difficult to determine. However, since douching is a widely accepted approach to vaginal hygiene, its incidence provides a clue. As many as 67 million females in the United States douche on a regular basis.[1,2]

EPIDEMIOLOGY OF INADEQUATE VAGINAL HYGIENE

The epidemiology of those who douche may also provide clues to the epidemiology of inadequate vaginal hygiene. At least two-thirds of black women douche, as opposed to 33% of whites.[3] The age group that douches most often (41%) is between 20 and 24. Conversely, only 31% of those aged 15 to 19 douche. Those who are impoverished douche almost twice as much as those who are not. Women without a high school degree douche four times more than those with 16 or more years of education.

ETIOLOGY OF INADEQUATE VAGINAL HYGIENE

Inadequate vaginal hygiene may be caused by internal vaginal secretions, seminal fluids deposited by the male, and/or residue remaining from various vaginal products (e.g., contraceptives, sexual lubricants, and cleansing agents).

MANIFESTATIONS OF INADEQUATE VAGINAL HYGIENE

Inadequate vaginal hygiene can result in vaginal and/or vulvar odors; however, vaginal odors also may be caused by infectious agents.[4]

TREATMENT OF INADEQUATE VAGINAL HYGIENE

Nonprescription Medications

The FDA Panel assigned to review vaginal products judged four ingredients to be safe and effective in removing vaginal discharge and secretions: docusate, nonoxynol-9, octoxynol-9, and sodium lauryl sulfate.[4] The FDA later withdrew this report, stating that these actions were cosmetic and would not be addressed further by the OTC review process.[5] Consequently, no nonprescription medications are indicated for providing a pharmacologic action in treating inadequate vaginal hygiene. (See "Nonpharmacologic Therapies.")

Nonpharmacologic Therapies: Douching

Douching—the irrigation of the vagina with a liquid possessing either cosmetic or medicinal actions—is a culturally acquired habit taught by or suggested by the mother or female role model in certain cultures.[6] Douching is often used to treat inadequate vaginal hygiene.[4,7] Several representative cosmetic-douche products are listed in Table 44.1. Douching equipment is considered to be a medical device by the FDA.[4]

As many as 37% of women (reportedly 20 to 67 million American women) douche; many do so once or twice weekly.[3,8,9] Douching provides a number of cosmetic benefits such as improving vaginal hygiene through mechanical cleansing actions, soothing and refreshing the vaginal vault, and deodorizing.

Females may douche with commercially available products or homemade solutions (e.g., vinegar and water).[10] Douche products for treating inadequate vaginal hygiene do not contain active ingredients per se and are regarded as cosmetic products by the FDA.[2]

Douching with commercially available douches is implicated in increased risk of tubal (ectopic) pregnancies and reduced fertility.[10–13] Douching also increases the patient's chances of developing pelvic inflammatory disease, perhaps by unbalancing local vaginal host defenses and subsequently facilitating the ascent of infectious agents to the upper genital tract.[2,14–17]

⚠ *Douching during pregnancy is dangerous because of the increased vascularity of the uterus.*[4] Potential complications include fatal air embolism, detachment of the placenta, rupture of the chorioamniotic membrane, intrauterine infection, and chemical damage to the fetus.

Women who wish to douche should observe the following FDA-recommended precautions[4]:

- Do not suspend the douche bag more than 3 feet above the vagina.
- Release the clamp of the douche bag prior to placing the nozzle in the vagina so any air in the tubing will be expelled from the tubing outside the vagina.
- The vaginal lips should not be pressed around the nozzle to allow free outflow of the douche solution. (Overfilling of the vagina may force fluid into the uterus and cause inflammation.)

Table 44.1. Representative Cosmetic Douche Products

PRODUCT	SELECTED INGREDIENTS[a]/COMMENTS
Massengill Disposable Douche Extra Mild Vinegar and Water	Purified water, sodium citrate, citric acid, vinegar
Massengill Disposable Douche Extra Cleansing Vinegar and Water	Purified water, sodium citrate, citric acid, vinegar, diazolidinyl urea, octoxynol-9, cetylpyridinium chloride, edatate disodium
Massengill Disposable Douche Baking Soda and Water	Purified water, sodium bicarbonate
Massengill Disposable Douche Country Flowers	Purified water, sodium citrate, citric acid, SD alcohol 40, diazolidinyl urea, octoxynol-9, fragrance, cetylpyridinium chloride, edatate disodium
Summer's Eve Disposable Douche	Purified water, citric acid, sodium benzoate, fragrance
Summer's Eve Disposable Douche Vinegar and Water	Purified water, sodium chloride, vinegar, benzoic acid
Vagi•Gard Medicated Douche	Octoxynol-9, purified water, lactic acid, aloe vera

[a]Concentrations of the ingredients in douche products are usually not provided by the manufacturers.

- Rinse and dry all reusable douche equipment prior to storage.
- When applying prepackaged disposable douches, gently insert the nozzle into the vagina. Only use enough pressure to allow solution to flow gently into the vagina.

If douching results in pain, soreness, itching, excessive dryness, or irritation, stop use of the douche product. If symptoms persist, see a physician. Douching does not prevent pregnancy.

VAGINAL FUNGAL INFECTIONS: VULVOVAGINAL CANDIDIASIS (VVC)

Vaginal infections may be caused by many different organisms. However, the vaginal fungal infection is the only type of vaginal infection the patient may self-treat. If the patient is not absolutely certain that her infection is fungal in origin, the pharmacist must advise that she see a physician to determine its etiology. For this reason this section is limited to the discussion of the vaginal fungal infection. The vaginal fungal infection is a mucosal infection most often caused by various *Candida* species.[18] It is also referred to as vulvovaginal candidiasis (VVC). Vaginal fungal infections may be spread during sexual activity, but this is not the primary mode of transmission. For this reason they are not included under problems related to sexual activity in Chapter 43.

PREVALENCE OF VAGINAL FUNGAL INFECTIONS

As many as 75% of females will experience at least one episode of VVC.[18] With an estimated 13 million cases annually in the United States, VVC is one of the most prevalent medical conditions in postpubertal females (some females experience more than one episode yearly).[18]

EPIDEMIOLOGY OF VAGINAL FUNGAL INFECTIONS

Vaginal fungal infections are precipitated by numerous factors that allow normal vaginal organisms (or organisms that reach the vagina from the GI tract) to increase excessively.

Age

Females who have not reached puberty or who have reached menopause—i.e., women whose levels of estrogen are reduced—seldom experience VVC.[18] VVC in a prepubertal female is uncommon and suggests a foreign body lodged in the vagina, sexual abuse, chemical irritation, or acute bacterial infection.[19,20]

Immune Status

Some patients with impaired cell-mediated immunity may not be able to combat candidal infections. This includes patients with AIDS and patients taking corticosteroids (e.g., posttransplantation).

Hormone Ingestion

Estrogen and progesterone reduce vaginal immune functions, specifically the secretion of IgG and IgA antibodies.[19] Thus oral contraceptives increase the risk of VVC, as do pregnancy and ingestion of hormone replacement products following menopause.[21]

Sexual Activity

Sexual transmission can introduce candidal organisms into the vagina.[18] Sexual activity with the use of a diaphragm increases the risk of vaginal *Candida* colonization, since a poorly maintained diaphragm may harbor *Candida*.[22]

Hygiene

Females may introduce gastrointestinal organisms into the vagina while carrying out post–bowel-movement hygiene.[18] Young children tend to cleanse from the bottoms forward, which increases the risk of VVC by contaminating the vagina with fecal candidal organisms. Females should be taught to cleanse from the vagina toward the anus, a backward motion.[19]

Diabetes Mellitus

Females with diabetes mellitus exhibit a prevalence of candidal infection 14% higher than women without diabetes.[23]

ETIOLOGY OF VAGINAL FUNGAL INFECTIONS

VVC is most often caused by *Candida albicans*.[24,25] This organism, a normal commensal resident of the genital and gastrointestinal tracts, is found in the vaginal cultures of 20 to 25% of asymptomatic females. *Candida albicans* boasts an exceptional tolerance for different temperatures and pH conditions.[26] This characteristic, and other factors, explain why it causes 85 to 90% of VVC.[18,27] The balance of VVC episodes are caused by *Candida glabrata* and *Candida tropicalis*.[28–31]

The *Candida* species are thought to colonize the vagina through disruption of the normal vaginal microflora. (Vaginal microflora normally present a biologic barrier to infection, preventing fungal species from gaining a toehold.) These organisms include *Lactobacillus, Peptostreptococcus, Streptococcus, Staphylococcus,* and other species.[32] The most striking example of this disruption is the high incidence of VVC following ingestion of broad-spectrum antibiotics.

MANIFESTATIONS OF VAGINAL FUNGAL INFECTIONS

Symptoms of candidal fungal infections include itching, burning, soreness, abnormal vaginal discharge, and **dys-**

pareunia (pain occurring during sexual intercourse), as well as erythema and inflammation of the vaginal and vulvar regions.[18] The discharge is odorless; the appearance may be that of a thick paste or look like cottage cheese.

SPECIFIC CONSIDERATIONS OF VAGINAL FUNGAL INFECTIONS

Classifying VVC by Recurrence

The factors that cause normal vaginal organisms to transform into infective invaders are not well understood. Individual sensitivity to organism load further clouds the issue. The typical patient has large numbers of pathogenic *Candida* and exhibits severe symptoms. However, some patients have few organisms, but complain of severe symptoms. Others have large numbers of organisms, but seem not to exhibit symptoms. For these reasons physicians hypothesize that different etiologies are responsible for sporadic versus recurrent VVC.

While the individual case of VVC is easily treated, recurrences occur in at least 5% of patients.[18] Since the number of recurrences helps determine etiology, physicians classify recurrence patterns in several categories.

SPORADIC VVC
Patients who have two episodes of VVC or fewer per year are said to have sporadic VVC. Episodes are further subclassified as primary or secondary sporadic VVC:

- Primary Sporadic VVC: Idiopathic, with no known cause
- Secondary Sporadic VVC: Infrequent and may be precipitated by pregnancy, ingestion of antibiotics, or wearing tight undergarments

RECURRENT VVC
Women who experience three or more episodes yearly are said to have recurrent VVC. Recurrent VVC is further subclassified as primary recurrent VVC and secondary VVC:

- Primary Recurrent VVC: Frequent idiopathic infections with no detectable cause[33]
- Secondary Recurrent VVC: Frequent recurrences resulting from AIDS, poorly controlled diabetes mellitus, administration of hormonal replacement therapy or oral contraceptives, and immunosuppression[18,31,34,35]

Physician Diagnosis of VVC

Physicians may diagnose the cause of VVC through several means[36]:

- A microscopic wet mount reveals *Trichomonas* as a motile protozoon. Application of potassium hydroxide to the slide allows microscopic detection of pseudohyphae and buds that indicate a fungal pathogen. Application of KOH also results in an amine odor when the pathogen is bacterial rather than fungal.
- A pH test on vaginal tissues indicates a bacterial or trichomonal cause if the pH is greater than 4.5 and a candidal etiology if the pH is less than 4.5.[36]

PROGNOSIS OF VAGINAL FUNGAL INFECTIONS

About one-half of patients with recurrent VVC experience the onset of a new infection within 5 to 90 days of successful treatment of the prior infection, while 5% will undergo repeated episodes.[37] Recurrences develop in some females despite their scrupulous avoidance of all known risk factors for the development of VVC.[18] Antifungal therapy is often curative for the ongoing episode, but ineffective in preventing future bouts of VVC.

TREATMENT OF VAGINAL FUNGAL INFECTIONS

Prior to the availability of nonprescription products to treat vaginal fungal infections, approximately 10 million of the 13 million cases in the United States each year were seen by physicians.[18] Since nonprescription products became available, that number has dropped. Thus there are millions of females who use nonprescription products for treatment of VVC each year.

Treatment Guidelines

A number of organisms produce vaginal infections that may be mistaken for fungal causes, including *Trichomonas vaginalis, Gardnerella vaginalis, Mycoplasma hominis,* and *Bacteroides*.[38] For this reason pharmacists should refer any vaginal infections unless there is absolute assurance that they are candidal in origin (as self-assessed by the patient who has had a prior, physician-diagnosed vaginal fungal infection). Product labels warn patients not to use vaginal antifungals unless they have had a previously diagnosed vaginal yeast infection. (See Patient Assessment Algorithm 44.1.) If the symptoms mirror symptoms experienced before, the patient can begin using nonprescription medications without physician consultation.

🔵 *If a vaginal-fungal-infection product does not work after the full course of therapy has been administered (1, 3, or 7 days depending on the product), the patient should consult a physician to check for resistant organisms or nonfungal pathogens.* Patients who experience frequent, recurring VVC should see a physician to evaluate the possibility of diabetes mellitus, allergy, immunodeficiency (including AIDS), or pregnancy.[39] Recurrence within about 2 months or shorter is cause for alarm.

Occasionally, a sex partner may harbor the infection. A moist, white scaling rash or redness under the foreskin of the penis, for example, may be fungal. If a sex partner exhibits symptoms, he or she should also receive therapy from a physician, since there is no nonprescription product for the male with a genital candidal infection.

Vaginal antifungal products are available as both vaginal suppositories (referred to as tablets by some companies) and cream. The product should be inserted or applied at night to increase contact time with vaginal mucosa (Fig. 44.1). The products do not stain, but a pad or minipad will help protect underclothing. *A tampon will absorb medication and should not be used with vaginal antifungal medications.*

Patient Assessment Algorithm 44.1. Fungal Vaginal Infection

```
┌─────────────────────────────────────────┐         ┌──────────────────────────────────────────┐
│ Has the patient previously had a          │   No    │              Refer to physician.           │
│ physician-diagnosed vaginal fungal        ├────────▶│                                            │
│ infection?                                 │         └──────────────────────────────────────────┘
└─────────────────────────────────────────┘
                    │ Yes
                    ▼
┌─────────────────────────────────────────┐         ┌──────────────────────────────────────────┐
│ Has the patient used a product for this   │   Yes   │              Refer to physician.           │
│ episode for the recommended number of     ├────────▶│                                            │
│ days without resolution?                   │         └──────────────────────────────────────────┘
└─────────────────────────────────────────┘
                    │ No
                    ▼
┌─────────────────────────────────────────┐         ┌──────────────────────────────────────────┐
│ Has the patient had a fungal infection     │   Yes   │              Refer to physician.           │
│ within the last 2 months?                  ├────────▶│                                            │
└─────────────────────────────────────────┘         └──────────────────────────────────────────┘
                    │ No
                    ▼
┌─────────────────────────────────────────┐         ┌──────────────────────────────────────────┐
│ Is the patient under the age of 12 years?  │   Yes   │              Refer to physician.           │
│                                            ├────────▶│                                            │
└─────────────────────────────────────────┘         └──────────────────────────────────────────┘
                    │ No
                    ▼
┌─────────────────────────────────────────┐         ┌──────────────────────────────────────────┐
│ Is the patient pregnant?                   │   Yes   │              Refer to physician.           │
│                                            ├────────▶│                                            │
└─────────────────────────────────────────┘         └──────────────────────────────────────────┘
                    │ No
                    ▼
┌─────────────────────────────────────────┐         ┌──────────────────────────────────────────┐
│ Does the patient have fever, chills,       │   Yes   │              Refer to physician.           │
│ nausea, vomiting, rash, back pain, a       ├────────▶│                                            │
│ foul-smelling discharge, or pain in        │         └──────────────────────────────────────────┘
│ either shoulder?                           │
└─────────────────────────────────────────┘
                    │ No
                    ▼
┌─────────────────────────────────────────┐
│ Recommend clotrimazole, miconazole,        │
│ butoconazole, or tioconazole.              │
└─────────────────────────────────────────┘
```

Reusable applicators should be washed with soap and water and air dried after each use to prevent reinfection. Prefilled, disposable applicators are preferred.

The multidose vaginal antifungals should be used for three or seven consecutive nights, even if menstrual flow begins during treatment. Patients should not douche during treatment to prevent washing out the antifungal.

Vaginal antifungals may contain ingredients that degrade condoms, diaphragms, or the cervical cap. If the patient contemplates use of these devices, the label of the antifungal must be examined carefully to ensure that it would not degrade the device. These contraceptives should not be used within 48 hours after application of a vaginal antifungal.

Vaginal antifungals are contraindicated in children under the age of 12 or during pregnancy since they are not proven safe in these patient groups. These products also are contraindicated for patients with fever (some packages state fever over 100°), chills, nausea, vomiting, rash, back pain, or a foul-smelling discharge—all symptoms that indicate more serious vaginal infections and/or STDs. One company also warns against use if the patient has pain in either shoulder, since some STDs (e.g., chlamydia) can cause referred pain in the shoulder.

Nonprescription Medications

Nonprescription treatment of VVC involves topical application of chemicals known as imidazoles (Table 44.2). These chemicals cure 80 to 90% of vaginal fungal infections.[39] Adverse reactions are mild, usually limited to vulvovaginal burning as a result of allergic contact dermatitis or irritant dermatitis. Currently available vaginal antifungals work in 1,

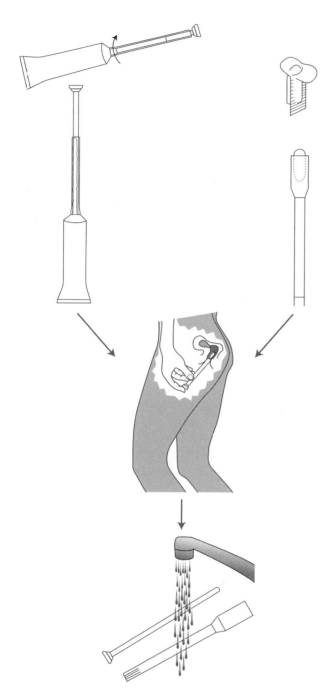

Figure 44.1. Use of vaginal antifungal creams (*left*) and suppositories (*right*): (1) Either fill applicator with cream or place one suppository in applicator. (2) Place applicator tip into vagina. (3) Disassemble and wash applicator.

3, or 7 days. Seven-day products require application for seven consecutive nights, which could hamper compliance. Thus the 3-day or 1-day products might be preferable because of the shorter duration of therapy. However, candidal organisms may persist in the vagina as long as 5 days after the onset of treatment. For this reason symptoms may not resolve in 1 day with a single-day product or in 3 days with 3-day products.[39] Products not proven safe and effective for treating vaginal fungal (yeast) infections should be avoided. See "Homeopathic Yeast Suppositories."

CLOTRIMAZOLE

Clotrimazole 1% cream and 100-mg inserts became an OTC product in late 1990, as Gyne-Lotrimin Cream and Inserts, Mycelex-7 Cream and Vaginal Tablets, and FemCare Cream and Vaginal Tablets. A combination pack contains seven tablets and a 7-g tube of cream to allow coverage of the external vulvae. A 3-day therapy known as Gyne-Lotrimin 3 became available in late 1996. Product containers do not carry warnings about use with condoms or diaphragms.

MICONAZOLE NITRATE

Miconazole 2% cream and 100-mg suppositories became an OTC product in early 1991, as Monistat 7 Cream (in a tube or in prefilled applicators) or Suppositories. A 3-day therapy became available as Monistat 3 in mid 1996. (See "A Pharmacist's Journal: Where's the Monistat?") A combination product contains 3 vaginal suppositories and a 9-g tube of cream to allow treatment of the external vulvae. Miconazole creams contain mineral oil; the suppositories contain hydrogenated vegetable oils. Thus the use of the products may weaken condoms and diaphragms and cause them to rupture.

BUTOCONAZOLE NITRATE

Butoconazole 2% cream was the first 3-day therapy for VVC, available as Femstat 3 Cream in early 1996. The product may damage condoms and diaphragms.

TIOCONAZOLE

Tioconazole 6.5% ointment was the first 1-day therapy for VVC. It entered the market as Vagistat-1 in early 1997, with the product Monistat 1 shortly added to the market. Its vehicle may damage condoms and diaphragms.

VAGINAL IRRITATION AND PRURITUS

Vaginal irritation is a nonspecific (poorly defined) term that includes minor symptoms such as pruritus or discomfort.

PREVALENCE OF VAGINAL IRRITATION AND PRURITUS

The prevalence of vaginal pruritus was found to be 11 to 25% in two studies.[40,41] However, in a survey, only 19.6% of females had ever used nonprescription vaginal antipruritics.[1]

EPIDEMIOLOGY OF VAGINAL IRRITATION AND PRURITUS

As many as 50% of postmenopausal women may experience vaginal discomfort (or some other urogenital problem).[42] Women who use products containing nonoxynol-9 experience a heightened incidence of vaginal irritation.[43–45] Use of polyurethane condoms may produce vaginal irritation.[46]

Table 44.2. Representative Vaginal Antifungal Products

PRODUCT	SELECTED INGREDIENTS/COMMENTS
Femstat 3 Disposable Applicators	Three prefilled applicators containing 100 mg each of butoconazole nitrate
Gyne-Lotrimin Cream	Clotrimazole 1% with 1 reusable applicator used for 7 days
Gyne-Lotrimin 3 Combination Pack	Three vaginal inserts containing 200 mg each of clotrimazole; also a 7-g tube of 1% cream
Monistat 1	One prefilled applicator containing tioconazole 300 mg
Monistat 3 Combination Pack	Three suppositories containing 200 mg each of miconazole nitrate; also a 9-g tube of 2% cream
Monistat 7 Vaginal Suppositories	Seven suppositories containing 100 mg each of miconazole nitrate with 1 applicator
Monistat 7 Vaginal Cream	Miconazole nitrate 2% with 1 applicator delivering 100 mg per dose for 7 days
Monistat 7 Disposable Applicators	Seven disposable applicators containing 100 mg each of miconazole nitrate
Monistat 7 Prefilled Applicators	Seven prefilled applicators containing 100 mg each of miconazole nitrate
Mycelex-3 Vaginal Cream	Butoconazole nitrate 2% (20-g tube) with three disposable applicators
Mycelex-7 Inserts	Seven inserts containing 100 mg each of clotrimazole with 1 applicator
Vagisil Homeopathic Suppositories	Pulsatilla 28X, Candida parapsilosis 28X, Candida albicans 28X (ingredients not proven safe or effective for vaginal candidal infections)
Vagistat-1	One prefilled applicator containing tioconazole 300 mg
Yeast•Gard Homeopathic Vaginal Suppositories	Pulsatilla 28X, Candida parapsilosis 28X, Candida albicans 28X (ingredients not proven safe or effective for vaginal candidal infections)

A Pharmacist's Journal

"Where's the Monistat?"

A woman wanted to return a box of Monistat 3 Vaginal Suppositories. As I talked with her, it became clear why she needed to return them. She had been told by her "cancer doctor" that she had a yeast infection. However, this time she told us what she had omitted before. The infec-tion was on her neck and under her breasts. She was understandably unable to apply a suppository in this manner. I sold her the correct product and advised that she use powder beneath her breasts and allow the skin to dry thoroughly following her bath/shower.

ETIOLOGY OF VAGINAL IRRITATION AND PRURITUS

The causes of vaginal itching and irritation are usually unknown; however, noninfective vaginal itch may be caused by lack of cleanliness or by an allergy to a specific ingredient in a topically applied vaginal product.[47]

TREATMENT OF VAGINAL IRRITATION AND PRURITUS

Treatment Guidelines

Patients should not self-treat vaginal irritation or pruritus that exceeds 1 week in duration.[4] Should the symptoms continue or should redness, swelling, or pain develop, the patient should stop self-treatment and consult a physician.

Nonprescription Medications

POVIDONE-IODINE

Povidone-iodine 0.15 to 0.3% in a douche was judged to be effective for minor vaginal irritations by the FDA OTC review panel, although the FDA later stated that further studies would be required to prove this claim; they lack of approval of safety/effectiveness as of this time.[4,5] This later FDA ruling was made as the agency withdrew the Advance Notice of Proposed Rulemaking for vaginal drug products, stating that it would refer further consideration to other OTC drug rulemaking processes. Povidone-iodine douches could conceivably allow overgrowth of pathogenic organisms, increasing the risk of infections.[48]

Several douches containing povidone-iodine are listed in Table 44.3. Some douche products require the female to place a small amount of concentrate in a container, dilute it, and place the douche nozzle on the container (Fig. 44.2). Other douche products are ready-to-use after the douche nozzle is attached (Fig. 44.3).

HYDROCORTISONE

Hydrocortisone 0.25 to 1% is effective for relieving pruritus of the genital areas.[49–51] However, products containing hydrocortisone must caution the patient to see a physician if they have a vaginal discharge since this may indicate the presence of an infection that would not respond to an anti-inflammatory.[50] Further, if symptoms persist for more than 7 days or clear up and recur within a few days, the patient should discontinue use and see a physician. Any product containing hydrocortisone (such as Gynecort Cream) could be used vaginally.

OTHER INGREDIENTS

Some products for vaginal application contain ingredients not yet approved by the FDA for such uses, including benzocaine, resorcinol, tripelennamine, diphenhydramine, and benzethonium chloride. Since they are of unknown safety/effectiveness, they should not be recommended.[52]

FOCUS ON...

HOMEOPATHIC YEAST SUPPOSITORIES

Homeopathic products such as Yeast•Gard are marketed for "vaginal yeast infections." One of the ingredients of these vaginal tablets is *Candida albicans,* homeopathically prepared to 28X, which the individual already has in abundance. Their method of action is based on a system of medicine in which the more diluted the product is, the stronger it is purported to become. (See Chapter 50, Homeopathy.) The FDA is powerless to force the companies to prove effectiveness of homeopathic remedies because of a loophole in federal law. Pharmacists should discourage the patients from purchasing these expensive placebos, which lack proof of efficacy. Rather, patients should be steered toward antifungal vaginal products that are proven to be safe and effective.

Table 44.3. Representative Products for Vaginal Irritation and Pruritus

PRODUCT	SELECTED INGREDIENTS/COMMENTS
Betadine Medicated Douche Concentrate	Povidone-iodine 10% (0.3% when diluted according to directions)
Betadine Medicated Douche Kit	Bottle of douche concentrate with a flexible plastic douche container and nozzle; contains povidone-iodine
Betadine Medicated Douche Pre-Mixed	Disposable bottles containing povidone-iodine 0.3%
Gynecort Cream Maximum Strength	Hydrocortisone 1%
Massengill Medicated Douche	6-ounce disposable bottle containing water and a separate small plastic bottle which is mixed with the water to form 0.3% povidone-iodine
Vagi•Gard Povidone-Iodine Medicated Douche Concentrate	Povidone-iodine 10% (0.3% when diluted according to directions)
Vagi•Gard Cream	Benzocaine 5%, benzalkonium chloride 0.13%
Vagisil Cream	Benzocaine 5%, dimethicone 1%, aloe
Vagisil Maximum Strength	Benzocaine 20%, dimethicone 1%
Vagisil Feminine Powder	Corn starch, aloe, mineral oil, magnesium stearate, silica, benzethonium chloride, fragrance

SUMMARY

Problems related to female genital conditions that can be addressed by nonprescription products include inadequate vaginal hygiene, vaginal fungal infections, and vaginal irritation and pruritus. Inadequate vaginal hygiene is often treated with the use of cosmetic douche products and douche

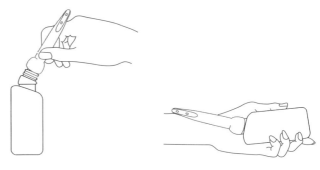

1. Attach nozzle to container.

2. Hold in palm.

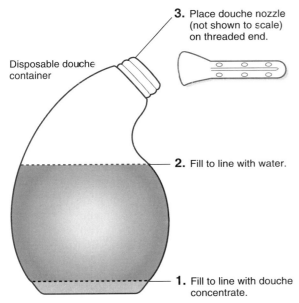

3. Place douche nozzle (not shown to scale) on threaded end.

Disposable douche container

2. Fill to line with water.

1. Fill to line with douche concentrate.

Figure 44.2. Use of typical, disposable-douche container packaged with separate bottle of douche concentrate: (1) Fill empty container to indicated line with douche concentrate. (2) Fill container with water to indicated line to dilute the concentrate. (3) Attach douche nozzle (not drawn to scale).

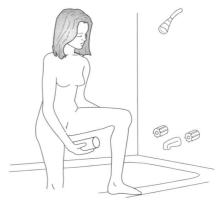

3. Shower method.

Figure 44.3. Use of typical, prefilled, disposable-douche container: (1) Attach nozzle to container. (2) Hold container in palm of hand. (3) Insert nozzle vaginally while on the toilet, in the shower (illustrated), or in the tub.

AT THE COUNTER

 A woman asks the pharmacist if she should see a physician for her fungal infection or if she can avoid a physician visit and use a nonprescription product.

Interview/Patient Assessment

The pharmacist discovers that the patient has never had a vaginal fungal infection, but that a friend suspects that she has one. She appears unwilling to describe the discharge, but says she is in extreme discomfort. Her computer profile lists Ortho-Novum 1/50–28.

Pharmacist's Analysis

1. What additional symptoms would indicate a need for physician referral?

2. Should she be referred to a physician for care?
3. What nonprescription products would be helpful?

Patient Counseling

Vaginal fungal infections are self-treatable if the patient can ascertain with assurance that the cause is fungal in origin. To do this, the patient must have had one prior physician-diagnosed vaginal fungal infection. After that confirmation, the symptoms are so similar on recurrence that the patient is capable of recognizing them as fungal. However, should the patient be under the age of 12; be pregnant; or suffer from fever, chills, nausea, vomiting, rash, back pain, or a foul-smelling discharge, she should see a physician. As this patient has never had a diagnosed vaginal fungal infection, she must make an appointment with a physician for confirmation of fungal etiology.

equipment, although this practice can result in an increased incidence of pelvic inflammatory disease.

Vaginal fungal infections, which are usually caused by a candidal organism, may arise when the female's immune status is lowered (e.g., from AIDS or corticosteroid administration), may be secondary to ingestion of oral contraceptives or other hormones, can result from improper hygiene following bowel movements, or affect patients with diabetes mellitus. These infections can be successfully treated with a 1-day, 3-day, or 7-day course of imidazoles, including clotrimazole, miconazole, butoconazole, and tioconazole.

Vaginal irritation and pruritus that does not exceed 1 week in duration may be treated with hydrocortisone topical products. After 1 week without resolution, patients should see a physician to rule out a serious cause of the problem.

References

1. Czerwinski BS. Adult feminine hygiene practices. Appl Nurs Res 9:123, 1996.
2. McGregor JA, Hammill HA. Contraception and sexually transmitted diseases: Interactions and opportunities. Am J Obstet Gynecol 168(6 Pt 2):2033, 1993.
3. Aral SO, Mosher WD, Cates W Jr. Vaginal douching among women of reproductive age in the United States, 1988. Am J Public Health 82:210, 1992.
4. Fed Reg 48:46694, 1983.
5. Fed Reg 59:5226, 1994.
6. Rosenberg MJ, Phillips RS, Holmes MD. Vaginal douching. Who and why? J Reprod Med 36:753, 1991.
7. Joesoef MR, et al. Douching and sexually transmitted diseases in pregnant women in Surabaya, Indonesia. Am J Obstet Gynecol 174(1 Pt 1):115, 1996.
8. Rosenberg MJ. (Untitled Letter). Obstet Gynecol 81:321, 1993.
9. Rosenberg MJ, Phillips RS. Does douching promote ascending infection? J Reprod Med 37:930, 1992.
10. Baird DD, et al. Vaginal douching and reduced fertility. Am J Public Health 86:844, 1996.
11. Scholes D, et al. Vaginal douching as a risk factor for acute pelvic inflammatory disease. Obstet Gynecol 81:601, 1993.
12. Critchlow CW, et al. Determinants of cervical ectopia and of cervicitis: Age, oral contraception, specific cervical infection, smoking, and douching. Am J Obstet Gynecol 173:534, 1995.
13. Kendrick JS, et al. Vaginal douching and the risk of ectopic pregnancy among black women. Am J Obstet Gynecol 176:991, 1997.
14. Zhang J, Thomas AG, Leybovich E. Vaginal douching and adverse health effects: A meta-analysis. Am J Public Health 87:1207, 1997.
15. Foxman B, Aral SO, Holmes KK. Interrelationships among douching practices, risky sexual practices, and history of self-reported sexually transmitted diseases in an urban population. Sex Transm Dis 25:90, 1998.
16. Jossens MO, et al. Risk factors for pelvic inflammatory disease. A case control study. Sex Transm Dis 23:239, 1996.
17. Abma JC, et al. Fertility, family planning, and women's health: New data from the 1995 National Survey of Family Growth. Vital Health Stat 23:1, 1997.
18. Fidel PL Jr, Sobel JD. Immunopathogenesis of recurrent vulvovaginal candidiasis. Clin Microbiol Rev 9:335, 1996.
19. Jones R. Childhood vulvovaginitis and vaginal discharge in general practice. Fam Pract 13:369, 1996.
20. Koumantakis EE, et al. Vulvovaginitis during childhood and adolescence. J Pediatr Adolesc Gynecol 10:39, 1997.
21. Spinillo A, et al. The impact of oral contraception on vulvovaginal candidiasis. Contraception 51:293, 1995.
22. Hooton TM, Roberts PL, Stamm WE. Effects of recent sexual activity and use of a diaphragm on the vaginal microflora. Clin Infect Dis 19:274, 1994.
23. Peer AK, et al. Vaginal yeast infections in diabetic women. S Afr Med J 83:727, 1993.
24. Nyirjesy P, et al. Chronic fungal vaginitis: The value of cultures. Am J Obstet Gynecol 173(3 Pt 1):820, 1995.
25. Cotch MF, et al. Epidemiology and outcomes associated with moderate to heavy *Candida* colonization during pregnancy. Vaginal Infections and Prematurity Study Group. Am J Obstet Gynecol 178:374, 1998.
26. Mendling W, Koldovsky U. Immunological investigations in vaginal mycoses. Mycoses 39:177, 1996.
27. Lockhart SR, et al. Most frequent scenario for recurrent *Candida* vaginitis is strain maintenance with "substrain shuffling": Demonstration by sequential DNA fingerprinting with probes Ca3, C1, and CARE2. J Clin Microbiol 34:767, 1996.
28. Geiger AM, Foxman B, Sobel JD. Chronic vulvovaginal candidiasis: Characteristics of women with *Candida albicans, C. glabrata* and no *Candida*. Genitourin Med 71:304, 1995.
29. White DJ, Johnson EM, Warnock DW. Management of persistent vulvovaginal candidosis due to azole-resistant *Candida glabrata*. Genitourin Med 69:112, 1993.
30. Mendling W, Koldovsky U. Immunological investigations in vaginal mycoses. Mycoses 39:177, 1996.
31. Fidel PL Jr, Sobel JD. Immunopathogenesis of recurrent vulvovaginal candidiasis. Clin Microbiol Rev 9:335, 1996.
32. Ross RA, Lee M-LT, Onderdonk AB. Effect of *Candida albicans* infection and clotrimazole treatment on vaginal microflora in vitro. Obstet Gynecol 86:925, 1995.
33. Maffei CM, et al. Phenotype and genotype of *Candida albicans* strains isolated from pregnant women with recurrent vaginitis. Mycopathologia 137:87, 1997.
34. Spinillo A, et al. Epidemiologic characteristics of women with idiopathic recurrent vulvovaginal candidiasis. Obstet Gynecol 81(5 Pt 1):721, 1993.
35. Corrigan EM, et al. Cellular immunity in recurrent vulvovaginal candidiasis. Clin Exp Immunol 111:574, 1998.
36. Ferris DG, et al. Office laboratory diagnosis of vaginitis. J Fam Pract 41:575, 1995.
37. Perera J, Clayton Y. Incidence, species distribution and antifungal sensitivity pattern of vaginal yeasts in Sri Lankan women. Mycoses 37:357, 1994.
38. Ferris DG, et al. Treatment of bacterial vaginosis: A comparison of oral metronidazole, metronidazole vaginal gel, and clindamycin vaginal cream. J Fam Pract 41:443, 1995.
39. Sobel JD. Controversial aspects in the management of vulvovaginal candidiasis. J Am Acad Dermatol 31(3 Pt 2):S10, 1994.
40. Jonsson M, et al. The silent suffering women—A population based study on the association between reported symptoms and past and present infections of the lower genital tract. Genitourin Med 71:158, 1995.
41. Molander U, et al. An epidemiological study of urinary incontinence and related urogenital symptoms in elderly women. Maturitas 12:51, 1990.

42. Milsom I. Rational prescribing for postmenopausal urogenital complaints. Drugs Aging 9:78, 1996.

43. Roddy RE, et al. A dosing study of nonoxynol-9 and genital irritation. Int J STD AIDS 4:165, 1993.

44. Poindexter AN 3rd, et al. Comparison of spermicides on vulvar, vaginal, and cervical mucosa. Contraception 53:147, 1996.

45. Stafford MK, et al. Safety study of nonoxynol-9 as a vaginal microbicide: Evidence of adverse effects. J Acquir Immune Defic Syndr Hum Retrovirol 17:327, 1998.

46. Farr G, et al. Safety, functionality and acceptability of a prototype polyurethane condom. Adv Contracept 13:439, 1997.

47. Dekker JH, et al. Vaginal symptoms of unknown aetiology: A study in Dutch general practice. Br J Gen Pract 43:239, 1993.

48. Onderdonk AB, et al. Quantitative and qualitative effects of douche preparations on vaginal microflora. Obstet Gynecol 80 (3 Pt 1):333, 1992.

49. Fed Reg 44:69768, 1979.

50. Fed Reg 48:5852, 1983.

51. Fed Reg 55:6932, 1990.

52. Currie JL, et al. Potential for an external vaginal antiitch cream containing benzocaine to cause methemoglobinemia in healthy women. Am J Obstet Gynecol 176:1006, 1997.

Nicotine Addiction

AT THE COUNTER

The pharmacist is approached by a male appearing to be in his late 20s who asks if Nicorette gum might work for him.

Interview/Patient Assessment

The pharmacist asks the patient to describe his smoking history. The patient states that he has been smoking about 15 cigarettes daily since he was in high school. He doesn't want to stop smoking, but he is forced to fly in connection with his job and wishes to use the product to prevent nicotine withdrawal during his hours in the airport and while on the plane. He has exercise-induced asthma for which he uses several inhalers both for maintenance and "breakthrough" symptoms.

Pharmacist's Analysis

1. Do nonprescription nicotine products allow the patient to stop smoking for only a short, specified time?

2. Which product is best for this patient, gum or a transdermal patch?
3. Will this patient's medications be affected?

Patient Counseling

The patient wishes to use nonprescription nicotine products for an unapproved indication. Their intended use is to augment cigarette withdrawal, not to serve as a bridge to allow the patient to continue the habit. Nonprescription nicotine products are inherently hazardous. They are appropriate only if their use will lead to cessation. Used in this manner, they are hazardous to the patient's health without conferring any health benefit. The pharmacist should caution the patient that there is no safe option for him while he is flying other than complete cessation of all nicotine products. If he cannot accomplish this, he may wish to chew gum on the flight or engage in another activity to distract his mind from the uncomfortable withdrawal symptoms.

If the patient persists in his desire to use the products, the pharmacist should caution him that dosages of his asthma medications may require adjustment.

Cigarette smoking (the most common form of nicotine addiction) is a self-induced phenomenon with deadly consequences. Because of the addictive nature of nicotine, recent federal programs focus on strategies to prevent youth from beginning cigarette smoking.

As a result of a number of studies of the impact of breathing "second-hand" smoke—smoke generated by others—restrictions on smoking have been implemented throughout the nation to lessen the deadly effects of environmental exposure to smoke. These restrictions have ignited acrimonious debate over the legitimacy of creating nonsmoking restaurants, workplaces, malls, etc. Nonetheless, even more Draconian proposals have surfaced such as refusing coronary bypass surgery to patients unless they discontinue smoking.[1]

Nicotine is an addictive substance that produces clear withdrawal symptoms when patients attempt to discontinue ingestion or inhalation. As such, cessation is extremely difficult for most patients. Many patients who earnestly wish to quit fail repeatedly. Each failed attempt may cause a cycle of self-reproach and shame. For this reason pharmacists should sympathize with (and congratulate) those patients who wish to cease smoking, whether the attempt is their first or the latest in a long string of attempts.

Nicotine addiction is not only caused by smoking. The abuse of smokeless tobacco products has also become a recognized health hazard. It is not as emotionally charged as cigarette smoking, since users do not expose others to noxious airborne chemicals. Nevertheless, the incidence of oral cancer and other adverse effects affirms that smokeless tobacco is not a safe alternative to cigarettes. Nonprescription products are not indicated for withdrawal from smokeless tobacco products. Nevertheless, smokeless tobacco addiction will also be discussed in this chapter.

The deadly use of tobacco products has also fueled a debate in pharmacy centers about the ethics of selling tobacco products. Many pharmacists believe that selling tobacco products is contradictory to the mission of pharmacy, which is to improve the health of patients. To this end, many pharmacies have ceased sales of tobacco.

The substantial dangers of tobacco products and the controversies over their use highlight the abuse of nicotine as one of the greatest public health challenges of the 21st century.

PREVALENCE OF NICOTINE ADDICTION

Smoking

The prevalence of cigarette use is decreasing, yet it remains dangerously high. As many as 25% of Americans smoke, ranging from 13.2% of Utah residents to 27.8% of Kentucky residents.[2,3] Specific long-term trend analysis illustrates the following[4]:

- Males with a high-school background or more smoke much less.
- Females with a high-school background or more smoke slightly less.

- Males with less than a high-school education have not changed their smoking habits appreciably.
- Females with less than a high-school education smoke in greatly increasing numbers.

It appears from the above data that the groups least likely to benefit from nonsmoking messages are those whose educational achievements are below the norm. Cigarettes are the most common drug that youth use daily; at least 18% of high-school seniors smoke.[5]

Using Smokeless Tobacco

Although used less than cigarettes, smokeless tobacco is also a significant health hazard. In surveys, as many as 7% of military, 10% of Indiana high-school juniors and seniors (both male and female), and 21% of Louisiana high-school athletes use smokeless tobacco products.[6-8] As many as 34% of adolescents in the southeastern United States have tried it, and 17% report that they consider themselves addicted to it.[9] Trend analysis reveals that chewing-tobacco use has decreased by 31% over the past 15 years, but use of snuff has increased by 52%.[10]

EPIDEMIOLOGY OF NICOTINE ADDICTION

Smoking

OCCUPATION

Smoking tends to be highly correlated with occupation, as illustrated by Table 45.1, which lists the percent of smokers in a cross-section of occupations. In general, a higher percent-

Table 45.1. Percentage of Smokers in Various Occupations

OCCUPATION	PERCENTAGE WHO SMOKE (1987–1990)
Roofers	57.8
Crane and tower operators	57.4
Machine feeders	55.4
Drywall installers	54.8
Bartenders	52.4
Construction laborers	47.1
Waiters and waitresses	46.6
Heavy-truck drivers	45.8
Nursing aides, orderlies, and attendants	36.9
Licensed practical nurses	31.8
Health aides (except nursing)	29.7
Dental assistants	22.8
Dietitians	22.5
Registered nurses	22.0
Elementary-school teachers	11.5
Pharmacists	10.5
Physical therapists	8.7
Dentists	7.4
Clergy	6.5
Physicians	5.5

Adapted from Nelson DE, et al. Cigarette smoking prevalence by occupation in the United States. J Occup Med 36:516, 1994.

age of blue-collar workers and individuals employed in service industries smoke than individuals with white-collar occupations.[11] (It is noteworthy that pharmacists have the fifth lowest smoking rate in the listing of 215 different occupations.) Predictably, the smoking rate is related to education, with better-educated individuals (those who tend to hold white-collar jobs) less likely to smoke.[11] High job stress and low level of job control, conditions more prevalent in blue-collar occupations, both increase the tendency to smoke.[11]

EDUCATIONAL BACKGROUND

As noted above, the number of years of education is strongly correlated with smoking. In one survey of females, the highest smoking rate was observed in females with only 9 to 11 years of education, while the lowest rate of all was seen in females who had 16 or more years of education.[12]

EMPLOYMENT STATUS

Workers who are unemployed are more likely to smoke than those who are either employed or not in the labor force by choice.[11]

GENDER

Women are less likely to be cigarette smokers than men, although the rates tend to differ by only 1 to 2 percentage points in the northeastern and western United States and 5 to 9% in the midwestern and southern United States.[11,13]

AGE

Smoking is perceived to be more common in older individuals, especially those who began smoking in the decades bracketing World War II.[11] However, the highest smoking rate is among 30 to 39 year olds, with a decline as the survey population ages.[13]

RACE

The prevalence of smoking in white youth is five times that of black Americans and two times that of Hispanic youth.[5] The ratios change with aging: black-American adults tend to have the highest smoking rates (31.3%), as opposed to whites (26.4%), Hispanics (25%), and Asian/Pacific Islanders (22.8%).[13]

GEOGRAPHIC REGION

More males smoke in the east south-central region of the United States (including Kentucky, Tennessee, Alabama, and Mississippi) than any other region.[13] Lowest rates occur in the Pacific region (e.g., Washington, Oregon, California, Alaska, and Hawaii).

Using Smokeless Tobacco

Smokeless tobacco is more often used by the young, those to whom it has been preferentially marketed. Whites are more likely to use smokeless tobacco products, as are athletes (both high school and professional).[8,14,15]

ETIOLOGY OF NICOTINE ADDICTION

The etiology of nicotine addiction cannot be discussed in the same manner as that of medical conditions with a genetic component (e.g., psoriasis) or conditions that arise as a result of chance exposure (e.g., insect bites).

Nicotine addiction is a result of a conscious decision to engage in self-damaging behavior. This behavior may be difficult to control, however, because of the many enticements and pressures to smoke.

Nicotine is highly addictive.[16] (See "Creating Addiction: Advertising and Peer Pressure.") When this chemical reaches the brain (5 to 8 seconds after smoking begins; 5 to 8 minutes after using chewing tobacco or after snuff usage starts), neurotransmitter disruption begins.[17] By mimicking acetylcholine and releasing norepinephrine and dopamine, it provides several perceived benefits such as initial stimulation, followed by calming.

Tolerance develops within a short period, so that the initial smoking level does not provide the calming effect. This forces the addict to increase use again and again. During the process of addiction, the individual develops additional acetylcholine receptors. If any attempt is made to stop smoking, acetylcholine activity increases dramatically, causing restlessness, irritability, and discontent. These withdrawal symptoms make cessation difficult.

MANIFESTATIONS OF NICOTINE ADDICTION

Smoking

Tobacco users exhibit several manifestations of nicotine addiction. One is a deeper voice than nonsmokers. The female voice may become so coarse and deep that it resembles that of a male. Smokers also experience a hacking, continuous cough. (See Chapter 15, The Common Cold and Related Conditions.) Smokers' body, hair, clothes, and breath may all have an unpleasant smoky odor.

The major visible manifestations of smoking are dermatologic. The fingers often are stained by smoking. The skin generally is prematurely aged because of the development of wrinkles (Fig. 45.1).[22] "Smoker's face" is medically described as follows:

- Prominent lines or wrinkles
- Prominent bony contours that give a gaunt appearance
- Slightly gray and atrophied skin
- Slightly orange, purple, and red blotchy discolorations on the skin

Smoking is additive with sun exposure. The combination of smoking and sun exposure produces wrinkling and aging that exceeds the effects of either alone.

FOCUS ON...

CREATING ADDICTION: ADVERTISING AND PEER PRESSURE

Advertising is responsible for the majority of nicotine abuse. Advertising forms perceptions of young people regarding the acceptability of smoking, the lifestyle of smokers, and the personality characteristics of smokers (e.g., rugged, individualistic, glamorous, and independent).[5,16] Marketing efforts have been directed specifically to young people in the past, especially with smokeless tobacco products.[18] Further, manufacturers design their products specifically to yield pharmacologic doses of nicotine for the purposes of creating addiction.[19,20]

Peer pressure is also important in initial use of smokeless tobacco products. The first use of tobacco products invariably occurs prior to high-school graduation. Eighty-two percent of smokers began their habit before age 18.[16] Various factors cause the abuse, including peer pressure in youth whose friends smoke.[5] The risk rises when young people also have low self-esteem and poor achievement in school. Statistics show that smoking rates among high-school dropouts are more than three times as high (43.3%) as those in students who graduated from high school and continued their education.[21] Peer pressure also exists to use smokeless tobacco. One study reported that 19.2% of boys in the ninth through twelfth grades use smokeless tobacco.

Using Smokeless Tobacco

Users of smokeless tobacco products often can be recognized by the visible "**quid**" (portion of chewing tobacco or snuff) located between the cheek and gum. Also, users of smokeless tobacco frequently need to spit out the saturated tobacco products, either into a "spit cup" or simply onto the ground. The patient also experiences halitosis.[23] The increased incidence of gingival recession in smokeless tobacco users causes their teeth to appear longer; caries are also more common and are frequently visible to others.[15]

SPECIFIC CONSIDERATIONS OF NICOTINE ADDICTION

Smoking

PASSIVE SMOKE

The nicotine-addicted smoker induces profound effects on his personal health. However, it has become clear that environmental smoke generated by others is a great health hazard to nonsmokers. This "passive smoke" contains over 4000 compounds.[24,25] Many have known toxicity such as benzene, xylenes, styrene, carbon monoxide, and ethylbenzene. The nation has taken severe steps to limit involuntary exposure to smoke such as prohibiting smoking in workplaces, campuses, restaurants, and other facilities. Taxes on nicotine products have also been increased as a disincentive.

Approximately 30% of nicotine-addicted mothers smoke when pregnant. At least 50% of children are exposed to cigarette smoke. Both prenatal and postnatal exposure to cigarette smoke results in profound adverse consequences on physical, mental, and behavioral growth and development.[24] Risks of sudden infant death syndrome, asthma, lower respiratory infections, and ear infections are all higher when

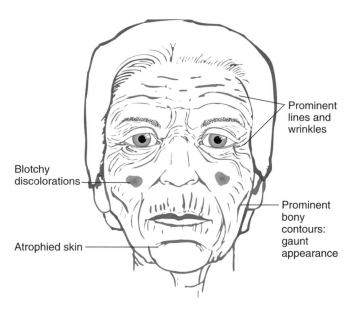

Figure 45.1. The "smoker's face." The skin may have an overall grayish discoloration with blotches of orange, purple, and red.

smokers share the house with a child. Children living with smokers have an increased risk of behavior problems, lower scores on various achievement and intelligence examinations, and are less likely to be promoted to the next grade.

BREAST-FEEDING

Breast-feeding exposes infants to noxious chemicals in the breast milk if the mother smokes.[24] Smoking also decreases milk "let-down," reduces milk supply, and limits weight gain of the infant.

Using Smokeless Tobacco: "Starter Products"

Tobacco companies manufacture flavored smokeless tobacco products with lower concentrations of nicotine. These flavored products are often the first used by the young addict and are referred to as "starter products."[7] As the patient ages, there is a tendency to graduate to more advanced forms of smokeless tobacco that contain higher concentrations of nicotine.

PROGNOSIS OF NICOTINE ADDICTION

Nicotine addiction results in abuse of products that deliver nicotine, usually cigarettes and smokeless tobacco. Therefore, an examination of the prognosis for nicotine addiction must include the prognosis of inhaling or ingesting the other components of nicotine-delivery systems.

Smoking

Smoking is responsible for more than 400,000 deaths each year in the United States, many caused by cancer (see "Complications of Nicotine Addiction" below). More Americans die from smoking-related conditions each year than die from

acquired immune deficiency syndrome (AIDS), car accidents, alcohol, homicide, illegal drugs, suicides, and fires combined.[16,22,26] British research indicates that smoking shortens smokers' lives an average of 23 years.[1] Fully 20% of those alive now will expire as a result of tobacco-related disease.[21] The best advice for smokers is to quit completely, but this advice is often difficult to follow. As a true addiction, nicotine abuse is difficult to control and can be compared with heroin or cocaine.[12]

Some smokers, especially females, continue smoking to prevent the average 5-pound weight gain associated with smoking cessation.[27–29] Withdrawal symptoms are unpleasant, too, causing equally high relapse rates in both adults and young people who try to quit.[5]

Using Smokeless Tobacco

Smokeless tobacco is a difficult addiction to conquer. In fact, many users graduate from low-dose smokeless tobacco products to high-dose products as tolerance develops.[30]

COMPLICATIONS OF NICOTINE ADDICTION

Smoking

Smoking is directly related to many serious—if not deadly—medical conditions. In addition to their own pain and suffering, smokers cost their employers 30% more than nonsmokers in lost productivity and health-related costs.[11] Male blue-collar workers, who have the highest smoking rate of any group or occupation, are often exposed to other hazardous substances in the workplace. Exposure to other hazards can cause their risk of lung cancers and other diseases to rise alarmingly.

CANCER

Cigarette smoke, the most common cause of preventable cancers, contains at least 40 carcinogenic compounds.[13,25]

tip *Environmental tobacco smoke breathed in passively—i.e., by nonsmokers (such as children)—has also been shown to be carcinogenic by many scientific organizations and federal agencies (e.g., the EPA).[11]* The primary cancer associated with tobacco smoke is carcinoma of the lung (the leading cause of cancer death for women in the United States).[31,32] However, other tumors are also induced by cigarettes, including esophageal, bladder, colorectal, laryngeal, nasal, and oral cancers.[12,33–35]

CARDIOVASCULAR AND CIRCULATORY COMPLICATIONS

Cigarette smoking is a strong predictor for myocardial infarction (tripling the risk), stroke, peripheral vascular disease, and aortic aneurysm.[22,29,36,37]

Cigarette smoking is a major risk factor for coronary heart disease and quitting is probably the single most important measure that can be taken to prevent this condition.[1] In the United States one-fourth of the deaths in those older than 60 occur as a result of coronary heart disease.[27] Coronary heart disease is also the leading cause of death and disability of women in the United States, causing 250,000 deaths per year.[29] Smoking as few as one to four cigarettes daily can triple the risk of coronary-related pathology.[29] *When smokers quit, the incidence of coronary artery disease declines to that of nonsmokers within 3 years.*[36]

RESPIRATORY PROBLEMS

Smoking damages or destroys pulmonary cilia and reduces or eliminates the mucokinesis method by which the body clears inhaled foreign substances from the airways.[25,35] Accordingly, smoking is strongly correlated with emphysema, chronic obstructive pulmonary disease, respiratory infection, and chronic bronchitis.[12,22]

INJURIES

Smokers are at higher risk of several types of injury:

- Cigarettes result in thousands of deaths and injuries from fires (the most common cause of smoking-related injuries) each year. Approximately 14% of the annual hospitalizations for burns are smoking related.[38]
- Smoking increases the risk of automobile accidents by 50%, perhaps because of the need to remove one hand from the wheel to light a cigarette, hold it, and remove it from the mouth. Further, when the smoker concentrates on these activities, the attention paid to driving must decrease.
- Smokers are at least twice as likely to experience an injury at the worksite.[38]

Smoking may increase the risk of injury for several reasons. Direct toxicity from carboxyhemoglobin (and perhaps carbon monoxide) reduces night vision (which has been demonstrated by lower scores on performance and vision tests).[38] Airborne smoke obstructs vision in vehicles and in the workplace. Smokers can become preoccupied with the act of smoking, including dealing with dropped embers. Smoking also induces cough, ophthalmic irritation, and blinking, all of which reduce attentiveness to other tasks.

STRESS

While many smokers claim that smoking reduces stress, the data are more complex. It appears that smokers may experience greater stress because of acute nicotine deprivation between cigarettes.[39] Smoking then reverses nicotine withdrawal, which is perceived by the individual as having reduced stress. *Individuals who smoke to relieve stress should be informed that nonsmokers report lower stress levels than smokers.*

PRENATAL COMPLICATIONS

Smoking during pregnancy increases the risks of miscarriage, **abruptio placentae** (premature detachment of the placenta), **placenta previa** (a portion of the placenta covering the mouth of the cervix or in close proximity), infertility, ectopic pregnancy, and perinatal mortality.[24] Also, low-birth-weight babies are more common in women who smoke because of a decrease in the delivery of oxygen and nutrients reaching the fetus.

OTHER COMPLICATIONS

Smoking increases the risk of cataracts.[38] Several substances in cigarettes (e.g., polonium-210 and benzene) induce myeloid leukemia.[31] Smokers and their children have greater risk of developing Crohn's disease.[40,41] Children whose parents smoke experience greater incidence of otitis media with effusion, upper respiratory tract infections, coughing, hearing defects, snoring, and sore throats.[25] Diabetics who smoke experience worse nephropathy than their nonsmoking cohorts.[42]

The smoker also must plan financially to be able to support the habit. In the worst case, the smoker may need to sacrifice in other areas such as food or clothing to support the addiction.

The social impact of smoking has gradually become more severe. Smokers are usually restricted to the outside of the workplace. Thus they are not able to socialize with non-smoking colleagues during smoke breaks. Further, standing outside on a winter day with below-freezing temperatures while finishing a cigarette may lead to a whole new set of problems such as frostbite.

Using Smokeless Tobacco

Smokeless tobacco results in the absorption of nicotine, leading to the development of coronary artery disease, cardiac ischemic events, hypertension, and cancer.[18,43,44] Smokeless tobacco also contains various carcinogens (e.g., nitrosamines).[31,45] As many as 1.5% of smokeless tobacco users will develop some type of oral lesion before the age of 17.[14] The patient may exhibit leukoplakia, an early oral mucosal change.[6] Oral cancer is more common in smokers and users of smokeless tobacco products (snuff, dip, chewing tobacco) than in individuals who do not use tobacco products. The incidence increases with the daily increase in minutes of use of either snuff or chewing tobacco. The smokeless tobacco user also experiences an increased risk of periodontal disease, with resultant loose teeth.[15,23,46] Snuff is associated with cancer of the cheek, gum, and pharynx.[10]

TREATMENT OF NICOTINE ADDICTION

Treatment Guidelines

Cessation of nicotine intake produces several withdrawal symptoms within a few hours—including tension, depression, irritability, difficulty in concentration, bradycardia, hypertension, EEG changes, decreased attentiveness, and impaired performance on job tasks that require a rapid reaction time.[47] Nonprescription nicotine products are meant to control the physical symptoms of withdrawal from smoking, allowing the patient to better acquire the mental discipline needed to cease. Nonprescription products are not labeled for cessation of smokeless tobacco use.

The approval of nonprescription nicotine was a novel FDA action, since traditionally nonprescription products must be safe and effective. As an addicting substance, nicotine is of questionable safety. However, nonprescription nicotine was approved for nonprescription sale because of the greater potential benefit of withdrawing from the more dangerous smoking habit. However, *nonprescription nicotine products are only indicated for smoking withdrawal*. As noted in Patient Assessment Algorithm 45.1, these products are not intended as a smoking substitute for those who wish to smoke, but cannot do so until a later time (e.g., during a long committee meeting or a plane flight).

Even with appropriate use of nonprescription products, patients may not be able to withdraw from smoking. These patients should be referred to a physician. Behavioral interventions may be helpful. As an alternative, the physician may prescribe Nicotrol Inhaler, a prescription device that delivers 4 mg of nicotine per cartridge. This product has been mentioned as a candidate for Rx-to-OTC switching, but it remains a prescription item as of this writing. Another approved prescription product for smoking cessation is bupropion sustained-release.[48]

Patient Assessment Algorithm 45.1. Nicotine Addiction

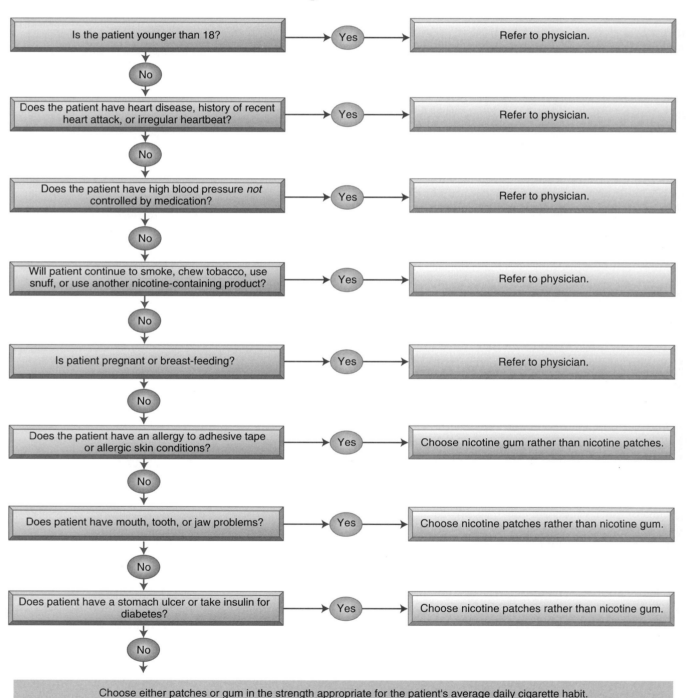

Nonprescription Medications

Drug manufacturers market two types of smoking cessation products, nicotine gum and nicotine patches (SmithKline Beecham markets NicoDerm CQ patches and Nicorette Gum; McNeil markets Nicotrol patches). As noted above, these products are only indicated for cessation from smoking (as opposed to smokeless tobacco use). Further, they contain nicotine—an addictive substance that is only to be used as labeled.

At one time manufacturers advertised products containing lobeline or silver acetate for smoking cessation. However, there was no evidence of their safety or efficacy, and all were removed from the market.

NICOTINE GUM

Nicotine gum became an FDA-approved nonprescription product (as the polacrilex salt of nicotine) in early 1996 as Nicorette 2 mg (for patients who smoke fewer than 25 cigarettes daily) or 4 mg (for patients who smoke more than 24 cigarettes a day).[49] There are ordinarily 20 cigarettes in a package.

The company produces a starter package and a refill package. Both contain an instructional booklet, but the starter package is recommended for initial use since it also contains a motivational/instructional audiotape and a personal code number that allows the purchaser to enroll in a company-sponsored program known as the Nicorette Stop Smoking Plan. After a phone interview via an 800 number, a patient will receive the following motivational materials:

- Week 1: A 12-week stop-smoking calendar, with a week-by-week plan to assist in smoking cessation
- Week 2: A newsletter with a motivational message
- Week 3: A postcard with a motivational message
- Week 6: A brochure with additional tips on quitting
- Week 9: A congratulations packet
- Week 12: An award certificate

Method of Use

The recommended schedule of Nicorette use is as follows:

- Weeks 1 through 6: Use one piece every 1 to 2 hours
- Weeks 7 through 9: Use one piece every 2 to 4 hours
- Weeks 10 through 12: Use one piece every 4 to 8 hours

To prevent toxicity, patients must not use more than 24 pieces daily. Patients should use at least 9 per day in the beginning to gain an adequate effect. (Heavy smokers may require more pieces per day at the outset to control the craving for nicotine.) *While using Nicorette, patients must refrain from using any other source of nicotine, including cigarettes, cigars, chewing tobacco, snuff, and nicotine patches (whether prescription or nonprescription).*

The use of Nicorette is optimized if the gum is chewed in a manner that gradually releases nicotine:

1. Chew the gum slowly several times. Stop chewing when a peppery taste or tingle in the mouth is apparent (usually after about 15 chews).
2. "Park" the gum by placing it between the cheek and gum and not chewing it.

3. When the peppery taste or tingle have almost disappeared, chew slowly a few more times, stopping when the peppery taste or tingle returns.
4. Park the gum in a different place in the mouth than used before.
5. Repeat the cycle of parking and chewing as described above until the gum fails to produce the peppery taste or tingle (usually after about 30 minutes), signifying that most of the nicotine has been utilized.

Precautions

Pharmacists should advise patients who purchase Nicorette to read the booklet accompanying the product thoroughly before beginning use.[49] Pharmacists should stress that Nicorette is not like ordinary chewing gum. All precautions associated with its use should be strictly adhered to.

Nicorette must not be stored or discarded where children or pets could find it. Also, if patients chew more than one piece at a time or chew them too rapidly, one after the other, nicotine overdose is possible, causing initial signs such as hiccups, heartburn, or stomach problems. These indicate that the patient should chew more slowly, but are not serious enough to call a physician. However, pharmacists should advise patients to call a physician if more serious symptoms of nicotine overdose occur (e.g., nausea, vomiting, dizziness, weakness, tachycardia). Adverse reactions may also include headache.

Patients should not eat or drink for 15 minutes before using Nicorette or while chewing the gum. Some foods and drinks (e.g., coffee, juices, wine, and soft drinks) reduce the effectiveness of Nicorette; these should not be ingested for 15 minutes prior to or during Nicorette use. Dosages of medications for asthma or depression may require adjustments while using Nicorette. The patient should ask a physician if the adjustment is necessary prior to using Nicorette.

Nicorette use should be stopped at the end of 12 weeks. Patients who have difficulty stopping Nicorette should see a physician.

Like any gum, nicotine polacrilex gum can cause dental fillings to loosen and can aggravate jaw, mouth, or tooth problems.

Nicorette is contraindicated in patients with heart disease, recent heart attack, or irregular heartbeat because of its ability to cause tachycardia. *Patients with poorly controlled hypertension should not use Nicorette because it increases blood pressure. Patients with stomach ulcers and diabetes requiring insulin should not use Nicorette because it both aggravates ulcers and contains sorbitol (which could affect blood glucose).*

Increased levels of acetylcholine produced when nicotine is in the circulation can cause bizarre dreams. Insomnia also may occur, but it usually resolves in 3 to 7 days. Patients may gain a few pounds the first 8 to 10 weeks of using Nicorette; pharmacists should urge them to modify eating habits rather than resume smoking.

Sale Requirements

Nicorette cannot be sold to patients under the age of 18; proof of age is required. Also, Nicorette cannot be placed in a vending machine or any other automatic dispensing location where proof of age cannot be verified.

NICOTINE TRANSDERMAL PATCHES

Nicotine patches switched from prescription to nonprescription status in 1996. Their once-a-day application gives them an advantage over nicotine gum.[50] Two brands of nicotine transdermal patches are available, Nicotrol (single strength) and NicoDerm CQ (three strengths).

Nicotrol delivers 15 mg of nicotine over 16 hours.[51] Nicotrol is available in a starter kit, containing instructions and an audiotape. Patients who complete an enclosed survey and mail it to the company will receive a Personal Quit Guide, individualized to help them stop smoking. Nicotrol can be used for a maximum of 6 weeks, after which patients must stop use. If it has been ineffective, a physician should be seen.

NicoDerm CQ is available in three strengths[52]:

- NicoDerm CQ Step 1 delivers 21 mg over 24 hours. The starting patch for patients who smoke more than 10 cigarettes a day, Step 1 should be used during weeks 1 to 6.
- NicoDerm CQ Step 2 delivers 14 mg over 24 hours. The starting patch for patients who smoke 10 cigarettes a day or fewer. Step 2 should be used during weeks 1 to 6 for those patients, and during weeks 7 to 8 for smokers who have completed Step 1.
- NicoDerm CQ Step 3 delivers 7 mg over 24 hours. It is used for weeks 7 to 8 for patients who started with Step 2 and for weeks 9 to 10 for patients who started with Step 1.

Packages of NicoDerm CQ also contain an instructional booklet, a motivational audio tape, and a personal code that allows the purchaser to enroll in the Committed Quitters Personalized Stop Smoking Plan. The benefits of NicoDerm CQ are similar to Nicorette, which is also marketed by SmithKline Beecham.

Method of Use

Patches should be applied to a clean, dry, hairless area of skin. Nicotrol instructions further specify the upper arm or hip. NicoDerm CQ instructions state that the skin cannot be burned, broken out, cut, or irritated in any way. In addition, there should be no soap or lotion on the skin that could hamper adherence. *Patients should use a new patch each time and should avoid previously used sites for at least 7 days.*

Pharmacists should advise patients to follow these steps when applying patches:

1. Remove the clear covering as directed.
2. Apply to the skin and hold the patch for 10 seconds to help secure it.
3. Wash hands to remove residual nicotine, which could cause ophthalmic and nasal irritation, stinging, or redness if it contacts the eyes or nasal mucosa.

Nicotrol is left on for only 16 hours. NicoDerm CQ may be kept on for either 16 or 24 hours. Patients who crave cigarettes when awakening in the morning should choose the 24-hour wearing time. If 24-hour wearing causes vivid dreams or other sleep disruptions, it should be removed at bedtime and only worn 16 hours.

Precautions

 *Patients must not use any other source of nicotine, including cigarettes, cigars, chewing tobacco, snuff, and nicotine gum while wearing a nicotine patch. **Nicotine patches are contraindicated in patients with heart disease, a recent history of myocardial infarction, or irregular heartbeat.** Patients with uncontrolled hypertension and patients taking medications for asthma or depression should not use patches without checking with their physician. Patients with allergies to adhesive tape or with skin problems (e.g., atopic dermatitis) should not use patches because of the increased risk of skin rashes. Patches should not be used by pregnant or nursing patients since they can increase the infant's heart rate.*

Patients should call a physician if symptoms of nicotine overdose occur (e.g., nausea, vomiting, dizziness, weakness, tachycardia), if irregular heartbeat or palpitations occur, or if skin redness caused by the patch does not abate after 4 days.

Nicotine transdermal patches must not be stored or discarded where children or pets can get them. Each package of NicoDerm CQ includes a disposal tray that helps prevent access to used patches.

Sale Requirements

Nicotine transdermal patches cannot be sold to patients under the age of 18; proof of age is required. Also, nicotine patches cannot be placed in a vending machine or any other automatic dispensing location where proof of age cannot be verified.

PREVENTION OF NICOTINE ADDICTION

The FDA, in a move intended to prevent nicotine addiction, ruled that cigarettes and smokeless tobacco are drugs delivered by devices (in the case of cigarettes).[16] The ruling allowed continued marketing, but specifically attacked sales to young people. Sales of tobacco products to individuals younger than 18 are prohibited, and retailers must verify age with a photographic identification. Free samples of these products are prohibited, and vending machine and self-service sales have been eliminated (except in establishments that permanently bar persons younger than 18). Advertising is restricted (e.g., only in adult-oriented magazines), and promotional items such as hats and tee shirts are prohibited. Sponsorship of sporting events, teams, and entries in the brand name of a tobacco product are also prohibited.

SUMMARY

The typical smoker is a poorly educated person working in a lower-level (blue-collar) occupation. Women are smoking in increasing numbers.

Abuse of nicotine is a destructive habit that results in in-

AT THE COUNTER

 A male patient who appears to be in his late 50s asks about nicotine cessation products. He specifically wants to know whether gum is better than patches.

Interview/Patient Assessment

The pharmacist ascertains that the patient has been smoking for 35 years, since he was 15 years old. He smokes approximately 20 cigarettes daily and an occasional cigar. He is a Type 2 diabetic, using Glucophage 850 mg twice daily and one injection of 45 units of NPH daily.

Pharmacist's Analysis

1. What is the significance of this patient's medical condition?
2. Is this patient free to use either a patch or gum?
3. What are his options in choosing a patch?

Patient Counseling

This patient's diabetes is an important factor in guiding therapy. Nicotine polacrilex gum is contraindicated in diabetics who use insulin. For this reason, the patient is restricted to nicotine patches for which he has no contraindications. The pharmacist may recommend Nicotrol or NicoDerm CQ. The Nicotrol therapy is shorter (6 weeks), but with NicoDerm CQ (10 weeks) the patient can taper off the patch. (Because he smokes more than 10 cigarettes daily, he should begin with NicoDerm Step 1.) The tapering nature of NicoDerm CQ is seen as an advantage by some, even though the therapy takes longer. The pharmacist should explain the two transdermal patch options to the patient and allow him to choose the better one for his particular situation. The pharmacist should also provide warnings about signs of toxicity that warrant a call to a physician and should caution against use of any nicotine product while using the patch. All steps in the use of the patch should be covered.

---

creased morbidity and mortality for those who engage in it and—in the case of smokers—for those who live and work around them because of the dangers of "second-hand" smoke. Cigarettes and, to a lesser extent, smokeless tobacco are known to cause numerous chronic and acute fatal diseases, including various cancers, cardiovascular and circulatory irregularities, respiratory problems, injuries, stress, prenatal complications, and various other medical conditions. In addition, smokers become visibly more aged, often carry a smoky odor, and are not allowed to smoke inside many workplaces.

Despite the evidence of the dangers of tobacco products, the addictive nature of nicotine ensures that even the most well-intentioned effort to stop smoking will produce unpleasant withdrawal symptoms. These symptoms often prevent cessation and result in relapse.

National prevention efforts now focus on beginning smokers, many of whom are younger and might not understand the nature of addiction. Nonprescription products—gum and patches—address the needs of patients who are already addicted to smoking by helping them stop smoking by easing or preventing nicotine withdrawal symptoms as they slowly reduce the use of the nonprescription products. The nicotine gum and patches can enable patients to deal with the mental aspects of smoking cessation. Nonprescription products are not labeled for smokeless tobacco; the pharmacist should counsel patients addicted to smokeless tobacco to visit a physician.

References

1. Jackson G. Risk factor management: The cardiologist's perspective. Br J Clin Pract Symp Suppl 77A:33, 1996.
2. Garfinkel L. Trends in cigarette smoking in the United States. Prev Med 26:447, 1997.
3. Anon. MMWR 45:962, 1996.
4. Escobedo LG, Peddicord JP. Smoking prevalence in US birth cohorts: The influence of gender and education. Am J Public Health 86:231, 1996.
5. Sells CW, Blum RW. Morbidity and mortality among US adolescents: An overview of data and trends. Am J Public Health 86:513, 1996.
6. Grasser JA, Childers E. Prevalence of smokeless tobacco use and clinical oral leukoplakia in a military population. Mil Med 162:401, 1997.
7. Christen AG. Smokeless tobacco usage: A growing and menacing addiction among Hoosier children and young adults. Indiana Med 89:176, 1996.
8. Davis TC, et al. Tobacco use among male high school athletes. J Adolesc Health 21:97, 1997.
9. Riley WT, et al. Perceived smokeless tobacco addiction among adolescents. Health Psychol 15:289, 1996.
10. Hoffman D, Djordjevic MV. Chemical composition and carcinogenicity of smokeless tobacco. Adv Dent Res 11:322, 1997.
11. Nelson DE, et al. Cigarette smoking prevalence by occupation in the United States. J Occup Med 36:516, 1994.
12. Kendrick JS, Merritt RK. Women and smoking: An update for the 1990s. Am J Obstet Gynecol 175:528, 1996.
13. Shopland DR, et al. Cigarette smoking among U.S. adults by state and region: Estimates from the current population survey. J Natl Cancer Inst 88:1748, 1996.
14. Tomar SL, et al. Oral mucosal smokeless tobacco lesions among adolescents in the United States. J Dent Res 76:1277, 1997.
15. Robertson PB, Walsh MM, Greene JC. Oral effects of smokeless tobacco use by professional baseball players. Adv Dent Res 11:307, 1997.

16. Fed Reg 61:44396, 1996.

17. Inaba DS, Cohen WE, Holstein ME. Uppers, Downers, All Arounders. 3rd ed. Ashland, OR: CNS Publications, 1997; p. 117.

18. Benowitz NL. Systemic absorption and effects of nicotine from smokeless tobacco. Adv Dent Res 11:336, 1997.

19. Kessler DA, et al. The legal and scientific basis for FDA's assertion of jurisdiction over cigarettes and smokeless tobacco. JAMA 277:405, 1997.

20. Burns D, et al. What should be the elements of any settlement with the tobacco industry? (Editorial) Tob Control 6:1, 1997.

21. Gritz ER. Reaching toward and beyond the year 2000 goals for cigarette smoking. Cancer 74:1423, 1994.

22. Smith JB, Fenske NA. Cutaneous manifestations and consequences of smoking. J Am Acad Dermatol 34:717, 1996.

23. Anon. Accessibility to minors of smokeless tobacco products—Broward County, Florida, March–June 1996. MMWR 45:1079, 1996.

24. Byrd RS, Howard CR. Children's passive and prenatal exposure to cigarette smoke. Pediatr Ann 24:640, 1995.

25. LeJeune HB, Cote DN. Passive smoking. J La State Med Soc 147:444, 1995.

26. Stellman SD, Resnicow K. Tobacco smoking, cancer and social class. IARC Sci Publ 138:229, 1997.

27. Schenck-Gustafsson K. Risk factors for cardiovascular disease in women: Assessment and management. Eur Heart J 17(Suppl D):2, 1996.

28. Baron JA. Beneficial effects of nicotine and cigarette smoking: The real, the possible and the spurious. Br Med Bull 52:58, 1996.

29. Wenger NK. Hypertension and other cardiovascular risk factors in women. Am J Hypertens 8:94S, 1995.

30. Henningfield JE, Fant RV, Tomar SL. Smokeless tobacco: An addicting drug. Adv Dent Res 11:330, 1997.

31. Hoffman D, Melikian AA, Wynder EL. Scientific challenges in environmental carcinogenesis. Prev Med 25:14, 1996.

32. Ernster VL. Female lung cancer. Annu Rev Public Health 17:97, 1996.

33. Droller MJ. Environment and the genitourinary tract. Otolaryngol Head Neck Surg 114:248, 1996.

34. Heineman EF, et al. Increased risk of colorectal cancer among smokers: Results of a 26-year follow-up of US veterans and a review. Int J Cancer 59:728, 1994.

35. Dye JA, Adler KB. Effects of cigarette smoke on epithelial cells of the respiratory tract. Thorax 49:825, 1994.

36. Wilson PWF. Established risk factors and coronary artery disease: The Framingham study. Am J Hypertens 7:7S, 1994.

37. Wynder EL. From the discovery of risk factors for coronary artery disease to the application of preventive measures. Am J Med Sci 310(Suppl 1):S119, 1995.

38. Sacks JJ, Nelson DE. Smoking and injuries: An overview. Prev Med 23:515, 1994.

39. Parrott AC. Smoking cessation leads to reduced stress, but why? Int J Addict 340:1509, 1995.

40. Lashner BA. Epidemiology of inflammatory bowel disease. Gastroenterol Clin North Am 24:467, 1995.

41. Birtwistle J. The role of cigarettes and nicotine in the onset and treatment of ulcerative colitis. Postgrad Med J 72:714, 1996.

42. Muhlhauser I. Cigarette smoking and diabetes: An update. Diabetic Med 11:336, 1994.

43. Winn DM. Epidemiology of cancer and other systemic effects associated with the use of smokeless tobacco. Adv Dent Res 11:313, 1997.

44. McGaw WT, Pan JT. Cancer of the gingiva, buccal mucosa, and palate. J Can Dent Assoc 62:146, 1996.

45. Perhsagen G. Smokeless tobacco. Br Med Bull 52:50, 1996.

46. Burgan SW. The role of tobacco use in periodontal diseases: A literature review. Gen Dent 45:449, 1997.

47. Sommese T, Patterson JC. Acute effects of cigarette smoking withdrawal: A review of the literature. Aviat Space Environ Med 66:164, 1995.

48. Goldstein MG. Bupropion sustained release and smoking cessation. J Clin Psychiatry 59(Suppl 4):66, 1998.

49. Trade Packages, Nicorette 2 mg and 4 mg: 1996.

50. Gourlay S. The pros and cons of transdermal nicotine therapy. Med J Aust 160:152, 1994.

51. Trade Package, Nicotrol: 1996.

52. Trade Packages, NicoDerm CQ Step 1, NicoDerm CQ Step 2, and NicoDerm CQ Step 3: 1996.

Diabetes Mellitus

AT THE COUNTER

 A patient asks the pharmacist for NPH Iletin II U-100 insulin. While the pharmacist removes the insulin from the refrigerator, the patient asks, "The last several days, I've been having itching around the injection sites. Should I change insulins?"

Interview/Patient Assessment

The pharmacist asks to see an injection site. The patient shows him an upper arm, on which the pharmacist can see several nonvesicular reddened areas. The patient says this is the latest site on which he is rotating injections. The pruritic spots blanch to the touch. From further questioning the patient, the pharmacist determines that the patient is a type 1 diabetic who has had the condition for 10 years.

Pharmacist's Analysis

1. What kind of reaction is this patient most likely to be having?

2. Would another type of insulin be less likely to produce this reaction? If so, which type(s)?

3. Is the patient able to choose another insulin without physician consultation?

The lesions appear to be caused by an allergic reaction to the patient's animal source insulin. This patient's insulin is the most allergenic available. As other options, the patient might use a human insulin.

Patient Counseling

Patients with diabetes should not change their insulin regimen without physician counseling and monitoring. Any change at all can result in unexpected bouts of hypoglycemia or hyperglycemia. (When changing insulin, patients are sometimes directed to check their blood glucose more frequently than when they are stabilized.) The pharmacist should advise the patient to ask the physician if a change is appropriate, so the physician will have a record of any change in therapy.

Diabetes mellitus is an umbrella term applied to several complicated medical conditions that are characterized by an abnormality of insulin production or utilization. The two most common types of diabetes will be described:

- Insulin-dependent diabetes mellitus (IDDM), or type 1 diabetes mellitus
- Non–insulin-dependent diabetes mellitus (NIDDM), or type 2 diabetes mellitus

Diabetes manifests in other forms such as maturity-onset diabetes in youth (MODY) and gestational diabetes, but they are beyond the scope of this chapter. Because of the complexities of IDDM (type 1) and NIDDM (type 2) diabetes mellitus and their treatment, readers are urged to consult other sources and therapeutics textbooks for additional information.

With most individuals, the beta-islet cells of the human pancreas produce a basal amount of plasma insulin, which prevents unduly high blood glucose while ensuring that the brain and other tissues that require constant glucose are adequately supplied (Fig. 46.1). The pancreas also produces insulin in a bolus or prandial mode, stimulated by food ingestion. Each bolus of insulin released into the blood stream ensures that the blood glucose does not rise too greatly in response to meals.

In IDDM (type 1), the pancreas does not produce the proper amounts of insulin. Therefore, ingested glucose cannot be moved into the cells that require it as a fuel. The body must turn to alternate fuel sources such as breaking down stored body fat. Glucose that is ingested but cannot enter cells gradually builds in the circulation, until it exceeds the renal threshold. At that point, the patient begins excreting glucose in the urine.

In NIDDM (type 2), the usual etiology is somewhat more complicated, involving such problems as weight gain, decreased activity, increased serum insulin levels, and insulin resistance.

Patients with IDDM (type 1) diabetes require daily injections of insulin, but patients with NIDDM (type 2) diabetes may be able to control the condition with diet and exercise. If this is not achieved, the patient may require oral medications or insulin.

Pharmacists can assist patients with diabetes in a number of ways, including teaching them to recognize adverse effects of insulin, explaining how to mix insulins, helping them choose syringes and syringe disposal methods, recommending administration devices, correcting hypoglycemia and hyperglycemia, and caring for their feet and skin.

Diabetes is an extremely expensive disease for patients, their insurers, governments, and employers; its direct and indirect costs (e.g., equipment, supplies, utilization of health facilities, and lost time from work) exceed $120 billion per year.[1,2] The pharmacist can help minimize these costs through various interventions such as suggesting that the patient make every effort to control the condition to prevent complications.

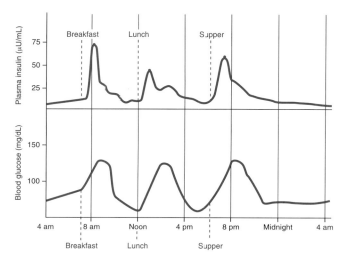

Figure 46.1. Blood glucose levels for an average patient (*below*) contrasted with plasma insulin levels (*above*).

INSULIN-DEPENDENT DIABETES MELLITUS (IDDM) (TYPE 1)

Type 1 diabetes mellitus is a polygenic condition also known as insulin-dependent diabetes mellitus (IDDM). Prior to the 1920s, a diagnosis of type 1 diabetes was tantamount to a death sentence because of the slow and progressive starvation stemming from the inability to use ingested glucose as a nutrient. At that time, therapies involved such Draconian measures as starvation, which prolonged the patient's life somewhat, albeit in a drastically reduced quality. Since the discovery of insulin, patients can now live a much more normal life with proper attention to all aspects of therapy. Unlike NIDDM, which can usually be controlled with strict attention to diet and exercise, IDDM requires lifetime insulin therapy, in addition to strict attention to diet and exercise.

PREVALENCE OF IDDM (TYPE 1)

At least 1.1 to 1.2 million residents of the United States have IDDM.[3] Of these, about 120,000 are children, with a prevalence of 1.6 per 1000.[4] New cases are diagnosed at the rate of over 10,000 per year.

EPIDEMIOLOGY OF IDDM (TYPE 1)

IDDM has a number of possible epidemiologic predictors, including genetics, environmental insults (e.g., viral infections, chemical exposure, diet), age, and ambient temperature. Researchers believe that a combination of these factors must be present to cause IDDM. For instance, IDDM patients have an underlying genetic defect. However, for the condition to develop, the patient must also experience certain triggering environmental factors such as viral infections.

Genetic Predisposition

Patients with IDDM have a genetic defect.[5] Several loci are thought to be responsible such as the HLA-DR and DQ genes on the short arm of chromosome number 6.

The risk of developing IDDM is 0.3 to 0.5% for the general population. However, if one has a first-degree relative with IDDM, the risk is at least 10 times higher.[3] Should one have a monozygotic (identical) twin with IDDM, the risk to the unaffected twin is 30 to 40%. The unaffected member of a set of dizygotic (fraternal) twins has a risk of 5 to 10%. The risk if one has an affected sibling, mother, or father is 6%, 2 to 3%, and 5 to 6%, respectively. Thus it is clear that many who have the genetic predisposition to develop IDDM do not do so.

Environmental Insult

While genetics is an important predictor of IDDM, at least 90% of newly diagnosed IDDM patients have no family history of the condition. Evidently, some type of environmental insult has triggered a process of islet cell destruction in all patients with IDDM.[3] The specific environmental trigger is difficult to discover for any one patient; however, investigators hypothesize that several offenders may be responsible such as viral infection, chemical exposure, or diet.[6]

VIRAL INFECTION

Such viral infections as mumps, coxsackie B, ECHO virus, and rubella may trigger the development of IDDM.[7,8] Perhaps the virus' molecular homologies also contain islet cell autoantigens, so viral infection would trigger production of antiislet autoantibodies that attack the individual's own pancreas.[7,8] Repeated viral infections accelerate the process until the majority of beta cells are destroyed.[9]

CHEMICAL EXPOSURE

Some physicians hypothesize that patients who develop IDDM may have been exposed to chemical toxins at some time from early gestation up to the postnatal period.[3]

DIET

Some researchers hypothesize that early introduction of cow's milk into the diet may cause IDDM because milk or other foods may contain islet autoantigens as a component of their molecular makeup.[3] This theory is not yet fully supported.

Age

About 1 out of every 300 people under 20 (approximately 0.33%) has IDDM.[5] The disease manifests most commonly in males aged 12 to 14 and females aged 10 to 12.[9,10]

Mean Ambient Temperature

Countries that have cooler mean temperatures year round have more cases of IDDM.[3] Further, for unknown reasons, initial symptoms of IDDM are most likely to appear during the winter.[3,4]

ETIOLOGY OF IDDM (TYPE 1)

In a genetically predisposed individual, the patient's own immune system is triggered to attack and destroy pancreatic beta-islet cells.[3] Thus, as described above, IDDM is thought to be caused by a combination of genetic and environmental factors, both of which must be present if the disease is to become active.

MANIFESTATIONS OF IDDM (TYPE 1)

IDDM presents with quite specific symptoms when it is first diagnosed. Patients begin to notice symptoms when the majority of beta cells have been obliterated.[7] At that time, glucose transport across cell membranes is greatly inhibited. Symptoms of IDDM before initiation of insulin treatment include the following[4]:

- **Polydipsia** (ingestion of large quantities of fluids): As the blood glucose rises (since insulin is unavailable to move it into cells), increased osmotic pressure draws water from the cells, dehydrating them, and triggering the thirst response.
- **Glucosuria** (presence of abnormally large amounts of glucose in the urine): As the blood glucose continues to rise, the massive amounts of glucose that cannot be used as fuel exceed the renal threshold, at which point glucose is excreted in the urine.
- **Polyuria** (excretion of large quantities of urine): As the body excretes glucose in the urine, osmotic pressure forces water that would normally be reabsorbed to remain in the urine, ensuring glucose solubility. Excretion of large quantities of urine further contributes to the polydipsia.
- **Polyphagia** (eating large quantities of food): The inability to utilize ingested carbohydrates as fuel leads to cellular and tissue starvation, triggering the patient to eat large quantities of food. Thus, despite the fact that the blood glucose may be greatly elevated, the patient is starving, which may be portrayed as "drowning in glucose, at the same time one is starving."
- **Weight Loss:** Despite the fact that the untreated IDDM patient ingests a great deal of food, family members may notice a paradoxical weight loss, not understanding that the patient is not able to properly utilize the food.
- **Ketosis** (accumulation of fat breakdown by-products in the blood) and acidosis: As the body continues to suffer caloric deprivation, it attempts to cope by breaking down stored fats. This causes the buildup of fat metabolism by-products in the blood such as acetoacetic acid. These products cause a loss of sodium, as well as a retention of hydrogen, leading to acidosis.

Pharmacists may help patients recognize the onset of IDDM by noticing the symptoms that are not dependent on lab tests: the "three P's"; polydipsia, polyuria, and polyphagia,

accompanied by weight loss.[4] Visual disturbances are also common during all of these conditions. See "Hyperglycemia."

The average time from onset of hyperglycemia symptoms until parents make an appointment and obtain a diagnosis is 7 days.[4] Diagnosis employs several examinations, one of the most common being the glucose tolerance test.[11] Patients who fail to see a physician will continue to deteriorate, experiencing dehydration, **Kussmaul breathing** (deep, rapid respirations), vomiting, central nervous system depression, somnolence, and eventually coma leading to death.[4]

PROGNOSIS OF IDDM (TYPE 1)

Although IDDM is an incurable condition, patients can live fully productive lives with proper attention to insulin, diet, and exercise. However, IDDM patients who do not properly monitor their condition have a reduced quality of life throughout its duration and also a reduced life expectancy.[3] Coronary artery disease (e.g., myocardial infarction) is a primary cause of early mortality.

COMPLICATIONS OF IDDM (TYPE 1)

The Diabetes Control and Complications Trial, a landmark 1993 study that explored the best methods to prevent complications of IDDM, clearly established that keeping patients' blood glucose normal lowers the risk of many complications (e.g., retinopathy, nephropathy, and neuropathy) through delaying their onset and slowing their progression.[12]

Patients with inadequate endogenous insulin cannot metabolize glucose normally because they are unable to move it into somatic tissues for use as a fuel source.[13] Thus glucose accumulates in the bloodstream, resulting in hyperglycemia. Prolonged hyperglycemia results in nonenzymatic irreversible glycosylation of various body substances.[7] Advanced glycosylation end products include cross-linked extracellular proteins, which will cause the affected basement membranes of blood vessels to thicken. Macromolecules then can begin to pass freely through them because of increased porosity, causing microvascular diseases that damage the retinas and kidneys.

Neuropathy

Inflammation and scarring of nerve tissues impairs conduction.[14] Patients might become unable to feel their feet, undergo painful or uncomfortable **paresthesias** (tingling or pricking sensations), and/or suffer impaired sexual ability.

Vascular Complications

Adverse effects on the circulation (e.g., stroke) usually do not begin to manifest until patients are in their 30s.[3] Patients may initially notice that minor wounds heal slowly.[14] Diabetes is a leading cause of amputation as a result of vascular insufficiency.[15]

Ophthalmic Complications

IDDM is the leading cause of total visual loss in all age groups from 20 to 74 in the United States.[3] Type 1 diabetics should have yearly visual exams for early detection of retinopathy.[14]

Renal Complications

IDDM is the most frequent cause of end-stage renal disease in the United States.[3] Patients should obtain yearly exams to detect early renal damage.[14]

Infection

Diabetics are prone to infection because of compromised circulation. For example, an 88-year-old female died from gas gangrene 4 days after giving herself an injection of insulin into the subcutaneous tissues of the arm.[16] Even a relatively minor infection (e.g., an ingrown toenail) can cause limb loss or death in diabetics.

Foot Problems

About 15% of diabetics will experience foot ulcers, which result from a combination of one or more of the following:

- Atherosclerosis
- Arterial insufficiency
- **Microangiopathy** (damage to small blood vessels)
- Peripheral neuropathy
- Impaired immune response[17]

These factors combine to increase the diabetic's susceptibility to infection, with feet a primary target. Diabetics are 15 to 40 times more likely to undergo lower limb amputation than the general public, with an infected foot ulcer a common cause.

Pharmacists can give diabetics many commonsense tips to avoid foot problems:

- Never self-treat corns, calluses, ingrown toenail, blisters, bunions, or warts on the feet.
- Inspect feet frequently for any sign of ulceration or infection and for changes in color, temperature, or shape. Obtain prompt physician treatment for any foot problem.
- Remind physicians to check the feet at each office visit.
- Wash the feet daily in lukewarm water (90 to 95°F). To prevent burns, avoid hot water soaks of the feet.
- Never enter a bathtub without first checking the temperature of the water with a hand.
- Never use any heating device or device for producing cold temperatures on the feet, including hot water bottles, heating pads, hot packs, and cold packs.
- Apply moisturizers to prevent the feet from becoming dry or cracked.
- Keep the feet as dry as possible between washings.
- Never walk barefoot (even indoors) or wear sandals. Always wear socks with shoes.

- To reduce the chance of ulcers, see an **orthotist** (an individual who can perform pressure analysis) for insoles that evenly distribute weight inside shoes.
- Do not wear new shoes more than 2 hours at a time. Inspect feet more frequently when breaking in new shoes.
- Never use nonprescription products containing salicylic acid, since they can cause damage to the feet resulting in amputation.
- Never use any type of razor, pumice stone, file, or other device to remove skin from the feet. An amputation may be necessary if the foot becomes infected.
- Do not smoke (smoking reduces blood flow to the feet).

Death Caused by Diabetic Ketoacidosis (DKA)

A major cause of death in diabetic adolescents, diabetic ketoacidosis (DKA) is related to a sustained rise in blood glucose, perhaps resulting from an illness (e.g., an illness that causes vomiting). While the brain does not require insulin to metabolize glucose, most other tissues do. In the absence of utilizable glucose, these tissues are then forced to utilize proteins and fats as fuel sources. Utilization of stored fats as fuels overloads the Krebs cycle, resulting in the accumulation of partially metabolized fat residues (ketoacids) in the bloodstream, a condition known as ketosis. ***Diabetic ketoacidosis is extremely dangerous and must be treated immediately, since coma and death can result.***[23]

TREATMENT OF IDDM (TYPE 1)

Pharmacists can provide invaluable assistance to the patient in treating diabetes. The following are just a few potential interventions: pharmacists should attempt to increase the patient's knowledge base regarding their medical condition; should provide advice regarding insulin, diet, and exercise; should help in the selection of the numerous products and devices used in diabetes management; and should help the patient prevent complications.

Treatment Guidelines

Without argument IDDM is the most serious medical condition for which nonprescription products are sold. From the point that this incurable disease is diagnosed, patients depend entirely on a constant supply of exogenous insulin.

The complications of hyperglycemia (e.g., microvascular and neurologic consequences) are largely prevented with proper metabolic control.[13] Ideally, the blood glucose of IDDM patients should be 80 to 120 mg/dL preprandially, 100 to 180 mg/dL 1 hour postprandially, and 80 to 140 mg/dL 2 hours postprandially.[15] From 2:00 am to 4:00 am the values should fall to between 70 to 120 mg/dL.[19] IDDM patients must constantly be aware of the impact on blood glucose of such vitally important factors as the timing and content of every meal and past and projected physical activity, plus other factors that affect glucose control, including stress and illness.[15] Merely giving a predetermined dosage of insulin without considering all the elements that affect blood glucose can result in unacceptable blood glucose values, both too high and too low.[13] Thus IDDM becomes a way of life in which patients must remain hypervigilant.

Intensive programs to normalize blood glucose offer great benefit to the type 1 diabetic. These intensive programs can encompass the following[18]:

- SMBG performed three to four times daily or more
- Meal planning in conjunction with a registered dietitian
- Regular exercise
- Continuous subcutaneous insulin infusion or multiple daily injections of insulin
- Instruction in prevention and treatment of hypoglycemia
- Continuing education, assessment, and support and reinforcement of goals

Nonprescription Medications

Pharmacists have responsibility for a wide variety of products and devices to help treat the patient with diabetes. They include products for treatment (insulin), devices for insulin injection (e.g., syringes and the paraphernalia for their proper disposal, and insulin pens), products to treat hypoglycemia, and devices for monitoring blood glucose.

INSULIN

Insulin, a complicated molecule containing 51 amino acids in two polypeptide chains, is the primary hormone responsible for glucose metabolism.[14,20,21] Secreted by the beta-islet cells of the pancreas in response to glucose in the blood, insulin facilitates the entrance of glucose into cells, which the cells use as a fuel. In the absence of insulin, glucose cannot be used as a fuel source, so that blood glucose remains high as the body is progressively more starved for fuel. The discovery of insulin in the early 1920s by Frederick Banting and Charles Best, and its purification by coworkers, was widely hailed as one of the greatest advances in the history of medicine, and won Banting, Best, J.B. Collip, and J.J.R. Macleod the 1923 Nobel Prize.

Nonprescription insulin is a mandatory medication for the IDDM patient. Failure to inject adequate insulin at the proper times can result in hyperglycemia, which can lead to deadly diabetic ketoacidosis. (See "Death Caused by Dia-

---

FOCUS ON...

CREATING NONSTANDARD INSULIN DOSES

Occasionally, a pediatrician, veterinarian, or other practitioner may ask a pharmacist to create a more-dilute insulin than 100 units/mL to facilitate the administration of small insulin doses. (See "A Pharmacist's Journal: This Cat Needs Insulin.") To create nonstandard insulin doses, follow the steps below, using sterile aseptic technique throughout and performing all activities in a laminar flow hood:

1. Determine the final concentration required, the number of doses or total volume required, and the type of insulin to be used. *For this example, assume 3 mLs of Regular U-40 insulin is needed for a patient who requires only 2 units of insulin per dose.*
2. Obtain the required amount of U-100 Regular insulin. *In this example, remove an amount of U-100 insulin equivalent to 3 mLs of U-40 insulin activity. (3 mLs of U-40 represents 120 units of insulin. Thus the pharmacist would remove 1.2 mL of U-100 insulin).*
3. Place the insulin in a sterile, pyrogen-free vial such as Sterilized Vials for Insulin Mixtures (Lilly).
4. Dilute the insulin with Sterile Diluting Fluid for Regular Iletin I, Regular Iletin II, and Humulin R to reach the final volume of 3 mL as requested. *In this example, 1.8 mL of diluent would be added.*
5. Place a maximum 30-day expiration date on the vial.

tip *When nonstandard insulins are prepared and dispensed, patients must be cautioned not to use a U-100 syringe, since the calibrations of U-100 syringes only pertain to U-100 insulin.* Instead, pharmacists should dispense allergy syringes, perhaps marking the required dose on the syringe barrels or making a drawing to guide the patient in dosing. All instructions should be in terms of "mL" since any instructions referring to units are irrelevant in the absence of a syringe that measures U-40 insulin in units.

---

betic Ketoacidosis [DKA].") However, even a moderate overdosage of insulin can produce hypoglycemia and lead to irreversible CNS damage and possibly death. For these reasons, **tip** *insulin can be considered to be the most necessary yet most dangerous nonprescription drug product available.*

Because of the serious nature of IDDM, insulin dosing is regulated by a physician. Patients must be cautioned never to alter their insulin regimen without physician approval. **tip** *Patients cannot freely change insulin type, concentration, or purity level.* They cannot switch from animal to human sources without careful monitoring. (See "Source.") Differences in diabetic control have even been observed when patients switch from one company's brand of human insulin to another company's brand.[22]

Nonprescription insulins are only available as 100 units/mL solutions or suspensions, otherwise known as U-100.[14] While 40 units/mL (U-40) and 80 units/mL (U-80) insulins were available until the 1970s (U-80) and 1980s (U-40), they were withdrawn in the United States to standardize the treatment of diabetes. When traveling to a foreign country, however, diabetics may find these other strengths. For this reason, **tip** *pharmacists should advise patients to carry an ample supply of the insulin currently being used when traveling.* If the patient requires a

A Pharmacist's Journal

"This Cat Needs Insulin."

A former student called me about a diabetic cat. The local veterinarian wished to give the cat U-40 Ultralente insulin in a dose of 9 units twice daily. The pharmacist (my former student) wanted to double-check calculations. We determined that a 2-week supply would be sufficient to mix at one time. Thus a total of 252 units, or 2.52 mL of U-100 would be needed. {(9 units)(2 times daily)(14 days)=252} To discover the final volume of the mixture, the pharmacist needed to carry out this calculation:

$$\frac{40 \text{ units}}{1 \text{ mL}} = \frac{252 \text{ units}}{x \text{ mL}} \quad X = 6.3 \text{ mL}$$

The amount of diluent required would be the total volume (6.3 mL) minus the volume occupied by the U-100 (2.52 mL), which equals 3.78 mL. Therefore, the pharmacist needed to employ aseptic technique in the laminar flow hood to dilute 2.52 mL of U-100 Ultralente with 3.78 mL of the appropriate diluting fluid in a sterile, nonpyrogenic vial. The pharmacist intended to sell the cat owner allergy syringes for dosing, with full explanation as to the volume needed.

nonstandard concentration of insulin, the pharmacist may prepare this. (See "Creating Nonstandard Insulin Doses.")

Insulin has no indication except treatment of diabetes. Its sale is restricted to pharmacies for this reason, even though it is a nonprescription medication. Pharmacists should refuse to sell insulin to anyone other than a diabetic or his or her caregivers. Depressed patients have been known to attempt suicide by means of self-injection of insulin.[23,24]

Insulin Administration

Humans manufacture insulin in pancreatic beta-islet cells. From there, endogenous insulin is delivered through the portal vein to the liver and periphery.[25] The means by which the type 1 diabetic must administer exogenous insulin are less efficient such as via subcutaneous injection. Subcutaneous injection is subject to considerable variation in the amount of insulin absorbed. For a given patient, absorption may vary day-to-day by as much as 25%.[19] Person-to-person variations are as high as 50%. The inability to mimic the body's natural method of insulin delivery leads to numerous difficulties that must be mastered by diabetics. IDDM patients generally are considered to be capable of insulin self-administration at age 7 to 8.[4]

Injection sites for insulin have been chosen carefully over many years to minimize the possibility of damage to nerves and other tissues and to provide adequate absorption (Fig. 46.2). (See "Injection Site Rotation.") Abdominal sites yield the most rapid absorption. Next, in descending order, are the arm, thigh, and buttocks.[14,19] Exercise increases blood flow and shortens the time of absorption; thus, patients should not administer to body parts that will be affected by exercise—such as the arm prior to weight lifting and the leg prior to jogging. Generally speaking, the abdomen is the preferred site.[15]

Insulin is normally administered approximately 30 minutes prior to a meal. This "lag time" allows the insulin to reach ef-

fective blood levels as the food is absorbed.[19] (See "Insulin Syringes" for details on syringes and administering insulin.)

Insulin Dosing

The typical IDDM patient injects approximately 0.4 to 1 unit of insulin per kilogram of body weight.[4,19] However, the patient may be given an algorithm or "sliding scale" in which the physician directs a certain amount of insulin to be given, depending on the blood glucose reading.

Classifications of Insulin

Insulins differ in several important characteristics such as time/action profile, source, and purity level. Table 46.1 lists insulins currently available in the United States, including their purity level, source, concentration, and manufacturer.

Time/Action Profile. The time/action profile of insulin is the most critical aspect of insulin dosing (aside from the dose given). To meet patients' varied requirements for time of onset, peak action, and duration, insulin is produced in the following basic formulations (Fig. 46.3):

- Regular. Regular insulin is the only insulin categorized as "rapid-acting." Because of its short duration when injected subcutaneously, several daily injections are necessary to provide proper glycemic control.[21] *As the only true solution of insulin, Regular is the only type of insulin that can be administered intravenously.*

- NPH. Neutral Protamine Hagedorn (NPH) insulin is created by adding protamine (extracted from salmon testes) and zinc to insulin. An intermediate-acting insulin suspension with a duration of approximately a day, NPH insulin is also referred to as Isophane insulin. Some patients are allergic to protamine.

- Lente. Lente insulin suspension is created by adding amorphous and crystalline zinc chloride to insulin, using specific buffering procedures. This insulin was also created to provide a duration of approximately a day.[21]

- Ultralente. Ultralente insulin suspension is created by adding crystalline zinc chloride to insulin using specific buffering procedures, producing the only sustained-action insulin.

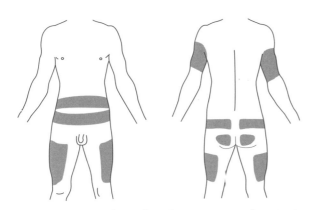

Figure 46.2. Potential sites for subcutaneous insulin injections.

Figure 46.3 and Table 46.2 illustrate the variation in onsets, peaks, and durations. (See "Source.") To help prevent patients from accidentally purchasing the wrong type of insulin, which could affect blood glucose levels for many hours, insulin is marked "R," "N," "L," or "U" (for Regular, NPH, Lente, and Ultralente).

As noted above, insulin absorption varies because of the nature of subcutaneous tissue injections. Absorption becomes even more uncertain as longer-acting insulin preparations are used. For this reason, Regular insulin causes the least variability in blood glucose.[19]

Source. Insulin comes from three sources:

- Isolated from beef pancreas (no longer available)
- Isolated from pork pancreas
- Produced biosynthetically (e.g., human insulin of recombinant DNA origin)[14]

Insulin from pork sources is made available as purified pork. The source of insulin can affect bioavailability.[21] For example, peak activities may occur sooner with human varieties of insulin.

Table 46.1. Types of Insulin Available in the United States

TRADE NAME	INSULIN TYPE	SOURCE	CONCENTRATION	MANUFACTURER
Short-acting insulins:				
Iletin I[a]	Regular	Beef/pork	U-100	Lilly
Iletin II	Regular	Purified pork	U-100	Lilly
Iletin II	Regular	Purified pork	U-500	Lilly
Humulin R	Regular	Human	U-100	Lilly
Regular[b]	Regular	Purified pork	U-100	Novo Nordisk
Novolin R	Regualr	Human	U-100	Novo Nordisk
Velosulin BR[c]	Regular	Human	U-100	Novo Nordisk
Insulin Lispro	N/A	Human (analog)	U-100	Lilly
Intermediate-acting insulins:				
Iletin I[a]	NPH	Beef/pork	U-100	Lilly
Iletin I[a]	Lente	Beef/pork	U-100	Lilly
Iletin II	NPH	Purified pork	U-100	Lilly
Iletin II	Lente	Purified pork	U-100	Lilly
Humulin N	NPH	Human	U-100	Lilly
Humulin L	Lente	Human	U-100	Lilly
NPH[b]	NPH	Purified pork	U-100	Novo Nordisk
Lente[b]	Lente	Purified pork	U-100	Novo Nordisk
Novolin N	NPH	Human	U-100	Novo Nordisk
Novolin L	Lente	Human	U-100	Novo Nordisk
Long-lasting insulin:				
Humulin U	Ultralente	Human	U-100	Lilly
Insulin mixtures:				
Humulin 70/30[d]	NPH/Regular	Human	U-100	Lilly
Humulin 50/50[e]	NPH/Regular	Human	U-100	Lilly
Novolin 70/30[d]	NPH/Regular	Human	U-100	Novo Nordisk

[a]Lilly ceased production of Iletin I in 1998; supplies were projected to be depleted in 1999.

[b]Novo Nordisk does not carry a trade name for their nonhuman insulins.

[c]Recommended for continuous subcutaneous insulin infusion.

[d]Product is 70% NPH and 30% Regular.

[e]Product is 50% NPH and 50% Regular.

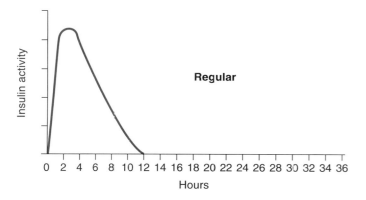

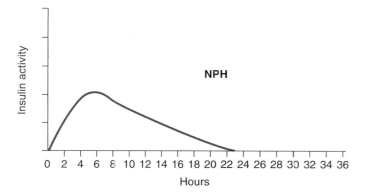

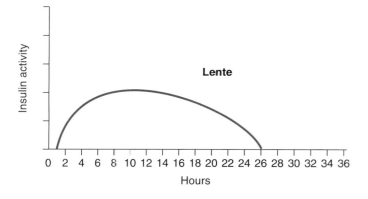

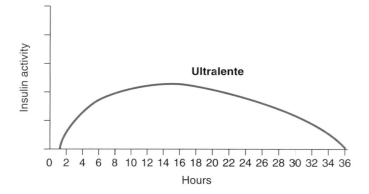

Figure 46.3. Approximate peaks and durations for Regular, NPH, Lente, and Ultralente insulin subcutaneous injections.

Table 46.2. Time/Action Profile of Subcutaneous Insulins

PRODUCT	ONSET (HOURS)	PEAK (HOURS)	DURATION (HOURS)
Animal Regular	0.5–2	3–4	6–8
Animal NPH	4–6	8–14	20–24
Animal Lente	4–6	8–14	20–24
Human Regular	0.5–1	2–3	4–6
Human NPH	2–4	4–10	14–18
Human Lente	3–4	4–12	16–20
Human Ultralente	6–10	12–16	20–30
Insulin Lispro	0.25	0.5–1.5	2

ANIMAL INSULINS. Although they have been used for decades, animal insulins have some theoretical disadvantages compared with human insulins. For instance, some investigators assert that circulating antibodies developed by some patients may bind with injected animal insulins, causing the insulin to be released at unpredictable times. When this occurs diabetes control becomes more difficult.

The most antigenic insulin is beef, since it differs from human by three amino acids. Pork differs by only one amino acid. Because of these characteristics, beef/pork mixtures (no longer available as of 1999) were most allergenic; pork is less antigenic than beef, and purified pork is the least antigenic nonhuman insulin. Unless a vial of nonhuman insulin specifically states "pork" or "purified pork," it is a mixture of 70% beef and 30% pork insulins. Most allergic reactions involve redness, burning, and pruritus at the injection site.[26]

HUMAN INSULINS. Human insulin was the first recombinant DNA product available in the United States.[27] To create human insulin, genetic engineers synthesized genes to produce human proinsulin, which are inserted into special strains of *Escherichia coli* (Eli Lilly Humulin products) or bakers' yeast (Novo Nordisk Novolin products).[21]

Human insulins are optimal for newly diagnosed patients since the availability of animal insulins has slowly decreased in recent years.[19] Further, pork insulin results in the formation of insulin antibodies; newly diagnosed patients initiated on human insulin will not develop these antibodies since exogenous human insulin is structurally identical to endogenous human insulin.[28]

Human insulin has no contraindications, so all patients could be switched to it under medical supervision. It is especially useful for pregnant type 1 diabetics and patients with type 2 diabetes, as well as those with insulin allergy, insulin lipoatrophy, and gestational diabetes.[28] (For a detailed discussion of type 2 diabetes see "Non–Insulin-Dependent Diabetes Mellitus [Type 2].")

Purity Level. Animal source insulins are purified through many chromatographic techniques.[21] (The marker used to designate insulin impurity is proinsulin, a nonactive polypeptide precursor to insulin.) Animal source insulins are available as standard or purified options. Older, less pure standard products contain approximately 10 parts per million of proinsulin; newer, purified products contain fewer than 10 parts per million, usually down to one part per million or fewer. Impurities known as "covalent insulin aggregates" may be responsible for allergies to insulin, so a patient with a local reaction to standard insulin may benefit from a physician-monitored switch to a purified or human insulin. Lilly designates standard insulins as Iletin I and purified pork products as Iletin II. NovoNordisk does not produce the standard insulins. Lilly ceased production of Iletin I insulins in 1998. Supplies were projected to be depleted in 1999.

Prescription Insulin and Insulin Analog. While the majority of patients using insulin purchase nonprescription varieties, this discussion would be incomplete without mention of two prescription versions.

U-500 INSULIN. Either type 1 or type 2 patients may develop a condition known as insulin resistance. It may be caused by infection, ketoacidosis, or the obesity of type 2 diabetes.[26] With this condition, normal doses of insulin produce a subnormal response.[21] Doses may require gradual increases to maintain glycemic control. Eventually, patients may experience discomfort from the volume of insulin required per injection into subcutaneous tissues. A prescription U-500 insulin can reduce the volume required by a factor of 5 (it is five times as concentrated as U-100). Manufactured by Lilly as an Iletin II product, this insulin is only available as a purified pork Regular insulin in 20-mL vials. Patients who might benefit from U-500 insulin include those with daily insulin requirements greater than 200 units.

The U-500 box and bottle are imprinted with warning stripes and a special precaution, "Warning—High Potency, Not for Ordinary Use." Patients should be warned not to use a U-100 syringe with U-500 insulin, since the markings would not reflect the actual amount of insulin. Rather, *a highly accurate 1 mL disposable allergy syringe should be used with U-500 insulin.* These syringes are not calibrated in units of insulin, but in 1/100 mL, which makes them the most accurate general purpose syringes readily available to the consumer.

INSULIN LISPRO. Conventional Regular human insulin contains insulin in the form of hexameric complexes. Before it can be absorbed, conventional insulins must dissociate into dimers and monomers of insulin, providing the lag time prior to action and the sustained peaks (e.g., as long as 2 to 3 hours for Regular human insulin). The lag time in action caused by sustained absorption from subcutaneous sites forces patients to inject as long as 30 minutes prior to a meal; the sustained time to peak often produces hypoglycemia after meals.[29] An insulin analog was developed through manipulation of amino acids to allow rapid dissociation of the hexamers directly to monomers. This analog, known as insulin lispro, is absorbed more rapidly, shortening the time of onset and time to peak action. Thus it may be injected only 15 minutes prior to a

meal. The product is known as Humalog, available in 10-mL vials and in cartridges for B-D Insulin Pens.[30]

Insulin Regimens

Insulin regimens are numerous. Historically, a common regimen for IDDM patients was to self-inject twice daily (e.g., 30 minutes before breakfast and dinner) or three times daily (30 minutes before breakfast, dinner, and bedtime).[4] However, these older, traditional regimens (also known as nonphysiologic regimens) have given way in many cases to newer regimens (known as physiologic regimens), which are designed to better mimic the human pancreatic release of endogenous insulin.[19] (The nonphysiologic regimens are now seen as adequate only for type 2 diabetes.) Several regimens are illustrated in Figure 46.4.

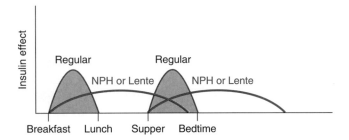

A. Twice-daily Regular and NPH or Lente mixtures

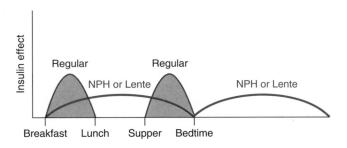

B. Regular and NPH or Lente at breakfast, Regular at supper, NPH or Lente at bedtime

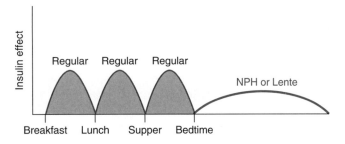

C. Regular before meals, NPH or Lente at bedtime

Figure 46.4. Several different insulin regimens that may be used in intensive insulin therapy.

Common regimens discussed below include the following:

- Split-mixed injections: twice-daily Regular and NPH/ Lente mixtures
- Split-mixed injection at breakfast, Regular at supper, and NPH or Lente at bedtime
- Three Regular preprandial injections and NPH or Lente at bedtime
- Three preprandial Regular injections and Ultralente preprandial injections twice daily
- Continuous subcutaneous insulin pump infusion (CSII)

Split-Mixed Injections: Twice-Daily Regular and NPH/Lente Mixtures. In this regimen, the most commonly used in the United States, either NPH or Lente (NPH/Lente) is mixed in the same vial or syringe with Regular insulin (see "Insulin Mixtures").[19] This mixture is administered prior to breakfast and supper, often 66% of the dose in the morning and the remainder in the supper dose (see Fig. 46.4). The Regular insulin controls the glucose ingested with breakfast and supper. Background NPH/Lente provides a basal ability to control glucose after the action of the Regular terminates.

The "dawn phenomenon," in which patients experience nocturnal hyperglycemia prior to breakfast because of premature dissipation of insulin activity, is a major disadvantage of this regimen. Attempting to increase the dose of supper NPH/Lente may cause patients to experience hypoglycemia during the night. For these reasons, patients may be switched to other regimens.

Split-Mixed Injection at Breakfast, Regular at Supper, and NPH or Lente at Bedtime. With this method, patients administer three injections daily: a mixture of Reg-

---

FOCUS ON . . .

INSULIN MIXTURES

Patients may be directed by an endocrinologist to administer a mixture of two insulins to better control blood glucose. The mixture is often Regular insulin, in combination with one of the intermediate-acting insulins.[4] This mixture may be administered using several methods:

- Patients may give two different injections in rapid succession.
- Several doses of insulin may be mixed together in the appropriate ratio in a sterile vial for withdrawal at a later time. Preferably, this should be done by the pharmacist, in a laminar flow hood, using sterile technique.
- Patients may use any one of several commercially available insulin mixtures.
- The insulins may be mixed together in the same syringe at the time of injection, so that only one injection is needed.

Making a mixture of insulins in the same syringe is a complicated process in which several steps must be followed carefully. To illustrate, the steps for mixing Regular and NPH follow[31]:

1. Wash hands.
2. *(tip)* Roll the NPH vial gently between the hands to mix the insulin. *To avoid getting air bubbles in the insulin and preserve insulin activity, never shake the vial.* Check to ensure that the insulin particles are evenly suspended. Discard any vial with clumps or aggregates that cannot be evenly resuspended.
3. Swab both vial tops with alcohol and wait until the alcohol is completely dried.
4. Draw into a syringe of appropriate size an amount of air equal to the amount of NPH that will be drawn into the syringe.
5. Insert the syringe into the vial of NPH and depress the syringe plunger to place the measured air into the vial.
6. Withdraw the syringe from the NPH vial without removing any insulin.
7. Draw into the syringe an amount of air equal to the amount of Regular that will be drawn into the syringe.
8. Insert the syringe into the vial of Regular and depress the syringe plunger to place the measured air into the vial.
9. Invert the vial of Regular and pull the plunger of the syringe down until the tip of the rubber on the syringe plunger is aligned exactly with the correct calibration for the amount of Regular required. *If the syringe contains air bubbles, reinject the insulin* *(tip)* *into the vial and withdraw the correct amount again.* At this point, most air bubbles should be gone. However, gently tapping the syringe will usually dislodge them. As they float toward the needle, they may be pushed back into the vial. Redraw the correct amount of Regular insulin until the measurement is correct.
10. Remove the syringe from the vial and place it into the top of the NPH vial.
11. Invert the vial and carefully pull the plunger down until the tip of the rubber on the syringe plunger is aligned exactly with the total number of units to be injected.
12. Even if bubbles are present, they may not be removed by reinjecting, or the vial will become contaminated.

The above steps have several objectives:

- Patients may obtain the exact ratio of Regular to modified insulin required by the physician.
- Air pressure in the vials is equalized without risking contamination of either vial.
- The possibility of NPH entering the vial of Regular insulin (by drawing Regular first) is eliminated. Should traces of the modifying agents (e.g., zinc, protamine) enter the vial of Regular, they potentially could bind with the unmodified Regular insulin, modifying it so that it loses its rapid-onset qualities.

Continued

ular and NPH or Lente prior to breakfast, Regular prior to supper, and NPH or Lente at bedtime (see Fig. 46.4). This regimen reduces the risk of nocturnal hyperglycemia seen with twice-daily Regular and NPH/Lente mixtures, while also minimizing nocturnal hypoglycemia.

Insulin Lispro may be mixed with Humulin N, but a decrease in the absorption rate should be expected.[34] When insulin lispro is mixed with Humulin U, however, no decrease in absorption occurs. Both mixtures should be given 15 minutes prior to a meal. There are no data on mixing insulin lispro with human insulins or with insulins from Novo Nordisk.

Three Regular Preprandial Injections and NPH or Lente Bedtime Injection. In this regimen, three Regular insulin injections are given **preprandially** (prior to meals) and one injection of NPH or Lente is given at bedtime (see Fig. 46.4). A great advantage to this regimen is the ability to alter the insulin dose upward or downward to match the projected size of the meal.

Three Preprandial Regular Injections and Ultralente Preprandial Injections Twice Daily. The use of Ultralente in this regimen provides a basal insulin availability while the preprandial Regular injections metabolize meals.

Continuous Subcutaneous Insulin Pump Infusion (CSII). Physicians have turned to insulin pumps as the ideal regimen, the regimen that most closely mimics the human pancreas. The patient carries a small battery-driven pump that can be programmed to deliver Regular insulin through a catheter placed into an area such as the periumbilical SQ tissues. The pump is periodically reloaded with insulin. Patients program a basal mode, delivered as serial Regular insulin micropulses as small as 0.1 unit. Basal delivery can be decreased between 12 am and 4 am to prevent nocturnal hypoglycemia and increased between 4 am and 8 am to prevent the dawn phenomenon.[19] The pump is also programmed to deliver three bolus preprandial insulin boluses. The patient can vary the specific bolus dose depending on the calorie content of the projected meal and the blood glucose. Typically, 50% of the total daily insulin dose will be basal, with the remainder being divided into the three preprandial doses.

CSII provides better glycemic control than periodic injections since Regular is the only insulin used. However, patients must be highly motivated and financially able to purchase the pump and its rechargeable batteries. Also, the injection site must be inspected frequently to ensure that it is not infected. Some insulins form monofilaments as they

In research, investigators have discovered that patients fail to follow these steps faithfully in many instances.[32] Studies showed that at least 71% of patients failed to eliminate air bubbles as suggested, 62% failed to add air correctly, 48% suspended NPH incorrectly, 27% swabbed the vial tops incorrectly, 23% cross-contaminated the vials, 15% did not draw the Regular first, and 14% did not manipulate the syringes and vials correctly. Thus pharmacists should demonstrate these procedures and should ask patients to perform them to correct their techniques.

Even health professionals often have difficulty obtaining the correct ratio when mixing insulins.[33] For this reason, pharmacists should be aware of the premixed insulins available in the United States, as listed in Table 46.1.

Mixtures of Regular and NPH are compatible.[28] Lente and Ultralente are also stable when mixed. Regular and Lente mixtures must be injected immediately or the effect of the Regular insulin will be lost. NPH is incompatible with Lente or Ultralente.

slowly pass through the pump tubing, eventually obstructing the lumen. Velosulin BR insulin is buffered to prevent formation of insulin filaments, and is recommended for CSII pumps.

Injection Devices

There are three types of injection devices commonly used. Insulin syringes are the most often utilized, but some patients find insulin pens to have specific advantages. Jet injectors are not common, but also possess unique advantages favored by some patients.

Insulin Syringes. Specially designed insulin syringes are used with U-100 insulin. Table 46.3 shows a listing of representative insulin syringes and their characteristics.

⚠ ***Diabetics should never use any syringe other than an insulin syringe with U-100 insulin, since noninsulin syringes are not marked with calibrations reflecting the actual number of units being injected.*** Deaths have resulted from using an incorrect syringe such as a patient who was sold 3-mL syringes by a pharmacist, administered an overdose, and died.[35] Also, insulin syringes should only be used to measure U-100 insulin. In one case, they were used to measure calcitonin-salmon by nurses who assumed a unit of insulin was also equal to a unit of calcitonin-salmon.[36] (See "A Pharmacist's Journal: I Need Insulin Syringes.")

INSULIN SYRINGE CALIBRATIONS. Insulin syringes are not calibrated in fractions of a milliliter. When insulin syringes do have a reference to milliliters, it is located only at the end of the plunger extension. Thus some 100 unit insulin syringes have the notation "1 cc" at the 100 unit mark. A 50 unit syringe may have a notation such as "1/2 cc" at the end of the barrel. However, these syringes will never have a notation such as 0.2 mL or 0.4 mL along the barrel. This prohibition is meant to clarify dosing for the diabetic, who measures insulin in units rather than mLs.

ACCURACY OF INSULIN SYRINGES. Patients should always choose the smallest capacity insulin syringe that will hold the required dose of insulin[35]:

Table 46.3. Representative Insulin Syringes

PRODUCT	COMMENTS
B-D Micro-Fine IV	28-gauge, 1/2-inch needle, available in 3/10-, 1/2-, and 1-mL sizes
B-D Ultra-Fine	29-gauge, 1/2-inch needle, available in 3/10-, 1/2-, and 1-mL sizes
B-D Ultra-Fine II Short Needle 1/2 cc	30-gauge, 5/16-inch needle, available in 3/10- and 1/2-mL sizes
Monoject Ultra Comfort	28- & 29-gauge needles; available in 3/10-, 1/2-, and 1-mL sizes
Monoject Safety Syringes	29-gauge needles; 1/2-inch needle, available in 1-mL size; needles have a safety shield to provide temporary protection from needle sticks during transport or permanent protection prior to discarding
Sure-Dose	28-gauge needles; 1/2-inch needle, available in 1/2- and 1-mL sizes
Sure-Dose Plus	29-gauge needles; 1/2-inch needle, available in 1/4-, 1/2-, and 1-mL sizes

A Pharmacist's Journal

"I Need Insulin Syringes."

Like many pharmacists in states that allow non-prescription sales of syringes, I have been highly sensitive over the years to patients who pretend that they are diabetic to obtain syringes for illicit purposes. In one memorable case, a young man asked for insulin syringes. I asked which type he wanted, and he said that it didn't matter. I explained that the syringes varied in accuracy and he should match the syringe to the specific dose of insulin he used. I then asked him, "What dose of insulin do you give?" His response betrayed his total lack of knowledge about diabetes: "Oh, about 100 milliliters." If syringes are nonprescription devices in the home state, the pharmacist must decide whether to sell them in these cases (perhaps stemming the spread of AIDS) or refuse to sell them (perhaps causing the user to utilize a used needle, contracting AIDS or another bloodborne pathogen).

- Patients injecting 51 to 100 units of insulin should use 1-mL syringes.
- Patients injecting 31 to 50 units of insulin should use 1/2-mL syringes.
- Patients injecting 26 to 30 units of insulin should use 3/10-mL syringes.
- Patients injecting 25 units or less should use a 0.25-mL syringe, which is graduated in 0.5 unit, the most accurate insulin syringe available.

Measuring of insulin doses with smaller syringes is easier than with larger syringes because smaller capacity syringes have narrower inner lumens, which allows the barrel to be lengthened and the graduations separated more widely, as illustrated in Table 46.4.

INSULIN SYRINGE NEEDLES. A syringe needle gauge is a primary predictor of injection pain. Fortunately, insulin needles are available as small as 30 gauge, a needle size that produces a nearly imperceptible insertion (a 31-gauge pen needle is available). Although most needles are 1/2 inch, some syringes are now available in a shorter length, which lessens the probability that the injection will enter muscular tissues.

Insulin syringes have variable accuracy for microdoses such as those required for infants (e.g., 2 units or less).[37] In these cases, the pharmacist may dilute the insulin to facilitate withdrawal of the proper dosage. See "Creating Nonstandard Insulin Doses."

INSULIN ADMINISTRATION USING SYRINGES. As illustrated in Figure 46.5, patients should follow the steps below to self-inject insulin using a syringe[35,38,39]:

1. Wash hands.
2. If the insulin is a suspension, roll the vial gently between the hands to mix the insulin. *To avoid getting air bubbles in the insulin and preserve insulin activity, never shake the vial.* Check to ensure that the insulin

Table 46.4. Capacities and Measurement Accuracy of Insulin Syringes

SYRINGE CAPACITY	APPROXIMATE LENGTH OF GRADUATIONS	ACCURACY OF MEASUREMENT
1 mL (100 units)	60 mm	1 graduation = 2 units (B-D, Sure-Dose) 1 graduation = 1 unit (Monoject)
1/2 mL (50 units)	51 mm	1 graduation = 1 unit
3/10 mL (30 units)	42 mm	1 graduation = 1 unit
1/4 mL (25 units)	45 mm	1 graduation = 1/2 unit

particles are evenly suspended. Discard any vial with clumps or aggregates that cannot be evenly resuspended.

3. Swab the top of the insulin vial with alcohol and wait until the alcohol is completely dried.

4. Draw into a syringe of appropriate size an amount of air equal to the amount of insulin that will be drawn into the syringe.

5. Insert the syringe into the vial of insulin and depress the syringe plunger to place the measured air into the vial.

6. Invert the vial of insulin and pull the plunger of the syringe down until the tip of the rubber on the syringe plunger is aligned exactly with the correct calibration for the amount of insulin required. *If the syringe contains air bubbles, reinject the insulin into the vial and withdraw the correct amount again.* At this point, most of the air bubbles should be gone. However, gently tapping the syringe will usually dislodge them. As they float toward the needle, they may be pushed back into the vial. Redraw the correct amount of insulin until the measurement is correct.

7. Clean the skin around the proposed injection site with alcohol.

8. Pinch the skin up to create a skinfold.

9. Push the needle through the skin at a 90° angle (most patients) or a 45° angle (thin patients and children) then depress the plunger.

10. Remove the needle and press a finger or fresh alcohol swab over the injection site.

The alcohol used during the injection process may be purchased as bottles of isopropyl or denatured ethyl alcohol and used with cotton balls. Alternatively, the patient may choose to use alcohol swabs premoistened with isopropyl alcohol (e.g., B-D Alcohol Swabs).

INSULIN SYRINGE DISPOSAL.   Syringe disposal can be a problem for diabetics, who must discard a device that has pierced the human body and should be treated using universal precautions to prevent bloodborne pathogens.

The problem of syringe disposal is heightened in the diabetic patient who employs intensive therapy—injecting three or more times daily—and accumulating as many as 90 or more syringes monthly.[40] The possible methods of syringe disposal are as follows:

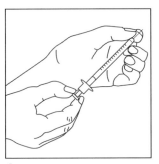

A. Draw air into syringe.

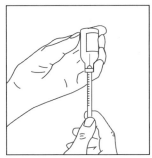

B. Inject air and withdraw insulin.

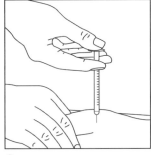

C. Inject at a 90° angle into a skinfold.

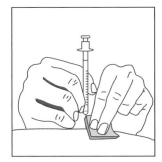

D. Withdraw the needle, pressing an alcohol swab over the site.

Figure 46.5. Before withdrawing and injecting insulin, patient washes hands, gently rolls vial between the hands (suspensions only), and swabs top of vial with alcohol. The patient then (**A**) draws air into syringe equal to amount of insulin to be withdrawn; (**B**) inverts vial and injects air into vial and then withdraws insulin dose; (**C**) pinches skin to create skinfold, inserts the needle into the skin at a 90° angle, and injects insulin by depressing plunger; and (**D**) removes the needle, pressing an alcohol swab over the injection site (see text for details).

• Disposal Containers. The American Diabetes Association (ADA) and the U.S. Environmental Protection Agency (EPA) advise placing used syringes into a solid container such as a plastic bleach bottle or laundry detergent bottle. However, these are not marked as containing potentially infectious materials nor do they have secure lids (as recommended by the EPA). A safer alternative product that more closely meets these guidelines is a syringe disposal container such as a "sharps" container ("sharps" is a general term for any device that could pierce the body such as lancets or syringes). One example is the B-D Home Sharps Container, a rigid plastic 1.4 quart container with a snap lock lid that will hold 70 to 100 syringes. Prominent external labels on the container display biohazard warnings.

- Needle Clippers. Some patients remove the needle from the syringe by bending the needle cover repeatedly until the needle breaks, a potentially hazardous technique because it is possible to accidentally puncture the skin. Other patients use wire clippers or pliers to clip the needle, but with this method the needle may be lost if it is allowed to drop to the floor after removal.[41] The American Diabetes Association recommends use of a device that retains clipped needles in an inaccessible compartment.[40] One such device is the B-D Safe-Clip, a plastic device with a small orifice just large enough to accommodate a needle. After inserting the needle, the patient closes the lid of the device, which clips the needle, rendering the syringe nonfunctional.[35] Syringes can then be disposed of without worry of abuse or injury, and the clipping device is disposed of when it is full. (The B-D Safe Clip holds up to a year's worth of clipped needles.) The B-D Safe Clip also carries a biohazard warning label.

SYRINGE REUSE.   To save money, some diabetics reuse their syringes. In addition to the lack of support for this practice in the literature, there are other compelling reasons against this practice[35]:

- Silicone used to lubricate the syringe plunger can enter an insulin vial with reuse, inactivating the insulin.
- Injections will become progressively more painful as the needle dulls.
- The plunger will not easily slide into the barrel with continued usage, making it harder to withdraw insulin and make the injection.
- Reuse can cause more inflammation at the injection site, perhaps related to reuse-associated contamination.

Manufacturers label insulin syringes as disposable, so any health professional advising reuse may be held liable for problems that occur from the practice.

SYRINGE INJECTION AIDS.   Patients may have difficulty in self-administering insulin with syringes. Some patients fear the needle or are apprehensive about piercing their skin. Several companies market injection aids that can ease the injection process somewhat. An example is the B-D Automatic Injector. The patient cocks the device by pulling up a latch bar until it clicks. He next places a preloaded syringe into an opening on top of the device, so that the syringe slides down into its barrel. The syringe body and needle are hidden inside of the device itself. The device is placed against the skin and triggered. The spring action pushes the syringe down-

ward so that the needle pierces the skin. The patient then depresses the syringe plunger to deliver the insulin.

Another syringe injection aid is the Monoject Injectomatic, which comes in one size to fit the 1-mL syringe and a second size to fit the 1/2-mL syringe. The device is a silver metal barrel that holds a syringe inside. The patient follows instructions for placing the preloaded syringe inside the Injectomatic. The device is cocked by pulling the top away from the bottom until it clicks. The cocked device is placed on the injection site, and the patient presses it downward, triggering it to cause the syringe's needle to pierce the skin. Then the patient injects the insulin and withdraws the syringe-device assembly.

Insulin Pens.   Insulin pens are insulin administration devices that allow patients to "dial a dose" and inject with a needle fitted onto the pen rather than through the use of separate syringes (Table 46.5).[9,42] Insulin pens have a number of benefits compared with syringes:

- The larger size makes it easier for patients with restricted mobility to administer doses of insulin.[13]
- They may be used with only one hand. (Syringes require both hands.)
- The dial-a-dose feature simplifies insulin measurement for patients with impaired sight.
- They are unobtrusive, resembling a regular ink pen when placed in one's pocket.

Many diabetics find insulin pens easier to use. However, patients must strictly adhere to all of the manufacturer's instructions. Failure to carry out all preinjection steps (such as priming the needle) can cause inaccurate dosing of the insulin. *Pharmacists must caution patients to read the instructions thoroughly and practice extensively before attempting the first injection.*[43] When cartridges of modified insulin are used, the patient should turn the cartridge upside down and then upright at least 10 times to obtain a uniform suspension.

Use of insulin pens is not without hazard. One patient noticed a hematoma at the injection site immediately following use of a pen.[44] An accidental intravenous injection had been made with a modified insulin, culminating in symptoms of hypoglycemia. *Immediate bleeding after the injection is a sign of impending hypoglycemia.*[44]

Jet Injectors.   Rather than using needles, these devices inject insulin into the skin with a jet of compressed gas that is smaller than even a 30-gauge needle.[45] Jet injectors (e.g., Vitajet Innova and the Medi-Jector Choice, both of which accept any 10-mL vial of insulin) are expensive (approximately $300 to $400), but patients with apprehension regarding needles may benefit from their use. In addition, absorption is more rapid with jet injection.

Injection Site Rotation
The abdomen is the preferred injection location for insulin because both hands may be used when injecting, the patient

Table 46.5. Representative Insulin Pens and Associated Products

PRODUCT	COMMENTS
B-D Pen	Pen that accepts 1.5-mL cartridges of insulin and disposable needles; patient dials a dose up to 30 units of insulin
B-D Ultra-Fine Original Pen Needles	Disposable needles used with the B-D Pen; 29 gauge, 0.5 inch
B-D Ultra-Fine III Short Pen Needles	Disposable needles used with the B-D Pen; 31 gauge, 5/16 inch
Humulin Cartridges	1.5-mL cartridges of insulin; available in Regular, NPH, and 70/30 (70% NPH and 30% Regular)
NovolinPen	Pen that accepts 1.5-mL cartridges of insulin and disposable needles, patient dials a dose up to 36 units of insulin
Novolin Prefilled	A 1.5-mL, prefilled, penlike syringe that delivers up to 58 units of insulin/dose; available in Regular, NPH, and 70/30 (70% NPH and 30% Regular); patient sets a dose in 2-unit increments by dialing a cap
Novolin PenFil	1.5-mL cartridges of insulin to fit the Novo family of pens; available in Regular, NPH, and 70/30 (70% NPH and 30% Regular)
Novolin PenNeedles	Disposable needles used with the Novo family of pens
NovoFine 30	Disposable needles used with the Novo family of pens, 30 gauge, 1/3-inch needle

cannot easily make an accidental injection into muscle, tendon, or nerves, and it has numerous possible injection sites. The abdomen can be divided into as many as 56 separate sites, with another 16 sites wrapping around the back, according to patient teaching handouts produced by a major United States insulin manufacturer. The front and back of the upper legs can allow the patient another 76 sites (approximately), the hips another 32 sites, and the upper arms another 66 sites[14] (see Fig. 46.2).

Patients should use a consistent pattern to rotate injection sites from day to day.[4,38] For instance, patients should use all of the sites in one location (e.g., abdomen) before moving to another location (e.g., leg). If more than one daily injection is required, authorities suggest using different locations such as the abdomen for the morning injection and the leg for the evening injection.

Younger children and adolescents sometimes settle on a favorite spot and inject there to the exclusion of other sites. Repeated injections of insulin can cause the local tissue to form a hard, egg-shaped area of hypertrophied subcutaneous fat, known as lipohypertrophy (a form of lipodystrophy). Overused areas are usually anesthetized because of scar tissue and fatty deposits, which lessens the already negligible pain of injection and reinforces their use. Patients with hypertrophied areas must be cautioned to use other sites since the growths do not allow proper insulin absorption and disrupt control of blood glucose.[4] Eventually, the growth may recede until it is flush with surrounding skin.

When insulins were less purified, patients who failed to rotate also developed another form of lipodystrophy known as lipoatrophy. The lipid layer of skin atrophied, appearing dimpled. This complication has become rare with increasing use of purified animal and human insulins.[19]

Insulin Degradation

Pharmacists should caution patients to never use insulin that has passed its expiration date. Further, each vial should be inspected before each injection. Regular insulin should always be clear, without any visible particles or sediment. Any vial of Regular not appearing crystal clear must be discarded. Modified insulins should appear evenly cloudy after gently rolling the vial between the hands.[20] Occasionally, the insulin may not resuspend, with large clumps at the bottom or suspended (Fig. 46.6). Also, the inside of the vial may appear frosted because of precipitation of insulin around the inner walls of the vial. In both of these cases, the vial must not be used, as the insulin will have lost full activity.[14]

Insulin Storage

Patients should keep all unused vials of insulin in the refrigerator, but not allow them to freeze. The vial(s) currently in use should be refrigerated whenever possible. When out of the refrigerator, insulin should be kept below 86°F and away from heat and light. Patients must not leave insulin in the car on hot days, since high temperatures can degrade the molecules.[14]

If necessary, patients can carry insulin in specially designed containers to keep the temperature acceptable. One such device is the Medicool, an insulated carrying case with a two-vial plastic cooler that is chilled in the refrigerator prior to travel. Medicool can keep insulin cool for 16 hours or more on warm days. Conversely, keeping the plastic cooler

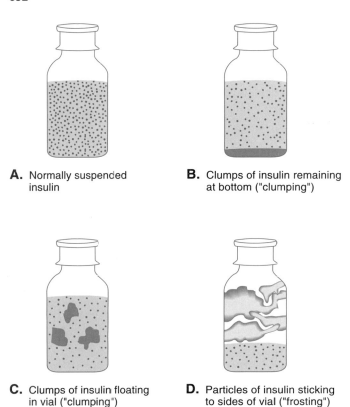

A. Normally suspended insulin

B. Clumps of insulin remaining at bottom ("clumping")

C. Clumps of insulin floating in vial ("clumping")

D. Particles of insulin sticking to sides of vial ("frosting")

Figure 46.6. Insulin should not be used unless it is **(A)** normally suspended. Insulins that cannot be completely suspended because of **(B)** clumps at the bottom of the vial, **(C)** suspended clumps, or **(D)** particles sticking to the inside of the vial must not be used.

at room temperature would help prevent freezing when the outside temperatures drop.

OTHER ASPECTS OF TREATMENT OF IDDM (TYPE 1)

The diabetic must manipulate insulin, diet, and exercise to ensure that the blood glucose remains precisely within well-defined limits. If insulin, diet, and/or exercise are not controlled well, the blood glucose may fall to unacceptable levels (hypoglycemia) or rise to dangerous levels (hyperglycemia). See Patient Assessment Algorithm 46.1.

Hypoglycemia

Hypoglycemia is a deadly consequence of diabetes. Should it continue for a sufficient duration, permanent central nervous system (CNS) damage or death may result.[25] Generally, the blood glucose should not drop below 80 mg/dL in adults and 100 mg/dL in children 5 years of age and under.[4] Blood glucose values below 55 mg/dL can result in brain dysfunction, impaired neurologic function, and compromised cognitive performance. All patients with diabetes should carry identifying materials such as wallet cards, bracelets, or necklaces that inform others of the medical condition and that advise about glucose administration if the patient is acting strangely or about calling for emergency care if the patient is unconscious.

Causes of Hypoglycemia. Hypoglycemia can be caused by failing to eat when scheduled, eating insufficient food, engaging in excessive exercise or unusual activities, or administration of excess insulin. Excessive ingestion of alcohol,

Patient Assessment Algorithm 46.1. The Diabetic Patient and Blood Glucose Extremes

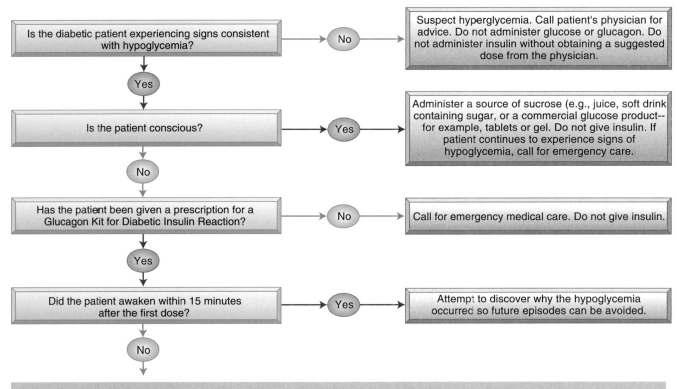

Is the diabetic patient experiencing signs consistent with hypoglycemia? — **No** → Suspect hyperglycemia. Call patient's physician for advice. Do not administer glucose or glucagon. Do not administer insulin without obtaining a suggested dose from the physician.

Yes ↓

Is the patient conscious? — **Yes** → Administer a source of sucrose (e.g., juice, soft drink containing sugar, or a commercial glucose product-- for example, tablets or gel. Do not give insulin. If patient continues to experience signs of hypoglycemia, call for emergency care.

No ↓

Has the patient been given a prescription for a Glucagon Kit for Diabetic Insulin Reaction? — **No** → Call for emergency medical care. Do not give insulin.

Yes ↓

Did the patient awaken within 15 minutes after the first dose? — **Yes** → Attempt to discover why the hypoglycemia occurred so future episodes can be avoided.

No ↓

Call for emergency care. Another dose of glucagon may be given while the patient is awaiting transport. Do not give insulin.

which reduces endogenous glucose production, can also result in hypoglycemia.[46]

Symptoms of Hypoglycemia.   Onset of hypoglycemic symptoms is usually sudden.[20] Symptoms of hypoglycemia can be subdivided into two categories (Fig. 46.7), the neurogenic (autonomic) and neuroglycopenic[46]:

- Neurogenic symptoms of hypoglycemia are caused by autonomic discharge, either adrengergic or cholinergic. **(tip)** *Neurogenic symptoms of hypoglycemia include headache, paresthesias, shaking, anxiety, sweating, palpitations, tachycardia, pallor, and hunger. Also, the skin may appear pale and moist.*
- Neuroglycopenic symptoms occur as the CNS becomes **(tip)** progressively more starved for glucose. *Neuroglycopenic symptoms of hypoglycemia include lack of coordination, difficulty concentrating, weakness, warmth, slurred speech, blurred vision, faintness, confusion, dizziness, disorientation, sleepiness, irritability, and irrational behaviors and can culminate in seizures, coma, and death.[4,46]*

⚠ *Treatment of Hypoglycemia.* **Hypoglycemia is an emergency situation requiring immediate correction.** Emergency medical technicians (EMTs) should be

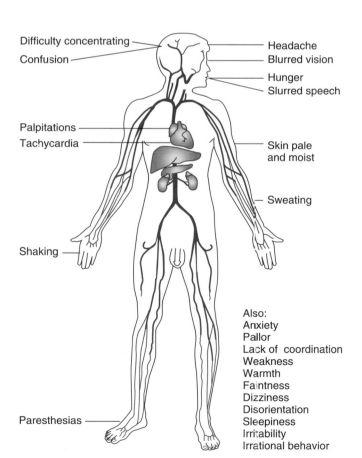

Figure 46.7. Manifestations of hypoglycemia.

Difficulty concentrating
Confusion
Palpitations
Tachycardia
Shaking
Paresthesias

Headache
Blurred vision
Hunger
Slurred speech
Skin pale and moist
Sweating

Also:
Anxiety
Pallor
Lack of coordination
Weakness
Warmth
Faintness
Dizziness
Disorientation
Sleepiness
Irritability
Irrational behavior

called immediately if a patient is unconscious because the CNS may not recover if hypoglycemia is prolonged.

Glucose is mandatory for the treatment of hypoglycemia. A conscious patient should be given a rapidly absorbed source of glucose such as table sugar or sucrose (four cubes), sweetened fruit juice or carbonated beverage (6 ounces), honey (1 to 2 tablespoons), or any of the other commercially available glucose sources. If a patient fails to resume normal mental status within a few minutes, EMTs should be called.

The typical pharmacy stocks several different forms of glucose (Table 46.6). Occasionally, a patient will enter the pharmacy in the rigors of hypoglycemia. Confusion arising **⚠** from the condition may hamper communication. *If the pharmacist suspects hypoglycemia, it is prudent to remove the product from the package for the patient and to offer any aid needed in ingesting tablets or ejecting gel into their oral cavity.* Restitution for the products should take a backseat to remedying hypoglycemia.

Some physicians will supply diabetic patients with a prescription for a Glucagon Kit for Diabetic Insulin Reaction. (Glucagon facilitates the release of glucose, which is stored as glycogen in the liver, raising the blood glucose.) When the product is dispensed, pharmacists must point out the method of use and suggest that the patient and all family members and coworkers become familiar with the product before it is needed.[14] The kit can be confusing to use because it contains a lyophilized vial of glucagon and a syringe containing sterile diluent. If the user is not entirely familiar with the product, the syringe could be injected without diluting the glucagon. In that case, the diluent would not affect blood glucose at all, and the patient would continue to be hypoglycemic. Patients (and others who might administer the medication) must be instructed to follow these steps:

1. Inject the syringe contents into the vial of glucagon, shaking the vial gently until the glucagon is entirely dissolved (Fig. 46.8).
2. Use the syringe to withdraw the glucagon.
3. Inject the glucagon into the buttock, arm, or thigh.

If the patient awakens, s/he must be given a glucose source. If the patient fails to awaken after 15 minutes, another dose may be given, but a physician should be called also to prepare for emergency transport to a hospital emergency room.

Hyperglycemia

A fasting blood glucose generally should not exceed 120 mg/dL; at other times, the blood glucose should not exceed 140 mg/dL.[4,18] Should an insulin dose be insufficient or forgotten, blood glucose will rise, causing hyperglycemia. **(tip)** *Symptoms of hyperglycemia include flushed and dry skin, drowsiness, fatigue, weakness, deep and labored breathing, vomiting, dry tongue, thirst, and abdominal pain (Fig. 46.9).[20] Ketones appear in the breath, causing a fruity, chemical smell.* These symptoms appear gradually in response to slowly rising blood glucose. Sustained hyperglycemia proceeds to diabetic ketoacidosis (DKA) if not properly treated.[4]

Table 46.6. Representative Products for Hypoglycemia Treatment

PRODUCT	COMMENTS
BD Glucose Tablets	Orange-flavored chewable tablets containing 5 g of glucose each; the patient may take 2 to 3 tablets as the usual dose; more or less may be needed depending on the severity of the reaction
Dex 4 Glucose Tablets	Grape, raspberry, orange, or lemon chewable tablets containing 4 g of glucose each
Glutose Liquid	A tube containing 25 g of lemon-flavored glucose
Glutose Tablets	Lemon-flavored chewable tablet containing 5 g of glucose each
Monojel Insulin Reaction Gel	Foil packet containing 25 g of glucose

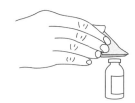

A. Swab top of glucagon vial

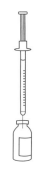

B. Inject contents of syringe

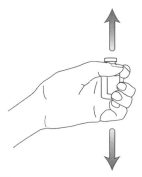

C. Shake bottle gently

Figure 46.8. When preparing glucagon for injection, the patient must remove the syringe containing diluent from the Glucagon Kit for Diabetic Insulin Reaction and then (**A**) swab the top of the vial containing unreconstituted glucagon, (**B**) add the diluent in the syringe to the glucagon vial, and (**C**) agitate the vial. The patient then withdraws the reconstituted glucagon from the vial and injects it as directed.

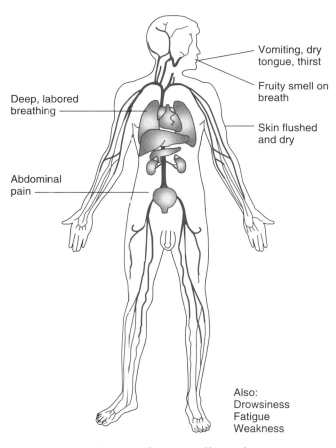

Vomiting, dry tongue, thirst

Fruity smell on breath

Deep, labored breathing

Skin flushed and dry

Abdominal pain

Also:
Drowsiness
Fatigue
Weakness

Figure 46.9. Manifestations of hyperglycemia.

Blood Glucose Monitoring

Glucose monitoring is an essential element of IDDM treatment. Patients with IDDM must continually balance insulin, exercise, and diet, and to do so properly they must know their blood glucose levels. Until the late 1970s, patients had to use urine glucose strips or tablets to monitor the control of diabetes.[c] These products (e.g., Clinitest, Diastix, and Clinistix), which were relatively poor reflections of blood glucose, have been replaced by self-monitoring blood glucose (SMBG) products. To perform blood glucose testing, patients lance a finger, place a drop of blood on a test strip, then either read a color change or insert the strip into a blood glucose meter.

Advantages and Disadvantages of Blood Glucose Testing (SMBG). SMBG is quick and accurate and can be performed almost anywhere since patients do not need to obtain a urine sample.[47] Although patients may have to draw blood samples as many as five times or more a day, this disadvantage is outweighed by the quality of information obtained.[9] With SMBG, patients can discover at any time how successful their treatment is by detecting hypoglycemia and hyperglycemia more rapidly than with urine tests.[47] Because of the many advantages of SMBG, as many as 55% of diabetics use this monitoring technique.

Blood Glucose Meters. The patient using SMBG first removes blood using any one of several lancet devices available (e.g., Auto Lancet, Glucolet, Penlet, Penlet II, Softclix, and Soft Touch). Some blood glucose test strips can be read visually without need for a meter, but the majority of patients opt to use test strips that are read by a blood glucose meter, because they are more accurate (Table 46.7). Although blood glucose meters are not difficult to use, they must be used correctly to yield reliable results that accurately identify the amount of glucose in the blood. In addition, blood glucose meters must be cleaned properly.[47] *Patients should be cautioned to keep the instruction manual provided*

with the monitor and to follow all of the manufacturer recommendations in it.

Blood glucose monitors are a dynamic market. Manufacturers introduce improved models constantly, attempting to make each new version more consumer-friendly. While this is laudable from the patient's point of view, it renders published information on blood glucose meters outdated soon after it is printed. Therefore, blood glucose monitor product summaries often include one or more obsolete models. Pharmacists should obtain the models currently on the shelf and use sample products and package inserts to become fully familiar with them. *Patients must be cautioned to purchase only the test strips recommended for the specific meter.*

Glycosylated Hemoglobin
Measurement of **glycosylated hemoglobin (HbA$_{1c}$)** (hemoglobin that has been altered by exposure to excess glucose, through a process known as nonenzymatic glycosylation) at least every 3 to 6 months allows physicians to obtain an estimate of patients' glucose control over the preceding 2 to 3 months.[9] HbA$_{1c}$ correlates with the likelihood of microvascular complications. Normal individuals should have a value of 4 to 6%; the goal for diabetics is less than 7%.[14] This procedure is carried out by a laboratory; however, the pharmacist should be able to interpret HbA$_{1c}$ values.

Urine Ketone Monitoring
Urine ketone testing is helpful when patients are ill, or when blood glucose values exceed 250 mg/dL.[4] The presence of

Table 46.7. Representative Blood Glucose Monitors

PRODUCT	COMMENTS
Boehringer Mannheim Accu-Chek Advantage	No cleaning required; 100-value memory; no wiping of test strips; 40 second results
Boehringer Mannheim Accu-Chek Easy	350-value memory; allows code markers such as "before exercise, after a meal," etc.; 15-second results
Boehringer Mannheim Accu-Chek Instant	12-second results
Boehringer Mannheim Accu-Chek III	20-value memory
ExacTech RSG Sensor	No calibration required
Glucometer Elite	20-value memory; 30-second results
Glucometer Encore	10-value memory; 15- to 60-second readings
LifeScan One Touch Profile	250-value memory; 45-second results; records up to 15 different activities along with blood glucose readings; averages results over 14 or 30 seconds; averages results by time of day or activity
LifeScan SureStep	10-value memory; provides extra assistance for the patient who wishes to be sure that he or she is testing correctly; 15-second results
LifeScan One Touch Basic	Records previous test result only; 45-second results
Precision QID System	Does not require cleaning; no optical window to be affected by dried blood, dirt, humidity, light

ketones (e.g., acetone, acetoacetic acid, and beta-hydroxy-butyric acid) in the urine indicates that the body has attempted to break down stored body fat to use as a fuel source.[20] Patients with ketones in the urine may require an upward adjustment in the dose of insulin to allow glucose to be used as the preferred fuel. The pharmacist sells products such as Ketostix for urine ketone monitoring.

Nonpharmacologic Therapies

Insulin is considered to be the cornerstone of type 1 diabetes mellitus treatment, but diet and exercise must also be in harmony to maintain normal blood glucose levels.[4]

DIET

The diabetic diet for the type 1 patient, which strictly controls all nutrients, is characteristically low in cholesterol, saturated fat, and sucrose and high in fiber.[4,9] An acceptable ratio is 30% fat, 55 to 60% carbohydrate, and 10 to 15% protein, with up to 40 g of fiber daily and with sodium levels not exceeding 3 g daily.[22,48,49] (The ADA has developed one of the most well-accepted diets.[50]) Diets for type 1 diabetics should be carefully planned by a nutritionist working with the patient's physician, with several goals in mind[22,51]:

- Maintain normal growth and weight
- Prevent obesity
- Prevent the patient from becoming hyperglycemic or hypoglycemic
- Prevent hyperlipidemia
- Control blood pressure
- Prevent future complications of diabetes (e.g., renal failure, cardiac complications, amputation, visual loss)

Should patients deviate from their diet, either hypoglycemia or hyperglycemia could result. Unfortunately, many patients deviate from the recommendations.[52,53]

Two dietary products available in pharmacies may help reduce the occurrence of nocturnal hypoglycemia associated with IDDM. Investigators have discovered that uncooked cornstarch provides a slow, steady absorption of carbohydrate lasting up to 9 hours. A product known as Zbar, a nonprescription medical food containing 5 g of uncooked cornstarch in combination with other ingredients, can prevent hypoglycemia without producing hyperglycemia.[54] NiteBite, a similar product, contains sucrose, protein, and uncooked cornstarch.[55]

EXERCISE

Exercise is not a major component of control of type 1 diabetes but aids in the development of cardiovascular fitness.[4] Furthermore, pharmacists might remind patients that because exercise can lower the need for insulin, they might need to ingest a preexercise light snack to prevent hypoglycemia.

PREVENTION OF IDDM (TYPE 1)

Before preventive steps can be instituted, individuals who are genetically predisposed for the development of IDDM must be identified. Patient identification can be accomplished by administering such examinations as islet cell antibodies and insulin autoantibodies to high-risk individuals (such as first-degree family members of IDDM patients).[56]

Once high-risk individuals are identified, measures to delay the onset of IDDM can be instituted such as administration of immune system suppressants (e.g., glucocorticoids, azathioprine, and cyclosporine).[3] Administering insulin to these at-risk patients also can help prevent IDDM perhaps by immunizing patients against insulin or allowing beta-islet cells to rest.

NON–INSULIN-DEPENDENT DIABETES MELLITUS (NIDDM) (TYPE 2)

Non–insulin-dependent diabetes mellitus (NIDDM), also known as type 2 diabetes mellitus, is dramatically different in many ways from type 1 diabetes. Both conditions share some clinical features such as hyperglycemia in the fasting and/or postprandial states, but the epidemiology, etiology, complications, prognoses, and treatments vary.[2] For instance, type 1 diabetes is incurable, but type 2 may disappear with diet and exercise. Also, type 1 diabetes usually manifests in childhood without regard to body weight, while type 2 usually manifests in the older, obese patient.

Certain features of therapy such as strict attention to diet and exercise are also common to both conditions. While insulin administration is mandatory for IDDM diabetes, it is merely a therapeutic option for NIDDM.

PREVALENCE OF NIDDM (TYPE 2)

NIDDM is the most common metabolic disorder.[2] Because NIDDM is related to age (see below) the prevalence is increasing steadily as the population ages. At least 10 to 13 million United States citizens suffer from type 2 diabetes mellitus (about 6 to 7% of the population).[2,3,57]

EPIDEMIOLOGY OF NIDDM (TYPE 2)

NIDDM has several strong epidemiologic subdivisions, including genetics, race, age, and body weight.

Genetics

A strong family history of NIDDM is predictive, in most cases revealing a strong genetic link.[2,58] Monozygotic twins have a 50 to 95% concordance rate for the condition. The risk of developing NIDDM is 10 times greater than the general population for monozygotic twins, 3.5 times greater for first-degree relatives, and 1.5 times greater for second-degree relatives of NIDDM patients.[2]

Race/Nationality

Certain racial/national groups are at extremely high risk of NIDDM, including Native Americans (such as the Pima Indians of Arizona), blacks, and Hispanics.[2,14] The prevalence in blacks is 10.2%, as compared with only 6.6% for whites.[1,59]

Age

Type 2 diabetes mellitus is strongly associated with increasing age, with an onset usually in the third or fourth decade of life.[60] Almost 15% of those over 65 suffer from NIDDM.[57,61]

Body Weight

Body weight is a strong predictor for the development of type 2 diabetes mellitus.[59] At least 80% of patients with type 2 diabetes weigh at least 20% more than their ideal body weight; most have been overweight for many years.[62] The cause of this association is unknown, although several mechanisms have been proposed. (See "Etiology.")

Other Factors

Type 2 diabetes mellitus is more likely to develop in patients who developed gestational diabetes or gave birth to a baby weighing over 9 pounds.[14]

ETIOLOGY OF NIDDM (TYPE 2)

Prior to the development of clinical symptoms, patients with type 2 diabetes typically follow a predictable pattern of pathogenesis:

1. Weight gain, especially in the abdomen
2. Decreased activity
3. **Hyperinsulinemia** (increased serum insulin levels)
4. Insulin resistance

Insulin resistance occurs when peripheral tissues lose the ability to respond to insulin. At some point, beta-pancreatic cells become incapable of compensating for the insulin resistance by raising the amount of endogenous insulin they are able to produce (Fig. 46.10).[2,57]

Insulin resistance is the primary defect of NIDDM that results in hyperglycemia. However, patients also usually experience a cluster of metabolic abnormalities such as elevations in triglycerides and lowered HDL cholesterol. This pernicious syndrome has been termed "Syndrome X."[60]

MANIFESTATIONS OF NIDDM (TYPE 2)

Generally, the manifestations of type 2 diabetes mirror those of type 1 diabetes, although they develop more slowly. For instance, the initial sign of the condition may be a need to urinate more frequently at night.[62] The patient may also notice paresthesias of the extremities, dermatologic or generalized pruritus, and recurrent gingival, skin, vaginal, and/or bladder infections.

PROGNOSIS OF NIDDM (TYPE 2)

NIDDM can be placed in remission if the patient achieves normal body weight. However, many cannot do so. The mortality rate for patients with type 2 diabetes is two to three times higher than that for age-matched patients without the

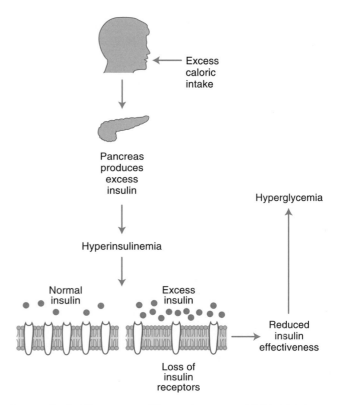

Figure 46.10. The genesis of hyperglycemia in NIDDM: The patient ingests excess calories, which causes the pancreas to produce excess insulin. Hyperinsulinemia causes loss of insulin receptors, reducing insulin effectiveness; reduced insulin effectiveness leads to hyperglycemia.

condition.[60] The primary cause of death is cardiovascular; heart disorders claim 50% of type 2 diabetics.

COMPLICATIONS OF NIDDM (TYPE 2)

Although the Diabetes Control and Complications Trial dealt with type 1 diabetes, the determination that excellent glycemic control may help prevent complications also applies to type 2 diabetes.[1,63] (See "Complications of IDDM [Type 1].") Even moderate hyperglycemia can produce long-term complications (e.g., neuropathy, nephropathy, retinopathy, and atherosclerotic disease) if it persists for sustained periods. The risks of hypertension, end-stage renal disease, lower extremity amputation, disability, and retinopathy are higher in blacks than whites.[1] At least 70% of patients suffer from neuropathy.[60]

TREATMENT OF NIDDM (TYPE 2)

Treatment Guidelines

Treatment of type 2 diabetes begins with control of diet and weight reduction. These steps reduce the problem of insulin resistance in most patients.[57,62] Indeed, many motivated NIDDM patients can be treated by diet alone, if it leads to weight loss.[60]

Oral prescription medications are typically considered as the next step in NIDDM therapy, especially with patients resistant to weight loss.[12,57] However, oral antidiabetics (e.g., sulfonylureas) do not alleviate the need to lose weight and may increase the risk of cardiovascular disease.[60] Also, patients who have attempted weight loss without success may find that oral antidiabetics are unsuccessful in controlling blood glucose. At this point in NIDDM treatment, insulin may be instituted, either alone or in conjunction with oral antidiabetics.

Nonprescription Medications

Approximately 40% of type 2 diabetics use insulin.[14] The particular regimen is variable, depending on the blood glucose. Generally, doses are somewhat lower than those used to control type 1 diabetes. See "Insulin" for a full discussion of this nonprescription medication.

Nonpharmacologic Therapies

The cornerstones of treatment for type 2 patients are therapies aimed at reduction of caloric intake and increased physical activity resulting in weight loss.[64] Since long-entrenched dietary habits and lifestyle issues are almost impossible for many patients to alter, various oral antidiabetic agents (beyond the scope of this chapter) may be prescribed.

PREVENTION OF NIDDM (TYPE 2)

Prevention of NIDDM consists of ingesting no more than a normal diet, which allows the individual to maintain a normal body weight.

SUMMARY

Diabetes mellitus is a broad term that encompasses several medical conditions. This chapter focuses on the two most common types, which are known as IDDM (type 1) and NIDDM (type 2) varieties.

Type 1 diabetes is a serious medical condition caused by a juxtaposition of genetic and environmental factors. Insulin is a vital part of therapy for type 1 diabetes; diet control and exercise are also therapeutic. Whichever method is used, the current trend is to control blood glucose so tightly that blood glucose remains within normal limits at all times. This technique can prevent many of the complications of diabetes.

Type 2 diabetes is caused by a combination of hyperinsulinemia and receptor changes on cell surfaces. Therapy begins with weight loss and exercise, but noncompliant patients may be placed on oral medications. Continued lack of compliance may necessitate eventual addition of insulin to the regimen.

Insulin may be administered with syringes, or through such innovative methods as insulin pens, jet injectors, or subcutaneous insulin pumps. When patients purchase insulin and associated products, pharmacists must be prepared to counsel on the use of syringe and injection devices. Pharmacists also should be prepared to discuss insulin mixing, injection site rotation, insulin storage, and related issues.

Pharmacists may assist diabetic patients by providing advice on use of insulin, its delivery devices, and devices for monitoring blood glucose. In addition, pharmacists may help diabetic patients understand the nature of diabetes, its complications, and other treatment aspects.

AT THE COUNTER

 A man about 55 to 60 asks the pharmacist for syringes.

Interview/Patient Assessment

The patient is a newly diagnosed type 2 diabetic who has been told to inject 20 units of Humulin N. He has never used a syringe before. He asks, "Can I use the syringes my wife uses for allergy shots?"

Pharmacist's Analysis

1. Are there dangers to the use of allergy syringes for U-100 insulin?
2. What size syringe should this patient be sold?
3. What ancillary instructions should he be given?

As a newly diagnosed diabetic, this patient requires considerable counseling from a number of health-care providers to competently use his insulin.

Patient Counseling

The patient should be cautioned not to use allergy syringes for insulin because allergy syringes are not calibrated in terms of units of insulin. The pharmacist should caution that insulin has a narrow therapeutic index with little margin for error, necessitating the use of syringes specifically designed for insulin injections.

For the sake of accuracy in measuring the dose, the patient should be sold syringes with a maximum capacity of 25 or 30 units. He should be shown how to disinfect the skin with alcohol swabs, given instructions for withdrawal from a vial of insulin, and instructed in the proper disposal of insulin syringes using either a clipping device or a home sharps container.

References

1. Ziemer DC, et al. Diabetes in urban black-Americans. III. Management of type II diabetes in a municipal hospital setting. Am J Med 101:25, 1996.
2. Kahn CR, Vincent D, Alessandro D. Genetics of non–insulin-dependent (type II) diabetes mellitus. Annu Rev Med 47:509, 1996.
3. Hoekelman RA. Juvenile diabetes: Prevention, control, and cure. Pediatr Ann 23:278, 1994.
4. Betschart J. Children and adolescents with diabetes. Nurs Clin North Am 28:35, 1993.
5. Maclaren N, Atkinson M. Is insulin-dependent diabetes mellitus environmentally induced? (Editorial). N Engl J Med 327:348, 1992.
6. Kelly HA, et al. Dramatic increase in incidence of insulin dependent diabetes mellitus in Western Australia. Med J Aust 161:426, 1994.
7. Maclaren N, et al. Early diagnosis and specific treatment of insulin-dependent diabetes. Ann NY Acad Sci 696:342, 1993.
8. Fohlman J, Friman G. Is juvenile diabetes a viral disease? Ann Med 25:569, 1993.
9. Lamb WH. Childhood diabetes. Br J Hosp Med 51:471, 1994.
10. Pray WS. Helping the type I diabetes patient. US Pharmacist 20(11):22, 1995.
11. Wiener K. The diagnosis of diabetes mellitus, including gestational diabetes. Ann Clin Biochem 29(Pt 5):481, 1992.
12. The Diabetes Control and Complications Trial Research Group. The effect of intensive treatment of diabetes on the development and progression of long-term complications in insulin-dependent diabetes mellitus. N Engl J Med 329:977, 1993.
13. Woollons S. Insulin pens for the management of diabetes. Prof Nurse 11:241, 1996.
14. Anderson RM, et al. Managing Your Diabetes. Indianapolis: Eli Lilly, 1994.
15. Nathan DM. Management of insulin-dependent diabetes mellitus. Drugs 44(Suppl 3):39, 1992.
16. Chin RL, Martinez R, Garmel G. Gas gangrene from subcutaneous insulin administration. Am J Emerg Med 11:622, 1993.
17. Shenaq SM, Klebuc MJA, Vargo D. How to help diabetic patients avoid amputation. Postgrad Med 96:177, 1994.
18. Anon. New standards of medical care for diabetes are issued by the American Diabetes Association (Editorial). Am Fam Physician 50:1134, 1994.
19. Hirsch IB, Farkas-Hirsch R. Type I diabetes and insulin therapy. Nurs Clin North Am 28:9, 1993.
20. Campbell RK. Diabetes and the Pharmacist. 2nd ed. Elkhart, IN: Ames Division, Miles Laboratories, 1986.
21. Galloway JA, Potvin JH, Shuman CR, eds. Diabetes Mellitus. 9th ed. Indianapolis: Eli Lilly, 1988.
22. Thom SL. Nutritional management of diabetes. Nurs Clin North Am 28:97, 1993.
23. Cooper AJ. Attempted suicide using insulin by a non diabetic: A case study demonstrating the acute and chronic consequences of prolonged hypoglycemia. Can J Psychiatry 39:103, 1994.
24. Fasching P, et al. Estimated glucose requirement following massive insulin overdose in a patient with type I diabetes. Diabetic Med 11:323, 1994.
25. Rosenbloom AL. Diabetes in childhood and adolescence. Pediatr Ann 23:282, 1994.
26. Grammer LC. Allergic reactions to insulin. Pharm Times 58(10):49, 1992.
27. Davidson JA, Ramirez LC, Selam JL. Transfer of patients with diabetes from semisynthetic human insulin to human insulin prepared by recombinant DNA technology using baker's yeast: A double-blind, randomized study. Clin Ther 13:557, 1991.
28. Campbell RK. The clinical use of insulin. US Pharmacist Diabetes Suppl 17(10):29, 1992.
29. Jehle PM, et al. The human insulin analog lispro improves insulin binding on circulating monocytes of intensively treated insulin-dependent diabetes mellitus patients. J Clin Endocrinol Metab 81:2319, 1996.
30. Anon. Humalog launch will be supported by direct mail and magazine promotions. Weekly Pharm Reports 45(27):2, 1996.
31. Anon. Mixing Insulins. Franklin Lakes, NJ: Becton Dickinson, 1995.
32. Newman KD, Weaver MT. Insulin measurement and preparation among diabetic patients at a county hospital. Nurse Pract 19:44, 1994.
33. Bell DS, et al. Dosage accuracy of self-mixed vs premixed insulin. Arch Intern Med 151:265, 1991.
34. Trade Package, Humalog: 1998.
35. Pray WS. Proper use of insulin syringes. US Pharmacist 18(12):76, 1993.
36. Cohen MR. Error 504: Insulin syringes are for measuring insulin. Hospital Pharmacy 28:1130, 1993.
37. Casella SJ, et al. Accuracy and precision of low-dose insulin administration. Pediatrics 91:1155, 1993.
38. Peragallo-Dittko V. Aspiration of the subcutaneous insulin injection: Clinical evaluation of needle size and amount of subcutaneous fat. Diabetes Educ 21:291, 1995.
39. Anon. Drawing and Injecting Insulin. Franklin Lakes, NJ: Becton Dickinson, 1993.
40. Turnberg WL, Lowen LD. Home syringe disposal: Practice and policy in Washington state. Diabetes Educ 20:489, 1994.
41. Ancona KG, et al. Insulin syringe disposal practices of pediatric patients with insulin-dependent diabetes mellitus. Clin Pediatr 33:232, 1994.
42. O'Hagan M, Greene SA. Pre-mixed insulin delivered by disposable pen in the management of children with diabetes. Diabetic Med 10:972, 1993.
43. Plevin S, Sadur C. Use of a prefilled insulin syringe (Novolin Prefilled) by patients with diabetes. Clin Ther 15:423, 1993.
44. Mueller-Schoop J. Accidental intravenous self-injection with insulin pen. Lancet 341:894, 1993.
45. Saudek CD. Future developments in insulin delivery systems. Diabetes Care 16(Suppl 3):122, 1993.
46. Cryer PE. Hypoglycemic unawareness in IDDM. Diabetes Care 16(Suppl 3):40, 1993.
47. Fleming DR. Accuracy of blood glucose monitoring for patients: What it is and how to achieve it. Diabetes Educ 20:495, 1994.
48. Mandel ED. The diabetic diet: A model for Americans. NJ Med 91:246, 1994.
49. Nuttall FQ. Carbohydrate and dietary management of individuals with insulin-requiring diabetes. Diabetes Care 16:1039, 1993.
50. Arnold MS, et al. Guidelines vs practice in the delivery of diabetes nutrition care. J Am Diet Assoc 93:34, 1993.
51. Thomas-Dobersen DA, Butler-Simon N, Fleshner M. Evaluation of a weight measurement intervention program in adoles-

cents with insulin-dependent diabetes mellitus. J Am Diet Assoc 93:535, 1993.

52. Humphreys M, et al. Are the nutritional recommendations for insulin-dependent diabetic patients being achieved? Diabetic Med 11:79, 1994.

53. Loghmani E, Rickard KA. Alternative snack system for children and teenagers with diabetes mellitus. J Am Diet Assoc 94:1145, 1994.

54. McCann B. Another medical food to be sold exclusively in drugstores. Drug Topics 140(13):87, 1996.

55. Snyder K. NiteBite designed to reduce nocturnal hypoglycemia. Drug Topics 140(18):65, 1996.

56. Robertson RP, Klein DJ. Treatment of diabetes mellitus. Diabetologica 35(Suppl 2):S8, 1992.

57. Surwit RS, Schneider MS. Role of stress in the etiology and treatment of diabetes mellitus. Psychosom Med 55:380, 1993.

58. Cook JTE, et al. Availability of type II diabetic families for detection of diabetes susceptibility genes. Diabetes 42:1536, 1993.

59. Shaten BJ, et al. Risk factors for the development of type II diabetes among men enrolled in the usual care group of the multiple risk factor intervention trial. Diabetes Care 16:1331, 1993.

60. Sinsel-Phillips P. Syndrome X. Nurse Pract 21:66, 1996.

61. Berger M, Jorgens V, Flatten G. Health care for persons with non–insulin-dependent diabetes mellitus. Ann Intern Med 124(1 Pt 2):153, 1996.

62. Randal J. Insulin key to diabetes but not full cure. FDA Consumer 26(4):15, 1992.

63. Wolffenbuttel BHR, Graal MB. New treatments for patients with type 2 diabetes mellitus. Postgrad Med J 72:657, 1996.

64. Lubbos H, Miller JL, Rose LI. Oral hypoglycemic agents in type II diabetes mellitus. Am Fam Physician 52:2075, 1995.

Dietary Inadequacy

Optimal nutrition throughout life is mandatory to maintain good health.[1] While proper nutrition must be maintained throughout life, it is especially critical in children, whose growth requires adequate levels of all nutrients. During the developmental years, dietary inadequacy can cause irreversible damage such as abnormal neurologic development.

Humans require many substances to achieve optimal nutrition, including macronutrients (such as, fat, carbohydrates, and protein), water, electrolytes, and various micronutrients (e.g., vitamins, minerals, trace elements, and ultratrace elements).[2] Improper nutrition can result in the development of one or more deficiency diseases such as beri-beri, scurvy, rickets, and pellagra. To prevent deficiency diseases, nutritionists and dietitians recommend a healthy diet with proper balance from all food groups (Fig. 47.1).

Dietary inadequacy can range from deficiency of a specific nutrient to overall malnutrition. Overall malnutrition involves protein and calories, as well as various micronutrient deficiencies.

A complete discussion of nutrition and nutritional deficiencies is beyond the scope of this chapter. Pharmacists should refer patients who require sophisticated nutritional information to a physician or a dietitian for advice. Pharmacists do field numerous questions about vitamins, minerals, and liquid nutritional products. Therefore, these products will be discussed in some detail.

Another type of nutritional supplement is the infant formula. Pharmacists do not often counsel patients about these products, since the infant's pediatrician makes the product recommendation. (See "Infant Formulas.")

PREVALENCE OF DIETARY INADEQUACY

Several factors influence dietary status, including the following:

- Standard of living
- Government assistance programs
- Addition of vitamins and minerals to certain foods

Because these factors vary so dramatically from country to country the prevalence of dietary inadequacy varies widely. In the United States general dietary inadequacies are uncommon in patients who are otherwise healthy because the standard of living is high, government assistance is widespread, and many foods are enriched.[1] Nevertheless, deficiencies of specific nutrients continue to be prevalent (e.g., calcium, iron, and folate in females, especially women of child-bearing age).

EPIDEMIOLOGY OF DIETARY INADEQUACY

Dietary inadequacy is a common phenomenon. Most United States citizens ingest inadequate fiber and water, for example. They also eat too few fruits and vegetables (while ingesting too much meat, sweetened snacks, and salty products such as corn chips). Most of these examples of dietary inadequacy do not present long-term problems. However, if the diet is sufficiently imbalanced, malnutrition can result.

Malnutrition affects several population subgroups, including the following:

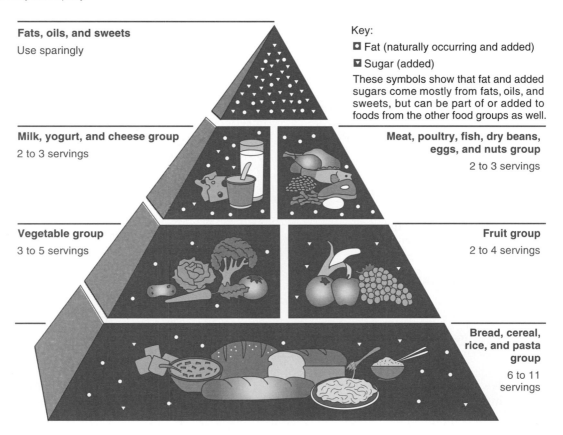

Figure 47.1. Food-guide pyramid developed by U.S. Departments of Agriculture and Health and Human Services to promote healthy diets.

- Elderly patients
- Patients with chronic illnesses (e.g., malabsorption syndromes, parenteral nutrition patients, and depressed patients)
- Patients with eating disorders (e.g., anorexia and bulimia)
- Alcoholics
- Low-income patients
- Patients who succumb to fad diets that ignore basic and sound nutritional precepts

ETIOLOGY OF DIETARY INADEQUACY

Dietary inadequacies that do not result from diseases or medications are rare, but when they occur they usually result from simple failure to follow sound nutritional guidelines. (See "Prevention of Dietary Inadequacy.") For older patients with dietary inadequacy, several factors are important in etiology:

FOCUS ON...

INFANT FORMULAS

The nutritional needs of infants differ widely, based on such variables as gestational age, birth weight, and growth rate.[3] While breast milk is considered the ideal food for infants, various problems do not allow some mothers to breast-feed (e.g., nipple abnormalities, insufficient milk production). Other mothers do not wish to breast-feed. Approximately 46% of infants ingest infant formulas as an alternative to breast-feeding.

There are many different brands of infant formulas that are useful for the infant with no special needs. Manufacturers also market products to meet specialized needs. The child's pediatrician or general practitioner provides a recommendation for formula in virtually all cases. The parent should be advised to follow this recommendation. The type of formula should not be changed without the physician's knowledge. For this reason the ability of the pharmacist to counsel patients about infant formulas is restricted, although the pharmacist may help the patient recognize lactose intolerance or cow's milk allergy.

Infant formulas must contain adequate fat; over half of the caloric content of breast milk and formulas is derived from fat. Protein is also a vital component of formula, being necessary to allow growth and development.

Carbohydrate is also a necessary component of infant formula, but if it is derived from lactose, some infants will exhibit lactose intolerance (see Chapter 9, Lactose Intolerance). For this reason lactose-free, soy-based formulas may be preferable. Formulas also contain vitamins and minerals to ensure proper development. Should the infant develop symptoms of cow's milk allergy when ingesting milk-based formulas (e.g., vomiting and diarrhea occurring within 1 hour of feeding, mucus in the stools, abdominal pain, and excessive gas), the formula should not be given again until the pediatrician is contacted. Soy-based products may also be preferable.

- Certain medications reduce appetite.[4]
- Medications that induce xerostomia make eating less efficient.
- Reduced ability to taste and smell reduces the appeal of foods.
- The ability to eat comfortably is affected by poorly fitting dentures and the associated gingival trauma, extensive dental work that may require surgery, periods of healing, and various intraoral injuries.

MANIFESTATIONS OF DIETARY INADEQUACY

Manifestations of vitamin and mineral deficiencies are described below in the discussion of specific micronutrients.

TREATMENT OF DIETARY INADEQUACY

Treatment Guidelines

Certain patients are likely to require nutritional supplementation. The prevalence of calcium, iron, and folate deficiencies in females (especially those who are periconceptual or lactating) is high, and the failure to supplement leads to well-known consequences (e.g., iron-deficiency anemia, osteoporosis, birth defects). Typically, however, patients who request a nutritional supplement have no real need for one. Exceptions are described in "Epidemiology of Dietary Inadequacy."

The only valid use for nutritional supplementation is the prevention of deficiency diseases. (There are limited exceptions such as the use of niacin to reduce cholesterol, but these require higher doses than recommended for self-care and should be coordinated by a physician). Most primary care physicians in the United States will never see an actual case of the classical vitamin deficiency diseases (e.g., scurvy, rickets, beri-beri, or pellagra).

The role of pharmacists in dietary supplementation has grown in importance since 1994 when Congress passed the Dietary Supplement Health and Education Act (DHSEA).[5] (See Patient Assessment Algorithm 47.1.) The net effect of the act was to weaken the power of the FDA over dietary supplements. The FDA now bears the full burden of proving that dietary supplements are unsafe, adulterated, falsely labeled, or misleadingly labeled. Unlike the manufacturers of prescription medications, the manufacturers of dietary supplements are not required to carry out these studies for submission to FDA prior to marketing, but may proceed to market. The DSHEA allows dietary-supplement manufacturers to make the following claims in their labeling related to diagnosis, treatment, or prevention of disease:

- The label can describe the general well-being that may be obtained from a nutrient or dietary ingredient.
- The label can describe the intended impact of a nutrient or dietary ingredient on the structure or function of part of the body in humans, characterizing the documented mechanism by which a nutrient or dietary ingredient acts to maintain such structure or function.

Patient Assessment Algorithm 47.1. Dietary Inadequacy

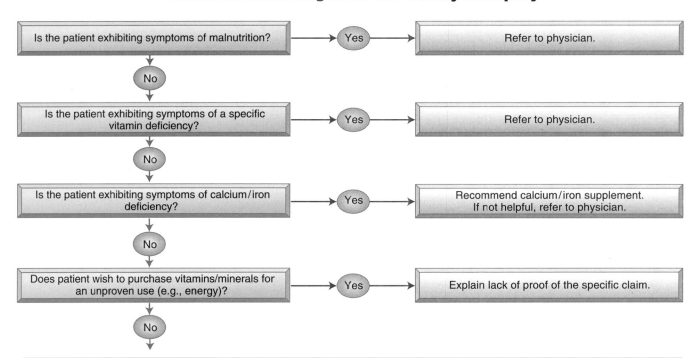

With no clear indication for the products, their use is questionable; if the patient wishes to purchase a multivitamin anyway, urge ingestion of a balanced diet and counsel the patient to take no more than one supplement tablet daily.

- The label can claim a benefit related to a classical nutrient deficiency disease, disclosing the prevalence of such disease in the United States.

The manufacturer's claims need only be backed by substantiation that they are truthful and not misleading. The packaging must also carry this warning, "This statement has not been evaluated by the Food and Drug Administration. This product is not intended to diagnose, treat, cure, or prevent any disease." *When a patient asks about a product that has this label, it is prudent for the pharmacist to tell patients the following: the role of the FDA is to sift through evidence in support of therapeutic claims and the FDA has not had an opportunity to evaluate the product they want to buy.*

Patients who request supplements should first be asked why they feel they need the supplement. Several popular answers and possible responses are as follows:

- "I just want to be sure I get everything I need." Pharmacists might explain that deficiency diseases are so rare in the United States that the risk is virtually nonexistent. Taking the vitamins as "diet insurance" is analogous to a patient who has never been diagnosed with hypertension taking an oral antihypertensive to ensure against the development of hypertension. Further, taking a medication that is not necessary could expose the patient to unneeded adverse reactions.
- "I'm not sure I'm eating well enough." Pharmacists might point out that there are many millions of people whose diets are borderline at best (such as many college students and teenagers), but they still obtain the microamounts of vitamins needed.
- "I feel better and more full of energy when I take them." Patients might be challenged to explore other factors that affect energy level such as work, sleep, and caffeine. No vitamin or mineral has ever been proven to give extra energy to patients who do not have a deficiency disease. (See "A Pharmacist's Journal: Which Vitamin Gives You Energy?")

Nonprescription Medications

LIQUID NUTRITIONALS
Liquid nutritionals are meal supplements that may be ingested with a meal or as a meal substitute.[6] Much of the advertising for these products targets older patients. Patients whose teeth are undergoing restoration or whose teeth are partially missing or totally absent suffer from impaired ability to chew food. The time required to eat may be appreciably prolonged. Also, elderly patients sometimes suffer from xerostomia caused by medications or certain medical conditions that dry the mouth, which also hampers food ingestion. An inability to cook or eat normally (e.g., depression, compromised mobility, tremor, or hemiplegia) also affects nutritional status.

Liquid nutritional products may help patients with compromised ability to cook and/or eat by providing a meal substitute in an easy-to-drink form. However, these products may prevent some patients from eating a variety of foods, as recommended for optimal health. Thus, whenever possible, patients should still strive to eat normal foods. Table 47.1 lists some lactose-free liquid nutritionals and their content.

VITAMINS
Annual vitamin sales in the United States exceed $3 billion.[7] Approximately one-third of Americans consume vitamin supplements each day.[8] Women are more likely to take vitamins than men, nonsmokers and former smokers are more likely than smokers, and light drinkers are more likely than heavy drinkers.[5] Likelihood of vitamin use also increases with age, income, and education.

The body normally carries out numerous chemical reactions that create energy and living tissues from ingested food and regulate genetic processes.[9] Vitamins—nutrients containing carbon that are required by humans in microamounts—function as enzymes or coenzymes to catalyze such chemical reactions as oxidation, reduction, group transfer, and antioxidation.[7] Inadequate microamounts needed by the body produce symptoms specific to each vitamin—the deficiency diseases. Exploration of the causes of deficiency

A Pharmacist's Journal

"Which Vitamin Gives You Energy?"

A middle-aged woman in the vitamin aisle asked me, "Which vitamin gives you energy?" I attempted to explain to her that an individual with normal vitamin status has the amount of energy they normally should, and I cautioned that extra vitamins do not provide energy but may produce toxicity. I then shared with her other causes of tiredness, including caffeine use and improper sleep habits. She listened patiently, but finally interrupted with, "Well, maybe vitamins won't give me energy, but I wasn't asking about myself. It's my dog. My poodle is tired all of the time." Of course, I advised her to have a veterinarian check the pet rather than attempting to administer human doses of vitamins.

Table 47.1. Representative Lactose-Free Liquid Nutritionals and Selected Information[a,b,c]

	BOOST	ENSURE	ENSURE PLUS	NUTRA START	RESOURCE STANDARD	RESOURCE PLUS	SUSTACAL HIGH PROTEIN FORMULA
Calories	240	250	355	210	250	355	240
Calories from fat	35	50	117	25	d	d	50
Total fat	4 g	6 g	13 g	2.5 g	8.8 g	12.6 g	6 g
Saturated fat	0.5 g	0.5 g	2 g	0.5 g	d	d	1 g
Cholesterol	5 mg	<5 mg	<5 mg	<5 mg	d	d	<5 mg
Sodium	130 mg	200 mg	250 mg	350 mg	210 mg	300 mg	220 mg
Potassium	400 mg	370 mg	460 mg	650 mg	380 mg	490 mg	d
Total carbohydrate	40 g	40 g	47 g	38 g	33.8 g	47.3 g	33 g
Dietary fiber	0 g	0 g	0 g	5 g	d	d	<1 g
Total protein	10 g	9 g	13 g	10 g	9.3 g	13 g	15 g

[a]All figures are for the standard 8-ounce size.

[b]All recommended daily amounts are based on a 2000-calorie daily diet.

[c]All products also contain assorted vitamins, minerals, and trace elements.

[d]Figures not provided on manufacturer's package.

diseases was the impetus for the discovery of the various vitamins.

Scientists have confirmed thirteen substances to be vitamins[10]:

- Fat-soluble vitamins: A, D, E, and K (their fat-soluble nature carries implications regarding toxicity)
- Water-soluble vitamins: the vitamin B complex (B_1, B_2, B_6, B_{12}, niacin, pantothenic acid, biotin, folic acid) and vitamin C

The different vitamins are found in a wide variety of foods. For most individuals in developed countries a well-rounded diet provides adequate vitamin intake. See "Vitamins in Common Foods" and "Recommended Daily Dietary Intakes."

Taken in excess, vitamins can exert pharmacologic effects beyond their micronutrient uses. For this reason they should only be taken when there is a good reason for it. Thus the discussion of each vitamin provides various symptoms of toxicity.

There is little chance that a previously unknown vitamin will be identified and added to the list of essential micronutrients. Patients who receive parenteral nutrition receive only the basic thirteen vitamins. No exotic deficiency disease, which would point to a heretofore undiscovered vitamin, has been reported for patients receiving total parenteral nutrition for years. This fact has important implications for the occasional claims of an essential new nutrient.

Patients are often misinformed, misguided, or confused about what vitamins can accomplish for them, the types of vitamins they should take, and what type of vitamin formulation is optimal. For example, some patients—notably many athletes—believe that vitamins will give them energy (a misconception since no vitamin can accomplish this). Patients also believe that certain vitamins can be particularly nutritious, thanks to ingenious advertising campaigns. (See "Antioxidant Vitamins.")

Some patients ask for organic, natural, or colloidal vitamins:

- Organic vitamins are supposedly free of artificial substances when grown and processed.
- Natural vitamins are obtained from a source found in nature as opposed to being synthesized (such as vitamin C from rose hips).
- Colloidal vitamins are alleged to be more available to the body and provide better nutrition than other vitamins.

None of these marketing schemes has validity. *Patients who need vitamin supplements do not obtain any special benefit from these special vitamins and may freely choose any supplement.*

Vitamin A

Vitamin A, also known as retinol, is critical for skeletal, dental, dermatologic, ophthalmic, and urologic systems.

Symptoms of Deficiency. The patient with vitamin A deficiency may notice dry eye as the initial symptom. Eventually, the patient may also complain of night blindness, photophobia, anorexia, impaired taste and smell, and difficulties with equilibrium.[7,10]

Specific Considerations. In recent years 10 to 15 cases have been reported in the United States each year in which vitamin A has produced toxic reactions, usually associated with intakes greater than 100,000 units daily.[12] Excessive vitamin A causes fatigue, malaise, lethargy, abdominal upset, throbbing headaches, irritability, night sweats, loss of body hair, brittle nails, insomnia, restlessness, anorexia, impaired growth in children, skin that is dry or scaly, hepatomegaly, splenomegaly, intracranial pressure, alopecia, joint pains, menstrual irregularities, and/or pain in the bones.[7,10,17] In one such case habitual daily ingestion of 25,000 units daily for 6 years resulted in fatal hepatotoxicity.[18] Large doses of vitamin A may produce teratogenicity.[5] Because of this the American Dietetic Association recommended that the first-trimester female avoid preformed vitamin A supplementation without clear evidence of vitamin A deficiency.

Carotenoids (e.g., beta-carotene), which are converted to vitamin A through the action of intestinal oxygenase, occur naturally in green leafy vegetables and yellow and orange fruits and vegetables.[19] Ingesting carotenoids as tablets avoids the toxicity associated with vitamin A, since they are converted to A quite slowly.[7,12] The skin (especially in the nasolabial folds and fat pads of the soles and palms) may develop a yellowish discoloration while taking these carotenoids that resolves when supplementation ceases.[12]

Vitamin D

"Vitamin D" is an umbrella term for substances such as vitamin D_2 (ergocalciferol) and vitamin D_3 (cholecalciferol). The former is a plant-derived chemical, while the latter is formed in human tissues when they are exposed to sunlight (hence its nickname the "sunshine vitamin").

Symptoms of Deficiency. Vitamin D is an essential factor in regulating the intracellular and extracellular levels of calcium.[7] Normally, the body increases

FOCUS ON...

VITAMINS IN COMMON FOODS

Foods contain a variety of nutrients such as vitamins, and each vitamin is found in many different types of foods. For this reason the basis of dietary adequacy is a balanced diet, containing adequate amounts of all of the suggested foods. The table presents several common foods and some of the nutrients they contain.

Vitamins in Common Foods[a]

FOOD	NUTRIENTS
Butter	A
Cabbage (raw)	C, K
Cantaloupe	A, C
Carrots	A
Cauliflower	K
Cheese	B_2
Citrus fruits	C
Eggs	A, B_2, Pantothenic Acid, B_{12}, Biotin, D, E
Enriched breads	B_1, Niacin
Fish	B_2, Niacin, B_6, Folic Acid
Fish liver oils	A, D
Green vegetables	A, B_1, B_2, Niacin
Green leafy vegetables	B_2, Folic Acid, K
Lettuce	E
Liver	A, B_2, Niacin, B_{12}, Biotin, E
Meat	B_1, Niacin, B_6, Pantothenic Acid, B_{12}, Folic Acid, E
Fortified milk	A, B_2, B_{12}, D, E
Nuts	B_1, Pantothenic Acid, Biotin, E
Peas	B_1
Potatoes	B_1, C
Poultry	B_2, Niacin, B_6, Folic Acid
Salmon	D
Soybeans	B_1
Strawberries	C
Sweet potatoes	A
Tomatoes	C
Tuna	D
Vegetables (as a group)	B_1, B_6, Biotin, E
Vegetable oils	E
Whole-grain breads	B_1, Niacin
Whole grain cereals	B_1, Niacin, B_6, Pantothenic Acid, E
Yeast	B_1, B_2, Niacin, B_6, Folic Acid
Yellow vegetables	A

[a]These listings are not exhaustive, in that some of the foods may contain other nutrients not listed; certain vitamins may also be found in foods other than those listed also.

absorption of calcium when stores are low or in times of increased need (e.g., lactation, pregnancy, and growth). Vitamin D deficiency prevents the body from increasing absorption. The deficiency of vitamin D is responsible for the condition known as rickets, a condition characterized by soft bones and deformed joints. In adults, deficiency causes osteomalacia, with unmineralized bone appearing on surfaces of bones.[20] Deficiency also can produce muscle weakness, limb pain, and impaired physical function.[21]

Vitamin D deficiency is most frequently seen in the following:

- Very young children
- Adolescents
- Elderly (those with age-related skin changes or impaired GI absorption and renal function)
- Patients who do not obtain adequate sunlight (e.g., females required by custom or religion to wear heavy veils when outdoors and elderly patients confined to bed)[20]
- Patients taking medications that interfere with vitamin D (e.g., phenytoin, phenobarbital)
- Patients with certain medical conditions (e.g., partial gastrectomy, renal disease, severe hepatic disease, malabsorption, and obesity)[21]

Specific Considerations. Vitamin D is a potent substance (it is used commercially to kill rodents).[20] Hypervitaminosis D in humans can cause anorexia, nausea, weakness, weight loss, polyuria, constipation, hypertension, vague aches, anemia, stiffness, kidney stones, calcification of tissues, acidosis, and fatal renal failure.[10] Vitamin D also acts as a hormone, a unique feature among vitamins.[9]

Vitamin E

Vitamin E, a group of compounds known collectively as the tocopherols, prevents oxidation of cell membrane fatty acids via attack by oxygen-free radicals and other chemicals.[9,22]

FOCUS ON...

RECOMMENDED DAILY DIETARY INTAKES

For each vitamin a Recommended Dietary Allowance (RDA) has been established by the FDA.[9] The RDA was intentionally set at a level above the minimum needed for optimal health in the prevention of deficiency diseases.[11] Thus an individual obtaining the RDA for each vitamin has an added margin of safety in case of several months of dietary inadequacy.[10] The table presents vitamins and their recommended daily dietary intakes.

Recommended Daily Dietary Intakes for Vitamins and Minerals for Healthy Patients

VITAMIN/MINERAL	PATIENT GROUP		
	ADULT MALE	ADULT FEMALE	CHILDREN AGED 1–14
A (measured as retinol equivalents)	1000 mcg	800 mcg	400–1000 mcg
B₁	1.2–1.5 mg	1–1.1 mg	0.7–1.4 mg
B₂	1.4–1.8 mg	1.2–1.3 mg	0.8–1.6 mg
Niacin	15–20 mg	13–15 mg	9–18 mg
B₆	1.4–2 mg	1.4–1.6 mg	0.9–1.8 mg
Pantothenic acid	4–10 mg	4–7 mg	3–7 mg
B₁₂	2 mcg	2 mcg	2–3 mcg
Biotin	30–100 mcg	50–100 mcg	65–200 mcg
Folate	150–200 mcg	150–180 mcg (400 if pregnant or of childbearing age)	100–400 mcg
C	50–60 mg	50–60 mg	45–50 mg
D (10 mcg = 400 international units or IU)	5–10 mcg	5–10 mcg	10 mcg
E (measured as alpha-tocopherol equivalents)	10 mg	8 mg	5–8 mg
K	45–80 mcg	45–65 mcg	15–100 mcg
Calcium	800–1200 mg	1200–1500 mg	800–1200 mg
Iron	10–12 mg	10–15 mg	10–12 mg
Phosphorus	800–1200 mg	800–1200 mg	800 mg
Magnesium	270–400 mg	280–300 mg	80–170 mg
Zinc	15 mg	12 mg	10 mg
Iodine	150 mg	150 mg	70–120 mg
Selenium	40–70 mg	45–55 mg	20–30 mg

Adapted from Issulbacher KJ, et al., eds. Harrison's Principles of Internal Medicine. 13th ed. New York: McGraw-Hill, 1994; p. 438.

Symptoms of Deficiency. Vitamin E deficiency, which is rare, produces few symptoms.[9] In one case a male patient who had undergone extensive small bowel surgery that required resection of a large portion of jejunum and ileum developed clinical hypovitaminosis E, with bilateral weakness of the hands of such severity that he could no longer grasp objects.[23] Weakness in the lower extremities resulted in gait unsteadiness and repeated episodes of falling. Nystagmus and loss of deep tendon reflexes were also noted.

Specific Considerations. Vitamin E has been promoted for numerous uses not approved by the FDA. Large trials of vitamin E have not yet confirmed any benefit in cardiovascular disease or cancer, although trials indicate it may augment the immune system.[22,24]

Excessive vitamin E intake can result in headache, nausea, tiredness, giddiness, oral inflammation, chapped lips, GI disturbances, muscular weakness, hypoglycemia, a tendency to bleed easily, degenerative changes, blurred vision (through interfering with vitamin A), and/or reduced sexual function.[9]

Vitamin K
Vitamin K encompasses several compounds:

- K_1, phylloquinone
- K_2, menaquinones
- K_3, menadione

Phylloquinone is obtained from a normal diet, and menaquinones are normally manufactured by intestinal bacteria, making deficiencies rare.[9,25]

Symptoms of Deficiency. Vitamin K is a cofactor in the synthesis of clotting factors II, VII, IX, and X, so that a deficiency results in **coagulopathies** (defects in coagulation).[26]

Specific Considerations. The newborn intestine does not become sufficiently colonized with bacteria to produce vitamin K until about 2 weeks of age. Thus mothers are often given vitamin K before childbirth to prevent hemorrhagic disease of the newborn.[9] Vitamin K as found in dietary sources has no known toxicity.

Vitamin B_1
Also known as thiamine (or thiamin), vitamin B_1 aids in metabolism of carbohydrates, assisting the function of the cardiovascular and nervous systems.

Symptoms of Deficiency. Deficiency is noted by the medical condition beri-beri. Thiamin deficiency is more common in the following patients:

- Patients who eat polished rice as the major dietary cereal product
- Alcoholics
- Patients with generalized intestinal malabsorption

Beri-beri symptoms include peripheral neuritis progressing to edema and cardiac failure.

Specific Considerations. Thiamin is excreted by the kidney quite readily, even with high doses, so it appears to be nontoxic.[27]

Vitamin B_2
Vitamin B_2, also called riboflavin, aids in cellular oxygen utilization.

Symptoms of Deficiency. Riboflavin deficiency generally is found in patients who exclude animal protein from the diet. Riboflavin is vital for dermatologic and ophthalmic health. Patients whose stores of riboflavin are exhausted may complain of cracks at the corners of the mouth (angular stomatitis), inflamed lips, sore tongue, and seborrheic dermatitis around the ears and/or nose, as well as the trunk and/or extremities.[9] Patients also may complain that light hurts the eyes.

Specific Considerations. High doses of riboflavin appear to be nontoxic.[28]

Vitamin B_6
Vitamin B_6, also known as pyridoxine, is essential for utilization of amino acids.[9]

Symptoms of Deficiency. Pyridoxine deficiency is not usually caused by poor nutrition, but instead results from a drug interaction such as ingestion of isoniazid or penicillamine. Pyridoxine deficiency leads to seborrheic dermatitis such as scaling around the nose, mouth, and eyes.[7] Infants accidentally administered a pyridoxine-free diet have exhibited weakness, ataxia, convulsive seizures, anemia, vomiting, nervous irritability, and abdominal pain.

Specific Considerations. Megadoses of B_6 taken in an attempt to reduce the severity of menstrual symptoms may result in severe sensory neuropathy and ataxia.[7]

Vitamin B_{12}
Vitamin B_{12}, also known as cyanocobalamin, and folic acid (discussed below) function to produce DNA in the cells.

Symptoms of Deficiency. Vitamin B_{12} deficiency may occur in vegetarians since this vitamin is mainly found in animal-derived foods.[5,29] However, if the vegetarian ingests eggs, milk, and cheese, the deficiency may be avoided. Cyanocobalamin deficiency slows DNA synthesis, reducing **hematopoiesis** (red blood cell formation). Thus the patient experiences anemia, leukopenia, and thrombocytopenia. Myelinated nerves deteriorate because of an inability to synthesize myelin. Patients may also exhibit glossitis, paresthesias, impaired muscle coordination, mental confusion, agitation, optic atrophy, hallucinations, and psychosis.[7]

Specific Considerations. Excessive B_{12} ingestion is apparently virtually free of risk.[7]

Niacin

Niacin, also known as nicotinic acid, maintains healthy tissue growth and the utilization of carbohydrate as energy and aids in the production of fats. The body is able to convert tryptophan as found in milk and eggs into niacin.[9] The biologically active form of nicotinic acid is the acid amide form, also known as nicotinamide. The vitamin is available in both the acid and acid amide forms.

Symptoms of Deficiency. Niacin deficiency is rare, but may be seen in alcoholics or those whose diet is high in corn (which is low in both niacin and tryptophan). If niacin is lacking, a condition known as pellagra develops. The body cannot properly utilize thiamine and riboflavin, leading to dermatologic, digestive, and CNS disorders.[9] Patients with niacin deficiency experience lassitude, anorexia, weakness, inability to digest properly, anxiety, irritability, and/or depression. Dermatitis manifests as thickening and scaling of skin. Mottled hyperpigmentation develops. Mucous membranes undergo inflammation, resulting in vaginitis, proctitis, urethritis, diarrhea, esophagitis, stomatitis, and/or glossitis. Left untreated, patients can develop delirium, disorientation, hallucinations, and dementia.

Specific Considerations. Excessive ingestion of the nicotinic acid form of the vitamin (as suggested for mental disorders) can cause flushing of the face and skin, gastric irritation leading to peptic ulcer, nausea, vomiting, diarrhea, pruritus, hepatotoxicity, tachycardia, hypertension, alopecia, skin rashes, gout, ulcers, and/or disorders of blood glucose regulation.[10] Nicotinic acid is sometimes taken by the lay public to help in cholesterol regulation by elevating HDL levels.[7] However, it should be taken cautiously by diabetics and by patients with gout. Further, the ingestion of nicotinic acid should be part of an overall physician-controlled cholesterol management program. Accordingly, pharmacists should suggest that patients wishing to use nicotinic acid first obtain a physician recommendation.

Pantothenic Acid

Pantothenic acid, converted by the body to coenzyme A, aids in the production of energy from food.

Symptoms of Deficiency. While a deficiency of pantothenic acid is theoretically possible, it is produced by intestinal bacteria, so that a clinically documented deficiency has yet to be reported.[9]

Specific Considerations. No adverse reactions have been reported with pantothenic acid ingestion.[30]

Biotin

Biotin, a sulfur-containing vitamin, aids in energy production through catalyzing the conversion of fats to fatty acids.[9]

Symptoms of Deficiency. Biotin deficiency may produce anorexia, nausea, vomiting, tongue inflammation, pallor, depression, alopecia, and dryness and scaliness of the skin.[31]

Specific Considerations No adverse reactions have been reported with biotin ingestion.[31]

Folic Acid

Also known as folacin or folate, folic acid works in conjunction with cyanocobalamin to produce DNA. Found in virtually all uncooked foods, folic acid prevents anemia.

Symptoms of Deficiency. Folate in foods may not be fully bioavailable for several reasons.[5] Heating foods can destroy folate, thus causing folate deficiency. (The actual amount of folate remaining depends on the extent of heat delivered to the foods.) Also, a substance in beans may inactivate folate.

Folic acid deficiency mimics cyanocobalamin (vitamin B_{12}) deficiency in the effects on hematopoiesis, but folate deficiency does not produce damage to myelin. Patients may exhibit cracks on the lips and at the corners of the mouth, anemia, and/or GI disorders.

Specific Considerations. Folic acid supplementation in the amount of 0.4 mg of folate daily reduces the risk of neural-tube-defect birth abnormalities such as spina bifida.[7] The U.S. Public Health Service has recommended its ingestion for all women of child-bearing age. Females who have previously experienced such a birth may need higher amounts of folic acid, but this should be recommended by a physician.[1] Large doses of folic acid may result in epileptic convulsions in patients taking phenytoin.[32] Doses of folic acid greater than 1 mg daily can mask symptoms of cyanocobalamin deficiency, allowing pernicious anemia to proceed unchecked.[33] Nonprescription products seldom exceed 400 micrograms of folic acid per daily dose.

Vitamin C

Vitamin C, also known as ascorbic acid, is vital in daily doses for maintenance of blood vessels, bones, and teeth.[9] Vitamin C also is vital in healing wounds since it aids in formation of collagen.

Symptoms of Deficiency. Scurvy is the deficiency disease associated with ascorbic acid. Symptoms include weakness, lassitude, irritability, joint and muscular aches and pains, capillary hemorrhage and pe-techiae, hemorrhage and spongy appearance of the gingiva, impaired growth and deformity in children, impaired wound healing, and/or decreased resistance to infection.[7,9] Hair follicles bleed, resulting in plugging with keratin, which in turn causes in-grown hairs to proliferate.

The risk of ascorbic acid deficiency is low for patients who eat at least one serving of a fresh fruit or vegetable daily. Although it is widely known that smoking reduces the plasma levels of vitamin C, physicians have not yet reported clinical scurvy in smokers who eat one serving of a fresh fruit or vegetable daily.[9] Nevertheless, the smoker's RDA is 100 mg daily rather than the 60 mg proposed for non-smokers.[34] The RDA for pregnant females is 70 mg daily, and for the lactating female it rises to 95 mg daily. Deficiency may also be seen in the following:

- Infants given fad diets such as cow's milk only
- Alcoholics
- Poor and/or undernourished persons
- Patients unable or unwilling to follow healthy dietary advice

Patients deficient in vitamin C may note early symptoms such as sore gums and bleeding beneath the skin.[9]

Specific Considerations. Single doses of vitamin C exceeding 2 g can produce abdominal bloating and diarrhea.[12,34] Excessive doses of vitamin C taken chronically can cause damage to growing bone, rebound scurvy (in those whose mothers took megadoses during pregnancy), and kidney stones. High doses of vitamin C can also interfere with vitamin B_{12}, converting some of that molecule to anti-B_{12} antibodies.[10] Oxalate excretion is increased, leading to renal stones.[7] For a discussion of vitamin C and the common cold see "Unproven Therapies and the Common Cold" in Chapter 15, The Common Cold and Related Conditions. See "The Effect of Vitamin C on the Common Cold" in this chapter for a more in-depth review.

MINERALS
Calcium

Calcium, an essential element for normal growth and maturation, comprises approximately 2% of total body weight.[41]

Symptoms of Deficiency. A major risk of calcium deficiency is osteoporosis, a disease of low bone mass that results in fragile bones and an increased risk of bone fractures.[42]

tip *More than half of American women will experience an osteoporotic fracture.* Most are caused by mild to moderate trauma such as falling while standing; hip and vertebral fractures are most common. Osteoporosis can be quantified by bone mineral density (BMD). The weight of evidence in-

---

FOCUS ON...

THE EFFECT OF VITAMIN C ON THE COMMON COLD

In 1970 Linus Pauling created a sensation by asserting in a best-selling book that vitamin C would prevent the common cold.[35] Research was carried out to verify this claim. Vitamin C has never been proven to prevent the common cold.[36] However, doses of 1 g daily may alleviate cold symptoms.[37,38] Other research indicates that doses up to 6 g per day may alleviate symptoms by 23%.[39,40] Results of research to this date do not provide clear evidence that a reduction in severity of symptoms by only 23% is clinically significant. The pharmacist should perhaps stress that normal doses of vitamin C are not dangerous to the average patient and might provide some benefit. However, making firm statements about the value of vitamin C in alleviating common cold symptoms cannot yet be supported by a wide body of literature.

---

dicates that the age-associated decrease in BMD can be largely prevented by exercise and early supplementation with calcium and slowed if older female patients ingest adequate calcium and vitamin D.[43] The average adult female only takes in 600 mg of calcium daily rather than the 1200 to 1500 mg recommended, while patients aged 1 to 14 and adult male patients (osteoporosis also occurs in males) should take in 800 to 1200 mg.[5]

Specific Considerations. An NIH panel has recommended that females alter their diet to increase the amount of calcium ingested above current RDAs.[5] One cup of skim milk, lowfat milk, or whole milk contains 280 to 290 mg of calcium. **tip** *Patients should avoid bone meal and dolomite as calcium sources because they may contain toxic amounts of lead.*

Vitamin D aids in the absorption of calcium, so many calcium supplements also contain D. **tip** *Vitamin D has a profound impact on the calcium supplement and should be recommended.* Most routine vitamin/mineral supplements contain 400 international units (IU) of vitamin D, which is equivalent to the 10 mcg required for most people. Should patients obtain more than this amount, the possibility of vitamin D toxicity arises. Thus patients who are presently consuming a vitamin supplement should not receive a calcium/vitamin D combination, and pharmacists should recommend a calcium product without vitamin D. Conversely, patients who are not presently taking another supplement might benefit from a calcium/vitamin D combination product. Table 47.2 lists several calcium supplements that contain vitamin D and several free of vitamin D.

Iron

Iron is an element mostly present in humans as a constituent of hemoglobin.[44]

Symptoms of Deficiency. Patients normally lose 0.5 to 1 mg of iron daily through exfoliation of dermatologic and gastrointestinal cells, biliary secretions, sweating, gastrointestinal blood loss, and urinary excretion. Some patients have enhanced losses such as women of reproductive age and

Table 47.2. Calcium Content of Representative Nonprescription Products

TRADE NAME	MG OF ELEMENTAL CALCIUM PER TABLET	UNITS OF VITAMIN D PER TABLET
OsCal 250+D	250	125
OsCal 500+D	500	125
OsCal 500	500	0
OsCal 500 Chewable	500	0
Caltrate 600	600	0
Caltrate 600+D	600	125
Calel D	500	200
Posture	600	0
Posture-D	600	125
Citracal	200	0
Citracal+D	315	200
Calcet	148.8	100
Tums 500 Calcium Supplement	500	0

Table 47.3. Iron Content of Representative Nonprescription Products

TRADE NAME	EQUIVALENT MG OF ELEMENTAL IRON PER TABLET/CAPSULE
Femiron	20
Ferralet	37
Fergon	36
Feosol Tablets	65
Feosol Capsules	50
Slow Fe	50
Ferro-Sequels	50 (+100 mg docusate Na)
Fero-Grad 500	105 (+ 500 mg C)

adolescent females who are growing and menstruating. An average menstrual period leeches 15 to 20 mg of iron from the female.[43] Pregnancy costs the average female 500 mg of iron, and lactation costs 0.5 to 1 mg of iron daily. Thus different people have different requirements for iron, ranging from 10 mg to 20 mg daily.[44] The average daily intake is 10 to 20 mg, but only about 5 to 10% of an ingested dose is absorbed. It is readily apparent that *the average female or male patient does not obtain sufficient iron*. Symptoms of iron deficiency anemia include pallor, fatigue, exhaustion, lassitude, dizziness, breathlessness, and headaches.[43]

Specific Considerations. Certain dietary substances (e.g., ascorbic acid and orange juice) convert iron from the ferric to ferrous form (via chemical reduction), facilitating its absorption.[44] Conversely, antacids, tannins from tea and phytic acid found in grain fibers, phosphates in eggs, and oxalates in vegetables can all impair absorption.[43] ***Pharmacists recommending an iron supplement should caution the patient to keep the product locked away from children, as iron supplements have become the major cause of poisoning deaths in children.*** Table 47.3 lists several representative iron-containing nonprescription products. When patients ingest iron supplements, as many as 5 to 20% experience such adverse effects as diarrhea or constipation, darkening of the stools, nausea, and abdominal pain.[45]

Fluorine
Fluorine is an essential mineral for maintaining strong teeth. (The role of fluorine in the prevention of caries is described in Chapter 3, "Plaque-Induced Diseases: Caries and Gin-

givitis.") Fluorine is not routinely added to vitamin-mineral supplements to avoid toxicity since the water in many towns already contains adequate fluoride.

Iodine
Iodine is an essential element for preventing goiter.

Symptoms of Deficiency. Goiter, the result of iodine deficiency, results from hyperplasia of the thyroid gland.

Specific Considerations. Iodine supplementation of salt and other foods has virtually eliminated goiter as a problem in the United States.

Other Micronutrients
In an attempt to cover all their nutritional bases, patients often supplement their diet with other micronutrients, including various trace elements (such as copper, manganese, zinc) and substances termed ultratrace elements (i.e., suspected dietary requirements less than 1 mg daily) such as aluminum, arsenic, boron, bromide, cadmium, chromium, fluoride, germanium, iodide, lead, lithium, molybdenum, nickel, rubidium, selenium, silicon, tin, and vanadium. Patients given long terms of total parenteral nutrition may require supplementation with iodide, manganese, molybdenum, selenium, zinc, copper, and chromium, but typical patients seen by pharmacists have no need to fear deficiencies of these elements.[46] Other ultratrace elements should not be ingested without physician advice. Lead, cadmium, nickel, arsenic, and boron, for example, exhibit well-known toxicities. *Patients should be cautioned against ingestion of ultratrace elements pending further information regarding safe dosing.*

PREVENTION OF DIETARY INADEQUACY

Proper health mandates ingestion of a balanced mixture of healthy foods.[47] (See "Vitamins in Common Foods" and "Recommended Daily Dietary Intakes.") As stated by the American Dietetic Association, "It is the position of the ADA that the best nutritional strategy for promoting optimal health and reducing the risk of chronic disease is to obtain adequate nutrients from a wide variety of foods. Vitamin and mineral supplementation is appropriate when well-accepted, peer-reviewed, scientific evidence shows safety and effectiveness."[5] The ADA notes that certain nutritionally vulnerable population subgroups (e.g., the elderly, young children, women of child-bearing age, pregnant or lactating females, alcoholics, and tobacco users) are often urged to use general multivitamin-mineral supplements, but cautions that "even modest amounts of multivitamin and mineral supplements may contribute to excessive intakes or imbalances."[5] For instance, the ADA believes that adult men and postmenopausal women are at little risk of iron deficiency and receive no real benefit from a general supplement containing iron while being exposed to iron's adverse reactions (e.g., gastrointestinal upset).

The U.S. Departments of Agriculture and Health and Human Services have developed a food-guide pyramid that simplifies the components of a healthy diet.[1] At the base of the pyramid is the bread, cereal, rice, and pasta group, for which six to eleven servings daily are recommended. Two to four servings of fruits and three to five of vegetables should be ingested daily. The group that includes meat, poultry, fish, dry beans, eggs, and nuts and the group including milk, yogurt, and cheese each require two to three servings daily. At the apex of the pyramid are the items to be used very sparingly (e.g., fats, oils, sweets). The agencies also elucidated the measurement of a serving. For instance, one serving of bread may be met by one slice of bread, 1/2 cup of cooked cereal, rice, or pasta, or 1 ounce of ready-to-eat cereal. The agencies stressed that teenage boys and active men should choose the high end of the suggested ranges (e.g., 11 servings of pasta), while children, teenage females, active women, and most men should choose servings in the middle of the range. Most women and some older adults should choose the lower end of the ranges.

Other dietary guidelines to prevent dietary inadequacy and promote health have been developed by the U.S. Department of Agriculture and Health and Human Services, including the following:

- Maintain a healthy weight.
- Carefully balance intake of fat, carbohydrate, protein, cholesterol, and polyunsaturated fats by eating a variety of foods.
- Ingest salt and other forms of sodium only in moderation.
- Restrict fat intake to no more than 15 to 30% of calories daily (approximately 65 g).
- Limit cholesterol intake to 0 to 300 mg/day.
- Limit saturated fat intake to 20 g/day.
- Ingest complex carbohydrates for 50 to 70% of the daily diet (approximately 300 g).
- Ingest protein for 10 to 15% of the daily diet (approximately 50 g).
- Limit alcohol consumption to no more than 5% of daily calories (equivalent to approximately 2 drinks).
- Avoid alternative dietary supplements in excess of the RDA.

SUMMARY

Proper nutrition, one of the cornerstones of health, usually can be achieved by ingesting a balanced diet consisting of required nutrients in the proper amounts. Liquid nutritionals, products that can be ingested by high-risk groups, can help attain proper nutrition.

The major controversies in nutrition involve vitamins and minerals. Deficiencies, which can result in the development of a recognized deficiency disease, are rare in patients eating

AT THE COUNTER

A female appearing to be in her late 50s asks the pharmacist about calcium products.

Interview/Patient Assessment

The patient is aware that she needs to obtain some calcium since she does not like milk or cheese. Her mother had osteoporosis. She is taking a vitamin/mineral supplement, but does not think it has enough calcium. She specifically wants to take OsCal 250+D. She has no underlying disease conditions and is taking Premarin 1.25 mg daily, alternating with Provera. She states that she is postmenopausal.

Pharmacist's Analysis

1. How much calcium should this patient ingest daily?
2. What is the significance of her vitamin/mineral supplement? Does it contain sufficient calcium?

3. Is OsCal 250+D the best choice for her?

Patient Counseling

This patient's failure to ingest sufficient calcium and her family history of osteoporosis indicate the possibility of calcium deficiency. She should ingest 1500 mg of calcium daily, since she is postmenopausal. Most standard vitamin/mineral supplements fall below this quantity of calcium, making a separate calcium supplement mandatory. However, most standard vitamin/mineral combinations already contain the RDA of vitamin D. Should she choose a calcium/vitamin D combination, she is at risk of hypervitaminosis D. Therefore OsCal 250+D is not a good choice for her. She should choose a vitamin D–free calcium supplement such as OsCal 500 or Caltrate 600.

a proper diet, so most primary-care practitioners will never see a patient with a deficiency disease (e.g., scurvy, rickets, beri-beri, pellagra). Supplementation of the thirteen vitamins is not required by most patients and, since some vitamins have known toxicity if taken in high doses, could lead to patient harm.

Certain groups require folic acid, such as pregnant females to prevent birth defects. However, the ingestion of folic acid should be monitored by a physician. Likewise, most women should consider supplementation with calcium and iron to prevent osteoporosis and anemia, perhaps after a physician carries out tests of mineral status.

The risk of deficiencies of iodine, magnesium, manganese, selenium, copper, zinc, phosphorus, and other trace elements is extremely low. Patients should be advised against routine supplementation with these substances unless a physician recommends them on the basis of lab tests that demonstrate a deficiency.

To prevent the improper use of vitamins and minerals, patients should be enlightened regarding myths associated with their use such as obtaining energy from vitamins, use of vitamin E to prevent heart attacks or increase potency, and ingestion of vitamin C to prevent the common cold.

References

1. U.S. Public Health Service. Nutrition in adults. Am Fam Physician 51 1485, 1995.
2. Turnlund JR. Future directions for establishing mineral/trace element requirements. J Nutr 124:1765S, 1994.
3. Pray WS. Infant formulas versus breast milk. U.S. Pharmacist 22(11):22, 1997.
4. Wood RJ, Suter PM, Russell RM. Mineral requirements of elderly people. Am J Clin Nutr 62:493, 1995.
5. Hunt JR. Position of the American Dietetic Association: Vitamin and mineral supplementation. J Am Diet Assoc 96:73, 1996.
6. Pray WS. Liquid nutritionals. US Pharm 22(7) (Spec Suppl):13, 1997.
7. Swain R, Kaplan B. Vitamins as therapy in the 1990s. J Am Board Fam Pract 8:206, 1995.
8. Olson JA. Vitamins: The tortuous path from needs to fantasies. J Nutr 124:1771S, 1994.
9. Herbert V. Nutrition Cultism, Facts and Fictions. Philadelphia: George F. Stickley, 1983.
10. Herbert V, Barrett S. Vitamins & "Health" Foods: The Great American Hustle. Philadelphia: George F. Stickley, 1985.
11. Jha P, et al. The antioxidant vitamins and cardiovascular disease. Ann Intern Med 123:860, 1995.
12. Meyers DG, Maloley PA, Weeks D. Safety of antioxidant vitamins. Arch Intern Med 156:925, 1996.
13. Johnson LE. The emerging role of vitamins as antioxidants. Arch Fam Med 3:809, 1994.
14. Diplock AT. Safety of antioxidant vitamins and B-carotene. Am J Clin Nutr 62:1510S, 1995.
15. Hennekens CH. Antioxidant vitamins and cancer. Am J Med 97:2S, 1994.
16. Hennekens CH, et al. Antioxidant vitamin-cardiovascular disease hypothesis is still promising, but still unproven: The need for randomized trials. Am J Clin Nutr 62:1377S, 1995.
17. Olson JA. Benefits and liabilities of vitamin A and carotenoids. J Nutr 126:1208S, 1996.
18. Kowalski TE, et al. Vitamin A hepatotoxicity: A cautionary note regarding 25,000 IU supplements. Am J Med 97:523, 1994.
19. Bates CJ. Vitamin A. Lancet 345:31, 1995.
20. Fraser DR. Vitamin D. Lancet 345:104, 1995.
21. Gloth, FM III, Tobin JD. Vitamin D deficiency in older people. J Am Geriatr Soc 43:822, 1995.
22. Meydani M. Vitamin E. Lancet 345:170, 1995.
23. Tanyel MCM, Mancano LD. Neurologic findings in vitamin E deficiency. Am Fam Physician 55:197, 1997.
24. Stampfer MJ, Rimm EB. Epidemiologic evidence for vitamin E in prevention of cardiovascular disease. Am J Clin Nutr 62:1365S, 1995.
25. Shearer MJ. Vitamin K. Lancet 345:229, 1995.
26. Lipsky JJ. Nutritional sources of vitamin K. Mayo Clin Proc 69:462, 1994.
27. Kurtzweil P. Vitamin B$_1$. FDA Consumer 25(2):35, 1991.
28. Kurtzweil P. Vitamin B$_2$. FDA Consumer 25(3):38, 1991.
29. Herbert V. Staging vitamin B-12 (cobalamin) status in vegetarians. Am J Clin Nutr 59:1213S, 1994.
30. Kurtzweil P. Pantothenic acid. FDA Consumer 25(9):38, 1991.
31. Kurtzweil P. Biotin. FDA Consumer 25(8):34, 1991.
32. Kurtzweil P. Folate. FDA Consumer 25(6):41, 1991.
33. Farley D. Dietary supplements. FDA Consumer 27(9):9, 1993.
34. Levine M, et al. Determination of optimal vitamin C requirements in humans. Am J Clin Nutr 62:1347S, 1995.
35. Hemila H. Vitamin C supplementation and the common cold—Was Linus Pauling right or wrong? Int J Vit Nutr Res 67:329, 1997.
36. Hemila H. Vitamin C intake and susceptibility to the common cold. Br J Nutr 77:59, 1997.
37. Hemila H. Vitamin C supplementation and common cold symptoms: Problems with inaccurate reviews. Nutrition 12:804, 1996.
38. Hemila H. Does vitamin C alleviate the symptoms of the common cold?—A review of current evidence. Scand J Infect Dis 26:1, 1994.
39. Hemila H. Vitamin C, the placebo effect, and the common cold: A case study of how preconceptions influence the analysis of results. J Clin Epidemiol 49:1079, 1996.
40. Hemila H, Herman ZS. Vitamin C and the common cold: A retrospective analysis of Chalmers' review. J Am Coll Nutr 14:116, 1995.
41. Gossel TA. Calcium supplements. US Pharm 16(4):26, 1991.
42. Ross PD. Osteoporosis. Arch Intern Med 156:1399, 1996.
43. Willis J. Please pass that woman some more calcium and iron. FDA Consumer 18(7):6, 1984.
44. Gossel TA. Iron supplements. US Pharm 17(2):22, 1992.
45. McEvoy GK, ed. AHFS Drug Information. Bethesda, MD: American Society of Health-System Pharmacists, 1998; p. 1153.
46. Nielsen FH. How should dietary guidelines be given for mineral elements with beneficial actions or suspected of being essential? J Nutr 126:2377S, 1996.
47. Mertz W. A balanced approach to nutrition for health: The need for biologically essential minerals and vitamins. J Am Diet Assoc 94:1259, 1994.
48. Isselbacher KJ, et al., eds. Harrison's Principles of Internal Medicine. 13th ed. New York: McGraw-Hill, 1994; p. 438.

Topics Related to Self-Care Therapies

Home Test Kits

A man asks the pharmacist for help, but appears reluctant to speak over the counter. The pharmacist leaves the prescription area and follows him to a quiet area of the pharmacy. The man says, "I think my kid is using drugs. Do you have a way I can find out?"

Interview/Patient Assessment

The pharmacist determines that the parent's concern stems from a variety of factors. The child, a 14-year-old male, is currently enrolled in a local high school that the pharmacist knows has many students with drug problems. The parent has noted increasing difficulty in getting the child to do his homework or chores. Also, the child is acting more aggressively toward his younger sister. He rides his bike for several hours most days and has been caught lying about his whereabouts. In addition, he has developed a new set of friends who are uncommunicative and stay in the child's room with the door closed. At recent teachers' conferences, the teachers shared concerns about the child's falling performance and surly attitude. The father is distraught, but has not noted obvious signs of drug abuse (e.g., needle tracks or nasal defects). The father does not know if the child is undergoing normal adolescent adjust-

ment reactions and does not want to alert authorities without some further proof of drug use.

Pharmacist's Analysis

1. Are the behaviors listed signs of possible drug abuse?
2. What is the significance of the absence of needle tracks or nasal septal defects?
3. How can the parent detect drug abuse in the child?

Patient Counseling

This child is certainly at the age where normal adolescent adjustment can produce parent-child conflicts. Unfortunately, these conflicts sometimes include drug abuse. The child's behaviors all point toward possible drug abuse when taken as a total picture. The earlier any abuse can be identified, the better the chances for altering the child's habits with proper professional intervention. The PDT-90 is a home testing kit that can detect possible use of five common recreational drugs. Preferably with the child's cooperation, the parent obtains a hair sample and submits it to the company. After a short waiting period, the parent calls the company to learn the results.

Home test kits for diabetes mellitus monitoring have been available for many decades. (See "Blood Glucose Monitoring" in Chapter 46, Diabetes Mellitus.) However, the market for other self-test devices was dormant until the introduction of the first home pregnancy test in 1977. Since that time home test kits have revolutionized the self-care area, allowing patients to detect and monitor a wide range of conditions. The annual market for home test kits is now estimated at more than 2 billion dollars.[1,2]

Several factors are driving the push for self-testing products. One is the increasing desire of patients to be personally involved in health, fitness, and preventive medicine.[3] Another is patients' desire to take health care into their own hands, at home if possible. Finally, patients often can save on health-care costs by avoiding visits to the clinic for professional testing (e.g., pregnancy).

The FDA Office of Device Evaluation evaluates all home test kits.[4] To be approved for consumer use, home test kits meet the following criteria:

- Assure 95 to 99% accuracy
- Allow safe and effective use with a low risk:benefit ratio
- Meet the same standards as professional kits
- Permit proper use, regardless of user intelligence and technique

- Offer quality-control features (e.g., detection of false positives and false negatives)
- Include simple, concise, and easy-to-use instructions, with figures where applicable
- Provide adequate warnings and precautions
- List all interfering substances, food, and medications on a sheet separate from the instructions
- Color-code reagents when practical to ensure correct use
- Conduct field tests to demonstrate that consumers can use the product as intended

The role of pharmacists in the use of home test kits is to help patients recognize their appropriate uses, understand the steps in proper use, and recognize the precautions and limitations of the kits. Because many tests yield incorrect results if patients are taking certain medications, pharmacists may need to provide the trade names or generic names of these medications so patients can better interpret the kit results.

Pharmacists may also point out the possibility of false-positive and false-negative results and the ramifications of each.[4] With a false-positive test patients who seek medical care may find that other tests do not yield a positive result (an expense of time and money but not dangerous). The false-negative test, however, can be extremely dangerous since patients may have an undeserved feeling of security. For instance, failing to visit a physician when one has colorectal cancer can result in death.

Pharmacists should also discuss general guidelines for use of home test kits with the patient or person who will administer the test[3,5]:

- Fully understand the intended use of the kit prior to purchase and understand that no kit provides 100% accuracy.
- Check the expiration date at the point of sale and again before use (if purchasing the kit for later use). The reagents may not function reliably past that point. Store the kit according to directions to keep it fully reactive to the expiration date.
- Many home test kits are temperature-sensitive. Avoid leaving them in the car while shopping or storing them in direct sunlight.
- Read all directions completely before use. Review all pictures and become familiar with the specific part of the kit to be used at each step. Know the sequence to be employed in carrying out the test.
- If any step is unclear, do not guess. Instead, call the pharmacist or call the manufacturer. (Generally, an 800 number appears on the package or in the labeling.)
- Follow all special instructions (diet, time of day to conduct the exam, physical activity, medication avoidance) exactly as directed.
- Never skip any step.
- If urine is to be collected and the kit does not include a container, wash a container thoroughly, rinsing out all soap traces with distilled water.
- Use a stopwatch or the second hand of a watch when a certain step must be timed; inaccurate timing can cause incorrect results.
- Read the package insert for the next step to follow if a certain test result appears (e.g., see a physician to confirm a positive pregnancy test).
- Should the test kit require interpretation of a color change, obtain help discovering color variations if necessary (e.g, the user has color-defective vision).
- Keep home test kits away from children and animals. (Some tests contain chemicals that may be toxic.) After use, discard any chemicals where children cannot get to them.

PREGNANCY

While some patients are trying to become pregnant, many other patients are trying to prevent pregnancy. Home pregnancy tests can allow both groups of patients to discover privately whether conception has occurred.

MANIFESTATIONS OF PREGNANCY

Pregnancy produces many changes in the female, but home test kits depend on detecting only one early manifestation of pregnancy. During pregnancy the placenta produces a hormone known as human chorionic gonadotropin (hCG), which is secreted in the urine.[2]

SPECIFIC CONSIDERATIONS OF SELF-DETECTION OF PREGNANCY

Current home pregnancy tests can detect pregnancy as early as the first day after the missed period.[1] There are numerous advantages of early detection. Women who discover pregnancy early have clearer options because early termination of pregnancy carries less complications than later. Women who wish to carry a pregnancy to term can also benefit from early pregnancy detection in many ways:

- The woman may decide to cease the use of drugs that affect the fetus, both legal (e.g., nicotine, caffeine, and alcohol) and illegal (e.g., marijuana, cocaine, crack, and amphetamines) substances.
- The woman's physician may choose alternative medications that are less toxic to the infant for women with chronic medical conditions (e.g., diabetes mellitus and asthma).
- The physician will be alerted so that medications that are clearly teratogenic will not be prescribed (e.g., Accutane, Cytotec).
- X-rays of the abdomen can be avoided.
- The due date can be calculated more accurately.
- Fertility treatments can be halted.
- Prenatal vitamin/mineral supplementation can be instituted (e.g., calcium and folic acid).

SELF-DETECTION OF PREGNANCY

Mechanism of Home Pregnancy Tests

Home pregnancy tests measure hCG produced by the **trophoblast** (tissue covering the blastocyst that also aids in nourishment of the embryo) of a fertilized ovum, which appears in the urine 1 to 2 weeks after implantation (Fig. 48.1).[1,6,7] During the subsequent 2 to 3 weeks, hCG levels rise sufficiently to allow detection (which would correspond roughly to the first day after a missed period). The method of detection is **monoclonal** (protein derived from a single cell clone) antibody reaction.[8]

Monoclonal antibodies are immunoglobulins, quite similar to antibodies normally produced by the body in response to any antigen.[3] However, each immunoglobulin is designed to bind to a specific target substance, so low concentrations of the target substances can be detected. In the case of home pregnancy test kits, any hCG present in the urine binds to the monoclonal antibodies in the kit, forming a complex that reacts with a second antibody, which contains an enzyme.[9] The enzyme produces a color change that indicates a negative (not pregnant) or positive (pregnant) test.

Home pregnancy tests have an accuracy of 99%.[10–13] The differences between the tests are very slight, one being the time required to yield a result (Table 48.1).

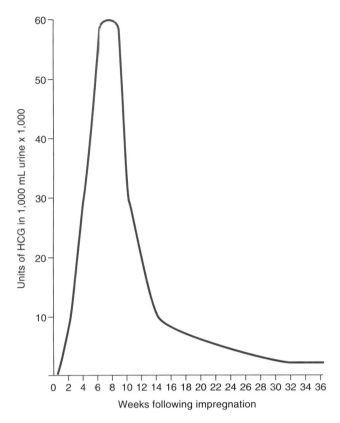

Figure 48.1. Levels of human chorionic gonadotropin (hCG) in urine following impregnation..

Table 48.1. Representative Home Pregnancy Tests and Recommended Reading Times	
PRODUCT	RECOMMENDED READING TIME
Answer Quick and Simple	2 minutes
Clearblue Easy	1 minute
Confirm	2 minutes
1 Step e•p•t	3 minutes
Fact Plus One Step	As soon as 1 minute
First Response 1-Step	2 minutes
Precise	3 minutes

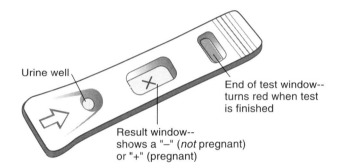

Figure 48.2. Simple one-step pregnancy test.

Using Home Pregnancy Tests

Home pregnancy tests have advanced from complicated kits using droppers, vials, and reagents to simple one-step tests (Fig. 48.2). (See "A Pharmacist's Journal: Home Pregnancy Tests.") Tests can be performed anytime after the missed period, at any time of the day. The current generation of tests require patients to proceed as follows:

1. Check the expiration date on the package to ensure it is still in date.
2. Read all directions thoroughly.
3. Remove the test kit from its foil pouch just prior to use.
4. Remove the cap covering the absorbent tip, if a cap is present.
5. Hold the stick in the urine stream for 5 to 10 seconds as directed to saturate the absorbent tip (for some test kits) or urinate into the urine well (for other tests); or, if preferred, collect urine in a clean, dry cup and expose the test stick to the urine as directed.
6. Lay the test stick on a flat surface and wait the recommended time.
7. Read the test results as directed.
8. Discard test stick. (It is not reusable.)

Precautions with Home Pregnancy Tests

Patients should be relatively certain about the date that menstrual flow should have begun. If patients miscalculate and test too early, the kit may not detect hCG that is actually present, which would be a false-negative result. *For this reason the female with a negative test result should test again a week later if menstrual flow has not yet begun.*[1] Unreliable results can occur for patients with an ovarian cyst or ectopic pregnancy.[12,13] A false positive may result if the female has suffered a miscarriage or given birth within the past 8 weeks, because of elevated hCG levels that remain.[10] Pergonal (menotropins for injection), Profasi (chorionic gonadotropin for injection), and other medications that either contain hCG or are used in combination with hCG also can produce false positives.

RESPONSE TO POSITIVE PREGNANCY-TEST-KIT RESULTS

With a positive result to a pregnancy home test kit, the patient should make an appointment with a general practitioner or obstetrician at her earliest convenience.

COMPROMISED FERTILITY

Infertility is defined medically as the inability to become pregnant after 1 full year of trying.[14] Some female patients with infertility are not completely infertile, but may conceive

A Pharmacist's Journal

Home Pregnancy Tests

Home pregnancy tests are frequently shoplifted because it can be embarrassing for some patients to be seen purchasing them. I was filling prescriptions one day when I noticed a young female picking up a pregnancy test. She slipped it up the sleeve of her coat, while glancing at me and making eye contact. I had never before seen such a brazen shoplifting episode and was ready to call store security. Then she walked the 12-foot distance to the pharmacy register and waited patiently. I walked to the register, whereupon she removed the hidden pregnancy test and paid for it. She confided, "I didn't want anyone to see me buy this."

In another case two young females were waiting at the register with a pregnancy test. As I approached them to sell the kit, they both ran off, leaving the kit on the counter. I placed it back in stock and moved back behind the pharmacy case. About 10 minutes later, the same two patients took the kit from the shelf and again approached the register. Somewhat leery, I moved to the register. They remained present this time. They said, "The reason we ran off before is that our homeroom teacher went by, and we didn't want her to know about this pregnancy."

if conditions are favorable. For this reason this section is titled "Compromised Fertility," indicating that nonprescription test kits can help the patient conceive. Since the kits are oriented toward detecting the female's ovulation, infertility caused by the male is not discussed in detail.

PREVALENCE OF COMPROMISED FERTILITY

As many as 5.3 million Americans of both genders are medically infertile.[14] In addition, a large percentage of females cannot become pregnant exactly when they wish, and at least 20% of females do not attain pregnancy in the first ovulation cycle attempted.[14]

EPIDEMIOLOGY OF COMPROMISED FERTILITY

Fertility declines with age. After age 30 the female slowly loses the ability to conceive. After age 40 fertility declines drastically.[14]

ETIOLOGY OF COMPROMISED FERTILITY

About 80% of infertility cases can be pinned to a specific cause. Half are the result of male factors (e.g., deficiency or lack of sperm, perhaps caused by prior mumps infection, or other problems such as prostate infection, alcohol, marijuana abuse, and nicotine). Half of infertility problems are the result of female factors, most directly caused by ovulation disorders.[14] Ovulation disorders are indicated by irregular or absent menstrual flow, which may be the result of stress, diet, or athletic training.

Sexually transmitted diseases are a major cause of infertility in women (and also in men).[14] Pelvic inflammatory disease, for example, blocks the passage of the ovum into the uterus (Fig. 48.3). Endometriosis and prior surgery for an ectopic pregnancy can also cause blockage.

SELF-DETECTION OF OVULATION

Ovulation prediction kits are useful for couples who experience compromised fertility because they allow females to better detect ovulation. Couples who know when ovulation occurs can time intercourse to coincide with optimal fertility, increasing the chances of impregnation.[15,16]

Mechanism of Ovulation Prediction Kits

Levels of luteinizing hormone (LH), a substance always found in the female's urine, rise sharply 24 to 36 hours prior to ovulation[1,2,17] (Fig. 48.4). In response to this phenomenon, known as the LH surge, an ovarian follicle will rupture, releasing a mature ovum.[3] Ovulation prediction kits detect the LH surge in the urine through the monoclonal antibody reaction.[1] A second antibody triggers a color change.[18] Females who perform the test for the recommended number of days should see a sudden development of color on the test strip a short period prior to ovulation. *Urine tests for LH may be more sensitive than serum tests.*[15]

Using Ovulation Prediction Kits

The average ovulation date is day 14 of the menstrual cycle (the first day of flow is day 1).[19] Ovulation prediction kits contain sufficient materials to test the urine for 5, 6, or 9 days

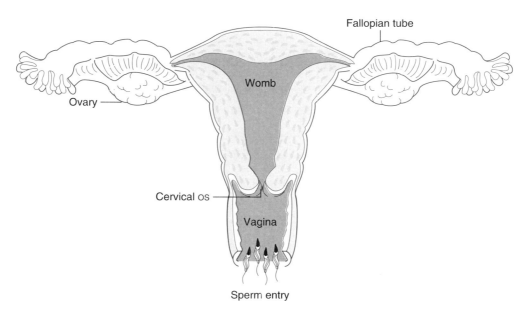

Figure 48.3. Simplified cross-section of the female reproductive system.

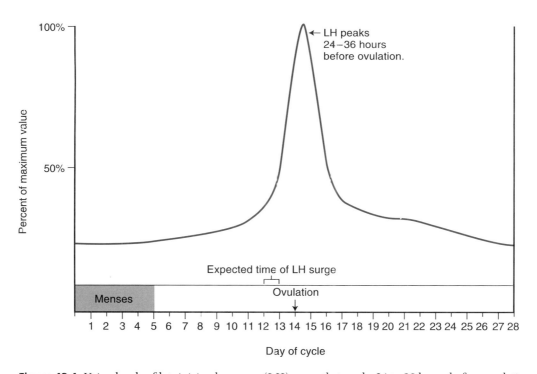

Figure 48.4. Urine levels of luteinizing hormone (LH) surge that peaks 24 to 36 hours before ovulation.

(Table 48.2). Patients should use the first test in the kit 2 to 3 days prior to the expected ovulation date.[20] Testing for 6 consecutive days will detect ovulation in about 66% of women; testing for 10 days increases the odds of success to 95%.[1] (Patients who run out of test material before detecting ovulation can purchase 3-day refills for some kits.[21])

To ensure reliable results, patients should reduce their fluid intake for about 2 hours prior to the test and should not urinate for 4 hours prior to drawing the sample.[21-23] The patient should use urine collected at

Table 48.2. Representative Ovulation Prediction Tests

First Response 1-Step Ovulation Predictor Test	5-day kit; predicts ovulation within 24–36 hours
One-Step Clearplan Easy	5-day kit; predicts ovulation within 24–36 hours
OvuQu ck 1 Step	6-day or 9-day kits available; predicts ovulation within 24–40 hours

the same time each day, to minimize the interference from using diluted versus concentrated urine. If urine is not used immediately, patients must follow the manufacturer's directions regarding refrigeration and warming to room temperature.

The exact directions on the ovulation prediction kits are variable because of the fact that there are two existing generations of kits. Older kits may contain glass vials with dried chemicals, filter droppers, test wells, and urine collection cups.[21] The patient must carry out as many as 13 steps in exact sequence such as placing urine into a vial, swirling and waiting for 3 minutes, pouring into a test well, and adding more chemical. However, with the newer stick tests, the patient simply holds the absorbent tip in the urine stream for 5 seconds and then reads the results after 5 minutes.[21]

Precautions with Ovulation Prediction Kits

Females who ovulate irregularly may not be able to detect ovulation with the kits.[1] Further, it is possible to begin using the product too late in the cycle and thus miss completely the LH surge.

Menopause and **polycystic ovary syndrome** (a condition thought to be caused by excessive androgens, which causes the female to develop hirsutism, infertility, ovarian enlargement, obesity, and menstrual irregularities) elevate LH levels and can cause false positives. Females who are less than 1 month past an abortion or already pregnant will obtain unreliable results.

Certain medications (e.g., clomiphene and menotropins) induce false positives with ovulation prediction kits.[1] If females are using clomiphene, they should not test until 1 day or more after it is discontinued.

A female who has used ovulation prediction kits for 3 months and failed to detect any ovulation should make an appointment with a physician, who may choose to refer her to a fertility specialist for in-depth examination.[3] Ovulation prediction test kits must not be used as contraceptive devices.[24] Their effectiveness has never been assessed when used for contraception.

RESPONSE TO POSITIVE OVULATION-PREDICTION-KIT RESULTS

The first strong color change on the test strip is the LH surge. Patients may discontinue testing, saving extra tests for the next month if they are needed. When the LH surge occurs, ovulation will usually occur within the succeeding 1 to 2 days.[3] Since sperm are capable of fertilizing an ovum for up to 72 hours following entry through the cervical os, couples should have frequent intercourse 2 days before ovulation, the day of ovulation, and the day following ovulation. The more acts of intercourse completed (especially within 24 hours of ovulation), the greater the chances of impregnation.

Colorectal cancer is a common but easily curable cancer if detected early. Fortunately, there are several home test kits to allow patients to test for **occult** (hidden) blood in the stool, an early warning of this condition.

PREVALENCE OF COLORECTAL CANCER

Colorectal cancer is second only to lung cancer in mortality rate in the United States.[25] At least one of every 25 Americans will develop this tumor—140,000 new cases each year.[26]

EPIDEMIOLOGY OF COLORECTAL CANCER

Colorectal cancer has a strong age link. Rare under age 40, it becomes progressively common as the age increases.[25] The risk doubles every 10 years after 40, reaching a peak in the 70s. It also occurs more commonly in patients with a family history of colorectal cancer or with a personal history of cancer, intestinal polyps, ulcerative colitis, or **Gardner's syndrome** (an inherited condition that causes the development of multiple polyps).

ETIOLOGY OF COLORECTAL CANCER

Colorectal cancer is more common in patients who consume animal fats in high amounts and neglect fiber intake.[27]

MANIFESTATIONS OF COLORECTAL CANCER

In most cases colorectal cancer produces no symptoms until it is quite advanced. The first detectable symptom is occult blood in the stool. If not treated, patients may experience weight loss, visible blood in the stool, a change in bowel habits, anorexia, pallor, and abdominal pain.[26,28]

SELF-DETECTION OF COLORECTAL CANCER

Early detection of colorectal cancer helps ensure successful treatment; at least 75% of the deaths could be prevented through early detection.[26,27,29] Further, the 5-year survival rate is higher than any other tumor if colorectal cancer is detected and treated early enough (Fig. 48.5).

The American Cancer Society suggests several steps to promptly detect colorectal cancer [26,30,31]:

- All patients 40 and over should have a digital exam from a physician.
- All patients aged 50 and over should have a yearly fecal occult blood test using a physician-supplied test kit.
- At the age of 50 every person should have a proctosigmoidoscopy, followed within several days by a second

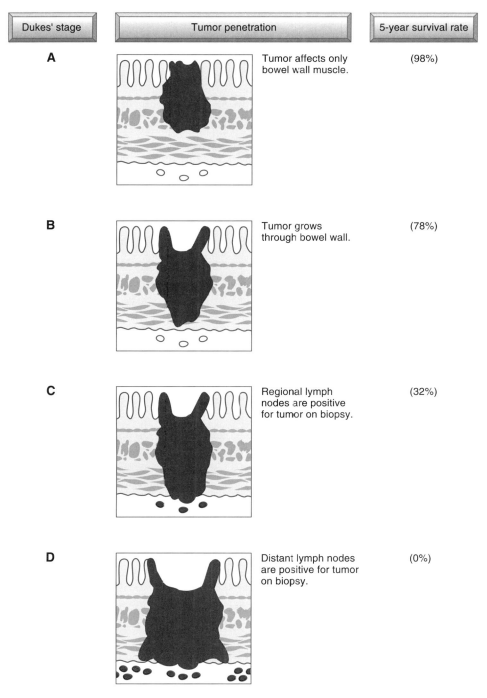

| Dukes' stage | Tumor penetration | 5-year survival rate |

A — Tumor affects only bowel wall muscle. — (98%)

B — Tumor grows through bowel wall. — (78%)

C — Regional lymph nodes are positive for tumor on biopsy. — (32%)

D — Distant lymph nodes are positive for tumor on biopsy. — (0%)

Figure 48.5. Dukes' staging system for colorectal carcinoma, with 5-year survival rates for each stage.

proctosigmoidoscopy to detect any tumors missed by the first. If both are negative, the two-test series should be repeated every 3 to 5 years.

tip *The American Cancer Society recommendations do not apply to patients who are exhibiting symptoms or who are at higher risk for colorectal cancer.* These patients must undergo far more intensive testing.

Home testing kits do not substitute for the digital exam or the proctosigmoidoscopy. They also do not substitute for a physician-supplied fecal occult blood kit. Their purpose is to serve as an early signal between the regularly scheduled exams recommended by the American Cancer Society. Realistically, many patients submit neither to the digital exam nor to the proctosigmoidoscopy, and they do not obtain physician-supplied fecal blood exams, so the nonprescription kits may be their only warning of colorectal cancer. (See "A Pharmacist's Journal: I Need a Digital.")

A Pharmacist's Journal

"I Need a Digital."

A pharmacist attending a continuing education lecture shared this incident. He was approached by a female patient, who said, "I need a digital." He walked with her to the digital thermometers. She appeared puzzled as he pointed them out, so he asked if that was what she wanted. She replied, "These don't look like digitals to me." He pointed out the digital fever thermometers and tried to explain the differences between them and the mercury thermometer, when she interrupted, "Why are you showing me these things?" He explained that these were the digital thermometers, to which she replied, "I don't want that, the doctor told me I need a digital rectal exam!" The pharmacist explained that this refers to the physician's digit being inserted rectally, rather than being a product she might purchase in a pharmacy.

Mechanism of Fecal Blood Detection Kits

Blood originating from the upper gastrointestinal tract will usually be found in the matrix of the stool, while blood originating as a result of colorectal cancer or other lower intestinal problems will usually be present only on the surface of the fecal bolus. Fecal blood detection kits detect blood that is shed from the stool into the water in the toilet bowl.

Since **heme** (the hemoglobin component that carries oxygen) in hemoglobin will oxidize certain reagents such as tetramethylbenzidine, the kits use a tetramethylbenzidine-impregnated pad, which will produce a blue-green color in the presence of heme.[3,27] Two kits are marketed at this time, ColoCare and EZ Detect.

Using Fecal Blood Detection Kits

The first tests available for patient self-detection of occult blood in the stool required the patient to apply stool to a pad with a stick and then apply a solution to the sample. The present generation of tests is far more simple. Patients simply place a test pad into the toilet following a bowel movement, while stool remains in the bowl.[1] (The test pads are printed on one side only, so the patient must drop the pad into the toilet with the printed side uppermost.) A positive test is indicated if blue and/or green color appears in the designated test area within 2 minutes (EZ Detect) or 30 seconds (Colo-Care). The pads are flushable.

The patient should ingest a high-roughage diet (e.g., vegetables, fruits, cereals, bran, and whole grain) for several days before testing to help ensure that necrotic areas bleed. Even with a high-roughage diet, one bowel movement may not contain blood since colorectal cancers bleed intermittently. To increase the effectiveness of fecal blood test kits, each kit contains three to five separate tests. Three consecutive bowel movements should be tested, even if the first two show negative results.

Avoidance of Unreliable Results with Fecal Blood Detection Kits

Fecal blood detection kits may give unreliable results in several circumstances.[32,33,34] (Because the two manufacturers list different precautions, the manufacturer's name appears after each precaution.) The false-positive result is less dangerous than the false negative, since patients will be prompted to see a physician. False negatives are potentially deadly, however, since patients with colorectal cancer will remain unwarned.

Dietary precautions:

- Do not eat red meat for two days prior to beginning and during the series of tests to prevent false positives. Also avoid raw or rare chicken, fish, and tuna (ColoCare).
- Avoid foods that cause discomfort or produce allergic reactions to prevent false positives (EZ Detect).

Medication precautions:

- For 2 days before the test and during the test period, avoid aspirin, NSAIDs, corticosteroids, reserpine, or other medications that can cause internal bleeding and could yield a false-positive result (ColoCare and EZ Detect).
- Avoid rectal products (e.g., ointments, suppositories, and foams) that may cause a false-positive reaction for 2 days prior to the test period and during the test (ColoCare and EZ Detect).
- Do not take more than 250 mg of vitamin C daily to avoid a false negative (ColoCare).
- Do not use laxatives containing mineral oil to avoid a false negative (ColoCare).

Medical condition precautions:

- Conditions that produce blood in the stool will produce a false-positive result for colorectal cancer such as abrasions of the GI tract, constipation, oral bleeding (e.g., gingivitis and dental extraction), nasal bleeding, esophageal varices, gastrointestinal bleeding (e.g., gastric ulcer, diverticulitis, and polyps), or fistulas.

- Patients are specifically cautioned not to test during menstrual flow or with bleeding hemorrhoids, either of which can produce a false-positive result (ColoCare and EZ Detect).

    Extraneous chemicals precautions:

- Toilet bowl cleaners, disinfectants, and deodorizers (e.g., Tidy-Bowl) may cause false positives. Patients should flush the bowl twice after removing any tablet or bottle from the tank and/or reservoir. If a noticeable color remains (from some colored toilet bowl products), the toilet should be flushed until it disappears (ColoCare and EZ Detect).
- Urine can alter the results unpredictably. Patients should urinate and flush the toilet before the bowel movement begins (EZ Detect).

Quality Control Features of Fecal Blood Detection Kits

The two fecal blood detection kits contain quality-control features. The ColoCare pad contains a large test area, with two smaller control areas at the bottom.[33] One test area should turn blue and/or green within 30 seconds of contacting water to help ensure that the chemicals on the pad are still reactive. If this control area does not change color, the test must not be used as a false negative may result. Another control area should remain colorless. Should it change color, some chemical in the toilet bowl is causing a false positive. The patient should flush the toilet more thoroughly to remove traces of toilet-bowl cleaners that remain. If the patient must discard one or more pads, another kit of three pads should be purchased to obtain the additional pads needed.

The EZ Detect kit has a different method to detect false positives and false negatives. The kit contains five test tissues and a small packet containing dry chemicals, the Positive Control Package.[34] One test tissue is used to test the toilet before the bowel movement. If a positive result appears, the patient should use another toilet to prevent false positives. If the patient does not see a positive result after the three consecutive bowel movements, the patient checks for false-negative conditions. First, the toilet is flushed. Next, the contents of the Positive Control Package are emptied into the toilet. After 1 minute, the final test tissue is dropped into the toilet. Color should appear within 2 minutes. If it does not, the patient may be experiencing false-negative results.

RESPONSE TO POSITIVE FECAL-BLOOD-DETECTION-KIT RESULTS

The patient who notices a positive response to a fecal blood detection kit must make an immediate appointment with a physician. If the physician's staff attempt to schedule a later appointment, the patient should be urged to stress the nature of the complaint.

URINARY TRACT INFECTIONS

The urinary tract infection (UTI) is a common problem that causes considerable morbidity and can cause death if not properly diagnosed and treated.

PREVALENCE OF URINARY TRACT INFECTIONS

Urinary tract infections are the cause of 7 million physician visits each year in the United States.[35] About 20% of females will develop at least one UTI at some time.

EPIDEMIOLOGY OF URINARY TRACT INFECTIONS

For men and women younger than 50, females are far more likely to contract UTIs because they have a shorter urethra than men (Fig. 48.6).[35] Thus enteric organisms originating from the bowel are more easily able to ascend their shorter urinary tract. However, because of prostate problems, men older than 50 have a greater likelihood of UTI than women.

Conditions that increase the risk of UTI include diabetes, neurologic deficits, urinary calculi or obstruction, and a history of prior urinary tract infections.[3,35,36] During pregnancy, 4 to 10% of females develop a UTI, and at least 25 to 30% of women develop bacteriuria in the postpartum period. Females who are sexually active are more likely to contract a UTI, and the use of diaphragms or vaginal spermicide further increases the risk.[37] The placement of a urinary catheter causes UTI in 5% of patients, and the risk rises by an additional 5% each day the catheter remains inserted. The suprapubic catheter also increases the risk of UTI. Patients who do not void when appropriate may also be more prone to UTI.[38]

ETIOLOGY OF URINARY TRACT INFECTIONS

Organisms that cause the UTI can reach the urinary tract through one of two methods[35]:

- In less than 5% of cases, bacteria reach the urinary tract via a systemic bacteremia or through the lymph channels.[36]
- In 95% of cases bacteria ascend from the urethra to the bladder, ureter, or kidney.

The most common urinary tract invader is *E. coli*, which causes 80% of infections.[35,39,40] Other organisms include *Staphylococcus saprophyticus* and *Enterococcus*. The organisms are thought to colonize the vaginal and/or urethral mucosa and often gain entrance to the urinary tract during sexual intercourse.

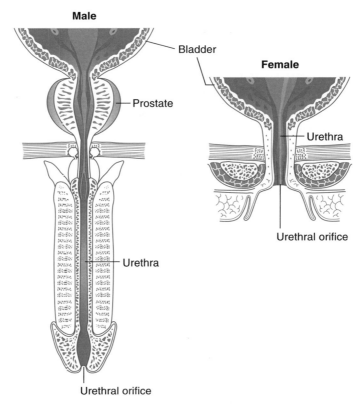

Figure 48.6. Female urethra is far shorter than the male's, which increases the risk of urinary tract infections.

MANIFESTATIONS OF URINARY TRACT INFECTIONS

Symptoms of a UTI include dysuria, urgency, frequency, and lower abdominal discomfort or pain.[3] (Many females have asymptomatic bacteriuria, however.[41]) If not treated, the UTI may cause sepsis and death.[35]

SELF-DETECTION OF URINARY TRACT INFECTIONS

Only one test is currently widely available for home testing for UTIs, the UTI Home Screening Test Kit, which provides sufficient materials to perform six tests. The directions below apply to this kit.

Mechanism of the Urinary Tract Infection Detection Kit

Nitrate taken in through dietary means is normally excreted through the urine as nitrate. However, in patients with a Gram-negative UTI, the bacteria convert nitrate to nitrite.[1,3] In the UTI Kit, arsanilic acid reacts with urinary nitrite to form a diazonium compound, which in turn reacts with another chemical in the kit to form a pink color.

The UTI kit detects 0.03 to 0.06 mg/100mL of nitrite ion in the urine.[42] A positive test requires a bacterial concentration of 10^5 per milliliter of urine. Urine must have had adequate bladder retention time to form nitrites, or a false-negative result might occur.

Using the Urinary Tract Infection Detection Kit

To obtain reliable results with the UTI urinary tract infection kit, patients should follow several steps[42]:

- Do not open the vial of test strips in a humid location such as a bathroom following a shower. One UTI strip should be removed quickly and the container top immediately replaced and closed tightly. If the test strip evaluation pad does not appear white, the strip should be discarded.
- Test the first morning urine or urine that has been retained in the bladder for 4 or more hours. Urine must be freshly collected in a clean, dry container. The test strip may also be passed through the urine stream.
- If the urine cannot be tested within 1 hour, it should be refrigerated immediately, but brought to room temperature prior to testing.
- Dip the test area of the strip into the urine, and tap it against the edge of the cup to remove excess urine.
- Wait 1 minute and compare the test strip to the color on the vial of test strips. A pink discoloration is indicative of a positive test. Any color change that occurs after 2 minutes should be ignored.

Precautions with the Urinary Tract Infection Detection Kit

False negatives or positives may occur with the UTI Test Kit for several reasons:

- The kit requires acidic urine, so any medication that alkalinizes the urine can block the reaction and cause a false negative. Vitamin C, fruit juices, and antibiotics, for instance, can yield false negatives.
- Phenazopyridine, rifampin, and other medications that discolor the urine may interfere with test interpretation, causing false positives or an inability to interpret the results.
- A false negative might result for patients who consume inadequate nitrates such as those patients on vegetarian diets. Thus ingestion of meats is critical for a successful test.
- Some organisms cannot convert nitrate to nitrite, causing false negatives.

RESPONSE TO POSITIVE URINARY-TRACT-INFECTION-DETECTION-KIT RESULTS

The patient with a positive response to a urinary tract infection detection kit should make an appointment with a physician at his/her earliest convenience, so a physician can prescribe an appropriate antibiotic or antibacterial product.

ABUSE OF ILLICIT DRUGS

Abuse of illicit drugs, a widespread problem in the United States, is perhaps the most commonly missed diagnosis in adolescents.[43] Also, drug abuse presents striking problems in the workplace, as substance abusers are more accident-prone and more likely to steal from coworkers.[44,45]

PREVALENCE OF ABUSE OF ILLICIT DRUGS

Perhaps 13 million Americans use illegal drugs.[44] About 10 million of these are marijuana users and 1.6 million are cocaine users. As many as 20% of children aged 12 to 17 admit current drug abuse in surveys.[46] At least 25% of high-school seniors use illicit drugs monthly, and 10% use illicit drugs daily. One-half of high-school seniors admit use of marijuana, two-thirds admit use of alcohol in the past month, and 17% have used cocaine.[43]

EPIDEMIOLOGY OF ABUSE OF ILLICIT DRUGS

Drug abuse crosses all strata of society. It is common in the young, who often wish to develop a reputation for risk behaviors in their peer group and who see it as a way to escape problems with parental relationships. Athletes abuse drugs to gain a competitive edge.[47]

MANIFESTATIONS OF ABUSE OF ILLICIT DRUGS

Drug use in teenagers sometimes causes cough, sore throat, red eyes, and fatigue.[43] School performance and family relationships often deteriorate. The abuser might avoid family activities and refuse to carry out chores. He or she could lose motivation, become depressed, undergo mood swings at unpredictable times, and develop a "conning" (such as lying, deceiving, and covering up) behavior in an attempt to continue substance abuse. The patient's affect may be blunted or absent. Eventually, legal problems may develop such as stealing, vandalism, shoplifting, and traffic offenses. Frequently, the peer group changes to include others who also display these behaviors. Characteristically, abusers avoid eye contact, exhibiting sadness or emptiness, when drugs or alcohol are discussed. Denial can be vocal, angry, and vehement.

HOME DETECTION OF ILLICIT DRUGS

There are several methods to detect past usage of illicit drugs, including urine and hair tests.[48] Urine tests, widely used by industry, have several disadvantages. Urine tests only detect usage within the last 2 to 3 days for most illicit drugs and do not provide an index of the degree of drug abuse over time.[46,49] Urine collection is objectionable to many non–drug users because of its offensive nature. Also, urine samples may be adulterated or substituted by the devious subject. If a positive urine test result is disputed, another sample covering the same time frame cannot be collected at a later date. Finally, some patients may be unable to empty the bladder because of stress.[50]

Because hair traps within it substances that were in the blood at the time the hair was formed in its follicle, hair analysis is gaining in popularity as an alternative to urine testing.[49,51] The chemical residues in hair cannot be removed by washing, bleaching, or carrying out any other hair-care routine. Since hair grows about 0.5 inch per month, a 1.5-inch sample detects use of drugs within the last 90 days. This surveillance window yields valuable information regarding the long-term use of illicit substances.[52] Also, hair analysis does not require offensive collection techniques. If a positive hair test is disputed, another sample can be tested. Hair analysis detected six times more drug abusers in one study than urine testing, especially cocaine users.[49] There is only one home test kit for hair to detect abuse of illicit drugs widely available at this time. The directions below will apply to this kit, known as the PDT-90 Personal Drug Testing Service.

Mechanism of the Drug Abuse Detection Kit

The PDT-90 requires that a sample of hair from the tested person be sent to the manufacturer. The amount of hair required is sufficiently small that it does not cause a cosmetic problem.[49,53] The company conducts a radioimmunoassay analysis of the hair for marijuana, cocaine (including crack cocaine), opiates (including heroin), methamphetamine, and PCP.[46] Before a positive result is reported, the company confirms with gas chromatography/mass spectrometry.

Using the Drug Abuse Detection Kit

Several steps must be followed carefully in using the PDT-90[46]:

- Prepare the PDT-90 test kit materials. Locate the hair sample collection package, which contains a sample acquisition card, a strip of foil, and an integrity seal.
- Obtain the consent of the person to be tested to collect a hair sample. The manufacturer does not recommend obtaining a sample without the cooperation of the individual, although a parent may be forced to snip hair from a sleeping or unconscious child.
- Remove the strip of foil (about 4.5 inches long by 1.5 inches wide) from the sample collection package. Fold the foil lengthwise to create a trough.
- Use a sharp pair of safety scissors to take the sample. Locate a small lock of hair that is 1/2 inch wide and one strand deep when held flat across the finger (Fig. 48.7). If the hair is braided, it should be undone prior to collecting.
- Cut the hair close to the scalp.
- Place the hair sample into the foil trough, with the cut ends extending 1/4 inch beyond a slanted end of the foil. If the hair is short or curly, it may be easier to wrap the foil around the hair before cutting it.
- Press the sides of the foil trough together, so the hair sample is trapped inside. Remaining hair may be wrapped around the foil.
- Place the sample in the Sample Acquisition Card. Remove the PDT-90 Code Card, containing a toll-free number and a confidential code number.
- Place the integrity seal on the Sample Acquisition Card, date it, and initial the card in the space provided.
- Mail the Sample Acquisition Card in an enclosed, first-class, postage-paid, return envelope.
- Call the toll-free number after 5 business days to obtain the testing results.

Precautions with the Drug Abuse Detection Kit

Hair collected secretively from a hair brush may not be from the desired person. Also, only the parent or custodial guardian of a child should submit samples.

RESPONSE TO POSITIVE DRUG-ABUSE-DETECTION-KIT RESULTS

Should the person submitting a sample of hair be notified of a positive result, several activities are advisable (among others):

- An appointment with another lab should be made to confirm the results of the home test.

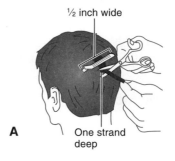
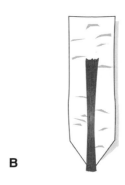
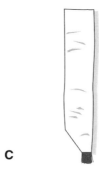

Figure 48.7. Using the PDT-90 drug-abuse detection kit. **A.** Hair sample should be 1/2 inch wide and one strand deep. **B.** Hair is placed in foil trough with the ends extending 1/4 inch. **C.** Sides of the trough are pressed together before sample is mailed to laboratory.

- If the person tested is a child, school authorities should be notified so the child can be observed for such activities as drug use during school hours or drug purchasing from known pushers.
- The child may need to be restricted in regard to after-school activities and visits with friends.
- An appointment with a family counselor might help the parents open lines of communication with the child.

ACQUIRED IMMUNODEFICIENCY SYNDROME (AIDS)

Acquired Immunodeficiency Syndrome (AIDS) is a medical condition often contracted through sexual activity. It is incurable and inevitably causes death. No vaccine is available at this time, and the medical regimens that have been instituted to control its progression are of variable help. For this reason much of the current public-health effort focuses on detection of patients who carry the virus that causes AIDS.

PREVALENCE OF AIDS

At least 1 million Americans are currently affected with type 1 human immunodeficiency virus (HIV-1), the causative agent of AIDS.[54] The silent nature of the initial infection allows victims to unknowingly spread the infection, particularly to sexual partners and those with whom they share apparatus for injecting illegal drugs. Eventual conversion of the carrier to AIDS signals the onset of the deadly disease. Detection of HIV-1 carriers allows them to modify their behaviors, which helps slow the epidemic.

EPIDEMIOLOGY OF AIDS

Certain population subgroups have experienced greater rises in cases of AIDS. The number of cases in females increased 10% in 1 year, as opposed to an increase of only 2.5% in men.[55] The problem is especially acute in minority females, with black-Americans and Hispanics making up 74% of females with AIDS, although they represent only 21% of total females.[55]

ETIOLOGY OF AIDS

AIDS is spread by contact with the blood or secretions of an infected individual. Sexual activity is a major method, but other patients are affected by sharing needles or through the injection of products such as blood fractions to treat hemophilia.

SELF-DETECTION OF AIDS

The FDA has undergone several changes of opinion regarding home testing for AIDS.[56] Initially the agency was concerned about the accuracy of the tests and the potentially deadly results of a false-negative test. (If a false negative were to occur, an infected patient could unwittingly spread the disease to uninfected sexual partners.) At this time the agency allows AIDS tests to be marketed in the hope that diagnosis will be easier and more accessible.[57] There are only two tests currently being marketed, the Home Access HIV-1 Test System and the Home Access Express HIV-1 Test System. (A test kit known as Confide was discontinued in 1997 because of poor sales.) The directions below refer to the Home Access products.

The company has produced "Silent Purchase Slips," which are 2.5″ × 2.5″ slips of paper that patients may find located by the products. The patient can tear off one slip and bring it to the pharmacist, indicating an intent to purchase either the Home Access or Home Access Express. These slips prevent patients from being forced to carry the product

through a busy pharmacy to the register. When patients present these slips, the pharmacist should discreetly obtain the product and immediately place it in a pharmacy bag to protect the purchaser from embarrassment. The pharmacist should also offer to counsel the patient regarding use of the kit, if the patient desires this service.

Mechanism of the HIV-1 Detection Kit

The Home Access kits use an initial test known as enzyme-linked immunoassay (ELISA) to test for antibodies to HIV-1. If the test is positive, the more specific immunofluorescence assay (IFA) is used. The accuracy matches that of professional tests.

Using the HIV-1 Detection Kit

The patient must correctly carry out several steps to obtain reliable results (Fig. 48.8)[58,59]:

- Locate the Blood Specimen Collection Card. Tear away the top sheet, which contains a confidential 11-digit Home Access Code Number.
- Read the informed-consent section of the booklet.
- Call the toll-free number included in the kit to register the

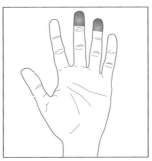

A. Preferred sites

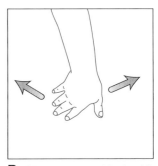

B. Shake back and forth while hand is hanging down.

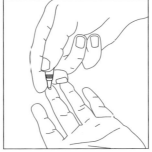

C. Trigger safety lancet.

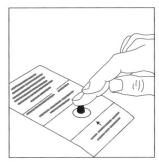

D. Allow blood to drop onto blood specimen collection card.

Figure 48.8. Using the Home Access HIV-1 detection kit. Patient **(A)** chooses soft pad of the middle or ring finger, **(B)** holds hand down and shakes it from side to side for 30 seconds, **(C)** triggers lancet, and **(D)** places drop of blood on the blood specimen collection card and then mails it to laboratory.

confidential 11-digit number. Making the call indicates that the patient has agreed to the informed-consent section of the booklet.

- Place the specimen collection kit on a clean, dry surface. The Blood Specimen Collection Card must be kept clean and dry.
- Wash and dry hands.
- Unfold the Blood Specimen Collection Card, exposing a printed circle where blood will be placed.
- Choose a puncture site on the soft pad of the fingertip. The little finger must not be used since sufficient blood may not be available. The middle or ring fingers are preferred. Callused areas should be avoided to ensure that an adequate amount of blood can be collected.
- Clean the puncture site with the alcohol pad included in the kit and dry with the gauze pad included in the kit.
- Hang hand by the side for 30 seconds and shake it back and forth vigorously several times to stimulate blood flow to the fingers.
- Place the hand on a table or countertop with the palm up to help avoid flinching or pulling away.
- Hold the lancet included in the kit between the first and second fingers of the other hand.
- Press the tip of the lancet against the target finger, using steady pressure to indent the skin in the selected location.
- Use the thumb to depress the lancet trigger, using steady pressure.
- Apply pressure to the finger near the puncture site. Allow large drops of blood to collect at the site. Use the thumb and first finger of the other hand to increase blood flow.
- Touch a large drop of blood to the circle of the Blood Specimen Collection Card. Additional drops may be placed around the edges of the primary drop to completely fill the circle.
- Examine the back of the card to ensure that blood has completely soaked through; if it has not, place more blood on the front of the card. If additional blood is needed, use the second lancet in the kit to create another puncture site.
- Place an adhesive bandage in the kit over the puncture site. Place the used lancet(s) in the lancet disposal container included in the kit.
- Write the Home Access Code Number on the Blood Specimen Collection Card.
- Allow 30 minutes for the blood to dry; place the Blood Specimen Collection Card inside the Specimen Return Pouch included in the kit.
- Seal the Specimen Return Pouch tightly and place it in a cardboard U.S. Mail envelope included in the kit (Home Access); or seal it in a cardboard envelope and place it in a FedEX Overnight envelope (Home Access Express).
- Call for results after 7 business days (Home Access) or 3 business days (Home Access Express).

Precautions with the HIV-1 Detection Kit

The HIV-1 Detection kit has several precautions associated with its use[58,59]:

- Hemophiliacs or patients taking anticoagulants should not use the kit.
- Lancets in the kit should only be used by the person testing himself or herself. Lancets should never be reused, and lancets used by another should never be used.
- Blood from the patient and that on the card to be mailed in should never be contacted by another person.
- If the blood specimen is not received within 10 days, it may not be tested because of perishability.
- The company has not investigated use of the test kit in patients under the age of 18 years.
- There are false negatives and false positives associated with the use of the kit.

RESPONSE TO POSITIVE HIV-1–DETECTION-KIT RESULTS

If a positive result is obtained with the HIV-1 detection kit, the patient should make an immediate appointment with a physician to order a confirming laboratory test. If the patient does not wish to do this, he or she should refrain from contact with other patients in which blood or other secretions might infect those patients.

HYPERCHOLESTEROLEMIA

Cardiovascular disease (CVD) has been identified as the world's leading public health issue by the World Health Organization.[60] Cholesterol is a major risk factor for CVD and for coronary heart disease (CHD), which is the leading cause of death in the United States.[61,62]

PREVALENCE OF HYPERCHOLESTEROLEMIA

As many as 35% of Americans have cholesterol levels that exceed those deemed safe.[63]

ETIOLOGY OF HYPERCHOLESTEROLEMIA

The majority of cholesterol is produced by the liver.[63] However, a certain amount is absorbed from foods rich in cholesterol such as eggs and whole-milk products.

MANIFESTATIONS OF HYPERCHOLESTEROLEMIA

Patients whose hypercholesterolemia presents the greatest risk are those who already have coronary heart disease or other atherosclerotic disease (e.g., carotid artery disease).[63] Total cholesterol is a combined figure reflecting two subtypes of lipoproteins. One, high-density lipoprotein (HDL), is known as "good cholesterol" since high levels denote reduced risk of CHD. However, low-density lipoproteins (LDLs) and very low density lipoproteins (VLDLs) both confer increased risk of CHD.

SELF-MONITORING HYPERCHOLESTEROLEMIA

The National Cholesterol Education Program recommends cholesterol and HDL measurements for all adults aged 20 or older at least once every 5 years and suggests that patients with high cholesterol levels have further evaluation and treatment.[64] Cholesterol values of less than 200 mg/dL are optimal. A value of 200 to 239 is borderline high, and a value of 240 or more is high. An HDL measurement of 35 mg/dL or less is too low and constitutes a CHD risk factor.[63]

(tip) Patients with borderline high or high cholesterol values or low HDL values should see a physician promptly. Effective interventions to lower cholesterol can have a profound impact on health. If cholesterol is lowered by 10%, the risk of coronary heart disease is lowered by 20%, and the risk of a fatal second myocardial infarction is lowered by 12%.[62,65]

Mechanism of the Cholesterol Monitoring Kit

At this time there is only one cholesterol monitoring kit available in the United States, the CholesTrak Home Cholesterol Test. The CholesTrak Kit is designed to meet the standards of the National Cholesterol Education Program.[1,66] Borderline high cholesterol levels will give a positive response to ensure that patients seek medical advice.

The CholesTrak test device is referred to as a "cassette." It uses a progressive enzymatic reaction to measure total cholesterol.[67] Two enzymes, cholesterol oxidase and cholesterol esterase, convert cholesterol to hydrogen peroxide. A second enzyme, horseradish peroxidase, reacts with hydrogen peroxide to produce a visible color band.

FOCUS ON...

BLOOD PRESSURE MONITORING

At least 50 million Americans are affected with hypertension.[70] Its importance as a predictor of cardiac events is well established.[71] However, physician-conducted blood-pressure readings have several disadvantages. The patient must pay for a physician appointment, the patient must have transportation to visit a physician's office (which may involve taking time off from work), and the results may not reflect actual blood pressures at home (some patients experience elevated blood pressure when it is performed by a professional—a phenomenon known as the "white coat" syndrome).[72]

Blood pressures performed by the patient at home do not have these disadvantages, being fairly inexpensive. They also allow the patient to take several blood pressures daily, in home or at work, under a variety of different conditions (e.g., when resting or exercising, at bedtime, after a meal). This increased accuracy provides a much better picture of the patient's diurnal blood pressure variations.

Home monitoring of blood pressure (HBP) also may increase the patient's compliance with therapy as s/he sees the actual effects of noncompliance on blood pressure.

The major questions about HBP monitoring is its accuracy, with HBP values being generally 10 mm Hg below office measurements. HBP is affected by such factors as cuff size, cuff position, and measurement technique (when an aneroid device is used), as well as the type of device used.

Home devices commonly sold for HBP are of several types[72]:

- Aneroid HBP monitors are the more accurate of the two common types. They also are less expensive, selling for $20 to $30.
- Electronic HBP monitors (also known as "digital" monitors since they provide a readout on a screen) are less accurate than aneroids, and they are more expensive, selling for $40 to $100. Their advantage is ease of use.
- Finger HBP monitors allow the patient to slip a small cuff over the finger. However, they suffer from several shortcomings: they cost over $100, their accuracy is impaired (since the finger is a longer distance from the heart, and the patient may also suffer impaired circulation), and they require the user to hold the finger at the exact level of the heart.

For the patient to correctly monitor blood pressures at home, pharmacists should advise them of several points[72]:

- Do not take the blood pressure just after completing physical activity.
- Do not continue to talk, smoke, or move about during a measurement.
- Do not discontinue, decrease, or increase any medications based on a home blood-pressure test result. Rather, contact a physician if the measurements are excessively low or high.
- Keep a written diary to note the date and time of day of each measurement.
- Hearing-impaired patients may not be able to hear heart sounds through an aneroid monitor; perhaps a digital device would be preferable.
- Digital models are affected by abnormal heart rates.
- Choose a cuff size that is appropriate for the arm size (e.g., regular, extra large, or pediatric).
- Have the blood pressure monitor checked at least once yearly by a physician to ensure continued accuracy.
- Rest quietly for 3 to 5 minutes before beginning the measurement.
- The arm should be raised to the level of the heart; when properly placed, the HBP cuff should be 1 inch above the elbow's inner bend.

Using the Cholesterol Monitoring Kit

Patients must first obtain a blood sample, placing two drops in a well at the bottom of the cassette. A blood filtration system separates the plasma from whole blood. After 2 minutes, the patient activates the enzymatic reaction by pulling a tab on the side of the cassette.[3] As the test develops, a purple color advances up a measuring device that resembles a thermometer.[63] The height of the peak of the color band is compared with a chart. The device measures cholesterol in a range from 125 to 400 mg/dL, producing a color change within 12 to 15 minutes.[68] The device can only be used once.

Precautions with the Cholesterol Monitoring Kit

Many variables affect serum cholesterol such as stress, illness, diet, exercise, and pregnancy.[1] For this reason patients are urged to test frequently rather than accept the results of one test.[69]

RESPONSE TO POSITIVE CHOLESTEROL-MONITORING-KIT RESULTS

The patient whose cholesterol measures high should make an appointment with a physician to have a physician-ordered cholesterol test. If this is also positive, the physician can supply information on diet and exercise to reduce the risk of cholesterol-related diseases.

OTHER HOME TESTING PRODUCTS

Home test kits may be forthcoming for breast cancer, streptococcal pharyngitis, and cervical carcinoma. Although the FDA is extremely careful in considering the ramifications of these kits prior to allowing their marketing, pharmacists can expect to see some of these self-test kits in the coming decade.

While this chapter is concerned primarily with home test kits, the patient may also purchase other devices that allow home monitoring of certain conditions such as home blood-pressure monitoring devices. (See "Blood Pressure Monitoring.")

SUMMARY

Consumers desire greater responsibility over their health care today. Home testing kits allow patients greater freedom in the medical process. The patient reads some kits directly; with other kits the patient self-collects a specimen, which then must be sent to the manufacturer for testing. (Self-testing for diabetes is discussed in Chapter 46.)

With home pregnancy tests patients test their urine for human chorionic gonadotropin (hCG) produced during pregnancy, perhaps permitting them to detect pregnancy earlier than if they were required to visit a physician. Early detection allows patients to modify behaviors that increase risks to the fetus such as smoking, consuming alcohol, and abusing drugs.

Ovulation prediction tests detect the urinary luteinizing hormone (LH), which surges prior to ovulation. This allows a couple with compromised fertility to time several acts of intercourse around the window of maximal fertility of the ovum, increasing the chances of conception.

Fecal blood detection kits provide a means to detect occult blood in the stool. Patients are often quite reluctant to submit to either a digital rectal exam or a colonoscopy. Home test kits minimize embarrassment, so patients will be more likely to test for—and thus detect—colorectal cancer. The earlier a physician is seen, the more likely treatment for colorectal cancer can be instituted.

Urinary tract infections (UTIs) are experienced by a large part of the population. Once symptoms begin, patients might wish to verify a UTI prior to contacting the physician. The nonprescription, self-test product detects urinary nitrite that has been produced by bacteria in the urinary tract.

Abuse of illicit drugs is a major national problem. Drug abuse can be detected by collecting a hair sample and sending it to a lab for analysis. With early knowledge of drug abuse, parents or caregivers can obtain counseling and other professional help for children, as well as watch their activities more closely.

AIDS is a growing problem in the United States. Two home AIDS test kits permit concerned patients to draw a blood specimen, which is sent to the manufacturer for testing. The results are obtained confidentially a short time later. With early detection of AIDS, infected individuals can modify risky behaviors (e.g., unprotected sexual intercourse and sharing needles while injecting illegal drugs).

High cholesterol is a major risk factor for cardiovascular heart disease. Lowering serum cholesterol can reduce the risk of deadly events such as myocardial infarction. The home cholesterol measurement kit provides a total cholesterol measurement. Patients who note an unacceptably high value might be prompted to visit a physician or dietitian to obtain advice on dietary modification or to make a physician appointment to discuss the use of cholesterol-lowering agents.

Home blood-pressure monitoring is an important means of monitoring hypertension. Pharmacists should advise patients in the purchase of home blood-pressure-monitoring devices and should discuss different measures to help increase the accuracy of their measurements.

Home testing kits are a trend that has grown in unexpected areas since the first home pregnancy test was introduced in 1977. Pharmacists should expect new and innovative products during the next decade.

AT THE COUNTER

A young couple is examining the home pregnancy tests with evident confusion. The pharmacist approaches, and the male states, "Why are there so many of these things. Which one is best?"

Interview/Patient Assessment

The pharmacist determines that the female's period should have started 2 to 3 days earlier, and she is wondering if she might be pregnant. She wants a product that is easy to use.

Pharmacist's Analysis

1. Are pregnancy test kits markedly different from each other?

2. Will the kits work this early in her pregnancy?
3. What directions should she be given?

Patient Counseling

The different home pregnancy test kits are very similar to each other. All detect pregnancy as early as the first day after a missed period, and she could use any product at this time. Some are available in a two-test option, so a negative test can be followed up a day or two later with the second test if the period has not yet begun. The tests are simple to use. The patient may need to do nothing more than expose a test area to urine flow and wait a specified time to read the test for a positive result. Several different kits should be pointed out to her, allowing her to choose a kit based on ease of use and cost.

References

1. Rheinstein PH, Thomas A. Home test kits and monitors. Am Fam Physician 52:293, 1995.
2. Newton GD. Monoclonal antibody-based self-testing products. Am Pharm NS33:22, 1993.
3. Munroe WP. Home diagnostic kits. Am Pharm NS34:50, 1994.
4. Hicks JM. Home testing: To do or not to do? Clin Chem 39:7, 1993.
5. Farley D. In-home tests make health care easier. FDA Consumer 28(10):25, 1994.
6. Daviaud J, et al. Reliability and feasibility of pregnancy home-use tests: Laboratory validation and diagnostic evaluation by 638 volunteers. Clin Chem 39:53, 1993.
7. Cole LA, et al. Selecting human chorionic gonadotropin immunoassays: Consideration of cross-reacting molecules in first-trimester pregnancy serum and urine. Am J Obstet Gynecol 168:1580, 1993.
8. Caiola SM. The pharmacist and home-use pregnancy tests. Am Pharm NS32:57, 1992.
9. Lewis R. Biotech devices. FDA Consumer 27(1):15, 1993.
10. Package Insert, 1 Step e•p•t: 1996.
11. Package Insert, Fact Plus One Step: 1996.
12. Package Insert, 1 Easy Step Advance: 1995.
13. Package Insert, Clearblue Easy: 1996.
14. Nordenberg T. Overcoming infertility. FDA Consumer 31(1):18, 1997.
15. Bischof P, Bianchi PG, Campana A. Comparison of a rapid, quantitative and automated assay for urinary luteinizing hormone (LH), with an LH detection test, for the prediction of ovulation. Hum Reprod 6:515, 1991.
16. Royston P. Identifying the fertile phase of the human menstrual cycle. Stat Med 10:221, 1991.
17. Miller PB, Soules MR. The usefulness of a urinary LH kit for ovulation prediction during menstrual cycles of normal women. Obstet Gynecol 87:13, 1996.
18. Martinez AR, et al. Reliability of home urinary LH tests for timing of insemination: A consumer's study. Hum Reprod 7:751, 1992.
19. Gossel TA, Mahalik MP. Ovulation and pregnancy testing products. US Pharm 18(7):37, 1993.
20. Moghissi KS. Ovulation detection. Endocrinol Metab Clin North Am 21:39, 1992.
21. Package Insert, First Response Ovulation Predictor Test: 1991.
22. Package Insert, Conceive 1-Step Ovulation Predictor: 1992.
23. Package Insert, Clearplan Easy Ovulation Predictor: (undated).
24. Farley D. Do-it-yourself medical testing. FDA Consumer 20(1):22, 1986.
25. Oldenski RJ, Flareau BJ. Colorectal cancer screening. Prim Care 19:621, 1992.
26. Pray WS. Understanding colonoscopy. US Pharm 18(7):26, 1993.
27. Gray SL. Fecal occult blood testing for colorectal cancer. Am Pharm NS32:50, 1992.
28. Gane EJ, Lane MR. Colonoscopy in unexplained lower gastrointestinal bleeding. NZ Med J 105:31, 1992.
29. Kronborg O. Population screening for colorectal cancer, the goals and means. Ann Med 23:373, 1991.
30. Park SI, Saxe JC, Weesner RE. Does use of the Coloscreen Self-Test improve patient compliance with fecal occult blood screening? Am J Gastroenterol 88:1391, 1993.
31. Weinrich SP, et al. Knowledge of colorectal cancer among older persons. Cancer Nurs 15:322, 1992.
32. Gregorio DI, Lolachi P, Hansen H. Detecting colorectal cancer with a large scale fecal occult blood testing program. Public Health Rep 107:331, 1992.
33. Package Insert, ColoCare: 1997.
34. Package Insert, EZ Detect: (undated).
35. Bacheller CD, Bernstein JM. Urinary tract infections. Med Clin North Am 81:719, 1997.
36. Wisinger DB. Urinary tract infection. Postgrad Med 100:229, 1996.

37. Hooton TM, et al. A prospective study of risk factors for symptomatic urinary tract infection in young women. N Engl J Med 335:468, 1996.
38. Wan J, Kaplinsky R, Greenfield S. Toilet habits of children evaluated for urinary tract infection. J Urol 154:797, 1995.
39. Yoshikawa TT, Norman DC. Approach to fever and infection in the nursing home. J Am Geriatr Soc 44:74, 1996.
40. Forland M. Urinary tract infection. Postgrad Med 93:71, 1993.
41. Nygaard IE, Johnson JM. Urinary tract infections in elderly women. Am Fam Physician 53:175, 1996.
42. Package Insert, UTI Urinary Tract Infection Urine Test Strips: 1996.
43. Macdonald DI. Diagnosis and treatment of adolescent substance abuse. Curr Prob Pediatr 19:395, 1989.
44. Floren AE. Urine drug screening and the family physician. Am Fam Physician 49:1441, 1994.
45. Walsh DC, Elinson L, Gostin L. Worksite drug testing. Annu Rev Public Health 13:197, 1992.
46. Package Insert, PDT-90 Personal Drug Testing Service: 1997.
47. Landry GL, Kokotailo PK. Drug screening in the athletic setting. Curr Prob Pediatr 24:344, 1994.
48. Fretthold DW. Drug-testing methods and reliability. J Psychoactive Drugs 22:419, 1990.
49. DuPont RL, Baumgartner WA. Drug testing by urine and hair analysis: Complementary features and scientific issues. Forensic Sci Int 70:63, 1995.
50. Klonoff DC, Jurow AH. Acute water intoxication as a complication of urine drug testing in the workplace. JAMA 265:84, 1991.
51. Henderson GL. Mechanisms of drug incorporation into hair. Forensic Sci Int 63:19, 1993.
52. Moeller MR, Fey P, Sachs H. Hair analysis as evidence in forensic cases. Forensic Sci Int 63:43, 1993.
53. Bost RO. Hair analysis-perspectives and limits of a proposed forensic method of proof: A review. Forensic Sci Int 63:31, 1993.
54. Frank AP, et al. Anonymous HIV testing using home collection and telemedicine counseling. Arch Intern Med 157:309, 1997.
55. Segal M. Women and AIDS. FDA Consumer 27(8):9, 1993.
56. Beall DP, Whyte JJ. Now that we can, should we? Investigating the wisdom of home HIV testing (Editorial). Md Med J 44:355, 1995.
57. Kubic M. New ways to prevent AIDS. FDA Consumer 31(1):7, 1997.
58. Package Insert: Home Access, 1996.
59. Package Insert: Home Access Express, 1996.
60. Seccombe DW. Cholesterol testing—A lifestyle focus for the nineties. Clin Biochem 26:17, 1993.
61. Anon. State-specific changes in cholesterol screening—Behavioral risk factor surveillance system, 1988–1991.
62. Yusuf S, et al. Primary and secondary prevention of myocardial infarction and strokes: An update of randomly allocated, controlled trials. J Hypertens Suppl 11:S61, 1993.
63. Larkin M. Lowering cholesterol. FDA Consumer 28(2):27, 1994.
64. Hulley SB, et al. Should we be measuring blood cholesterol levels in young adults? JAMA 269:1416, 1993.
65. Flaker GC, Singh VN. Prevention of myocardial reinfarction. Postgrad Med 94:94, 1993.
66. McNamara JR, et al. Multicenter evaluation of a patient-administered test for blood glucose measurement. Prev Med 25:583, 1996.
67. Allen MP, et al. A noninstrumented quantitative test system and its application for determining cholesterol concentration in whole blood. Clin Chem 36:1591, 1990.
68. Anon. First OTC test kit for blood cholesterol. FDA Consumer 27(5):4, 1993.
69. Noble D. Home test for cholesterol. Anal Chem 65:1037A, 1993.
70. Merrick RD, et al. Factors influencing the accuracy of home blood pressure measurement. South Med J 90:1110, 1997.
71. Sakuma M, et al. Reproducibility of home blood pressure measurements over a 1-year period. Am J Hypertens 10(7 Pt 1):798, 1997.
72. Kriesand T, Cohen IM. Home blood pressure monitoring. Am Fam Physician 54:537, 1996.

Precautions in Self-Care

AT THE COUNTER

A male in his early 20s asks the pharmacist for help with an ingrown toenail. He is in obvious pain, grimacing and limping when walking.

Interview/Patient Assessment

The patient relates a history of ingrown toenails dating back to high school, when he began wearing western-style boots. At first, he took care of the problem by himself, using scissors to excise the toenail. However, this time he says he waited too late and cannot get the toenail out. He remembers hearing about a product that claimed to relieve ingrown toenails and wonders if it will help him remove the toenail on his own.

Pharmacist's Analysis

1. What is the status of products for ingrown toenails?
2. Should the patient be allowed to excise the toenail on his own?

3. What risk factors might this patient modify to help prevent recurrences?

Patient Counseling

Ingrown toenail is not a problem the patient can remedy without professional care. Attempts to remove the toenail could leave a piece of nail embedded in the skin, which in turn could act as a focus for continuing debility and infection. The nonprescription product, misleadingly trade-named Outgro, cannot allow the toenail to "outgrow." The pharmacist should urge him to make an appointment with a podiatrist or physician, either of which may opt to surgically remove the ingrown nail section; in addition, an antibiotic might be prescribed to help combat infection in the nail. The pharmacist also should warn the patient that tight toe boxes such as those in "cowboy" boots are a significant risk factor. Finally, the pharmacist should counsel him on the method of cutting the toenails straight across, rather than tapering them downward toward the nail tips.

Retail pharmacy is eternally trapped in an uncomfortable dichotomy. Are retail pharmacists medical professionals or merchants? Are the two roles mutually exclusive? Pharmacists can often fulfill both roles simultaneously by recommending safe and effective products that also provide a good profit margin. However, the availability—and demand—for unproven therapies (often high-profit-margin products) creates a substantial challenge for pharmacists.

Many conditions must be seen by a physician, dentist, or other professional, requiring pharmacists to refer patients and sacrifice potential profit from nonprescription product sales. Products that purport to be effective for conditions that should not be self-treated may be sold by pharmacists, despite clear indications from the FDA that they are unsafe. Unfortunately, pharmacists more interested in profit than professional ethics may choose to sell these products, despite lack of evidence of safety and/or efficacy. In a landmark investigative feature, reporters from a prestigious American news magazine scanned pharmacy shelves and found many such products, a fact used to issue a scathing indictment against pharmacy in general.[1] For example, although the spokesperson for a major chain claimed that it would not sell banned products, reporters had purchased those very products from the chain.

Many articles in pharmacy journals promote products that lack proof of safety and/or efficacy. Other professionals have taken notice of these ethical dilemmas. In one case a registered dietitian protested a magazine's article claiming that pharmacists should become alternative nutritional practitioners to make an additional $3000 to $5000 monthly.[2] The

dietitian characterized this blatant appeal to the business side of pharmacy as a "breach of professional ethics." (See "Pharmacy Ethics.")

In this era of professional triage, the retail pharmacist must choose between self-interest and patient care. Pharmacists committed to providing optimal care to patients should be aware of conditions that must be referred and should be familiar with the dangerous and/or ineffective therapies that are currently being promoted to patients.

PART 1: CONDITIONS THAT SHOULD NOT BE SELF-TREATED

For various reasons, consumers assume that serious conditions are self-treatable. Misleading product trade names and seductive advertising campaigns are responsible for some of these misperceptions. In most cases the FDA OTC review has put an end to these potentially dangerous situations, but pharmacists continually must address such questions as, "Where is the Q-Vel for leg cramps?" and "I need Outgro for my ingrown toenail."

Part 1 of this chapter addresses several conditions that should be referred to other professionals for evaluation. These specific conditions are included because products lacking evidence of safety and/or efficacy have been promoted for them for decades. In addition, this textbook mentions conditions that should not be self-treated in several other chapters such as toothache (see Chapter 4, Oral Problems) and serious otic conditions (e.g., ear pain; see Chapter 28, Otic Conditions).

NAUSEA/VOMITING

For many years vomiting was the advertised indication for a popular product containing phosphorated carbohydrate (e.g., Emetrol), a claim that has never been proven to the satisfaction of the FDA. The manufacturer has changed the labeling so it now asserts effectiveness for nausea—also an unproven claim as of this writing.

Nausea, the feeling that one is about to vomit, usually arises from the throat and stomach.[5,6] Nausea may be accompanied by hypersalivation, tachycardia, and increased swallowing. Vomiting is a forceful oral expulsion of stomach contents.[5] Both are thought to protect the human from ingested poisons. Nausea serves as an early warning to stop eating a food that the body perceives as toxic. Nausea also produces a learned aversion to the food so that it is rejected when seen, smelled, or tasted in the future. Vomiting removes the material from the stomach prior to its full absorption to limit the extent of toxin exposure.

Nausea is unpleasant but harmless. However, vomiting can produce esophageal tears and hemorrhage, rib fracture, gastric herniation, and muscular strain.[5] Consequently, vomiting should not be allowed to continue unchecked. **⚠ *Aspirating vomitus can cause death.*** Patients who aspirate vomitus require swift medical intervention.

Vomiting is not a medical condition in its own right, but a symptom of underlying pathology. It is seen as a symptom of serious medical conditions such as thyrotoxicosis, acquired immune deficiency syndrome (AIDS), and toxic shock syndrome and is an adverse reaction of numerous medications (e.g., digitalis and chemotherapeutic agents).[7–10] Vomiting also may indicate pregnancy. Vomiting, too, may be self-induced as part of the bulimia syndrome. Therefore, underlying causes must be explored by recommending physician referral. Merely suppressing the symptom is counterproductive and allows the primary condition to continue unrecognized, as happened with a series of patients who were given dimenhydrinate for vomiting: use of dimenhydrinate delayed

---

FOCUS ON...

"PHARMACY ETHICS"

Pharmacy has long been concerned with the problem of medical treatments whose worth is unproven. As early as 1848, the Philadelphia College of Pharmacy agreed that certain principles should govern the conduct of pharmacists. Among them was "Whilst the College does not at present feel authorized to require its members to abandon the sale of secret or quack medicines, they earnestly recommend the propriety of discouraging their employment, when called upon for an opinion as to their merits."[3]

The 1852 Code of Ethics of the American Pharmaceutical Association admonished members to "discountenance quackery and dishonorable competition," while the 1922 version urged members to "discourage the use of objectionable nostrums."[3] The latter further noted, "The Pharmacist should hold the health and safety of his patrons to be of first consideration; he should make no attempt to prescribe or treat diseases or strive to sell drugs or remedies of any kind simply for the sake of profit. . . . He should not accept agencies for objectionable nostrums nor allow his name to be used in connection with advertisements or correspondence for furthering their sale."[3]

These views continued through the 1952, 1969, and 1981 revisions of the APhA Code of Ethics. The latest American Pharmaceutical Association Code of Ethics, adopted in 1994, states the following: " . . . a pharmacist has moral obligations in response to the gift of trust received from society. In return for this gift, a pharmacist promises to help individuals achieve optimum benefit from their medications, to be committed to their welfare, and to maintain their trust." The 1994 Code of Ethics continues: "A pharmacist places concern for the well-being of the patient at the center of professional practice." "A pharmacist has a duty to tell the truth and to act with conviction of conscience."[3]

State pharmacy organizations may also address the issue of ethics in sales of unproven products. For instance, the 1997 Oklahoma Pharmacy Lawbook contains this statement, "[The pharmacist] will not lend his support or his name to the promotion or exploitation of objectionable or unworthy products, nor will he participate in any advertising or promotional program which would tend to lower the honor and dignity of his profession."[4]

While some Codes of Ethics are more specific than others, all speak to some extent about dealing honestly with patients. When certain therapies lack proof of safety or efficacy, the pharmacist should honestly communicate this fact to the patients, who are then better informed prior to their purchase.

---

diagnosis of such conditions as asthma, pelvic inflammatory disease, and urinary tract infection by as much as 12 hours.[11]

Parents often wish to treat nausea and vomiting in infants and children. The differential diagnosis varies by age. For instance, for children from birth to 1 month, congenital disorders, reflux, sepsis, diaphragmatic hernia, malrotation, and motility disorders should be considered.[11–13] For children from 1 month to 2 years, colic, gastroenteritis, appendicitis, adhesions, and malrotation are simply a few of the possible causes.

Motion sickness is the sole self-treatable cause of vomiting. The pharmacist can easily recognize this etiology through judicious questioning because of its close relationship to travel, whether by automobile, boat, or plane. (See Chapter 6, Motion Sickness.)

NOCTURNAL LEG CRAMPS

Nocturnal leg cramps are usually felt in the lower leg.[14] (Leg cramps are also known as "charley horses.") This painful condition is often produced when patients awaken and stretch. The calf shortens as the toes are extended, which produces an involuntary knotting of the muscle. Nocturnal leg cramps may be sporadic or so frequent that they disrupt sleep. The cramps are more common in patients who exercise without carrying out warm-up activities and in patients who are overweight.

🔵 *To stop the cramping, the patient should stand on both feet and raise the front of the foot on the affected leg while supporting weight on the heel.* The patient may also remain in bed and pull the toes up smoothly toward the knee. Both interventions stretch the calf muscle.

Several years ago, a number of products containing quinine were alleged to be effective for nocturnal leg cramps. Their widespread advertising continued for many years until the FDA finally banned the sale of all nonprescription quinine-containing products because of the risk of severe toxicity. Prescription products may eventually be removed from the market also.

Pharmacists can teach patients preventive exercises for nocturnal leg cramps:

1. With shoes off, stand facing a wall 2 to 3 feet away.
2. With arms extended, lean toward the wall.
3. Keeping heels in contact with the floor, bend arms to lean farther into the wall, until a pulling sensation is felt in each calf.
4. Hold the position for 10 seconds, and then straighten arms.
5. Rest 5 seconds.
6. Repeat the stretch several times to finish the first session.
7. Repeat the exercise session three times a day.

BOILS

The **furuncle** (boil) is a subcutaneous abscess around a hair follicle.[15] Its causative agent is usually *Staphylococcus aureus*. (Patients often inoculate themselves through organisms residing in the nasal passages.) The boil continues to mature until it discharges a plug, which allows the pain and inflammation to regress quickly. A boil may extend beneath the skin, however, and infect other sites, which could result in the formation of a lesion known as a carbuncle. Patients with either furuncles or carbuncles should be referred to a physician for specific antibiotic or antibacterial therapy. Products (e.g., Boil-Ease) were advertised to cure boils for many years, but advertising now promises only to relieve the pain of boils. However, pharmacists should refer patients to a physician

🔵 rather than recommending this product. *Nonprescription therapy for boils is ineffective and can prolong the time until a patient consults a physician.*[16]

NAIL FUNGI

When fungi infect the nail, they cannot be treated with nonprescription products (see Chapter 35, Fungal Skin Infec-

tions). One product (Fungi-Nail) was advertised for years as being effective in curing fungal nail infections; although it no longer makes that claim, it has retained its misleading name. Patients with fungal nail infections should be referred.

THUMB/FINGER SUCKING

Thumb or finger sucking can occur with patients of all ages, from the fetus to adulthood.[17] Usually, children discontinue the practice by the age of 4 years because of peer pressure. However, some continue later, which can result in open bite, overbite, narrowing of the dental arches, temporomandibular joint disorder (TMJ), abnormal facial growth, and incorrect lip and tongue postures. (These conditions are more likely if thumb or finger sucking continues after the permanent teeth have erupted.) The practice can also cause nail infections, irritant dermatitis, and rotational finger deformities. Products have been sold for many years that claim to stop thumb sucking (e.g., Thum). They contain bitter chemicals—such as cayenne pepper, sucrose octaacetate, or dentatonium benzoate—which are applied to the preferred thumb and/or finger(s). These bitter chemicals supposedly produce an aversion to placing the digit(s) in the mouth, but have never been proven effective. While the ingredients are not dangerous, patients should be referred rather than allowed to use them.

NAILBITING

Nailbiting technically is an intentional act of self-mutilation, which is usually free of long-lasting effects.[17] However, patients may experience **paronychia** (inflammation of the tissues adjacent to the nail), chronic subungual infection, periungual warts, and/or **pterygium** (an abnormal growth of the cuticle over the proximal nail plate). In extreme cases the nail may be lost. In addition, the teeth may undergo apical root resorption and small fractures can occur in the incisors as a result of chronic, excessive pressure. Products sold for nailbiting—the same products as those for thumb/finger sucking—are ineffective for this condition. Therefore, patients who wish to stop nailbiting should be referred to a physician.

INGROWN TOENAIL

Ingrown nails are the most frequently seen nail condition.[18] Common in adolescent males, they result from continual lateral pressure on the toes, which causes excessive contact between the edge of the nail and the soft tissues of the nail fold. Because the nail cannot fit normally into its groove, a callus forms, which further tightens the nail's growth space. The nail is forced to perforate the nail groove as it grows in this confined area. Ingrown nails can cause pain, inflammation, bacterial infection, ulceration, and difficulty in walking.

Patients with ingrown nails must visit a physician or podiatrist for surgical treatment. Nonprescription products (e.g.,

Outgro) claimed to help the ingrown toenail grow correctly, but have not been proven effective. The indication has been changed by the manufacturer to relief of pain of ingrown toenail, but the pharmacist should refer patients rather than recommending this product.

Patients may prevent ingrown nails by not trimming toenails shorter than the tips of the toes. Furthermore, shoes should fit properly to avoid the formation of the callus that begins the ingrown toenail. Shoes that push toes together are especially troublesome.

PART 2: DANGEROUS AND/OR INEFFECTIVE THERAPIES

Legitimate medicine applies a standard methodology to determine the safety and effectiveness of medications and therapies. These standard procedures must be fully utilized before prescription products are allowed to reach the market. Legitimate nonprescription products and devices also must undergo this intense scrutiny prior to marketing. The standard procedures follow accepted and conventional methods of scientific inquiry:

- Safety of medications must be demonstrated by administration first to animals or other models and then to healthy humans and to humans with the medical condition to be treated.
- Effectiveness of medications must be demonstrated through the use of multiple studies employing double-blinding and placebo controls; the studies must have sufficient sample sizes to ensure that properly applied statistical methodologies demonstrate a significant benefit.

Properly applying these scientific standards yields a body of prescription medications and therapies that physicians can prescribe with confidence and another body of nonprescription products and devices that the pharmacist can recommend with confidence. No medication or therapy is without possible adverse reactions, of course. Thus physicians must balance risk to the patient to potential benefit when prescribing. Likewise, pharmacists must also balance potential risk to potential benefit when recommending nonprescription products for self-treatable disorders.

On the other side of the counter, there are many thousands of products and devices that do not meet any standards of legitimate science, but are sold today in pharmacies; in nonpharmacy retail outlets; by mail via the Internet; and through person-to-person, multilevel, marketing schemes. Their efficacy has never been studied with properly controlled scientific scrutiny. Further, their safety has never been fully assessed. Although some of these products and devices might survive acceptable tests of safety and effectiveness, many would not. Without scientific evidence of safety and effectiveness, it is ethical and prudent to avoid them.

The practice of recommending therapies of unproven

safety and/or efficacy is often referred to as "quackery" by medical professionals, and those who promote and recommend these questionable products and devices are often referred to as "quacks" (one who pretends to be able to cure a disease or health problem).[19] Those who recommend and sell these therapies often do so under the guise of "alternative medicine" or "complementary medicine."

This chapter lists and describes representative, common, dangerous, and/or ineffective therapies. Unfortunately, this selection only scratches the surface. For each example listed, hundreds of others are offered to the public.

THE CONSEQUENCES OF USING DANGEROUS AND/OR INEFFECTIVE THERAPIES

While selling dangerous and/or ineffective therapies can enrich sellers, it can negatively affect victims in numerous ways.

Economic Losses

Worldwide, many people turn to unproven therapies (estimates range to 50%).[20,21] In the United States, an estimated 34% of adults use unconventional medical therapies and 3% choose herbal medicines.[20] Americans make hundreds of millions of visits each year to alternative care practitioners at a cost as high as 100 billion dollars.[19,22] These figures exceed the annual number of visits to primary-care physicians in the United States and also the costs of all hospitalizations in this country.

Direct Hazards

Therapies lacking full legitimate scientific evaluation present many health hazards to unwary patients, resulting from toxicities and drug-nutrient interactions.[23] For example, a 17-year-old female diagnosed with herpes simplex keratouveitis of the right eye and a visual acuity of 20/30 was prescribed tapering doses of prednisolone ophthalmic drops.[24] However, a friend suggested that she discontinue legitimate therapy and begin using an herbal ophthalmic drop sold by a local herbalist. She experienced pain and redness while using the herbal drops, and a checkup after 2 weeks revealed that her visual acuity had decreased to 20/200 and that she had developed a large corneal ulcer. The herbal ophthalmic drop was found to be contaminated with *Klebsiella* and *Pseudomonas*. Its "active ingredients" were euphrasia and plantain, two herbs with no scientifically demonstrated benefit in treating ophthalmic problems. Eventually, with legitimate therapy her visual acuity improved to 20/60, but did not match the pretreatment levels; she retained extensive scarring.

Many other examples of dangerous products and devices and their associated hazards will be provided in this chapter.

Indirect Hazards

Ineffective products may also be indirectly hazardous because they can give a false sense of security to patients. Many patients turn to unproven products rather than to legitimate medical care because of advertising claims, friends' recommendations, and reluctance or inability to seek medical attention.[25] Use of ineffective products and/or devices can allow a tumor to continue to grow, for instance, or a serious underlying disease to proceed unchecked. By the time the deluded patient finally contacts a legitimate, health-care provider, it may be too late to prevent extensive morbidity or even death.[23] In one case a patient diagnosed with precancerous cervical cells refused the advice of her gynecologist and opted to visit a naturopath. She was given bromelain vaginal swabs and vaginal suppositories containing vitamin A, zinc chloride, and bloodroot.[26] None of these interventions would be of value in her disease condition.

Another example of indirect hazards was discovered in a lawsuit against General Nutrition Center, a major retailer of health foods. The company had labeled oil of evening primrose as a preventive for a wide range of diseases, including hypertension, arthritis, and multiple sclerosis.[27] They pled guilty to promoting these claims in newspapers, on talk shows, and through oral representations by employees to purchasers. Patients prone to those conditions might have been misled into thinking that the product would replace a physician's monitoring.

In one report, an 18-year-old female with a lesion of the leg avoided physicians while consulting nonphysician healers who used secret potions and injections.[28] After 11 years, when she visited a physician for pain, an infected, necrotic lesion measuring 14 × 19 cm was present. A cough and diffuse chest pain with radiation suggested metastatic disease. A biopsy revealed fibrosarcoma, but the patient refused surgery. She died 6 weeks later. The authors of the report stressed that early resection of the tumor combined with radiotherapy might have cured the condition, but the medical malpractice of the nonphysician healers prevented proper care.

Another type of indirect hazard lies in the false hope given to terminally ill patients.[29] Patients informed of a terminal illness pass through several stages: denial, anger, bargaining, depression, and acceptance. Use of ineffective therapy prolongs the time the patient spends in denial, perhaps preventing the victim from moving to a healthier acceptance of the condition.

HOW TO RECOGNIZE DANGEROUS AND/OR INEFFECTIVE THERAPIES

Promoters and sellers of dangerous and/or ineffective therapies have a simple strategy to convince unwary patients[29]:

- Offer to cure diseases that undergo periods of waxing and waning symptoms.
- Intervene during a period when the condition has been worsening.
- Apply the dangerous and/or ineffective treatment.
- If the condition improves or stabilizes, take credit. Then reduce the dose or discontinue "therapy."

- If the condition worsens with initial application or with discontinuation after a "success," claim that the dosage was stopped too soon, that the dosage must be increased, or that treatment must last longer. Also claim that any worsening indicates that the body is throwing off toxins.
- Whenever the patient improves, claim another success.
- If the patient dies, claim that he or she should have come in sooner.

How can one recognize the illegitimate practitioner? Fortunately, there are numerous clues.

No Legitimate Medical Credentials

While professionals with medical, dental, nursing and pharmacy degrees occasionally do promote dangerous and/or ineffective therapies, the vast majority of sellers do not have any legitimate medical degree. For example, a scientist from Kenya without medical training has claimed to have found a cure for AIDS in Pearl Omega, an herbal mixture.[30] When promoters do pretend to have a legitimate medical degree, it is often issued by a nonaccredited diploma mill that issues mail-order diplomas. The salespersons also often boast membership in medical organizations that are nonexistent or of questionable integrity.[31]

Perception of Nontoxicity

Nonphysician healers often convince patients that traditional medicines are highly toxic and have many adverse reactions. In contrast, many dangerous and/or ineffective therapies are described as being free of adverse effects.

Aura of Natural Medicine

Illegitimate healers often stress that their system is *natural* such as those who utilize herbs, electrical impulses, waves, or radiations.[32] They claim that utilization of these *natural* methods allows the body to exert its own restorative processes. They may also plant the fear that commercially available food is somehow "unnatural," which is a falsehood.[33] (The purpose is to make patients believe that ingestion of food has caused many of their problems.)

Empowerment: Appealing to Patients' Desire for Autonomy

Many patients wish to control their own future, a desire that extends to medical treatment. The current term is "empowerment" of the patient, which often translates into patients refusing to listen to their legitimate health-care providers and turning to nonphysician healers.[34]

Overblown Claims

Promoters often claim that product(s) can cure an extremely wide variety of medical conditions, ranging from infective to carcinogenic, from genetic to environmental, "all in one simple 4-ounce bottle."[31,35] Even though these different types of conditions have virtually nothing in common, the magical product somehow has the power to attack all of their numerous etiologies.[1]

Appeal to Easy Answers

The professional ethics of legitimate medicine requires informed consent. However, many patients become noncompliant when told that a particular therapy is slow to produce results, may cause adverse reactions, and may only have a 50% cure rate. Cancer patients may completely abandon legitimate therapy on hearing the particulars of their regimen.[19] Nonphysician healers are not bound by professional ethics and are free to promise a complete cure of any condition within a matter of days, without adverse reactions (e.g., "Doctor's Diet Cures Arthritis").[34]

This pitch—understandably quite attractive to many unwary patients—may even come from medical professionals with legitimate credentials. For example, a California physician and his partner promoted a product known as "Immunostim" to those with terminal diseases, promising a cure for $26,000.[36] The product, injected intravenously, was found to contain the same ingredients as toilet-bowl cleaners, dishwashing detergents, and disinfectants. Treatments were described by patients as very painful, causing burning pain when extravasation occurred. The injected vein often closed permanently following the treatment, with only a hard knot remaining. As a result of this scam, the physician's medical license was revoked; the partner served 5 years in the San Diego county jail.

Absolute Assurance

Medical professionals are ethically and legally required to inform patients about the possibility that a certain product may not be effective. However, illegitimate practitioners are free to promise extraordinary results with absolute assurance—including a complete cure—to those who are willing to buy the product. This "magical thinking" usually includes such key words as "amazing," "miraculous," and "painless."[37] The confidence of promoters in their own "cures" may inhibit victims from any serious questioning. Typically, if a patient voices concerns, the promoter takes personal offense, accusing the patient of lacking trust.[38] This tactic generally disarms the patient, who then often purchases the product to please the seller.

Simplicity

Illegitimate medical impostors offer simple explanations for disease such as the assertion that all diseases spring from the liver, and then they follow with simple treatments such as the myth that proper nutrition can cure cancer.[38,39]

Testimonials and Anecdotal Evidence

Nonmedical healers lack standard scientific proof of efficacy for their unproven products. However, marketers are fully aware of the potency of the testimonial. If a sports figure, movie star, or any other popular or widely respected person recommends a specific product, people assume that it must work. The authority figure lends an undeserved air of authority to the product being endorsed.[40]

Disparagement of Legitimate Medicine

Nonphysician healers must plant a seed of doubt or distrust in the victim's mind toward legitimate medicine. They do this by claiming that scientists have discovered secret cures for AIDS or cancer, for example, and have hidden them from the public to ensure that doctor's incomes are not reduced. They also might claim that the medical community is "out to get them."[30,31,39] (This latter claim is one of the few verifiable statements of nonphysician healers.)

Selling Directly to the Consumer

Legitimate medications are recommended or prescribed by legitimate medical practitioners, such as pharmacists and physicians. Nonphysician healers lack medical credentials and therefore must market directly to the public, not through legitimate medical organizations. Dangerous and/or ineffective therapies are commonly promoted through talk shows, television "infomercials," books, magazines, and the tabloid press.[31]

Using the Internet

Use of the Internet to reach consumers with unproven medical therapies has risen alarmingly. Unfortunately, most of the people writing home pages and offering medical products on the Internet lack any medical training. Many thousands of unproven and dangerous therapies are sold on the Internet every day, making it the new "lawless frontier" as far as medical topics are concerned. Until the FDA or FTC manage to control this incredibly dangerous situation, the pharmacist and other trained medical professionals are the last lines of defense against medically unproven and fraudulent products.[41]

One example of Internet medical dangers is that of a man who purchased what he assumed was absinthe liquer from an **aromatherapy** (an unproven therapy employing various odors to cure diseases) site.[42] However, the liquid he purchased electronically was actually oil of wormwood. He ingested 10 mL, and within several hours medical complications began, including tonic and clonic seizures, congestive heart failure, and acute renal failure, all of which resolved after hospitalization and extensive diagnostic testing and treatment. The authors cautioned that sales of potent herbal medicines via the Internet could cause many such instances of "Internet-mediated toxic diseases."

As another example of Internet medical "advice," one site offers information on psoriasis.[43] It touts the praises of a spa pool in Turkey, where psoriasis patients may go to be treated. In the pool are thousands of tiny carp, known as "strikers, jabbers, and lickers." The Internet site sports a testimonial from a purported patient who describes the effect of the strikers in eating the upper layers of skin, the jabbers in puncturing the skin, and the lickers in sealing the holes made by the jabbers. After 9 days, the testimonial says, it may have cured his psoriasis. This site, not unexpectedly, is sponsored by a travel company, which provided an address for the unwary to schedule a booking to be eaten by the "little doctor fish of Kangal."

NONHERBAL SUPPLEMENTS LACKING PROOF OF SAFETY/EFFICACY

Herbal supplements usually lack evidence of safety and efficacy. Their use is so pervasive that they are discussed in a separate chapter. (See Chapter 51, Herbal Supplements.)

Bee Pollen

Beekeepers sometimes collect the pollen that falls from bees as they return to their hives. Because this plant pollen was carried by a bee for a few minutes, nonphysician healers claim that patients can gain the energy of the bee by ingesting it.[44] *However, patients with allergies, asthma, and allergic rhinitis have suffered numerous adverse effects from taking bee pollen tablets, including anaphylaxis and death.*[45]

Bioflavinoids

Bioflavinoids—such as rutin and hesperidin—are substances that for decades have been alleged to reduce capillary permeability and fragility.[46] No study has ever proven any of the claims for these chemicals, and their safety is unknown.

Cholestin

The manufacturers claimed that Cholestin, a dietary supplement derived from yeast fermented on rice, lowers cholesterol by 25 to 40 points in 8 weeks.[47] The company defended the labeling for lowering cholesterol by stating that it is not recommended to treat a condition, but solely to help maintain a healthy cholesterol level. The FDA disagreed with the company, stating that Cholestin was discovered to contain lovastatin, found in the prescription product Mevacor. As such, Cholestin was found to be an unapproved drug marketed in violation of the federal Food, Drug, and Cosmetic Act.[48] The decision barred the company from marketing Cholestin, although it may remain available in some locations where stocks were not depleted.

Chromium Picolinate

Chromium picolinate is variously referred to as a weight-loss ingredient or as one that helps body builders increase muscle mass. Research, however, has failed to confirm these findings. The supplement has caused GI disturbances (e.g., flatulence, loose stools, constipation) and many have been responsible for rare cases of anemia and renal failure.[49]

DHEA

DHEA, considered a wonder drug for those who wish to add muscle mass or feel better, contains dehydroepiandrosterone, a precursor to both androgens and estrogens.[50] Because it is listed as a dietary supplement, DHEA can be sold without restriction in any pharmacy or health-food store. Patients taking DHEA can experience adverse effects identical to those of anabolic steroids: Females report male pattern baldness, hirsutism in the beard area, and deepening of the voice, while males may undergo feminization (e.g., breast growth, high voice). Hirsutism in the beard area and deepening of the voice in females may be irreversible. Potentially, DHEA could stimulate the dissemination of cancer of the prostate, breast, or endometrium. Patients should be urged to avoid the product.

Germanium

Germanium is a toxic element that is not essential for health, although supporters claim it prevents Alzheimer's disease.[35] 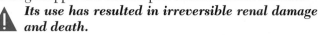 *Its use has resulted in irreversible renal damage and death.*

Hydrogen Peroxide

Hydrogen peroxide in industrial grade concentrations has been illegally sold for the treatment and cure of AIDS, cancer, acne, gum disease, athlete's foot, colic, headache, and varicose veins.[51] *Patients must dilute it prior to drinking, but accidental ingestion of the undiluted product has caused several deaths.*[52-54]

Kombucha Mushroom

Patients have been caught in the fad of the "magic mushroom," also known as "Kombucha tea." According to popular lore, a patient is given a "mushroom" starter, a gray organic gel smelling of vinegar, about 6 inches in diameter and perhaps 1/2 inch thick.[55] After fermenting the mushroom in sugared tea for 7 days, the patient lifts the object from the top of the tea, discarding it. This exposes a baby membrane "mushroom" beneath, which must be given away to keep the "magic" working. (The concept is similar to starter yeasts or friendship bread that has been passed around for generations.) Patients report that ingesting the tea cures cancer, decreases blood pressure, increases energy, reduces acne, increases the sex drive, alleviates constipation, etc. (Actual methods of use may vary somewhat from this description because of the lack of standardized directions and word-of-mouth information passage.)

In actuality, Kombucha "mushroom" is not a mushroom but a symbiotic growth of yeasts and bacteria, which forms a permeable membrane.[55] Organisms growing in it include *Acetobacter ketogenum* and *Pichia fermentans*. Since it is passed from person to person like a chain letter, its organisms may be toxic.

The full spectrum of adverse reactions of drinking this mix of bacteria and yeasts is unknown. There have been several reports of hepatotoxicity reported with this practice, however.[56]

At least one death has occurred, and a number of hospitalizations have been reported.[56]

Melatonin

Melatonin is a hormone made naturally by the human pineal gland.[57] It is purported to be effective as an antiaging chemical, in preventing jet lag, and in inducing sleep. However, appropriate studies of melatonin have not been undertaken.[58] Further, its adverse reaction profile is unknown, although reports indicate the possibility of sedation, headache, and abdominal cramps. Since it is an endogenous hormone, it remains to be seen whether ingestion of exogenous product will reduce endogenous secretion, as happens with corticosteroids. With an individual's normal secretions disrupted, internal melatonin secretion might not normalize.

RNA/DNA

Promoters claim that oral ingestion of RNA and DNA rejuvenates cells, slows aging, aids memory, and prevents wrinkles—all claims without evidence.[35] RNA and DNA are proteins that are destroyed by oral ingestion in any case.[56]

Shark Cartilage

Shark cartilage is purported to be an anticancer remedy. The basis for its use is as follows: Sharks are said to be immune from cancer, so something in the shark must be an anticancer chemical. Therefore, if humans ingest an amount of cartilage from sharks, they also will gain immunity from cancer.[59]

Logic breaks down at several places in this delusionary system. For instance, how can the proteinaceous cartilage preferentially become toxic to malignant cells while exerting no toxicity on normal cells? Why should the cartilage be the magic ingredient rather than another component of the shark? The most compelling argument against shark cartilage is the absolute lack of data to prove any health benefit from its ingestion. Finally, sharks *do* contract cancer, sometimes in the cartilage itself.

Tryptophan

Tryptophan is an amino acid that is thought to enhance sleep.[60] However, either because of the amino acid itself or an impurity, over 1500 users developed a painful hematologic and connective tissue disease known as eosinophilia-myalgia syndrome. Thirty-eight of these victims died. The supplement was banned shortly thereafter. This incident points out graphically the dangers of ingesting products of unknown safety.

SPECIFIC DANGEROUS AND/OR INEFFECTIVE THERAPIES

Naturopathy

Naturopathy is a study that pulls together numerous unproven therapies to concoct a medical philosophy of treat-

ment. Elements included in naturopathy are botanicals, homeopathy, nutritional supplements, acupuncture, minor surgery, and spinal manipulation.[32]

Iridology

Nonphysician healers cannot order legitimate medical diagnostic examinations, nor can they order laboratory tests. Thus they are forced to rely on noninvasive methods by which to make otherwise healthy people unsure about their health. Iridology is one such unproven diagnostic practice. Its adherents section the human iris into areas, each of which reflects a different area of the body. Iridologists are supposedly able to examine the proper location on the iris and detect pathology in the liver, vagina, scapula, spleen, heart, nose, or any one of dozens of other anatomic locations, without even looking at the body part itself.[61] Once the diseases are diagnosed, the iridologist can steer customers to dietary supplements—perhaps monthly or weekly purchases of hundreds of dollars of unneeded products.

Research has confirmed that these nonphysician diagnosticians cannot detect disease when presented with irises in a controlled manner. Nonetheless, some pharmacists practice iridology to augment their income, and medically untrained lay people utilize iridologic exams to provide advice on sophisticated medical diseases in thousands of communities across the country.

Chelation Therapy

Chelation therapy is an unproven method of treatment for coronary artery disease, carotid artery disease, and generalized atherosclerosis through the intravenous injection of chelating substances such as the sodium salt of ethylene diamine tetra-acetic acid (EDTA).[32,62] This therapy lacks any controlled trials to prove its effectiveness. Further, it may be hazardous because of the invasive nature of injections.

Athletics-Oriented Quackery

Because athletes (professional and amateur) are often quite concerned about health, they are easy targets for illegitimate practitioners. Athletes are often urged to gain the competitive edge over other athletes by purchasing amino acids, growth hormone, anabolic steroid alternatives, trace minerals, herbs, glandular products, vitamin-mineral supplements, and "stack-packs," which are a variety of these items packaged together.[19] Some athletes ingest gamma hydroxy butyrate (GHB), which is alleged to be a synthetic steroid that will bulk up muscles. ***However, GHB can cause nausea, uncontrollable shaking, coma, and death.***[63,64]

Acupuncture

Acupuncture is the oriental practice of piercing the skin with needles to treat disorders.[65,66] Traditional Chinese medicine has its own system of anatomy and physiology. For instance, acupuncture sites are based on the supposed existence of energy channels or meridians that run over the body. Acupuncture is said to correct the flow of energy through these channels. The energy channels have no basis in anatomy as recognized in medicine practiced in the United States; they cannot be located on dissection.

Some pharmacies have formed partnerships with acupuncturists to treat patients such as those with AIDS and other serious medical conditions.[67] Since the practice is not part of legitimate medicine in the United States, pharmacists should exercise extreme caution in giving it the stamp of approval through alliances such as these.

Magnetism

Magnets have had a long history as tools of nonphysician healers.[32] Magnets are sold in many forms today, with seductive claims that are completely lacking in scientific evidence:

- Magnets are included in pressurized adhesive dots placed over arthritic areas.[35]
- Impotence is supposedly cured by men's underwear containing a magnet.
- A magnetic suppository is available to cure hemorrhoids.

Kirlian Photography

Nonphysician healers have claimed for many years that the human body is surrounded by an invisible aura that supposedly consists of the energy from the body projecting into the spaces around the human. While the aura is invisible and cannot be detected by legitimate science, some healers claim to be able to *see* the aura and to see changes in it that indicate disease. Kirlian photography is an unproven method used to take a "photograph" of the aura to reveal "disturbances in the body's electromagnetic circulatory system."[68]

Kirlian photography is somewhat misnamed since it does not use a camera. Instead, light-sensitive paper is used to generate an image of a patient with the use of a high-voltage, high-frequency, alternating electric field.[59] This process produces bright colors and haloes. Research has demonstrated that these illusory haloes around the patient are due to voltage, moisture, exposure time, and the amount of pressure the patient applies to the paper. They do not change in the presence of disease, nor do they change as the disease abates and health returns. Kirlian photography is therefore of unproven benefit as a diagnostic tool.

Ear Candling

Ear candles (or cones) are promoted to help remove earwax from the ears. Patients (or caregivers) place one end of a hollow wax tube in the ear and light the other end. As the "candle burns," it supposedly liquefies the ear wax and creates a type of suction, drawing the earwax out of the ear. While numerous Internet sites sell ear candles directly to patients, they are an unapproved medical device, and the FDA has seized various shipments.[70]

COMBATTING THE MOVEMENT TOWARD DANGEROUS AND/OR INEFFECTIVE THERAPIES

The fight against unproven medical products and devices is difficult because of the massive numbers of promoters and the multitude of sales pitches used. The fight became much more difficult in 1994, when the dietary supplement industry (driven by the nation's 10,000 health-food stores) pressured Congress to pass the Dietary Supplement and Health Education Act of 1994.[56,71] By tying the hands of the FDA, this unprecedented piece of legislation allows products to be marketed with no testing for efficacy, allows companies to escape from providing any proof of product safety, ensures that companies do not need to manufacture products according to any standards, allows claims for altering the body's structure or function, and does not require FDA approval for packaging or marketing claims.

Thus the legislation ignores the fact that any dietary supplement can be contaminated at several points.[72] If it is an herb, for example, pickers may choose the toxic parts of the plant or choose the entirely wrong plants.[56] (See Chapter 51, Herbal Supplements.) Insecticides, heavy metals, and fungicides may adulterate crude herbs during production and processing. Fungal growth may occur during storage or shipping, leading to contamination with mycotoxins. Minerals and other plants may be added solely to increase weight and thereby increase profits. Heavy metals can be added to make the color more appealing, and medications may be added to make the product more efficacious. The lack of manufacturing standards ensures that these practices and problems will remain undetected.

Companies who wish to market a product that might affect the structure or function of the body are required to notify the FDA, to have evidence that the claim would be truthful, and to include this statement on the label: "This statement has not been evaluated by the Food and Drug Administration. This product is not intended to diagnose, treat, cure, or prevent any disease." Unfortunately, the amount of evidence the company must have is unspecified. Further, products or ingredients that have no dietary value at all are covered under this law such as St. John's Wort, gingko, and ginseng.[60]

The burden of proof is now on the already overworked FDA to prove that many hundreds of claims made by dietary supplements are truthful.[19] This situation has led to this 1992 quotation from an FDA Commissioner, "I can tell you, and it is not secret, that in terms of safety of dietary supplements, FDA is not doing very much today. It is really 'buyer beware!' which Dr. Kessler (a former FDA Commissioner) and many of us have said."[19]

The situation is exacerbated by the fact that any person may label himself as a "nutritionist." Also, some individuals who claim to have valid degrees have obtained them from unaccredited programs.

Unproven products are highly advertised because of the substantial profit potential of these products. They are advertised on radio and television (including local cable channels), in newspapers and magazines, and in local store bulletin boards. They are sold through unsolicited mailers and catalogs and via multilevel marketing schemes. The average-sized town in the United States has several health-food stores, and the average mall has one or more (usually staffed by clerks without medical training). Internet sites return many hundreds of "hits" for unproven therapies (e.g., herbs), the majority of which are oriented toward selling the products to casual Web surfers.[73–75] Patients are bombarded by vast amounts of advertising with one goal: promoting the purchase of products with unsubstantiated claims and unknown safety.

Undercover shoppers for a popular consumer magazine discovered that the operators of a health-food store promised cures for cancer, including cures from honeysuckle crystals, shark cartilage, coenzyme Q10, garlic, and beta-carotene.[56] (See "A Pharmacist's Journal: I Don't Want to Go to My Doctor Anymore.")

The editors of Consumer Reports characterized the knowledge of pharmacists in regard to herbal supplements as: "Pharmacists . . . [are] . . . often clueless about the supplements sold in their drugstores. Schools of pharmacy usually don't teach courses about the uses of herbal remedies."[56] Indeed, a survey revealed that some pharmacy schools do not offer any instruction in herbal medicine; in others; it is covered only in an elective course.[76] (See Chapter 51, Herbal Supplements.)

A leading physician spokesman against unproven medical products offered a document on his Internet home page: "Unethical Behavior of Pharmacists."[77] In this document he pointed out the conflict of interest pharmacists face because they depend on the sale of questionable products for an income. (See "A Pharmacist's Journal: I'm Paying You $60,000 a Year!") He further characterized pharmacists as greedy and lacking the ethical duty to act in the best interest of the patient in regard to quackery. Many tens of thousands of Web surfers read this document. Its criticisms should give pharmacists who are selling unapproved products food for thought.

The pharmacist can combat the trend toward the use of unproven products by the following means:

- Refusing to stock unproven products
- Discussing with patients who inquire about these products why they cannot find them in that business location
- Reading the advertising for unproven products to be able to offer logical, well-reasoned arguments against them
- Scanning the medical literature to discover episodes of morbidity and mortality associated with unproven medical products
- Talking to church assemblies, civic organizations, schools, and other groups of lay people to caution them against the use of dangerous and/or ineffective therapies
- Talking to groups of medical professionals to caution them about dangerous and/or ineffective therapies
- Writing to local newspapers to counter the unqualified claims made in advertising and/or in articles for unproven products
- Advertising one's own practice as one that is "more concerned with your health" than with unqualified health claims

SUMMARY

The pharmacist has an ethical and legal responsibility to recommend nonprescription products that are proven safe and effective. Despite this, articles in professional journals constantly extol the business wisdom of stocking large numbers

A Pharmacist's Journal

"I Don't Want to Go to My Doctor Anymore."

A patient complained to the pharmacist that a health-food-store owner was giving dangerous advice. State authorities were notified and sent an enforcement agent with a hidden microphone to the store posing as a customer. The agent presented a medical complaint to which the store owner counseled, "Stop going to the doctors and using their medicine, I can cure you in 6 months with my dietary supplements."

What was the complaint the health-food-store owner promised to cure? The agent said that he had been diagnosed with prostate cancer and the doctor's medicine was making his hair fall out. Then it had metastasized to his brain and he didn't know if the doctors knew what they were doing. Prosecution was under consideration at the time I spoke with law enforcement about the case.

A Pharmacist's Journal

"I'm Paying You $60,000 a Year!"

A student who was well acquainted with the dangers of unproven medical therapies was interviewing for a potential job in an independent pharmacy. During the interview she noted large stocks of products lacking in proof of safety and/or efficacy. She asked the owner, "If I come to work here, will I be expected to recommend nonprescription products with which I disagree?" The owner answered, "Look, I'm paying you $60,000 a year plus benefits. I expect you to sell products, not turn down sales. Why would you do anything else?" She attempted to explain her philosophy that patients would appreciate the integrity involved in refusing to sell products and would bring their prescriptions to the store to experience the same integrity. The pharmacist-owner was not willing to concede her point, and she declined the job offer.

AT THE COUNTER

A patient approaches the pharmacist to ask for an opinion about a product purchased at a health-food store. The product is a solution labeled "Liver & Gall Bladder Formula," containing 10 ingredients unfamiliar to the pharmacist such as "Carduus marianus 2x."

Interview/Patient Assessment

The pharmacist discovers that the patient was experiencing abdominal pain with blood in the stools and that a physician advised further lab tests. However, the patient was afraid to undergo the tests and was sure that nothing was really wrong. He then visited a local health-food store, where the person in charge conducted an iridologic exam, discovering that his liver and gall bladder were disoriented and diseased. He was then advised to use this product three to five times daily for a complete cure.

Pharmacist's Analysis

1. What is the value of the iridologic exam carried out by the health-food-store owner?

2. Should the patient take the homeopathic product? (See Chapter 50, Homeopathy.)
3. What should the pharmacist advise about the physician's suggested course of action?

Patient Counseling

This patient is typical of individuals who neglect proper medical care and place their health in the hands of people who may have no medical training at all. The pharmacist should attempt to convince the patient that the iridologic exam is of unproven benefit in diagnosing any disease. Further, the product purchased is of unknown safety and efficacy and should be returned so a refund can be issued. In no case should it be taken. The patient must be urged to return to the physician immediately so proper diagnostic examinations can be conducted. If the patient has a colorectal carcinoma, for instance, following the advice of a nonphysician healer and ignoring the advice of a physician could be deadly.

---

of products lacking proof of safety and efficacy. As a critical aspect of pharmaceutical care, the pharmacist should resist the urge to sell products that are unproven.

Products have been sold for many conditions that are not self-treatable. Patients should be referred to a medical practitioner when they experience nausea or vomiting (unless related to motion sickness), nocturnal leg cramps, boils or other skin infections, nail or scalp fungi, thumb or finger sucking, nailbiting, and ingrown toenails. Nonprescription products with misleading names may persuade the patient that they are effective for these conditions, but the pharmacist must point out their lack of safety and/or efficacy.

Dangerous and/or ineffective therapies abound, and many promoters present persuasive arguments for the use of these therapies. Unfortunately, when untrained individuals attempt to diagnose and/or treat health problems with unproven (and possibly unsafe) products, patients may experience severe morbidity or death. Various forms of dangerous and/or ineffective therapies include nonherbal dietary supplements lacking evidence of efficacy (e.g., bee pollen and chromium picolinate); unsafe therapies such as ear candling and DHEA; and other therapies such as naturopathy, iridology, chelation therapy, acupuncture, magnetism, and kirlian photography.

When patients ask about these and other products or practices, the pharmacist should seize the opportunity to counsel caution with their use. Pharmacists should urge patients to seek legitimate medical care from a professional licensed to diagnose and to recommend either nonprescription or prescription products.

References

1. Podolsky D, et al. Questionable medicine. U.S. News & World Report 118(19):101, 1995.
2. Peterson D. Alternative nutritional treatments 'unproven' (Letter). Am Drugg 214(4): 8, 1997.
3. Buerki RA, Vottero LD. Ethical Responsibility in Pharmacy Practice. Madison, WI: American Institute of the History of Pharmacy, 1994; pp. 147–162.
4. Anon. Oklahoma Pharmacy Lawbook. Oklahoma City: The Oklahoma State Board of Pharmacy, 1997; p. 29.
5. Andrews PLR. Physiology of nausea and vomiting. Br J Anaesth 69(7 Suppl 1):2S, 1992.
6. Hogan CM. Advances in the management of nausea and vomiting. Nurs Clin North Am 25:475, 1990.
7. Harper MB. Vomiting, nausea, and abdominal pain: Unrecognized signs of thyrotoxicosis. J Fam Pract 29:382, 1989.
8. Szucs R. Case of the season: Nausea and vomiting in a patient with the acquired immunodeficiency syndrome. Semin Roentgenol 26:195, 1991.
9. Westfall MD, Lumpkin J. A 33-year-old white female with abdominal pain, nausea, vomiting and hypotension. J Emerg Med 11:271, 1993.
10. Favero AD, et al. Assessment of nausea. Eur J Clin Pharmacol 38:115, 1990.
11. Anquist KW, et al. Diagnostic delay after dimenhydrinate use in vomiting children. Can Med Assoc J 145:965, 1991.
12. Alford BA, McIlhenny J. The child with acute abdominal pain and vomiting. Radiol Clin North Am 30:441, 1992.
13. Swischuk LE. Acute-onset vomiting in a 15-day-old infant. Pediatr Emerg Care 8:359, 1992.
14. Pray WS. Nocturnal leg cramps: The dangers of quinine therapy. US Pharm 17(6):17, 1992.
15. Pray WS. Boils: Why professional care is a must. US Pharm 19(6):29, 1994.
16. Anon. Unapproved over-the-counter (OTC) drugs still marketed? FDA Med Bull 26(1):4, 1996.
17. Pray WS. Adverse effects of finger sucking and nailbiting. US Pharm 18(12):43, 1993.
18. Pray WS. Therapy for ingrown toenails. US Pharm 19(10):20, 1994.
19. Short SH. Health quackery: Our role as professionals. J Am Diet Assoc 94:607, 1994.
20. Woolf GM, et al. Acute hepatitis associated with the Chinese herbal product Jin Bu Huan. Ann Intern Med 121:729, 1994.
21. Fleischer AB, et al. Alternative therapies commonly used within a population of patients with psoriasis. Cutis 58:216, 1996.
22. Jarvis W. The cost of quackery (Letter). FDA Consumer 20(2):7, 1986.
23. Anon. Position of the American Dietetic Association: Food and nutrition misinformation. J Am Diet Assoc 95:705, 1995.
24. Hufnagel TJ, Schein OD. Suppurative keratitis from herbal ocular preparation. Am J Ophthalmol 113:722, 1992.
25. Gelb L. Hope or Hoax? Unproven cancer treatments. FDA Consumer 26(2):10, 1992.
26. Cowley G, et al. Going mainstream. Newsweek 125(26):56, 1995.
27. Anon. GNC pleads guilty to misbranding. FDA Consumer 21(1):4, 1987.
28. Nores J-M, et al. Malpractice by nonphysician healers. NY State J Med 87:473, 1987.
29. Skelly FJ. Beyond conventional medicine. Am Med News 30, 1989 (November 10).
30. Dodd R. Patients sue "AIDS-cure" Kenyan scientist. Lancet 347:1688, 1996.
31. Cagle E. The billion dollar hoax. Am Drugg 201(1): 39, 1990.
32. Wardwell WI. Alternative medicine in the United States. Soc Sci Med 38:1061, 1994.
33. Bidlack WR, Meskin MS. Nutritional quackery: Selling health misinformation. Calif Pharm 36(8):34, 1989.
34. Panush RS. Alternative medicine: Science or superstition (Editorial)? J Rheumatol 21:8, 1994.
35. Napier K. Unproven medical treatments lure elderly. FDA Consumer 28(2):33, 1994.
36. Kurtzweil P. A 'washed-up' snake-oil scheme. FDA Consumer 30(7):30, 1996.
37. Lasswell AB, Leddy T. Nutrition misinformation: How to protect your patients. RI Med J 69:263, 1986.
38. O'Connor G. Confidence trick. Med J Aust 147:456, 1987.
39. Jarvis W. Helping your patients deal with questionable cancer treatments. CA Cancer J Clin 36:293, 1986.
40. Montgomery MR. Advances in medical fraud: Chelation therapy replaces laetrile. J Fla Med Assoc 73:681, 1986.
41. Mannix M. Have I got a deal for you! U.S. News World Rep 123(16):59, 1997.
42. Weisbord SD, Soule JB, Kimmel PL. Poison on line—Acute renal failure caused by oil of wormwood purchased through the Internet. N Engl J Med 337:825, 1997.
43. Anon. Psoriasis treatment—The little fish of Kangul. http://www.holidaybank.co.uk/special/thermali/t0295a.htm.
44. Larkin T. Bee pollen as a health food. FDA Consumer 18(3):21, 1984.
45. Fischer JM, Schwinghammer T. What is bee pollen and what are its uses? US Pharm 8(4):25, 1983.
46. Johnson SC. What is vitamin P and what are the indications for its use? US Pharm 13(8):23, 1988.
47. Snyder K. New dietary supplement sparks debate. Drug Topics 141(8):23, 1997.
48. Anon. Pharmanex Cholestin. Wkly Pharm Reports 47(21):1, (May 25) 1998.
49. Chavez ML. Chromium picolinate. Hosp Pharm 32:1466, 1997.
50. Anon. Dehydroepiandrosterone (DHEA). Med Lett Drugs Ther 38:91, 1996.
51. Dickson KF, Caravati EM. Hydrogen peroxide exposure— 325 exposures reported to a regional poison control center. J Toxicol Clin Toxicol 32:705, 1994.

52. Lambert V. Peroxide pusher shut down. FDA Consumer 26(9):43, 1992.

53. Anon. Sale of peroxy products halted. FDA Consumer 24(10):38, 1990.

54. Anon. Hydrogen peroxide warning. FDA Consumer 23(6):2, 1989.

55. Perron AD, Patterson JA, Yanofsky NN. Kombucha "mushroom" toxicity (Letter). Ann Emerg Med 26:660, 1995.

56. Anon. Herbal roulette. Consumer Reports 60(11):698, 1995.

57. Thomas KE, Barnes CL. Melatonin—Safe and effective? US Pharm 21(1):80, 1996.

58. Lin AYF. Is melatonin effective in alleviating jet lag? Pharm Times 62(2):10, 1996.

59. Markman M. Shark cartilage: The laetrile of the 1990s. Cleve Clin J Med 63:179, 1996.

60. Barrett S. Notes on the tryptophan disaster. Skeptical Inquirer 19(4):6, 1996.

61. Simon A, Worthen DM, Mitas JA II. An evaluation of iridology. JAMA 242:1385, 1979.

62. Cicero LA. Is there any merit to chelation as a treatment for coronary artery disease? Drug Topics 141(5):60, 1997.

63. Henkel J. Gym owner jailed for GHB sales. FDA Consumer 31(3):34, 1997.

64. Kurtzweil P. Drug trafficker jailed. FDA Consumer 29(7):30, 1995.

65. Lewith GT. Acupuncture. Practitioner 230:1057, 1986.

66. Prance SE, et al. Research on traditional Chinese acupuncture— Science or Myth: A review. J Royal Soc Med 81:588, 1988.

67. Slezak M. Practicing on pins and needles. Am Drugg 213(11): 26, 1996.

68. Royal DF, Royal FF. Homeopathy: How it relates to modern medicine. Am J Pain Mgt 2:55, 1992.

69. Dodes JE, Schissel MJ. Quacks among us. NY State Dent J 61:16, 1995.

70. Anon. Ear candles. FDA Consumer 29(2): 35, 1995.

71. Anon. Fraud or find? Nutr Action Newsletter 24(7):8, 1997.

72. But PP-H. Need for correct identification of herbs in herbal poisoning (Letter). Lancet 341:637, 1993.

73. Latner AW. Natural medicine on the net: The wild west lives again. Pharm Times 62(11):31, 1996.

74. Keoun B. Cancer patients find quackery on the web. J Natl Cancer Inst 88:1263, 1996.

75. Snyder K. FDA evaluating Internet ads for drugs and devices. Drug Topics 140(23):130, 1996.

76. Miller LG, Murray WJ. Herbal instruction in United States pharmacy schools. Am J Pharm Ed 61:160, 1997.

77. Barrett S. Unethical behavior of pharmacists. Quackwatch (www.quackwatch.com), 1997.

Homeopathy

Homeopathy is a different branch of medicine from that studied by pharmacy students. Its theories are directly opposed to the dose-response relationship of traditional pharmacology. The practice of homeopathy includes a large range of nonprescription drug products, all of which are exempt from providing any proof of efficacy to the FDA through a loophole in the Food, Drug and Cosmetic (FDC) Act of 1938. Because of this situation, pharmacists are confronted with a wide variety of homeopathic products, some of which purport to cure serious medical conditions, but have never been tested for efficacy using the tools of legitimate scientific inquiry.

To properly counsel patients, pharmacists must understand the fundamental precepts of homeopathy and the medical claims it makes and must be familiar with the lack of legitimacy of its claims and the risks of recommending homeopathic products.

HOMEOPATHY OVERVIEW

In the early 1800s a German physician, Samuel Hahnemann, became disillusioned by the medical practice of that time, which included the application of blistering agents, the use of leeches, and the frequent administration of emetics and laxatives.[1,2] He called this type of medicine "allopathy." In response, he developed his own branch of medicine to which he gave the name "homeopathy." According to his new medical science, he would enable practitioners to diagnose and treat all diseases. Homeopathy rests on several fundamental principles, the Law of Similars, the Law of Infinitesimals, and the process of succussion.[3]

The Law of Similars

Traditional, legitimate medicine teaches certain pharmacologic principles such as treatment using a substance that will act against the disease process. For instance, to treat an allergy with traditional medicine, antihistamine or decongestant is administered. To treat fatigue, caffeine might be given. Likewise, to treat excess stomach acid, an agent that reduces acid production or neutralizes the acid is administered. Homeopathy, however, does not adhere to fundamental pharmacology.[4]

One of the cornerstones of homeopathy is the Law of Similars in which Hahnemann alleged that in disease the body is not in its normal state and needs help to reach homeostasis. To accomplish this, a medication that produces the same symptoms the patient is experiencing must be administered (Table 50.1). For instance, cockroach extract, histamine, and crushed bees are homeopathic remedies for allergies. Bronchial cancer extract is administered to patients with bronchial cancer. Caffeine is a homeopathic remedy for insomnia. Vaginal suppositories containing *Candida* are a homeopathic remedy for vaginal candidiasis. A homeopathic product prepared from a patient's urine was given to a patient suffering from hyperactivity.[5]

The Law of Similars seems to be counterproductive in that administration of cockroach extract to a patient with cockroach allergy would logically be expected to worsen the allergy. Homeopathy is protected from this type of reaction through a second Hahnemannian law, the law of Infinitesimals.

The Law of Infinitesimals

Traditional pharmacology adheres to the dose-response model in which increasing doses of medications exert stronger effects. Homeopathy inverts this well-accepted model to assert the exact reverse: the more diluted the medication is, the stronger it becomes.[6,7] Thus the homeopath begins with original liquid or powder, and dilutes 1 part to 99 of solvent. This dilution is known as 1C. Then one drop is removed and mixed again with 99 drops of solvent and becomes a 2C dilution (1/10,000). Homeopathic remedies may be as diluted as 60C.

The problem with the law of infinitesimals arises when one considers the scientific realities of Avogadro's number. According to this universally accepted basic law, there are only 6.023×10^{23} molecules in one mole of substance. Should the homeopath dilute past 12C (a 1×10^{-25} dilution), there are no remaining molecules of active ingredient.[8] Thus the typical homeopathic remedy is nothing more than an expensive placebo containing water or lactose with no active ingredient. Accordingly, it becomes clear how a patient who has diarrhea can be given a medication that causes diarrhea. There is no pharmacologic activity remaining in homeopathic remedies, allowing the original disease process to continue unabated.

Nonprescription homeopathic products are labeled with the dilution used. For instance, a homeopathic infant colic remedy lists some of its ingredients as "natrum sulphuricum 3x, magnesia phosphorica 3x."

The Process of Succussion

Hahnemann also developed the theory that medications are inert when they are in their native state. Thus he alleged that an herbal product would have no effect unless its hidden, dynamic powers were released. This would be accomplished by a process of succussion carried out at each stage of the dilution process. Succussion was a term Hahnemann coined for rubbing or shaking of the powder or liquid. He alleged that shaking the diluted medication would "potentize" or "dynamize" the medications, releasing hidden healing forces. Homeopaths suggest that the water with which the product is diluted somehow uses the molecules of medication as a template, taking on the characteristics of the medication, perhaps through some unproven transfer of energy. This assertion has no grounding in chemistry, but is the basis for asserting that successive dilutions actually strengthen a homeopathic remedy.

THE DICHOTOMY OF HOMEOPATHY AND TRADITIONAL MEDICINE

The pharmacist is well grounded in the proven precepts of traditional medicine. The theories of homeopathy, specifically

Table 50.1. Various Homeopathic Remedies Lacking Proof of Efficacy

MEDICAL PROBLEM	HOMEOPATHIC REMEDY	PURPORTED JUSTIFICATION FOR USAGE
Bronchial cancer	Actual extracts from bronchial cancer	Rationale not provided
Vomiting	Ipecac, nuc vomica	Cause vomiting
Homesickness	Red pepper	Produces feeling of homesickness
Cystitis, burned skin	Cantharidin (Spanish fly)	Potent vesicant
Broken love affair	Table salt	Allows one to express emotions
Asthma	Cockroach extract	Causes allergies
Past exposure to X-rays	Radium bromide	Removes effects of radiation
Allergies	Honey bee extract, histamine, milk, chocolate, wheat, beef, yeast	Produces or worsens allergies
Reaction to DPT immunization	Diphtheritic membrane	Unlocks cellular mechanism that was disturbed
Idiopathic thrombocytic purpura	Spleen sarcode	Directs body's energy to be focused in the splenic tissues
Insomnia	Crude coffee	Causes insomnia
Suicidal depression	Metallic gold	Rationale not provided
Rhinitis, Sinusitis	Nasal mucus, extracts from infected sinus	Rationale not provided
Infant fever	Belladonna suppositories	Rationale not provided
Degenerative arthritis	Poison ivy, embryo, placenta	Rationales not provided
Salmonella food poisoning	Arsenic trioxide	Rationale not provided
Vertigo	Petroleum, ambergris	Causes vertigo in "provings"
Multiple sclerosis	Poliomyelitis	Rationale not provided
Rectal polyps	Extracts from rectal polyps	Rationale not provided
Psoriasis	Extract from psoriasis lesions	Rationale not provided
Tuberculosis	Extracts from tuberculosis lesions	Rationale not provided
Attention deficit/hyperactivity disorder	The child's own urine	Rationale not provided

Adapted from Pray WS. The challenge to professionalism presented by homeopathy. Am J Pharm ED 60:198, 1996.

designed to be an alternative to legitimate medicine, are incompatible with accepted mechanisms of pharmacology. In fact, they are so far removed from traditional medicine as to render them mutually exclusive. For instance, medications become more potent in one of two opposite ways:

- Traditional medicine: increase the dose.
- Homeopathy: decrease the dose and succuss the product.

  Likewise, disease may be treated using one of two models:

- Traditional medicine: administer medications proven to be beneficial for the disease in controlled scientific studies, using medications that directly combat the pathogen, the underlying disease process, or its symptoms.
- Homeopathy: administer medications that are not required to prove efficacy through controlled scientific

studies, using medications that cause the same symptoms as those observed in the patient.

Pharmacists cannot switch from one of these irreconcilable belief systems to the other and provide consistent treatment for patients. Further, giving equal weight to both does not allow pharmacists to maintain scientific credibility among other health professionals. Thus pharmacists who choose homeopathy should embrace it fully, discarding all traditional medicines in the pharmacy, and vice versa.

SCIENTIFIC STUDIES OF HOMEOPATHY

To provide further information for the reader, it is useful to examine brief summaries of reports that both support and fail to support homeopathy. The reports included are representative rather than exhaustive.

The Problem of Negative Bias in Publications

Homeopathy must prove that its theories actually produce patient benefit. Homeopathy would perhaps be more well accepted if sufficient studies exhibited that it actually performs as advertised. For it to become accepted as a completely novel branch of medicine, a full body of work is needed. While any legitimate medication (e.g., ranitidine) has many thousands of well-conducted studies verifying its effectiveness, the entire science of homeopathy is characterized by a startlingly empty body of research. Instead, there is meager evidence that its products perform as claimed. The lack of adequate publications over the 200 years since its inception is puzzling, but may be partly because of negative publication bias. Briefly, if an experimenter does not obtain the results expected, the publication is not submitted. For instance, homeopathic supporters whose studies conclude that homeopathic products are ineffective may never submit them, opting to design another study that will finally demonstrate efficacy.

Reports That Support Homeopathy

CONTROLLED TRIALS

A meta-analysis of 89 randomized trials of homeopathy demonstrated possible benefit, but did not yield evidence that homeopathy was effective for any clinical condition in particular.[9]

Another meta-analysis of 107 controlled trials demonstrated that a positive trend for homeopathy existed, but the authors cautioned that most trials were of low quality in terms of methodologic structure and also reminded readers of the unknown role of negative publication bias.[10]

FOCUS ON...

HOMEOPATHY: WHAT SHOULD THE PHARMACIST DO?

Abraham Lincoln was once petitioned by homeopathy supporters to allow homeopathic medicines to be included in the United States Army Dispensary. His refusal was worded, "The application is dismissed. You cannot fertilize with flatus."[29] Ambrose Bierce, in *The Devil's Dictionary,* defined "homeopath" as "the humorist of the medical profession."[30] These quotes speak directly to the laughable aspects of homeopathy. However, the use of alternative medicine, and homeopathy, can have serious repercussions on health.

British investigators related the cases of four patients with insulin-dependent diabetes mellitus who stopped their insulin in favor of alternative approaches such as faith healing, prayer, unusual diets, and vitamin/trace element supplementation.[31] As a result three developed ketoacidosis (which was life-threatening in one), one experienced weight loss and hyperglycemia, and one developed serious retinopathy. The authors used these as a framework for the exploration of such alternative diabetic treatments as homeopathy.

Alternative medicine is a delusional system wherein a predator makes promises that cannot be fulfilled through any method known to legitimate science. The victim cooperates in the predator's schemes, perhaps discontinuing legitimate medical care.

As one of many alternative medical schemes, homeopathy consists of administering placebos to patients—albeit incredibly expensive placebos. Specific objections to homeopathy include the following:

- As mentioned in the text, two of the fundamental doctrines of homeopathy (e.g., dilutions becoming stronger; treating with a substance that causes the same symptoms) are implausible at best and flatly contradict the principles of pharmacology as taught to all pharmacy students.
- Hahnemann's incredible thought that medications in their crude stage are inert led him to further state that repeated grinding or pounding (succussion) would "potentize" the drugs. Of course, medications in their crude states can be incredibly potent. Anyone who has mistakenly ingested a plant containing a cardioactive medication has discovered this fact. Thus the entire framework behind succussion and dilution rests on an impossible assumption.
- Hahnemann asserted that disease is not caused by any external force, but is solely the result of ill-defined spiritual changes in the body. Thus classical homeopathy denies that microorganisms cause disease. In homeopathic colleges, bacteriology classes were omitted. One wonders how many of Hahnemann's mistaken delusions must be disproven before homeopathy is exposed as the sham it is.
- Among Hahnemann's many delusions was the astounding belief that there are really only three chronic diseases (which he refers to as miasmas): sycosis (fig-wort disease), syphilis, and psora. He developed the thought that psora was the cause of all chronic illnesses (except venereal diseases). This antique line of reasoning exposes Hahnemann's 200-year-old lack of sophistication when compared with modern medicine. Similarly, the entire body of homeopathy is the product of an unsophisticated mind that sought to reduce the complexity of medicine to a few simple truths. Unfortunately, each of its truths are falsehoods.
- In any legitimate branch of medicine, many dozens of great leaders elucidated different principles and practices. However, homeopathy has only its single founder, whose delusions of grandeur allowed him to believe that he had developed a system of medicine that could diagnose and treat any disease.
- Hahnemann himself stated that homeopathy demands administration of an ingredient that causes similar symptoms. He specifically spoke against giving the *same* product as that causing the symptoms, referring to it as isopathy, and asserted that it would actually aggravate the disease. Some companies have transgressed this by marketing *nosodes.* As shown in Table 50.1, various nosodes are created from body constituents

Continued

Several reports seem to indicate that homeopathy might be beneficial in specific conditions, although many more would be needed to prove compelling evidence of efficacy. Children aged 6 months to 5 years with acute diarrhea were given homeopathic medicine, which reduced the duration of diarrhea when compared with the placebo group.[11] A homeopathic after-bite gel seemed to reduce the extent of erythema following mosquito bites when compared with the vehicle in two studies.[12,13] A meta-analysis of homeopathy in reducing the duration of ileus after abdominal or gynecologic surgery indicated that a reduction in the duration of ileus might occur with homeopathy.[14] Patients given homeopathic treatment recovered from influenza symptoms more rapidly than those given placebo.[15]

CASE REPORTS

A patient with migraine was controlled by a homeopathic remedy.[16] In a small series of 12 adults, homeopathy seemed to improve depression and anxiety, although the treatment was not blinded or placebo-controlled.[17] A patient with lung cancer survived longer than expected when given homeopathic treatment and extract of mistletoe.[18]

Reports That Do Not Support Homeopathy

CONTROLLED TRIALS

Researchers reviewed forty randomized trials of homeopathy, most of which included double-blinding.[19] They concluded that homeopathy was not effective.

Homeopathic products were no better than placebo in treating plantar warts in a well-designed, double-blind, placebo-controlled trial.[20] Homeopathic treatments were no better than placebo in treating rheumatoid arthritis in a double-blind, placebo-controlled trial.[21]

In a randomized, placebo-controlled, double-blinded study 175 children given homeopathic medicine or placebo did not exhibit any difference in symptom severity or need for adenoidectomy and tonsillectomy.[22]

such as bronchial cancer, tuberculosis lesions, stool, or pus. Other companies market suppositories for vaginal yeast that actually contain vaginal yeast. These products are being sold under the disguise of homeopathy, which exempts them from federal legislation. As part of the entire picture of homeopathy, their use must be strongly discouraged.

- Followers of homeopathy point to the large numbers of followers it has gained in many countries. Unfortunately, quantity does not equal quality. If anything, the large number of adherents simply highlights the deplorable state of scientific education in those countries. After all, large numbers of people believe in UFOs, astrology, psychic hot lines, alien abductions, crystal power, ghosts, and Atlantis. No amount of wishful thinking can make these illegitimate belief systems any more valid than they make homeopathy.

- A fundamental tenet of homeopathy was the requirement that the homeopathic practitioner spend large amounts of time with each patient, individually formulating a remedy, which might contain a dozen ingredients or more. The various "shotgun" nonprescription products sold as homeopathic remedies allow the lay person to purchase and use them without ever consulting a homeopathic practitioner. Thus their manufacturers evidently subscribe to a non-Hahnemannian view that a fixed combination can be created for mass sales. This violation of homeopathy should cause the FDA to demand their recall.

- Hahnemann envisioned homeopathy as something only open to actual medical physicians, who would add it to their armamentarium of potential treatments. Today, however, homeopathy is practiced by nonphysicians such as pharmacists, nurses, dentists, veterinarians, acupuncturists, chiropractors, and physicians' assistants. (An article in the dental literature deplores the use of homeopathy in dentistry.[32]) Even worse, any person who wishes (even those working in health-food stores with no medical training whatsoever) may freely diagnose diseases and recommend homeopathic treatments.

- The current FDA compliance policy for homeopathic drugs contains the following, "A product's compliance with requirements of the Homeopathic Pharmacopeia of the United States. . . . does not establish that it has been shown by appropriate means to be safe, effective, and not misbranded for its intended use."[33] Legitimate medicines must submit to safety and efficacy testing; homeopathic remedies are not required to do so.

In light of these many questionable aspects of homeopathy, pharmacists must confront the issue head-on. The following are several possible approaches:

- Refuse to stock any homeopathic remedy.
- Describe the shortcomings of homeopathy with potential purchasers.
- Refer patients with serious complaints to legitimate medical professionals.
- Recommend a nonprescription ingredient that is safe and effective, when appropriate.
- When given the opportunity to speak to lay audiences, enlighten the attendees on the lack of logic and rationality behind homeopathy.

In a randomized, double-blinded, placebo-controlled trial of homeopathy versus placebo, patients recovering from oral surgery experienced the same degree of pain regardless of whether they received the homeopathic product or a placebo.[23]

CASE REPORTS

A 37-year-old patient with a giant melanoma neglected follow-up treatment, opting instead to visit a homeopath, whose treatment of her was characterized as negligence by the authors.[24] A group of 34 patients with minor burns were given a popular homeopathic remedy for burns, Cantharis; results were not statistically different from placebo.[25] An infant with atopic eczema treated with homeopathic medicines developed erythema and limb edema, which resolved when conventional treatment was instituted.[26]

The Double Standard for Homeopathic Products

The lack of studies to prove the effectiveness of homeopathy becomes less puzzling when one considers the legal status of homeopathic products. When the FDC Act of 1938 was passed, Senator Royal Copeland (D-NY; a 1921 graduate of Hahnemann College in Philadelphia and a leading homeopathic practitioner) inserted a stipulation that homeopathic remedies not be required to be proven effective.[4] This move has been characterized as a "fraud perpetrated on the public with the government's blessing, thanks to the abuse of political power of Sen. Royal Copeland . . . "[27] As a result manufacturers of homeopathic products need not conduct any research to prove effectiveness. This double standard with regard to homeopathic products does not provide a level playing field for medications sold to unsuspecting patients. Various scientists have petitioned the FDA to institute standards of efficacy for homeopathic products, but this step has not yet been taken.[28] (See "Homeopathy: What Should the Pharmacist Do?")

SAFETY OF HOMEOPATHIC PRODUCTS

One would presume that many homeopathic medications would be safe simply because they contain few if any molecules of active ingredient. However, there is accumulating evidence that they are not. Homeopathic products have caused direct hazards to patients, including allergic dermatitis in a patient allergic to dichromate in a homeopathic product, acute pancreatitis from another remedy, and caries and lactose intolerance from the diluents.[4]

A lawsuit against several pharmacy chains filed in the interests of the general public accused Longs Drugs Stores and Payless Drug Stores of deceptive advertising of homeopathic products.[34] As it was settled out of court, all terms are confidential. Other lawsuits seek to prevent manufacturers and retailers from selling and advertising the products unless a statement is added to assert that the products "have not been found to be effective for the treatment of any disease."

SUMMARY

Homeopathy is an alternative medical model that does not use the pharmacologic principles taught in pharmacy school. Homeopathic theories—which have not been proven sound—include the idea that disease should be treated by administering a medication that produces the same symptoms as those observed in the patient, the practice of diluting medications to make them more effective, and the practice of repeatedly shaking a medication to release its hidden energies. Pharmacists must choose to follow either traditional medicine or homeopathy. The basic principles on which each rests are incompatible with each other, and they cannot be reconciled.

References

1. Pray WS. A challenge to the credibility of homeopathy. Am J Pain Mgt 2:63, 1992.
2. Perez CB, Tomsko PL. Homeopathy and the treatment of mental illness in the 19th century. Hosp Community Psychiatry 45:1030, 1994.
3. Bayley C. Homeopathy J Med Philos 18:129, 1993.
4. Pray WS. The challenge to professionalism presented by homeopathy. Am J Pharm Ed 60:198, 1996.
5. Royal DF, Royal FF. Homeopathy: How it relates to modern medicine. Am J Pain Mgt 2:55, 1992.
6. Morgan PP. Homeopathy—Will its theory every hold water? Can Med Assoc J 146:1719, 1992.
7. Stehlin I. Homeopathy—Real medicine or empty promises? FDA Consumer 30(10):15, 1996.
8. Beckerich MJ. Appetoff: Another diet fad. Vet Hum Toxicol 31:540, 1989.
9. Linde K, et al. Are the clinical effects of homeopathy placebo effects? A meta-analysis of placebo-controlled trials. Lancet 350:834, 1997.
10. Kleijnen J, Knipschild P, ter Riet G. Clinical trials of homoeopathy. BMJ 302:316, 1991.
11. Jacobs J, et al. Treatment of acute childhood diarrhea with homeopathic medicine: A randomized clinical trial in Nicaragua. Pediatrics 93:719, 1994.
12. Hill N, et al. A placebo controlled clinical trial investigating the efficacy of a homeopathic after-bite gel in reducing mosquito bite induced erythema. Eur J Clin Pharmacol 49:103, 1995.
13. Hill N, Stam C, van Haselen RA. The efficacy of Prrikweg gel in the treatment of insect bites: A double-blind, placebo-controlled clinical trial. Pharm World Sci 18:35, 1996.
14. Barnes J, Resch KL, Ernst E. Homeopathy for postoperative ileus? A meta-analysis. J Clin Gastroenterol 25:628, 1997.
15. Ferley JP, et al. A controlled evaluation of a homoeopathic preparation in the treatment of influenza-like syndromes. Br J Clin Pharmacol 27:329, 1989.
16. Whitmarsh TE. When conventional treatment is not enough: A case of migraine without aura responding to homeopathy. J Altern Complement Med 3:159, 1997.
17. Davidson JR, et al. Homeopathic treatment of depression and anxiety. Altern Ther Health Med 3:46, 1997.
18. Bradley GW, Clover A. Apparent response of small cell lung cancer to an extract of mistletoe and homoeopathic treatment. Thorax 44:1047, 1989.
19. Hill C, Doyon F. Review of randomized trials of homoeopathy. Rev Epidemiol Sante Publique 38:139, 1990.
20. Labrecque M, et al. Homeopathic treatment of plantar warts. Can Med Assoc J 146:1749, 1992.
21. Andrade LE, et al. A randomized controlled trial to evaluate the effectiveness of homeopathy in rheumatoid arthritis. Scand J Rheumatol 20:204, 1991.
22. de Lange de Klerk ES, et al. Effect of homoeopathic

medicines on daily burden of symptoms in children with recurrent upper respiratory tract infections. BMJ 309:1329, 1994.

23. Lokken P, et al. Effect of homoeopathy on pain and other events after acute trauma: Placebo controlled trial with bilateral oral surgery. BMJ 310:1439, 1995.

24. Benmeir P, et al. Giant melanoma of the inner thigh: A homeopathic life-threatening negligence. Ann Plast Surg 27:583, 1991.

25. Leaman AM, Gorman D. Cantharis in the early treatment of minor burns. Arch Emerg Med 6:259, 1989.

26. Goodyear HM, Harper JI. Atopic eczema, hyponatremia, and hypoalbuminaemia. Arch Dis Child 65:231, 1990.

27. Jarvis W. Health fraud leader speaks out on homeopathy (Letter). FDA Consumer 31(3):6, 1997.

28. Der Marderosian AH. Understanding homeopathy. J Am Pharm Assoc NS36:317, 1996.

29. Gerring D. Is there a future for homeopathy? (Letter) Can Med Assoc J 133:182, 1985.

30. Gevitz N. Sectarian medicine. JAMA 257:1636, 1987.

31. Gill GV, et al. Diabetes and alternative medicine: Cause for concern. Diabetic Med 11:210, 1994.

32. Schissel MJ, Dodes JE. Dentistry and alternative therapy. N Y State Dent J 63:32, 1997.

33. Anon. Food and Drug Administration. Conditions under which homeopathic drugs may be marketed. Compliance Policy Guides (Chapter 32). Guide 7132.15: 1, 1988.

34. Anon. Homeopathy suits settled. Drug Topics 149(17):7, 1996.

Herbal Supplements

Herbal medicine involves several misconceptions on the part of the public. Chief among these is the widespread myth that herbs are somehow safer than traditional medicine. The herbal industry has managed to convince consumers of the myth of "beneficial nature and the natural products she provides." While many herbs may be consumed in small amounts without harm, consumers often do not know that many plants found in nature are highly toxic. Further, the FDA has cautioned that toxicity information on most marketed herbs is completely lacking. Although most people who use herbal supplements escape injury, there are isolated reports of death and serious injury arising from ingestion of herbs. Further, virtually all products sold as dietary supplements have no recognized role in nutrition.[1]

The herbal industry is huge and poorly regulated. Even sales figures are sometimes contradictory. For instance, sales of herbal products were estimated at $1.7 billion in 1994 in one reference, while another reference stated that in 1995 annual sales were $106.7 million, up 35% from the previous year.[2,3] Yet another reference cited figures of $772 million in 1995 and projected sales of $1.6 billion by 2001.[4] These incongruent figures notwithstanding, it is true that herbal product sales are growing exponentially each year.

CHARACTERISTICS OF PATIENTS WHO USE HERBS

Customers of two health-food stores were surveyed about their patronage of those establishments.[5] Most purchased herbs, and the most commonly purchased herbs were ginseng, garlic, and gingko. Patients visiting the health-food stores were mainly white (94.1%) and female (75.7%) and had one or more years of college education (70.6%).

LACK OF MANUFACTURING STANDARDS FOR HERBAL SUPPLEMENTS

Herbal manufacturers are not required to perform any testing or quality control on the products they sell.[6] As a result, neither the retailer nor the consumer can be assured that the plant's active ingredients are actually in the product (assuming the plant has any active ingredient in the first place), whether the herbs are bioavailable, whether other substances are in the product, whether the product is safe, or whether there is any variation in the product from lot-to-lot. See "Combating the Movement Toward Dangerous and/or Ineffective Therapies" in Chapter 49 for a full discussion of the Congressional Act that removed normal manufacturing standards for herbs.

The FDA is only able to act against herbal supplements on a case-by-case basis because of its limited resources.[7] For instance, reports of serious reactions may be needed for the agency to examine a particular herb. One FDA official stated, "Keeping track of herbs is an impossible task. The herb industry is the least organized of the food industries. Herbs are

sold at a multitude of small outlets, and it's very difficult to find out who sells what and how much is being sold."[7] Further, as one pharmacist noted in a letter to the editor of a national pharmacy journal, " . . . health-food store clerks and grocery store clerks can make any claims they want about the efficacy of their products. We can't [because of] that little thing called liability."[8] For this reason, pharmacists may be the only source of objective information for patients who learn about herbal medicinals through advertising and discussions with nonmedical salespeople, family, and friends. For example, pharmacists should carefully point out the disclaimer on dietary supplements that make health claims: "This statement has not been evaluated by the Food and Drug Administration. This product is not intended to diagnose, treat, cure, or prevent any disease."

USES OF HERBAL SUPPLEMENTS

The various herbs and their purported uses comprise a vast body of information that fills entire books. Unfortunately, there is a general lack of accepted scientific evidence for the efficacy and safety of most of the traditional uses of virtually all herbs.

This chapter presents a summary of some herbs and their purported uses, but prudent pharmacists will exercise extreme caution in making these herbal recommendations. For instance, the male patient with an enlarged prostate would benefit more from a physician referral than a trial of an unproven herbal product (e.g., saw palmetto). Likewise, pharmacists should caution against patients discontinuing physician-prescribed antihypertensives in favor of arnica, which is of unproven benefit. (See "Former FDA Commissioner Blasts Pharmacy.")

VARIOUS HERBS AND THEIR PURPORTED USES

Patients often request advice regarding herbal products such as those listed in Table 51.1. Lay publications provide advice on purported uses, but, increasingly, pharmacy-related sources also offer suggestions for recommending herbs and provide doses for the herbs. This text will describe various herbs and their purported uses, although the herbs lack FDA approval for safety and efficacy for those uses.

Many patients consume herbal teas in a misguided attempt to obtain medical benefit and/or as a supposedly safer alternative to caffeine. (See "Herbal Teas.") Although some herbal teas are safe, patients generally are not sufficiently informed to choose safe teas from the great variety of herbal teas available.[12,13]

Unless otherwise stated, the information concerning purported uses is taken from literature published by a major pharmacy chain, a major producer of herbal products, a popular textbook about herbs, or a major marketer of continuing education in herbal products.[14–17] These references reflect the sources consulted by practicing pharmacists.

Legitimate medical sources were consulted for each herb by instituting a Medline search for the years 1983 to 1998. Each search called forth every abstracted article published in English, using human subjects. All articles were perused in compiling the herbal descriptions below.

Doubtless many thousands of patients use herbs and do not suffer injury. However, there are also many reports of patients who have experienced injury from the use of these products. The following descriptions also present adverse reactions as they have been published in the medical literature.

This text cannot provide safe dosages for the herbs. At the present time, there are no FDA-approved uses for these herbs. Therefore, providing a dose is irrational. Further, there is often little agreement in popular references about which doses are safe or effective.

For each herb, the genus and species of the plant supposedly contained in the bottle is provided, since manufacturers sometimes list the ingredients of multiherb concoctions with the Latin name.

This text can only list some of the more common herbs. However, there are numerous examples of little-known herbs causing severe adverse reactions such as interstitial renal fibrosis or lead toxicity.[18,19]

The Food and Drug Administration may be able to exert more control over dietary supplements in the future. The agency has proposed to allow structure or function claims such as "promoting cardiovascular health" or "supporting immune system function."[20] At the same time, the agency would require evidence for disease claims (e.g., claims to allow the consumer to diagnose, treat, prevent, or cure a disease).

FOCUS ON...

FORMER FDA COMMISSIONER BLASTS PHARMACY

David Kessler, a physician, dean of the Yale Medical School and former Commissioner of the FDA, was asked to address the issue of consumer safety at a national symposium in 1998.[9,10] He took the occasion to relate that he had visited a neighborhood chain drugstore and said, "There, next to the pharmacy counter, not just in any of the aisles, but right there underneath the pharmacist . . . I counted 26 different displays for dietary supplements making claims." The claims included such unproven statements, as "mood enhancer," "immune enhancer," "improves memory and concentration," and "improves leg health." (See "A Pharmacist's Journal: Where's the Medicine for Varicose Veins?")

Dr. Kessler also stated, "I wonder whether many pharmacists really have given up their roles as health professionals, as pharmacists. "[10] "Maybe they are no longer in control of the store; they are just behind the counter and anything in front of that counter goes."[9] Dr. Kessler also noted the past perception that patients could enter any pharmacy and buy a product that functioned as the label promised, and he then elaborated, "You now see an erosion of that in the pharmacy. The goal is not to go down to the lower denominators, but to take all products, including these herbal and dietary supplements, back up to the standards we have fought for during the past century." In light of this indictment, it is noteworthy that a leading hospital pharmacist has argued against including homeopathic products and herbal items on the formulary of any hospital, since it might encourage physicians to prescribe them.[11]

A Pharmacist's Journal

"Where's the Medicine for Varicose Veins?"

A man in his 40s who weighed about 230 pounds and was about 6 feet, 3 to 4 inches tall approached me as I was in the nutritional supplements aisle. "Where's the medicine for varicose veins?" he asked. I asked what medicine he was using, and he responded, "I don't remember the name, but it's good for varicose veins." He explained that he had varicose veins, "not the little ones, but the real big ones, that I've had for about 20 years." I asked if they caused problems, and he stated, "They're stinging right now, from my knees to my ankles. My mom had them, too." I asked if

he had ever seen a physician for them, and he assured me that he didn't need to because this new medicine was helping. I mentioned the possibility of surgery when he might become tired of treating them himself, but he didn't want to speak about that. I took 2 to 3 minutes explaining the benefits of support hosiery, but he didn't want that, either. He finally found the product he had been using, Venastat, containing 300 mg of horse-chestnut seed extract per capsule. This was his third box. He assured me that it worked well, despite the fact that horse chestnut has never been proven safe or effective for any indication, including varicose veins.

Table 51.1. Representative Herbal Products

PRODUCT	SELECTED INGREDIENTS
Circulation Complex	Horse chestnut seed extract 30 mg, ginko 60 mg, butcher's broom 40 mg, ginger root 40 mg, rutin 40 mg
Garlique	Garlic powder 400 mg
Ginkoba	Gingko biloba 40 mg
Ginsana	Ginseng extract 100 mg
Harmonex	St. John's wort 450 mg, Siberan ginseng 90 mg
Kira	St. John's wort extract LI 160 300 mg (0.3% hypericin)
Kwai	Allicin 600 mg equivalent to 300 mg fresh garlic
Kyolic	Aged garlic extract 600 mg
Movana	St. John's wort extract WS-5572 300 mg
PhytoEstrogen Complex	Vitamin E 50 mg, soy germ concentrate 350 mg, chasteberry 25 mg, kudzu root 15 mg, Korean ginseng 15 mg, Mexican wild yam extract 15 mg, boron 0.75 mg, arrowroot 6.25 mg
Propalmex	Zinc 7.5 mg, saw palmetto berry extract 160 mg, pumpkin seed extract 40 mg
Venastat	Horse chestnut seed extract 300 mg

Alfalfa (Medicago sativa)

Alfalfa is purported to be effective in lowering cholesterol and functions as a laxative, diuretic, and antifungal. A medicagenic acid derivative isolated from alfalfa exhibited fungistatic activity in a limited animal study.[21] Alfalfa seeds in a dose of 40 g three times daily also decreased total cholesterol by 26% and LDL cholesterol by 30% in a noncontrolled study using only 15 patients.[22] Alfalfa seeds contain an amino acid that has caused pancytopenia and systemic lupus erythematosus in monkeys.[23] Alfalfa also enhances tumor development.[24] Until controlled studies establish effectiveness, alfalfa supplements should not be recommended.

Arnica (Arnica montana)

Arnica has popularly been used for improving blood circulation and blood pressure, reducing inflammation, and as an antibiotic. Only one study was found supporting the use of arnica in improving blood circulation; it involved in vitro work with thromboxane.[25] This limited study did not present clinical applications, nor did it include any controlled human testing. Its conclusions therefore cannot be generalized to the statement that arnica would be useful in humans.

Investigators have elucidated a possible mechanism of arnica in reducing inflammation, inhibition of a specific transcription factor by helenalin, one of the sesquiterpene lactones found in arnica.[26] However, when administered to patients undergoing impacted wisdom tooth removal, arnica actually increased the pain level and degree of inflammation when compared with placebo, so that the purported mechanism may not exist.[27] When homeopathic arnica was compared with placebo in treating pain and infection after total hysterectomy, there was no difference between the groups, leading the authors to conclude that homeopathic arnica was of no benefit in postoperative recovery.[28] Several of the constituents of arnica, especially helenalin and jaceosidin, were found to be cytotoxic against certain carcinoma cell lines, but this cytotoxicity would present potential hazards to normal human cells as well.[29] In fact, arnica has produced fatal cardiotoxicity when taken internally because of the presence of its sesquiterpene lactones (e.g., helenalin).[23]

Topical arnica also causes contact eczema.[30,31] Arnica belongs to the Compositae family, which also contains chamomile, feverfew, tansy, yarrow, marguerite, aster, sunflower, laurel, chrysanthemums, and pyrethrins, so the patient allergic to pyrethrins (as found in nonprescription pediculicides) or the others should avoid the arnica.[32–34]

There is no evidence to support the purported uses of arnica, but examples of local allergy and systemic toxicity exist. For this reason, the prudent pharmacist should not recommend arnica.

Bilberry (Vaccinium myrtillus)

Bilberry is a general term for a variety of blueberries, or huckleberries. It is alleged to help acute, nonspecific diarrhea when administered as a tea and to relieve oral and pharyngeal inflammation when used topically. It is also used to prevent cancer and to improve night vision, angina, varicose veins, hemorrhoids, lower limb venous insufficiency, and liver injury. Leaf infusions are used for diabetes.[35] Components known as anthocyanidins or proanthocyanidins may be responsible for any benefit.

An in vitro study seemed to demonstrate anticarcinogenic activity of the proanthocyanidin component of bilberry, but this finding awaits further work and human testing.[36]

Bilberry supplements appear to be safe for use, but the lack of evidence for any proven benefit in the surveyed medical literature argues against their use for such serious conditions as diabetes and angina, which should be supervised by a physician.

Black Cohosh (*Cimicifuga racemosa*)

According to unsubstantiated Internet sources, black cohosh acts to help coughing, diarrhea, irregular menstruation, angina, arthritis, asthma, bronchitis, birth pains, cholera, convulsions, gonorrhea, and many other medical conditions.

No evidence of efficacy for any indication was found in the literature search for black cohosh, although one of its components reduced levels of luteinizing hormone in a noncontrolled study.[37]

Despite this, a black cohosh product (Remifemin) was introduced in 1997 for women undergoing menopause. The pharmacy publication revealed that advertisements for the product in a popular lay publication would include a testimonial from a leading pharmacognocist, asserting that the herb was found to be safe in German studies (despite the fact that the product is neither proven safe nor effective in this country).[38] In fact, it can cause gastrointestinal problems, vertigo, hypotension, nausea, headache, impaired vision, vomiting, and impaired circulation.[38]

Black cohosh is alleged to be active for many serious conditions that should instead be treated under physician care. The pharmacist should refer the patient who wishes to treat a serious medical condition with black cohosh to the physician.

Blue Cohosh (*Caulophyllum thalictroides*)

Blue cohosh is available through Internet sources, allegedly to treat menstrual cramps by acting as a uterine antispasmodic and to ease childbirth pains or speed childbirth. It is also said to induce menstrual flow and to act as a diuretic.

The literature review did not yield any research on blue cohosh for any medical indication. However, it did report the case of a newborn infant whose mother had ingested blue cohosh to promote uterine contractions.[39] The child experienced acute myocardial infarction, profound congestive heart failure, and shock. He recovered after several weeks. The authors blamed toxic glycosides present in blue cohosh for the problems. The pharmacist should never recommend this herb, which is neither proven safe nor effective for any medical indication.

Borage (*Borago officinalis*)

Borage seed oil contains gamma linoleic acid, which is said to decrease the inflammation and injury of arthritis, prevent

cancer, improve PMS symptoms, improve eczema, prevent viral infection, lower blood pressure, help prevent infections, improve diabetic neuropathy, and reduce weight.

In a double-blind, placebo-controlled trial with a small sample size, borage oil reduced a rise in blood pressure and heart rate induced by stress.[40] Borage oil was found to augment cardiovascular responses to negative pressure in a group of 9 patients, although the clinical significance of this finding is not clear.[41]

Borage oil applied topically reduced symptoms of seborrheic dermatitis in a group of 37 patients, but did not clearly suppress growth of Malassezia furfur in another study.[42,43]

Borage seed oil providing a dose of 1.1 g daily improved rheumatoid arthritis in an uncontrolled study group of 7 patients; in another more well-controlled study, it relieved such rheumatoid arthritis symptoms as tender and swollen joints.[44,45]

Patients with cystic fibrosis given 1500 mg of borage oil daily for 4 weeks experienced increased vital capacity in an uncontrolled study.[46]

Borage and borage oil appear to be of low toxicity. However, there is little information in the surveyed medical literature that substantiates the claims made for it. The patient with serious conditions such as arthritis, hypertension, and diabetic neuropathy is better advised to see a physician.

Cat's Claw (*Uncaria tomentosa, U. guianensis*)

Cat's claw bark has been recommended as a contraceptive and for the treatment of gastric ulcer, inflammation, rheumatoid arthritis, and cancer. It is said to augment the immune system in cancer patients and to serve as an antitumor agent.

One study of cat's claw seemed to indicate a protective effect against antimutagenesis, although it used in vitro research and the results of a study on only one patient's urine.[47] There is very little else in the surveyed medical literature to indicate medical usefulness of cat's claw.

The literature does not support the many purported uses of cat's claw. Patients who ask about its use are better referred to a physician.

Cayenne (*Capsicum frutescens, C. annuum*)

Cayenne contains capsaicin and other related compounds. Applied externally, it is proven safe and effective as a counterirritant (see Chapter 20).[48] However, it is also recommended for many unproven uses such as reducing the incidence of peptic ulcer disease and helping heal gastric lesions, as well as serving as a carminative and stimulant. Capsaicin was hypothesized to be of use as an anticarcinogenic agent, based on in vitro research.[49]

The effects of cayenne as red pepper have been studied in healthy humans. Rather than providing any gastrointestinal benefit when given internally, it was found to cause gastric-cell exfoliation and mucosal microbleeding.[50] In another study, 20 g of chili powder slowed gastric emptying but shortened whole gut transit time.[51]

Cayenne is usually considered to be nontoxic, but exposure can cause contact dermatitis, and in vitro tests on human buccal mucosal cells demonstrated cytotoxicity when exposed to *Capsicum frutescens* extract.[52]

Cayenne is a popular spice used by many millions of people every day. Its adverse reaction incidence is quite low. However, it is implicated in food allergy and food intolerance.[53] Further, it should not be recommended for any serious medical condition such as peptic ulcer in light of the paucity of medical evidence to support these uses.

Chamomile (*Chamaemelum nobile, Matricaria recutita*)

Chamomile is allegedly active as an antiinflammatory, antispasmodic, sedative, hypnotic, and analgesic.[54] One of its constituents, chamazulene, was found to inhibit leukotriene synthesis, which might contribute to an antiinflammatory effect, although this was in vitro research.[55] Another constituent of oil of chamomile partially inhibited degranulation of mast cells in rats; the significance of this finding in humans is unknown.[56]

In an attempt to prevent oral mucositis attributed to 5-fluorouracil, researchers administered a chamomile mouthwash, but it was not efficacious.[57]

As a member of the Compositae family, chamomile may cause allergic reactions in those allergic to such other members as feverfew, tansy, chrysanthemums, arnica, and yarrow, as well as ragweed, daisies, and asters (see "Arnica").[6,32] An 8-year-old boy was given chamomile tea infusion for the first time and developed an anaphylactic reaction; a 35-year-old woman died of anaphylactic shock after ingesting a small quantity of chamomile tea.[6,58] The authors hypothesized that previous sensitization to mugwort (another member of the Compositae) caused the cross-sensitization. Although washing one's eyes with chamomile tea is a folk remedy for conjunctivitis and other ocular problems, this use is hazardous and has caused eyelid angioedema and further conjunctivitis.[59]

Chamomile is not proven to have the various actions ascribed to it. In light of the potentially deadly allergic reactions in those not previously known to be sensitive to chamomile (because of the large number of cross-sensitizing plants), it should not be recommended for use by patients.

Chaparral (*Lerrea tridentata*)

Chaparral has been sold as a blood purifier and cancer cure, but was never proven efficacious for any use. Despite this, many thousands of people purchased it. The uncontrolled sales of chaparral had deadly consequences. *Chaparral has caused numerous cases of acute cholestatic hepatitis, jaundice, cirrhosis, and acute liver failure; one patient required a transplant.[60–67] Chaparral also causes serious kidney damage such as cystic renal disease and cystic adenocarcinoma.[68]* Chaparral has no possible benefit, especially one that could justify the lethal risk of ingestion. *Pharmacists must not stock this herb and must advise against its use at any time.*

Chasteberry (*Vitex agnus castus*)

Chasteberry is an herb touted on various Internet sites as a tonic for menstrual problems. It is sold in pharmacies and health-food stores as oral tablets.

The medical literature survey did not contain evidence of efficacy for chasteberry for any problem. However, in one report, a woman using it experienced abnormal levels of serum gonadotropin and ovarian hormones. Her symptoms resembled mild ovarian stimulation during the luteal phase of the menstrual cycle.[69] The authors advised against use of chasteberry to promote normal ovarian function.

Coltsfoot (*Tussilago farfara*)

Coltsfoot, sometimes taken in tea form to help coughing and respiratory problems, has caused cancer in laboratory studies.[70] Further, an 18-month-old boy given what was assumed to be coltsfoot tea for 15 months to "aid in the child's healthy development" developed venoocclusive disease resulting in portal hypertension and severe ascites that resolved after 2 months.[71] Unfortunately, the parents collected their own herb and incorrectly collected Alpendost (*Adenostyles alliariae*), which contains toxic pyrrolizidine alkaloids. While this report does not involve coltsfoot tea, it illustrates vividly the dangers inherent in collection of one's own herbs. There is no evidence of efficacy for coltsfoot in the surveyed medical literature in any case.

Comfrey (*Symphytum officinale*)

Comfrey has traditionally been recommended as a general healing agent for such conditions as gout, arthritis, and infections. *However, this plant contains pyrrolizidine alkaloids, which have been implicated in liver disease, liver cancer, and lung cancer, and has caused death.[72–76] Comfrey obstructs hepatic circulation (a condition known as venoocclusive disease) and also produces hepatic carcinoma.[7,77] In one case, a newborn may have suffered hepatic damage because of the mother's ingestion of comfrey tea.[6]*

Cranberry Fruit (*Vaccinium macrocarpon*)

Cranberry fruit is thought to acidify the urine, thereby reducing the risk of urinary tract infections. It is also allegedly of benefit in reducing the odor of urine.

Evidence for cranberry in urinary tract infections is contradictory. One small study indicated that it might inhibit bacterial adherence.[78] Others indicate that the herb may be of benefit through lowering urinary pH, although some studies fail to show this effect.[79–83]

While cranberry fruit is generally considered to be nontoxic, one case-control study demonstrated that people living in close proximity to a cranberry cultivation facility experienced twice the risk of brain cancer as those who did not.[84]

Cranberry fruit or juice carries an extremely low risk of toxicity and may be of benefit in prevention of urinary tract infections. However, the pharmacist must stress that the patient who suspects a present urinary tract infection should consult a physician.

Devil's Claw (*Harpagophytum procumbens*)

This herb is recommended as an antiinflammatory, analgesic and for tendinitis, anorexia, and stomach problems. Its safety and benefits are not addressed in the surveyed medical literature. Therefore, it should not be recommended; nonprescription products proven safe and effective as antiinflammatories, analgesics, and gastric remedies may be recommended instead.

Dong Quai (*Angelica sinensis, A. polymorpha*)

Dong quai (also sometimes labeled as Tang kuei) is an oriental herb alleged to treat gynecologic problems (such as menstrual irregularities); to be a tonic to purify the blood; and to help control hypertension, rheumatism, constipation, and anemia.[85,86]

A double-blind, placebo-controlled trial discovered that Dong quai was no more helpful than placebo in relieving several symptoms of menopause, including such hallmark problems as the number of vasomotor flushes.[87]

Dong quai contains coumarin derivatives such as psoralens, which can induce photodermatitis.[23]

There is a lack of evidence of effectiveness of Dong quai for any indication in the surveyed medical literature. This fact, coupled with the possibility of photodermatitis, should cause the pharmacist to recommend against its use. Instead, the patient should be referred to a physician who can prescribe appropriate therapy for rheumatism, hypertension, and the other serious medical conditions for which patients might attempt to self-medicate with Dong quai.

Echinacea (*Echinacea angustifolia, E. purpurea, E. pallida*)

Echinacea is thought to stimulate the immune system, thereby reducing the severity of cold and flu symptoms.[88] It is also alleged to help treat urinary tract infection, upper respiratory infections (e.g., tonsillitis, otitis media, sore throat, whooping cough), and *Candida albicans* infections.

Evidence for the efficacy of Echinacea in the surveyed medical literature is less than conclusive.[89] In several in vitro studies, *E. purpura* seemed to stimulate lymphokine production, enhance natural-killer-cell activity, and stimulate cytokine production by macrophages, thereby boosting cell-mediated immunity.[90–93] However, in another study, Echinacea did not produce any change in either cytokine production or leukocyte numbers.[94]

In two studies, Echinacea was given to patients with colorectal cancers and hepatocellular carcinomas.[95,96] However, the herb was given in a regimen that also included cyclophosphamide and "thymostimulin," so the effects of the Echinacea alone cannot be easily determined.

Echinacea may produce allergic reactions in patients with a preexisting allergy to sunflower and related plants.[6] One patient developed severe anaphylaxis.[97] The authors of that report cautioned against the use of Echinacea, since anaphylaxis may occur with first-time use because of cross-sensitization with other plants.

Echinacea has moved into the mainstream, with the introduction of Celestial Seasonings Herbal Comfort Lozenges with Echinacea. In light of the general paucity of controlled trials in humans demonstrating any beneficial effect from Echinacea, and considering the possibility of severe allergic reactions with first-time use, pharmacists should only recommend it with caution.

Elderberry (*Sambucus canadensis, S. nigra*)

Elderberry has been traditionally used for its diuretic, laxative, and astringent effects. It is also said to boost the immune system and help prevent influenza.

Elderberry extract shortened the time to recovery from influenza when administered in a double-blind, placebo-controlled trial.[98] However, further research to replicate these results has not yet been carried out.

Elderberry contains dangerous components that have caused toxicity when ingested as juice. The safety of elderberry tablets has yet to be studied in an adequate trial. Because of the general lack of evidence for efficacy of elderberry for any of its purported uses, it should not be recommended.

Eleuthero, Siberian Ginseng (*Eleutherococcus senticosus*)

Siberian ginseng is recommended for fortifying the person's capacity for work, improving the ability to concentrate, preventing colds and flu, helping during chronic fatigue syndrome, and providing support during radiation or chemotherapy.

The only article in the surveyed medical literature addressing medical effectiveness of Siberian ginseng was a study in which mice were given the herb during a period of major environmental stress.[99] Siberian ginseng significantly increased their aggressive behaviors, but there was no change in either stamina or longevity.

In one case, a 74-year-old man stabilized on digoxin was discovered to have unexpectedly elevated serum levels.[100] When he confessed to taking Siberian ginseng, the herb was subsequently found to be the culprit. Ceasing use allowed digoxin levels to normalize. He resumed the herb, and the levels rose again.

Since there is no evidence to support its use, and since there is at least one potentially dangerous drug interaction, pharmacists should advise against the use of Siberian ginseng.

Evening Primrose Oil (*Oenothera biennis*)

Evening primrose oil has a high content of essential fatty acids, which are allegedly effective for a wide range of disorders:

- Breast pain[101]
- Premenstrual syndrome, menopausal symptoms[102,103]
- Weight loss
- Skin conditions: psoriasis, dry skin, scaly skin, eczema, acne

- High cholesterol
- Rheumatoid arthritis[104]
- Raynaud's disease
- Sjögren's syndrome[105]
- Asthma
- Diabetic neuropathy[106]
- Liver damage
- Attention deficit/hyperactivity disorder
- Ulcerative colitis

Evening primrose oil given to women suffering from breast pain did not function any better than expected from the placebo effect.[107] Evening primrose oil did not prevent recurrence of breast cysts in a well-controlled trial of 200 female patients when compared with placebo.[108]

Evening primrose oil reduced symptoms of premenstrual syndrome in several well-controlled studies, but a systematic literature review of all studies conducted led authors to the conclusion that there was little evidence to support its use.[109,110] A well-controlled trial failed to demonstrate any benefit in PMS.[111] The herb was no more effective than placebo in reducing the flushing associated with menopause in a well-controlled study.[112]

Evening primrose oil given to 100 women with substantial obesity failed to produce any clinically significant weight loss.[113]

Evening primrose oil given to patients with chronic hand dermatitis and atopic dermatitis in two well-controlled studies failed to produce any effect.[114,115] In another study, the herb failed to improve either eczema or asthma in a well-controlled trial of children with one or both conditions.[116] However, when given to patients with atopic dermatitis in other studies, evening primrose oil improved the eczema significantly when compared with placebo.[117–120]

Evening primrose oil given to psoriatic patients in a well-controlled trial did not produce clinical improvement, nor were patients able to reduce their dosages of nonsteroidal, antiinflammatory medications while taking it.[121] It was also ineffective in improving psoriasis in another well-controlled trial.[122]

Patients with hypertriglyceridemia given evening primrose oil did not experience a lowering of serum lipoproteins in one study.[123] In another, it failed to reduce serum cholesterol, HDL cholesterol, or triglyceride mean values.[124]

When 20 patients with active rheumatoid arthritis were given evening primrose oil, there was no effect on the number of tender joints, number of swollen joints, duration of morning stiffness, or the patient's self-estimation of pain.[125] In another study, evening primrose oil performed no better than placebo in improving rheumatoid arthritis.[126] Other researchers noticed that evening primrose oil might have effects on eicosanoid precursors that would actually worsen the condition.[127] One study seemed to show benefit for evening primrose oil in reducing the morning stiffness of rheumatoid arthritis at 3 months, but the olive oil placebo reduced the pain at 6 months, pointing out the dangers of drawing con-

clusion from relatively short-term therapy in a condition that normally undergoes periodic exacerbations and remissions.[128]

Evening primrose oil given to patients with Raynaud's syndrome in a well-controlled study produced symptomatic benefit, although objective assessments of blood flow did not change.[129]

Evening primrose oil did not improve dry eye of Sjögren's syndrome significantly when compared with placebo.[130]

Two well-controlled studies of evening primrose oil in asthmatics failed to elicit any beneficial effect on asthma.[131,132]

Patients with chronic hepatitis B given evening primrose oil exhibited no improvement in biochemical or histologic indicators of hepatic damage.[133]

In two double-blind, placebo-controlled trials, evening primrose oil was not of significant benefit in children with attention deficit/hyperactivity disorder.[134,135]

Investigators administered evening primrose oil to patients suffering from ulcerative colitis in a well-controlled study and found that it improved stool consistency when compared with placebo.[136]

Evening primrose oil seemed to reduce the edema of pregnancy in a placebo-controlled, partially double-blinded trial.[137]

Although its toxicity profile is evidently low, careful scrutiny of all included studies involving evening primrose oil demonstrates convincingly that it has little, if any therapeutic benefit. Many of the conditions for which it was studied failed to improve and should be treated by a physician in any case, rather than through self-administration of an herb that is neither proven safe nor effective. The prudent pharmacist would refer the patient to a physician when serious conditions are present (e.g., asthma, atopic dermatitis, liver damage).

Eyebright (*Euphrasia*)

Eyebright is an herb allegedly effective for ophthalmic problems, although the literature search failed to reveal evidence of eyebright efficacy in any condition. In one case, a 17-year-old female patient with herpes simplex keratitis of the right eye was to receive corticosteroid eyedrops.[138] Instead she visited a local herbalist, who sold her an eyedrop containing eyebright and plantain. As a result of this therapy, which was neither proven safe nor effective, she developed suppurative keratitis; the product was also contaminated with multiple pathogenic organisms. She developed extensive scarring and visual loss that only partly resolved when she resumed legitimate medical therapy.

Feverfew (*Tanacetum parthenium*, *Chrysanthemum parthenium*)

Feverfew has been recommended for use in fever, for migraine headache, and as an arthritis remedy. It may also possess antithrombotic potential and antiinflammatory actions.[139–143] It contains sesquiterpene lactones of which parthenolide is the most well known.[144]

In Canada, a major manufacturer of nonprescription products began sales of migraine prophylaxis products containing feverfew in 1996.[145] Feverfew given to migraine sufferers in a well-controlled trial reduced the number and severity of attacks and vomiting, although the duration of the attacks did not change.[146] Any beneficial effect may be caused by an ability of feverfew to affect platelet aggregation.[147,148] However, in another well-controlled trial, feverfew did not change the frequency or severity of migraine attacks.[149]

Feverfew given to rheumatoid arthritis sufferers in a well-controlled trial failed to improve either laboratory or clinical variables.[150]

Feverfew cross-reacts with the Compositae family of plants, so should be avoided by those with an allergy to any of its members.[34,151,152] (See "Arnica" above for a complete listing.) Feverfew also causes oral ulcerations and swollen tongue and may affect hemostasis.[153,154]

Feverfew is not clearly of benefit in any condition and may cause severe allergic reactions in first-time users. The patient with migraine or rheumatoid arthritis should instead be referred to a physician for more appropriate therapy.

Garlic (*Allium sativum*)

Garlic allegedly has many actions, including lowering cholesterol, helping cardiovascular problems, acting as an antibacterial, antifungal, anthelmintic, hypotensive, anticarcinogenic, and antiviral.[155–162]

One review of trials of garlic in cardiovascular problems concluded that its use would not be justified; however, a later meta-analysis of its potential in hypercholesterolemia came to the opposite conclusion.[163,164] Additional research demonstrated that some of its constituents (allicin, adenosine, and paraffinic polysulfides) possessed antiplatelet actions; it also improved thrombocyte aggregation and epidermal microcirculation.[165–169] Garlic did not produce changes in blood coagulation or fibrinolysis in one study.[170]

The ability of garlic to lower total cholesterol did not differ significantly from placebo in one study, but it was effective in others.[171–175] It did not affect blood lipids or blood coagulation in another study.[176]

Garlic was active against several bacteria and fungi during in vitro testing, and several of its components (e.g., ajoene, allicin) also exhibited antiviral activity.[177–178]

Garlic self-administered in one patient with severe hepatopulmonary syndrome who refused a liver transplant may have produced partial relief of symptoms.[179]

Garlic may be responsible for a decrease in the incidence of stomach cancer noticed in one survey of Chinese citizens, although a similar study failed to demonstrate any benefit for garlic in prevention of lung cancer in the Netherlands.[180–181] A possible link of *Helicobacter pylori* to gastric carcinoma led researchers to explore the activity of garlic against the organism.[182] It was found to possess activity against *Helicobacter pylori* in in vitro tests. Garlic consumption was not found to alter the incidence of female breast cancer.[183] A major review of the role of garlic in cancer concluded that conclusive evidence of its effectiveness was lacking.[184]

Patients may develop an allergy to garlic, which cross-reacts with onion, leek, and chives.[185–188]

⚠ ***Topical garlic is unsafe. In one case, a naturopathic "physician" prescribed garlic in a petroleum jelly plaster.[189] The child sustained partial thickness burns as a result.*** (For precautions regarding naturopathy and other unproven medical practices, see Chapter 49, Precautions in Self-Care.) People who handle garlic during food preparation or use the home remedy of rubbing garlic on the skin for fungal infections often develop contact dermatitis.[190,191] This practice should be discouraged.

Garlic taken orally during pregnancy can be detected in amniotic fluid.[192] The effects of this on the fetus are unknown.

Garlic is a food flavoring agent used safely by many millions of people every day. As such, it is undoubtedly safe for the majority of users to ingest. However, the literature concerning its reported medical uses is self-contradictory. Should the pharmacist wish to recommend it, its toxicity is so low that it would not be harmful in moderate doses. However, patients whose medical conditions are potentially serious (e.g., cancer, infections, high cholesterol) are better managed by a physician.

Germander (*Teucrium chamaedrys*)

⚠ Germander was alleged to be a weight loss aid. ***Germander tea has caused many cases of acute hepatitis, with at least one fatality.[193,194] In some cases, discontinuation of the herb allowed jaundice to disappear within 8 weeks, but patient readministration allowed hepatitis to recur.[195,196] The herb is banned in France; it should neither be stocked nor recommended.***

Ginger (*Zingiber officinale*)

Ginger is a traditional remedy for motion sickness and is purported to relieve stomach problems and morning sickness of pregnancy.[197]

Two well-controlled studies demonstrated efficacy of ginger in decreasing the incidence of postoperative nausea and vomiting, while another failed to do so.[198–200] It also decreased experimentally induced vertigo.[201] Ginger improved symptoms of hyperemesis gravidarum in a well-controlled trial.[202]

In another, it reduced the tendency to vomit and cold sweating in naval cadets during heavy seas.[203] However, ginger was not of benefit in affecting either the vestibular or oculomotor systems, both of which are critical in the genesis of motion sickness; it also did not alter gastric function during experimentally induced motion sickness.[204,205]

Ginger administered to seven patients with rheumatic disorders produced pain relief, although the trial was neither placebo controlled nor double-blinded.[206]

Ginger did not affect platelet function when administered to healthy volunteers, but did do so in another study.[207,208]

While ginger has been discussed as a possible migraine remedy, there are no studies extant that can be used to recommend it.[209]

Ginger is a contact allergen, so patients should not prepare it from the raw plant or its components.[187,210]

Ginger is a common food component used by many people every day without adverse effect. While it is probably not a good choice for migraine or serious causes of nausea and vomiting, it may possess activity in motion sickness. The patient who cannot tolerate antihistamines may benefit from this herb, should the pharmacist wish to recommend it. However, the dose is unknown since the product is not approved by the Food and Drug Administration for this use.

Gingko (*Gingko biloba*)

Gingko allegedly improves memory, concentration, dementia, and depression through its purported effects in improving cerebral blood flow.[211–213] It is also said to improve vertigo, tinnitus, and intermittent claudication and to act as an antimicrobial, antiinflammatory, and vasodilating agent.

A well-controlled trial of gingko in eight healthy female volunteers demonstrated no benefit in several psychologic examinations, but memory was significantly improved.[214] When gingko was given to patients aged over 50 with mild to moderate memory impairment, it improved cognitive function and speed of response on a computerized task.[215] Gingko also seemed to improve patients with acute ischemic stroke.[216] A German extract of gingko improved attention and memory for patients with Alzheimer's dementia in a dose of 240 mg per day.[217] Gingko also improved mental performance in patients with dementia in another widely publicized, well-controlled study.[218]

Investigators reviewed the results of 40 trials of gingko in improving cerebral insufficiency (most trials using 120 mg of gingko extract daily) and found many methodologic flaws such as small sample sizes in 32 of the trials.[219] The authors also pointed out the dangers of publication bias in which negative results are often not reported. They concluded that further studies of the efficacy of gingko would be needed before it could be recommended with confidence.

In one well-controlled trial, gingko was superior to placebo in improving peripheral arteriopathy, allowing patients to walk farther.[220] In another, it decreased erythrocyte aggregation in 10 subjects, but did not affect platelets.[221]

A gingko sesquiterpene known as bilobalide was found to inhibit *Pneumocystis carinii* in rats, leading the authors to conclude that it might be of use in prophylaxis against that organism and in treating the infections it produces.[222]

Gingko was given to patients with severe tinnitus, but had no effect.[223]

Gingko is usually safe, but may cause gastrointestinal upset, headache, and allergic skin reactions.[211,224] Gingko has been linked to bilateral subdural hematoma.[211] It can interact with anticoagulants to prolong bleeding time.[54]

Overwhelming evidence to support the use of gingko is not yet available. However, its safety is such that the pharmacist might recommend it for minor problems (general memory improvement). If the patient has a serious medical problem, referral is a more logical option than recommending self-treatment with gingko.

Ginseng, Asian Ginseng (*Panax ginseng*)

Ginseng allegedly acts as a general tonic for the fatigued or debilitated patient, improves stamina and sexual health, helps the healing process, lowers blood pressure, acts as an athletic ergogenic aid, and makes people work more efficiently, among other unproven uses.[225–228]

Ginseng's potential as an ergogenic aid was examined in a double-blind, placebo-controlled trial in which the duration of subjects during graded maximal aerobic exercise was assessed.[229] Ginseng did not affect any standard measure of exercise performance. In another study, ginseng did not improve the performance of patients riding a cycle ergometer.[230]

Ginseng was found to exert a steroid effect on T-cell–mediated immunity in research using a small group of four healthy volunteers, and it also enhanced cellular immune function in another study, although any actual clinical effect is unclear.[92,231] In another study, a saponin extracted from ginseng enhanced the immune function of lymphocytes in elderly patients.[232]

Two retrospective studies examined consumption of ginseng in relation to cancer risk of Koreans.[233,234] Ginseng extract and powder appeared to reduce the risk of cancer (e.g., lip, oral cavity, pharynx, colorectal, esophageal) in both genders.

An extract of ginseng and gingko reduced diastolic blood pressure and heart rate in a small uncontrolled trial.[235] The herb also produced a slight contraction of renal veins of rabbits and relaxed the pulmonary artery.[236]

Ginseng elevated the mood, improved psychologic performance, and reduced the fasting blood glucose of 36 patients with non–insulin-dependent diabetes mellitus in a well-controlled trial.[237]

When given to a small group of geriatric patients in a well-controlled trial, ginseng failed to act as an aid to treatment or rehabilitation.[238] However, in a well-controlled trial of ginseng plus vitamins versus multivitamins alone, ginseng improved the quality of life in 501 patients living in large Mexican cities.[239]

Ginseng enhanced clearance of alcohol from the blood in a small noncontrolled study.[240]

Ginseng has been known to produce hypertension, estrogenic effects, swollen and painful breasts, and vaginal bleeding.[153] A 28-year-old woman ingested a large quantity of ginseng extracted with ethanol, experiencing severe headache.[241]

A cerebral arteriogram revealed cerebral arteritis. In another case, a topical face cream with ginseng produced postmenopausal bleeding, perhaps caused by estrogenic actions on vaginal tissues.[242] Chinese researchers illustrated the dangers of using herbal medicines by pointing out that ginseng may become adulterated during the collection process with other herbs containing such toxic chemicals as scopolamine.[243]

The various studies of ginseng are often flawed and contradictory. In light of the possibility of adverse reactions with its use, ginseng should not be recommended until more adequate proof of efficacy for some condition is presented.

Goldenseal (*Hydrastis canadensis*)

Goldenseal is alleged to help treat respiratory tract conditions, influenza, inflammation of the mucosa, gastritis, traveler's diarrhea, heavy menstrual flow, ophthalmic problems, dyspepsia, and skin wounds.

There is little evidence that can be located to support any medical use of goldenseal. On the other hand, it may produce cardiac and vascular irregularities. It should not be recommended.

Gotu Kola (*Centella asiatica*)

Gotu kola allegedly aids in improving memory, helping venous insufficiency, and relieving stress, circulation, fatigue, mental confusion, night cramps, and edema.[244]

Investigators administered gotu kola extract to patients with lower limb venous insufficiency in a well-controlled study.[245] It relieved heaviness of the lower limbs and edema and improved venous distensibility. In another study, it reduced the number of circulating endothelial cells in patients with postphlebitic syndrome.[246] It also improved capillary permeability in patients with venous hypertension in a small uncontrolled study.[247] Patients with venous hypertension experienced improvement of capillary filtration and ankle edema when given gotu kola.[248]

Crude extract of gotu kola seemed to inhibit tumor cells in an in vivo study, but the applicability of this to humans is unknown.[249] Gotu kola also stimulated collagen synthesis in in vitro research.[250]

One of the ingredients of gotu kola, madecassol, has been used for wound healing and prevention of scarring. However, madecassol and other constituents of gotu kola (asiaticoside, asitic acid, and madecassic acid) cause contact dermatitis and should be avoided.[251–253]

Although a few preliminary studies show promise for gotu kola, it should not be recommended for serious conditions until more evidence accumulates regarding efficacy and safety when self-administered without physician supervision.

Grape Seed (*Vitis vinifera*)

Grape seed has purported benefits in assisting blood flow, treating capillary fragility and permeability in diabetes mellitus, and exerting antiinflammatory effects.

There is no evidence for the purported effects of grape seed. Further, the safety of consumption is unknown. Unless evidence for efficacy develops, it should not be recommended.

Green Leaf Tea (*Camellia sinensis*)

Green tea supposedly acts to lower cholesterol, prevent cancer and dental caries, and treat atherosclerosis and hypertension.

Green tea may reduce the risk of cancer in smokers, based on a study in which the frequency of sisterchromatid exchange was reduced by consuming it.[254]

Caffeine consumption in pregnancy can increase the risk of birth defects and may increase the risk of sudden infant death syndrome.[255]

Green leaf tea infusions were found to inhibit the utilization of thiamin in one study and increased the urinary loss of niacin.[256]

There is no clear evidence for any therapeutic benefit from green tea. Further, in pregnancy, it can cause adverse effects on the fetus. Until it is proven safe for a therapeutic use, it should not be recommended.

Hawthorn Berries (*Cratageus monogyna, C. laevigata*)

Hawthorn is said to prevent coronary complications and conditions, heart failure, hypertension, angina, and arteriosclerosis.[257]

There is little evidence from the literature review for effectiveness of hawthorn in cardiac conditions. In any case, any condition related to possible cardiac pathology is serious. The pharmacist must suggest referral to a physician rather than self-treatment with hawthorn berries.

Horse Chestnut (*Aesculus hippocastanum*)

Horse chestnut is allegedly active in treating varicose veins. (See "A Pharmacist's Journal: Where's the Medicine for Varicose Veins?")

In one partially controlled study and two other placebo-controlled studies, horse chestnut reduced lower leg edema in patients with chronic venous insufficiency.[258–260]

Horse chestnut is a sensitizer and causes allergic reactions during the spring.[261] Further, patients may exhibit cross-sensitization to horse chestnut, latex, avocado, banana, and passion fruits.[262]

Jin Bu Huan

This oriental herb is an example of products heavily promoted to certain ethnic groups. It has only been available in the U.S. since the mid 1980s. Its reported uses are as a sedative and analgesic.[263]

There are several reports of hepatotoxicity, including acute hepatitis, jaundice, vomiting, hepatomegaly, fatigue, and fever from the use of jin bu huan.[263–265] In three children, unintentional overdoses resulted in central nervous system depression, respiratory depression, and life-threatening bradycardia.[263,266]

The contents of the packaging of jin bu huan misrepresent the actual ingredients, which causes delays in identifying the toxic principles.[267]

⚠ *Jin bu huan has a toxicity profile that renders it unacceptable for patient use. It must not be stocked in the pharmacy.*

Kava Kava (*Piper methysticum*)

Kava kava (also referred to as simply kava), a plant used for intoxicant properties in the Pacific islands, allegedly alleviates nervous anxiety, stress, and restlessness; enhances sleep; and acts as a sedative.[268,269]

In one well-controlled study, kava improved anxiety.[270] There is little additional evidence in the medical literature to support the use of kava.

Kava causes scaling eruptions of the skin in those who consume it, perhaps through interference with cholesterol metabolism.[271,272] It also reduces visual function.[273] When Aboriginal heavy kava users were studied, it was found that they were more likely to have poor health, be underweight, have low levels of albumin and plasma protein, exhibit hematuria, and have decreased platelet and lymphocyte counts.[274] They also exhibited shortness of breath and decreased lung volumes; all of the findings caused the authors of the study to call for initiatives to reduce the consumption of kava.

The literature on efficacy of kava is virtually nonexistent. On the other hand, there are several reports of adverse effects. There is no reason for a patient to risk the adverse effects of kava by using it. It should not be recommended.

Licorice (*Glycyrrhiza glabra*)

Licorice is alleged to treat upper respiratory tract conditions, gastritis, duodenal ulcers, bronchitis, and insufficiency of the adrenocortical gland.

In an in vitro study, licorice seemed to exert an antiviral effect, although the clinical significance is unknown.[275] A preliminary study also showed promise for chronic hepatitis B.[276]

Licorice may act as an antioxidant, as suggested by one study where it inhibited LDL oxidation in rats and in an additional in vitro study.[277,278]

Licorice is not without ill effects (e.g., sodium retention, fluid retention), because of the steroidlike activity (which causes apparent mineralocorticoid excess or pseudoaldosteronism) and potential potassium depletion caused by glycyrrhizinic acid and/or 18-beta-glycyrrhetinic acid.[279–285] A 35-year-old man who ingested one to two bags of licorice tablets each day for 2 years (the equivalent of 20 to 40 g daily) experienced acute myopathy as a result of this effect; another case of myopathy caused by licorice has been reported.[279,286] Other patients have experienced hypokalemic rhabdomyolysis.[287,288] Still other patients experienced hypertension, hypokalemia, and/or low plasma renin as a result of licorice ingestion.[289,290] A 15-year-old boy developed hypertensive

encephalopathy that required 5 months for recovery after ingesting 500 g of licorice candy.[291]

In light of the many incidents of severe adverse reactions caused by licorice, ingestion of licorice as a dietary supplement seems extremely unwise. Pharmacists should not recommend it.

Lobelia (*Lobelia inflata*)

Lobelia has allegedly been of use in helping patients withdraw from nicotine addiction and as a respiratory stimulant. It was found by the FDA to be lacking in safety and efficacy for this use.[292,293]

Lobelia can cause bronchodilation, reduced breathing, ⚠ hypotension, sweating, coma, and death.[6,70] *Lobelia teas are quite toxic, producing nausea, vomiting, diarrhea, breathing problems, convulsions, coma, and death.*[7,294] In one case, a renal transplant recipient was given lobelia by a girlfriend while hospitalized, subsequently experiencing disorientation, confusion, agitation, pressured speech, and visual hallucinations.[295] Further, he was found to have hypertension and tachycardia.

Lobelia is a potentially toxic herb with no proven therapeutic benefit. It should not be recommended for self-treatment of any condition.

Ma Huang, Chinese Ephedra (*Ephedra sinica*)

⚠ *Ma huang, a popular dieting and energy boosting product, contains ephedrine and has caused heart attack, acute hepatitis, liver failure, hypertension, strokes, seizures, psychosis, dizziness, muscle damage, nerve damage, amnesia, palpitations, and irregular heartbeat.*[6,70,296] *Its use has resulted in 15 deaths, some in high school students, which has forced restrictions on its sale.* It should neither be stocked in pharmacies or recommended for self-treatment.

Milk Thistle (*Silybum marianum*)

Milk thistle is purported to help prevent or treat toxic liver damage such as cirrhosis or other conditions through a hypothesized inhibition of Kupffer cells.[297,298]

An active ingredient of milk thistle, silymarin, may have increased survival in patients with alcoholic cirrhosis, based on a small-scale, well-controlled study.[299] It may also have exerted an anticarcinogenic effect in in vitro work on prostate carcinoma cells and breast cancer cells.[300,301] Another active ingredient, silibinin, was reported to enhance the motility of human neutrophils.[302]

Any of the preliminary research of milk thistle begs a more important question: If a patient has existing liver disease, or expects at some time to have liver disease, why use milk thistle rather than making an immediate physician appointment? Hepatic disease is not a condition that can be self-treated, certainly not with the use of an unproven herb such as milk thistle. The pharmacist can be of great service to patients by asking for the reason for proposed purchase of milk thistle, followed by a referral for liver function tests when appropriate.

Nettle (*Urtica dioica*)

Nettle root is sold for its alleged ability to improve urinary and prostate function. In one study, authors hypothesized that steroids contained in nettle root extract suppress prostate cell metabolism and growth.[303] Nettle was also found to inhibit binding of sex hormone-binding globulin to its receptor on human prostatic membrane, which is a possible mechanism for activity in benign prostatic hypertrophy.[304,305] However, nettle causes allergy in some patients.[306] In summary, prostatic and urinary problems should be seen by a physician rather than being self-treated with a substance of unknown effectiveness such as nettle.

Passion Flower (*Passiflora alata, P. incarnata*)

Passion flower is said to be a natural calming agent, soothing the patient and providing relaxation after a stressful day. However, there is a paucity of information available to confirm these hypotheses. Further, the plant causes allergic reactions.[307] Finally, five patients with altered consciousness caused by passion flower were admitted to a hospital, prompting the authors of the report to question nonprescription sales of herbal products that might have sedative effects.[308] The risk of sedation with unsupervised use is too high for the pharmacist to recommend passion flower for patients.

Pennyroyal (*Hedeoma pulegioides*)

⚠ *Pennyroyal oil is occasionally taken to induce abortion. However, it is a deadly hepatotoxic agent.*[309] In one case, a 24-year-old female died after ingesting it.[70] Two infants given home-brewed mint tea for colic developed fatal hepatic and neurologic injuries from the toxic contaminant pennyroyal oil.[310] Those seeking pennyroyal oil must be informed by the pharmacist that its toxicity can cause death and that it should never be considered for use as an abortifacient agent.

Peppermint (*Mentha piperita*)

Peppermint has traditionally been used to aid the gastrointestinal tract, gall bladder, and bile ducts.

A combination product containing peppermint oil and caraway oil was administered to patients with non-ulcer dyspepsia in a well-controlled study, and it yielded benefit for degree of pain, frequency of pain, and severity of the disorder.[311] Peppermint oil added to barium sulfate suspension reduced the incidence of colonic spasm during barium enema.[312] Peppermint oil given to patients with irritable bowel syndrome reduced severity of abdominal pain, abdominal distension, stool frequency, borborygmi, and flatulence.[313] Peppermint oil reduced the severity of postoperative nausea in a study comparing it to placebo.[314]

Peppermint oil taken orally can increase the incidence of gastroesophageal reflux through interfering with the action of the lower esophageal sphincter. It is also a common allergen when used in toothpastes.[315] Excessive ingestion can also induce stomatitis.[316]

Although peppermint oil is probably safe for most users, those wishing to use it for treatment of conditions involving the gastrointestinal tract, gall bladder, or bile ducts should be questioned closely to uncover serious medical problems that warrant a physician referral.

Plantain (*Plantago lanceolata*)

Plantain is alleged to act as a digestive aid and laxative.[317] However, the medical literature speaks mainly of its allergenicity.[318–320]

Some plantain supplements actually contain digitalis, which could be cardiotoxic.[321] The FDA warned patients to stop using certain brands (a list is available by calling 1-800-FDA-4010) and suggested that any adverse reaction caused by plantain be reported to the FDA MedWatch adverse event reporting line at 1-800-FDA-1088.

Poke Root (*Phytolacca americana*)

Poke root is a well-known folk remedy used as a tonic and constitutional strengthener. However, those who drink the tea made from poke root occasionally develop toxic symptoms. A single cup of poke root tea caused bloody diarrhea, gastroenteritis, and severe hypotension in one case.[77] Those wishing to use this old home remedy must be strongly persuaded not to do so, since there is no proven therapeutic benefit to its use.

Pygeum (*Pygeum africanum*)

Pygeum allegedly helps maintain a healthy prostate gland.[322]

Pygeum improved benign prostatic hypertrophy symptoms (e.g., urine flow, residual urine after attempting to empty the bladder, and nocturia) in a double-blind trial of 134 patients.[323]

The evidence needed for the pharmacist to recommend pygeum for prostate problems is too sketchy at present. Benign prostatic hypertrophy should be checked by a physician.

Red Clover (*Trifolium pratense*)

Red clover is alleged through Internet sources to be effective in cleaning the bloodstream; relieving colds, bronchial problems, spasmodic cough, and nervous tension; stimulating digestion and appetite; relieving constipation; and curing cancer and acoustic tumors.

A patient seeking a less expensive alternative treatment for psoriasis purchased a red clover extract, one of the ingredients of which is cascara sagrada.[324] As a result, this patient developed pseudomelanosis coli, a benign discoloration of the colon.

The literature failed to reveal any research on red clover for any medical use. Since its safety and efficacy are both unknown, it should not be recommended.

Sassafras (*Sassafras albidum*)

Sassafras and saffrole, a component found in it, are both hepatocarcinogens.[7,77] Sassafras also causes diaphoresis, which may result in diagnostic checkups to identify the cause until consumption of sassafras tea is finally identified as the culprit.[325]

The risk of carcinogenicity with sassafras is unacceptable in light of the fact that there is no medical use for which it is proven effective. It should not be recommended.

Saw Palmetto (*Serenoa repens*)

Saw palmetto is widely believed to be active in improving benign prostatic hypertrophy and to act as an antiandrogenic agent, as well as a diuretic, urinary antiseptic, and antiinflammatory, among other effects.[326] While some trials show promise, others have been disappointing.[327–329]

Saw palmetto administered to 20 patients did not affect plasma hormone levels in one study, but exerted an antiestrogenic effect in another.[330,331]

Saw palmetto occasionally causes nausea and abdominal pain.[332]

The usefulness of saw palmetto in prostate problems is not well documented. Further, only a physician can diagnose the cause of a prostatic disorder. The risks of a patient with prostate carcinoma attempting to boost urine output with saw palmetto are quite real. It should not be recommended for a self-diagnosed urinary tract condition. Rather, the patient should be urged to consult a physician.

St. John's Wort (*Hypericum perforatum*)

St. John's wort underwent a great deal of marketing hype beginning in 1997 and continuing through 1999. It allegedly acted to improve mild to moderate depression, as well as relieving anxiety, excitability, and menopausal neurosis. One alternative medical journal even suggested its use in severe depression.[333]

Some studies have examined the efficacy of St. John's wort or its alleged active ingredient, hypericum. It has improved mild depression in several studies.[334–337] In two incompletely controlled studies, hypericum may have reduced the severity of seasonal affective disorder.[338,339] In another, a meta-analysis of randomized clinical trials revealed that hypericum may provide relief of mild to moderate depression.[340] However, the authors of yet another study concluded that most trials of hypericum suffer from flaws in methodology.[341]

St. John's wort causes gastrointestinal irritation, allergic reactions, tiredness, restlessness, tachycardia, convulsions, shortness of breath, dizziness, disorientation, hypersensitivity, photodermatitis, and fatal liver failure.[153,342–344] Photosensitivity reactions manifest as inflammation of the skin and mucous membranes.[345]

Depression is a serious condition, with the possibility of the patient harming others or becoming suicidal. Patients with self-diagnosed depression or physician-diagnosed depression must be carefully monitored. Pharmacists can do them a real disservice by recommending self-treatment with

St. John's wort.[345] Rather, the pharmacist's professional obligation is to refer the depressed patient for proper counseling through a local mental health care practitioner.

Tonka Beans (*Coumarouna odorata*)

A 25-year-old woman drank a tea containing tonka beans, melilot, and woodruff (in combination with other ingredients).[7] Those three substances contain coumarins, which produced abnormal menstrual bleeding in the patient. Any form of tonka bean should not be used by patients.

Valerian (*Valeriana officinalis*)

Valerian is an herb that has been recommended for restlessness, insomnia, nervousness, cramping, and dysmenorrhea.

Valerian may exert a mild hypnotic effect, apparently caused by cytotoxic valepotriates and sesquiterpenes.[346–349]

The toxicity of valerian appears to be low in overdose situations.[350] However, 23 patients taking a mixture of valerian, hyoscine, and cyproheptadine known as "Sleep Qik" developed hepatotoxicity, central nervous system depression, and anticholinergic toxicity.[351]

Insomnia is a medical condition that may require sophisticated examination (See Chapter 24, Sleep Disturbances). For this reason, the patient should be referred to a physician rather than advised to begin self-therapy with valerian.

Yohimbine (*Pausinystalia yohimbe*)

Yohimbine is a prescription product, yet patients may freely purchase nonprescription products in which the major alkaloid is yohimbine.[352] Often, yohimbine is included in products as a male potency aid or illegally sold to promise an "herbal high."[353]

Studies of yohimbine as aid to erections are mixed, with some demonstrating efficacy while others do not.[354–356]

The FDA has documented such health hazards as hypotension or hypertension, weakness, nervous stimulation, paralysis, fatigue, stomach disorders, renal failure, seizures, and death.[6] Yohimbine also has properties as a monoamine oxidase inhibitor, sharing the well-known adverse reactions and drug interactions of that group of prescription medications.

In one user, yohimbine caused cutaneous drug eruption, progressive renal failure, and lupuslike syndrome.[357] In a study examining the efficacy of yohimbine for narcolepsy, it was also found to produce insomnia, diarrhea, dyspepsia, flushing, and tremor.[358]

Erectile dysfunction should be referred to a physician for evaluation. The adverse reaction profile of yohimbine is unacceptable to advise self-treatment.

HERBAL TEAS

Many of the herbs mentioned in this chapter are available in tea form. Their toxicities persist. Further, their effectiveness is no greater in tea form than in tablet form. They are especially hazardous when patients turn to them instead of legitimate medical therapy. In one case, a 17-month-old girl was diagnosed with juvenile rheumatoid arthritis.[359] The parents ceased gold therapy, which had produced a remission. Instead, they consulted a naturopath, whose treatments consisted of lentils, herbal teas, and spasm drops. Her arthritis flared, with active synovitis of the large and small joints. Her parents refused intraarticular injections, and the naturopath was allowed to institute electromagnetic therapy. The parents demanded she be allowed to continue this therapy, insisting that she had improved, in the face of the actual fact that she had lost 10% of her body weight and developed marasma and lethargy; life-threatening starvation necessitated hospitalization. She was lost to follow-up after discharge, illustrating the disheartening nature of overreliance on unproven therapy and absolute refusal to accept legitimate medical wisdom.

DIETER'S TEAS

Herbal mixtures sold with false claims to help in weight loss often contain such dangerous ingredients as senna, aloe, buckthorn, rhubarb, cascara, castor oil, and other herbal laxatives. These "teas," which can cause diarrhea, vomiting, nausea, stomach cramps, chronic constipation, and fainting, have been implicated in the deaths of four young women with eating disorders.[360,361] Dieter's teas are based on the false premise that regular laxative use results in weight loss. They are ineffective in preventing caloric absorption since they act on the colon rather than the small intestine, where caloric absorption occurs. Examples of such products are Laci Le Beau Super Dieter's Tea and Thermo Slim Tea. In one case, a patient who used herbal stimulant products for decades experienced severe pain and constipation; loss of colon function necessitated surgical removal of the colon.[360]

An FDA Advisory Committee recommended that herbal products such as teas containing stimulant laxatives carry the following warning: "NOTICE: Contains [insert names of herbs] that can act as stimulant laxatives. Prolonged steeping time can increase the risk of adverse laxative effects, including nausea, vomiting, abdominal cramps, and diarrhea. Chronic use of laxatives can impair colon function. Use of laxatives may be hazardous in the presence of abdominal pain, nausea, vomiting, or rectal bleeding. Laxative-induced diarrhea does not significantly reduce absorption of food calories. Acute or chronic diarrhea may result in serious injury or death." The FDA has urged pharmacists to report adverse reactions to these or similar products to FDA's MedWatch hotline at 1–800-FDA-1088.

SUMMARY

Herbal medicines are seen as a sure route to profitability by many pharmacists. Sales figures for these products confirm that many millions of patients purchase herbal supplements. Although most patients can consume herbal supplements without harm, the lack of manufacturing standards for herbal medicinals raises cautions for the prudent pharmacist.

Health-food stores that sell herbal medicines usually are not staffed by medically trained personnel. Thus the standards of medical ethics do not apply to them. Further, these salespersons do not have the responsibility for medical malpractice associated with a medical degree. Pharmacists are different. The standard of medical ethics requires pharmacists to render care to patients without doing harm. (See "Pharmacy Ethics" in Chapter 49.)

Because herbal medicinals are of questionable effectiveness (lacking well-established scientific studies to prove efficacy), any benefit they might provide is unknown in most cases, while in some cases they present clear hazards. Consequently, recommending herbal supplements is a practice fraught with danger for both patients and pharmacists. Pharmacists who do wish to recommend herbal products must be diligent in searching out studies proving efficacy and cases demonstrating toxicities so informed decisions can be made.

References

1. Anon. Dietary supplements: A regulatory battle. NABP Newsletter 23(3):21, 1994.
2. Anon. Herbs march on. Drug Topics 139(9):18, 1995.
3. Miller LG, Murray WJ. Herbal instruction in United States pharmacy schools. Am J Pharm Educ 61:160, 1997.
4. Heller A. Herbs & pharmacy: A natural alliance. Pharm Times 62(11):75, 1996.
5. Eliason BX, et al. Dietary supplement users: Demographics, product use, and medical system interaction. J Am Board Fam Pract 10:265, 1997.
6. Anon. Herbal roulette. Consumer Reports 60(11):698, 1995.
7. Snider S. Herbal teas and toxicity. FDA Consumer 25(4):31, 1991.
8. Anon. The all-important dollar (Letter). Drug Topics 140(22):11, 1996.
9. Anon. Pharmacists' role in selling dietary supplements questioned. Wkly Pharm Reports 47(11):3, 1998.
10. Smith EA. Take high road. Drug Topics 142(7):3, 1998.
11. Beal FC. Herbals and homeopathic remedies as formulary items? Am J Health-Syst Pharm 55:1266, 1998.
12. Anon. Contaminated tea destroyed. FDA Consumer 29(8):32, 1995.
13. Huxtable RJ. The myth of beneficent nature: The risks of herbal preparations. Ann Intern Med 117:165, 1992.
14. Anon. Vitamins, Minerals, Herbs, & Other Nutrients. Bentonville: Wal-Mart Corporation, (undated).
15. Anon. Pharmacist Herbal Education Guide. 1997, Rexall Sundown, Inc. (no location given).
16. Schirmer GP. Alternative Medicine. Bedford, TX: Med2000, 1998.
17. Foster S. Herbs For Your Health. Loveland, CO: Interweave Press, 1996.
18. Vanherweghem J-L, et al. Rapidly progressive interstitial renal fibrosis in young women: Association with slimming regimen including Chinese herbs. Lancet 341:387, 1993.

19. Markowitz SB, et al. Lead poisoning due to hai ge fen. The porphyrin content of individual erythrocytes. JAMA 271:932, 1994.

20. Anon. Supplement structure/function v. disease claims distinction. Wkly Pharm Reports 47(18):3, 1998.

21. Zehavi U, Polacheck I. Saponins as antimycotic agents: Glycosides of medicagenic acid. Adv Exp Med Biol 404:535, 1996.

22. Molgaard J, von Schenck H, Olsson AG. Alfalfa seeds lower low density lipoprotein cholesterol and apolipoprotein B concentrations in patients with type II hyperlipoproteinemia. Atherosclerosis 65:173, 1987.

23. Williamson JS, Wyandt CM. Herbal therapies: Fact and fiction. Drug Topics 141(15):78, 1997.

24. Jacobs LR. Relationship between dietary fiber and cancer: Metabolic, physiologic, and cellular mechanisms. Proc Soc Exp Biol Med 183:299, 1986.

25. Schroder H, et al. Helenalin and 11 alpha, 13-dihydrohelenalin, two constituents from Arnica montana L., inhibit human platelet function via thiol-dependent pathways. Thromb Res 57:839, 1990.

26. Lyss G, et al. Helenalin, an anti-inflammatory sesquiterpene lactone from Arnica, selectively inhibits transcription factor NF-kappaB. Biol Chem 378:951, 1997.

27. Kaziro GS. Metronidazole (Flagyl) and Arnica Montana in the prevention of post-surgical complications, a comparative placebo controlled clinical trial. Br J Oral Maxillofac Surg 22:42, 1984.

28. Hart O, et al. Double-blind, placebo-controlled, randomized clinical trial of homeopathic arnica C30 for pain and infection after total abdominal hysterectomy. J R Soc Med 90:73, 1997.

29. Woerdenbag HJ, et al. Cytotoxicity of flavonoids and sesquiterpene lactones from Arnica species against the GLC4 and the COLO 320 cell lines. Planta Med 60:434, 1994.

30. Pirker C, et al. Cross-reactivity with Tagetes in Arnica contact eczema. Contact Dermatitis 26:217, 1992.

31. Spettoli E, et al. Contact dermatitis caused by sesquiterpene lactones. Am J Contact Dermat 9:49, 1998.

32. Hausen BM. A 6-year experience with Compositae mix. Am J Contact Dermat 7:94, 1996.

33. Paulsen E, et al. Compositae dermatitis in a Danish dermatology department in one year (I). Results of routine patch testing with the sesquiterpene lactone mix supplemented with aimed patch testing with extracts and sesquiterpene lactones of Compositae plants. Contact Dermatitis 29:6, 1993.

34. Hausen BM, Osmundsen PE. Contact allergy to parthenolide in Tanacetum parthenium (L.) Schulz-Bip. (feverfew, Asteraceae) and cross-reactions to related sesquiterpene lactone containing Compositae species. Acta Derm Venereol 63:308, 1983.

35. Cignarella A, et al. Novel lipid-lowering properties of Vaccinium myrtilus L. leaves, a traditional antidiabetic treatment, in several models of rat dyslipidemia: A comparison with ciprofibrate. Throm Res 84:311, 1996.

36. Bomser J, et al. In vitro anticancer activity of fruit extracts from Vaccinium species. Planta Med 62:212, 1996.

37. Duker EM, et al. Effects of extracts from Cimicifuga racemosa on gonadotropin release in menopausal women and ovariectomized rats. Planta Med 57:420, 1991.

38. Anon. Rimefemin black cohosh for menopause. Wkly Pharm Reports 46(44):3, 1997.

39. Jones TK, Lawson BM. Profound neonatal congestive heart failure caused by maternal consumption of blue cohosh herbal medication. J Pediatr 132(3 Pt 1):550, 1998.

40. Mills DE, et al. Dietary fatty acid supplementation alters stress reactivity and performance in man. J Hum Hypertens 3:111, 1989.

41. Mills DE, et al. Alteration of baroreflex control of forearm vascular resistance by dietary fatty acids. Am J Physiol 259(6 Pt 2):R1164, 1990.

42. Tollesson A, Frithz A. Transepidermal water loss and water content in the stratum corneum in infantile seborrheic dermatitis. Acta Derm Venereol 73:18, 1993.

43. Tollesson A, Frithz A, Stenlund K. Malassezia furfur in infantile seborrheic dermatitis. Pediatr Dermatol 14:423, 1997.

44. Pullman-Mooar S, et al. Alteration of the cellular fatty acid profile and the production of eicosanoids in human monocytes by gamma-linolenic acid. Arthritis Rheum 33:1526, 1990.

45. Leventhal LJ, Boyce EG, Zurier RB. Treatment of rheumatoid arthritis with gammalinoleic acid. Ann Intern Med 119:867, 1993.

46. Christophe A, et al. Effect of administration of gamma-linoleic acid on the fatty acid composition of serum phospholipids and cholesteryl esters in patients with cystic fibrosis. Ann Nutr Metab 38:40, 1994.

47. Rizzi R, et al. Mutagenic and antimutagenic activities of Uncaria tomentosa and its extracts. J Ethnopharmacol 38:63, 1993.

48. Cordell GA, Araujo OE. Capsaicin: Identification, nomenclature, and pharmacotherapy. Ann Pharmacother 27:330, 1993.

49. Modly CE, et al. Capsaicin as an in vitro inhibitor of benzo(a)pyrene metabolism and its DNA binding in human and murine keratinocytes. Drug Metab Dispos 14:413, 1986.

50. Myers BM, Smith JL, Graham DY. Effect of red pepper and black pepper on the stomach. Am J Gastroenterol 82:211, 1987.

51. Horowitz M, et al. The effect of chili on gastrointestinal transit. J Gastroenterol Hepatol 7:52, 1992.

52. van Wyk CW, et al. Effect of chili (Capsicum frutescens) extract on proliferation of oral mucosal fibroblasts. Indian J Exp Biol 33:244, 1995.

53. Jensen Jarolim E, et al. Hot spices influence permeability of human intestinal epithelial monolayers. J Nutr 128:577, 1998.

54. Nemecz G. Chamomile. US Pharm 23(3):104, 1998.

55. Safayhi H, et al. Chamazulene: An antioxidant-type inhibitor of leukotriene B4 formation. Planta Med 60:410, 1994.

56. Miller T, et al. Effects of some components of the essential oil of chamomile, Chamomila recutita, on histamine release from rat mast cells. Planta Med 62:60, 1996.

57. Fidler P, et al. Prospective evaluation of a chamomile mouthwash for prevention of 5-FU–induced oral stomatitis. Cancer 77:522, 1996.

58. Subiza J, et al. Anaphylactic reaction after the ingestion of chamomile tea: A study of cross-reactivity with other composite pollens. J Allergy Clin Immunol 84:353, 1989.

59. Subiza J, et al. Allergic conjunctivitis to chamomile tea. Ann Allergy 65:127, 1990.

60. Anon. Chaparral dangerous. FDA Consumer 27(2):4, 1993.

61. Alderman S, et al. Cholestatic hepatitis after ingestion of chaparral leaf: Confirmation by endoscopic retrograde cholangiopancreatography and liver biopsy. J Clin Gastroenterol 19:242, 1994.

62. Sheikh NM, Philen RM, Love LA. Chaparral-associated hepatotoxicity. Arch Intern Med 157:913, 1997.

63. Batchelor WB, Heathcote J, Wanless IR. Chaparral-induced hepatic injury. Am J Gastroenterol 90:831, 1995.

64. Gordon DW, et al. Chaparral ingestion: The broadening spectrum of liver injury caused by herbal medications. JAMA 273:489, 1995.

65. Smith AY, et al. Cystic renal cell carcinoma and acquired renal cystic disease associated with consumption of chaparral tea: A case report. J Urol 152 (6 Pt 1):2089, 1994.

66. Anon. Chaparral-induced toxic hepatitis—California and Texas, 1992. MMWR 41:812, 1992.

67. Katz M, Saibil F. Herbal hepatitis: Subacute hepatic necrosis secondary to chaparral leaf. J Clin Gastroenterol 12:203, 1990.

68. Napier K. Unproven medical treatments lure elderly. FDA Consumer 28(2):33, 1994.

69. Cahill DJ, et al. Multiple follicular development associated with herbal medicine. Hum Reprod 9:1469, 1994.

70. Hager M, et al. Herbal warning. Newsweek 127(19):60, 1996.

71. Sperl W, et al. Reversible hepatic veno-occlusive disease in an infant after consumption of pyrrolizidine-containing herbal tea. Eur J Pediatr 154:112, 1995.

72. Couet CE, Crews C, Hanley AB. Analysis, separation, and bioassay of pyrrolizidine alkaloids from comfrey (Symphytum officinale). Nat Toxins 4:163, 1996.

73. Abbott PJ. Comfrey: Assessing the low-dose health risk. Med J Aust 149:11, 1988.

74. Yeong ML, et al. Hepatic veno-occlusive disease associated with comfrey ingestion. J Gastroenterol Hepatol 5:211, 1990.

75. McDermott WV, Ridker PM. The Budd-Chiari syndrome and hepatic veno-occlusive disease. Recognition and treatment. Arch Surg 125:525, 1990.

76. Ridker PM, et al. Hepatic venocclusive disease associated with the consumption of pyrrolizidine-containing dietary supplements. Gastroenterology 88:1050, 1985.

77. Anon. Many herbal teas are toxic. Am Pharm NS28:230, 1988.

78. Sobota AE. Inhibition of bacterial adherence by cranberry juice: Potential use for the treatment of urinary tract infections. J Urol 131:1013, 1984.

79. Jackson B, Hicks LE. Effect of cranberry juice on urinary pH in older adults. Home Health Nurs 15:198, 1997.

80. Tsukada K, et al. Cranberry juice and its impact on peri-stomal skin conditions for urostomy patients. Ostomy Wound Manage 40:60, 1994.

81. Avorn J, et al. Reduction of bacteriuria and pyuria after ingestion of cranberry juice. JAMA 271:751, 1994.

82. Fleet JC. New support for a folk remedy: Cranberry juice reduces bacteriuria and pyuria in elderly women. Nutr Rev 52:168, 1994.

83. Nazarko L. Infection control. The therapeutic uses of cranberry juice. Nurs Stand 9:33, 1995.

84. Aschengrau A, et al. Cancer risk and residential proximity to cranberry cultivation in Massachusetts. Am J Public Health 86:1289, 1996.

85. Zhu DP. Dong quai. Am J Chin Med 15:117, 1987.

86. Shaw CR. The perimenopausal hot flash: Epidemiology, physiology, and treatment. Nurse Pract 22:55, 1997.

87. Hirata JD, et al. Does dong quai have estrogenic effects in postmenopausal women? A double-blind, placebo-controlled trial. Fertil Steril 68:981, 1997.

88. Combest WL, Nemecz G. Echinacea. US Pharmacist 22(10):126, 1997.

89. Melchart D, et al. Results of five randomized studies on the immunomodulatory activity of preparations of Echinacea. J Altern Complement Med 1:145, 1995.

90. Coeugniet EG, Elek E. Immunomodulation with Viscum album and Echinacea purpurea extracts. Onkologie 10(Suppl 3):27, 1987.

91. Burger RA, et al. Echinacea-induced cytokine production by human macrophages. Int J Immunopharmacol 19:371, 1997.

92. See DM, et al. In vitro effects of Echinacea and ginseng on natural killer and antibody-dependent cell cytotoxicity in healthy subjects and chronic fatigue syndrome or acquired immunodeficiency syndrome patients. Immunopharmacology 35:229, 1997.

93. Roesler J, et al. Application of purified polysaccharides from cell cultures of the plant Echinacea purpurea to test subjects mediates activation of the phagocyte system. Int J Immunopharmacol 13:931, 1991.

94. Elsasser Beile U, et al. Cytokine production in leukocyte culture during therapy with Echinacea extract. J Clin Lab Anal 10:441, 1996.

95. Lersch C, et al. Nonspecific immunostimulation with low doses of cyclophosphamide (LDCY), thymostimulin, and Echinacea purpurea extracts (echinacin) in patients with far advanced colorectal cancers: Preliminary results. Cancer Invest 10:343, 1992.

96. Lersch C, et al. Stimulation of the immune response in outpatients with hepatocellular carcinomas by low doses of cyclophosphamide (LDCY), Echinacea purpurea extracts (echinacin) and thymostimulin. Arch Geschwulstforsch 60:379, 1990.

97. Mullins RJ. Echinacea-associated anaphylaxis. Med J Aust 168:170, 1998.

98. Zakay RZ, et al. Inhibition of several strains of influenza virus in vitro and reduction of symptoms by an elderberry extract (Sambucus nigra L.) during an outbreak of influenza B Panama. J Altern Complement Med 1:361, 1995.

99. Lewis WH, Zenger VE, Lynch RG. No adaptogen response of mice to ginseng and Eleutherococcus infusions. J Ethnopharmacol 8:209, 1983.

100. McRae S. Elevated serum digoxin levels in a patient taking digoxin and Siberian ginseng. CMAJ 155:293, 1996.

101. Pye JK, Mansel RE, Hughes LE. Clinical experience of drug treatments for mastalgia. Lancet 2:373, 1985.

102. Simpson LO. The etiopathogenesis of premenstrual syndrome as a consequence of altered blood rheology: A new hypothesis. Med Hypotheses 25:189, 1988.

103. Campbell EM, et al. Premenstrual symptoms in general practice patients: Prevalence and treatment. J Reprod Med 42:637, 1997.

104. Mera SL. Diet and disease. Br J Biomed Sci 51:189, 1994.

105. Horrobin DF. Essential fatty acid and prostaglandin metabolism in Sjogren's syndrome, systemic sclerosis and rheumatoid arthritis. Scand J Rheumatol Suppl 61:242, 1986.

106. Cameron NE, Cotter MA. Metabolic and vascular factors in the pathogenesis of diabetic neuropathy. Diabetes 46(Suppl 2):S31, 1997.

107. Wetzig NR. Mastalgia: A 3 year Australian study. Aust N Z J Surg 64:329, 1994.

108. Mansel RE, et al. A randomized trial of dietary intervention with essential fatty acids in patients with categorized cysts. Ann N Y Acad Sci 586:288, 1990.

109. Horrobin DF. The role of essential fatty acids and prostaglandins in the premenstrual syndrome. J Reprod Med 28:465, 1983.

110. Budeiri D, Li Wan Po A, Dornan JC. Is evening primrose oil of value in the treatment of premenstrual syndrome? Control Clin Trials 17:60, 1996.

111. Khoo SK, Munro C, Battistutta D. Evening primrose oil and treatment of premenstrual syndrome. Med J Aust 153:189, 1990.

112. Chenoy R, et al. Effect of oral gamolenic acid from evening primrose oil on menopausal flushing. BMJ 308:501, 1994.

113. Haslett C, et al. A double-blind evaluation of evening primrose oil as an antiobesity agent. Int J Obes 7:549, 1983.

114. Whitaker DK, Cilliers J, de Beer C. Evening primrose oil (Epogam) in the treatment of chronic hand dermatitis: Disappointing therapeutic results. Dermatology 193:115, 1996.

115. Bamford JT, Gibson RW, Renier CM. Atopic eczema unresponsive to evening primrose oil (linoleic and gamma-linoleic acids). J Am Acad Dermatol 13:959, 1985.

116. Hederos CA, Berg A. Epogam evening primrose oil treatment in atopic dermatitis and asthma. Arch Dis Child 75:494, 1996.

117. Bordoni A, et al. Evening primrose oil (Efamol) in the treatment of children with atopic eczema. Drugs Exp Clin Res 14:291, 1988.

118. Biagi PL, et al. A long-term study on the use of evening primrose oil (Efamol) in atopic children. Drugs Exp Clin Res 14:285, 1988.

119. Kerscher MJ, Korting HC. Treatment of atopic eczema with evening primrose oil: Rationale and clinical results. Clin Invest 70:167, 1992.

120. Wright S. Atopic dermatitis and essential fatty acids: A biochemical basis for atopy? Acta Derm Venereol Suppl 114:143, 1985.

121. Veale DJ, et al. A double-blind placebo controlled trial of Efamol Marine on skin and joint symptoms of psoriatic arthritis. Br J Rheumatol 33:954, 1994.

122. Oliwiecki S, Burton JL. Evening primrose oil and marine oil in the treatment of psoriasis. Clin Exp Dermatol 19:127, 1994.

123. Boberg M, Vessby B, Selinus I. Effects of dietary supplementation with n-6 and n-3 long-chain polyunsaturated fatty acids on serum lipoproteins and platelet function in hypertriglyceridaemic patients. Acta Med Scand 220:153, 1986.

124. Viikari J, Lehtonen A. Effect of primrose oil on serum lipids and blood pressure in hyperlipidemic subjects. Int J Clin Pharmacol Ther Toxicol 24:668, 1986.

125. Hansen TM, et al. Treatment of rheumatoid arthritis with prostaglandin E1 precursors cis-linoleic acid and gamma-linoleic acid. Scand J Rheumatol 12:85, 1983.

126. Jantti J, et al. Evening primrose oil and olive oil in treatment of rheumatoid arthritis. Clin Rheumatol 8:238, 1989.

127. Jantti J, et al. Evening primrose oil in rheumatoid arthritis: Changes in serum lipids and fatty acids. Ann Rheum Dis 48:124, 1989.

128. Brzeski M, Madhok R, Capell HA. Evening primrose oil in patients with rheumatoid arthritis and side-effects of non-steroidal anti-inflammatory drugs. Br J Rheumatol 30:370, 1991.

129. Belch JJ, et al. Evening primrose oil (Efamol) in the treatment of Raynaud's phenomenon: A double-blind study. Thromb Haemost 54:490, 1985.

130. Oxholm P, et al. Patients with primary Sjogren's syndrome treated for two months with evening primrose oil. Scand J Rheumatol 15:103, 1986.

131. Stenius-Aarniala B, et al. Evening primrose oil and fish oil are ineffective as supplementary treatment of bronchial asthma. Ann Allergy 62:534, 1989.

132. Ebden P, et al. A study of evening primrose seed oil in atopic asthma. Prostaglandins Leukot Essent Fatty Acids 35:69, 1989.

133. Jenkins AP, Green AT, Thompson RP. Essential fatty acid supplementation in chronic hepatitis B. Aliment Pharmacol Ther 10:665, 1996.

134. Aman MG, Mitchell EA, Turbott SH. The effects of essential fatty acid supplementation by Efamol in hyperactive children. J Abnorm Child Psychol 15:75, 1987.

135. Arnold LE, et al. Gamma-linoleic acid for attention-deficit hyperactivity disorder: Placebo-controlled comparison to D-amphetamine. Biol Psychiatry 25:222, 1989.

136. Greenfield SM, et al. A randomized controlled study of evening primrose oil and fish oil in ulcerative colitis. Aliment Pharmacol Ther 7:159, 1993.

137. D'Almeida A, et al. Effects of a combination of evening primrose oil (gamma linoleic acid) and fish oil (eicosapentaenoic + docahexaenoic acid) versus magnesium, and versus placebo in preventing pre-eclampsia. Women Health 19:117, 1992.

138. Hufnagel TJ, Schein OD. Suppurative keratitis from herbal ocular preparation. Am J Ophthalmol 113:722, 1992.

139. Loesche W, et al. Feverfew—An antithrombotic drug? Folia Haematol Int Mag Klin Morphol Blutforsch 115:181, 1988.

140. O'Neill LA, Barrett ML, Lewis GP. Extracts of feverfew inhibit mitogen-induced human peripheral blood mononuclear cell proliferation and cytokine mediated responses: A cytotoxic effect. Br J Clin Pharmacol 23:81, 1987.

141. Heptinstall S, et al. Inhibition of platelet behaviour by feverfew: A mechanism of action involving sulphydryl groups. Folia Haematol Int Mag Klin Morphol Blutforsch 115:447, 1988.

142. Losche W, et al. An extract of feverfew inhibits interactions of human platelets with collagen substrates. Throm Res 48:511, 1987.

143. Loesche W, et al. Effects of an extract of feverfew (Tanacetum parthenium) on arachidonic acid metabolism in human blood platelets. Biomed Biochim Acta 47:S241, 1988.

144. Nemecz G, Combest WL. Feverfew. US Pharmacist 22(11): 122, 1997.

145. Cottrell K. Herbal products begin to attract the attention of brand-name drug companies. CMAJ 155:216, 1996.

146. Murphy JJ, Heptinstall S, Mitchell JR. Randomised double-blind placebo-controlled trial of feverfew in migraine prevention. Lancet 2:189, 1988.

147. Groenewegen WA, Heptinstall S. A comparison of the effects of an extract of feverfew and parthenolide, a component of feverfew, on human platelet activity in-vitro. J Pharm Pharmacol 42:553, 1990.

148. Groenewegen WA, Knight DW, Heptinstall S. Compounds extracted from feverfew that have anti-secretory activity contain an alpha-methylene butyrolactone unit. J Pharm Pharmacol 38:709, 1986.

149. Johnson ES, et al. Efficacy of feverfew as prophylactic treatment of migraine. Br Med J (Clin Res Ed) 291:569, 1985.

150. Pattrick M, Heptinstall S, Doherty M. Feverfew in rheumatoid arthritis: A double-blind, placebo controlled study. Ann Rheum Dis 48:547, 1989.

151. Fernandez de Corres L. Contact dermatitis from Frullania, Compositae and other plants. Contact Dermatitis 11:74, 1984.

152. Sriramarao P, Rao PV. Allergenic cross-reactivity between Parthenium and ragweed pollen allergens. Int Arch Allergy Immunol 100:79, 1993.

153. Anon. Herbal medicines—Safe and effective? Drug Ther Bull 24(25):97, 1986.

154. Gianni L, Dreitlein WB. Some popular OTC herbals can interact with anticoagulant therapy. US Pharmacist 23(5):80, 1998.

155. Kendler BS. Garlic (Allium sativum) and onion (Allium cepa): A review of their relationship to cardiovascular disease. Prev Med 16:670, 1987.

156. Augusti KT. Therapeutic values of onion (Allium cepa L.) and garlic (Allium sativum L.). Indian J Exp Biol 34:634, 1996.

157. Adetumbi MA, Lau BH. Allium sativum (garlic)—A natural antibiotic. Med Hypotheses 12:227, 1983.

158. Ernst E. Cardiovascular effects of garlic (Allium sativum): A review. Pharmatherapeutica 5:83, 1987.

159. Dausch JG, Nixon DW. Garlic: A review of its relationship to malignant disease. Prev Med 19:346, 1990.

160. Fewick GR, Hanley AB. The genus Allum—Part 1. Crit Rev Food Sci Nutr 22:199, 1985.

161. Sendl A. Comparative pharmacological investigations of Allim ursinum and Allium sativum. Planta Med 58:1, 1992.

162. Agarwal KC. Therapeutic actions of garlic constituents. Med Res 16:111, 1996.

163. Kleijnen J, Knipschild P, ter Riet G. Garlic, onions and cardiovascular risk factors. A review of the evidence from human experiments with emphasis on commercially available preparations. Br J Clin Pharmacol 28:535, 1989.

164. Warshafsky S, Kamer RS, Sivak SL. Effect of garlic on total serum cholesterol. A meta-analysis. Ann Intern Med 119 (7 Pt 1):599, 1993.

165. Makheja AN, Bailey JM. Antiplatelet constituents of garlic and onion. Agents Actions 29:3, 1990.

166. Mayeux PR, et al. The pharmacological effects of allicin, a constituent of garlic oil. Agents Actions 25:182, 1988.

167. Srivastava KC. Evidence for the mechanism by which garlic inhibits platelet aggregation. Prostaglandins Leukot Med 22:313, 1986.

168. Srivastava KC, Tyagi OD. Effects of a garlic-derived principle (ajoene) on aggregation and arachidonic acid metabolism in human blood platelets. Prostaglandins Leukot Essent Fatty Acids 49:587, 1993.

169. Kiesewetter H, et al. Effect of garlic on thrombocyte aggregation, microcirculation, and other risk factors. Int J Clin Pharmacol Ther Toxicol 29:151, 1991.

170. Nagda KK, et al. Effect of onion and garlic on blood coagulation and fibrinolysis in vitro. Indian J Physiol Pharmacol 27:141, 1983.

171. Neil HA, et al. Garlic powder in the treatment of moderate hyperlipidaemia: A controlled trial and meta-analysis. J R Coll Physicians Lond 30:329, 1996.

172. Jain AK, et al. Can garlic reduce levels of serum lipids? A controlled clinical study. Am J Med 94:632, 1993.

173. Bakhsh R, Chugtai MI. Influence of garlic on serum cholesterol, serum triglycerides, serum total lipids and serum glucose in human subjects. Nahrung 28:159, 1984.

174. Gadkari JV, Joshi VD. Effect of ingestion of raw garlic on serum cholesterol level, clotting time and fibrinolytic activity in normal subjects. J Postgrad Med 37:128, 1991.

175. Vorberg G, Schneider B. Therapy with garlic: Results of a placebo-controlled, double-blind study. Br J Clin Pract Symp Suppl 69:7, 1990.

176. Luley C, et al. Lack of efficacy of dried garlic inpatients with hyperlipoproteinemia. Arzneimittelforschung 36:766, 1986.

177. Elnima EI, et al. The antimicrobial activity of garlic and onion extracts. Pharmazie 38:747, 1983.

178. Weber ND, et al. In vitro virucidal effects of Allium sativum (garlic) extract and compounds. Planta Med 58:417, 1992.

179. Caldwell SH, et al. Ancient remedies revisited: Does Allium sativum (garlic) palliate the hepatopulmonary syndrome? J Clin Gastroenterol 15:248, 1992.

180. You WC, et al. Allium vegetables and reduced risk of stomach cancer. J Natl Cancer Inst 81:162, 1989.

181. Dorant E, van den Brandt PA, Goldbohm RA. A prospective cohort study on Allium vegetable consumption, garlic supplement use, and the risk of lung carcinoma in The Netherlands. Cancer Res 54:6148, 1994.

182. Sivam GP, et al. Helicobacter pylori—In vitro susceptibility to garlic (Allium sativum) extract. Nutr Cancer 27:118, 1997.

183. Dorant E, van den Brandt PA, Goldbohm RA. Allium vegetable consumption, garlic supplement intake, and female breast carcinoma incidence. Breast Cancer Res Treat 33:163, 1995.

184. Dorant E, et al. Garlic and its significance for the prevention of cancer in humans: A critical review. Br J Cancer 67:424, 1993.

185. Papageorgiou C, et al. Allergic contact dermatitis to garlic (Allium sativum L.). Identification of the allergens: The role of mono-, di-, and trisulfides present in garlic. A comparative study in man and animal (guinea-pig). Arch Dermatol Res 275:229, 1983.

186. Anibarro B, Fontela JL, De La Hoz F. Occupational asthma induced by garlic dust. J Allergy Clin Immunol 100(6 Pt 1):734, 1997.

187. Kanerva L, Estlander T, Jolanki R. Occupational allergic contact dermatitis from spices. Contact Dermatitis 35:157, 1996.

188. Fenwick GR, Hanley AB. The genus Allium—Part 3. Crit Rev Food Sci Nutr 23:1, 1985.

189. Parish RA, McIntire S, Heimbach DM. Garlic burns: A naturopathic remedy gone awry. Pediatr Emerg Care 3:258, 1987.

190. Lee TY, Lam TH. Contact dermatitis due to topical treatment with garlic in Hong Kong. Contact Dermatitis 24:193, 1991.

191. Delaney TA, Donnelly AM. Garlic dermatitis. Australas J Dermatol 37:109, 1996.

192. Mennella JA, Johnson A, Beauchamp GK. Garlic ingestion by pregnant women alters the odor of amniotic fluid. Chem Senses 20:207, 1995.

193. Mostefa-Kara N, et al. Fatal hepatitis after herbal tea. Lancet 340:674, 1992.

194. Latner AW. Natural medicine on the net: The wild west lives again. Pharm Times 62(11):31, 1996.

195. Larrey D, et al. Hepatitis after germander (Teucrium chamaedrys) administration: Another instance of herbal medicine hepatotoxicity. Ann Intern Med 117:129, 1992.

196. Laliberte L, Villeneuve JP. Hepatitis after the use of germander, a herbal remedy. CMAJ 154:1689, 1996.

197. Aikins Murphy P. Alternative therapies for nausea and vomiting of pregnancy. Obstet Gynecol 91:149, 1998.

198. Phillips S, Ruggier R, Hutchinson SE. Zingiber officinale (ginger)—An antiemetic for day case surgery. Anaesthesia 48:715, 1993.

199. Bone ME, et al. Ginger root—A new antiemetic. The effect of ginger root on postoperative nausea and vomiting after major gynaecological surgery. Anaesthesia 45:669, 1990.

200. Arfeen Z, et al. A double-blind randomized controlled trial of ginger for the prevention of postoperative nausea and vomiting. Anaesth Intensive Care 23:449, 1995.

201. Grontved A, Hentzer E. Vertigo-reducing effect of ginger root. A controlled clinical study. ORL J Otorhinolaryngol Relat Spec 48:282, 1986.

202. Fischer-Rasmussen W, et al. Ginger treatment of hyperemesis gravidarum. Eur J Obstet Gynecol Reprod Biol 38:19, 1991.

203. Grontved A, et al. Ginger root against seasickness. A controlled trial on the open sea. Acta Otolaryngol 105:45, 1988.

204. Holtmann S, et al. The anti-motion sickness mechanisms of ginger. A comparative study with placebo and dimenhydrinate. Acta Otolaryngol 108:168, 1989.

205. Stewart JJ, et al. Effects of ginger on motion sickness susceptibility and gastric function. Pharmacology 42:111, 1991.

206. Srivastava KC, Mustafa T. Ginger (Zingiber officinale) and rheumatic disorders. Med Hypotheses 29:25, 1989.

207. Lumb AB. Effect of dried ginger on human platelet function. Thromb Haemost 71:110, 1994.

208. Verma SK, et al. Effect of ginger on platelet aggregation in man. Indian J Med Res 98:240, 1993.

209. Mustafa T, Srivastava KC. Ginger (Zingiber officinale) in migraine headache. J Ethnopharmacol 29:267, 1990.

210. Futrell JM, Rietschel RL. Spice allergy evaluated by results of patch tests. Cutis 52:288, 1993.

211. Nemecz G, Combest WL. Ginkgo biloba. US Pharm 22(9):144, 1997.

212. Chavez ML, Chavez PI. Gingko. I. History, use, and pharmacologic properties. Hosp Pharm 33:658, 1998.

213. Itil T, Martorano D. Natural substances in psychiatry (Gingko biloba in dementia). Psychopharmacol Bull 31:147, 1995.

214. Subham Z, Hindmarch I. The psychopharmacological effects of Gingko biloba extract in normal healthy volunteers. Int J Clin Pharmacol Res 4:89, 1984.

215. Rai GS, Shovlin C, Wesnes KA. A double-blind, placebo controlled study of Gingko biloba extract ('tanakan') in elderly outpatients with mild to moderate memory impairment. Curr Med Res Opin 12:350, 1991.

216. Garg RK, Nag D, Agrawal A. A double blind placebo controlled trial of gingko biloba extract in acute cerebral ischaemia. J Assoc Physicians India 43:760, 1995.

217. Maurer K, et al. Clinical efficacy of Gingko biloba special extract EGb 761 in dementia of the Alzheimer type. J Psychiatr Res 31:645, 1997.

218. Anon. Gingko biloba extract improves mental performance in dementias. Wkly Pharm Reports 46(43):4, 1997.

219. Kleijnen J, Knipschild P. Gingko biloba for cerebral insufficiency. Br J Clin Pharmacol 34:352, 1992.

220. Bauer U. 6-Month double-blind randomised clinical trial of Gingko biloba extract versus placebo in two parallel groups in patients suffering from peripheral arterial insufficiency. Arzneimittelforschung 34:716, 1984.

221. Jung F, et al. Effect of Gingko biloba on fluidity of blood and peripheral microcirculation in volunteers. Arzneimittelforschung 40:589, 1990.

222. Atzori C, et al. Activity of bilobalide, a sesquiterpene from Gingko biloba, on Pneumocystis carinii. Antimicrob Agents Chemother 37:1492, 1993.

223. Holgers KM, Axelsson A, Pringle I. Gingko biloba extract for the treatment of tinnitus. Audiology 33:85, 1994.

224. Tomb RR, Foussereau J, Sell Y. Mini-epidemic of contact dermatitis from gingko tree fruit (Gingko biloba L.). Contact Dermatitis 19:281, 1988.

225. Kwan CY. Vascular effects of selected antihypertensive drugs derived from traditional medicinal herbs. Clin Exp Pharmacol Physiol 22(Suppl 1):S297, 1995.

226. Chong SK, Oberholzer VG. Ginseng—Is there a use in clinical medicine? Postgrad Med J 64:841, 1988.

227. Bahrke MS, Morgan WP. Evaluation of the ergogenic properties of ginseng. Sports Med 18:229, 1994.

228. Beltz SD, Doering PL. Efficacy of nutritional supplements used by athletes. Clin Pharm 12:900, 1993.

229. Engels HJ, Wirth JC. No ergogenic effects of ginseng (Panax ginseng C.A. Meyer) during graded maximal aerobic exercise. J Am Diet Assoc 97:1110, 1997.

230. Morris AC, et al. No ergogenic effect of ginseng ingestion. Int J Sport Nutr 6:263, 1996.

231. Chong SK, et al. In vitro effect of Panax ginseng on phytohaemagglutinin-induced lymphocyte transformation. Int Arch Allergy Appl Immunol 73:216, 1984.

232. Liu J, et al. Stimulatory effect of saponin from Panax ginseng on immune function of lymphocytes in the elderly. Mech Ageing Dev 83:43, 1995.

233. Yun TK, Choi SY. A case-control study of ginseng intake and cancer. Int J Epidemiol 19:871, 1990.

234. Yun TK, Choi SY. Preventive effect of ginseng intake against human cancers: A case-control study on 1987 pairs. Cancer Epidemiol Biomarkers Prev 4:401, 1995.

235. Kiesewetter H, et al. Hemorrheological and circulatory effects of Gincosan. Int J Clin Pharmacol Ther Toxicol 30:97, 1992.

236. Chen X, Gillis CN, Moalli R. Vascular effects of ginsenosides in vitro. Br J Pharmacol 82:485, 1984.

237. Sotaniemi EA, Haapakoski E, Rautio A. Ginseng therapy in non–insulin-dependent diabetic patients. Diabetes Care 18:1373, 1995.

238. Thommessen B, Laake K. No identifiable effect of ginseng (Gericomplex) as an adjuvant in the treatment of geriatric patients. Aging 8:417, 1996.

239. Case Marasco A, et al. Double-blind study of a multivitamin complex supplemented with ginseng extract. Drugs Exp Clin Res 22:323, 1996.

240. Lee FC, et al. Effects of Panax ginseng on blood alcohol clearance in man. Clin Exp Pharmacol Physiol 14:543, 1987.

241. Ryu SJ, Chien YY. Ginseng-associated cerebral arteritis. Neurology 45:829, 1995.

242. Hopkins MP, Androff L, Benninghoff AS. Ginseng face cream and unexplained vaginal bleeding. Am J Obstet Gynecol 159:1121, 1988.

243. Chan TY. Anticholinergic poisoning due to Chinese herbal medicines. Vet Hum Toxicol 37:156, 1995.

244. Arpaia MR, et al. Effects of Centella asiatica extract on mucopolysaccharide metabolism in subjects with varicose veins. Int J Clin Pharmacol Res 10:229, 1990.

245. Pointel JP, et al. Titrated extract of Centella asiatica (TECA) in the treatment of venous insufficiency of the lower limbs. Angiology 38(1 Pt 1):46, 1987.

246. Montecchio GP, et al. Centella asiatica triterpenic fraction (CATTF) reduces the number of circulating endothelial cells

in subjects with post phlebitic syndrome. Haematologica 76:256, 1991.

247. Belcaro GV, Grimaldi R, Guidi G. Improvement of capillary permeability in patients with venous hypertension after treatment with TTFCA. Angiology 41:533, 1990.

248. Belcaro GV, Rulo A, Grimaldi R. Capillary filtration and ankle edema in patients with venous hypertension treated with TTFCA. Angiology 41:12, 1990.

249. Babu TD, Kuttan G, Padikkala J. Cytotoxic and anti-tumour properties of certain taxa of Umbelliferae with special reference to Centella asiatica (L.) Urban. J Ethnopharmacol 48:53, 1995.

250. Maquart FX, et al. Stimulation of collagen synthesis in fibroplast cultures by a triterpene extracted from Centella asiatica. Connect Tissue Res 24:107, 1990.

251. Eun HC, Lee AY. Contact dermatitis due to madecassol. Contact Dermatitis 13:310, 1985.

252. Hausen BM. Centella asiatica (Indian pennywort), an effective therapeutic but a weak sensitizer. Contact Dermatitis 29:175, 1993.

253. Gonzalo Garijo MA, Revenga Arranz F, Bobadilla Gonzalez P. Allergic contact dermatitis due to Centella asiatica: A new case. Allergol Immunopathol 24:132, 1996

254. Shim JS, et al. Chemopreventive effect of green tea (Camellia sinensis) among cigarette smokers. Cancer Epidemiol Biomarkers Prev 4:387, 1995.

255. Ford RP, et al. Heavy caffeine intake in pregnancy and sudden infant death syndrome. New Zealand Cot Death Study Group. Arch Dis Child 78:9, 1998.

256. Wang RS, Kies C. Niacin, thiamin, iron and protein status of humans as affected by the consumption of tea (Camellia sinensis) infusions. Plant Foods Hum Nutr 41:337, 1991.

257. Kendler BS. Recent nutritional approaches to the prevention and therapy of cardiovascular disease. Prog Cardiovasc Nurs 12:3, 1997.

258. Diehm C, et al. Comparison of leg compression stocking and oral horse-chestnut seed extract therapy in patients with chronic venous insufficiency. Lancet 347:292, 1996.

259. Rehn D, et al. Comparative clinical efficacy and tolerability of oxerutins and horse chestnut extract in patients with chronic venous insufficiency. Arzneimittelforschung 46:483, 1996.

260. Diehm C, et al. Medical edema protection—Clinical benefit in patients with chronic deep vein incompetency. A placebo controlled double blind study. Vasa 21:188, 1992.

261. Randolph C, Fraser B. Latex hypersensitivity in a horse farmer. Allergy Asthma Proc 17:89, 1996.

262. Popp W, et al. Horse chestnut (Aesculus hippocastanum) pollen: A frequent cause of allergic sensitization in urban children. Allergy 47(4 Pt 2):380, 1992.

263. Anon. Jin bu huan toxicity in adults—Los Angeles 1993. MMWR 42:920, 1993.

264. Picciotto A, et al. Chronic hepatitis induced by jin bu huan. J Hepatol 28:165, 1998

265. Woolf GM, et al. Acute hepatitis associated with the Chinese herbal product Jin Bu Huan. Ann Intern Med 121:729, 1994.

266. Anon. Jin bu huan toxicity in children. MMWR 42:633, 1993.

267. Horowitz RS, et al. The clinical spectrum of jin bu huan toxicity. Arch Intern Med 156:899, 1996.

268. Singh YN. Kava: An overview. J Ethnopharmacol 37:13, 1992.

269. Norton SA. Herbal medicines in Hawaii from tradition to convention. Hawaii Med J 57:382, 1998.

270. Volz HP, Kieser M. Kava-kava extract WS 1490 versus placebo in anxiety disorders—A randomized placebo-controlled 25-week outpatient trial. Pharmacopsychiatry 30:1, 1997.

271. Norton SA, Ruze P. Kava dermopathy. J Am Acad Dermatol 31:89, 1994.

272. Ruze P. Kava-induced dermopathy: A niacin deficiency? Lancet 335:1442, 1990.

273. Garner LF, Klinger JD. Some visual effects caused by the beverage kava. J Ethnopharmacol 13:307, 1985.

274. Mathews JD, et al. Effects of the heavy usage of kava on physical health: Summary of a pilot survey in an aboriginal community. Med J Aust 148:548, 1988.

275. Badam L. In vitro antiviral activity of indigenous glycyrrhizin, licorice and glycyrrhizic acid (Sigma) on Japanese encephalitis virus. J Commun Dis 29:91, 1997.

276. Sato H, et al. Therapeutic basis of glycyrrhizin on chronic hepatitis B. Antiviral Res 30:171, 1996.

277. Fuhrman B, et al. Licorice extract and its major polyphenol glabridin protect low-density lipoprotein against lipid peroxidation: In vitro and ex vivo studies in humans and in atherosclerotic apolipoprotein E–deficient mice. Am J Clin Nutr 66:267, 1997.

278. Vaya J, Belinky PA, Aviram M. Antioxidant constituents from licorice roots: Isolation, structure elucidation and antioxidative capacity toward LDL oxidation. Free Radic Biol Med 23:302, 1997.

279. Corsi FM, et al. Acute hypokalemic myopathy due to chronic licorice ingestion: Report of a case. Ital J Neurol Sci 4:493, 1983.

280. White PC, Mune T, Agarwal AK. 11 Beta-hydroxysteroid dehydrogenase and the syndrome of apparent mineralocorticoid excess. Endocr Rev 18:135, 1997.

281. Walker BR, Edwards CR. Licorice-induced hypertension and syndromes of apparent mineralocorticoid excess. Endocrinol Metab Clin North Am 23:359, 1994.

282. Kato H, et al. 3-Monoglucuronyl-glycyrrhetinic acid is a major metabolite that causes licorice-induced psuedoaldosteronism. J Clin Endocrinol Metab 80:1929, 1995.

283. Forslund T, et al. Effects of licorice on plasma atrial natriuretic peptide in healthy volunteers. J Intern Med 225:95, 1989.

284. Biglieri EG. My engagement with steroids: A review. Steroids 60:52, 1995.

285. Benediktsson R, Edwards CR. Apparent mineralocorticoid excess. J Hum Hypertens 8:371, 1994.

286. Cibelli G, et al. Hypokalemic myopathy associated with liquorice ingestion. Ital J Neurol Sci 5:463, 1984.

287. Heidemann HT, Kreuzfelder E. Hypokalemic rhabdomyolysis with myoglobinuria due to licorice ingestion and diuretic treatment. Klin Wochenschr 61:303, 1983.

288. Barrella M, et al. Hypokalemic rhabdomyolysis associated with liquorice ingestion: Report of an atypical case. Ital J Neurol Sci 18:217, 1997.

289. Cugini P, et al. Hypertension in licorice abuse: A case report. G Ital Cardiol 13:126, 1983.

290. Beretta-Piccoli C, et al. Body-sodium and blood volume in a patient with licorice-induced hypertension. J Hypertens 3:19, 1985.

291. van der Zwan A. Hypertension encephalopathy after liquorice ingestion. Clin Neurol Neurosurg 95:35, 1993.

292. Nunn-Thompson CL, Simon PA. Pharmacotherapy for smoking cessation. Clin Pharm 8:710, 1989.

293. Fed Reg 58:31236, 1993.

294. Hecht A, et al. Toxic tea—Part II. FDA Consumer 20(8):40, 1986.

295. Henry ML, et al. Herbal overdose in a renal transplant recipient. Res & Staff Physician 35(1):88, 1989.

296. Nadir A, et al. Acute hepatitis associated with the use of a Chinese herbal product, ma-huang. Am J Gastroenterol 91:1436, 1996.

297. Flora K, et al. Milk thistle (Silybum marianum) for the therapy of liver disease. Am J Gastroenterol 93:139, 1998.

298. Dehmlow C, Erhard J, de Groot H. Inhibition of Kupffer cell functions as an explanation for the hepatoprotective properties of silibinin. Hepatology 23:749, 1996.

299. Ferenci P, et al. Randomized controlled trial of silymarin treatment in patients with cirrhosis of the liver. J Hepatol 9:105, 1989.

300. Zi X, et al. A flavonoid antioxidant, silymarin, inhibits activation of erbB1 signaling and induces cyclin-dependent kinase inhibitors, G1 arrest, and anticarcinogenic effects in human prostate carcinoma DU145 cells. Cancer Res 58:1920, 1998.

301. Zi X. Anticarcinogenic effect of a flavonoid antioxidant, silymarin, in human breast cancer cells MDA-MB 468: Induction of GI arrest through an increase in Cip1/p21 concomitant with a decrease in kinase activity of cyclin-dependent kinases and associated cyclins. Clin Cancer Res 4:1055, 1998.

302. Kalmar L, et al. Silibinin (Legalon-70) enhances the motility of human neutrophils immobilized by formyl-tripeptide calcium ionophore, lymphokine and by normal human serum. Agents Actions 29:239, 1990.

303. Hirano T, Homma M, Ola K. Effects of stinging nettle root extracts and their steroidal components on the Na+,K(+)-ATPase of the benign prostatic hyperplasia. Planta Med 60:30, 1994.

304. Hryb DJ, et al. The effect of extracts of the roots of the stinging nettle (Urtica dioica) on the interaction of SHBG with its receptor on human prostatic membranes. Planta Med 61:31, 1995.

305. Schottner M, Gansser D, Spiteller G. Lignans from the roots of Urtica dioica and their metabolites bind to human sex hormone binding globulin (SHBG). Planta Med 63:529, 1997.

306. Bousquet J, et al. Allergy in the Mediterranean area. II: Cross-allergenicity among Urticaceae pollens (Parietaria and Urtica). Clin Allergy 16:57, 1986.

307. Giavina Bianchi PF Jr, et al. Occupational respiratory allergic disease induced by Passiflora alata and Rhamnus purshiana. Ann Allergy Asthma Immunol 79:449, 1997.

308. Solbakken AM, Rorbakken G, Gundersen T. Nature medicine as intoxicant. Tidsskr Nor Laegeforen 117:1140, 1997.

309. Anderson IB, et al. Pennyroyal toxicity: Measurement of toxic metabolite levels in two cases and review of the literature. Ann Intern Med 124:726, 1996.

310. Bakerink JA, et al. Multiple organ failure after ingestion of pennyroyal oil from herbal tea in two infants. Pediatrics 98:944, 1996.

311. May B, et al. Efficacy of a fixed peppermint oil/caraway oil combination in non-ulcer dyspepsia. Arzneimittelforschung 46:1149, 1996.

312. Sparks MJ, et al. Does peppermint oil relieve spasm during barium enema? Br J Radiol 68:841, 1995.

313. Liu JH, et al. Enteric-coated peppermint-oil capsules in the treatment of irritable bowel syndrome: a prospective, randomized trial. J Gastroenterol 32:765, 1997.

314. Tate S. Peppermint oil: A treatment for postoperative nausea. J Adv Nurs 26:543, 1997.

315. Sainio EL, Kanerva L. Contact allergens in toothpastes and a review of their hypersensitivity. Contact Dermatitis 33:100, 1995.

316. Rogers SN, Pahor AL. A form of stomatitis induced by excessive peppermint consumption. Dent Update 22:36, 1995.

317. Fintelman V. Modern phytotherapy and its uses in gastrointestinal conditions. Planta Med 57:S48, 1991.

318. Mehta V, Wheeler AW. IgE-mediated sensitization to English plantain pollen in seasonal respiratory allergy: Identification and partial characterisation of its allergenic components. Int Arch Allergy Appl Immunol 96:211, 1991.

319. Granel C, et al. Plantain allergy (Plantago lancelota): Assessment of diagnostic tests. Allergol Immunopathol 21:158, 1993.

320. Clarke PS. Improved diagnosis and treatment of allergic rhinitis by the use of nasal provocation tests. Ann Allergy 60:57, 1988.

321. Anon. Not bananas. Drug Topics 141(13):24, 1997.

322. Paubert Braquet M, et al. Effect of Pygeum africanum extract on A23187-stimulated production of lipoxygenase metabolites from human polymorphonuclear cells. J Lipid Mediat Cell Signal 9:285, 1994.

323. Krzeski T, et al. Combined extracts of Urtica dioica and Pygeum africanum in the treatment of benign prostatic hyperplasia: Double-blind comparison of two doses. Clin Ther 15:1011, 1993.

324. Bertram PD. Melanosis coli: A consequence of "alternative therapy: for psoriasis (Letter). Am J Gastroenterol 88:971, 1993.

325. Haines JD Jr. Sassafras tea and diaphoresis. Postgrad Med 90:75, 1991.

326. Shimada J, Tyler VE, McLaughlin JL. Biologically active acylglycerides from the berries of saw-palmetto (Serenoa repens). J Nat PROD 60:417, 1997.

327. Grasso M, et al. Comparative effects of alfuzosin versus Serenoa repens in the treatment of symptomatic benign prostatic hyperplasia. Arch Esp Urol 48:97, 1995.

328. Di Silverio F, et al. Plant extracts in BPH. Minerva Urol Nefrol 45:143, 1993.

329. Paubert Braquet M, et al. Effect of the lipidosterolic extract of Serenoa repens (Permixon) and its major components on basic fibroplast growth factor-induced proliferation of cultures of human prostate biopsies. Eur Urol 33:340, 1998.

330. Casarosa C, Cosci Di Coscio M, Fratta M. Lack of effects of a lyposterolic extract of Serenoa repens on plasma levels of testosterone, follicle, stimulating hormone, and luteinizing hormone. Clin Ther 10:585, 1988.

331. Di Silverio F, et al. Evidence that Serenoa repens extract displays an antiestrogenic activity in prostatic tissue of benign prostatic hypertrophy patients. Eur Urol 21:309, 1992.

332. Plosker GL, Brogden RN. Serenoa repens (Permixon). A review of its pharmacology and therapeutic efficacy in benign prostatic hyperplasia. Drugs Aging 9:379, 1996.

333. Miller AL. St. John's Wort (Hypericum perforatum): Clinical effects on depression and other conditions. Altern Med Rev 3:18, 1998.

334. Sommer H, Harrer G. Placebo-controlled double-blind study examining the effectiveness of an hypericum preparation in 105 mildly depressed patients. J Geriatr Psychiatry Neurol 7(Suppl 1):S9, 1994.

335. Vorbach EU, Hubner WD, Arnoldt KH. Effectiveness and tolerance of the hypericum extract LI 160 in comparison with imipramine: Randomized double-blind study with 135 outpatients. J Geriatr Psychiatry Neurol 7(Suppl 1):S19, 1994.

336. Hansgen KD, Vesper J, Ploch M. Multicenter double-blind study examining the antidepressant effectiveness of the hypericum extract LI 160. J Geriatr Psychiatry Neurol 7(Suppl 1):S15, 1994.

337. Hubner WD, Lande S, Podzuweit J. Hypericum treatment of mild depression with somatic symptoms. J Geriatr Psychiatry Neurol 7(Suppl 1):S12, 1994.

338. Kasper S. Treatment of seasonal affective disorder (SAD) with hypericum extract. Pharmacopsychiatry 30(Suppl 2):89, 1997.

339. Martinez B, et al. Hypericum in the treatment of seasonal affective disorders. J Geriatr Psychiatry Neurol 7(Suppl 1):S29, 1994.

340. Linde K, et al. St John's wort for depression—An overview and meta-analysis of randomised clinical trials. BMJ 313:253, 1996.

341. Volz HP. Controlled clinical trials of hypericum extracts in depressed patients—An overview. Pharmacopsychiatry 30 (Suppl 2):72, 1997.

342. Brockmoller J, et al. Hypericin and pseudohypericin: Pharmacokinetics and effects of photosensitivity in humans. Pharmacopsychiatry 30(Suppl 2):94, 1997.

343. Woelk H, Burkard G, Grunwald J. Benefits ands risks of the hypericum extract LI 160: Drug monitoring study with 3250 patients. J Geriatr Psychiatry Neurol 7(Suppl 1):S34, 1994.

344. Anon. Dietary supplement adverse event. Wkly Pharm Reports 47(11):1, 1998.

345. Wincor MZ, Gutierrez MA. St. John's wort and the treatment of depression. US Pharm 22(8):88, 1997.

346. Balderer G, Borbely AA. Effect of valerian on human sleep. Psychopharmacology 87:406, 1985.

347. Lindahl O, Lindwall L. Double blind study of a valerian preparation. Pharmacol Biochem Behav 32:1065, 1989.

348. Houghton PJ. The biological activity of Valerian and related plants. J Ethnopharmacol 22:121, 1988.

349. Schulz H, Stolz C, Muller J. The effect of valerian extract on sleep polygraphy in poor sleepers: A pilot study. Pharmacopsychiatry 27:147, 1994.

350. Willey LB, et al. Valerian overdose. Vet Hum Toxicol 37:364, 1995.

351. Chan TY, Tang CH, Critchley JA. Poisoning due to an over-the-counter hypnotic, Sleep Qik (hyoscine, cyproheptadine, valerian). Postgrad Med J 71:227, 1995.

352. Short SH. Health quackery: Our role as professionals. J Am Diet Assoc 94:607, 1994.

353. Riley AJ. Yohimbine in the treatment of erectile disorder. Br J Clin Pract 48:133, 1994.

354. Rowland DL, Kallan K, Slob AK. Yohimbine, erectile capacity, and sexual response in men. Arch Sex Behav 26:49, 1997.

355. Carey MP, Johnson BT. Effectiveness of yohimbine in the treatment of erectile disorder: Four meta-analytic integrations. Arch Sex Behav 25:341, 1996.

356. Mann K, et al. Effects of yohimbine on sexual experiences and nocturnal penile tumescence and rigidity in erectile dysfunction. Arch Sex Behav 25:1, 1996.

357. Sandler B, Aronson P. Yohimbine-induced cutaneous drug eruption, progressive renal failure, and lupus-like syndrome. Urology 41:343, 1993.

358. Wooten V. Effectiveness of yohimbine in treating narcolepsy. South Med J 87:1065, 1994.

359. Southwood TR, et al. Unconventional remedies used for patients with juvenile arthritis. Pediatrics 85:150, 1990.

360. Kurtzweil P. Dieter's brews make tea time a dangerous affair. FDA Consumer 31(5):6, 1997.

361. Anon. California issues senna warning. Drug Topics 141(3):8, 1997.

FDA-Labeled Lower Age Limits for

Use of Nonprescription Products

This appendix provides the age limits for use of nonprescription products. For instance, if an age limit is 6 years, it becomes safe to recommend that product when a child reaches the age of 6. However, data for use in children who have not yet reached their sixth birthday is lacking.

When the FDA monographs do not specifically mention a lower age cutoff, the general age limit of 2 years applies (e.g., antacids and antiflatulents). Further information is provided in the relevant chapter of this book. *If the federal publication noted as a reference indicates that the publication is other than a final rule (e.g., tentative final monograph, notice of proposed rulemaking, or proposed rule), the information below may change.*

ORAL AND GASTROINTESTINAL CONDITIONS

PLAQUE-INDUCED DISEASES: CARIES AND GINGIVITIS

- Anticavity rinses, treatment gels: Under 12 years only with supervision; not under the age of 6 without physician or dentist supervision[1]
- Fluoride toothpastes: Under 6 years only with supervision; not under the age of 2 years[1]

ORAL PROBLEMS

- Carbamide peroxide, hydrogen peroxide: 2 years; under 12 only with supervision[2]
- Sodium perborate monohydrate: 6 years; under 12 only with supervision[2]
- Gingival analgesics (teething): 4 months[2]
- Gingival analgesics (oral irritation): 2 years[2]
- Hypersensitive teeth: 12 years[2]
- Canker sore products: 2 years[2]

GASTRIC DISTRESS (H2-BLOCKERS): 12 YEARS[3]

MOTION SICKNESS (ANTIEMETIC PRODUCTS)[4]

- Meclizine: 12 years
- Cyclizine: 6 years
- Dimenhydrinate: 2 years

CONSTIPATION (LAXATIVES)[5]

- Ingredients safe down to the age of 2 include malt soup extract, polycarbophil, glycerin suppositories, sorbitol, lubricant enemas, magnesium citrate, magnesium hydroxide, magnesium sulfate, sodium phosphate/biphosphate enemas, casanthranol, cascara, and castor oil.
- Ingredients not to recommend under 5 include oral sodium phosphate/biphosphate products.
- Ingredients not to recommend under 6 include celluloses, psyllium, oral lubricants, bisacodyl (oral and suppositories), and aloe.
- Ingredients not to recommend under 12 include bran, senna, and carbon-dioxide laxatives.

DIARRHEA

- Antidiarrheals: 3 years[6]
- Antidiarrheals containing loperamide: 6 years[7]

PINWORM PRODUCTS (ANTHELMINTIC PRODUCTS): 2 YEARS OR 25 POUNDS[8]

HEMORRHOIDS (HEMORRHOID PRODUCTS): 12 YEARS[9]

RESPIRATORY CONDITIONS

ALLERGIC RHINITIS

- Antihistamines: 6 years[10]
- Cromolyn sodium nasal solution: 6 years[11]

THE COMMON COLD AND RELATED CONDITIONS

- Sprays and inhalers containing nasal decongestants[12]:
  —Ingredients safe down to the age of 2 include phenylephrine 0.125%, xylometazoline 0.05%, oxymetazoline 0.025%
  —Ingredients not to recommend under age 6 include

oxymetazoline 0.05%, phenylephrine 0.25%, and propylhexedrine.

—Ingredients not to recommend under 12 years include naphazoline 0.05%, phenylephrine 0.5% and 1%, and xylometazoline 0.1%.

- Oral nasal decongestants: 2 years[12]
- Sore throat products: 2 years[2]
- Oral and topical antitussives, expectorants: 2 years[13]
- Antitussives containing diphenhydramine, codeine: 6 years[13]

ASTHMA (ANTIASTHMATICS)[14]

- Oral ephedrine products: 12 years
- Inhalation epinephrine products: 4 years

PAIN CONDITIONS

HEADACHE AND OTHER MINOR PAINS (INTERNAL ANALGESICS): 2 YEARS[15]

- Extended release internal analgesics containing acetaminophen: 12 years[16]
- Products containing ibuprofen (tablets, caplets): 12 years[17]
- Products containing ibuprofen (junior strength tablets): 6 years[18]
- Products containing ibuprofen (oral suspension): 2 years[19]
- Products containing naproxen: 12 years[20]
- Products containing ketoprofen: 16 years[21]

INJURIES TO MUSCLES, LIGAMENTS, AND TENDONS (EXTERNAL ANALGESICS): 2 YEARS[22]

MISCELLANEOUS INTERNAL PROBLEMS

OBESITY

- Appetite suppressants: 12 years[23]
- Products containing phenylpropanolamine: 18 years[24]

FATIGUE AND DROWSINESS (STIMULANTS): 12 YEARS[25]

SLEEP DISTURBANCES (SLEEP AIDS): 12 YEARS[26]

POISONING EMERGENCIES (ANTIDOTES CONTAINING IPECAC SYRUP): 6 MONTHS[27]

FEVER: 2 YEARS[15]

OPHTHALMIC/OTIC CONDITIONS

OPHTHALMIC CONDITIONS (COMBINATION PRODUCTS CONTAINING OPHTHALMIC VASOCONSTRICTORS/ANTIHISTAMINES): 6 YEARS[28]

OTIC CONDITIONS (EXCESSIVE EARWAX PRODUCTS): 12 YEARS[29]

DERMATOLOGIC CONDITIONS

SUN-INDUCED SKIN DAMAGE (SUNSCREENS): 6 MONTHS[30]

FUNGAL SKIN INFECTIONS (ANTIFUNGALS): 2 YEARS[31]

SKIN HYPERPIGMENTATION (HYPOPIGMENTATION PRODUCTS): 12 YEARS[32]

CONTACT DERMATITIS AND POISON IVY/OAK/SUMAC (PRODUCTS FOR ALLERGIC SKIN REACTIONS): 2 YEARS[22]

- Products containing hydrocortisone: 2 years[33]
- Products containing bentoquatam: 6 years[34]

HAIR LOSS (PRODUCTS CONTAINING MINOXIDIL): 18 YEARS[35,36]

MISCELLANEOUS MEDICAL CONDITIONS AND SITUATIONS

FEMALE GENITAL CONDITIONS (VAGINAL ANTIMONILIAL PRODUCTS): 12 YEARS[37]

NICOTINE ADDITION (NICOTINE GUM/PATCHES): 18 YEARS[38,39]

References

1. Anticaries drug products for over-the-counter human use; Final monograph; Final rule. Fed Reg 60:52474, 1995.
2. Oral health care drug products for over-the-counter human use; Tentative final monograph; Notice of proposed rulemaking. Fed Reg 56:48302,1991.
3. Axid AR, Mylanta•AR, Pepcid AC, Tagamet HB, Zantac 75 Stock Packages. 1995, 1996; Eli Lilly & Company; Johnson & Johnson•Merck; SmithKline Beecham, Glaxo Wellcome.
4. Antiemetic drug products for over-the-counter human use; Final rule. Fed Reg 52:15886, 1987.
5. Laxative drug products for over-the-counter human use; tentative final monograph. Fed Reg 50:2124, 1985.
6. Antidiarrheal drug products for over-the-counter human use; Tentative final monograph; Proposed rulemaking. Fed Reg 51:16138, 1986.
7. Imodium A-D Stock Package. 1995; McNeil Consumer Products.
8. Anthelmintic drug products for over-the-counter human use; Final monograph. Fed Reg 51:27756,1986.
9. Anorectal drug products for over-the-counter human use; Final monograph; final rule. Fed Reg 55:31776, 1990.
10. Cold, cough, allergy, bronchodilator, and antiasthmatic drug products for over-the-counter human use; Final monograph for OTC antihistamine drugs products; Final rule. Fed Reg 57:58356, 1992.
11. Nasalcrom Stock Package. 1997; McNeil Consumer Products.
12. Final monograph for OTC nasal decongestant drug products; Final rule. Fed Reg 59:43386, 1994.
13. Cold, cough, allergy, bronchodilator, and antiasthmatic drug products for over-the-counter human use; Final monograph for OTC antitussive drug products; Final rule. Fed Reg 52:30042, 1987.
14. Cold, cough, allergy, bronchodilator, and antiasthmatic drug products for over-the-counter human use; Final monograph for OTC bronchodilator drug products. Fed Reg 51:35326, 1986.
15. Internal analgesic, antipyretic, and antirheumatic drug products for over-the-counter human use; Tentative final monograph; Notice of proposed rulemaking. Fed Reg 53:46204, 1988.
16. Tylenol Extended Relief Stock Package. 1997; McNeil Consumer Products.
17. Advil Stock Package. 1995; Whitehall Laboratories.
18. Motrin Junior Strength Stock Package. 1997; McNeil Consumer Products.
19. Children's Motrin Oral Suspension Stock Package. 1997; McNeil Consumer Products.
20. Aleve Stock Package. 1995; Procter & Gamble.
21. Actron, Orudis KT Stock Packages. 1997; Bayer Corporation, Whitehall-Robins Healthcare.
22. External analgesic drug products for over-the-counter human use; Tentative final monograph. Fed Reg 48:5852, 1983.
23. Weight control drug products for over-the-counter human use; Establishment of a monograph. Fed Reg 47:8466, 1982.
24. Over-the-counter drug products containing phenylpropanolamine; Required Labeling; Proposed rule. Fed Reg 61:5912, 1996.
25. Stimulant drug products for over-the-counter human use; Final monograph; Final rule. Fed Reg 53:6100, 1988.
26. Nighttime sleep-aid drug products for over-the-counter human use; Final monograph, Final rule. Fed Reg 54:6814, 1989.
27. Poison treatment drug products for over-the-counter human use; Tentative final monograph. Fed Reg 50:2244, 1985.
28. Naphcon A, Opcon-A, Vasocon-A Stock Packages. 1995; Alcon Laboratories, Bausch & Lomb, CIBA Vision Ophthalmics.
29. Topical otic drug products for over-the-counter human use; Final monograph; Final rule. Fed Reg 51:28656, 1986.
30. Sunscreen drug products for over-the-counter human use; Tentative final monograph; Proposed rule. Fed Reg 58:28164, 1993.
31. Topical antifungal drug products, final monograph; Final rule. Fed Reg 58:49890, 1993.
32. Skin bleaching drug products for over-the-counter human use; Tentative final monograph. Fed Reg 47:39108, 1982.
33. External analgesic drug products for over-the-counter human use; Amendment of tentative final monograph; Notice of proposed rulemaking. Fed Reg 55:6932, 1990.
34. Ivy Block Stock Package. 1997; EnviroDerm Pharmaceuticals.
35. Rogaine for Men Stock Package. 1997; Upjohn.
36. Rogaine for Women Stock Package. 1997; Upjohn.
37. Femstat 3, Gyne-Lotrimin, Monistat, Vagistat-1 Stock Packages. 1995; Procter & Gamble, Schering-Plough Health-Care, Advanced Care Products, Bristol-Myers Squibb.
38. Nicorette Gum Stock Package. 1997; SmithKline Beecham.
39. Nicotrol, NicoDerm CQ Stock Packages. 1997; McNeil Consumer Products, SmithKline Beecham.

FDA-Labeled Time Limits for Use of Nonprescription Products

This appendix presents the time beyond which the patient should not use a nonprescription product without consulting a physician or other medical professional such as a dentist or podiatrist.

When the FDA monographs do not specifically mention a lower time cutoff, the ingredient or product group is not mentioned in this table (e.g., motion sickness products and allergic rhinitis products). Further information is provided in the relevant chapter of this book. *If the reference noted indicates that it is other than a final rule (e.g., tentative final monograph, notice of proposed rulemaking, or proposed rule), the information below may change.*

ORAL AND GASTROINTESTINAL CONDITIONS

ORAL PROBLEMS

- Oral mucosal injury products: 7 days[1]
- Gingival analgesics: 7 days[2]
- Hypersensitive teeth: 4 weeks without dentist diagnosis[2]
- Canker sore products: 7 days[2]

GASTRIC DISTRESS

- Antacids: 2 weeks[3]
- H2-blockers: 2 weeks[4]
- Hangover relief products: 2 days[5]

CONSTIPATION (LAXATIVES): 7 DAYS[6]

DIARRHEA (ANTIDIARRHEALS): 2 DAYS[7]

PINWORM (ANTHELMINTIC PRODUCTS): TAKE ONE TIME AS A SINGLE DOSE. DO NOT REPEAT TREATMENT.[8]

HEMORRHOIDS (HEMORRHOID PRODUCTS): 7 DAYS[9]

RESPIRATORY CONDITIONS

THE COMMON COLD AND RELATED CONDITIONS

- Sprays and inhalers containing nasal decongestants:
  —Products not containing l-desoxyephedrine: 3 days[10]
  —Products containing l-desoxyephedrine: 7 days[11]
- Oral nasal decongestants: 7 days[10]
- Sore throat products: 2 days; if it persists for more than 7 days, seek physician care[2]
- Oral and topical antitussives, expectorants: 7 days[12]

ASTHMA (ANTIASTHMATICS)[13]

- Oral ephedrine products: Do not continue to use this product, but seek medical assistance immediately if symptoms are not relieved within 1 hour or become worse.
- Inhalation epinephrine products: Do not continue to use this product, but seek immediate medical attention if symptoms are not relieved in 20 minutes or if they worsen.

PAIN CONDITIONS

HEADACHE AND OTHER MINOR PAINS (INTERNAL ANALGESICS)[14]

- Adult pain: 10 days
- Pain in a child:
  —Products containing acetaminophen, aspirin: 5 days[14]
  —Products containing ibuprofen: 3 days[15]
- Salicylates when used for long-term aspirin regimens: See your doctor for other uses of this product, but do not use for more than 10 days without consulting your doctor because serious side effects may occur.[14]
- Migraine: 48 hours[16]

INJURIES TO MUSCLES, LIGAMENTS, AND TENDONS (EXTERNAL ANALGESICS): 7 DAYS[17]

MISCELLANEOUS INTERNAL PROBLEMS

OBESITY (APPETITE SUPPRESSANTS): 3 MONTHS[18]

FATIGUE AND DROWSINESS (STIMULANTS): FOR OCCASIONAL USE ONLY[19]

SLEEP DISTURBANCES (SLEEP AIDS): 14 DAYS[20]

FEVER: 3 DAYS [14]

OPHTHALMIC/OTIC CONDITIONS

OPHTHALMIC CONDITIONS

- Tear replacement products: 72 hours[21]
- Corneal edema: No self-treatment allowed unless physician diagnosis[21]
- Ophthalmic vasoconstrictors: 72 hours[21]
- Combination products containing ophthalmic vasoconstrictors/antihistamines: 72 hours[22]

OTIC CONDITIONS (EXCESSIVE EARWAX PRODUCTS): 4 DAYS[23]

DERMATOLOGIC CONDITIONS

HYPERPROLIFERATIVE SKIN DISORDERS (PRODUCTS CONTAINING COAL TAR): DO NOT USE FOR PROLONGED PERIODS WITHOUT CONSULTING A PHYSICIAN[24]

ARTHROPOD STING AND BITE ANALGESICS: 7 DAYS (EXTERNAL ANALGESICS)[17]

MINOR WOUNDS

- Products containing topical antimicrobials, antibiotics: 7 days[25,26]
- First-aid antiseptics: 7 days[27]
- Health-care antiseptic products: 72 hours[28]

BURNS (BURN PRODUCTS): 7 DAYS (EXTERNAL ANALGESICS)[17]

FUNGAL SKIN INFECTIONS (ANTIFUNGALS)[29]

- Athlete's foot and ringworm: 4 weeks
- Jock itch: 2 weeks

WARTS (WART REMOVAL PRODUCTS): 12 WEEKS[30]

CONTACT DERMATITIS AND POISON IVY/OAK/SUMAC (PRODUCTS FOR ALLERGIC SKIN REACTIONS)

- External analgesics: 7 days[17]
- Hydrocortisone: 7 days[31]
- Astringents: 7 days[32]

DIAPER RASH (TOPICAL ANTIMICROBIAL PRODUCTS): 7 DAYS[33]

SKIN HYPERPIGMENTATION (HYPOPIGMENTATION PRODUCTS): 3 MONTHS[34]

FOOT PROBLEMS (CALLUS/CORN REMOVERS): 14 DAYS[35]

HAIR LOSS

- Products containing 2% minoxidil for men: 12 months[36]
- Products containing 5% minoxidil for men: 4 months[37]
- Products containing 2% minoxidil for women: 8 months[38]

MISCELLANEOUS MEDICAL CONDITIONS AND SITUATIONS

FEMALE GENITAL CONDITIONS

- Vaginal fungal infections (vaginal antimonilial products): 1, 3, or 7 days as indicated on package; recurrent vaginal yeast infections are a sign of HIV infection.[39]
- Vaginal irritation and pruritus (products containing hydrocortisone for minor vaginal irritation): 7 days[40]

NICOTINE ADDICTION

- Nicotine gum: 12 weeks[41]
- Nicotine patches
  —Nicotrol: 6 weeks[42]

—NicoDerm CQ: 8 weeks (light smokers who begin with Step 2); 10 weeks (heavy smokers who begin with Step 1)[43]

References

1. Oral mucosal injury drug products for over-the-counter human use; Tentative final monograph. Fed Reg 48:33984, 1983.
2. Oral health care drug products for over-the-counter human use; Tentative final monograph; Notice of proposed rulemaking. Fed Reg 56:48302,1991.
3. Antacid and antiflatulent products. Fed Reg 39:19862, 1974.
4. Axid AR, Mylanta•AR, Pepcid AC, Tagamet HB, Zantac 75 Stock Packages. 1995, 1996; Eli Lilly & Company; Johnson & Johnson•Merck; SmithKline Beecham, Glaxo Wellcome.
5. Internal analgesic, antipyretic, and antirheumatic drug products for over-the-counter human use; Proposed amendment to the tentative final monograph; Notice of proposed rulemaking. Fed Reg 56:66762, 1991.
6. Laxative drug products for over-the-counter human use; tentative final monograph. Fed Reg 50:2124, 1985.
7. Antidiarrheal drug products for over-the-counter human use; Tentative final monograph; Proposed rulemaking. Fed Reg 51:16138, 1986.
8. Anthelmintic drug products for over-the-counter human use; Final monograph. Fed Reg 51:27756,1986.
9. Anorectal drug products for over-the-counter human use; Final monograph; Final rule. Fed Reg 55:31776, 1990.
10. Final monograph for OTC nasal decongestant drug products; Final rule. Fed Reg 59:43386, 1994.
11. Cold, cough, allergy, bronchodilator, and antiasthmatic drug products for over-the-counter human use; OTC nasal decongestant drug products; Partial stay of final rule; enforcement policy. Fed Reg 61:9570, 1996.
12. Cold, cough, allergy, bronchodilator, and antiasthmatic drug products for over-the-counter human use; Final monograph for OTC antitussive drug products; Final rule. Fed Reg 52:30042, 1987.
13. Cold, cough, allergy, bronchodilator, and antiasthmatic drug products for over-the-counter human use; Final monograph for OTC bronchodilator drug products. Fed Reg 51:35326, 1986.
14. Internal analgesic, antipyretic, and antirheumatic drug products for over-the-counter human use; Tentative final monograph; Notice of proposed rulemaking. Fed Reg 53:46204, 1988.
15. Children's Advil, Children's Motrin Stock Packages. 1997; Whitehall-Robins Healthcare, McNeil Consumer Products.
16. Excedrin Migraine Stock Package. 1998; Bristol-Myers Products.
17. External analgesic drug products for over-the-counter human use; Tentative final monograph. Fed Reg 48:5852, 1983.
18. Weight control drug products for over-the-counter human use; Establishment of a monograph. Fed Reg 47:8466, 1982.
19. Stimulant drug products for over-the-counter human use; Final monograph; Final rule. Fed Reg 53:6100, 1988.
20. Nighttime sleep-aid drug products for over-the-counter human use; Final monograph, Final rule. Fed Reg 54:6814, 1989.
21. Ophthalmic drug products for over-the-counter human use; Final monograph; Final rule. Fed Reg 53:7076, 1988.
22. Naphcon A, Opcon-A, Vasocon-A Stock Packages. 1995; Alcon Laboratories, Bausch & Lomb, CIBA Vision Ophthalmics.
23. Topical otic drug products for over-the-counter human use; Final monograph; Final rule. Fed Reg 51:28656, 1986.
24. Dandruff, seborrheic dermatitis, and psoriasis drug products for over-the-counter human use; Final rule. Fed Reg 56:63554, 1991.
25. Topical antimicrobial drug products for over-the-counter human use; Final monograph for OTC first aid antibiotic drug products; Final rule. Fed Reg 52:47312, 1987.
26. Topical antimicrobial drug products for over-the-counter human use; Proposed rule. Fed Reg 61:5918, 1996.
27. Topical antimicrobial drug products for over-the-counter human use; Tentative final monograph for first aid antiseptic drug products. Fed Reg 56:33644, 1991.
28. Tentative final monograph for health-care antiseptic drug products; Proposed rule. Fed Reg 59:31402, 1994.
29. Topical antifungal drug products, Final monograph; Final rule. Fed Reg 58:49890, 1993.
30. Wart remover drug products for over-the-counter human use; Final monograph; Final rule. Fed Reg 55:33246, 1990.
31. External analgesic drug products for over-the-counter human use; Amendment of tentative final monograph; Notice of proposed rulemaking. Fed Reg 55:6932, 1990.
32. Skin protectant drug products for over-the-counter human use; Astringent drug products; Final rule. Fed Reg 58:54458, 1993.
33. Topical antimicrobial drug products for over-the-counter human use; Proposed rule for diaper rash drug products. Fed Reg 55:25246, 1990.
34. Skin bleaching drug products for over-the-counter human use; Tentative final monograph. Fed Reg 47:39108, 1982.
35. Corn and callus remover drug products for over-the-counter human use; Final monograph; Final Rule. Fed Reg 55:33258, 1990.
36. Rogaine for Men Stock Package. 1997; Upjohn.
37. Rogaine Extra Strength for Men Stock Package. 1998; Upjohn.
38. Rogaine for Women Stock Package. 1997; Upjohn.
39. Femstat 3, Gyne-Lotrimin, Monistat, Vagistat-1 Stock Packages. 1995; Procter & Gamble, Schering-Plough HealthCare; Advanced Care Products, Bristol-Myers Squibb.
40. Vaginal drug products for over-the-counter human use; Withdrawal of advance notice of proposed rulemaking. Fed Reg 59:5226, 1994.
41. Nicorette Gum Stock Package. 1997; SmithKline Beecham.
42. Nicotrol Stock Package. 1997; McNeil Consumer Products.
43. NicoDerm CQ Stock Package. 1997; SmithKline Beecham.

FDA-Labeled Contraindications for

Use of Nonprescription Products

This appendix delineates the various contraindications required by the FDA on nonprescription products for various conditions.

In addition to the contraindications discussed below, many nonprescription products are contraindicated during pregnancy and breast-feeding. While the pregnancy/breast-feeding warnings on some products are even more restrictive, virtually all nonprescription products carry this general warning: As with any drug, if you are pregnant or nursing a baby, seek the advice of a health professional before using this product.

ORAL AND GASTROINTESTINAL CONDITIONS

ORAL PROBLEMS

- Oral mucosal analgesics containing benzocaine or butacaine sulfate: Do not use this product if you have a history of allergy to local anesthetics such as procaine, butacaine, benzocaine, or other "caine" anesthetics.[1]
- Teething products: Fever and nasal congestion are not symptoms of teething and may indicate the presence of infection. Consult a physician if they persist.[1]

GASTRIC DISTRESS

- Antacids[2]:
  —For products containing more than 50 mEq of magnesium or 25 mEq of potassium per maximum recommended daily dose: Do not use this product except under the advice and supervision of a physician if you have kidney disease.
  —For products containing more than 5 mEq of sodium per maximum recommended daily dose: Do not use this product except under the advice and supervision of a physician if you are on a sodium-restricted diet.
- H2-Blockers: If you have trouble swallowing or persistent abdominal pain, see your doctor promptly. You may have a serious condition that may need a different treatment.[3]
- Products for overindulgence in food and beverages containing bismuth subsalicylate: Children and teenagers who have or are recovering from chicken pox, flu symptoms, or flu should NOT use this product. If nausea, vom-

iting, or fever occur, consult a physician because these symptoms could be an early sign of Reye syndrome, a rare but serious illness.[4]

MOTION SICKNESS (ANTIEMETICS)

Do not take this product, unless directed by a doctor, if you have a breathing problem such as emphysema or chronic bronchitis, or if you have glaucoma or difficulty in urination due to enlargement of the prostate gland.[5]

CONSTIPATION (LAXATIVES)[6]

- General category contraindications: Only for occasional constipation. Do not use when abdominal pain, nausea, or vomiting are present, unless directed by a doctor. If you have noticed a sudden change in bowel habits that persists over a period of 2 weeks, consult a physician before using a laxative. Rectal bleeding or failure to have a bowel movement following use of a laxative may indicate a serious condition. Discontinue use and see a physician. If the product contains more than 5 mEq of sodium in the maximum recommended daily dose: Do not use if on a low-sodium diet unless advised by a physician. If the product contains more than 25 mEq of potassium or 50 mEq of magnesium per recommended daily dose: Do not use if you have kidney disease unless advised by a physician.
- Saline laxatives containing phosphates: Do not use this product if you have kidney disease, heart problems, or are dehydrated, or for more than 3 days, without asking a doctor.[7]
- Products containing lubricants: Pregnancy, bedridden patients, persons with difficulty swallowing.
- Enteric-coated tablets containing bisacodyl: Do not give to people who cannot swallow without chewing.

DIARRHEA (PRODUCTS CONTAINING LOPERAMIDE)

Do not use if diarrhea is accompanied by a high fever (greater than 101°F), or if blood or mucus is present in the stool, or if you have had a rash or other allergic reaction to loperamide HCl. If you are taking antibiotics, or have a history of liver disease, consult a physician before using this product.[8]

PINWORM (ANTHELMINTIC PRODUCTS CONTAINING PYRANTEL PAMOATE)

If you are pregnant or have liver disease, do not take this product unless directed by a physician. If any other worms than pinworms are present before or after treatment, consult a doctor.[9]

HEMORRHOIDS (HEMORRHOID PRODUCTS)

In case of bleeding, consult a physician promptly.[10]

- Products containing ephedrine, epinephrine, or phenylephrine: Do not use this product if you have heart disease, high blood pressure, thyroid disease, diabetes, or difficulty in urination due to enlargement of the prostate gland, unless directed by a physician.
- Products containing resorcinol: Do not use on open wounds near the anus.

RESPIRATORY CONDITIONS

ALLERGIC RHINITIS

- Products containing antihistamines: Do not take this product, unless directed by a physician, if you have a breathing problem such as emphysema or chronic bronchitis, or if you have glaucoma or difficulty in urination due to enlargement of the prostate gland.[11]
- Nasal solutions containing cromolyn sodium: Ask a doctor before use if you have fever, discolored nasal discharge, sinus pain, or wheezing. Do not use this product to treat sinus infection, asthma, or cold symptoms.[12]

THE COMMON COLD AND RELATED CONDITIONS

- Sprays containing nasal decongestants: Do not use if you have heart disease, high blood pressure, thyroid disease, diabetes, or difficulty in urination due to enlargement of the prostate gland unless directed by a doctor.[13]
- Oral nasal decongestants: If symptoms do not improve or are accompanied by fever, consult a doctor. Do not use if you have heart disease, high blood pressure, thyroid disease, diabetes, or difficulty in urination due to enlargement of the prostate gland, unless directed by a doctor.[13]
- Products containing phenylpropanolamine: Do not take if you have heart or thyroid disease, high blood pressure, or an enlarged prostate gland, unless directed by a doctor.[14]
- Sore throat topical products: Do not use products if the sore throat is severe, accompanied by fever, headache, rash, swelling, nausea, and/or vomiting.[1]

- Sore throat internal analgesics: Do not use products if the sore throat is severe, accompanied by fever, headache, rash, nausea, and/or vomiting.[15]
- Oral and topical antitussives, expectorants[16,17]:
  —General category contraindications: A persistent cough may be the sign of a serious condition. If cough persists for more than 1 week, tends to recur, or is accompanied by fever, rash, or persistent headache, consult a physician. Do not take this product for persistent or chronic cough such as occurs with smoking, asthma, emphysema, or if cough is accompanied by excessive phlegm (mucus) unless directed by a physician.
  —Products containing codeine: Do not take this product if you have pulmonary disease or shortness of breath unless directed by a physician.

ASTHMA (ANTIASTHMATICS)

Do not use if you have heart disease, high blood pressure, thyroid disease, diabetes mellitus, or difficulty in urination due to enlargement of the prostate gland, without physician supervision. Do not use if you have ever been hospitalized for asthma or are taking any prescription drug for asthma unless directed by a physician.[18]

PAIN CONDITIONS

HEADACHE AND OTHER MINOR PAINS (INTERNAL ANALGESICS)

Do not take if the area is red or swollen.[19]

- Alcohol warning: If you generally consume 3 or more alcohol-containing drinks per day, you should consult your doctor for advice on when and how you should take this product and other pain relievers.[20]
  —Products containing acetaminophen: If you drink three or more alcoholic beverages daily, ask your doctor whether you should take this product or other pain relievers. This product may increase your risk of liver damage.[21]
  —Products containing aspirin, carbaspirin calcium, choline salicylate, ibuprofen, ketoprofen, magnesium salicylate, naproxen sodium, or sodium salicylate: If you drink three or more alcoholic beverages daily, ask your doctor whether you should take this product or other pain relievers. This product may increase your risk of stomach bleeding.[21]
- Pain in a child: Do not give this product to children for the pain of arthritis unless directed by a physician.[19]
- Products containing salicylates: Do not take if you have stomach problems (such as heartburn, upset stomach, or stomach pain) that persist or recur, or if you have ulcers or bleeding problems, unless directed by a doctor. Do not take if allergic to salicylates (including aspirin) or

if asthmatic unless directed by a physician. Products in a chewable dosage form: Do not take for 7 days after tonsillectomy or oral surgery.[19]

- Products containing magnesium salicylate in a high enough quantity that a patient could take more than 50 mEq of magnesium in the recommended daily dose: Do not take if you have kidney disease unless directed by a physician.
  —Proposed revised warning for oral and rectal aspirin products: Children and teenagers who have or are recovering from chicken pox, flu symptoms, or flu should NOT use this product. If nausea, vomiting, or fever occur, consult a doctor because these symptoms could be an early sign of Reye syndrome, a rare but serious illness.[22]

- Products containing ibuprofen, naproxen sodium, or ketoprofen (tablets, caplets): Warning: Aspirin Sensitive Patients. Do not take this product if you have had a severe allergic reaction to aspirin—e.g., asthma, swelling, shock, or hives—because even though this product contains no aspirin or salicylates, cross-reactions may occur in patients allergic to aspirin. As with aspirin and acetaminophen, if you have any condition that requires you to take prescription drugs or if you have had any problems or serious side effects from taking any nonprescription pain reliever, do not take this product without first discussing it with your doctor. **IT IS ESPECIALLY IMPORTANT NOT TO USE IBUPROFEN DURING THE LAST 3 MONTHS OF PREGNANCY UNLESS SPECIFICALLY DIRECTED TO DO SO BY A DOCTOR BECAUSE IT MAY CAUSE PROBLEMS IN THE UNBORN CHILD OR COMPLICATIONS DURING DELIVERY.**[20]

- Products containing ibuprofen (junior strength tablets, oral suspension): Warnings: Aspirin Sensitive Children. This product contains no aspirin, but may cause a severe allergic reaction in people allergic to aspirin. Do not use this product if your child has had an allergic reaction to aspirin such as asthma, swelling, shock, or hives. Do not use for stomach pain unless directed by a doctor. Do not use if your child is dehydrated (significant fluid loss) due to continued vomiting, diarrhea, or lack of fluid intake. Call your doctor if your child is under a doctor's care for any serious condition or is taking any other drug; or if your child has problems or serious side effects from taking fever reducers or pain relievers.[23]

MENSTRUAL DISCOMFORT (PRODUCTS CONTAINING AMMONIUM CHLORIDE)

Do not use if you have kidney or liver disease.[24]

INJURIES TO MUSCLES, LIGAMENTS, AND TENDONS (PRODUCTS CONTAINING COUNTER-IRRITANTS)

Do not apply to wounds or damaged skin.[25]

MISCELLANEOUS INTERNAL PROBLEMS

OBESITY (APPETITE SUPPRESSANTS CONTAINING PHENYLPROPANOLAMINE)

Do not take if you have heart or thyroid disease, high blood pressure, or an enlarged prostate gland, unless directed by a doctor.[14]

SLEEP DISTURBANCES (SLEEP AIDS)

Do not take this product, unless directed by a doctor, if you have a breathing problem such as emphysema or chronic bronchitis, or if you have glaucoma or difficulty in urination due to enlargement of the prostate gland.[26]

POISONING EMERGENCIES (PRODUCTS CONTAINING ACTIVATED CHARCOAL OR SYRUP OF IPECAC)

Do not use in persons who are not fully conscious. Do not use this product, unless directed by a health professional, if turpentine, corrosives, such as alkalies (lye) and strong acids, or petroleum distillates, such as kerosene, gasoline, paint thinner, cleaning fluid, or furniture polish, have been ingested.[27]

FEVER: SEE INTERNAL ANALGESIC PRODUCTS.

OPHTHALMIC/OTIC CONDITIONS

OPHTHALMIC CONDITIONS

- Products containing mercury as a preservative: Do not use this product if you are sensitive to mercury.[28]
- Products containing ophthalmic vasoconstrictors: If you have narrow angle glaucoma, do not use this product except under the advice and supervision of a physician.[29]
- Combination products containing ophthalmic vasoconstrictors/antihistamines: Do not use if you have heart disease, high blood pressure, difficulty in urination, or narrow angle glaucoma unless directed by a physician.[30]

OTIC CONDITIONS (EXCESSIVE EARWAX PRODUCTS)

Do not use if you have ear drainage, discharge, ear pain, irritation, a rash in the ear, or are dizzy. Do not use if you have an injury or perforation of the ear drum or after ear surgery, unless directed by a physician.[31]

DERMATOLOGIC CONDITIONS

HYPERPROLIFERATIVE SKIN DISORDERS (PRODUCTS FOR SEBORRHEIC DERMATITIS, PSORIASIS)

If condition covers a large area of the body, consult your physician before using this product.[32]

MINOR WOUNDS[33,34]

- Products containing antibiotics, alcohols: In case of deep or puncture wounds, animal bites, or serious burns, consult a physician.
- Products containing topical antibiotics: Do not treat a wound larger than may be covered by the amount of product that covers the tip of the finger.
- Topical antibiotics containing bacitracin, bacitracin zinc, neomycin, neomycin sulfate, polymyxin B, polymyxin B sulfate: Do not use this product if you are allergic to any of the ingredients.[35,36]

FUNGAL SKIN INFECTIONS (ANTIFUNGALS)

This product is not effective on the scalp or nails. Do not use on diaper rash.[37]

WARTS: (WART REMOVAL PRODUCTS)

Do not use the products on irritated skin, or on any area that is infected or reddened. Do not use on moles, birthmarks, warts with hair growing from them, genital warts, or any wart on the face or mucous membranes. Do not use this product if you are a diabetic, or if you have poor blood circulation.[38]

CONTACT DERMATITIS AND POISON IVY/OAK/SUMAC (PRODUCTS FOR ALLERGIC SKIN REACTIONS)

- Products containing diphenhydramine: Do not use on chicken pox, poison ivy, sunburn, large areas of the body, or on broken, blistered, or oozing skin.[39]
- Products containing hydrocortisone: For use in any condition not part of the FDA-approved labeling: Other uses of this product should only be under the advice and supervision of a physician.[40]
- Products containing bentoquatam: Do not use if you are allergic to any ingredients. Do not use if you already have a rash from poison ivy, poison oak, or poison sumac.[41]

DIAPER DERMATITIS (TOPICAL ANTIMICROBIAL POWDERS)

Do not use on broken skin.[42]

FOOT PROBLEMS (CALLUS/CORN REMOVERS)

Do not use if diabetic or if you have poor circulation.[43]

HAIR LOSS (PRODUCTS CONTAINING MINOXIDIL)

Do not use if you have no family history of hair loss; hair loss is sudden and/or patchy; scalp is red, inflamed, infected, irritated, or painful; you do not know the reason for your hair loss; you use other topical prescription products on your scalp. Do not use if your hair loss is associated with childbirth.[44]

MISCELLANEOUS MEDICAL CONDITIONS AND SITUATIONS

FEMALE GENITAL CONDITIONS

- Vaginal fungal infections (vaginal antimonilial products): If this is the first time you have had vaginal or vulvar itch and discomfort, consult your doctor. If you are pregnant or think you may be pregnant, do not use this product except under the advice and supervision of a doctor. Do not use if you have fever higher than 100°F orally. Do not use if you have pain, in either the lower abdomen, back, or either shoulder. Do not use if you have a vaginal discharge that smells bad.[45]
- Vaginal antipruritics containing hydrocortisone: Do not use if you have a vaginal discharge.[40]

NICOTINE ADDICTION (PRODUCTS CONTAINING NICOTINE)

Nicotine can increase your baby's heart rate. First try to stop smoking without the product. Ask your doctor before use if you have heart disease, have recently had a heart attack, experience irregular heartbeat, or have high blood pressure not controlled by medication.[46,47]

- Nicotine gum: Ask your doctor before use if you have stomach ulcer.[46]
- Nicotine patches: Ask your doctor before use if you are allergic to adhesive tape or have skin problems.[47]

References

1. Oral health care drug products for over-the-counter human use; Tentative final monograph; Notice of proposed rulemaking. Fed Reg 56:48302,1991.
2. Antacid and antiflatulent products. Fed Reg 39:19862, 1974.
3. Axid AR, Mylanta•AR, Pepcid AC, Tagamet HB, Zantac 75 Stock Packages. 1995, 1996; Eli Lilly & Company; Johnson & Johnson•Merck; SmithKline Beecham, Glaxo Wellcome.
4. Orally administered drug products for relief of symptoms associated with overindulgence in food and drink for over-the-counter human use; Proposed amendment to the tentative final monograph; Proposed rule. Fed Reg 58:26886, 1993.

5. Antiemetic drug products for over-the-counter human use; Amendment of final monograph. Fed Reg 59:16981, 1994.

6. Laxative drug products for over-the-counter human use; tentative final monograph. Fed Reg 50:2124, 1985.

7. Laxative drug products for over-the-counter human use; Proposed amendment to the tentative final monograph. Fed Reg 63:27886, 1998.

8. Imodium A-D Caplets Stock Package. 1997; McNeil Consumer Products.

9. Anthelmintic drug products for over-the-counter human use; Final monograph. Fed Reg 51:27756, 1986.

10. Anorectal drug products for over-the-counter human use; Final monograph; Final rule. Fed Reg 55:31776, 1990.

11. Cold, cough, allergy, bronchodilator, and antiasthmatic drug products for over-the-counter human use; Final monograph for OTC antihistamine drug products; Final rule. Fed Reg 57:58356, 1992.

12. Nasalcrom Stock Package. 1997; McNeil Consumer Products.

13. Final monograph for OTC nasal decongestant drug products; Final rule. Fed Reg 59:43386, 1994.

14. Over-the-counter drug products containing phenylpropanolamine; Required labeling; Proposed rule. Fed Reg 61:5912, 1996.

15. Internal analgesic, antipyretic, and antirheumatic drug products for over-the-counter human use; Tentative final monograph; Notice of proposed rulemaking. Fed Reg 53:46204, 1988.

16. Cold, cough, allergy, bronchodilator, and antiasthmatic drug products for over-the-counter human use; Final monograph for OTC antitussive drug products; Final rule. Fed Reg 52:30042, 1987.

17. Cold, cough, allergy, bronchodilator, and antiasthmatic drug products for over-the-counter human use; Expectorant drug products for over-the-counter human use; Final monograph; Final rule. Fed Reg 54:8494, 1989.

18. Cold, cough, allergy, bronchodilator, and antiasthmatic drug products for over-the-counter human use; Final monograph for OTC bronchodilator drug products. Fed Reg 51:35326, 1986.

19. Internal analgesic, antipyretic, and antirheumatic drug products for over-the-counter human use; Tentative final monograph; Notice of proposed rulemaking. Fed Reg 53:46204, 1988.

20. Actron, Advil Aleve, Orudis KT Stock Packages. 1997; Bayer Corporation, Whitehall Laboratories, Procter & Gamble.

21. Over-the-counter drug products containing analgesic/antipyretic active ingredients for internal use; Required alcohol warning. Fed Reg 62:61041, 1997.

22. Labeling of oral and rectal over-the-counter drug products containing aspirin and nonaspirin salicylates; Proposed rule. Fed Reg 58:54228, 1993.

23. Motrin Junior Strength, Children's Motrin Oral Suspension Stock Packages. 1997; McNeil Consumer Products.

24. Orally administered menstrual drug products for over-the-counter human use; Tentative final monograph; Notice of proposed rulemaking. Fed Reg 53:46194, 1988.

25. External analgesic drug products for over-the-counter human use; Tentative final monograph. Fed Reg 48:5852, 1983.

26. Antiemetic drug products; Nighttime sleep-aid drug products; Notices of proposed rulemaking. Fed Reg 58:45217, 1993.

27. Poison treatment drug products for over-the-counter human use; Tentative final monograph. Fed Reg 50:2244, 1985.

28. Ophthalmic drug products for over-the-counter human use; Final monograph; Final rule. Fed Reg 53:7076, 1988.

29. Ophthalmic drug products for over-the-counter human use: Proposed amendment of final monograph. Fed Reg 63:8888, 1998.

30. Naphcon A, Opcon-A, Vasocon-A Stock Packages. 1995; Alcon Laboratories, Bausch & Lomb, CIBA Vision Ophthalmics.

31. Topical otic drug products for over-the-counter human use; Final monograph; Final rule. Fed Reg 51:28656, 1986.

32. Dandruff, seborrheic dermatitis, and psoriasis drug products for over-the-counter human use; Final rule. Fed Reg 56:63554, 1991.

33. Topical antimicrobial drug products for over-the-counter human use; Final monograph for OTC first aid antibiotic drug products; Final rule. Fed Reg 52:47312, 1987.

34. Alcohol drug products for topical antimicrobial over-the-counter human use; Establishment of a monograph; and reopening of administrative record. Fed Reg 47:22324, 1982.

35. Topical antimicrobial drug products for over-the-counter human use; Proposed rule. Fed Reg 61:5918, 1996.

36. Topical antimicrobial drug products for over-the-counter human use; Amendment of final monograph for OTC first aid antibiotic drug products. Fed Reg 61:58471, 1996.

37. Topical antifungal drug products, final monograph; Final rule. Fed Reg 58:49890, 1993.

38. Wart remover drug products for over-the-counter human use; Final monograph; Final rule. Fed Reg 55:33246, 1990.

39. Labeling of diphenhydramine-containing drug products for over-the-counter human use. Fed Reg 62:45767, 1997.

40. External analgesic drug products for over-the-counter human use; Amendment of tentative final monograph; Notice of proposed rulemaking. Fed Reg 55:6932, 1990.

41. Ivy Block Stock Package. 1997; EnviroDerm Pharmaceuticals.

42. Topical antimicrobial drug products for over-the-counter human use; Proposed rule for diaper rash drug products. Fed Reg 55:25246, 1990.

43. Corn and callus remover drug products for over-the-counter human use; Final monograph; Final Rule. Fed Reg 55:33258, 1990.

44. Rogaine for Men, Rogaine for Women Stock Packages. 1997; Upjohn.

45. Femstat 3, Gyne-Lotrimin, Monistat, Vagistat-1 Stock Packages. 1995; Procter & Gamble, Schering-Plough HealthCare; Advanced Care Products, Bristol-Myers Squibb.

46. Nicorette Gum Stock Package. 1997; SmithKline Beecham.

47. Nicotrol, NicoDerm CQ Stock Packages. 1997; McNeil Consumer Products, SmithKline Beecham.

FDA-Labeled Drug Interactions and Concurrent Use Precautions with Nonprescription Products

This appendix includes drug interaction warnings as required by FDA-approved labeling. This appendix also includes alcohol and food warnings when the FDA requires such labels.

ORAL AND GASTROINTESTINAL CONDITIONS

GASTRIC DISTRESS

- Antacids: Antacids may interact with certain prescription drugs. If you are presently taking a prescription drug, do not take this product without checking with your physician or other health professional.[1]
- Products containing cimetidine: Consult your doctor if you are taking theophylline (oral asthma medicine), warfarin (blood thinning medicine), or phenytoin (seizure medicine) before taking (a cimetidine-containing product).[2]

MOTION SICKNESS (ANTIEMETICS)[3]

- Products containing cyclizine or meclizine: May cause drowsiness; alcohol, sedatives, and tranquilizers may increase the drowsiness effect. Do not take this product if you are taking sedatives or tranquilizers without first consulting your doctor.
- Products containing dimenhydrinate or diphenhydramine. Same as meclizine and cyclizine, except it must say MARKED drowsiness in the first sentence.

CONSTIPATION (LAXATIVES)[4]

- Products containing mineral oil: Do not take this product if you are currently taking a stool softener laxative. Do not take with meals.
- Oral tablets containing bisacodyl: Do not take within 1 hour after taking an antacid or milk.
- Suppositories containing carbon dioxide: Do not lubricate this laxative with mineral oil or petrolatum prior to rectal insertion.

- Products containing emollients: Do not take this product if you are presently taking mineral oil, unless directed by a doctor.

DIARRHEA (PRODUCTS CONTAINING BISMUTH SUBSALICYLATE)

This product contains salicylate. Do not take this product with other salicylate-containing products such as aspirin unless directed by a doctor. If you are taking a drug for anticoagulation (thinning blood), diabetes, gout, or arthritis, do not take this product unless directed by a doctor.[5]

HEMORRHOIDS (HEMORRHOID PRODUCTS)[6]

- Products containing ephedrine, epinephrine, or phenylephrine: Do not use this product if you are presently taking a prescription drug for high blood pressure or depression, without first consulting your physician.
- Products containing aluminum hydroxide gel or kaolin: Remove petrolatum or greasy ointment before using this product because they interfere with the ability of this product to adhere properly to the skin area.

RESPIRATORY CONDITIONS

ALLERGIC RHINITIS

- Products containing antihistamines: Alcohol, sedatives, and tranquilizers may increase the drowsiness effect. Avoid alcoholic beverages while taking this product. Do not take this product if you are taking sedatives or tranquilizers without first consulting your doctor.[7]
- Products containing diphenhydramine: Do not use with any other product containing diphenhydramine, including one applied topically.[8]
- Products containing phenylpropanolamine: See drug interactions listed under the common cold.

THE COMMON COLD AND RELATED CONDITIONS

- Oral nasal decongestants: Do not take this product if you are now taking a prescription monoamine oxidase inhibitor (MAOI) (certain drugs for depression, psychiatric or emotional conditions, or Parkinson's disease), or for 2 weeks after stopping the MAOI drug.[9]
  - Products containing phenylpropanolamine: Do not use with any allergy, asthma, cough-cold, nasal decongestant, or weight control product (containing phenylpropanolamine, phenylephrine, pseudoephedrine, or ephedrine), or any prescription drug, unless directed by a doctor.[10]
- Oral antitussives containing dextromethorphan: Do not take this product if you are now taking a prescription monoamine oxidase inhibitor (MAOI) (certain drugs for depression, psychiatric or emotional conditions, or Parkinson's disease), or for 2 weeks after stopping the MAOI drug.[11]
- Oral antitussives containing codeine: Do not give this product to children who are taking other drugs, unless directed by a physician.[12]

ASTHMA (ANTIASTHMATICS)

Do not take this product if you are now taking a prescription monoamine oxidase inhibitor (MAOI) (certain drugs for depression, psychiatric or emotional conditions, or Parkinson's disease), or for 2 weeks after stopping the MAOI drug.[13]

PAIN CONDITIONS

HEADACHE AND OTHER MINOR PAINS (INTERNAL ANALGESICS)[14]

- Alcohol warning: If you generally consume 3 or more alcohol-containing drinks per day, you should consult your doctor for advice on when and how you should take this product and other pain relievers.[15]
  - Products containing acetaminophen: If you drink three or more alcoholic beverages daily, ask your doctor whether you should take this product or other pain relievers. This product may increase your risk of liver damage.[16]
  - Products containing aspirin, carbaspirin calcium, choline salicylate, ibuprofen, ketoprofen, magnesium salicylate, naproxen sodium, or sodium salicylate: If you drink three or more alcoholic beverages daily, ask your doctor whether you should take this product or other pain relievers. This product may increase your risk of stomach bleeding.[16]
- Products containing salicylates: Do not take this product if you are taking a prescription drug for anticoagulation (thinning blood), diabetes, gout, or arthritis, except under a physician's supervision.
- Products containing ibuprofen (tablets, caplets): Al-

though ibuprofen is indicated for the same conditions as aspirin and acetaminophen, it should not be taken with them except under a doctor's direction.[17]
- Products containing ibuprofen (junior strength tablets, oral suspension): Do not use with any other product that contains ibuprofen, or any other pain reducer/fever reducer, unless directed by a doctor.[18]
- Products containing naproxen sodium: Although naproxen sodium is indicated for the same conditions as aspirin, ibuprofen, and acetaminophen, it should not be taken with them or other naproxen-containing products except under a doctor's direction.[19]
- Products containing ketoprofen: Do not use with any other pain reliever/fever reducer or with any other product containing ketoprofen.[20]

MISCELLANEOUS INTERNAL PROBLEMS

OBESITY (APPETITE SUPPRESSANTS CONTAINING PHENYLPROPANOLAMINE)

Do not use with a monoamine oxidase inhibitor (MAOI) (certain drugs for depression, psychiatric or emotional conditions, or Parkinson's disease), or for 2 weeks after stopping the MAOI drug. Do not use with any allergy, asthma, cough-cold, nasal decongestant, or weight control product (containing phenylpropanolamine, phenylephrine, pseudoephedrine, or ephedrine), or any prescription drug, unless directed by a doctor.[10]

FATIGUE AND DROWSINESS (STIMULANTS)

The recommended dose of this product contains about as much caffeine as a cup of coffee. Limit the use of caffeine-containing medications, foods, or beverages while taking this product because too much caffeine can cause nervousness, irritability. sleeplessness and, occasionally, rapid heart beat.[21]

SLEEP DISTURBANCES (SLEEP AIDS)

Avoid alcoholic beverages while taking this product. Do not take this product if you are taking sedatives or tranquilizers, without first consulting your physician.[22]

- Products containing diphenhydramine: Do not use with any other product containing diphenhydramine, including one applied topically.[8]

POISONING EMERGENCIES (PRODUCTS CONTAINING SYRUP OF IPECAC)

Do not administer milk with this product. Activated charcoal will adsorb ipecac syrup. Do not give activated charcoal until after the patient has vomited, unless directed by a health professional.[23]

DERMATOLOGIC CONDITIONS

HYPERPROLIFERATIVE SKIN DISORDERS (PRODUCTS CONTAINING COAL TAR)

Do not use this product with other forms of psoriasis therapy such as ultraviolet radiation or prescription drugs, unless directed to do so by a physician.[24]

ACNE

Using other topical acne medications at the same time or immediately following use of this product may increase dryness or irritation of the skin. If this occurs, only one medication should be used unless directed by a physician.[25]

CONTACT DERMATITIS AND POISON IVY/OAK/SUMAC (PRODUCTS FOR ALLERGIC SKIN REACTIONS)

Products containing diphenhydramine: Do not use with any other product containing diphenhydramine, even one taken by mouth.[8]

HAIR LOSS (PRODUCTS CONTAINING MINOXIDIL)

Do not use if you use other topical prescription products on the scalp.[26]

MISCELLANEOUS MEDICAL CONDITIONS AND SITUATIONS

NICOTINE ADDICTION

- Nicotine gum: Do not use if you continue to smoke, chew tobacco, use snuff, or use a nicotine patch or other nicotine-containing products. Ask your doctor before use if you take insulin for diabetes.[27]
- Nicotine patches: Do not use if you continue to smoke, chew tobacco, use snuff, or use nicotine gum or other nicotine-containing products.[28]

References

1. Antacid drug products; Rule. Fed Reg 58:45204, 1993.
2. Tagamet HB Stock Package. 1997; SmithKline Beecham.
3. Antiemetic drug products for over-the-counter human use; Final rule. Fed Reg 52:15886, 1987.
4. Laxative drug products for over-the-counter human use; tentative final monograph. Fed Reg 50:2124, 1985.
5. Antidiarrheal drug products for over-the-counter human use; Tentative final monograph; Proposed rulemaking. Fed Reg 51:16138, 1986.
6. Anorectal drug products for over-the-counter human use; Final monograph; Final rule. Fed Reg 55:31776, 1990.
7. Cold, cough, allergy, bronchodilator, and antiasthmatic drug products for over-the-counter human use; Final monograph for OTC antihistamine drugs products; Final rule. Fed Reg 57:58356, 1992.
8. Labeling of diphenhydramine-containing drug products for over-the-counter human use. Fed Reg 62:45767, 1997.
9. Final monograph for OTC nasal decongestant drug products; Final rule. Fed Reg 59:43386, 1994.
10. Over-the-counter drug products containing phenylpropanolamine; Required labeling; Final rule. Fed Reg 61:5912, 1996FR 2/14/96.
11. Cold, cough, allergy, bronchodilator, and antiasthmatic drug products for over-the-counter human use; Amendment of final monograph for OTC antitussive drug products. Fed Reg 58:54232, 1993.
12. Cold, cough, allergy, bronchodilator, and antiasthmatic drug products for over-the-counter human use; Final monograph for OTC antitussive drug products; Final rule. Fed Reg 52:30042, 1987.
13. Cold, cough, allergy, bronchodilator, and antiasthmatic drug products for over-the-counter human use; Amendment of final monograph for OTC bronchodilator drug products. Fed Reg 58:54238, 1993.
14. Internal analgesic, antipyretic, and antirheumatic drug products for over-the-counter human use; Tentative final monograph; Notice of proposed rulemaking. Fed Reg 53:46204, 1988.
15. Actron, Advil, Aleve, Orudis KT Stock Packages. 1997; Bayer Corporation, Whitehall Laboratories, Procter & Gamble.
16. Over-the-counter drug products containing analgesic/antipyretic active ingredients for internal use; Required alcohol warning. Fed Reg 62:61041, 1997.
17. Advil, Motrin IB Stock Packages. 1997; Whitehall Laboratories., McNeil Consumer Products.
18. Children's Motrin Oral Suspension, Motrin Junior Strength Stock Packages. 1997; McNeil Consumer Products.
19. Aleve Stock Package. 1995; Procter & Gamble.
20. Actron, Orudis KT Stock Packages. 1997; Bayer Corporation, Whitehall-Robins Healthcare.
21. Stimulant drug products for over-the-counter human use; Final monograph; Final rule. Fed Reg 53:6100, 1988.
22. Nighttime sleep-aid drug products for over-the-counter human use; Final monograph, Final rule. Fed Reg 54:6814, 1989.
23. Poison treatment drug products for over-the-counter human use; Tentative final monograph. Fed Reg 50:2244, 1985.
24. Dandruff, seborrheic dermatitis, and psoriasis drug products for over-the-counter human use; Final rule. Fed Reg 56:63554, 1991.
25. Topical acne drug products for over-the-counter human use; Final rule. Fed Reg 56:41008, 1991.
26. Rogaine for Men, Rogaine for Women Stock Packages. 1997; Upjohn.
27. Nicorette Gum Stock Package. 1997; SmithKline Beecham.
28. Nicotrol, NicoDerm CQ Stock Packages. 1997; McNeil Consumer Products, SmithKline Beecham.

Miscellaneous FDA-Labeled Precautions with Use of Nonprescription Products

This appendix includes miscellaneous FDA-required use precautions for nonprescription products. If the FDA currently feels that precautions dealing with the product group are adequately covered through labeling for drug interactions, age limitations, time limitations, and contraindications (see Appendices 1 through 4), no miscellaneous precautions are required.

ORAL AND GASTROINTESTINAL CONDITIONS

PLAQUE-INDUCED DISEASES: CARIES AND GINGIVITIS

- Products containing stannous fluoride: This product may produce surface staining of the teeth. Adequate toothbrushing may prevent these stains, which are not harmful or permanent and may be removed by your dentist.[1]
- Anticavity rinses: Do not swallow the rinse. Do not eat or drink for 30 minutes after rinsing. Instruct children under 12 years of age in good rinsing habits (to minimize swallowing).[1]
- Anticaries gels, pastes, or powders: If you accidentally swallow more than used for brushing, seek professional assistance or contact a Poison Control Center immediately.[2]

ORAL PROBLEMS

- Gingival protectants, oral mucosal cleansing products, oral mucosal analgesics: If sore mouth symptoms do not improve in 7 days; if irritation, pain, or redness persists or worsens; or if swelling, rash, or fever develops, see your dentist or doctor.[3]
- Products containing sodium perborate monohydrate: Do not swallow.[3]
- Hypersensitive teeth: Sensitive teeth may indicate a serious problem that may need prompt care by a dentist. See your dentist if the problem persists or worsens.[3]

GASTRIC DISTRESS (ANTACIDS)

- For products that cause constipation in 5% or more of persons who take the maximum recommended dose: May cause constipation.[4]

- For products that cause laxation in 5% or more of persons who take the maximum recommended dose: May have laxative effect.[4]
- For products containing sodium bicarbonate in a dosage form intended for dissolution in a liquid prior to administration: STOMACH WARNING—To avoid serious injury, do not take until (tablet or powder) is completely dissolved. It is very important not to take this product when overly full from food or drink. Consult a physician if severe stomach pain occurs after taking this product.[5] (First two sentences must be in bold print, using all capital letters)

MOTION SICKNESS (ANTIEMETICS)

Use caution when driving a motor vehicle or operating heavy machinery.[6]

CONSTIPATION (LAXATIVES)

- Products containing methylcellulose, psyllium, polycarbophil, guar gum, and other water-soluble gums: Warnings—Taking this product without adequate fluid may cause it to swell and block your throat or esophagus and may cause choking. Do not take this product if you have difficulty in swallowing. If you experience chest pain, vomiting, or difficulty in swallowing or breathing after taking this product, seek immediate medical attention. Take this product with at least 8 ounces (a full glass) of water or other fluid. Taking this product without enough liquid may cause choking.[7]
- Saline laxatives: Drink a full glass (8 ounces) of liquid with each dose.[8] Do not exceed recommended dose unless directed by a doctor. Serious side effects may occur from excess dosage.[9]
- Saline laxatives containing phosphate[10]:
  —Oral use: Taking more than the recommended dose in 24 hours can be harmful.
  —Rectal use: Using more than one enema in 24 hours can be harmful.
- Products containing magnesium citrate: Store at temperatures between 46 and 86°F.[8]

- Enteric-coated tablets containing bisacodyl: Do not chew tablets. This product may cause abdominal discomfort, faintness, and cramps.[8]
- Suppositories containing bisacodyl: This product may cause abdominal discomfort, faintness, rectal burning, and mild cramps.[8]
- Suppositories containing carbon dioxide: Moisten suppository by placing it under a water tap for 30 seconds or in a cup of water for at least 10 seconds before insertion.[8]
- Suppositories containing glycerin: May cause rectal discomfort or a burning sensation.[8]

PINWORM (ANTHELMINTIC PRODUCTS CONTAINING PYRANTEL PAMOATE)

Abdominal cramps, nausea, vomiting, diarrhea, headache, or dizziness sometimes occur after taking this drug. If any of these conditions persist, consult a doctor. Take only according to directions and do not exceed the recommended dosage unless directed by a doctor. When one individual in a household has pinworms, the entire household should be treated unless otherwise advised. If any symptoms or pinworms are still present after treatment, consult a doctor.[11]

HEMORRHOIDS (HEMORRHOID PRODUCTS)

Do not exceed the recommended daily dosage unless directed by a physician.[12]

- Products for external use only: Do not put this product into the rectum by using fingers or any mechanical device or applicator.
- Products for intrarectal use to be used with a special applicator (e.g., intrarectal tube): Do not use this product with an applicator if the introduction of the applicator into the rectum causes additional pain. Consult a physician promptly. Lubricate applicator well, then gently insert into the rectum.
- Products for external use containing a local anesthetic, menthol, or resorcinol: Certain persons can develop allergic reactions to ingredients in this product. If the symptom being treated does not subside or if redness, irritation, swelling, pain, or other symptoms develop or increase, discontinue use and consult a physician.
- Products containing ephedrine: Some users of this product may experience nervousness, tremor, sleeplessness, nausea, and loss of appetite. If these symptoms persist or become worse, consult your physician.
- Products containing hydrocortisone labeled for external anal itching: Do not exceed the recommended daily dosage unless directed by a physician. In case of bleeding, consult a physician promptly. Do not put this product into the rectum by using fingers or any mechanical device or applicator.[13]

- Products formulated as suppositories: Remove wrapper before inserting into the rectum.[12]

RESPIRATORY CONDITIONS

ALLERGIC RHINITIS

- Products containing antihistamines: May cause excitability, especially in children.[14]
- All antihistamines except diphenhydramine and doxylamine: May cause drowsiness. Use caution when driving a motor vehicle or operating machinery.[14]
- Products containing diphenhydramine and doxylamine: May cause marked drowsiness. Use caution when driving a motor vehicle or operating machinery.[14]
- Products containing phenindamine: May cause nervousness and insomnia in some individuals.[14]
- Nasal solutions containing cromolyn sodium: Brief stinging or sneezing may occur right after use. Do not share this bottle with anyone else as this may spread germs. Stop using this product if your symptoms worsen; you have new symptoms; your symptoms do not begin to improve within 2 weeks. See your doctor because these could be signs of a serious illness.[15]

THE COMMON COLD AND RELATED CONDITIONS

- Sprays and inhalers containing nasal decongestants: Do not exceed recommended dosage. Frequent or prolonged use may cause nasal congestion to recur or worsen. If symptoms persist, consult a physician. This product may cause temporary discomfort such as burning, stinging, sneezing, or an increase in nasal discharge. The use of this container by more than one person may spread infection.[16]
- Products containing naphazoline 0.05%: Do not use this product in children under 12 because it may cause sedation if swallowed.
- Inhalers containing l-desoxyephedrine and propylhexedrine: This inhaler is effective for a minimum of 3 months after first use (Author's note: The Federal Register uses the word "minimum" and this is found on the products, although it would be more logical as a "maximum" time of effectiveness for the products after opening them). Keep inhaler tightly closed.[16]
- Oral nasal decongestants: Do not exceed recommended dosage. If nervousness, dizziness, or sleeplessness occur, discontinue use and consult a physician.[16]
  —Products containing phenylpropanolamine: Do not take more than 75 milligrams per day (24 hours). Taking more can be harmful. Stop using if you develop nervousness, dizziness, sleeplessness, headache, or palpitations. If symptoms continue, ask a physician.[17]

- Sore throat products: Only for occasional minor sore throat pain.[3]
- Oral Antitussives
  —Products containing codeine: May cause or aggravate constipation. A special measuring device should be used to give an accurate dose of this product to children under 6 years of age. Giving a higher dose than recommended by a doctor could result in serious side effects for your child.[18]
- Topical antitussives containing camphor/menthol in an ointment: For external use only. Do not take by mouth or place in nostrils.[18]
- Topical antitussives containing camphor/menthol for steam inhalation use: For steam inhalation only. Do not take by mouth.[18]

ASTHMA (ANTIASTHMATICS)

Do not use this product unless a diagnosis of asthma has been made by a physician.[19]

- Oral products containing ephedrine: Some users of this product may experience nervousness, tremor, sleeplessness, nausea, and loss of appetite. If these symptoms persist or worsen, consult your physician.
- Inhalation products containing epinephrine: Do not use more frequently or at higher doses than recommended unless directed by a physician. Excessive use may cause nervousness and rapid heart beat, and, possibly, adverse effects on the heart. The use of this product by children should be supervised by an adult.
- Products to be used in a nebulizer: Do not use this product if it is brown in color or cloudy.

PAIN CONDITIONS

HEADACHE AND OTHER MINOR PAINS (INTERNAL ANALGESICS)

If pain or fever persists or gets worse, if new symptoms occur, or if redness or swelling is present, consult a doctor because these could be signs of a serious condition.[20]

- Products containing salicylates: If ringing in the ears or a loss of hearing occurs, consult a doctor before taking any more of this product.[20] IMPORTANT: See your doctor before taking this product for your heart or for other new uses of aspirin, because serious side effects could occur with self-treatment.[21]
  —Products containing salicylates in solid dosage forms: Adults: Drink a full glass of water with each dose. Children 2 to under 12 years of age: Drink water with each dose.[20]
- Products containing acetaminophen: Do not exceed recommended dosage; in an overdose situation, prompt

medical attention is critical for adults as well as for children even if you do not notice any signs or symptoms.[20]

- Products containing naproxen sodium: Consult a doctor if more than mild heartburn, upset stomach, or stomach pain occurs with use of this product or if even mild symptoms persist.[22]
- Products containing ketoprofen: Ask a doctor after use if stomach pain occurs with use of this product.[23]

MENSTRUAL DISCOMFORT (PRODUCTS CONTAINING AMMONIUM CHLORIDE)

This drug may cause nausea, vomiting, and gastrointestinal distress.[24]

INJURIES TO MUSCLES, LIGAMENTS, AND TENDONS (EXTERNAL ANALGESICS)

For external use only. Avoid contact with the eyes. If condition worsens, or if symptoms persist for more than 7 days or clear up and occur again within a few days, discontinue use of this product and consult a physician.[25]

- External analgesic products containing counter-irritants: Do not bandage tightly.
- External analgesic products containing dibucaine, lidocaine, or tetracaine: Do not use in large quantities, particularly over raw surfaces or blistered areas.
- External analgesic products containing phenol: Do not apply over large areas of the body or bandage.
- External analgesic products containing resorcinol: Do not apply over large areas of the body.

MISCELLANEOUS INTERNAL PROBLEMS

OBESITY (APPETITE SUPPRESSANTS CONTAINING PHENYLPROPANOLAMINE)

Do not take more than 75 milligrams per day (24 hours). Taking more can be harmful. Stop using if you develop nervousness, dizziness, sleeplessness, headache, or palpitations. If symptoms continue, ask a physician.[17]

FATIGUE AND DROWSINESS (STIMULANTS)

For occasional use only. Not intended for use as a substitute for sleep. If fatigue or drowsiness persists or continues to recur, consult a physician.[26]

SLEEP DISTURBANCES (SLEEP AIDS)

Insomnia may be a symptom of serious underlying medical illness.[27]

POISONING EMERGENCIES (PRODUCTS CONTAINING SYRUP OF IPECAC OR ACTIVATED CHARCOAL)

If possible, call a Poison Control Center, emergency medical facility, or health professional for help before using this product. If help cannot be reached quickly, follow the directions on the container. Read the warnings and directions as soon as you buy this product. Insert emergency phone number(s) in the space provided on the label. Keep patient active and moving. Save the container of poison. If previous attempts to contact a poison control center, emergency medical facility, or health professional were unsuccessful, continue trying.[28]

- Products containing activated charcoal: Do not give activated charcoal until the patient has vomited unless directed by health care personnel.
- Kits containing both activated charcoal and syrup of ipecac: When professional advice is not available, first give ipecac syrup to induce vomiting; after vomiting has occurred, give activated charcoal to help adsorb any remaining toxic substance.[28]

OPHTHALMIC/OTIC CONDITIONS

OPHTHALMIC CONDITIONS

To avoid contamination, do not touch tip of container to any surface. Replace cap after using.[29]

- Products supplied in single-use containers: Do not reuse. Once opened, discard.[29]
- Products containing ophthalmic astringents, ophthalmic demulcents, ophthalmic emollients, ophthalmic vasoconstrictors, ophthalmic vasoconstrictor/antihistamine combinations: If you experience eye pain, changes in vision, continued redness or irritation of the eye, or if the condition worsens or persists for more than 72 hours, discontinue use and consult a physician.[29,30]
- Products containing ophthalmic hypertonicity agents: Do not use this product except under the advice and supervision of a physician. If you experience eye pain, changes in vision, continued redness or irritation of the eye, or if the condition worsens or persists, discontinue use and consult a physician. This product may cause temporary burning and irritation on being instilled into the eye.[29]
- Products containing ophthalmic astringents, ophthalmic demulcents, ophthalmic hypertonicity products, ophthalmic vasoconstrictors: If solution changes color or becomes cloudy, do not use.[29]
- Products containing ophthalmic vasoconstrictors, ophthalmic vasoconstrictor/antihistamine combinations: Overuse of this product may produce increased redness of the eye.[29,30] Pupils may become dilated (enlarged).[31]
- Eyewashes: If you experience eye pain, changes in vision, continued redness or irritation of the eye, or if the condition worsens or persists, consult a physician. Obtain immediate medical treatment for all open wounds in or near the eyes.[29]
  —Eyewashes intended for use with an eyecup: Rinse cup with clean water immediately before each use. Avoid contamination of rim and inside surfaces of cup. Rinse cup with clean water after each use.[29]

OTIC CONDITIONS (EXCESSIVE EARWAX PRODUCTS)

Tip of applicator should not enter ear canal. Avoid contact with the eyes.[32]

DERMATOLOGIC CONDITIONS

HYPERPROLIFERATIVE SKIN DISORDERS

For external use only. Avoid contact with the eyes. If contact occurs, rinse eyes thoroughly with water. If condition worsens or does not improve after regular use of this product as directed, consult a physician.[33]

- Products containing coal tar: Use caution in exposing skin to sunlight after applying this product. It may increase your tendency to sunburn for up to 24 hours after application.[33]
- Products containing coal tar in cream, lotion, or ointment form to be applied and left on the skin: Do not use this product in or around the rectum or in the genital area or groin except on the advice of a physician.

ARTHROPOD STINGS AND BITES (PEDICULICIDES CONTAINING SYNERGIZED PYRETHRINS)

Use with caution on persons allergic to ragweed. For external use only. Do not use near the eyes or permit contact with mucous membranes. If product gets into the eyes, immediately flush with water. Consult a doctor if infestation of the eyebrows or eyelashes occurs. If skin irritation or infection is present or develops, discontinue use and consult a doctor. Allow product to remain on area for 10 minutes but no longer. Wash area thoroughly with warm water and soap or shampoo. A second treatment must be made in 7 to 10 days to kill any newly hatched lice.[34]

MINOR WOUNDS

- Products containing topical antimicrobials, antibiotics: For external use only. Do not use in the eyes or apply over large areas of the body. Stop use and consult a physician if the condition persists or gets worse.[35,36]

- Topical antibiotic products containing bacitracin, bacitracin zinc, neomycin, neomycin sulfate, polymyxin B, and/or polymyxin B sulfate: Stop use and consult a physician if the condition persists or gets worse, or if a rash or other allergic reaction develops.[37]
- Products containing alcohols: For external use only. Do not use in or near the eyes. Flammable, keep away from fire or flame.[38]
  —Products containing isopropyl alcohol: Use only in a well-ventilated area; fumes may be toxic.[38]
- Products containing camphorated metacresol, camphor + phenol, or phenol alone: Do not bandage.[36]

SUN-INDUCED SKIN DAMAGE (PRODUCTS CONTAINING SUNSCREENS)

SUN ALERT: The sun causes skin damage. Regular use of sunscreens over the years may reduce the chance of skin damage, some types of skin cancer, and other harmful effects due to the sun. For external use only, not to be swallowed. Avoid contact with the eyes. If contact occurs, rinse eyes thoroughly with water. Discontinue use if signs of irritation or rash appear. If irritation or rash persists, consult a physician. Reapply after 40 minutes (if water resistant) or 80 minutes (if very water resistant) of swimming or excessive sweating or any time after towel drying. Children under 2 years of age should use sunscreen products with a minimum SPF of 4.[39]

- For products that do not satisfy the water resistant testing procedures: Reapply after swimming, excessive sweating, or any time after towel drying.[39]

ACNE

Because excessive drying of the skin may occur, start with one application daily, then gradually increase to two or three times daily if needed or as directed by a physician. If bothersome dryness or peeling occurs, reduce application to once a day or every other day.[40]

- Products containing sulfur: Do not get into eyes. If excessive skin irritation develops or increases, discontinue use and consult a physician.
- Products containing resorcinol combined with sulfur: Apply to affected areas only. Do not use on broken skin or apply to large areas of the body.
- Products containing benzoyl peroxide: Warning—When using this product, avoid unnecessary sun exposure and use a sunscreen. If going outside, use a sunscreen. Allow this product to dry, then follow directions on the sunscreen labeling. If irritation or sensitivity develops, discontinue use of both products and consult a physician.[41]
- For new users, optional labeling: Apply product sparingly to one or two small affected areas during the first 3 days. If no discomfort occurs, follow the directions stated elsewhere on this label.

FUNGAL SKIN INFECTIONS (ANTIFUNGALS)

For external use only. Avoid contact with the eyes. If irritation occurs, discontinue use and consult a physician. Do not use for diaper rash.[42]

WARTS (WART REMOVAL PRODUCTS)

For external use only. If discomfort persists, see your physician.[43]

- Products with volatile vehicles: Cap bottle tightly and store at room temperature away from heat.
- Products with flammable vehicles: Keep away from fire or flame.
- Products with collodion vehicles: If product gets into the eye, flush with water for 15 minutes. Avoid inhaling vapors.

CONTACT DERMATITIS AND POISON IVY/OAK/SUMAC (PRODUCTS FOR ALLERGIC SKIN REACTIONS)

- Products containing colloidal oatmeal: Take special care to avoid slipping when getting into and out of the tub.[44]
- Products containing astringents: Avoid the eyes.
- Products containing aluminum acetate as a compress or wet dressing: Do not cover compress or wet dressing with plastic to prevent evaporation.[45]
- Products containing hydrocortisone: If condition worsens, or if symptoms persist for more than 7 days or clear up and occur again within a few days, stop use of this product and do not begin use of any other hydrocortisone product unless you have consulted a doctor. For external use only. Avoid contact with the eyes. Do not use for treatment of diaper rash.[13]
- Products containing bentoquatam (Ivy Block is the only product containing bentoquatam, as of this writing): For external use only. Ivy Block contains alcohol. Keep away from fire or flame. Ivy Block will remain flammable until it dries on the skin. Cap bottle tightly and store at room temperature. Keep away from heat.[46]

DIAPER DERMATITIS

- Products containing topical antimicrobials: For external use only. Avoid contact with the eyes. If condition worsens, consult a physician.[47]
- Topical antimicrobial powder products: Keep powder away from child's face to avoid inhalation, which can cause breathing problems.
- Skin protectant diaper rash products: Apply powder close to the body away from child's face. Carefully shake the powder into the diaper or into the hand and apply to the diaper area.[48]

SKIN HYPERPIGMENTATION (HYPOPIGMENTATION PRODUCTS)

Avoid contact with the eyes. Some users of this product may experience a mild skin irritation. If skin irritation becomes severe, stop use and consult a physician. Sun exposure should be limited by using a sunscreen agent, a sun blocking agent, or protective clothing to cover bleached skin when using and after using this product to prevent darkening from recurring.[49]

- Products containing a sunscreen: This product is not for use in the prevention of sunburn.

FOOT PROBLEMS (CALLUS/CORN REMOVERS)

For external use only. Do not use this product on irritated skin, or on any area that is infected or reddened. If discomfort persists, see your physician or podiatrist.[50]

- Products containing a flammable vehicle: Keep away from fire or flame.
- Products formulated in a volatile vehicle: Cap bottle tightly and store at room temperature away from heat.
- Products in collodion-like vehicles: If product gets into the eye, flush with water for 15 minutes. Avoid inhaling vapors.

HAIR LOSS (PRODUCTS CONTAINING MINOXIDIL)

Continued use is necessary to increase and keep your hair regrowth or hair loss will begin again. Stop use and see a doctor if you get chest pain, rapid heartbeat, faintness, or dizziness; sudden, unexplained weight gain; swollen hands or feet; redness or irritation. Avoid contact with the eyes. In case of accidental contact (with the eyes), rinse with large amounts of cool tap water. In case of accidental ingestion, seek professional assistance or contact a poison control center immediately.[51]

MISCELLANEOUS MEDICAL CONDITIONS AND SITUATIONS

PROBLEMS RELATED TO SEXUAL ACTIVITY

- Male genital desensitizers: Premature ejaculation may be due to a condition requiring medical supervision. If this product, used as directed, does not provide relief, discontinue use and consult a physician. Avoid contact with the eyes. If you or your partner develop a rash or irritation, such as burning or itching, discontinue use. If symptoms persist, consult a physician. Wash product off after intercourse.[52]
- Contraceptive products containing vaginal spermicides: If douching is desired, always wait at least 6 hours after intercourse before douching. If you or your partner develop

ops irritation, such as burning or itching in the genital area, stop using this product. If irritation continues, contact your physician.[53,54]

FEMALE GENITAL CONDITIONS

- Douching products: Do not press the lips of the vagina around the nozzle. Overfilling the vagina may force fluid into the uterus (womb) and cause inflammation. Douching does not prevent pregnancy. If douching results in pain, soreness, itching, excessive dryness, or irritation, stop douching. If symptoms persist, consult a physician.[55,56]
- Products containing docusate or sodium lauryl sulfate for douching: Avoid prolonged contact with the skin and avoid contact with the eyes. If vaginal itching, redness, swelling, or pain develop, stop douching. Consult your physician if these symptoms persist.[55]
- Vaginal antimonilial products: If your symptoms return within 2 months or if you have infections that do not clear up easily with proper treatment, consult your doctor. You could be pregnant or there could be a serious underlying medical cause for your infections, including diabetes or a damaged immune system (including damage from infection with HIV—the virus that causes AIDS). For vaginal use only. Do not use in eyes or take by mouth. Do not use tampons while using this medication.[57]
- Antimonilial suppositories: Antimonilial suppositories contain hydrogenated vegetable oil, which may weaken latex in condoms or diaphragms. Do not rely on condoms or diaphragms to prevent sexually transmitted disease while using suppositories.

NICOTINE ADDICTION (PRODUCTS CONTAINING NICOTINE)

Keep this out of reach of children and pets. Stop use and see your doctor if you have irregular heartbeat or palpitations or if you have symptoms of nicotine overdose such as nausea, vomiting, dizziness, weakness, and rapid heartbeat.[58,59]

- Nicotine gum: Stop use and see your doctor if you have mouth, teeth, or jaw problems.[58]
- Nicotine patches: Used patches have enough nicotine to poison children and pets. Fold sticky ends together and discard away from children and pets. For accidental overdose, seek professional help or contact a poison control center immediately. Stop use and see your doctor if you have skin redness caused by the patch that does not go away after 4 days, or if your skin swells or you get a rash.[59]

References

1. Anticaries drug products for over-the-counter human use; Final monograph; Final rule. Fed Reg 60:52474, 1995.

2. Anticaries drug products for over-the-counter human use; Final monograph; Technical amendment; Partial delay of effective date. Fed Reg 61:52285, 1996.

3. Oral health care drug products for over-the-counter human use; Tentative final monograph; Notice of proposed rulemaking. Fed Reg 56:48302,1991.

4. Antacid and antiflatulent products. Fed Reg 39:19862, 1974.

5. Antacid drug products for over-the-counter human use; Amendment to antacid final monograph; Proposed rule. Fed Reg 59:5060, 1994.

6. Antiemetic drug products for over-the-counter human use; Final rule. Fed Reg 52:15886, 1987.

7. Warning statement for over-the-counter drugs containing water-soluble gums; Rule. Fed Reg 58:45194, 1993.

8. Laxative drug products for over-the-counter human use; tentative final monograph. Fed Reg 50:2124, 1985.

9. Laxative drug products for over-the-counter human use; Proposed amendment to the tentative final monograph. Fed Reg 59:15139, 1994.

10. Package size limitation for sodium phosphates oral solution and warning and direction statements for oral and rectal sodium phosphates for over-the-counter laxative use. Fed Reg 63:27836, 1998.

11. Anthelmintic drug products for over-the-counter human use; Final monograph. Fed Reg 51:27756,1986.

12. Anorectal drug products for over-the-counter human use; Final monograph; Final rule. Fed Reg 55:31776, 1990.

13. Hydrocortisone; Marketing status as an external analgesic drug product for over-the-counter human use; Notice of enforcement policy. Fed Reg 56:43025, 1991.

14. Cold, cough, allergy, bronchodilator, and antiasthmatic drug products for over-the-counter human use; Final monograph for OTC antihistamine drugs products; Final rule. Fed Reg 57:58356, 1992.

15. Nasalcrom Stock Package. 1997; McNeil Consumer Products.

16. Final monograph for OTC nasal decongestant drug products; Final rule. Fed Reg 59:43386, 1994.

17. Over-the-counter drug products containing phenylpropanolamine; Required labeling; Proposed rule. Fed Reg 61:5912, 1996.

18. Cold, cough, allergy, bronchodilator, and antiasthmatic drug products for over-the-counter human use; Final monograph for OTC antitussive drug products; Final rule. Fed Reg 52:30042, 1987.

19. Cold, cough, allergy, bronchodilator, and antiasthmatic drug products for over-the-counter human use; Final monograph for OTC bronchodilator drug products. Fed Reg 51:35326, 1986.

20. Internal analgesic, antipyretic, and antirheumatic drug products for over-the-counter human use; Tentative final monograph; Notice of proposed rulemaking. Fed Reg 53:46204, 1988.

21. Labeling for over-the-counter oral drug products containing aspirin, buffered aspirin, or aspirin in combination with an antacid; Proposed rule. Fed Reg 58:54224, 1993.

22. Aleve Stock Package. 1995; Procter & Gamble.

23. Actron, Orudis KT Stock Packages. 1997; Bayer Corporation, Whitehall-Robins Healthcare.

24. Orally administered menstrual drug products for over-the-counter human use; Tentative final monograph; Notice of proposed rulemaking. Fed Reg 53:46194, 1988.

25. External analgesic drug products for over-the-counter human use; Tentative final monograph. Fed Reg 48:5852, 1983.

26. Stimulant drug products for over-the-counter human use; Final monograph; Final rule. Fed Reg 53:6100, 1988.

27. Nighttime sleep-aid drug products for over-the-counter human use; Final monograph, Final rule. Fed Reg 54:6814, 1989.

28. Poison treatment drug products for over-the-counter human use; Tentative final monograph. Fed Reg 50:2244, 1985.

29. Ophthalmic drug products for over-the-counter human use; Final monograph; Final rule. Fed Reg 53:7076, 1988.

30. Naphcon A, Opcon-A, Vasocon-A Stock Packages. 1995; Alcon Laboratories, Bausch & Lomb, CIBA Vision Ophthalmics.

31. Ophthalmic drug products for over-the-counter human use: Proposed amendment of final monograph. Fed Reg 63:8888, 1998.

32. Topical otic drug products for over-the-counter human use; Final monograph; Final rule. Fed Reg 51:28656, 1986.

33. Dandruff, seborrheic dermatitis, and psoriasis drug products for over-the-counter human use; Final rule. Fed Reg 56:63554, 1991.

34. Pediculicide drug products for over-the-counter human use; Tentative final monograph; Notice of proposed rulemaking. Fed Reg 54:13480, 1989.

35. Topical antimicrobial drug products for over-the-counter human use; Final monograph for OTC first aid antibiotic drug products; Final rule. Fed Reg 52:47312, 1987.

36. Topical antimicrobial drug products for over-the-counter human use; Tentative final monograph for first aid antiseptic drug products. Fed Reg 56:33644, 1991.

37. Topical antimicrobial drug products for over-the-counter human use; Amendment of final monograph for OTC first aid antibiotic products. Fed Reg 61:58471, 1996.

38. Alcohol drug products for topical antimicrobial over-the-counter human use; Establishment of a monograph; and reopening of administrative record. Fed Reg 47:22324, 1982.

39. Sunscreen drug products for over-the-counter human use; Tentative final monograph; Proposed rule. Fed Reg 58: 28164, 1993.

40. Topical acne drug products for over-the-counter human use; Final rule. Fed Reg 56:41008, 1991.

41. Topical drug products containing benzoyl peroxide; Required labeling; Proposed rule. Fed Reg 60:9554, 1995.

42. Topical antifungal drug products, Final monograph; Final rule. Fed Reg 58:49890, 1993.

43. Wart remover drug products for over-the-counter human use; Final monograph; Final rule. Fed Reg 55:33246, 1990.

44. Skin protectant and external analgesic drug products for over-the-counter human use; Proposed rulemaking for poison ivy, poison oak, poison sumac, and insect bites drug products. Fed Reg 54:40808, 1989.

45. Skin protectant drug products for over-the-counter human use; Astringent drug products; Final rule. Fed Reg 58:54458, 1993.

46. Ivy Block Stock Package. 1997; EnviroDerm Pharmaceuticals.

47. Topical antimicrobial drug products for over-the-counter human use; Proposed rule for diaper rash drug products. Fed Reg 55:25246, 1990.

48. Skin protectant drug products for over-the-counter human

use; Diaper rash products; Proposed rule. Fed Reg 55:25204, 1990.

49. Skin bleaching drug products for over-the-counter human use; Tentative final monograph. Fed Reg 47:39108, 1982.

50. Corn and callus remover drug products for over-the-counter human use; Final monograph; Final Rule. Fed Reg 55:33258, 1990.

51. Rogaine for Men, Rogaine for Women Stock Packages. 1997; Upjohn.

52. Male genital desensitizing drug products for over-the-counter human use; Final monograph; Final rule. Fed Reg 57:27654, 1992.

53. Vaginal contraceptive drug products for over-the-counter human use; Establishment of a monograph; Proposed rulemaking. Fed Reg 45:82014, 1980.

54. Vaginal contraceptive drug products for over-the-counter human use; Proposed rule. Fed Reg 60:6892, 1995.

55. Vaginal drug products for over-the-counter human use; Establishment of a monograph; Advance notice of proposed rulemaking. Fed Reg 48:46694, 1983.

56. Vaginal drug products for over-the-counter human use; Withdrawal of advance notice of proposed rulemaking. Fed Reg 59:5226, 1994.

57. Femstat 3, Gyne-Lotrimin, Monistat, Vagistat-1 Stock Packages. 1995; Procter & Gamble, Schering-Plough HealthCare; Advanced Care Products, Bristol-Myers Squibb.

58. Nicorette Gum Stock Package. 1997; SmithKline Beecham.

59. Nicotrol, NicoDerm CQ Stock Packages. 1997; McNeil Consumer Products, SmithKline Beecham.

Index

Page numbers in italics denote figures; those followed by a "t" denote tables.